Pediatric and Adolescent Gynecology

Pediatric and Adolescent Gynecology

JOSEPH S. SANFILIPPO, M.D.
Professor of Obstetrics and Gynecology
University of Louisville School of Medicine
Director, Reproductive Biology
Director, Pediatric Adolescent Gynecology
Chairman, Obstetrics and Gynecology
Norton Hospital
Louisville, Kentucky

Associate Editors:

DAVID MURAM, M.D.
Associate Professor of Obstetrics and
   Gynecology
University of Tennessee–Memphis
Director, Division of Gynecology
Director, Pediatric and Adolescent Gynecology
Le Bonheur Children's Medical Center and St.
   Jude Children's Research Hospital
Memphis, Tennessee

PETER A. LEE, M.D.
Professor of Pediatrics
University of Pittsburgh School of Medicine
Director of NIH General Clinical Research
   Center
Children's Hospital of Pittsburgh
Pittsburgh, Pennsylvania

JOHN DEWHURST, F.R.C.O.G., F.R.C.S
Emeritus Professor
University of London
Queen Charlotte's and Chelsea Hospital
London, England

W.B. SAUNDERS COMPANY
A Division of Harcourt Brace & Company
Philadelphia   London   Toronto   Montreal   Sydney   Tokyo

W.B. SAUNDERS COMPANY
A Division of
Harcourt Brace & Company

The Curtis Center
Independence Square West
Philadelphia, Pennsylvania 19106

Library of Congress Cataloging-in-Publication Data

Pediatric and adolescent gynecology / editor,
Joseph S. Sanfilippo;
associate editors, David Muram, Peter A. Lee, John Dewhurst.

p.   cm.

ISBN 0–7216–3971–2

1. Pediatric gynecology.   2. Adolescent gynecology.
  I. Sanfilippo, J. S. (Joseph S.)
  [DNLM: 1. Genital Diseases, Female—in adolescence.
  WS 360 P3707 1994]

RJ478.P43 1994   618.92′098—dc20

DNLM/DLC   93–162

Pediatric and Adolescent Gynecology   ISBN 0–7216–3971–2

Printed in the United States of America

Last digit is the print number: 9   8   7   6   5   4   3   2   1

To our families,
Pat, Angela, Andrea, and Luke;
Helen, Leeat, Fred, and Talia;
Karin, Kristen, and Dan;
and Hazel,
for their unending support and enthusiasm
for our contributions to the field of pediatric and adolescent gynecology,
as we move on to new vistas of care
for our special patients.

Contributors

SARAH BERGA, M.D.
Assistant Professor of Obstetrics, Gynecology, Reproductive Science, and Psychiatry, University of Pittsburgh School of Medicine; Magee–Women's Hospital, Pittsburgh, Pennsylvania
Abnormal Sexual Differentiation and Hypogonadism: Management and Therapy

KUNWAR P. BHATNAGAR, Ph.D.
Professor of Anatomy, Department of Anatomical Sciences and Neurobiology, University of Louisville School of Medicine, Louisville, Kentucky
Embryology and Normal Anatomy

ROBERT T. BROWN, M.D.
Professor of Clinical Pediatrics and Clinical Obstetrics and Gynecology, and Director, Division of Adolescent Medicine, College of Medicine, Ohio State University; Chief, Section of Adolescent Health Services, Children's Hospital, Columbus, Ohio
Adolescent Sexuality

JOSÉ F. CARA, M.D.
Assistant Professor of Pediatrics, University of Chicago Pritzker School of Medicine; Section of Pediatric Endocrinology, Wyler Children's Hospital; Director, Chicago Children's Diabetes Center, Chicago, Illinois
Androgens and the Adolescent Girl

ANTHONY CASALE, M.D.
Associate Professor of Surgery, University of Louisville School of Medicine; Associate in Pediatrics, Department of Pediatrics, Director of Pediatric Urology, University of Louisville School of Medicine; Pediatric Urologist, The Commission for Handicapped Children, Louisville, Kentucky
Urologic Problems

BARBARA A. CROMER, M.D.
Associate Professor of Pediatrics and Associate Director, Division of Adolescent Medicine, College of Medicine, Ohio State University; Associate, Section of Adolescent Health Services, Children's Hospital, Columbus, Ohio
Adolescent Sexuality

JOHN DEWHURST, F.R.C.O.G., F.R.C.S.
Emeritus Professor, University of London, Queen Charlotte's and Chelsea Hospital, London, England
Rectovaginal Fistulae and Associated Anomalies

MILENA DORTA, M.D.
Senior Fellow, Department of Obstetrics and Gynecology, University of Milan; Resident in Obstetrics and Gynecology, University of Milan School of Medicine, Milan, Italy
Diagnostic Imaging

D. KEITH EDMONDS, F.R.C.O.G., F.R.A.C.O.G.
Consultant, Queen Charlotte's and Chelsea Hospital, London, England
Sexual Developmental Anomalies and Their Reconstruction: Upper and Lower Tracts

vii

THOMAS E. ELKINS, M.D.
Abe Mickal Professor and Head, Department of Obstetrics and Gynecology, School of Medicine in New Orleans, Louisiana State University, New Orleans, Louisiana
Reproductive Health Care Needs of the Developmentally Disabled

LUIGI FEDELE, M.D.
Associate Professor of Obstetrics and Gynecology, University of Milan; Associate Director, Department of Obstetrics and Gynecology, University of Milan School of Medicine, Milan, Italy
Diagnostic Imaging

THOMAS P. FOLEY, Jr., M.D.
Professor of Pediatrics, University of Pittsburgh School of Medicine; Director, Division of Endocrinology, Metabolism and Diabetes Mellitus, Children's Hospital of Pittsburgh, Pittsburgh, Pennsylvania
Effects of the Thyroid on Gonadal and Reproductive Function

GILBERT B. FORBES, M.D.
Professor of Pediatrics and Biophysics, University of Rochester School of Medicine and Dentistry; Staff Pediatrician, Strong Memorial Hospital, Rochester, New York
Nutrition, Growth, and Development

DENISE FORD-NEPA, Ph.D.
Consultant, Department of Child and Adolescent Psychiatry, Memphis, Tennessee
Depression and Suicide

DIANE FRANCOEUR, M.D.
Lecturer, Department of Obstetrics and Gynecology, University of Montreal, Montreal, Quebec, Canada
Urologic Problems

GITA P. GIDWANI, M.D.
Staff Physician, Departments of Gynecology and Pediatric and Adolescent Medicine, Cleveland Clinic Foundation, Cleveland, Ohio
Dysmenorrhea and Pelvic Pain

S. PAIGE HERTWECK, M.D.
Assistant Professor, Department of Obstetrics and Gynecology, University of Louisville School of Medicine; Co-Director, Pediatric Adolescent Gynecology Fellowship, Louisville, Kentucky
Vaginal Bleeding in Childhood and Menstrual Disorders in Adolescence

MICHAEL L. HICKS, M.D.
Assistant Professor of Obstetrics and Gynecology, Case Western Reserve University, Cleveland, Ohio; Staff Gynecologic Oncologist, Henry Ford Hospital, Detroit, Michigan
Oncologic Problems

RAYMOND L. HINTZ, M.D.
Professor of Pediatrics, Stanford University Medical Center; Head, Division of Endocrinology, Lucile Salter Packard Children's Hospital at Stanford, Stanford, California
Abnormalities in Growth

BARBARA R. HOSTETLER, M.D.
Instructor, Department of Obstetrics and Gynecology, University of Tennessee–Memphis, Memphis, Tennessee
Appendices

CLAUDETTE E. JONES, M.D.
Instructor, Department of Obstetrics and Gynecology, Section of Pediatric and Adolescent Gynecology, University of Tennessee–Memphis, Memphis, Tennessee
Vulvovaginitis

MARSHA KAY, M.D.
Clinical Associate, Department of Pediatrics, Section of Pediatric Gastroenterology and Nutrition, Cleveland Clinic Foundation, Cleveland, Ohio
Dysmenorrhea and Pelvic Pain

PAUL KING, M.D.
Clinical Assistant Professor of Child and Adolescent Psychiatry, University of Tennessee–Memphis; Medical Director of Adolescent Services, Charter Lakeside Hospital, Memphis, Tennessee
Adolescent Drug Abuse

HOWARD E. KULIN, M.D.
Professor of Pediatrics, Pennsylvania State University College of Medicine; Chief, Division of Pediatric Endocrinology, University Hospital, The Milton S. Hershey Medical Center, Hershey, Pennsylvania
Neuroendocrinology of Puberty

PETER A. LEE, M.D.
Professor of Pediatrics, University of Pittsburgh School of Medicine; Director of NIH General Clinical Research Center, Children's Hospital of Pittsburgh, Pittsburgh, Pennsylvania
Neuroendocrinology of Puberty; Pubertal Disorders: Precocious and Delayed

Puberty; Abnormal Sexual Differentiation and Hypogonadism: Management and Therapy

PAUL G. McDONOUGH, M.D.
Professor of Obstetrics and Gynecology, Medical College of Georgia, Augusta, Georgia
Future Perspectives

KRISTI MORGAN MULCHAHEY, M.D.
Private Practice, Atlanta, Georgia
Sexually Transmitted Diseases in Childhood

DAVID MURAM, M.D.
Associate Professor of Obstetrics and Gynecology, University of Tennessee–Memphis; Director, Division of Gynecology, Director, Pediatric and Adolescent Gynecology, Le Bonheur Children's Medical Center and St. Jude Children's Research Hospital, Memphis, Tennessee
Vulvovaginitis; Vaginal Bleeding in Childhood and Menstrual Disorders in Adolescence; Sexually Transmitted Diseases in Adolescence; HIV Infection in Adolescents; Child Sexual Abuse; Delayed Consequences of Childhood Malignancies; Reproductive Health Care Needs of the Developmentally Disabled

LOUIS ST. L. O'DEA, M.B., B.Ch., B.A.O., F.R.C.P.(C).
Assistant Professor of Medicine, Faculty of Medicine, McGill University; Associate Physician, Departments of Medicine and Obstetrics–Gynecology, Montreal General Hospital, and Assistant Physician, Department of Obstetrics–Gynecology, Royal Victoria Hospital, Montreal, Quebec, Canada
Pubertal Disorders: Precocious and Delayed Puberty

GEETA N. PANDYA, D.(Obst.), R.C.O.G., M.R.C.O.G., C.F.P.(Lon.), F.R.C.O.G.
Consultant, Gynecologic Endocrinology, Jaslok Hospital and Research Centre and Breach Candy Hospital and Research Centre, Bombay, India
Puberty Aberrancy in the Third World

M. STEVEN PIVER, M.D.
Clinical Professor and Director of the Division of Gynecologic Oncology, State University of New York at Buffalo; Chief, Department of Gynecologic Oncology, Roswell Park Cancer Institute, Buffalo, New York
Oncologic Problems

LEO PLOUFFE, Jr., M.D.
Associate Professor of Obstetrics and Gynecology, Section of Reproductive Endocrinology and Infertility, Director of Pediatric and Adolescent Gynecology Program, Augusta, Georgia
Future Perspectives

SUSAN F. POKORNY, M.D.
Assistant Professor of Obstetrics and Gynecology and Pediatrics, Baylor College of Medicine; Chief of Gynecology, Texas Children's Hospital, and Director of Obstetrics and Gynecology Outpatient Clinics, Ben Taub General Hospital, Houston, Texas
Genital Examination of Prepubertal and Peripubertal Females

WILLIAM J. POKORNY, M.D.
Professor, Department of Surgery, Chief, Pediatric Surgery, Baylor College of Medicine, Houston, Texas
Surgically Correctable Congenital Anomalies: Diagnosis and Management

PAULINE S. POWERS, M.D.
Professor of Psychiatry and Behavioral Medicine, College of Medicine, University of South Florida; Attending Psychiatrist, University of South Florida Psychiatry Center, and Courtesy Staff Privileges, Tampa General Hospital and University Community Hospital, Tampa, Florida
Eating Disorders

FREDERICK J. RAU, M.D.
Assistant Clinical Professor of Obstetrics and Gynecology and Pediatrics, University of Connecticut School of Medicine, Farmington; Director, Child and Adolescent Gynecology Clinic, Newington Children's Hospital, Newington, and Staff Physician, Obstetrics and Gynecology and Pediatrics, Hartford Hospital, Hartford, Connecticut
Vulvovaginitis

ROBERT W. REBAR, M.D.
George B. Riley Professor and Director, Department of Obstetrics and Gynecology, University of Cincinnati College of Medicine; Clinical Chief, Obstetrics and Gynecology, University Hospital, Cincinnati, Ohio
Sports-Related Problems in Reproductive Function

EDWARD O. REITER, M.D.
Professor of Pediatrics, Tufts University School of Medicine, Boston; Chairman, De-

partment of Pediatrics, Baystate Medical Center, Springfield, Massachusetts
Neuroendocrinology of Puberty

ALAN RETIK, M.D.
Professor of Surgery, Urology; Harvard Medical School; Chief, Division of Urology, Children's Hospital, Boston, Massachusetts
Urologic Problems

C. MARJORIE RIDLEY, M.D.
Honorary Consultant Dermatologist, St. Thomas's Hospital, London, United Kingdom
Vulvar Disorders

MARY E. RIMSZA, M.D.
Professor of Pediatrics, University of Arizona College of Medicine, Tucson; Chairman, Department of Pediatrics, Maricopa Medical Center, Phoenix, Arizona
Genital Trauma

ROBERT L. ROSENFIELD, M.D.
Professor of Pediatrics and Medicine, University of Chicago Pritzker School of Medicine; Chief, Section of Pediatric Endocrinology, Wyler Children's Hospital, Chicago, Illinois
Androgens and the Adolescent Girl

STEVEN S. ROTHENBERG, M.D.
Clinical Assistant Professor of Surgery, University of Colorado; Pediatric Surgeon, Presbyterian/St. Luke's Medical Center, Denver, Colorado
Surgically Correctable Congenital Anomalies: Diagnosis and Management

JOSEPH S. SANFILIPPO, M.D.
Professor of Obstetrics and Gynecology, University of Louisville School of Medicine; Director, Reproductive Biology, Director, Pediatric Adolescent Gynecology, Chairman, Obstetrics and Gynecology, Norton Hospital, Louisville, Kentucky
Vaginal Bleeding in Childhood and Menstrual Disorders in Adolescence; Chronic Pelvic Pain: Medical and Surgical Approach

KENNETH SCHIKLER, M.D.
Associate Professor of Pediatrics, University of Louisville School of Medicine; Director, Pediatric Rheumatology, and Director, Adolescent Medicine, Kosair Children's Hospital, Louisville, Kentucky
Expressive Therapy

LEE P. SHULMAN, M.D.
Assistant Professor, Department of Obstetrics and Gynecology, University of Tennessee–Memphis; Division of Reproductive Genetics, Attending Physician, Regional Medical Center, Memphis, Tennessee
Molecular Biology and Genetic Aspects

SELMA F. SIEGEL, M.D.
Assistant Professor of Pediatrics, Division of Pediatric Endocrinology, University of Pittsburgh School of Medicine; Staff Pediatrician, Children's Hospital of Pittsburgh and Magee–Women's Hospital, Pittsburgh, Pennsylvania
Pubertal Disorders: Precocious and Delayed Puberty; Abnormal Sexual Differentiation and Hypogonadism: Management and Therapy

PATRICIA S. SIMMONS, M.D.
Associate Professor of Pediatrics, Mayo Medical School; Department of Pediatrics and Adolescent Medicine, Mayo Clinic and Foundation, Rochester, Minnesota
Breast Disorders

JOE LEIGH SIMPSON, M.D.
Professor and Chairman, Department of Obstetrics and Gynecology, University of Tennessee–Memphis, Memphis, Tennessee
Disorders of Abnormal Sexual Differentiation

RAMONA I. SLUPIK, M.D.
Assistant Professor, Department of Obstetrics and Gynecology; Northwestern University Medical School; Chief, Pediatric and Adolescent Gynecology, Children's Memorial Hospital, Chicago, Illinois
Contraception

STEVEN R. SMITH, J.D., M.A.
Dean, Cleveland-Marshall College of Law, Cleveland State University, Cleveland, Ohio
Treating Minors

DENNIS STYNE, M.D.
Professor and Chair, Department of Pediatrics, University of California–Davis, School of Medicine, Davis, California
Normal Growth and Pubertal Development

PATRICK J. SWEENEY, M.D., M.P.H., Ph.D.
Professor of Obstetrics and Gynecology, Brown University; Director of Ambulatory Care, Women and Infants Hospital of Rhode Island, Providence, Rhode Island
Adolescent Pregnancy

EDWIN M. THORPE, Jr., M.D.
Assistant Professor, Department of Obstetrics and Gynecology, University of Tennessee, Memphis, Tennessee
Sexually Transmitted Diseases in Adolescence; HIV Infection in Adolescents

LISA A. TURNER-SCHIKLER, M.A., A.T.R.
Adjunct Clinical Faculty Field Supervisor, Department of Expressive Therapies, University of Louisville; Expressive Therapist, Kosair Children's Hospital, Louisville, Kentucky
Expressive Therapy

STEPHEN S. WACHTEL, Ph.D.
Professor of Obstetrics and Gynecology, Division of Reproductive Genetics, University of Tennessee–Memphis, Memphis, Tennessee
Molecular Biology and Genetic Aspects

Foreword

It is a pleasure to have been asked to write a foreword for this excellent textbook on pediatric and adolescent gynecology. This area of health care, focusing on a segment of the female population, has been underserved not only by the medical profession but also by third-party payers. Policy-makers have failed by not allocating adequate funds to care for this patient population. The medical profession has been deficient both by not transmitting information to patients and by not accepting the social responsibility of becoming involved in public information services.

To have Professor Sir John Dewhurst write the prologue is an honor. Sir John has trained many physicians on both sides of the Atlantic in this special area of medicine.

This book has been divided into three parts: Growth and Development, Medical Problems, and Surgical Problems. Dr. Peter Lee, who is Professor of Pediatrics at the University of Pittsburgh, has seen to it that the growth and development section includes chapters on molecular biology, genetics, anatomy, embryology, normal growth and development, and the special interest of the Pittsburgh Group, the neuroendocrinology of puberty. The authors have made a scientific subject easy to read and have included a great deal of information.

The medical problems of this age group from a gynecologic perspective are well covered under the editing of Dr. David Muram of the University of Tennessee. His expertise in the area of sexual abuse and sexually transmitted diseases is well known and certainly outstanding, but to be able to find, in one section of a text, material that ranges from androgens in the adolescent to depression and suicide is unusual. The medical problems found in this age group are well documented and addressed in a fashion that is easily understandable.

The third part of this book, the section on surgical problems, has been edited by Professor Sir John Dewhurst. The contributions by various authors are understandable even by the nonsurgically oriented clinician.

Other texts have been devoted to pediatric and adolescent gynecology, but none has been approached in this integrated fashion, with each portion relating to the others. I congratulate Dr. Sanfilippo on having developed the theme and surrounded himself with three excellent associate editors. If indeed gynecologic care begins in the pediatric and adolescent age group, then all of us are better off for having this text as a reference to enhance management of gynecologic problems in the female pediatric and adolescent patient.

ALVIN F. GOLDFARB, M.D.

Professor of Obstetrics and Gynecology and Director of Educational Programs, Jefferson Medical College; Executive Director, North American Society for Pediatric and Adolescent Gynecology, Philadelphia, Pennsylvania

Preface

Pediatric and adolescent gynecology is a subspecialized area of gynecology focusing on patients from neonatal life to age 21 years. The problems encountered are often unique to this age group. Medical and surgical management of this patient population requires particular expertise. It is the major objective of this textbook to provide the clinician with a composite text, ranging from explanation of the physiology of normal puberty to the succinct, well-organized, and thorough evaluation of sexual abuse. The clinical challenges found in Third World countries are also included. In essence, a distinct effort has been made to address every aspect of the subspecialty area. How does one approach the sexually abused child? What questions are appropriate to ask? What constitutes normal genital anatomy? How does one document the findings? These questions and many others are addressed in the textbook. A sincere effort to present *normal* versus *abnormal*, e.g., normal pubertal development versus abnormal development, is a recurring theme throughout the text. The intricate aspects of molecular biology as applied to pediatric and adolescent gynecology are conveyed. The more commonly observed problems, such as vulvovaginitities, are approached in a differential diagnosis manner, allowing the clinician to determine the proper diagnosis and proceed with management.

We have presented a compilation of new and exciting developments within the discipline that include areas such as expressive (art) therapy and sports-related gynecologic problems in the adolescent. The culmination of our effort is manifested in the chapter "Future Perspectives," which gives the clinician a glimpse into the future. It is the specific objective of the editors of Pediatric and Adolescent Gynecology to provide a compact compilation of current literature appropriate to the many medical and surgical problems encountered by clinicians who provide care for pediatric and adolescent gynecologic patients.

JOSEPH S. SANFILIPPO
LOUISVILLE, KENTUCKY

Contents

SECTION I

Prologue: A Short History of Pediatric and Adolescent Gynecology 1

Associate Editor • John Dewhurst

SECTION II

Growth and Development 5

Associate Editor • Peter A. Lee

CHAPTER 1

Embryology and Normal Anatomy 6

Kunwar P. Bhatnagar

CHAPTER 2

Normal Growth and Pubertal Development 20

Dennis Styne

CHAPTER 3

Abnormalities in Growth 34

Raymond L. Hintz

CHAPTER 4

Neuroendocrinology of Puberty 44

Peter A. Lee, Edward O. Reiter, and Howard E. Kulin

CHAPTER 5

Pubertal Disorders: Precocious and Delayed Puberty 53
Louis St. L. O'Dea, Selma F. Siegel, and Peter A. Lee

CHAPTER 6

Disorders of Abnormal Sexual Differentiation 77
Joe Leigh Simpson

CHAPTER 7

Abnormal Sexual Differentiation and Hypogonadism:
Management and Therapy 104
Selma F. Siegel, Sarah Berga, and Peter A. Lee

CHAPTER 8

Nutrition, Growth, and Development 128
Gilbert B. Forbes

CHAPTER 9

Effects of the Thyroid on Gonadal and
Reproductive Function 139
Thomas P. Foley, Jr.

CHAPTER 10

Molecular Biology and Genetic Aspects 151
Lee P. Shulman and Stephen S. Wachtel

SECTION III

Medical Problems **169**
Associate Editor • David Muram

CHAPTER 11

Genital Examination of Prepubertal and
Peripubertal Females 170
Susan F. Pokorny

CHAPTER 12

Vulvovaginitis 187
Frederick J. Rau, Claudette E. Jones, and David Muram

CHAPTER 13

Vulvar Disorders 203
C. Marjorie Ridley

CHAPTER 14

Vaginal Bleeding in Childhood and Menstrual
Disorders in Adolescence 222
David Muram, Joseph S. Sanfilippo, and S. Paige Hertweck

CHAPTER 15

Dysmenorrhea and Pelvic Pain 233
Gita P. Gidwani and Marsha Kay

CHAPTER 16

Androgens and the Adolescent Girl 250
José F. Cara and Robert L. Rosenfield

CHAPTER 17

Adolescent Sexuality 278
Robert T. Brown and Barbara A. Cromer

CHAPTER 18

Contraception 289
Ramona I. Slupik

CHAPTER 19

Adolescent Pregnancy 299
Patrick J. Sweeney

CHAPTER 20

Sexually Transmitted Diseases in Childhood 310
Kristi Morgan Mulchahey

CHAPTER 21

Sexually Transmitted Diseases in Adolescence 336
Edwin M. Thorpe, Jr., and David Muram

CHAPTER 22

HIV Infection in Adolescents 356
Edwin M. Thorpe, Jr., and David Muram

CHAPTER 23

Child Sexual Abuse 365
David Muram

CHAPTER 24

Expressive Therapy 383
Lisa A. Turner-Schikler and Kenneth Schikler

CHAPTER 25

Eating Disorders 397
Pauline S. Powers

CHAPTER 26

Depression and Suicide 417
Denise Ford-Nepa

CHAPTER 27

Adolescent Drug Abuse 432
Paul King

CHAPTER 28

Diagnostic Imaging 441
Luigi Fedele and Milena Dorta

CHAPTER 29

Delayed Consequences of Childhood Malignancies 467
David Muram

CHAPTER 30

Sports-Related Problems in Reproductive Function 478
Robert W. Rebar

CHAPTER 31

Reproductive Health Care Needs of the
Developmentally Disabled 490
David Muram and Thomas E. Elkins

CHAPTER 32

Treating Minors 499
Steven R. Smith

CHAPTER 33

Puberty Aberrancy in the Third World 513
Geeta N. Pandya

SECTION IV
Surgical Problems 527
Associate Editor • John Dewhurst

CHAPTER 34

Genital Trauma 528
Mary E. Rimsza

CHAPTER 35

Sexual Developmental Anomalies and Their
Reconstruction: Upper and Lower Tracts 535
D. Keith Edmonds

CHAPTER 36

Urologic Problems 567
Diane Francoeur, Anthony Casale, and Alan Retik

CHAPTER 37

Breast Disorders 583
Patricia S. Simmons

CHAPTER 38

Oncologic Problems 601
Michael L. Hicks and M. Steven Piver

CHAPTER 39

Surgically Correctable Congenital Anomalies:
Diagnosis and Management 616
Steven S. Rothenberg and William J. Pokorny

CHAPTER 40

Rectovaginal Fistulae and Associated Anomalies 630
John Dewhurst

CHAPTER 41

Chronic Pelvic Pain: Medical and Surgical Approach 635
Joseph S. Sanfilippo

CHAPTER 42

Future Perspectives 654
Leo Plouffe, Jr., and Paul G. McDonough

APPENDICES

Barbara R. Hostetler

Appendix A

Growth Charts 667

Appendix B

Tanner Staging 676

Appendix C

Normal Laboratory Values 677

Appendix D

Temperature Conversion 681

Appendix E

Commonly Used Medications 682

Appendix F

Oral Contraceptives: Combination, Sequential, and
Microdose Progestins 689

Index 691

Pediatric and Adolescent Gynecology

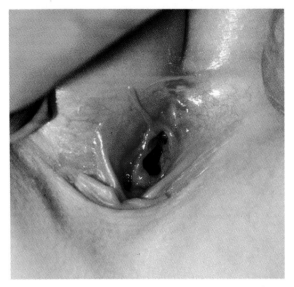

FIGURE 13–1 ••• Hymenal polyp noted on gynecologic examination of a newborn.

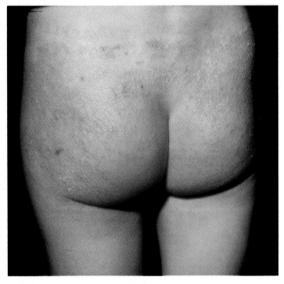

FIGURE 13–2 ••• Diaper dermatitis. Note the clear demarcation of the diaper area with the irritation.

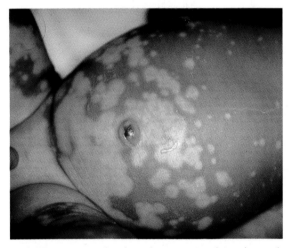

FIGURE 13–4 ••• Seborrheic dermatitis involving the trunk and vulvar area.

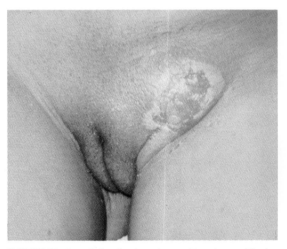

FIGURE 13–6 ••• Infantile gluteal granuloma located in the left inguinal area.

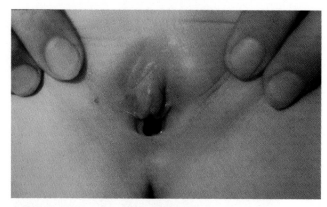

FIGURE 13–7 ••• *D,* An intact hymen and introitus with lateral displacement of the adherent area.

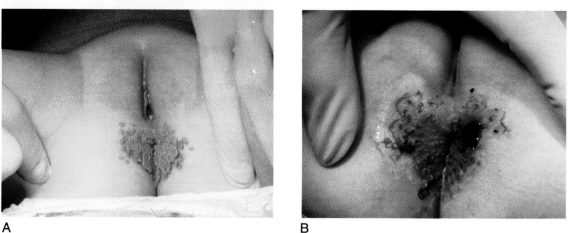

A   B

FIGURE 13–8 ••• *A,* A 24-month-old female with recurrent condylomata acuminata refractory to medical therapy. *B,* Same patient during intraoperative CO_2 laser treatment of the condylomata.

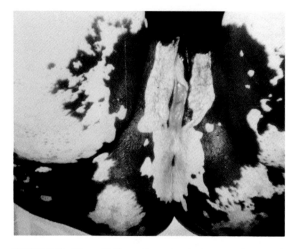

FIGURE 13–13 ••• Vitiligo. Note the depigmented areas of the vulva.

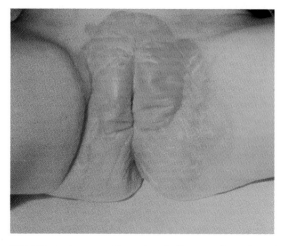

FIGURE 13–15 ••• Epidermolysis bullosa involving the vulvar area.

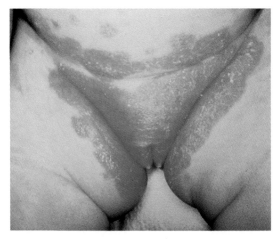

FIGURE 13–17 ••• Psoriasis involving the vulvovaginal area.

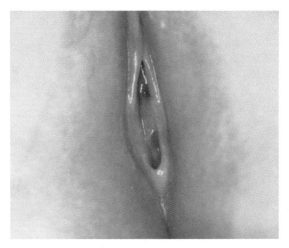

FIGURE 14–1 ••• Acute vulvovaginitis. Note the typical area of distribution.

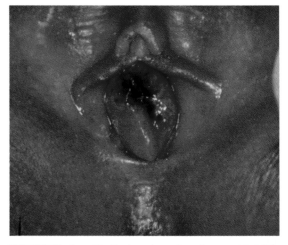

FIGURE 14–5 ••• Urethral prolapse in a 6-year-old child.

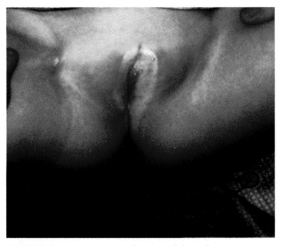

FIGURE 14–6 ••• Lichen sclerosus of the vulva in a 6-year-old child.

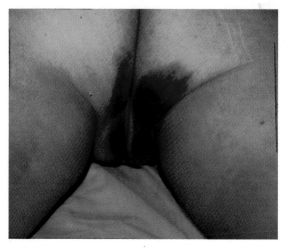

FIGURE 34–1 ••• Labial bruising extending onto the buttocks secondary to a straddle injury.

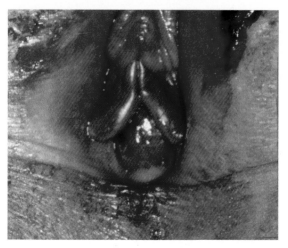

FIGURE 34–2 ••• Vulvar hematoma.

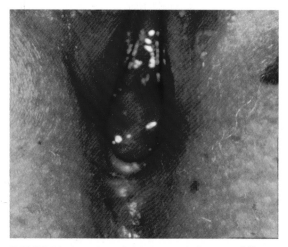

FIGURE 34–3 ••• Superficial tear secondary to a fall onto a stick.

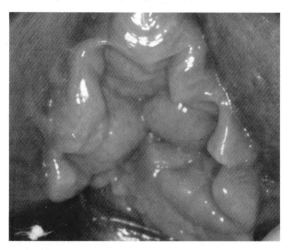

FIGURE 34–4 ••• Scarring of the posterior fourchette secondary to accidental trauma.

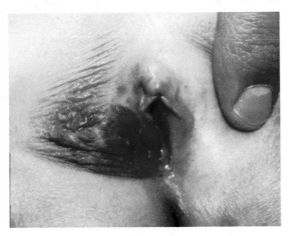

FIGURE 34–5 ••• Vaginal-hymenal tear secondary to sexual abuse. Note the disruption of the hymen at the lower margin of the photograph.

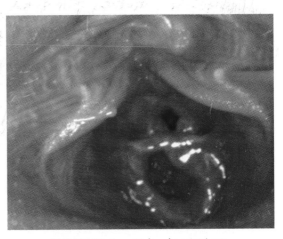

FIGURE 34–6 ••• Vulvar hemangioma.

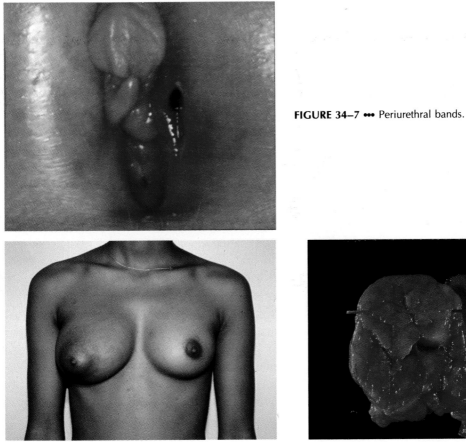

FIGURE 34–7 ••• Periurethral bands.

A   B

FIGURE 37–3 ••• *A,* Unilateral fibroadenoma. *B,* Surgical specimen of a fibroadenoma.

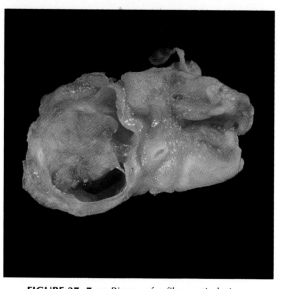

FIGURE 37–7 ••• Biopsy of a fibrocystic lesion.

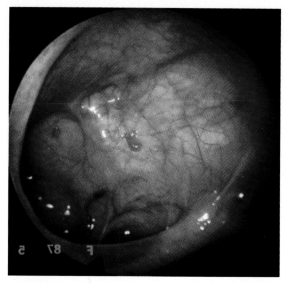

FIGURE 41–3 ••• Endometriosis as represented by polypoid structures (American Fertility Society stage I).

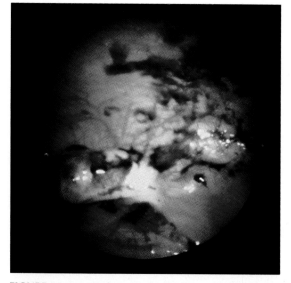

FIGURE 41–4 ••• Endometriosis, American Fertility Society stage IV. This is indicative of extensive endometriosis in association with retrograde menstruation secondary to outflow tract obstruction.

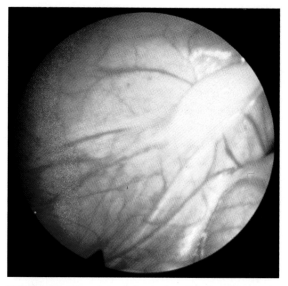

FIGURE 41–16 ••• Intraabdominal testicle in a 22-month-old male.

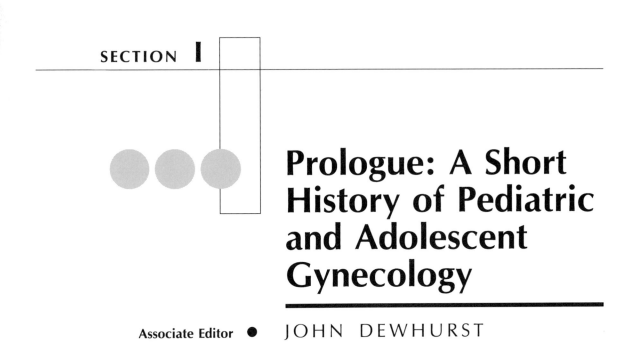

Prologue: A Short History of Pediatric and Adolescent Gynecology

Associate Editor ● JOHN DEWHURST

It often seems that a new development in medicine is introduced in more than one country at around the same time. The origin of pediatric and adolescent gynecology has been no exception. We know that there were pioneers in Czechoslovakia and the United States, and perhaps there were others elsewhere whose early contributions to the subject have remained unrecognized.

In Prague, Professor Peter conceived the idea of setting up an independent outpatient clinic in pediatric gynecology; this became a reality on September 12, 1940. His clinic was probably the first to be established in Europe. In the United States, Dr. Goodrich Shauffler published the first book on pediatric gynecology in 1941. It is clear that his experience in the subject preceded the publication of this book by a number of years, indicating the probability that he and Professor Peter, although separated by thousands of miles, began their practice of pediatric gynecology at approximately the same time and thus should be considered its founders.

At this time Europe, of course, was at war, and the effects of the turmoil, which were widespread and devastating, continued for some years after the conflict ended. Prague suffered greatly, as did many other cities, and it was not until 1962 that a pediatric faculty was established at Charles University in Prague, with Professor Peter as its first Professor of Gynecology and Obstetrics; these subjects were included in the pediatric curriculum.

By this time in the United States, not only had Schauffler's book reached its fourth edition, but other physicians were also showing a keen interest in the gynecologic disorders of children. These included Dr. Elsie Carrington and Dr. Stewart Taylor, each of whom contributed to the literature by including a chapter devoted to the subspecialty in their published textbooks. Another early writer was Dr. Warren Lang of Philadelphia. Dr. Leon Israel, also of Philadelphia, saw the potential importance of the subject and supported its development.

The most important early American contributor, however, was Dr. John Huffman, whose work, *The Gynecology of Childhood and Adolescence,* appeared in 1958. This was a detailed account of childhood gynecologic disorders that undoubtedly stimulated many clinicians, not only in the United States but also in Europe, to pay more attention to these early years. This book was not Huffman's only contribution to the subject; he also produced many original articles for scholarly journals and was in demand as a speaker at a number of European conferences. He was joined at these meetings by Dr. Vincent Capraro of Buffalo, New York, who had independently established a regular pediatric gynecologic clinic in his hospital.

It was my privilege to accompany Drs. Huffman and Capraro to these meetings, and we became lifelong friends. My own interest in the subject had begun during the 1950s and was a natural development of an earlier interest in intersexuality. Realizing, as have all pediatric gynecologists since, that the subject required a cooperative approach, I was fortunate to collaborate with two admirable colleagues: Professor Robert Zachary, a pediatric surgeon, and Dr. Ronald Gordon, a pediatric physician. We worked closely together, and in 1963, I was able to publish *The Gynaecological Disorders of Infants and Children,* which was then only the third book on the subject. It is curious that an interest in intersexuality also led Dr. Howard Jones, a distinguished American gynecologist, to develop a wider interest in childhood gynecology and to publish, in collaboration with Dr. R. H. Heller, the fourth book on the topic in 1966.

Interest grew on both sides of the Atlantic, but it was in Europe that the subject was to become officially organized. After one or two local conferences had been held, the Fédération Internationale de Gynécologie Infantile et Juvénile (FIGIJ) was formed at the First International Symposium in Lausanne in 1971. FIGIJ's President and founder was Dr. Robert Contamin from Grenobles, and its Secretary General was Dr. Irmi Rey-Stocker who continued to guide it for many years. National societies were formed and accepted as members of the Fédération. Soon afterward the Fédération became a corporate member of the International Federation of Gynecology and Obstetrics (FIGO).

Many gynecologists from Europe and elsewhere who had already developed an interest in these disorders were represented at early meetings. Prominent among them were Dr. Vessaly (Prague), who had succeeded Professor Peter; Professor Widholm (Helsinki), Dr. Sersiron (Paris), Dr. Huber (Innsbruck), Professor Matsumoto (Tokyo), Dr. Gurucharri (Buenos Aires), Professor Haspels (Utrecht), Dr. Creatsas (Athens), and Professor Rauramo (Turku, Finland), who became President in 1973. He was succeeded as President by Professor Christian Lauritzen of Ulm, Federal German Republic, who has presided over the Federation's activities since that time.

During the 1970s, worldwide interest was demonstrated by the venues for International Federation meetings in Bordeaux; Lausanne; Florence; Tokyo; Punta del Este, Uruguay; and Athens. Canada kept to the forefront of the specialty with excellent programs in Vancouver under Fred Bryans, in Toronto under Carol Cowell, and in Ottawa under Jay Spence.

In spite of this spreading international interest, the United States was surprisingly slow to progress during these years, although a number of individuals continued to be active. These included Dr. Albert Altchek, who organized several postgraduate courses in New York; Vincent Capraro, who continued to accept foreign postgraduates for training in Buffalo; and in Boston, Donald Goldstein and S. Jean Emans; somewhat later there were Gita Gidwani of Cleveland and

David Muram of Memphis, who set up pediatric gynecologic units after working in Britain. For a period of time, pediatric gynecology was included in the postgraduate courses associated with the annual meetings of the American College of Obstetricians and Gynecologists (ACOG).

Two individuals who were regular speakers at these postgraduate courses— Dr. Paul McDonough and Dr. Alvin Goldfarb—played a prominent part in the organization of pediatric and adolescent gynecology meetings in North America. Initial discussions were held at the ACOG Annual Meeting in Dallas in April 1982 with a view to the establishment of a North American chapter that would become part of FIGIJ. This became a reality when the 8th International Symposium was held in Washington, DC in August 1986. There have been several North American meetings since that time.

An important endeavor planned at the Washington meeting also became a reality: the reestablishment of a journal. An earlier journal entitled *Pediatric and Adolescent Gynecology* had been started in 1983, but support for it did not flourish, and the project was never completely successful. The proposal at the Washington meeting was to seek support for launching another journal, *Adolescent and Pediatric Gynecology*, the first issue of which appeared in 1988. The journal has enjoyed considerable success under its editors, Dr. Joseph Sanfilippo and Dr. Paul McDonough.

Enthusiasm and interest continue to expand, as evidenced at many important meetings. The 9th World Congress was held in Bombay in 1989, and the 10th was held in Paris in 1992. European meetings have been held in Florence (1987) and Rhodes (1988); a European Congress was held in 1990 in Dresden, and the FIGIJ met in Paris in 1992.

Great strides have clearly been made since the 1940s. What will the future hold?

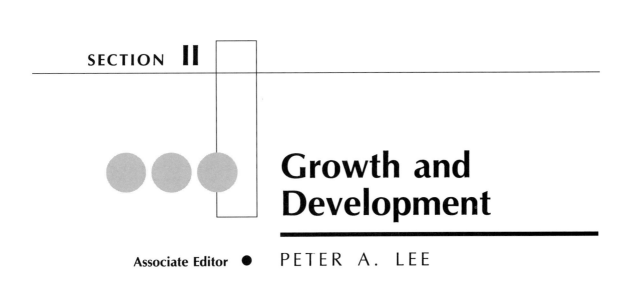

Growth and Development

Associate Editor ● P E T E R A . L E E

CHAPTER 1

Embryology and Normal Anatomy

KUNWAR P. BHATNAGAR

Ovaries are not necessary for primary female sexual development. In embryos with no gonads or ovaries, most of the internal and external genitalia develop like those in females. Conversely, testes are essential for male sexual development. In the early embryo three sets of renal excretory organs develop: the pronephros, the mesonephros, and the metanephros. In the male, the mesonephros and its duct, the mesonephric (wolffian) duct, develop into the ductal structures of the internal male reproductive tract, whereas in the female only nonfunctional remnants develop from the regressing mesonephric duct. In the female, the paramesonephric (müllerian) duct, another paired structure, develops lateral to the mesonephric duct and forms the major internal female reproductive organs, whereas in the male the paramesonephric duct regresses, leaving a few nonfunctional remnants. Thus, although the gonads differentiate into the ovaries in the female, the uterine tubes, the uterus, and the upper portion of the vagina develop independently of ovarian influence. In the constitutive development of the external genitalia in the female, the undifferentiated fetal external genitalia become the vulva. The developmental history of the female genital system is systematically presented in this chapter.

PRIMORDIAL GERM CELLS

The primordial germ cells are relatively large cells, 12 to 20 μm in diameter, with vesicular, centrally located nuclei and distinct nuclear membranes.[1] Yolk granules persist in these cells much longer than in the somatic cells and become a diagnostic feature. The cytoplasm is rich in glycogen. Spindle-shaped germ cells are seen in the interstitial tissue, whereas the germ cells resting beneath or between the coelomic epithelial cells are round or oval. These sex cells are first recognized in the 13-somite, 4-week human embryo, when as many as 30 of them are seen in the endoderm and the splanchnic mesoderm near the base of the allantois and the adjacent yolk sac. These primordial germ cells are believed to be derived from the endoderm. Migrating through the dorsal mesentery, they reach the medial mesonephric ridges, the sites for gonadal development. These sex cells become incorporated into the primary sex cords during the sixth week. Some of them may not reach the sex cords, and such ectopically oriented primordial germ cells may be the source for extragonadal teratomas and seminoma-like tumors.[2]

The ultrastructural characteristics of the germ cell are unique.[1] A few pseudopodia extend from the germ cell surface. The round nucleus contains one or two nucleoli, finely dispersed chromatin, and numerous nuclear pores. In the cytoplasm are seen juxtanuclear Golgi complexes, centrioles, ribosomes, round mitochondria with vesicular cristae, some elements of rough endoplasmic reticulum, lysosome-like granules, lipid droplets, and pinocytotic vesicles (Fig. 1–1). Glycogen particle aggregates and monofilament bundles are con-

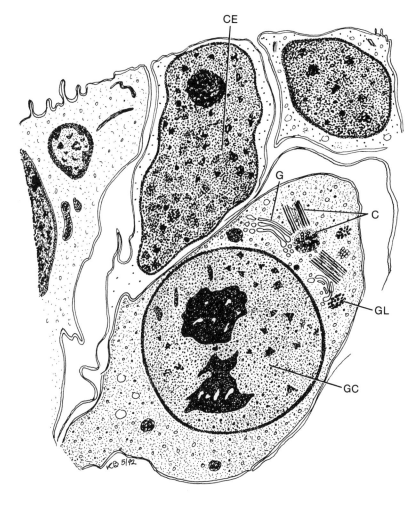

CE

G

C

GL

GC

KB 5/92

FIGURE 1–1 ••• A diagrammatic illustration of the ultrastructure of a human primordial germ cell (GC) located beneath the coelomic epithelium (CE). The nucleus is round and contains two irregular and prominent nucleoli. The juxtanuclear cytoplasm shows the Golgi complex (G), centrioles (C), and glycogen particles (GL). (Modified from Fukuda T. Ultrastructure of primordial germ cells in human embryo. Virchows Arch [Cell Pathol] 1976; 20:85–89.)

spicuous. Microtubules and chromatoid bodies are not observed. Occasional desmosomes are noted between germ cells and the surrounding coelomic epithelial or interstitial cells.

ULTRASTRUCTURE OF THE MATURE HUMAN OOCYTE

The normal mature human oocyte (Fig. 1–2) is large and is enveloped by follicular cells. The nucleus is large, spherical, and eccentric in location with a large nucleolus. Chromatin is mostly dispersed, and nuclear pores are numerous. A cluster of fine filaments is attached to the nuclear envelope. Attached to the nucleus is an aggregate of cytoplasmic organelles that corresponds to Balbiani's vitelline body[3, 4]; this consists of multiple Golgi complexes; a single stack of annulate lamellae; randomly distributed mitochondria; lipid droplets; dilated, smooth-surfaced endoplasmic re-

ticulum; a centrosome; fine filaments; small aggregates of dense amorphous material; dispersed or aggregated vesicles; short and irregular tubules; multivesicular bodies; and a few membrane-attached and free ribosomes (see Fig. 1–2). The rest of the cytoplasm has a uniform texture with fewer of the organelles. The entire circumference of the subplasmalemmal cytoplasm of the oocyte and the cytocortical region of the first polar body shows a heavy population of cortical granules.[5] Microvilli cover the entire oocyte surface, with the exception of the region in contact with the first polar body. The metaphase II spindle is characteristically organized.[5]

DEVELOPMENT OF THE FEMALE INTERNAL ORGANS

As stated earlier, female sexual development does not depend on the presence of

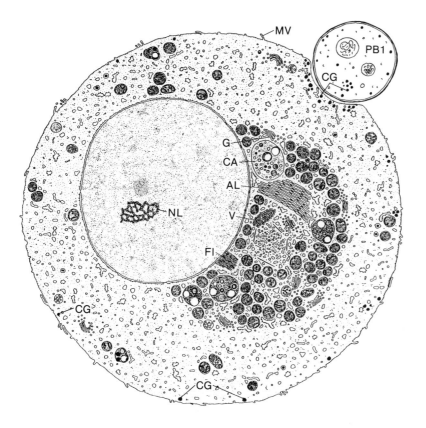

FIGURE 1–2 ••• A diagrammatic illustration of the ultrastructure of a normal human oocyte in contact with the first polar body. Notice the cluster of cell organelles in the paranuclear complex of Balbiani's body (vitelline body). AL, Annulate lamellae; CA, compound aggregates; CG, cortical granules; FI, filaments; G, Golgi complexes; MV, microvilli; NL, nucleolus; PB1, first polar body; V, vesicles. (Modified from Lentz TL. Cell Fine Structure. An Atlas of Drawings of Whole-Cell Structure. Philadelphia: WB Saunders, 1971; and VanBlerkom J. Occurrence and developmental consequences of aberrant cellular organization in meiotically mature human oocytes after exogenous ovarian hyperstimulation. J Electron Microsc Technol 1990; 16:324–346.)

ovaries. The gonad, in an undifferentiated stage, begins to develop in the fifth week as a region of multilayered coelomic epithelium on the entire medial aspect of the gonadal (mesonephric) ridge. The coelomic epithelium is only one to two cells thick elsewhere on the mesonephric ridge. Primary sex cords, consisting of finger-like extensions of the epithelial cords, grow into the mesenchyme. An outer cortex and an inner medulla result. In embryos with 46,XX chromosomes, the cortex develops into the ovary, and the medulla regresses. In male embryos, this is reversed, with the medulla differentiating into the testis and the cortex regressing. A tunica albuginea develops in both sexes, but in the female it develops at a later stage and is a much thinner layer than in males.

The developing ovary differentiates slowly. Very few primary sex cords invade the medulla, and nearly all of them remain in the cortex. After the regression of the medulla, the primary sex cord clusters surround the primordial ova, which at this time are differentiated as primary oocytes that are in the prophase of the first meiotic division. The

follicular cells proliferate from the coelomic epithelium. A full complement of primary oocytes—estimated to be 2 million—are present in the ovaries of a newborn. Regression occurs during childhood, and by puberty some 40,000 primary oocytes are said to remain.[6] Of these, only approximately 400 will develop into secondary oocytes by completing the first meiotic division, one by one, shortly before ovulation each month. Virtually always, only one follicle matures and ruptures at midcycle each month. This continues until about 51.4 years of age, which is the average age when menopause occurs.[5]

During the early fetal period, the ovaries are juxtarenal. They gradually descend into the lesser pelvis. Rarely, when the gubernaculum fails to unite with the uterine fundus, the ovarian and round ligaments become continuous, fail to lengthen, and as a result pull the ovary into the labia majora. In the newborn the ovaries are triangular in a cross section made centrally through the longest plane and are rounded at the ends.[7–9] Surface furrows disappear within months after birth.[9]

Mesonephric (Wolffian) Ducts and Formation of Nonfunctional Remnants

The urogenital organs develop from the intermediate mesoderm (Fig. 1–3). They are closely associated with each other during early development. The fetal renal excretory system consists of three organs that develop chronologically into the pronephros, the mesonephros, and the metanephros.[6] Only the mesonephros and its duct participate in the formation of the female genital ducts (Table 1–1). Excluding the most cranial one or two tubules and the associated mesonephric, or wolffian, duct, some five or six cranial mesonephric tubules form the epoöphoron, a vestigial structure associated with the ovary. The more caudal mesonephric tubules give rise to

TABLE 1–1 ••• HOMOLOGIES OF THE FEMALE GENITAL SYSTEM*[6, 8, 10, 11]

Female	Undifferentiated	Male
Oocytes	Primordial germ cells	Spermatozoa
Ovary	Gonad	Testis
Proper ovarian ligament and round ligament of the uterus	Gubernaculum	Gubernaculum testis
Epoöphorantic (Gartner's) duct	Mesonephric (wolffian) duct	Duct of epididymis and ductus deferens (distal)
No homologue		Ductus deferens (proximal); ejaculatory duct and seminal vesicle
Appendices vesiculosae (?)	Mesonephric tubules	Appendix of epididymis (?)
Epoöphoron		Efferent ductules
		Lobules of epididymis
Paroöphoron		Paradidymis (tubuli)
		Paradidymis
		Aberrant ductules
Ostium abdominale of uterine tube	Paramesonephric (müllerian) duct	Appendix of testis
Uterus		No homologue
Vagina (? lower portion)		Prostatic utricle
Vagina (upper portion)		No homologue
Urethra	Urogenital sinus	Urethra (except navicular fossa)
Greater vestibular glands		Bulbourethral glands
Urethral and paraurethral glands		Prostate gland
		Remaining urethra and glands
Vestibule	—	
Labia minora	Genital folds	Penis, urethral surface
Clitoris	Genital tubercle	Remaining penis
		Urethra in the glans
Labia majora	Labioscrotal swellings	Scrotum
Hymen	Sinus tubercle	Seminal colliculus
Urachus (median umbilical ligament)	Allantois	Urachus (median umbilical ligament)
Rectum and upper anal canal	Dorsal cloaca	Rectum and upper anal canal
Most of the bladder and the urethra	Ventral cloaca	Most of the bladder; part of prostatic urethra
Ureter, pelvis, calices, and collecting tubules	Metanephric diverticulum (ureteric bud)	Ureter, pelvis, calices, and collecting tubules
Broad ligament	Peritoneal fold	No homologue
	Generalized mesoderm	
Mesovarium		Mesorchium
Corpus cavernosum clitoridis		Corpus cavernosum penis
Bulbs of the vestibule		Bulb of the penis
Mons pubis		No named homologue; this region is similar to the mons pubis of the female†

*Corresponding male structures are also given for comparison.
†In the *Nomina Anatomica*,[11] the term *mons pubis* has been listed both as a general surface feature, as well as under the female external genitalia. No such listing occurs with the scrotum. On the basis of surface anatomy, the mons pubis (the rounded fleshy prominence over the symphysis pubis) should be a valid landmark in both sexes. The question remains whether males have either a mons pubis or at least its homologue. *Mons veneris* is the name of the prominence in the female. *Mons martialis* is the term suggested for this yet-to-be-specified region in the male.

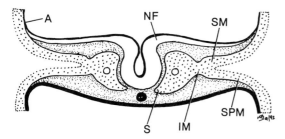

FIGURE 1–3 ••• Cross section of an early 3-week embryo showing the three divisions of the mesoderm. A, Amnion; IM, intermediate mesoderm; NF, neural fold; S, somite; SM, somatic mesoderm, SPM, splanchnic mesoderm. (Redrawn from Moore KL. The Developing Human. Clinically Oriented Embryology. 4th ed. Philadelphia: WB Saunders, 1988.)

the paroöphoron, an inconsistent group of coiled tubules seen between the layers of the mesosalpinx. The paroöphoron usually disappears before adulthood. Additionally, one or more stalked, oval, pea-sized cysts known as the *appendices vesiculosae epoöphorontis* (hydatids of Morgagni) are found near the epoöphoron and close to the ostium of the uterine tube. The vestigial remains of the lower portion of the mesonephric (wolffian) duct may be identified laterally on the upper half of the vagina as a minute tube or fibrous cord, the epoöphorantic duct (duct of Gartner). Occasionally, this duct may form into a cyst (Figs. 1–4, 1–5).

Paramesonephric (Müllerian) Ducts and Formation of the Uterine Tubes and Uterus

The paired paramesonephric ducts develop as an invagination of the coelomic epithelium on the lateral aspect of the cranial end of the mesonephric ridge. The caudal end of this ridge grows blindly, acquires a lumen subsequently as it lengthens, and remains lateral to the mesonephric duct (see Figs. 1–4, 1–5). At the caudal end of the mesonephros, the paramesonephric duct turns medially and, crossing ventrally to the mesonephric duct, enters the genital cord where it bends caudally, juxtaposed with its companion on the opposite side by the third month of gestation. The blind ends of the two ducts produce an elevation on the dorsal wall of the urogenital sinus, the sinus (müllerian) tubercle. Each duct consists of vertical cranial and caudal segments with an intermediate horizontal section (Fig. 1–6). The cranial segment forms the uterine tube, with its coelomic invagination forming the ostium of the tube; the caudal vertical segments fuse to form the uterovaginal primordium, which develops into the lower uterine segment and, while enlarging, incorporates the horizontal aspects to give rise to the fundus and the body of the uterus. The endometrial stroma and myometrium develop from the surrounding mesenchyme.

Adnexa

The ovary traverses a short distance while descending to occupy its place in the ovarian fossa. It does not enter the inguinal canal. Through the mesovarium the ovary is attached to the medial aspect of the mesonephric fold. The inguinal fold attaches it to the ventral abdominal wall. A gubernaculum develops in the inguinal fold and later attaches to the uterus laterally near the entrance of the uterine tube. The lower part of the gubernaculum becomes the round ligament of the uterus, whereas the upper part becomes the ovarian ligament. The processus vaginalis peritonei (saccus vaginalis) also develops as a temporary peritoneal evagination. Usually its prolongation into the inguinal canal is completely obliterated. When patent (known as the *canal of Nuck*), it may form the sac of a potential inguinal hernia. The urethral and paraurethral glands remain rudimentary. The greater vestibular glands develop from the urogenital sinus.

Accessory Structures and Congenital Malformations

Supernumerary ovaries have been reported to occur in the mesovarium, in the broad ligament, and, very rarely, in association with a third uterine tube. Bilateral absence of ovaries is rare. Unilateral absence has been reported associated with the absence of the corresponding uterine tube. Divided ovaries are common. Ectopically, an ovary can be drawn through the inguinal canal into the labia majora.

The uterus, fallopian tubes, and vagina are often absent in those with severe congenital malformations such as in sympodia or sirenomelia. Unilateral absence of the parameso-

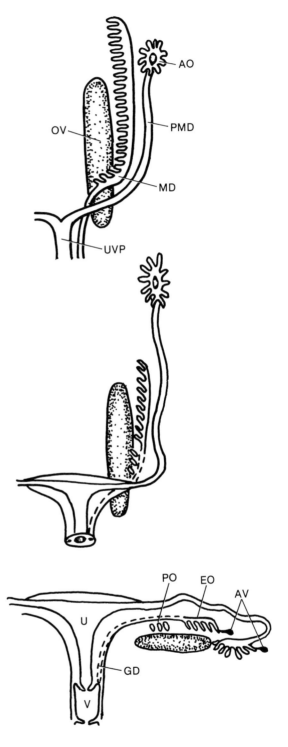

FIGURE 1–4 ••• Transformation of the mesonephric (wolffian) and paramesonephric (müllerian) ducts into definitive structures. AO, Abdominal ostium; AV, appendices vesiculosae (hydatids of Morgagni); EO, epoöphoron; GD, Gartner's duct; MD, mesonephric (wolffian) duct; OV, ovary; PMD, paramesonephric (müllerian) duct; PO, paroöphoron; U, uterus; UVP, uterovaginal primordium; V, vagina. (Modified from Anson BJ [ed]. Morris' Human Anatomy. 12th ed. New York: McGraw-Hill, 1966. Modified with permission of McGraw-Hill, Inc.)

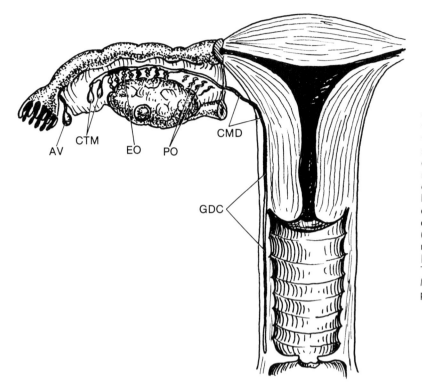

FIGURE 1–5 ••• Persisting remnants of the mesonephric (wolffian) duct at puberty drawn in relation to the uterine tubes, uterus, and vagina. AV, Appendices vesiculosae; CMD, cranial mesonephric duct remnants; CTM, cranial mesonephric tubules; EO, epoöphoron (cranial mesonephric tubule remnants); GDC, Gartner's duct cysts (caudal mesonephric duct remnants); PO, paroöphoron (caudal mesonephric tubule remnants). (Modified from Anson BJ [ed]. Morris' Human Anatomy. Treatise. 12th ed. New York: McGraw-Hill, 1966. Modified with permission of McGraw-Hill, Inc.)

nephric duct, resulting in severe anomalies, has been reported. The anomalies of the female genital system result from faulty union or lack of the two paramesonephric (müllerian) ducts. This may result in either incomplete or complete duplication of the uterus combined with duplication of the vagina. Many variations between the two extremes are seen. The bi-

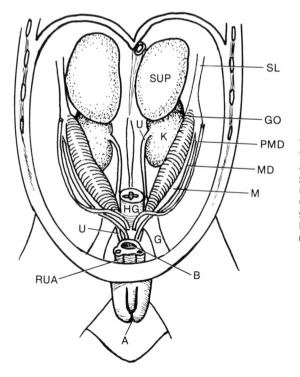

FIGURE 1–6 ••• Dissection of a 26-mm human embryo at the end of the embryonic period (about 56 days) showing the developing mesonephric and paramesonephric ducts. A, Anus; B, bladder; G, gubernaculum in inguinal fold; GO, gonad; HG, hindgut; K, kidney; M, mesonephros; MD, mesonephric duct; PMD, paramesonephric duct; RUA, right umbilical artery; SL, atrophying suspensory ligament; SUP, suprarenal gland; U, ureter. (Redrawn from Hamilton WJ, Boyd JD, Mossman HW. Human Embryology. 4th ed. Baltimore: Williams & Wilkins, 1972.)

cornuate uterus is a common condition in which a single vagina and cervix occur with duplication of the body of the uterus.

Hypospadias in the female, in which the urethra opens in the vagina, is quite different from that in the male. Epispadias in females is very rare and is similar to that in males. Usually there is an associated bifid clitoris and prepuce. A deep groove separates the two halves, and the urethral orifice may be in the clitoris or ventral to it.

Errors in sexual development result in ambiguous genitalia. These may be the result of defective genetic direction, steroidogenesis, abnormal hormonal influences, or dyssynchrony during organogenesis. These disorders are discussed in Chapter 6.

DEVELOPMENT OF THE FEMALE EXTERNAL GENITALIA

The mons pubis, the rounded fleshy prominence over the symphysis pubis, is formed from subcutaneous adipose tissue. It remains devoid of hair until puberty, when it becomes covered by coarse hair limited above by a horizontal boundary.

The external genitalia initially develop in an undifferentiated state, and it is not possible to identify the sex externally before 12 weeks of gestation (Fig. 1–7, Table 1–2). At the end of the embryonic period (about 8 weeks), the genital tubercle appears as a surface elevation at the cranial end of the cloacal membrane and lengthens into the phallus (Figs. 1–8, 1–9). Within it, the urethral plate grows toward the tip. The lower end of the plate abuts against the ectoderm-lined primary urethral groove, which concomitantly develops along the caudal surface of the phallus. The margins of the groove are the genital folds that surround the urogenital membrane and proximally terminate near the ventral end of the anus. The urogenital membrane ruptures at about 6 weeks, providing a common perineal space (the future vestibule) for the urinary and genital openings at the base of the phallus, bounded by the genital folds, which develop into labia minora. Two genital (labioscrotal) swellings form laterally and become the labia majora. The vestibule develops from the remains of the urogenital sinus. The urethral meatus, vaginal opening, the ducts of the greater and lesser vestibular glands, and the bulbs of the vestibule are found in the floor of the vestibule (Fig. 1–10).

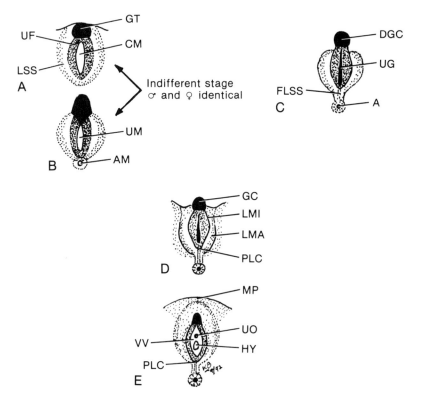

FIGURE 1–7 ••• A series of diagrams illustrating the developing female external genitalia. A, B, The undifferentiated stages, 4 to 8 weeks. C–E, At 9, 11, and 12 weeks, respectively. A, Anus; AM, anal membrane; CM, cloacal membrane; DGC, developing glans clitoridis; FLSS, fused labioscrotal swellings; GC, glans clitoridis; GT, genital tubercle; HY, hymen; LMA, labia majora; LMI, labia minora; LSS, labioscrotal swelling; MP, mons pubis; PLC, posterior labial commissure; UF, urogenital fold; UG, urethral groove; UM, urogenital membrane; UO, urethral orifice; VV, vestibule of vagina. (Redrawn from Moore KL. The Developing Human. Clinically Oriented Embryology. 4th ed. Philadelphia: WB Saunders, 1988.)

TABLE 1–2 ••• CHRONOLOGIC APPEARANCE OF THE VARIOUS COMPONENTS
OF THE GENITAL SYSTEM

Fertilization Age	Crown-to-Rump Length (mm)	Developmental Event
Days		
Zero time	—	Chromosomal sex established
24–25	2.5–4.5 (13–20 somites)	Primordial germ cells; genital tubercle develops at the cranial end of the cloacal membrane
33–36	7.0–9.0	Undifferentiated gonad
41–43	11.0–14.0	Primordial germ cells incorporated in the primary sex cords; paramesonephric (müllerian) duct; nipples; urorectal septum fuses with the cloacal membrane; urogenital membrane ruptures (15-mm embryo)
56	27.0–31.0	Anal membrane ruptures; despite the fetus's human resemblance, the external genitalia still have an ambiguous appearance
Weeks		
10	61	Ovary and vagina differentiate
12	87	External genitalia distinguished
16	140	Primordial follicles
18	160	Clitoris relatively large
Perinatal period	—	Hymen ruptures
Newborn	—	2 million primary oocytes in the ovaries
Childhood puberty	—	Regression of primary oocytes; some 40,000 remain at puberty
Reproductive period (about 15–50 years)	—	Only about 400 secondary oocytes are expelled, one at a time, at ovulation
After menopause	—	Reproductive organs gradually regress

Data from Moore KL. The Developing Human. Clinically Oriented Embryology. 4th ed. Philadelphia: WB Saunders, 1988.

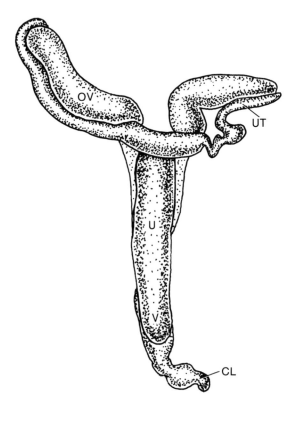

FIGURE 1–8 ••• The female internal genitalia at 13 weeks (crown–rump length, 101 mm). CL, Clitoris; OV, ovary; U, uterus; UT, uterine tube; V, vagina. (Redrawn from England MA. Color Atlas of Life Before Birth. Normal Fetal Development. London: Mosby-Year Book Europe Ltd., 1983.)

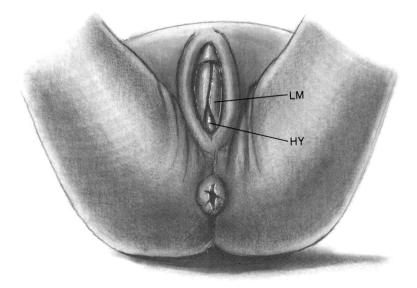

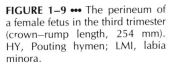

FIGURE 1–9 ••• The perineum of a female fetus in the third trimester (crown–rump length, 254 mm). HY, Pouting hymen; LMI, labia minora.

The phallus, which in the early stages is longer in the female than in the male, forms the clitoris. The prepuce develops first as a ridge proximal to the glans and extending forward. Over the dorsum and the sides of the glans clitoridis, the shallow preputial sac is formed, but the ventral side remains free. Only in this manner does preputial development differ from the male homologue. The homologies of the external (and internal) genital organs are shown in Table 1–1.[8, 10, 11]

DEVELOPMENT OF THE VAGINA AND HYMEN

In the tenth week of gestation an epithelial proliferation from the dorsal lining of the urogenital sinus begins in the region of the sinus tubercle. The hymen develops later at this site of proliferation. It is not known whether the proliferating epithelium is derived from the sinus tubercle or from the mesonephric duct. The proliferating epithelium extends cranially and forms a solid flattened plate inside the tubular uterovaginal primordium. The fibromuscular vagina develops from this solid plate by recanalization in a caudocranial direction. The caudal end of the paramesonephric duct recedes until its junction with the sinus epithelium reaches the cervical canal. Vaginal fornices develop from the upper end of the vaginal plate, growing around the cervix. At the lower end, the plate around the hymenal orifice forms the hymen by trapping a thin layer of mesoderm. The walls of the vagina are seen

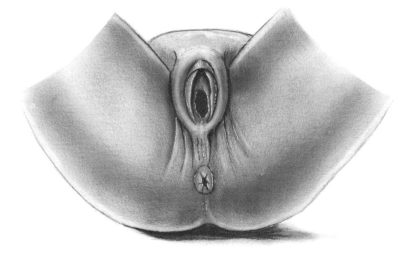

FIGURE 1–10 ••• Perineum of a newborn female.

through the hymenal orifice; the rugae in the lower part of the anterior wall of the vagina immediately beneath the urethra are more prominent in young females and in virgins.

The hymen is lined on its superior (vaginal) surface by the vaginal epithelium and by the sinus epithelium on its inferior (vestibular) surface. In later development the inferior hymenal surface and most of the vestibule are lined by an epithelium similar to that of the vagina. The urogenital sinus shortens to form the vaginal vestibule, which opens on the surface between the genital folds. The vaginal epithelium hypertrophies greatly in the fetus under the influence of maternal hormones but remains unproliferated after birth and through childhood.

The hymen, a fold of vascularized mucous membrane, lies within the vaginal orifice and separates the vagina from the vestibule. It shows great variations in thickness and in the size and shape of the hymenal opening. The more commonly observed hymenal variations are described and illustrated in Table 1–3.

GENITAL SYSTEM OF THE FEMALE NEWBORN AND THE CHILD

The average weight of a full-term newborn infant is about 3300 gm (7 lb), and the average crown-to-heel length is about 50 cm (20 in). In general, the newborn female is slightly smaller and weighs less than the newborn male.[9] Water constitutes 80% of the total body weight, compared with 60% at puberty. The newborn has 45% of water as extracellular fluid and 35% as intracellular fluid (compared with 17% and 43% respectively, at puberty). The development of the various components of the female genital system is given in Table 1–2.

In the newborn, the relatively large labia majora are bound inferiorly by a posterior labial commissure. Superiorly they merge into the mons pubis (see footnote in Table 1–1). The labia minora are relatively larger at birth. The clitoris is also relatively larger and more prominent in the newborn than in the adult. The hymen in late fetal life and at birth consists of a membranous fold, which may protrude between the labia minora (see Fig. 1–9). The vaginal orifice has a circumference of about 5 cm and can permit speculum examination of the vagina. During early childhood the orifice is more deeply positioned. The rugae of the anterior vaginal wall are prominent and are seen through the vaginal orifice (Fig. 1–11; see Table 1–3). The vaginal wall is thin until puberty and has a much redder appearance than in the adult. At puberty, Döderlein's bacillus (*Lactobacillus acidophilus*), a large gram-positive microorganism, appears in the

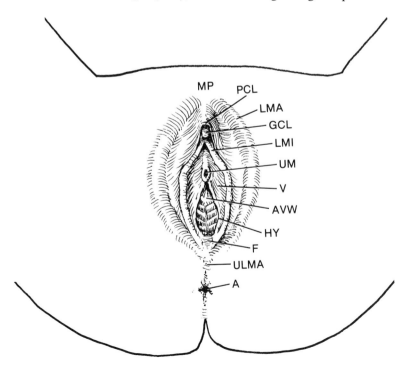

FIGURE 1–11 ••• Illustration of the perineum of a 10-year-old female with labia separated. A, Anus; AVW, anterior vaginal wall; F, fourchette; GCL, glans clitoridis; HY, hymen; LMA, labia majora; LMI, labia minora; MP, mons pubis; PCL, prepuce of the clitoris; ULMA, union of labia majora, posterior commissure; UM, urethral meatus; V, vestibule. (Redrawn from Snell RS. Atlas of Clinical Anatomy, Boston: Little, Brown, 1978.)

TABLE 1–3 ••• COMMONLY OBSERVED HYMENAL TYPES*

Hymen	Hymenal Opening(s)	Illustrations†
i. Annular; circular; lunar	Circular or moon-shaped	GC UM LM HY
ii. Bifenestratus; biforis	Two side-by-side openings with an intervening septum between them	
iii. Crescentic	Half moon–shaped	
iv. Cribriform; fenestrated	Many small openings	
v. Denticular; fringed	Serrate-edged (as in a parous condition)	
vi. Falciform	Sickle-shaped	
vii. Imperforate	None; vaginal orifice completely closed	
viii. Infundibuliform	Centrally open with sloping sides	
ix. Septate	Opening divided by a narrow septum	
x. Subseptate	Opening partially blocked by a septum growing out of one edge but not reaching the other	

*After coitus the remnants of the torn hymen are known as hymenal caruncles.

†All illustrations (i–x) depict the hymenal condition in a 3-year-old child. The labia minora (LM) are pulled widely apart; the hymenal openings (HY) are diagrammatically exaggerated. GC, glans clitoridis; UM, urinary meatus.

Data partly from Anson BJ (ed). Morris' Human Anatomy. 12th ed. New York: McGraw-Hill, 1966, p 1523.

vagina and breaks down glycogen in desquamated cells to form lactic acid. This protective phenomenon changes the pH of vaginal secretions from alkaline to acidic, thus reducing the incidence of vaginitis. Mucous glands are absent in the vagina; cervical gland mucus keeps the vagina moist. Pubic hair appears at puberty; the labia minora remain devoid of hair.

The vaginal vestibule is the cleft between the labia minora into which open the urethra, the vagina, and many lesser vestibular glands (Fig. 1–12). The greater vestibular glands open by a duct in the groove between the hymen and a labium minus at the posterior or inferior aspect of the vaginal orifice. Between the vaginal orifice and the frenulum of the labia minora is a shallow vestibular fossa. The hymen surrounds the vaginal orifice, which ap-

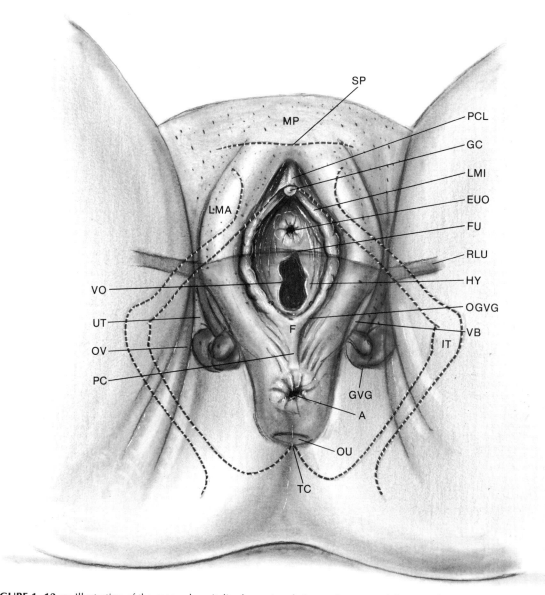

FIGURE 1–12 ••• Illustration of the external genitalia shown in relation to the uterus, fallopian tubes, and ovaries, and the bony pelvis in a 10-year-old female. These internal structures are shown superimposed from an examining physician's view. A, Anus; EUO, external urethral opening; F, fourchette; FU, fundus uteri; GC, glans clitoridis; GVG, greater vestibular gland; HY, hymen; IT, ischial tuberosity; LMA, labia majora; LMI, labia minora; MP, mons pubis; OGVG, opening of the greater vestibular gland; OU, ostium uteri; OV, ovary; PC, posterior commissure; PCL, prepuce of the clitoris; RLU, round ligament of the uterus, SP, pubic symphysis; TC, tip of coccyx; UT, fallopian (uterine) tube; VB, vestibular bulb; VO, vaginal orifice. (Modified from Anson BJ [ed]. Morris' Human Anatomy. 12th ed. New York: McGraw-Hill, 1966. Modified with permission of McGraw-Hill, Inc.)

pears as an opening into it. As stated earlier, the hymen shows great variation (see Table 1–3). The bulbs of the vestibule, the homologue of the corpus spongiosum penis, are paired, erectile bodies on both sides of the vaginal orifice and are united in front of it by a commissura bulborum or pars intermedia. Posteriorly they are in contact with the greater vestibular glands, and their anterior ends are joined to one another by a commissure and to the glans clitoridis by two bands of erectile tissue.

The form, size, position, and histologic appearance of the internal genital organs vary greatly from between birth and the attainment of puberty (Table 1–4).[9] Before birth, the uterus projects above the lesser pelvis, and the cervix is much larger than the fundus. The

TABLE 1–4 ••• DATA ON THE INTERNAL ORGANS[9]

	Ovaries	Fallopian Tubes	Uterus	Vagina†
Combined weight				
In the newborn	0.3 gm	—	3–4 gm	—
First 6 weeks postnatally	0.6 gm	—	—	—
Increase between birth and adulthood	5.0 gm*	—	—	—
Size				
At birth	1.5–3.0 cm long, 4.0–8.0 cm wide and thick	3.0 cm long, 5.0 mm wide	2.5–5.0 cm long, 2.0 cm wide, 1.3 cm thick	2.5–3.5 cm long, 1.5 cm wide; only potential cavity
In the adult	2.5–3.5 cm long, 2.0 cm wide, 1.0 cm thick	7.5 cm long, 5.0 cm wide, 2.5 cm thick	10.0 cm long	Anterior wall, 7.5 cm long; posterior wall, 9.0 cm long; circumference, about 4–5 cm†
Long axis				
At birth	Vertical	—	—	—
During descent after birth	Horizontal	—	—	—
In ovarian fossa	Vertical	—	—	—
Epithelium				
Fetal	—	—	—	Greatly hypertrophied
During childhood	—	—	—	Remains inactive, growing slowly

*The ovaries weigh 11.3 gm at maturity, a 32-fold increase from the birth weight.[10]
†The stated circumference of the orifice is about 5 cm.[9]

uterus is piriform at puberty and weighs 14 to 17 gm. Usually the fundus is below the superior pelvic aperture, but its position depends on the contents of the bladder and the rectum. The organ is somewhat enlarged during menstruation because of increased vascularity. The ovaries are very large in the fetus, extending nearly the entire length of the uterine tubes (see Fig. 1–8).[7] After birth, subsequent development reduces their overall dimension, and they reach the adult size at puberty.

References

1. Fukuda T. Ultrastructure of primordial germ cells in human embryo. Virchows Arch [Cell Pathol] 1976; 20:85–89.
2. Turner JH, Bloodworth JMB Jr. The testis. In: Bloodworth JMB Jr (ed). Endocrine Pathology. Baltimore: Williams and Wilkins, 1968, pp 430–477.
3. Hertig AT. The primary human oocyte: Some observations on the fine structure of Balbiani's vitelline body and the origin of the annulate lamellae. Am J Anat 1968; 122:107–138.
4. Lentz TL. Cell Fine Structure. An Atlas of Drawings of Whole-Cell Structure. Philadelphia: WB Saunders, 1971, p 269.
5. VanBlerkom J. Occurrence and developmental consequences of aberrant cellular organization in meiotically mature human oocytes after exogenous ovarian hyperstimulation. J Electron Microsc Technol 1990; 16:324–346.
6. Moore KL. The Developing Human. Clinically Oriented Embryology. 4th ed. Philadelphia: WB Saunders, 1988.
7. England MA. Color Atlas of Life Before Birth. Normal Fetal Development. Chicago: Year Book Medical, 1983.
8. Williams PL, Warwick R, Dyson M, Bannister LH. Gray's Anatomy. 37th ed. Edinburgh: Churchill Livingstone, 1989.
9. Crelin ES. Functional Anatomy of the Newborn. New Haven, CT: Yale University Press, 1973.
10. Anson BJ (ed). Morris' Human Anatomy. A Complete Systematic Treatise. 12th ed. New York: McGraw Hill, 1966.
11. International Anatomical Nomenclature Committee. Nomina Anatomica. 5th ed. Baltimore: Williams & Wilkins, 1983.

CHAPTER 2

Normal Growth and Pubertal Development

DENNIS STYNE

Growth encompasses many physical and psychological concepts. This chapter will address the physical aspects and the endocrinologic factors that control growth and development, focusing particularly on growth in stature and secondary sexual development in normal girls. Although diseases affecting growth and pubertal development will not be considered, the appropriate historical and physical evaluation of patients with such problems is presented.

GROWTH

Fetal Growth

In the transition from a single fertilized ovum to an approximately 3.5-kg newborn, the fetus manifests a spectacular growth rate.[1] For example, peak growth velocity in the fetus approaches 12 cm/month (approximately 12 times the peak growth velocity during the pubertal growth spurt) at 4 to 6 months of gestation. Fetal growth rate then decreases toward term. This negative regulation is presumably due to limitations of space within the uterine environment (Fig. 2–1).[2] A brief increase in growth rate occurs in the months after parturition; this has been suggested to be catch-up growth following release from uterine constraints. Weight velocity increases later than growth velocity in the fetus, usually after 30 weeks of gestation, as most adipose tissue is added during the third trimester.

Fetal size is more closely related to maternal factors than to paternal influences. The birth size of singletons is proportional to maternal size rather than paternal size. This relationship is noted among members of most Western societies but is most clearly demonstrated in the 2.4-kg mean birth weight reported in pygmies, whose maternal stature rarely exceeds five feet. (The differing standards of nutrition in that group compared with those in Western society, as well as alterations in insulin-like growth factor [IGF] physiology, may also play a role.) Multiple births reduce the space available in the uterus, and twins, triplets, etc., are smaller for gestational age than age-matched singletons.

Genetic influences also affect birth weight. Male term newborns weigh, on average, 150 gm more than females at term. Numerous syndromes characterized by disorders of chromosomal number (e.g., trisomies) or structure (e.g., abnormalities of the X chromosome) lead to poor fetal growth and low birth weight.

Placental adequacy is of prime importance in fetal growth. The placenta accounts for 20% of total pregnancy weight in normal situations. Maternal toxemia, hypertension, and severe diabetes mellitus decrease placental blood flow and fetal growth. Cigarette smoking and abuse of certain drugs will likewise decrease fetal growth. Uterine circulation will be impaired by placental infarction, infection, or the development of fistulae, hemangiomas, etc.

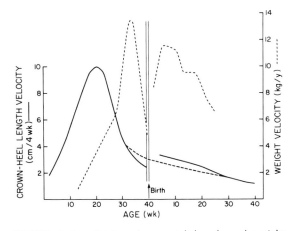

FIGURE 2–1 ••• Fetal and neonatal length and weight velocity curves. The solid line indicates growth velocity in centimeters per 4 weeks, with a peak occurring at mid gestation. The dashed line denotes what growth velocity would have been if uterine restraint were eliminated, thereby allowing increased growth in utero to term and less "catch-up" growth after release from the uterine environment in the neonatal period. Weight velocity is indicated by the dotted line. (Data from Tanner JM. Fetus into Man. Cambridge, MA: Harvard University Press, 1978. Reproduced from Underwood LE, Van Wyk JJ. Normal and abnormal growth. In: Wilson JD, Foster DW [eds]. Williams' Textbook of Endocrinology. 7th ed. Philadelphia: WB Saunders, 1985.)

Infections such as toxoplasmosis, rubella, cytomegalovirus, herpes, and syphilis are well-described causes of decreased fetal growth and birth weight.

Birth order exerts an effect on fetal growth, as first-born infants weigh an average of 100 gm less than subsequent siblings. Furthermore, maternal age over 35 years reduces birth weight; this factor may also relate to parity.

The endocrine control of prenatal growth is not yet clear. Most evidence suggests that neither growth hormone nor thyroid hormone is necessary for normal prenatal growth in length, but insulin-like growth factor II (IGF II) may be of importance in normal fetal growth and development. Furthermore, the presence of adequate amounts of insulin is necessary for normal fetal growth, and when insulin is present in excess amounts, fetal growth is increased.

Growth in Infancy

During the first postnatal year, a normal child will double its birth weight and increase its length 50% over the initial measurement at birth. Thus the growth rate of postnatal infants is greater than at any other age with the exception of fetal life. Male infants have more advanced osseous development than females and have a more rapid growth rate than females for the 3 to 6 months after birth. This coincides with the episodic increases in testosterone secretion characteristic of male infants, and elevated levels of this anabolic hormone may increase growth rate.

Although the birth weights of most healthy infants tend to cluster about the population mean, during the 2 years after birth, infants settle into a growth rate percentile that will remain consistent until puberty.[3, 4] Thus two thirds of children will cross percentile lines on the growth chart by 18 months of age, with one half of this group reaching higher percentiles and one half reaching lower percentiles than their percentile at birth. Those destined genetically to achieve taller stature but born with a birth weight below average (perhaps because of a smaller mother) will increase their growth velocity until a stature above average is reached. Conversely, those born with above average birth length but with a genetic endowment to achieve a shorter than average stature will have a lower than average growth rate during this period. Among these children, those who ultimately decrease their position on the curves to the lower percentiles may have constitutional delay in growth.

Prematurely born infants who are an appropriate size for gestational age will "catch up" to their appropriate position on the curve, and by 2 years of postnatal age, most will reach a stable percentile that they will occupy for the rest of their childhood. Infants who are small for gestational age as a result of inadequate intrauterine nutrition or growth exhibit less (or no) catch-up growth and remain below the mean for most of their childhood.

Growth in Childhood

Presently most physicians evaluating growth in the United States use charts derived from a survey of children's heights using National Center for Health Statistics (NCHS) data (Figs. 2–2, 2–3.).[5] However, other available charts are based on theoretical constructs that explain different aspects of growth. For example, Tanner and Davies have constructed growth curves utilizing longitudinal data de-

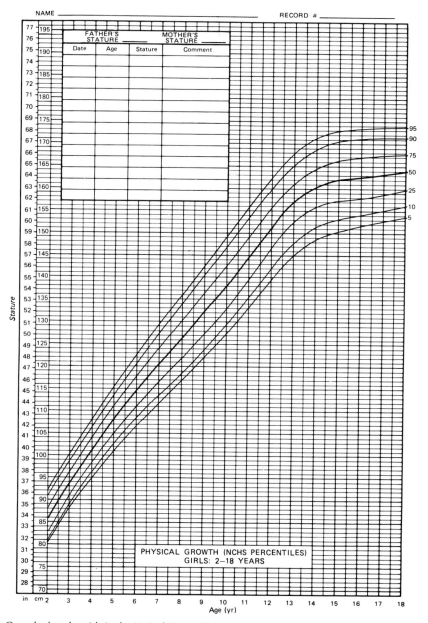

**FIGURE 2–2 ••• ** Growth chart for girls in the United States. This is a distance chart displaying height at a given chronologic age. The fact that the lower limit of the curve is set at the fifth percentile is arbitrary and does not mean per se that a child below the fifth percentile requires medical evaluation. (Data from 1976 study of the National Center for Health Statistics, Hyattsville, MD; and Hamill PVV, et al. Physical growth: National Center for Health Statistics percentiles. Am J Clin Nutr 1979; 32:607. Reproduced from Styne DM. Growth. In: Greenspan FP [ed]. Basic and Clinical Endocrinology. 3rd ed. Los Altos, CA: Lange Medical Publishers, 1991. Redrawn by Appleton & Lange and reprinted with permission of Ross Laboratories, Columbus, OH 43216 and Appleton & Lange, San Mateo, CA. © 1991, Ross Laboratories.)

rived from the NCHS and calculated data from theoretical growth curves.[6]

Karlberg separates phases of infant, childhood, and pubertal (ICP) growth from overall growth in the ICP growth curves (Fig. 2–4).[7] The "infancy" period is considered to be a manifestation of the continuation of the decreasing growth rate observed in the fetus after mid gestation. Thus, there is a very high growth rate during the first 12 to 18 months, but a consistent downward trend until the infancy influence on total growth disappears, usually between 18 and 48 months. The infancy period is considered to be growth hormone independent.

The "childhood" component then becomes prominent at about 3 to 4 years of age and is characterized by the onset of growth hormone–responsive growth. However, there is an overlap of these two phases of growth hormone–independent and growth hormone–dependent growth. Thus, at 6 to 12 months of age, many children demonstrate an increase in growth rate (the infancy childhood growth spurt) that is growth hormone dependent and is absent in growth hormone–deficient patients; it is the cumulative growth of the infancy and the childhood phases that cause this spurt. After the infantile period ends, growth rate is relatively stable, with a slow deceleration of linear growth and weight gain during childhood until the onset of puberty. A mid-childhood growth spurt has been described at about 7 years of age in 60% of children; this causes an upward inflection of the stable growth rate of childhood.[8]

It is possible to revise the "percentile" height of a child based on the parents' heights. Tanner proposed charts to perform this adjustment in British children. Himes et al.[9] developed tables to determine whether a child's height percentile should be revised upward or downward as a result of the influence of parents' heights.

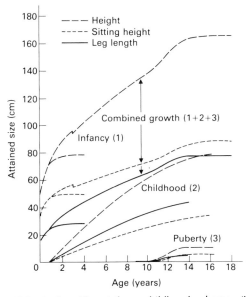

FIGURE 2–4 ••• The infancy-childhood-puberty (ICP) model for girls for attained height, sitting height, and leg length. The mean functions are plotted for each component as well as for the mean combined growth. The average age at peak velocity was used to time the function for the mean puberty component. (From Karlberg J, Fryer JG, Engstrom I, Karlberg P. Analysis of linear growth using a mathematical model. II. From 3 to 21 years of age. Acta Paediatr Scand (Suppl) 1987; 337:13.)

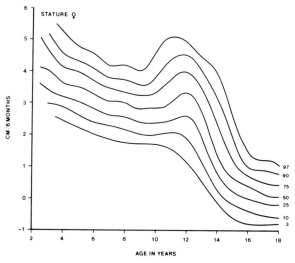

FIGURE 2–3 ••• Growth velocity chart for girls in the United States showing the amount of growth achieved over a 6-month period. Note the pubertal growth spurt and the lower limit of the third percentile. (From Roche AF, Himes JH. Incremental growth charts. Am J Clin Nutr 1980; 33:2041. © American Society for Clinical Nutrition.)

Incremental growth charts plot growth per period of time versus age of the child. Roche and Himes present growth per 6 months on a chart indicating the mean and various percentiles of growth rate for age.[10] Plotting data on their chart demonstrates deviations from the normal growth rate much more quickly than plotting on standard height-versus-age charts.

Several methods are available to predict final height with accuracy. The Bayley-Pinneau charts found in Greulich and Pyle's atlas of bone ages use height and bone age to predict final height in children with a bone age over 6 years.[11] The Roche-Wainer-Thissen (RWT) method uses recumbent length, bone age, midparental height, and weight to predict final height in children over 2 years of age.[12] Lastly, the height adjusted for pubertal onset (HAPO) method is based on the ICP growth charts.[7]

Growth in Puberty

Adolescent Growth Spurt

During the pubertal period, growth in stature occurs at a rate greater than at any postnatal period after infancy. The striking pubertal growth spurt has been divided into three stages by Tanner et al.[13]:

1. Age at takeoff: the time of minimal growth velocity in peripuberty.
2. Peak height velocity (PHV): the time of most rapid growth.
3. The stage of decreased velocity and cessation of growth at epiphyseal fusion.

Because boys reach PHV approximately 2 years later than girls, they are taller at takeoff than girls; peak height velocity occurs during stage 5 of puberty in more than 95% of boys. On the average, males grow 28 cm and females 25 cm between takeoff and cessation of growth. The mean height difference of 13 cm between adult males and adult females results from two factors: the taller height of boys at age of takeoff, and the greater male gain in height during the spurt.[14]

The pubertal growth spurt is an early pubertal event in girls. In fact, it is the first manifestation of puberty in most girls, although breast development is much more obvious. Peak height velocity occurs in 50% of girls during Tanner breast stage III, although about one fourth experience it in stage II and one fourth in stage IV. There is limited growth potential in a postmenarchal girl, because girls reach PHV before menarche and growth rate decelerates thereafter.

Measurement of Growth

Measurement of stature is the cheapest procedure available in the clinician's office and of exceptional importance. Clinical evaluation of gynecologic and endocrinologic disorders often requires accurate measurement of growth. Failing to measure a child limits the assessment of the health of the child. With no measurement taken, a growth deficiency may be missed for several visits, and diagnosis of a systemic disorder that may cause such a growth failure as its first outward manifestation may be delayed. Inaccurate measurements are responsible for numerous incorrect referrals for short stature. Alternating measurements with and without shoes on or allowing various degrees of slouching causes many such errors.

An accurate measurement of infant length is difficult to obtain and always requires two adults. The child must be laid on a flat surface with a device that has one plane perpendicular to the backboard at the top of the child's head and another plane parallel to the first at the child's feet. The two planes should be at a 90-degree angle to a ruler on which the child's height is read. A device known as an Infantometer operates as described. Errors occur with the most common method used for infant measurements, which calls for a single observer to make a mark on the paper covering the examining table at the foot of the child and another at the head so that the distance between the marks can be measured. Unfortunately, the paper is pliant, and the distance between the mark at the head and the mark at the feet will vary. If the paper crumples during the measuring procedure, the distance may deviate even more. Any movement of the child will make such measurements useless.

The measurement of a child more than 2 years of age is taken with the child standing. The change from lying to standing measurements is responsible for a large number of inappropriate referrals as a result of the 1- to 2-cm decrease in height that occurs when changing from lying to standing measurements; the type of measurement should be indicated on the chart next to the numeric value for children of this age so that this mistake will not occur. The clinician must measure the child with the shoes off; if the child is measured in shoes one time and then without them the next time, a 2- to 4-cm variation in height velocity is guaranteed.

The device used to measure standing height must be a variation of a stadiometer (Fig. 2–5). The child must hold his or her back against a wall or a hard surface with the back straight and the heels and back pressed posteriorly to the surface. The head is level. The bare feet must be on a horizontal plane made of a hard surface, considered to be the lower border of the measurement; the top or upper border of the distance of height must be delineated by a firm plate completely parallel to the plane of the feet, and the measurement must be read off a stationary ruler that is at right angles to the planes at the feet and head. A Harpenden stadiometer is the most accurate of such devices, but even a homemade apparatus that follows the above guidelines will give accurate measurements. Unfortunately, a device attached to the office scale is used in many pediatric offices. The plate at the top of the pole is rarely parallel to the floor and usually can move up and down, thereby fallaciously decreasing and increasing the measurement; with no way to straighten the patient's back,

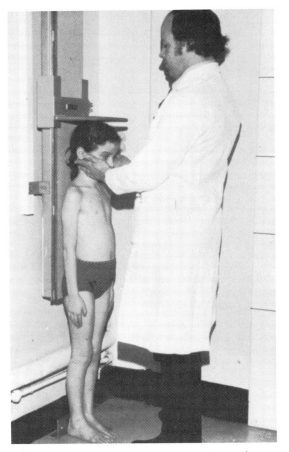

FIGURE 2–5 ••• Measuring stature using a Harpenden stadiometer. The head is held with the external auricular meatus and outer canthus of the eye in a horizontal plane. Upward pressure is applied to the mastoid processes in order to encourage the child to stand up straight and thus eliminate changes in posture and bearing. The counter to the right of the moving platform is read when the child has taken a deep breath and exhaled. This equipment can be obtained from Jeritax Inc., Carlstadt, NJ. (From Hindmarsh PC, Brook CGD. Normal growth and its endocrine control. In: Brook CGD [ed]. Clinical Paediatric Endocrinology. 2nd ed. Oxford: Blackwell Scientific Publications, 1989, p 59.)

the child may slouch, thereby decreasing the measurement.

We suggest that the observer make all measurements in the metric system. The tendency to round off numbers becomes troublesome when an inch is the unit of measure; an inaccuracy of 1 or ½ inch as a result of rounding off is a more serious error than a mistake of 1 or ½ cm; a ½-inch (1.25-cm) rounding error over a 6 month period can mean the difference between a growth rate of 4 cm/year, which is abnormal, and 6.5 cm/year, which is normal in mid childhood. After the measurement is ob-

tained, it must be displayed graphically on the growth chart. An abnormality of stature or growth is more obvious on a graph than when written as a number on a table, although the exact measurement should be recorded on the chart in tabular form as well. A decrease in growth rate in which the child "falls away" from the curve becomes obvious on the graph. Height velocity charts demonstrating growth per 6 months or per year make variations in growth rate extremely obvious earlier than is apparent on height versus age growth charts. These charts are readily available.[10]

Growth charts are also available for some disease states, and more are being developed. For example, achondroplasia and Turner and Down syndromes growth charts are available to assess the progress of a child with these conditions compared with the expected pattern. It is important, therefore, to realize that children with one of these syndromes can have another complicating, possibly treatable, condition that can further impair their growth. A patient with Down syndrome may have hypothyroidism, which will make him or her extremely short (for a Down patient) if the condition remains untreated.

The upper-to-lower segment (U:L) ratio is useful in determining causes of growth deviations. The U:L segment ratio is defined as the length from the top of the pubic ramus to the top of the head, divided by the distance from the top of the pubic ramus to the floor. Because of the elongation of the extremities during puberty, the U:L segment ratio changes markedly during the peripubertal and early pubertal periods. The gain in length of the legs is similar to the gain in the upper torso as a result of growth of the spine, although the increase in length of the legs occurs before the growth of the trunk. Thus there is an increase in sitting height during puberty. The mean U:L ratio of white adults is 0.92 ± 0.4 and that of black adults is 0.85; there are no differences in U:L ratio between the sexes.[14] Eunuchoid proportions are found in hypogonadal patients as a result of delayed epiphyseal fusion, leading to lengthened extremities, a decreased U:L ratio, and an increased height span.

Assessment of Growth

The evaluation of a patient with a growth abnormality must start with a comprehensive history. The prenatal history, including the health of the mother and exposure to toxins or drugs, may explain some cause of growth deficiency. The birth history, including difficulties of delivery, evidence of anoxia, and length and weight at birth, can point to acquired hormonal deficiencies or small-for-gestational age syndromes. The height of all family members and their age at pubertal onset will point to genetic tendencies toward short stature or constitutional delay in puberty. A review of systems should be performed to determine symptoms that may lead to a diagnosis of diseases of those systems. For example, headaches or visual deficiencies can suggest a CNS problem; nocturia or enuresis may suggest diabetes insipidus; gastrointestinal symptoms may point to coeliac disease, which may suppress growth rate during childhood and delay puberty; and pulmonary, renal, or cardiac symptoms may suggest an avenue of investigation for diagnosis of the cause of short stature.

A detailed, complete physical examination is necessary in the evaluation of every patient with a growth disorder. A search for midline defects of the skull, face, optic nerves, or palate, which can be related to hypothalamic deficiencies, is essential. Detection of signs of chronic disease that can lead to poor nutrition or energy imbalance will direct the examiner toward a likely diagnosis.

ENDOCRINE CONTROL OF THE PUBERTAL GROWTH SPURT

The pubertal growth spurt is controlled by multiple factors. In boys, it is created by the concerted action of testosterone and thyroid and growth hormones; patients lacking one or all of these hormones do not have a pubertal growth spurt. The adolescent growth spurt in girls depends on both estradiol and growth hormone, although ovarian and adrenal androgens may have a small effect. Secretion of growth hormone (GH) increases with pubertal development as a result of increased GH pulse amplitude, although frequency is not increased. Increased sex steroid secretion is one of the major factors responsible for increasing growth hormone secretion. Girls with precocious puberty demonstrate increased GH secretion compared with girls in normal prepuberty, and this increase accounts for part of their increased growth rate.[14]

The concentration of plasma insulin-like growth factor I (IGF I) rises during puberty to reach concentrations higher than at any other age; this peak occurs earlier in girls than in boys. This rise in IGF I is related to increased GH secretion, and both are temporally associated with the pubertal growth spurt. Plasma IGF I concentrations are high for chronologic age in sexual precocity and low for chronologic age in constitutional delay in puberty. Sex steroids indirectly increase the concentration of IGF I through increased secretion of GH and appear to directly increase IGF I production within the growing cartilage of the long bones.[14, 15]

There is no pubertal growth spurt in children with severe primary or secondary hypogonadism. In the presence of deficient adrenal androgen secretion, children with chronic adrenal insufficiency usually have a normal growth spurt, indicating the minimal role of adrenal androgens in stimulating normal pubertal growth. Hypopituitary patients with GH and gonadotropin deficiency do not have an adolescent growth spurt when only one replacement hormone is administered; both GH and sex steroids (stimulated by gonadotropins) are necessary. Phenotypic females with 46,XY genotypes who have the complete form of familial androgen insensitivity (testicular feminization), despite virtually complete insensitivity to androgens (but not to estrogen), have a pubertal growth spurt, thereby demonstrating a role for estrogen in the adolescent growth spurt.

Bone Age

Skeletal development is a better reflection of physiologic maturity than chronologic age. For example, bone age is closely correlated with menarche and is better correlated with the onset of secondary sexual development in delayed puberty than is chronologic age. Bone age is determined by the comparison of radiographs of the hand, knee, or elbow with standards of maturation in a normal population as presented in photographic atlases such as that of Greulich and Pyle, which is used most frequently in the United States.[11] Ossification centers appear in early life and then mold to fit with surrounding bones, and finally the epiphyses or growth plates fuse with their shafts. A delay or advancement in bone age is expressed in standard deviations from the mean reading for chronologic age: if the bone age is more than two standard deviations delayed or advanced from the mean for chronologic age, the deviation is significant. Increased accuracy in the technique is demonstrated by radiologists who are most familiar with this type of assessment; unfortunately, most general radiologists who are not associated with a pediatric center do not assess bone age very often, and their readings may not be correct. Bone age, height, and chronologic age are used for the prediction of final adult height from the Bayley-Pinneau tables or the RWT or HAPO techniques.[7] Because osseous maturation is more advanced in females than in males of the same chronologic age, separate standards are used for boys and girls. For example, bone ages of 11 years in girls and 13 years in boys (bone ages of early puberty in each sex) represent equivalent stages of bone maturation. While bone age determinations can assist with the diagnostic process in various conditions, they do not by themselves indicate a diagnosis.

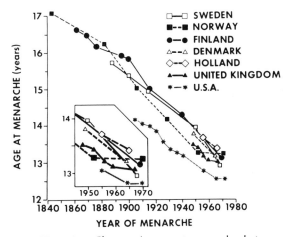

FIGURE 2–6 ••• Changes in age at menarche between 1840 and 1978. (From Tanner JM, Eveleth PB. Onset of puberty. In: Berenberg SR [ed]. Puberty: Biologic and Social Components. Leiden, The Netherlands, HE Stenfert Kroese Publishers, 1975, p 256. Reprinted by permission of Kluwer Academic Press.)

Body Composition

Changes in body composition occur during puberty and are a reflection of much of the dichotomy in physique between men and women. While lean body mass, skeletal mass, and body fat are equal in prepubertal boys and girls, by the end of puberty, men have 1.5 times the lean body mass and almost 1.5 times the skeletal mass of women, whereas women have twice as much body fat as men. Abdominal fat accumulates in girls with progression through pubertal development and leads to the differences in the generalized distribution of fat found in males (central fat, or apple shaped) compared with females (lower body fat predominance, or pear shaped). The discrepancy in adult strength between males and females is partly a result of the fact that males have twice as many muscle cells and partly a result of the greater cell size of muscles in males.

PUBERTAL DEVELOPMENT

Timing of Puberty

The average age of menarche in industrialized European countries has decreased between 2 and 3 months per decade during the past 150 years (Fig. 2–6).[1, 15] However, this trend ceased in developed countries such as the United States around 1940. Although menarche is a middle pubertal event, it is used as an indication of the general trend of pubertal development. According to the most recent survey by the NCHS, the age of menarche in the United States is 12.8 years.[5]

Socioeconomic conditions, nutritional status, and general health and well being influence the age of onset and the progression of pubertal development. Genetic factors also affect the age of puberty, as demonstrated by the similar age of menarche in members of an ethnic population and in mother-daughter pairs. Secondary sexual development occurs earlier in black females compared with white females in the United States; there is no apparent effect of social or economic factors on this relationship. In countries where standards of living have not improved over the past century, the age of onset of puberty may not have changed during the past 100 years.

Other influences also affect the age of puberty. Delayed puberty is a feature of chronic disease and malnutrition. Strenuous physical activity in girls can delay or arrest puberty, especially when associated with a thin habitus. Moderate obesity (up to 30% above normal weight for age) is associated with earlier menarche, although delayed menarche is common in severe obesity.[16]

When socioeconomic and environmental factors lead to good nutrition and general health, the age of onset of puberty in normal children is determined largely by genetic factors.

Physical and Hormonal Changes in Puberty

Secondary Sexual Characteristics

An objective method to describe the maturation of secondary sexual characteristics is important if the observer is to discern whether progression through puberty begins at a normal age and/or occurs at a normal rate (Fig. 2–7).[17] The standards proposed by Tanner have been universally accepted.[18]

Development of the breast is mainly controlled by estrogens secreted by the ovaries, while the growth of pubic and axillary hair is primarily under the influence of androgens secreted by the ovary and the adrenal. The classification of the stages of breast development depends on specific characteristics common to all females but does not include size or inherent shape of the breast, which are determined by genetic and nutritional factors. Initial breast development may be unilateral for several months and may cause concern to girls or their parents. An adolescent girl may unnecessarily undergo a breast (bud) biopsy because this fact was overlooked. Changes in areola papilla diameter are an indication of pubertal development. Papillary diameter does not increase much (3 to 4 mm) during pubic hair development stages I through III or breast development stages I through III but does increase after stage III, providing an objective method of differentiating stage IV from V.[19] Final papillary diameter is approximately 9 mm (Table 2–1).

In normal girls the stage of breast development is usually equal to the stage of pubic hair development. However, because two different endocrine organs cause these two physical manifestations, the stage of breast development should be classified separately from that of pubic hair development to increase accu-

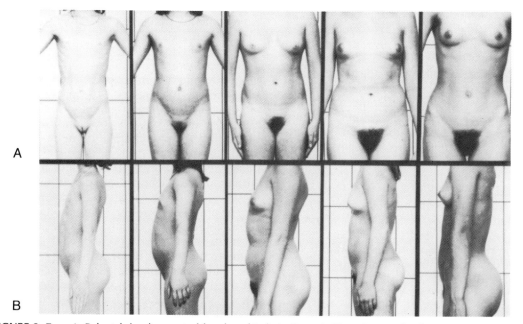

FIGURE 2–7 ••• *A,* Pubertal development of female pubic hair. Stage 1: There is no pubic hair. Stage 2: There is sparse growth of long, slightly pigmented, downy hair, straight or only slightly curled, primarily along the labia. Stage 3: The hair is considerably darker, coarser, and more curled and spreads sparsely over the junction of the pubes. Stage 4: The hair, now adult in type, covers a smaller area than in the adult and does not extend onto the thighs. Stage 5: The hair is adult in quantity and type, with extension onto the thighs. *B,* Pubertal development of female breasts. Stage 1: The breasts are preadolescent. There is elevation of the papilla only. Stage 2: Breast bud stage. A small mound is formed by the elevation of the breast and papilla, and the areolar diameter enlarges. Stage 3: There is further enlargement of breasts and areola with no separation of their contours. Stage 4: There is a projection of the areola and papilla to form a secondary mound above the level of the breast. Stage 5: The breasts resemble those of a mature female as the areola has recessed to the general contour of the breast. (From Brook CGD, Stanhope R. Normal puberty: Physical characteristics and endocrinology. In: Brook CGD [ed]. Clinical Paediatric Endocrinology. 2nd ed. Oxford: Blackwell Scientific Publications, 1989, p 172.)

TABLE 2–1 ••• CROSS-SECTIONAL AND LONGITUDINAL PAPILLARY DIAMETER AT EACH STAGE OF PUBERTAL DEVELOPMENT

	Nipple Size (mm)*	
Stage	*Cross-Sectional*	*Longitudinal*
BI	2.89 (0.81)	3.00 (0.77)
BII	3.28 (0.89)	3.37 (0.96)
BIII	4.07 (1.32)	4.72 (1.40)†
BIV	7.74 (1.64)†	7.25 (1.46)†
BV	9.94 (1.38)†	9.41 (1.45)†
PH1	2.95 (1.02)	3.14 (1.31)
PH2	3.32 (0.91)	3.69 (1.34)
PH3	4.11 (1.54)	4.44 (1.17)†
PH4	7.15 (1.81)†	6.54 (1.47)†
PH5	9.66 (1.59)†	8.98 (1.56)†

*Results are means ± SD (in parentheses).
†Significantly different from previous state, $P <.05$.
From Rhone RD. Papilla (nipple) development during female puberty. J Adolesc Health Care 1982; 2:217.

racy. Dulling of the surface of the vaginal mucosa from its prepubertal reddish appearance occurs as a result of estrogen stimulation, and secretion of clear or whitish discharge increases in the months before menarche. The vaginal pH decreases as menarche approaches. Thickening, protrusion, and rugation of the labia majora and minora occur during puberty. Thickening of the hymen has been described as preceding other physical changes of pubertal development.[20]

The corpus of the uterus increases during puberty from its initial tubular shape and a size approximately equal to that of the cervix to a bulbous shape with lengthening. The length of the uterus increases from 2 to 3 cm to 5 to 8 cm (about two times the length of the cervix). During prepuberty, the ovaries measure 0.7 to 0.9 cm on ultrasound but increase to 2 to 10 cm after puberty.

The limits of two standard deviations from the mean age at onset of puberty encompass 95% of normal children and are customarily accepted as the normal range in most studies. Unfortunately, one large study on the attainment of stages of puberty in the United States started with subjects at 12 years of age and therefore was only useful in determining the upper limits of normal pubertal development, not the lower limits.[20a] Nonetheless, assumptions can be made using British data.[19] Some sign of puberty is present in 95% of normal American girls between 8 and 13 years of age (mean, 10.5), whereas 95% of boys enter puberty between 9 and 14 years of age (mean, 11.5). British girls complete secondary sexual

development in a mean of 4.2 years, with a range of 1.5 to 6 years; the mean for boys is 3.5 years, with a range of 2 to 4.5 years (Fig. 2–8). Black American girls are advanced in their secondary sexual development compared with white American girls.

Prepubertal boys and girls have similar heights at the same age, but the earlier pubertal development in girls leads to a female predominance in stature in early puberty. This is followed by the male growth spurt, which leads to the taller stature of men than women.

Hormonal Changes in Puberty

Gonadotropins. During the first 1 to 2 years after birth, plasma levels of luteinizing hormone (LH) and follicle-stimulating hormone (FSH) increase in episodes of secretion leading to high peak concentrations similar to adult values (Table 2–2). The plasma concentrations of FSH and LH remain low thereafter until the onset of puberty (Fig. 2–9).

The peripubertal period is the time of hormonal change that precedes the signs of sexual maturation. During this stage, increased release of LH in response to intravenous gonadotropin-releasing hormone (GnRH) is demonstrable, and augmented release of pulsatile LH occurs during sleep. Ultrasensitive assays demonstrate episodic LH secretion at night in late prepubertal boys but infrequent secretion during the day; the amplitude of such peaks increases, and daytime secretion appears with

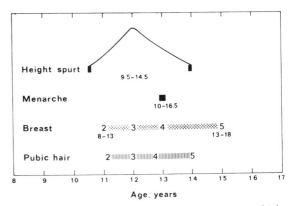

FIGURE 2–8 ••• A graphic depiction of the ages at which normal pubertal development occurs in girls. The data are from Great Britain and the ages are about 6 months older than those of girls in the United States, but the general pattern of development is constant between the countries. (From Marshall WA, Tanner JM. Variation in the pattern of pubertal changes in girls. Arch Dis Child 1969; 44:291–303.)

TABLE 2–2 ••• SERUM CONCENTRATIONS FOR FOLLICLE-STIMULATING HORMONE (FSH), LUTEINIZING HORMONE (LH), ESTRADIOL, AND DEHYDROEPIANDROSTERONE (DHEA)

Tanner Stage	FSH (mIU/ml)	LH (mIU/ml)	Estradiol (pg/ml)	DHEA (ng/dl)
Stage 1	0.9–5.1	1.8–9.2	<1.0	19–302
Stage 2	1.4–7.0	2.0–16.6	7–37	45–1904
Stage 3	2.4–7.7	5.6–13.6	9–59	125–1730
Stage 4	1.5–11.2	7–14.4	10–156	153–1321
Adult:				
Follicular	3–20	5–25	30–100	162–1620

From Speroff L, Glass RH, Kase NG. Abnormal puberty and growth problems. In: Clinical Gynecologic Endocrinology and Infertility. 4th ed. Baltimore: Williams & Wilkins, 1989.

the progression of pubertal development. In girls, FSH levels increase during the early stages of puberty and LH levels tend to increase in the later stages; in boys, FSH levels increase progressively through puberty, while LH levels rise early and slowly reach a plateau. It must be emphasized that the episodic nature of LH and FSH secretion makes the measurement of individual samples insensitive as an indicator of pubertal development.[21]

The increase in biologically active LH at the onset of puberty appears greater than the increase in immunologically active LH. Although the explanation for this discordance is uncertain, it may be related to a qualitative change in the degree of glycosylation of the LH molecule, in addition to technical factors such as the purity of the LH standard, the quality of the radiolabeled LH, and the specificity of the antiserum.[22]

Testosterone. In females, the peripheral

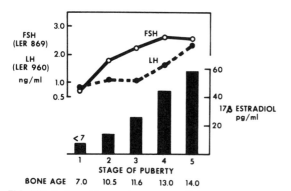

FIGURE 2–9 ••• Mean plasma estradiol, FSH, and LH concentrations in prepubertal and pubertal females by pubertal stage of maturation. Bone age is expressed in years. (From Grumbach MM. Onset of puberty. In: Berenberg SR [ed]. Puberty: Biologic and Social Components. Leiden, The Netherlands, HE Stenfert Kroese Publishers, 1975, pp 1–21. Reprinted by permission of Kluwer Academic Press.)

conversion of ovarian and adrenal androstenedione accounts for most of the circulating testosterone. Prepubertal boys and girls have plasma testosterone concentrations of less than 10 ng/dl. Although there is a great increase in testosterone in boys during puberty, there is a smaller but definite increase in concentrations of testosterone in girls between pubertal stages I and IV.

Estrogens. The major estrogen, estradiol (E_2), is secreted by the ovary, with a small contribution to total circulating levels from the extraglandular conversion of testosterone and androstenedione. Estrone (E_1) arises from extraglandular conversion of estradiol and from ovarian and adrenal androstenedione.

In the fetus and the term neonate, serum values of estrogen are extremely high (approximately 5000 pg/ml at term) because of the conversion of fetal and maternal C-19 steroid precursors to estrogen by the placenta. The fetal ovary has the capacity to secrete estrogen by mid gestation, but the contribution of the fetal ovary is minimal, as the fetal adrenal-placental unit produces much more estrogen. Breast budding in term male and female infants is the physical manifestation of these high concentrations of circulating estrogen, but this soon resolves in all but a few newborns, who may be destined to develop premature thelarche. Plasma levels of placentally derived estrogen decrease precipitously in the first few days after delivery.

There are episodic peaks of LH and FSH in the months after birth. Plasma estrogens rise as a result of these gonadotropin peaks but gradually fall during the first year and remain low until puberty; estradiol falls to <7 pg/ml and estrone to <20 pg/ml.[21] In girls, estradiol increases steadily through the stages of puberty until maturity, when concentrations of 50 pg/ml are reached in the early to mid follicular

TABLE 2–3 ••• MEAN SERUM CONCENTRATIONS OF DHEAS DURING CHILDHOOD

CHRONOLOGIC AGE (yr)	1–6	6–8	8–10	10–12	12–14	14–16	16–20
Girls (μg/dl)	24.7 ± 11.1	30.4 ± 7.6	117.3 ± 41.7	112.7 ± 16.4	168.9 ± 19.3	253.5 ± 41.3	232.5 ± 49.8

BONE AGE (yr)	1–6	6–8	8–10	10–12	12–14	14–16	16–20
Girls (μg/dl)	2.5 ± 2.5	27.2 ± 9.6	—	112.9 ± 27.6	159.7 ± 26.3	261.0 ± 45.0	145.3 ± 32.2

From Reiter EO, Fuldauer VG, Root AW. Secretion of the adrenal androgen, dehydroepiandrosterone sulfate, during normal infancy, childhood, and adolescence, in sick infants, and in children with endocrinologic abnormalities. J Pediatr 1977; 90:766.

stage and concentrations of 150 pg/ml or more in the late follicular phase; estrone rises early in pubertal development but reaches a plateau by mid puberty.

Adrenal Androgens. Both boys and girls demonstrate a progressive increase in the plasma Δ-5 steroids, dehydroepiandrosterone (DHEA) and dehydroepiandrosterone sulfate (DHEAS), that is initiated by 8 years of age (skeletal age of 6 to 8 years) and continues through ages 13 to 15 years (Table 2–3).[23] This increase in the secretion of adrenal androgens is known as *adrenarche*. Although the factors causing adrenarche are unknown, it is clear that adrenocorticotropic hormone (ACTH) is necessary for the process. This increase in the secretion of adrenal androgens precedes the increased secretion of gonadal sex steroids (gonadarche) and the increased pulsatile secretion of gonadotropins by approximately 2 years. Plasma DHEAS levels show less variation than DHEA levels and are a useful biochemical marker of adrenarche.

Inhibin. Inhibin, a dimeric glycoprotein secreted by Sertoli cells and granulosa cells, exerts a specific negative feedback action on the secretion of FSH from the pituitary gland. The production of inhibin is stimulated by FSH. Inhibin appears to play a role in the feedback regulation of FSH secretion during puberty in males and during the development of ovarian follicles in females. This is the time at which Sertoli cells and granulosa cells, the target cells for FSH, divide. Plasma inhibin-like immunoactivity increases in both boys and girls undergoing puberty.

Sex Hormone–Binding Globulin. Between 97% and 99% of circulating testosterone and estradiol is reversibly bound to sex hormone–binding globulin (SHBG); only the free steroid is the physiologically active moiety. SHBG is a glycoprotein hormone of mass 90,000 to 100,000 d, consisting of heterogenous monomers and possessing one steroid-binding site per dimeric molecule. Levels of SHBG are approximately equal in boys and girls before puberty. A decrease in SHBG occurs with advancing prepubertal age, which leads to an increase in the free sex steroids. During puberty there is a small decrease in SHBG levels in girls but a greater decrease in boys, so that adult males have half the SHBG concentration of adult females. While the plasma concentration of testosterone is 20 times greater in men than in women, the concentration of free testosterone is 40 times greater because of the differences in SHBG.[24]

Prolactin. Prepubertal boys have mean plasma prolactin concentrations of 6.0 ± 0.5 ng/ml (± standard error), and girls have concentrations of 7.2 ± 0.5 ng/ml.[25] Because of elevations of estradiol concentrations, late pubertal girls and adult women have higher concentrations (8.5 ± 1.5 ng/ml) of prolactin, whereas mean concentrations in adult men (5.2 ± 0.5 ng/ml) are similar to those in prepubertal children.

Growth Hormone. GH is a 191–amino acid protein that increases linear growth via the stimulation of IGF I, increases gluconeogenesis, and exerts antiinsulin effects as well as lipolytic effects. During puberty there is an increase in the amplitude of GH pulsatile secretion as a result of sex steroid secretion. GH circulates in association with a binding protein that has the amino acid sequence of the extracellular domain of the GH receptor.

GH is released from the pituitary gland after stimulation by hypothalamic growth hormone–releasing factor (GHRF) and is inhibited by somatostatin release–inhibiting factor (SRIF). During most of the day, GH concentrations are low, but several peaks occur during the day, most notably during electroencephalogram (EEG) sleep stages 3 to 4. Thus random sampling for GH concentrations is of no value. Stimulatory tests utilizing alpha-adrenergic agents, beta-adrenergic blocking agents, hypoglycemia, or GHRF are necessary to diagnose GH deficiency.

IGF I (Somatomedin). IGF I is the growth factor most closely associated with linear growth. It is GH dependent and circulates associated with binding proteins, of which more than six are presently identified. IGF I and IGF binding protein 3 (IGFBP 3) decrease with GH deficiency and increase with GH replacement.[15] Both factors may be used as an aid in the diagnosis of GH deficiency. IGF I increases during puberty to values higher than those of prepubertal or adult subjects, remains elevated past the time of peak height velocity, and then falls to normal adult levels. The increase in testosterone in males and in estradiol in females correlates with the rise in IGF I, but sex steroids have not been implicated as the sole direct cause of the increase in serum IGF I. GH secretion approximately doubles during puberty as a result of increased sex steroid secretion; thus, at least one effect of estrogen and testosterone on IGF I generation is mediated indirectly via augmented release of growth hormone. Children with true precocious puberty have plasma IGF I values characteristic of children in the same stage of normal puberty rather than of children of the same chronologic age.[26] After several months of therapy with a superactive gonadotropin-releasing hormone agonist, IGF I values in patients with precocious puberty decrease along with the secretion of GH.[27]

Menarche. There is a high incidence of anovulatory cycles in the first years after menarche, and even 5 years later, girls may be anovulatory. It is possible to become pregnant well before the end of puberty, and in fact, pregnancy can occur even before the first menstrual period.

Constitutional Delay in Puberty

A familial tendency toward delay in physiologic development is more a variation of normal than a true disease. In the United States, delayed puberty is usually of more concern to boys and their parents than to girls and their parents. However, a girl more than 13 years old with no evidence of pubertal development requires evaluation. If there are no signs or symptoms of CNS disease, chronic conditions, or interference with nutrition and if the child seems healthy in general, constitutional delay in puberty should be considered. Affected children are usually short and have

been shorter than average their whole childhood, although their growth rate remains within normal velocity for bone age. In 50% of such cases, there is a family history of delay in a parent or sibling. Skeletal development is delayed two or more standard deviations as a sine qua non of the diagnosis. Sex steroid and gonadotropin values are prepubertal, as are serum chemistry levels and IGF I concentrations. In fact, this disorder in the tempo of development cannot be reliably diagnosed by any given test but instead is confirmed after normal pubertal development occurs at an advanced age. If the patient's psychological state and educational situation are affected, and if constitutional delay seems unlikely, low-dose estrogen may be offered for a 3-month period to advance physical development cosmetically and improve self-esteem. A more detailed discussion of constitutional delay in growth and puberty is given in Chapter 5.

References

1. Styne DM. Growth. In: Greenspan FS (ed). Basic and Clinical Endocrinology. 3rd ed. Los Altos, CA: Lange Medical Publishers, 1990, pp 147–176.
2. Underwood LE, Van Wyk JJ. Normal and aberrant growth. In Wilson JD, Foster DW (eds). Williams' Textbook of Endocrinology. 7th ed. Philadelphia: WB Saunders, 1985, pp 155–205.
3. Smith DW. Growth and Its Disorders: Basics and Standards, Approach and Classifications, Growth Deficiency Disorders, Growth Excess Disorders, Obesity. Vol XV. Philadelphia: WB Saunders, 1977.
4. Tanner JM, Whitehouse BH, Takaishi M. Standards from birth to maturity for height, weight, height velocity, and weight velocity, British children, 1965. Arch Dis Child 1966; 41:454–471, 613–635.
5. Hamill PVV, Drizd TA, Johnson CL, et al. Physical growth: National Center for Health Statistics percentiles. Am J Clin Nutr 1979; 32:607.
6. Tanner JM, Davies PSW. Clinical longitudinal standard for height and height velocity for North American children. J Pediatr 1985; 107:317.
7. Karlberg J. On the construction of the infancy-childhood-puberty growth standard. Acta Paediatr Scand (Suppl) 1989; 356:26–37.
8. Karlberg J, Fryer JG, Engstrom I, et al. Analysis of linear growth using a mathematical model. II. From 3 to 21 years of age. Acta Paediatr Scand (Suppl) 1987; 337:12–29.
9. Himes JH, Roche AF, Thissen D. Parent specific adjustments for assessment of recumbent length and stature. Monographs in Paediatrics. Vol 13. Basel, Switzerland: Karger, 1981.
10. Roche AF, Himes JH. Incremental growth charts. Am J Clin Nutr 1980; 333:2041.
11. Greulich WS, Pyle SI. Radiographic Atlas of Skeletal Development of the Hand and Wrist. 2nd ed. Stanford, CA: Stanford University Press, 1959.
12. Roche AF, Wainer H, Thissen D. The RWT method

for the prediction of adult stature. Pediatrics 1975; 56:1026.

13. Tanner JM, Whitehouse RH, Marubini E, Resele LF. The adolescent growth spurt of boys and girls of the Harpenden Growth Study. Ann Hum Biol 1976; 3:109.

14. Attie MK, Ramirez NR, Conte FA, et al. The pubertal growth spurt in eight patients with true precocious puberty and growth hormone deficiency: Evidence for a direct role of sex steroids. J Clin Endocrinol Metab 1990; 71:975–983.

15. McKusick VA. Heritable Disorders of Connective Tissue. 4th ed. St. Louis: CV Mosby, 1972, pp 73–74.

16. Grumbach MM, Styne DM. Puberty: Ontogeny, neuroendocrinology, physiology, and disorders. In: Wilson JD, Foster DW (eds). Williams' Textbook of Endocrinology. 8th ed. Philadelphia: WB Saunders, 1991.

17. Hartz AJ, Barboriak PN, Wong A. The association of obesity with infertility and related menstrual abnormalities in women. Int J Obes 1979; 3:57–73.

18. Tanner JM. Trend toward earlier menarche in London, Oslo, Copenhagen, the Netherlands and Hungary. Nature 1973; 243:95.

19. Marshall WA, Tanner JM. Variation in the pattern of pubertal changes in girls. Arch Dis Child 1969; 44:291.

20. Rohn RD. Papilla (nipple) development during female puberty. J Adolesc Health Care 1982; 2:217.

20a. Harlan WR, Harlan EA, Grillo GP. Secondary sex characteristics of girls 12 to 17 years of age. The U.S. Health Examination Survey. J Pediatr 1980; 96:1074–1078.

21. Wheeler MD. Physical changes of puberty. Endocrinol Metab Clin North Am 1990; 20:1–14.

22. Forest MG. Pituitary gonadotropin and sex steroid secretion during the first two years of life. In: Grumbach MM, Sizonenko PC, Aubert ML (eds). Control of the Onset of Puberty. Baltimore: Williams & Wilkins, 1990, pp 451–478.

23. Beitins IZ, Padmanabhan V. Bioactivity of gonadotropins. Endocrinol Metab Clin North Am 1990; 20:85–120.

24. Reiter EO, Fuldauer VG, Root AW. Secretion of the adrenal androgen, dehydroepiandrosterone sulfate, during normal infancy, childhood, and adolescence, in sick infants, and in children with endocrinologic abnormalities. J Pediatr 1977; 90:766.

25. Bartsch W, Horst HJ, Derwah KM. Interrelationships between sex hormone-binding globulin and 17β-estradiol, testosterone, 5α-dihydrotestosterone, thyroxine, and triiodothyronine in prepubertal and pubertal girls. J Clin Endocrinol Metab 1980; 50:1053–1056.

26. Aubert ML, Sizonenko PC, Kaplan SL, et al. The ontogenesis of human prolactin from fetal life to puberty. In: Crosignani PG, Robyn C (eds). Prolactin and Human Reproduction. New York: Academic Press, 1977, pp 9–20.

27. Harris DA, Van Vliet G, Egli CA, et al. Somatomedin-C in normal puberty and in true precocious puberty before and after treatment with a potent luteinizing hormone releasing hormone agonist. J Clin Endocrinol Metab 1985; 61:152–159.

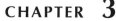

CHAPTER 3

Abnormalities in Growth

RAYMOND L. HINTZ

CONTROL OF GROWTH

The control of growth is a complex process involving many hormonal and nonhormonal components (Fig. 3–1). Many of the hormonal components of growth are controlled via the hypothalamic-pituitary axis.[1] Thus, the secretion of growth hormone (GH), which leads to the release of insulin-like growth factors (IGFs), is under the control of the hypothalamic neuropeptide hormones growth hormone-releasing factor (GRF) and somatostatin or somatotropin release–inhibiting factor (SRIF). Similarly, the secretion of thyrotropin-stimulating hormone (TSH), follicle-stimulating hormone (FSH), luteinizing hormone (LH), and adrenocorticotropic hormone (ACTH), all of which play major roles in the control of growth, is itself under the control of hypothalamic neurohormones. In addition, the secretion of insulin, which is not directly under pituitary control, plays an important role in the control of cellular growth.[2]

Many nonhormonal factors play a significant role in the control of growth. Foremost among these is nutrition, as without substrate no cell could grow or divide. There are also underlying genetic factors that determine the potential for growth, not only for the whole organism, but also for each organ and tissue. There are many tissue growth factors, such as epidermal growth factor (EGF) and nerve growth factor (NGF), whose roles in the overall control of growth are only beginning to be understood.[3] The interaction of these hormonal and nonhormonal factors leads to normal growth and development, and it is abnormalities of these mechanisms that lead to disorders in growth.

The Growth Hormone– Insulin-like Growth Factor Axis

Growth Hormone

GH is a 191–amino acid polypeptide secreted by somatotropes located in the anterior pituitary gland. Neurohormones control these cells through the hypophysial-portal system, and both an effector and an inhibitor of GH secretion exist.[4] Present data indicate that GRF is responsible for the rapid pulses of GH secretion seen mainly during the nighttime hours and in response to meals and exercise, while the inhibitor of growth hormone secretion, SRIF, appears to be responsible for the underlying tone of GH secretion. There are two major forms of GH that are synthesized, stored, and secreted by the somatotropes.[5] The most abundant form (making up approximately 90% of the total) is the 22-kd molecular weight form. In addition, there is an alternative splicing of the GH messenger RNA (mRNA), which leads to a minor (20 kd) form of GH whose physiologic role is unknown.

It has been known for some time that GH secretion, like that of many other polypeptide hormones, is pulsatile.[6] In addition, GH has a striking predilection for secretion in association with sleep. A large number of brain centers and neurotransmitters have been implicated in the control of GH. In addition, there

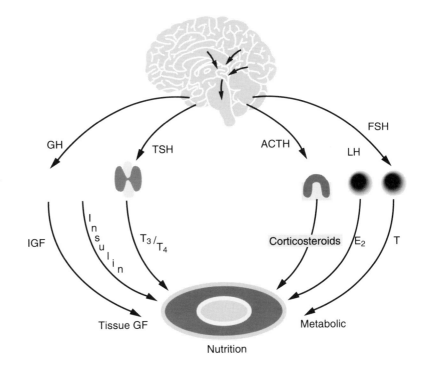

FIGURE 3–1 ••• Control of cellular growth.

is evidence that one of the growth hormone–stimulated peptides, insulin-like growth factor I (IGF I), plays a feedback role at the level of both the hypothalamus and the somatotropes regulating the secretion of GH.[7]

The secretion of GH leads to a complex chain of events (Fig. 3–2) that ultimately results in stimulation of growth at the endocrine level. After GH is released into the blood stream, a large proportion of it binds to a specific GH-binding protein.[8] Recent advances have led to a better understanding of the molecular character of this GH-binding protein, and it is now clear that it represents the extracellular portion of the GH receptor site. Like many receptors for polypeptide hormones, the receptor site for GH consists of three polypeptide domains: an extracellular domain, which contains all of the three-dimensional structure necessary for the recognition of the hormone; a transmembrane domain that is highly hydrophobic; and an intracellular domain, which contains the three-dimensional structure necessary to lead to the biologic action within the cell. In humans it appears that there is a proteolytic cleavage of the extracellular domain of the GH receptor, which leads to a soluble, circulating polypeptide that plays a major role in protein binding of GH in the serum. The exact biologic role of this binding protein is unclear, but it does

seem that it will serve as a useful index to the level of GH receptor in the body. GH receptors are widely distributed throughout tissues in the body, and it is the binding of the GH ligand to these GH receptors that leads to the biologic events within the cells. Of the many

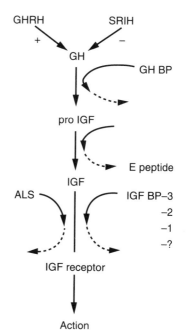

FIGURE 3–2 ••• The chain of growth hormone action.

direct biologic events that are ascribed to GH action, one of the most important is clearly the control of the production of IGF I.

Insulin-like Growth Factors

IGF mRNA is widely distributed throughout the body and is under GH control not only in the liver, as would have been predicted by the original somatomedin hypothesis, but in other tissues as well.[9] There are two distinctly different types of IGFs; these are known as IGF I and IGF II. These IGFs bear a strong homology to each other and to insulin. Of the two polypeptides, IGF I is the most closely related to GH secretion and action. There are two predicted forms of IGF I prohormone, and thus far only one predicted prohormone for IGF II. All of these prohormone forms contain long carboxyterminal extensions beyond the known structure of the active hormone; these are known as E regions. It appears that under normal circumstances, these E regions are cleaved off very efficiently before IGF is secreted. However, in certain circumstances such as renal failure and tumor-associated hypoglycemia, both circulating prohormone forms and E peptide segments have been demonstrated.[10]

IGFs circulate tightly bound to proteins known as IGF-binding proteins (IGFBPs).[11] In most normal circumstances there is little or no free IGF I or IGF II polypeptide circulating. Six distinct but homologous IGFBPs are now

known; these are summarized in Table 3–1. By far the most abundant form in normal serum is IGFBP 3, which is a glycosylated protein of approximately 40 kd molecular weight. The combined IGF peptide–IGFBP 3 complex binds to yet another protein known as acid labile subunit (ALS) to form a 150-kd, three-subunit protein complex that is the major circulating form of the IGFs. This 150-kd complex contains well over 90% of the total IGF in the serum in most circumstances. A smaller proportion of the IGFs in serum circulate bound to the other forms of IGFBP (IGFBP 1, 2, 4, 5, and 6). In addition, these other IGFBPs are major components in certain body fluids (e.g., IGFBP 1 in amniotic fluid, IGFBP 2 in joint fluid, and IGFBP 5 in cerebrospinal fluid). The exact biologic purpose of this complex system in controlling the amount and distribution of IGFs in the serum and body fluids is unclear. However, it does result in prolongation of the circulating time of IGFs in plasma and may play a role in modulating the delivery of the IGF peptides to the cellular receptor sites.

Biologic Actions

Just as there is more than one form of IGF, there is more than one form of IGF receptor identified on the surface of cells.[12] The type 1 IGF receptor has the strongest affinity for IGF I and a less strong binding affinity for IGF II

TABLE 3–1 ••• INSULIN-LIKE GROWTH FACTOR BINDING PROTEINS*

Designation	Characteristics	Source	N-terminal Amino Acid (Human)
IGFBP 1	GH independent Insulin dependent High in fetal life	Amniotic fluid Hep G-2 media	APWQ*CAPC*SAEKLAL
IGFBP 2	GH independent Insulin dependent High in fetal life	Joint fluid MDBK media BRL 3A media	EVLFR*CPPC*TPERLA
IGFBP 3	GH dependent Insulin independent Major IGFBP in serum postnatally	Serum (150-kd complex)	GASSGGLGPVVR*CEP*
IGFBP 4	"Inhibitory" IGFBP	Serum Osteosarcoma	DEAIH*CPPC*SEEKLA
IGFBP 5	High in joint fluid	Serum CSF Human bone extract	LGSFVH*CEPC*DEKAL
IGFBP 6	CSF binding protein	Serum CSF Transformed and fetal fibroblasts	ALAR*CPGC*GQVQAGC

*The homologous *C**C* regions of the N-terminal amino acid sequences are italicized.
IGFBP, insulin-like growth factor binding proteins; GH, growth hormone; CSF, cerebrospinal fluid.

and insulin. This type 1 receptor resembles the insulin receptor in its subunit construction and amino acid sequence and appears to have been teleologically derived from the insulin receptor. The type 2 IGF receptor has its highest affinity for IGF II and somewhat less binding attraction for IGF I. Unlike the type 1 receptor and the insulin receptor, the type 2 IGF receptor has no affinity for insulin itself. The molecular corollary of this observation is that there is no structural relationship between the type 2 receptor and either the type 1 receptor or the insulin receptor. Instead, the type 2 receptor appears to be a bifunctional receptor with ligand specificity for both IGF peptides and for mannose-6-phosphate. The role of the type 2 receptor in the control of growth is unclear and controversial. Most of the observed biologic actions of GH with respect to control of growth appear to be subserved by the chain of action initiated by GH. This leads to the production of IGF I and its delivery to the IGF type 1 receptor sites in the tissues (see Fig. 3–2). It is this chain of action that has been most clearly linked to the anabolic and growth-promoting events associated with GH in humans.

Thyroid Hormone

Thyroid hormone also plays an extremely important role in the control of growth. Like the GH-IGF axis, there is a hypothalamic mechanism of control, with the neurohormone thyrotropin-stimulating hormone (TRH) being secreted by specialized neurons into the hypophyseal portal system, leading to the release of the pituitary hormone, TSH.[13] Release of TSH leads to the production and release of the final hormones in the chain, triiodothyronine (T_3) and thyroxine (T_4). Like the IGFs, the thyroid hormones are almost totally bound to plasma proteins, which control the half-life and tissue delivery of the thyroid hormones. Thyroid hormone action is subserved by the thyroid hormone receptor site, which is widely distributed throughout cells in the body. This receptor site is located intracellularly, similar to that of steroid hormones, and the ligand-T_3 complex binds to chromatin and DNA to initiate mRNA synthesis. Without thyroid hormone action through its receptor sites, GH and IGFs are unable to stimulate anabolic and growth responses. Furthermore, there is a close interaction of thyroid hormone with GH

secretion.[14] In the presence of hypothyroidism, GH secretion from the pituitary gland is decreased in response to both pharmacologic and physiologic stimulation.

Sex Hormone

The sex hormones, estrogen and androgen, play an extremely important role in the control of growth during puberty. The secretion of these hormones is relatively low after the perinatal period until there is an increase in the gonadotropins (LH and FSH) prior to the clinical onset of puberty.[15] The secretion of estrogens and androgens under the control of the pituitary gonadotropins leads to the development of the secondary sex characteristics that are closely associated with the events of puberty. Estrogens and androgens have been associated with growth-stimulating actions both directly and indirectly. Both androgens and estrogens have been shown to influence the secretion of GH at the time of puberty.[16] This increase in GH secretion at the time of puberty is thought to play a major part in the pubertal growth spurt. Direct end-organ effects of both androgens and estrogens have also been demonstrated in a variety of experimental systems. In addition to these, steroid hormones also play a major role in bone maturation and the ultimate disappearance of the epiphyseal centers.[17] This event results in the cessation of linear growth at the end of puberty. Like the thyroid hormones, the sex hormones appear to act by diffusing into the cell and binding to the specific steroid/TSH receptor sites. The binding of androgens and estrogens to their respective receptor sites initiates changes in the three-dimensional structure that allow the interaction of these activated receptors with chromatin and the chromosomal DNA. This interaction leads to the production of specific mRNA and secretion of specific proteins leading to the biologic action observed.[18]

Adrenal Hormones

In addition to the other hormonal factors reviewed, it is clear that adrenal hormones also play a role in the control of growth. Adrenal androgens appear to have an important adjunctal role in the events of puberty and act in concert with androgens from the testes and ovaries, resulting in growth stimulation, both by direct and indirect means, and bone maturation.[19] In addition, the adrenal glucocorticoids appear to have a bimodal action in the control of growth. Experimental evidence suggests that a minimal level of glucocorticoids is necessary for cells to function, grow, and divide. On the other hand, many observations have shown that an excess of glucocorticoids causes cells to be unresponsive to the other hormonal growth-stimulating agents discussed earlier.[20]

Associated Factors

In addition to the hormonal factors controlling growth, there are many extremely important nonhumoral factors. It is intuitively obvious that without adequate nutrition, and therefore without adequate substrate for cells, no effective growth can occur. This is seen most clearly in the clinical disorders of kwashiorkor and marasmus,[21] but it is also manifested in many more subtle clinical disorders.

Genetics also plays an extremely important role in determining final height. The potential for ultimate growth attainment for three related primates—the gorilla, the human, and the chimpanzee—are genetically determined. On a more subtle level, it is clear that the differences in stature among humans depends to a large extent on differing genetic constitutions. So far the best, albeit a relatively crude, way of determining these underlying genetic factors is to look at the parental and familial heights.[22]

Tissue growth factors such as EGF clearly play a critical although largely unknown role in the control of growth in the organism.[3] A compilation of these tissue growth factors is given in Table 3–2. Further work will be necessary to relate these individual growth factors to clinical growth disorders.

Finally, the role of systemic disease in the growth of children and adolescents cannot be overemphasized. Even in the presence of normal hormonal, nutritional, and genetic factors, underlying systemic disease such as inflammatory bowel disease can interfere with growth potential.[23] The existence of short or tall stature in a patient is an important clue to the underlying condition of the patient.

SHORT STATURE

As might be expected from the multiplicity of control mechanisms for growth, there are

TABLE 3–2 ••• FAMILIES OF TISSUE GROWTH FACTORS

Insulin related
  Insulin-like growth factor-I (IGF I)
  Insulin-like growth factor-II (IGF II)
  Nerve growth factor (NGF)
Epidermal growth factor related
  Epidermal growth factor (EGF)
  Transforming growth factor-α (TGF-α)
Transforming growth factor-β related
  Transforming growth factor-β (TGF-β)
  Müllerian inhibiting factor (MIF)
  Inhibin
  Activin
Platelet-derived growth factor
Fibroblast growth factor
Cytokines
  Erythropoietin
  Granulocyte/monocyte–colony stimulating factor (GM-CSF)
  Granulocyte-CSF (G-CSF)
  Monocyte-CSF (M-CSF)
  Multi-CSF
Interleukins
  Interferon (IL) 1 through 9
  Tumor necrosis factor (TNF)
Interferons

many causes of short stature. These causes are summarized in Table 3–3.

Nonpathologic Short Stature

Clinically significant short stature is defined as height below the third percentile for age as

TABLE 3–3 ••• CAUSES OF SHORT STATURE

Nonpathologic causes of short stature (NVSS)
  Constitutional delay
  Familial
  Nutritional
GH-related causes
  GH deficiency
  GH resistance syndrome (Laron's syndrome)
Hypothyroidism
Sex hormone–related causes
  Delayed puberty
  Hypogonadotropic hypogonadism (Kallmann's syndrome)
Glucocorticoid excess
  Cushing's disease
  Pharmacologic administration
Genetic causes
  Chromosomal
    Turner syndrome (45,X and variants)
    Down syndrome (trisomy 21)
  Syndromes
    Pseudohypoparathyroidism
    Prader-Willi syndrome
    Lawrence-Moon-Biedl syndrome
    Skeletal dysplasias
    Miscellaneous (Russel-Silver, Seckel, etc.)

compared with relevant standards. Using this definition, it is clear that the majority of children with short stature do not have underlying hormonal or genetic disease. These children are frequently referred to as having normal variant short stature (NVSS). Many of these children come from families with a history of short stature (familial short stature). Others are from families with average height but have delayed bone aging and so could be classified as having constitutional delay. However, the reality in clinical practice is that many children have a combination of these features, and subcategorization of NVSS is often not very helpful. Hidden within this large number of basically normal children are some who may have clinically significant disorders. As a group, children with NVSS have a lower mean secretion of GH[24] and lower mean levels of circulating IGF I than age-matched controls. This has led to the suggestion that some of these children have subtle abnormalities in GH secretion and/or action and may benefit from treatment with GH. In addition to NVSS, nutritional disorders, including maternal deprivation, anorexia, and bulimia, can certainly lead to short stature.

GH-Related Short Stature

Clinical abnormalities of growth hormone secretion or action are clearly associated with short stature. The most apparent of these is GH deficiency, in which there is either a disorder of the hypothalamic control of GH secretion or an inability of the pituitary to secrete GH.[25] The consequences of classic GH deficiency are reflected not only in low levels of circulating GH as assessed by both physiologic and pharmacologic stimulation, but also in extremely low levels of IGF I and a consequent decrease in growth rate. These children almost invariably respond to GH treatment with a marked increase in growth rate.[26] An interesting although rare disorder of the chain of GH action is Laron's syndrome (also known as GH resistance syndrome). This disorder, originally described in Oriental Jews,[27] is now known to be more widely distributed ethnically and geographically.[28] Laron's syndrome consists of a group of genetic disorders of the GH receptor in which the GH receptor is unable to bind GH. This results in an increase in circulating GH levels as a result of a lack of IGF feedback, a decrease in the level of circulating GH-

binding protein derived from the GH receptor, markedly decreased levels of IGF I, and extremely poor growth rates. Early results suggest that children with Laron's syndrome respond to treatment with synthetic IGF I.[29] It is possible that more subtle abnormalities of the GH-binding protein or the GH receptor are underlying causes in a number of the undiagnosed cases of poor growth.

Thyroid Hormone–Related Short Stature

Because of the important role of thyroid hormone in both the secretion and endocrine actions of GH, it is clear that any degree of hypothyroidism will lead to a decrease in growth rate and, eventually, short stature.[30] Figure 3–3 demonstrates the remarkable decrease in growth rate seen with severe hypothyroidism and the rapid increase of growth rate after appropriate therapy is instituted. Some patients with severe hypothyroidism actually present with a peculiar form of preco-

ACQUIRED HYPOTHYROIDISM

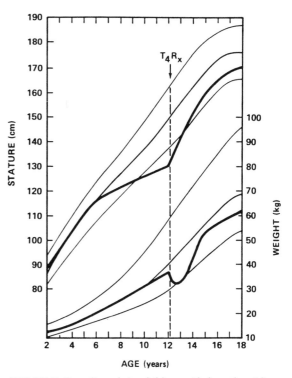

FIGURE 3–3 ••• Growth in children with hypothyroidism before and after treatment.

cious puberty known as *overlap syndrome,*[31] in which there is premature activation of gonadotropins, apparently associated with the high levels of TRH secretion by the hypothalamus. However, treatment of hypothyroidism can lead to the rapid onset of true puberty, which leads to an accelerated advance in bone age and may compromise final height despite the institution of thyroid therapy.

Sex Hormone–Related Short Stature

Short stature can also occur as a result of inadequate sex hormone secretion. This is most commonly seen in boys who have delayed puberty, but some girls also have a significant delay in puberty. Treatment with short courses of androgen has been used in boys with severely delayed puberty.[32] Many times this delay in puberty is physiologic, but it can also be associated with hypogonadotropic hypogonadism in both boys and girls. These patients may present in early puberty with short stature, which is due to the lack of sex hormone secretion and resultant pubertal growth spurt, but their final adult height may not be short. A relatively common form of hypogonadotropic hypogonadism, both in boys and girls, is Kallmann's syndrome, in which the hypogonadotropic hypogonadism is associated with anosmia.[33] These patients can be treated with sex steroids, as appropriate.

Adrenal Hormone–Related Short Stature

Short stature can also be associated with hypersecretion of glucocorticoids caused by an increase in ACTH secretion (Cushing's disease)[34] or by a functional adrenal tumor. Treatment consists of controlling excess glucocorticoid secretion. Of course, the most common cause of glucocorticoid excess leading to growth failure is pharmacologic doses of glucocorticoids used to treat steroid-responsive diseases. In these patients the obvious treatment, decreasing or stopping the glucocorticoid therapy, may be very difficult to accomplish because of exacerbation of the underlying disease state.

Genetic Causes of Short Stature

In girls, by far the most common genetic disorder leading to short stature is Turner syndrome.[35] The mechanism by which Turner syndrome leads to short stature is not yet clear, but it does not appear to be directly GH related. These girls have relatively poor growth rates during childhood, which leads to a progressive decrease in their average height when compared with that of normal girls of the same age (Fig. 3–4). In addition, they fail to enter puberty because of the ovarian failure associated with Turner syndrome, and thus they achieve very short adult stature (average height, approximately 4'7″ [140 cm]). Treatment with GH has had some success in increasing growth rates and final height in girls with Turner syndrome.[36] Although most of these children will have delayed puberty, a significant percentage do have sufficient estrogen secretion from their ovaries to develop secondary sex characteristics and even to menstruate. Thus any physician dealing with a girl who is significantly short and has no other established diagnosis should always perform a chromosome study, regardless of the presence or absence of secondary sex characteristics.

Other genetic causes of severe short stature include Down syndrome, pseudohypoparathyroidism, Lawrence-Moon-Biedl syndrome, Weaver's syndrome, and Prader-Willi syndrome.

TALL STATURE

Just as is the case with short stature, there are many causes of tall stature. These are given in Table 3–4.

Nonpathologic Causes of Tall Stature

Most children with clinically significant tall stature (above the 97th percentile of height for age) do not have a defined disease, and most are from tall families or genetic groups. However, studies of these children have suggested that as a group they may have higher rates of GH secretion and higher levels of IGF I.[37] These findings suggest that at least one of the underlying reasons for normal variant tall stature is a genetically determined increase in GH

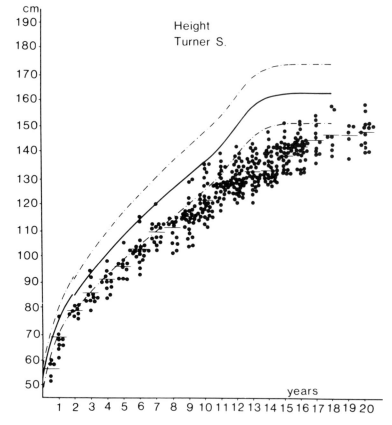

FIGURE 3–4 ••• Growth in children with Turner syndrome. (From Ranke MB, Pfluger H, Rosendahl W, et al. Turner syndrome: Spontaneous growth in 150 cases and review of the literature. Eur J Pediatr 1983; 141:81–88.)

secretion and/or action. Another common cause of relatively tall stature is obesity. Studies of obesity in childhood have demonstrated that almost all patients are above the 50th percentile of height for age, regardless of their genetic background, and a high proportion are above the 97th percentile. For not fully defined neuroendocrine reasons, these obese children have relatively low GH secretion as determined both by physiologic and pharmacologic stimulation.[38]

GH-Related Causes of Tall Stature

There are well-documented instances of pituitary tumors causing excess GH secretion leading to tall stature; these include the famous Alton Giant.[39] However, these tumors are a rare cause of tall stature in most endocrinologists' experience. It is important to exclude this possibility in rapidly growing children, and determination of serum IGF I level is probably an adequate screen for pituitary secretion of excess GH.

Thyroid-Related Causes of Tall Stature

In addition to GH-related causes, hyperthyroidism has been associated with tall stature in

TABLE 3–4 ••• CAUSES OF TALL STATURE

Nonpathologic causes of tall stature
  Genetic/familial
  Obesity
Pituitary gigantism
Hyperthyroidism
Sex hormone–related causes
  Precocious puberty
  Hypogonadotropic hypogonadism
Adrenal hormone–related causes
  Precocious adrenarche
  Adrenogenital syndrome
  Adrenal tumors
Genetic causes of tall stature
  Disorder of sex chromosomes
    Klinefelter's syndrome (47,XXY)
    Extra Y (47,XYY, 48,XYYY, etc.)
  Genetic syndromes
    Marfan's syndrome
    Homocystinuria
    Cerebral gigantism (Sotos's syndrome)
    Weaver's syndrome

childhood.[40] These patients may grow rapidly under the influence of high levels of thyroid hormone, but their epiphyseal centers also mature faster so that they finish their growth prematurely.

Sex Hormone–Related Causes of Tall Stature

Precocious puberty is well known to be associated with relatively tall stature for age[41] and is the best clinical illustration of the role of sex hormone secretion in growth. The disorder of precocious puberty is covered in more detail in Chapter 5. Somewhat paradoxically, delayed puberty caused by hypogonadotropic gonadotropism or Kallmann's syndrome can also be associated with tall stature. The explanation is that although these children grow relatively slowly during the time that other children their age are undergoing their pubertal growth spurt, they continue to grow long after the majority of children have completed puberty and eventually attain a tall stature. In fact, even children with physiologic delayed puberty can be tall for age, as illustrated by the growth data on the eighteenth century German poet Friedrich Schiller.[42]

Adrenal Hormone–Related Tall Stature

Adrenal causes of tall stature in childhood are also commonly seen. Children with precocious adrenarche, in which there is an increased secretion of adrenal androgens early in childhood associated with the other events in puberty, can have rapid growth rates and develop clinically significant tall stature. Children with adrenogenital syndrome can also present with tall stature along with signs of adrenal stimulation and early development of secondary sex characteristics.[43] Of course, this syndrome of early development and relatively tall stature for age can also be seen with functional adrenal tumors causing androgen secretion. Children with tall stature resulting from hypersecretion of androgens experience early epiphyseal fusion and attain only short or low-normal adult height.

Genetic Causes of Tall Stature

Genetic influences on the nonpathologic causes of tall stature, including familial- and the race-related causes, have been discussed earlier. In addition, Klinefelter's syndrome (47,XXY), as well as a genetic male with extra Y chromosomes (47,XYY, 48,XYYY, etc.) can also present with tall stature.[44] Marfan's syndrome, homocysteinuria, and cerebral gigantism are also relatively common genetic syndromes associated with tall stature.

References

1. Lechan RM. Neuroendocrinology of pituitary hormone regulation. Endocrinol Metab Clin North Am 1987; 16:475–501.
2. Susa JB, Widness JA, Hintz RL, et al. Somatomedins and insulin in diabetic pregnancies: Effects on fetal macrosomia in the human and rhesus monkey. J Clin Endocrinol Metab 1984; 58:1099.
3. Hintz RL. Growth factors. Curr Opin Pediatr 1990; 2:786–793.
4. Reichlin S. Neuroendocrinology. In: Wilson JD, Foster DW (eds). Williams' Textbook of Endocrinology. 8th ed. Philadelphia, WB Saunders, 1992, pp 135–219.
5. Baumann G. Growth hormone heterogeneity: Genes, isohormones, variants, and binding proteins. Endocr Rev 1991; 12:424–449.
6. Tannenbaum GS. Neuroendocrine control of growth hormone secretion. Acta Paediatr Scand Suppl 1991; 372:5–16.
7. Berelowitz M, Szabo M, Frohman LA, et al. Somatomedin-C mediates growth hormone negative feedback by effects on both the hypothalamus and the pituitary. Science 1981; 212:1279–1281.
8. Leung DW, Spencer SA, Cachianes G, et al. Growth hormone receptor and serum binding protein: Purification, cloning and expression. Nature 1987; 330:537–543.
9. Holly JMP, Wass JAH. Insulin-like growth factors; autocrine, paracrine or endocrine? New perspectives of the somatomedin hypotheses in the light of recent developments. J Endocrinol 1989; 122:611–618.
10. Powell DR, Lee PDK, Chang D, et al. Antiserum developed for the E peptide region of human IGF-IA prohormone recognizes a 13–19 kilodalton serum protein. J Clin Endocrinol 1987; 65:868–875.
11. Hintz RL. The role of growth hormone and insulin-like growth factor binding proteins. Horm Res 1990; 33:105–110.
12. Rosenfeld RG, Hintz RL. Somatomedin receptors: Structure, function and regulation. In: Conn PM (ed). The Receptors. Vol III. New York: Academic Press, 1986, pp 281–329.
13. Morley JE. Neuroendocrine control of thyrotropin secretion. Endocr Rev 1981; 2:396–436.
14. Frasier SD. A review of growth hormone stimulation tests in children. Pediatrics 1974; 53:929–937.
15. August GP, Grumbach MM, Kaplan SL. Hormonal changes in puberty. III. Correlation of plasma testosterone, LH, FSH, testicular size and bone age with male pubertal development. J Clin Endocrinol Metab 1972; 34:319–326.
16. Rose SB, Municchi G, Barnes KM, et al. Spontaneous growth hormone secretion increases during puberty in

normal girls and boys. J Clin Endocrinol Metab 1991; 73:428–35.

17. Greulich WW, Pyle SI. Radiographic Atlas of Skeletal Development of the Hand and Wrist. 2nd ed. Stanford, CA: Stanford University Press, 1959.

18. O'Malley BW, Tsai SY, Bagchi M, et al. Molecular mechanisms of action of a steroid hormone receptor. Recent Prog Horm Res 1991; 47:1–24.

19. Tanner JM. Growth and endocrinology of the adolescent. In: Gardner L (ed). Endocrine and Genetic Diseases of Childhood and Adolescence. 2nd ed. Philadelphia: WB Saunders, 1975, pp 14–64.

20. Solomon IL, Schoen EJ. Juvenile Cushing syndrome manifested primarily by growth failure. Am J Dis Child 1976; 130:200–202.

21. Hintz RL, Suskind R, Amatayakul K, et al. Somatomedin and growth hormone in children with protein calorie malnutrition. J Pediatr 1978; 92:153–156.

22. Tanner JM, Goldstein H, Whitehouse RH. Standards for children's height at ages 2–9 years allowing for height of parents. Arch Dis Child 1970; 45:755–762.

23. Sobel EH, Silverman FN, Lee CM Jr. Chronic regional enteritis and growth retardation. Am J Dis Child 1962; 103:569–576.

24. Albertsson-Wikland K, Hall K. Growth hormone treatment in short children: relationship between growth and serum insulin-like growth factor-I and -II levels. J Clin Endocrinol Metab 1987; 65:671–678.

25. Jorgensen JO. Human growth hormone deficiency replacement therapy: Pharmocological and clinical aspects. Endocr Rev 1991; 12:189–207.

26. Kaplan SL, Underwood LE, August GP, et al. Clinical studies with recombinant-DNA derived methionyl-hGH in GH deficient children. Lancet 1986; 1:697–700.

27. Laron Z, Kowadlo-Silbergeld A, Eshet R, Pertzelan A. Growth hormone resistance. Ann Clin Res 1980; 12:269–277.

28. Fielder PJ, Guevara-Aguirre J, Rosenbloom AL, et al. Expression of serum insulin-like growth factors, IGF binding proteins, and the growth hormone-binding protein in heterozygote relatives of Ecuadorian GH-receptor deficiency patients. J Clin Endocrinol Metab 1992; 74:743–750.

29. Walker JL, Ginalska-Malinowska M, Romer TE, et al. Effects of infusion of IGF-I in a child with growth hormone insensitivity syndrome (Laron dwarfism). N Engl J Med 1991; 324:1483–1488.

30. Rivkees SA, Bode HH, Crawford JD. Long-term growth in juvenile acquired hypothyroidism: The failure to acheive normal stature. N Engl J Med 1988; 318:599–602.

31. Van Wyk JJ, Grumbach MM. Syndrome of precocious menstruation and galactorrhea in juvenile hypothyroidism: An example of hormonal overlap in pituitary feedback. J Pediatr 1960; 57:416–435.

32. Wilson DM, Kei J, Hintz RL, Rosenfeld RG. Effects of testosterone enanthate treatment for pubertal delay. Am J Dis Child 1988; 142:96–99.

33. White BJ, Rogol AD, Brown KS, et al. The syndrome of anosmia with hypogonadotropic hypogonadism: a genetic study of 18 new families and a review. Am J Med Genet 1983; 15:417–435.

34. McArthur RG, Cloutier MD, Hayles AB, Sprague RE. Cushing's disease in children. Findings in 13 cases. Mayo Clin Proc 1972; 47:318–326.

35. Ranke MB, Pfluger H, Rosendahl W, et al. Turner syndrome: Spontaneous growth in 150 cases and review of the literature. Eur J Pediatr 1983; 141:81–88.

36. Rosenfeld RG, Hintz RL, Johanson AJ, Sherman B. Growth hormone therapy in Turner syndrome. In: Rosenfeld RG, Grumbach MM (eds). Turner Syndrome. New York: Marcel Dekker, 1990, pp 393–403.

37. Albertsson-Wikland K, Rosberg S. Analysis of 24-hour growth hormone profiles in childhood: Relation to growth. J Clin Endocrinol Metab 1988; 67:493–500.

38. Veldhuis JD, Iranmanexh A, Ho KK, et al. Dual defects in pulsatile growth hormone secretion and clearance subserve the hyposomatotropism of obesity in man. J Clin Endocrinol Metab 1991; 72:51–59.

39. Behrens LH, Barr DP. Hyperpituitarism beginning in infancy. The Alton giant. Endocrinology 1932; 16:120–128.

40. Sotos JF, Romsche CM. Gigantism and acromegaly. In: Gardner L (ed). Endocrine and Genetic Diseases of Childhood and Adolescence. 2nd ed. Philadelphia: WB Saunders, 1975, pp 158–187.

41. Rosenfield RL. Puberty and its disorders in girls. Endocrinol Metab Clin North Am 1991; 20:15–42.

42. Tanner JM. A History of the Study of Human Growth. Cambridge, England: Cambridge University Press, 1981, pp 106–112.

43. White PC, New MI, Dupont B. Congenital adrenal hyperplasia. N Engl J Med 1987; 316:1519–1524, 1580–1586.

44. Robinson A, Lubs HA, Bergsma D. Summary of clinical findings: Profiles of children with 47,XXY, 47,XYY, and 47,XXX karyotypes. Birth Defects 1982; 18:1–5.

CHAPTER 4

Neuroendocrinology of Puberty

PETER A. LEE

EDWARD O. REITER

HOWARD E. KULIN

Puberty is the transitional period between childhood and adulthood, between the first signs of sexual maturation and physical and reproductive maturity. During this period, the primary sexual characteristics (genitals and gonads) mature, the secondary sexual characteristics (sexual hair and breasts) appear and mature, and a dramatic growth spurt occurs. Profound psychological changes take place, leading to mental and emotional maturity.

The changes of puberty result from a rise in sex steroid secretion, primarily estradiol in females and testosterone in males. The increased activity of the ovary, including follicular maturation and steroidogenesis, follows increased stimulation by the pituitary gonadotropins, luteinizing hormone (LH), and follicle-stimulating hormone (FSH). In turn, the synthesis and release of LH and FSH are the result of increased hypothalamic gonadotropin-releasing hormone (GnRH) stimulation.

The hypothalamus is capable of producing and secreting ample GnRH to maintain full function of pituitary gonadotropes at any time after birth. Likewise, neither the pituitary gland nor the gonads are rate limiting in the maturational process. The gonad in the prepubertal child will respond and mature when stimulated at any point during childhood. The juvenile pituitary can be upregulated at any age when appropriately stimulated. The control of puberty, then, is above the level of the hypothalamus; puberty begins when the hypothalamus is stimulated to release increased amounts of GnRH from the gonadostat.

NEUROENDOCRINE SYSTEM

The neuroendocrine (CNS-hypothalamic-pituitary) portions of this hormone axis (Fig. 4–1) consist of three principal components present in all mammalian species:[1–4]

1. Suprahypothalamic sites, higher cortical centers, and the limbic system, which influence production and release of the decapeptide GnRH by neurons within the hypothalamus.

2. The arcuate nucleus of the medial basal hypothalamus, which controls GnRH release in intermittent bursts from the median eminence into the hypothalamic-hypophyseal portal circulation. This periodic, oscillatory release coincides with signals from this nucleus and from associated transducer neurosecretory neurons. The pulse generator may actually be the composite of interconnected GnRH-secreting neurons. The magnitude of the intermittent bursts increases markedly with the onset of puberty.[5]

3. The gonadotropes in the pituitary, which respond to regular episodic GnRH stimulation with a similar rhythmic release of LH and FSH into the petrosal sinus.

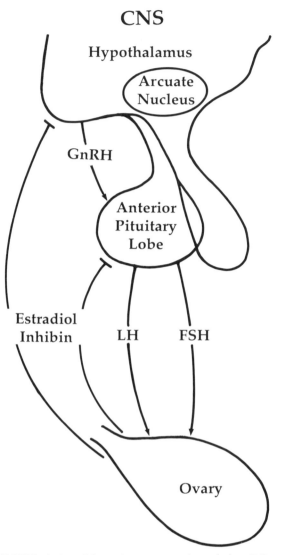

CNS

Hypothalamus

Arcuate Nucleus

GnRH

Anterior Pituitary Lobe

Estradiol Inhibin

LH   FSH

Ovary

FIGURE 4–1 ••• Schematic representation of the CNS-hypothalamic-pituitary-ovarian axis. Neurotransmitters from higher centers of the CNS may stimulate or inhibit pulsatile release of gonadotropin-releasing hormone (GnRH). GnRH pulses stimulate gonadotropin pulsatile release. Feedback from the ovary to the hypothalamus may be negative or positive. LH, Luteinizing hormone; FSH, follicle-stimulating hormone.

Within each of the components of the gonadotropin-gonadal axis, target cells containing hormone-specific receptors receive and mediate input. Between components there are a variety of stimulatory and inhibitory control mechanisms. The end result of the neuroendocrine component is the activation by gonadotropins of specific target receptors within the gonad, stimulating synthesis and secretion of gonadal steroids and peptides and maturation of germinal tissue.

OVERVIEW

Pubertal maturation is but one phase in a developmental continuum that begins with sexual differentiation during the first trimester of fetal life and continues through advanced age. The mechanism for pubertal maturation actually begins with a significant upsurge of the gonadotropin secretion that initially develops during fetal life, persists during infancy, and then becomes relatively quiescent during the middle childhood years (Fig. 4–2).[1–4] The hypothalamic-pituitary-gonadal axis differentiates and functions during the last half of fetal life and in early infancy at a level similar to that seen in adult life.

The characteristic release pattern of gonadotropin secretion is intermittent and is a response to the episodic release of GnRH from the arcuate nucleus of the hypothalamus (Fig. 4–3). During the childhood years, this hormonal axis functions at a very low level, reflected in small secretory bursts that can be detected only by the most sensitive assays.[6–8] At the onset of puberty, the pulsatile release of GnRH increases, resulting in more dramatic spikes of circulating levels of gonadotropins. This phenomenon represents a reactivation of the increased GnRH secretion that had first developed during fetal life.[9] Responses of LH and FSH to exogenous GnRH (Fig. 4–4) reflect the extent of endogenous GnRH priming of the gonadotropes; hence, greater responses are obtained from pubertal patients.

Thus, puberty is not the initiation of a new secretory process, but rather an amplification of existing hormonal events. The factors that restrain gonadotropin secretion during the prepubertal years and the process that removes this restraint, allowing secretion to resume during puberty, are unknown. However, it is clear that undefined CNS input from suprahypothalamic sites primarily controls the sequence of downregulation and reactivation.[4]

REGULATION OF GONADOTROPIN SECRETION

Negative Feedback

The process by which suppressive input from one portion of the hypothalamic-pituitary-gonadal axis inhibits the activity of another portion is referred to as *negative feedback*. The

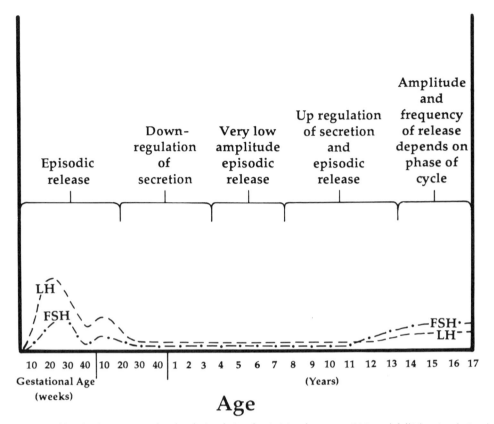

FIGURE 4–2 ••• Profile of relative mean levels of circulating luteinizing hormone (LH) and follicle-stimulating hormone (FSH) during fetal life, infancy, childhood, and puberty. Episodic release, first apparent before birth, persists into early infancy, becomes less frequent during childhood, and then resurges to stimulate puberty.

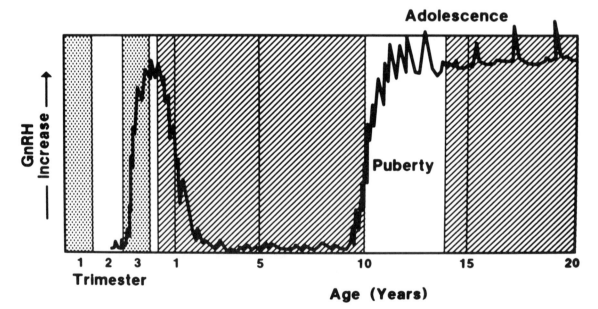

FIGURE 4–3 ••• Diagrammatic representation of the ontogeny of gonadotropin-releasing hormone (GnRH) secretion from fetal life to adolescence. Note the prepubertal nadir and upswing of GnRH secretory activity at the onset of puberty. This is followed by irregular luteinizing hormone (LH) surges during adolescence in girls. (From Yen SSC. The hypothalamic control of pituitary hormone secretion. In: Yen SSC, Jaffe RB [eds]. Reproductive Endocrinology. 3rd ed. Philadelphia: WB Saunders, 1991.)

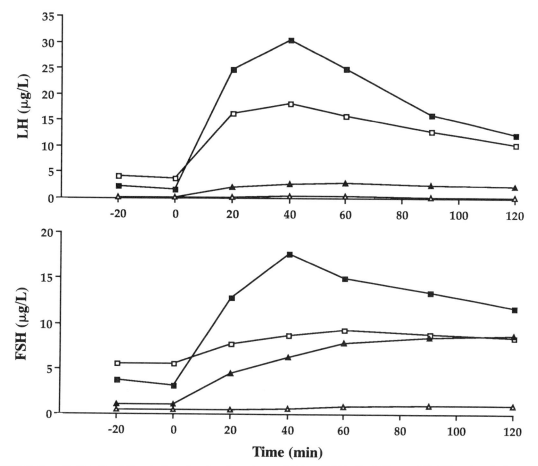

FIGURE 4–4 ••• GnRH stimulation testing showing the release of LH and FSH after 100 μg of GnRH at time 0. Responses are depicted for a 6-year-old girl with central sexual precocity (■), a 14-year-old girl with normal pubertal development (□), a 5-year-old prepubertal girl (△), and a 16-year-old girl (▲) with hypothalamic-pituitary destruction secondary to a craniopharyngioma, after treatment.

primary example is the effect of the gonadally produced sex steroids and peptide hormones of the germinal epithelium causing a diminution of hypothalamic GnRH release and a decrease of pituitary gonadotropin secretion. In addition, the direct effects of pituitary gonadotropins on the production and release of hypothalamic GnRH are known as *short-loop feedback systems*, while the direct inhibiting effect of GnRH on its further synthesis and secretion by the same or adjacent arcuate nucleus neurons is an *ultrashort-loop feedback*.

Negative feedback lowers gonadotropin secretion during the latter half of gestation, causes diminution of gonadotropin secretion after the neonatal period, is part of the maturational process that alters the regulation of gonadotropin secretion during puberty, and maintains the homeostasis of gonadotropin production in adults.[1–4] Sex steroid–induced gonadotropin suppression appears to occur at both the hypothalamic and the pituitary levels, although in higher mammals it may occur primarily at the pituitary level.[10]

Positive Feedback

In addition to having the inhibiting effects of sex steroids on gonadotropin secretion, both males and females have the potential for an acute release of gonadotropins after a sudden rise of estradiol. This enhancement of gonadotropin secretion is known as *positive feedback*[1–4] and is physiologically significant, as the midcycle gonadotropin surge is an obligatory part of the ovulatory portion of the menstrual cycle in women. The capacity for positive feedback is attained in the later stages of pubertal maturation.

Modulators of Hypothalamic GnRH Activity

Control of the onset of puberty resides in the system that allows or stimulates greater episodic GnRH secretion. GnRH synthesis, secretion, and feedback control by sex steroids are regulated by a variety of modulators secreted by neurons that control GnRH release from the arcuate nucleus. These modulators include catecholamines, noradrenaline, dopamine, opiates, and neuroactive amino acids such as glutamate and aspartate, but not melatonin.[1, 4, 5, 10]

PITUITARY GONADOTROPIN SECRETION

LH and FSH are secreted in discrete bursts separated by intervals without secretory activity.[6, 7, 11] Both the frequency and the amplitude of the pulses appear to be modulated by GnRH and sex steroid influences at the pituitary. The intervals between pulses vary considerably during different phases of the menstrual cycle and apparently are related to variations in the levels of estrogen and progesterone.[12]

Developmental Changes

The fetal pituitary begins to synthesize FSH and LH, as is evident in storage granules, by 8 weeks of gestation, with secretion beginning by 12 weeks.[9] By midgestation, levels within the pituitary and in the circulation gradually increase to the very high levels characteristic of agonadal adults, suggesting the lack of a negative feedback mechanism. After midgestation there is a decline in fetal levels that persists until birth; this decline provides evidence of maturation of negative feedback control.

Birth produces an abrupt cessation of the placental source of sex steroids. Concomitant with the decrease in the levels of sex steroids and the diminution of negative feedback, LH and FSH concentrations rise and fluctuate considerably during the first 4 to 6 weeks of life (see Fig. 4–2). Higher gonadotropin levels are accompanied by increased estradiol levels among female infants and by dramatically elevated testosterone levels in males.[13] Available evidence suggests that gonadotropin secretion during the neonatal period, as well as during fetal life, is episodic and under controlling influences that are similar to those seen at later ages.

Concentrations of gonadotropins gradually decrease to the low levels characteristic of childhood, presumably as restraint of GnRH secretion occurs. Levels typical of childhood are seen in females by 2 years of age. FSH levels are relatively higher than LH levels in females and are higher in females than in age-matched males. Levels remain low until the start of pubertal secretion, a resurgence of the GnRH-driven episodic release that is first apparent during fetal life.

Episodic and Circadian Variation

During childhood, normal gonadotropin secretion involves both episodic fluctuation of release and a sleep-related circadian rhythm.[6, 7] The onset of puberty is marked by a dramatic increase in amplitude of gonadotropin pulses and an accentuation of a circadian variation that is minimally detectable, but clearly present, before puberty (Fig. 4–5).[1–4] In the prepubertal child, there is a diurnal pattern resulting from a moderate sleep-enhanced episodic secretion. This configuration can be demonstrated for LH and, less noticeably, for FSH in blood and urine samples. The accentuation of this sleep enhancement of gonadotropin secretion, particularly an increased amplitude of pulsatile LH release, is characteristic of pubertal physiology.

With progression into the pubertal process, the episodic release gradually extends throughout the sleep period (see Fig. 4–5). Eventually, nocturnal accentuation becomes less prominent as the amplitude of the pulsations becomes more pronounced and the pulsations extend throughout the 24-hour day (i.e., the typical adult pattern). After maturation, as during pubertal development, both the amplitude and the frequency of gonadotropin pulses (and thus the mean circulating levels) are regulated by GnRH and sex steroid interaction at the pituitary level.[14]

There are important sex differences in pubertal gonadotropin secretion; ratios of LH and FSH responses to GnRH stimulation at the onset of puberty differ between males and females.[15] Also, ratios of bioactive and immunoactive gonadotropins change with puberty and may also differ between the sexes.[16] In the mature female, LH pulses occur every 60 to 90 minutes in the follicular and early luteal

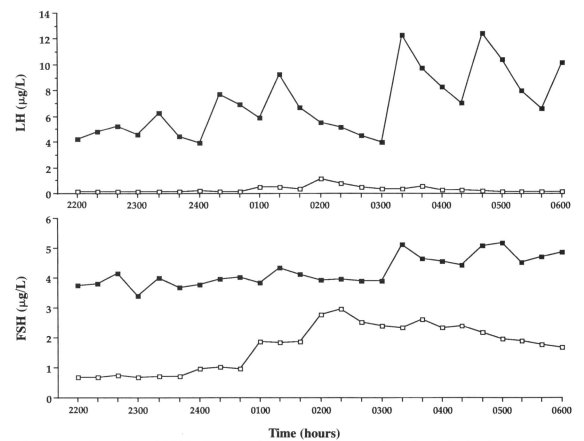

FIGURE 4–5 ••• Serum LH and FSH levels measured by fluoroimmunoassay of samples obtained at 20-minute intervals between 10 PM and 6 AM from a 7-year-old prepubertal female (□) and a 13-year-old pubertal, premenarchial female (■). Note the episodic release, particularly of LH in the pubertal girl.

phases of the menstrual cycle. During the middle and late luteal phases, the occurrence of LH pulses diminishes to every 3 to 4 hours.[12]

Children with true or central precocious puberty display the more mature pattern of episodic and circadian variation.[4, 17] Indeed, the intermittent nature of the GnRH stimulus is critical to upregulate and maintain pubertal or adult LH and FSH synthesis and release. If the intermittent pattern is disrupted by persistently high levels of GnRH at the pituitary level (as with continual GnRH infusion or by injection of long-acting GnRH analogues), gonadotropin synthesis and secretion are downregulated, and a hypogonadotropic or prepubertal state is created.[4, 17–19]

Prepubertal Period of Hormonal Quiescence

The factors or neurohormonal systems responsible for the period of suppressed repro-

ductive system activity during childhood, after a period of increased gonadotropin levels during fetal and early infant life, are not well understood. Before it was recognized that this system was functionally capable in the fetus, it was assumed that differentiation was not complete until puberty.

Negative Feedback During Childhood

As negative feedback mechanisms were studied and it became apparent that patients with primary hypogonadism may have markedly elevated gonadotropin levels even during childhood, a sex steroid–dependent mechanism for the midchildhood quiescent period was hypothesized.[1, 4, 10, 20] This theory suggests that the inhibition of hypothalamic GnRH release and the decrease in pituitary gonadotropin secretion after infancy are the result of progressively increased sensitivity of the hypothalamus and pituitary gland to the negative feedback inhibition of sex steroids. This varying set-point regulation feature of negative feedback control has been called a *gonadostat*.[1, 4] This regulatory mechanism, although operative during later fetal life, becomes more important during late infancy.

During the prepubertal years, the hypothalamic-pituitary-gonadal negative feedback control system becomes highly sensitive to the suppressive effect of even the very low levels of circulating sex steroids present in prepubertal children. Both before and after childhood, considerably higher levels of sex steroids are required to suppress gonadotropin secretion. The elevated gonadotropin concentrations during the first few years of life in agonadal patients are evidence that low levels of hormones secreted by the normal prepubertal gonad inhibit a more highly sensitive gonadotropin secretion. As puberty commences, the arcuate nucleus in the hypothalamus and the gonadotropes in the pituitary progressively become less sensitive to the inhibitory effects of sex steroids, resulting in greater GnRH release and gonadotropin secretion.[1, 4, 10, 21]

CNS Control of Prepubertal Restraint

The clinical basis of the theory that control is not just the result of a change in feedback sensitivity is found in the fact that the pattern of gonadotropin secretion from birth to adulthood is qualitatively similar for agonadal patients and normal individuals.[20, 22] Gonadotropin levels are higher during the first years of life; a dramatic decrease occurs during childhood, followed by an increase at puberty. Throughout this time, agonadal patients have quantitatively greater levels of gonadotropins. Because agonadal children evidence a diminution of gonadotropin secretion similar to that seen in normal individuals during the childhood years,[18, 22] an additional mechanism was proposed to fully explain the decrease in gonadotropin levels during childhood. It was hypothesized that a sex steroid–independent mechanism adjusted the stimulatory and inhibitory influences, including sex steroids, on the arcuate nucleus in the hypothalamus or suprahypothalamic centers. This sex steroid–independent mechanism appears to reside in higher CNS centers.[1, 4, 5] CNS inhibitory influences restrict gonadotropins during childhood and

prompt increased secretion at pubertal age, independent of gonadal sex steroid secretion.

The makeup of this CNS controlling system has not been determined. However, it is clear that aberrations within the CNS can interrupt the inhibitory mechanism and lead to premature reactivation of gonadotropin secretion. Central (gonadotropin-stimulated) precocious puberty (see Fig. 4–4) occurs in children with a variety of suprahypothalamic tumors and after CNS radiation (often concomitantly with radiation-induced damage resulting in growth hormone or other pituitary hormone deficiencies). The apparent impairment of the CNS inhibitory system results in the untimely appearance of the augmented, pulsatile gonadotropin secretion representative of puberty.[14, 17–19]

From median eminence effluent in monkeys, it has been shown not only that the hypothalamus releases low levels of GnRH during the prepubertal years and greater amounts (with more frequent pulses of greater amplitude) after puberty, but also that prepubertal monkeys release greater amounts of GnRH and gonadotropin when stimulated with an excitatory neuroamine, *N*-methyl-D-aspartate.[4, 23] This confirms the potential for adult levels of GnRH production during prepubertal years, identifying the hypothalamus, pituitary, and gonad as components of the system that are capable and ready to operate at any time. This supports the hypothesis that suprahypothalamic neuroregulatory factors are primary in the regulation of quiescent childhood secretion and the timing of the onset of puberty.[1, 4]

TIMING OF THE ONSET OF PUBERTY

Although it is generally agreed that the CNS (hypothalamus) controls the time of the onset of puberty, specific mechanisms are not well understood. The secular changes in the average age of menarche over the decades from 1890 to 1980 suggest that improvements in nutritional status, general health, and socioeconomic conditions are significant factors. Nutritional status as an influence seems clear, as puberty occurs earlier among moderately overweight girls and is delayed in those with malnutrition and who have undergone voluntary weight loss. The fact that metabolic alterations involving utilization of alternative energy stores occur during maturation is suggested by the finding that fasting juvenile primates use amino acids and fatty acids earlier than fasting adult primates. Opiate inhibitory effects on GnRH release, although clear among adults, have not been shown to be significant during puberty.

THE MATURE REPRODUCTIVE SYSTEM

Midcycle Gonadotropin Surge and Positive Feedback

The midcycle LH and FSH surge is the result of positive feedback induced by estradiol of adequate concentration for an ample time (>36 hours) at the end of the follicular phase of the menstrual cycle. This does not occur before midpuberty because the negative feedback system is highly sensitive, not because the pituitary is incapable of secreting bursts of gonadotropins. The hormonal milieu also requires (1) FSH priming of the ovarian follicle so that it is able to secrete enough estradiol for an adequate time and (2) GnRH priming of the pituitary so that it contains an adequate pool of releasable gonadotropins to produce a surge.[1, 4]

If the midcycle surge acts via GnRH release and not directly at the level of the pituitary, adequate estrogen must have been present to sensitize the pituitary to GnRH stimulation, and GnRH-secreting neurons must contain adequate stores to respond to the estradiol stimulation with an acute release of GnRH. As mentioned, the negative feedback system at this time must be insensitive enough to allow GnRH and gonadotropin levels to increase rather than fall as the estradiol levels are rising.

The cyclicity of gonadotropins and estrogen-induced positive feedback have been demonstrated by midpuberty, but the positive feedback loop does not appear to be completely mature at this stage.[24] The ovary is not adequately responsive or is insufficiently primed to secrete enough estradiol for long enough periods of time to induce an LH surge, even though the pituitary contains sufficient stores of readily releasable gonadotropin. This may explain why, during the first few years after menarche, the majority of cycles are anovulatory.[25, 26]

Regulation and Function of the Gonad

During infancy the ovary responds to the relatively greater gonadotropin secretion char- acteristic of this stage with follicular maturation and estrogen secretion.[1, 4, 27] Estrogen secretion may be evident by breast development, which is not uncommon at this time.[28] The higher circulating levels of LH, FSH, and estradiol during infancy fall within months to the low levels characteristic of the physiologically normal hypogonadotropic state of childhood. Before puberty, mean estradiol levels are usually less than 10 pg/ml and are not different from those in male children or hypogonadal individuals. However, there may be brief periods of increased gonadotropin stimulation and ovarian response. In fact, there may be more stimulation, at least intermittently, than generally assumed, although this has not been detected by random hormone sampling and assay methods. Indeed, throughout this period there is activity within the ovary, with limited follicular growth and regression.[27] This may result in the development of follicular cysts, which may occasionally secrete sufficient estrogen to stimulate pubertal development temporarily.[29]

The pubertal increase in estrogen secretion begins gradually at least as early as age 7 years. Although this increase is difficult to demonstrate by measuring estradiol levels, uterine growth is apparent before the onset of breast development. Significantly increased estradiol concentrations are present by the age of 10 years, and mean levels gradually increase with pubertal progression, although wide fluctuations are apparent by midpuberty and persist, as expected, after menarche.

In addition to the sex steroids secreted by the ovary that exert a negative feedback effect on the hypothalamus and pituitary, there is also a family of gonadally produced glycoproteins, the inhibins, that regulate gonadotropin secretion, apparently primarily via an FSH inhibitory action.[30, 31] The granulosa cells produce inhibin in the presence of LH and FSH. Circulating levels of inhibin progressively rise during pubertal maturation. Levels in males rise to a higher level during puberty than do those in females.[32] The influence of inhibin on GnRH, LH, and FSH secretion is not well understood, and its significance in relation to the maturing hypothalamic-pituitary-gonadal axis is not known.

References

1. Reiter EO, Grumbach MM. Neuroendocrine control mechanisms and the onset of puberty. Annu Rev Physiol 1982; 44:595.

2. Lee PA. Pubertal neuroendocrine maturation. Early differentiation and stages of development. Adolesc Pediatr Gynecol 1988; 1:3.

3. Lee PA. Neuroendocrinology of puberty. Semin Reprod Endocrinol 1988; 6:13.

4. Grumbach MM, Styne DM. Puberty. Ontogeny, neuroendocrinology, physiology and disorders. In: Wilson JD, Foster DW (eds). Williams' Textbook of Endocrinology. 8th ed. Philadelphia: WB Saunders, 1992; p. 1139.

5. Knobil E. The GnRH pulse generator. Am J Obstet Gynecol 1990; 153:1721.

6. Wu FCW, Butler GE, Kelnar CJH, Sellar RE. Patterns of pulsatile luteinizing hormone secretion before and during the onset of puberty in boys: A study using an immunoradiometric assay. J Clin Endocrinol Metab 1990; 70:629.

7. Wu FCW, Butler GE, Kelnar CJH, et al. Patterns of pulsatile luteinizing hormone and follicle-stimulating hormone secretion in prepubertal (midchildhood) boys and girls and patients with idiopathic hypogonadotropic hypogonadism (Kallmann's syndrome): A study using an ultrasensitive time-resolved immunofluorometric assay. J Clin Endocrinol Metab 1991; 72:1229.

8. Drop SLS, de Muinck Keizer-Scharama SMPF. Pubertal development and gonadal function. Curr Opinion Pediatr 1991; 3:701.

9. Kaplan SL, Grumbach MM, Aubert ML. The ontogenesis of pituitary hormones and hypothalamic factors in the human fetus: Maturation of central nervous system regulation of anterior pituitary function. Rec Prog Horm Res 1976; 32:161.

10. Plant TM. Puberty in primates. In: Knobil E, Neill JD (eds). The Physiology of Reproduction. New York: Raven Press, 1988; p 1763.

11. Veldhuis JD, Johnson ML. A novel general biophysical model for simulating episodic endocrine gland signaling. Am J Physiol 1988; 255:749.

12. Filicori M, Butler JP, Crowley WF. Neuroendocrine regulation of the corpus luteum in the human. J Clin Invest 1984; 74:1638.

13. Winter JSD, Fairman C, Hobson WB, et al. Pituitary gonadal regulation in infancy. I. Patterns of serum gonadotropin concentrations from birth to four years of age in man and chimpanzee. J Clin Endocrinol Metab 1975; 40:545.

14. Reichlin S. Neuroendocrinology. In: Wilson JD, Foster DW (eds). Williams' Textbook of Endocrinology. 8th ed. Philadelphia: WB Saunders, 1991; p 178.

15. Oerter KE, Uriarte MM, Rose SR, et al. Gonadotropin secretory dynamics during puberty in normal girls and boys. J Clin Endocrinol Metab 1990; 71:1251.

16. Hassing JM, Padmanabhan V, Kelch RP, et al. Differential regulation of serum immunoreactive luteinizing hormone and bioactive follicle-stimulating hormone by testosterone in early pubertal boys. J Clin Endocrinol Metab 1990; 70:1082.

17. Kaplan SL, Grumbach MM. Pathophysiology and treatment of sexual precocity. J Clin Endocrinol Metab 1990; 71:785.

18. Rosenfield RL. Puberty and its disorders in girls. Endocrinol Metab Clin North Am 1991; 20:15.

19. Wheeler MD, Styne DM. The treatment of precocious puberty. Endocrinol Metab Clin North Am 1991; 20:183.

20. Dunkel L, Alfthan H, Stenman UH, Perheentupa J. Gonadal control of pulsatile secretion of luteinizing hormone and follicle-stimulating hormone in prepubertal boys evaluated by ultrasensitive time-resolved immunofluorometric assays. J Clin Endocrinol Metab 1990; 70:107.

21. Grumbach MM, Kaplan SL. The neuroendocrinology of human puberty: An ontogenetic perspective. In: Grumbach MM, Sizonenko PC, Aubert ML (eds). Control of the Onset of Puberty. Baltimore: Williams & Wilkins, 1990; p 1.

22. Conte FA, Grumbach MM, Kaplan SL. A diphasic pattern of gonadotropin secretion in patients with the syndrome of gonadal dysgenesis. J Clin Endocrinol Metab 1975; 40:670.

23. Medmurthy R, Dichek HL, Plant TM, et al. Stimulation of gonadotropin secretion in prepubertal monkeys after hypothalamic excitation with aspartate and glutamate. J Clin Endocrinol Metab 1990; 71:1390.

24. Reiter EO, Kulin HE, Hamwood SM. The absence of positive feedback between estrogen and luteinizing hormone in sexually immature girls. Pediatr Res 1974; 8:740.

25. Apter D, Vihko R. Serum pregnenolone, progesterone, 17-hydroxyprogesterone, testosterone and 5-dihydrotestosterone during female puberty. J Clin Endocrinol Metab 1977; 45:1039.

26. Winter JSD, Faiman C. Pituitary-gonadal relations in female children and adolescents. Pediatr Res 1973; 7:948.

27. Peters H, Byskov AG, Grinsted J. Follicular growth in fetal and prepubertal ovaries of humans and other primates. J Clin Endocrinol Metab 1978; 7:469.

28. Mills JL, Stolley PD, Davies J, et al. Premature thelarche: Natural history and etiologic investigation. Am J Dis Child 1981; 135:743.

29. Towne BH, Mahour GH, Wooley MM, et al. Ovarian cysts and tumors in infancy and childhood. J Pediatr Surg 1975; 10:311.

30. Ying SY. Inhibins, activins, and follistatins: Gonadal proteins modulating the secretion of follicle-stimulating hormone. Endocr Rev 1988; 9:267.

31. Skinner MK. Cell-cell interactions in the testis. Endocr Rev 1991; 12:45.

32. Burger HG, McLachlan RI, Bangah M, et al. Serum inhibin concentrations rise throughout normal male and female puberty. J Clin Endocrinol Metab 1988; 67:689.

CHAPTER 5

Pubertal Disorders: Precocious and Delayed Puberty

LOUIS St. L. O'DEA

SELMA F. SIEGEL

PETER A. LEE

As discussed in Chapter 4, puberty is initiated by the reactivation of integrated hypothalamic-pituitary-gonadal axis activity, which is relatively quiescent between early infancy and puberty.[1] The inhibitory influences maintaining latency of the axis during childhood remain unidentified, as do the stimulatory influences for the reinitiation process. The somatic manifestations of the initiation of puberty—secondary sexual characteristics and increased physical growth—are the result of increased levels of gonadal steroids. Changes in linear growth and body composition are mediated both directly and indirectly by sex steroid hormones. Although sex steroids directly stimulate growth, much of this growth promotion results from stimulation of greater amplitude growth hormone (GH) secretion by rising estrogen levels and, in turn, the effect of GH on insulin-like growth factor I (IGF-I) production.[2, 3]

Therefore, sexual maturation and physical growth are intimately related during adolescence. The statistical norms for the age of onset of puberty and for the rate of progression through its stages differ among countries and even among different ethnic groups and social classes within a population. Generally, puberty begins between the ages of 8 and 13 years in girls and 9 and 14 years in boys. Abnormalities of this process of sexual maturation may be classified as (1) premature or precocious, (2) late or delayed, or (3) dysynchronous (e.g., when physical changes are not followed by the onset of menses after an appropriate interval).

PRECOCIOUS PUBERTY

Precocious puberty in girls is defined as the onset of the physical changes of puberty before 8 years of age. Usually the first indication noticed is breast development, followed by growth acceleration. Menarche occurring before 10 years of age is also considered precocious. In boys, the onset of puberty, testicular enlargement, or pubic hair prior to 9 years of age is considered precocious. Precocious puberty can be classified as (1) gonadotropin-releasing hormone (GnRH)–driven precocious puberty, also designated central (CPP), true, or gonadotropin-dependent precocious puberty; (2) GnRH-independent precocious puberty, also termed peripheral or gonadotropin-independent precocious puberty (GIP) or precocious pseudopuberty (PPP); or (3) incomplete precocious puberty (IPP) or isolated partial early development (e.g., premature thelarche and premature pubarche). Nonprogressive precocious puberty is the occurrence

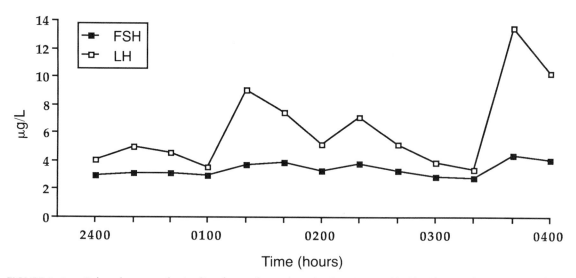

FIGURE 5–1 ••• Pubertal pattern of episodic release of gonadotropins in a 6-year-old girl with central precocious puberty.

of signs and symptoms consistent with CPP but with failure to progress. Isosexual development is that appropriate for the sex of the individual.

Central Precocious Puberty

GnRH-driven precocious puberty is physiologically normal pubertal development, albeit at an inappropriately early age. This GnRH-dependent precocious puberty is due to premature activation of the hypothalamic-pituitary-gonadal (HPG) axis with pubertal pituitary gonadotropin secretion. Amplification of pulsatile gonadotropin secretion along with sleep enhancement (Fig. 5–1) and an accentuation of gonadotropin response, particularly luteinizing hormone (LH), to exogenous GnRH are manifestations of this activation

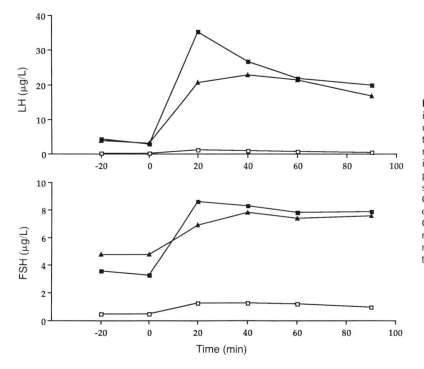

FIGURE 5–2 ••• Plasma luteinizing hormone (LH) and follicle-stimulating hormone (FSH) responses to gonadotropin-releasing hormone (GnRH) stimulation testing in a girl with central precocious puberty showing a pubertal response at diagnosis and before GnRH analogue therapy (■), lack of response during suppression of GnRH analogue therapy (□), and recovery of pubertal response 6 months after discontinuation of therapy (▲).

(Fig. 5–2). GnRH-driven precocious puberty may be idiopathic, associated with CNS abnormalities, or the result of prolonged untimely exposure to sex steroids, which accelerate the maturation of the HPG axis. The origins of CPP are listed in Table 5–1.

Therefore, central isosexual precocious puberty is characterized by normal pubertal changes in secondary sexual characteristics (i.e., in girls, breast and pubic hair development) (Fig. 5–3). Accelerated growth velocity and advanced skeletal maturation are observed. A pubertal gonadotropin response to exogenous GnRH stimulation at an inappropriately early age is observed. In girls, menarche and cyclical menstrual bleeding may follow.

Origins of Central Precocious Puberty

Isosexual CPP occurs more commonly in girls than in boys. The cause among girls is more often unclear and thus categorized as idiopathic and attributed to premature enhancement of the hypothalamic GnRH pulsatile release (see Fig. 5–1). The familial form of idiopathic precocious puberty is more common in boys but has been reported in girls.[4, 5]

CPP may be associated with a variety of CNS abnormalities, including hypothalamic hamartomas that arise from the tuber cinereum.[6] Only when these embryonic tumors are pedunculated can surgical excision be considered feasible.[7] Removal of pedunculated ham-

---

TABLE 5–1 ••• ORIGINS OF PRECOCIOUS PUBERTY

I. Central GnRH-dependent precocious puberty
  A. Idiopathic, including familial
  B. CNS dysfunction
    1. Congenital defects
      a. Septo-optic dysplasia
    2. Destruction from tumors
      a. Craniopharyngiomas
      b. Dysgerminomas
      c. Ependymomas
      d. Ganglioneuromas
      e. Optic gliomas
    3. Destruction from other space-occupying lesions
      a. Arachnoid cysts
      b. Suprasellar cysts
    4. Excessive exposure to sex steroids
      a. Congenital adrenal hyperplasia
      b. McCune-Albright syndrome
    5. Excessive pressure
      a. Hydrocephalus
    6. Infection/inflammation
      a. Brain abscess
      b. Encephalitis
      c. Granulomas
      d. Meningitis
    7. Injury
      a. Head trauma
      b. Irradiation
    8. Redundant GnRH-secreting tissues
      a. Hypothalamic hamartomas
    9. Syndromes/phakomatoses
      a. Neurofibromatosis (with or without optic gliomas)
      b. Prader-Willi syndrome
      c. Tuberous sclerosis

II. Peripheral (GnRH-independent) precocious puberty
  A. Exogenous sex steroids/gonadotropins
  B. Chronic primary hypothyroidism
  C. Ovarian tumors
    1. Granulosa cell
    2. Granulosa–theca cell
    3. Mixed germ cell
    4. Cystadenoma
    5. Gonadoblastoma
    6. Lipoid
  D. Ovarian cysts
  E. Feminizing adrenal tumors
  F. McCune-Albright syndrome
III. Incomplete precocious puberty
  A. Premature breast development
    1. Premature thelarche
    2. Initial presentation: precocious puberty
    3. Nonprogressive precocious puberty
    4. Exogenous sex steroids
  B. Premature pubarche
    1. Premature adrenarche
    2. Congenital adrenal hyperplasia
    3. Adrenal tumors
    4. Ovarian tumors
      a. Arrhenoblastoma (Sertoli-Leydig)
      b. Lipoid tumors
  C. Isolated vaginal bleeding
    1. Exogenous sex steroids
    2. Foreign body
    3. Hemorrhagic cystitis
    4. Hypothyroidism
    5. McCune-Albright syndrome
    6. Ovarian cyst
    7. Sexual abuse/child abuse
    8. Trauma
    9. Tumor
      a. Rhabdomyosarcoma
      b. Clear cell
      c. Endodermal carcinoma
      d. Mesonephric carcinoma
    10. Urethral prolapse
    11. Vulvovaginitis

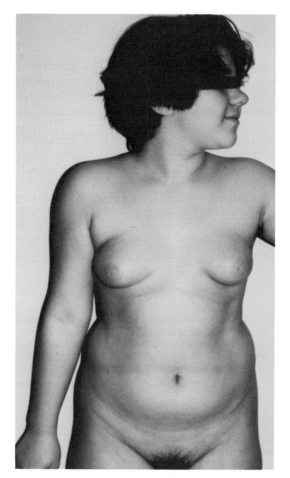

FIGURE 5–3 ••• A 9-year-old girl with central (GnRH-driven) precocious puberty. Puberty began at 6 years of age. Gonadotropin levels for this patient are shown in Figures 5–1 and 5–2.

artomas, which have been shown to contain neurons and neurofibers that immunohisto-chemically stain for GnRH, can be expected to result in regression of the precocious pubertal development.[6, 8] Tumors that are not pedunculated, however, present a much greater surgical risk without the prospect of complete cure and pubertal regression. With improved imaging techniques, it has become apparent that more cases of idiopathic precocious puberty are due to hypothalamic hamartomas than were previously demonstrable.[9] Rapidly progressing CPP occurring in a child less than 2 years of age suggests this etiology. However, regardless of the age of the patient, when there are no neurologic symptoms or signs at presentation, it is unlikely that such symptoms will subsequently develop.[10]

Other tumors associated with precocious pu-

berty include optic gliomas, which may occur in association with neurofibromatosis.[11] Previous CNS radiation therapy, or prophylaxis for intracranial tumors or other malignancies, is associated with CPP. Such children may have concomitant growth hormone deficiency.[12] Previous head trauma, CNS infections, and arachnoid cysts have also been identified with CPP. Although septo-optic dysplasia is more commonly associated with hypopituitarism, it may also occur with sexual precocity.[13] Finally, CPP that occurs secondary to prolonged excessive sex steroid exposure (indicated by extreme bone age advancement) may be a consequence of congenital adrenal hyperplasia, adrenal tumors, or ovarian tumors.[14] Treatment of CPP is discussed later in this chapter.

GnRH-Independent Precocious Puberty

GIP (precocious pseudopuberty) is pubertal development resulting from sex steroid exposure other than that mediated by pituitary gonadotropins, and therefore, it is GnRH/gonadotropin independent. This form may present with some or all of the physical changes found in CPP. Causes include inappropriate sex steroid hormone secretion and exposure to exogenous steroids (see Table 5–1). Because pituitary gonadotropins are not stimulated and in fact may be suppressed by the autonomous or exogenous steroids, circulating LH and follicle-stimulating hormone (FSH) concentrations are low, at prepubertal levels. In girls, this type of precocity may occur in either an isosexual (feminization) or a heterosexual (virilization) form. Breast development or vaginal bleeding suggests increased estrogen stimulation, whereas pubic hair, acne, genital enlargement, and adult-type body odor suggest increased androgenic hormone effect.

Origins of GnRH-Independent Precocious Puberty

Because GIP is defined as precocity occurring independent of pituitary gonadotropin secretion, LH and FSH levels are within the prepubertal or suppressed range. Causes are diverse and primarily include inappropriate sex steroid exposure from endogenous and exogenous sources and, more rarely, gonadal activation by nonpituitary gonadotropins or other peptide hormones.

Ovarian tumors are uncommon and rarely present with sexual precocity.[15] Stromal tumors and granulosa or granulosa-thecal cell tumors are associated with precocious puberty.[16] Mixed germ cell–sex cord–stromal tumors may present with isosexual precocity and are usually benign, but malignant transformation has been described.[17] Presenting features may consist of rapid progression of breast development, vaginal bleeding, or abdominal pain. On physical examination, a palpable abdominal mass and dulling of the vaginal mucosa may be detected. Estradiol levels are often excessively elevated, while gonadotropin levels are undetectable. Imaging studies using ultrasound, computed tomography (CT), or magnetic resonance imaging (MRI) are helpful in confirming the diagnosis of an ovarian lesion. The treatment of choice is surgical resection. Regression of secondary sexual characteristics often occurs following removal of the tumor.

Other rare ovarian tumors, such as cystadenomas, gonadoblastomas, and lipoid tumors of the ovary, may produce estrogen, androgen, or both. Children with Peutz-Jeghers syndrome have a particular predisposition to tumors of the gonad, requiring regular evaluation for this possibility. Other functioning ovarian tumors include epitheliomas and dysgerminomas.

Functional ovarian cysts may occur in prepubertal girls.[18] Such cysts can secrete estrogen, which may cause premature breast development or vaginal bleeding. Sexual maturation is not progressive and can be expected to wane. The vaginal bleeding is often due to estrogen withdrawal secondary to spontaneous regression of the cyst. Small cysts are not uncommon in the prepubertal ovary; usually one to two such cysts are present in each ovary, ranging in size from 5 to 7 mm.[19] When an isolated, functioning ovarian cyst is identified by ultrasound, no therapy is indicated unless rupture is considered a threat. Clinical observation and a repeat ultrasound in 2 to 3 months will likely verify regression.

The classic McCune-Albright condition is characterized by the triad of polyostotic fibrous dysplasia, café au lait spots with irregular margins, and endocrinopathies, most commonly GIP (Fig. 5–4), but this autonomous form of precocious puberty may be found with only one of the other two typical findings. This syndrome is more common in girls but does occur in boys. Other autonomous endocrinopathies, including hyperthyroidism, acromegaly, hyperparathyroidism, and Cushing's syn-

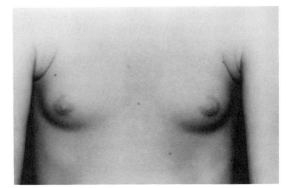

FIGURE 5–4 ••• Breast development in a 5-year-old girl with McCune-Albright syndrome, an autonomous form of peripheral precocious puberty characterized by low gonadotropin levels and episodically elevated estradiol levels.

drome, can occur. Autonomous ovarian function is often associated with ovarian cysts.[20] Normal menses, fertility, and normal adult height may subsequently occur in these patients.[21] The molecular basis of this syndrome is postulated to be a mutation in the G_s protein leading to persistent activation of adenylate cyclase and increased intracellular cyclic adenosine monophosphate (cAMP) levels.[22, 23]

Feminizing adrenal tumors are rare causes of GIP.[24] Most adrenal sex steroid–producing tumors also secrete glucocorticoids and androgens, so such patients present with virilization or evidence of Cushing's syndrome.

Exogenous medications such as oral contraceptives, topical estrogens, or postmenopausal estrogen agents or the overuse of vaginal estrogen creams in prepubertal girls can induce early pubertal development.

PPP associated with hypothyroidism may manifest with breast development, with or without galactorrhea, and vaginal bleeding. Although the mechanism by which hypothyroidism induces PPP is unclear, hyperprolactinemia, elevated thyroid-stimulating hormone (TSH) levels, and elevated α subunit levels are present. Pituitary hypertrophy may be demonstrated on CT scans, with regression occurring after thyroid replacement therapy. Pelvic ultrasound may show ovarian cysts, but the nature of the relationship is unclear.

Incomplete Precocity

Incomplete early puberty consists of partial sexual development, including isolated breast development (premature thelarche), isolated pubic hair development (premature pubarche or adrenarche), and isolated vaginal bleeding (premature menarche). It is characterized by partial, often transient and minimal, pubertal development in the absence of the other stigmata of puberty. There may be slow progression, no change, or waning (as in premature thelarche during infancy) of the physical findings.

Premature Thelarche

Premature thelarche is defined as isolated early pubertal breast development. The unilateral or bilateral breast development is nonprogressive and is not associated with areolar development. Most frequently, premature thelarche occurs before age 2 years (Fig. 5–5), a period of relative but decreasing activity of the hypothalamic-pituitary-ovarian (HPO) axis. Patient history may show persistence of breast tissue since early infancy or even birth. Other constitutional changes of puberty, such as sexual hair, acne, and accelerated growth velocity,

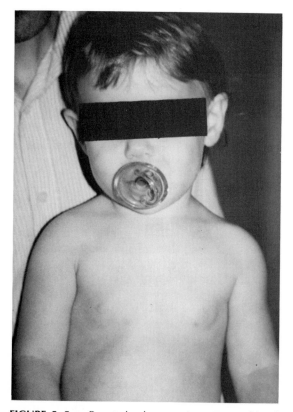

FIGURE 5–5 ••• Breast development in a 1-year-old girl with premature thelarche. Height and growth rates were normal for age.

may be absent. Skeletal maturation is not advanced for chronologic age.

Estradiol levels are low or minimally elevated. However, some evidence of estrogen stimulation may be found on vaginal smear. LH levels are prepubertal, whereas immunoactive and bioactive FSH levels may be normal or somewhat elevated for age.[25] The prepubertal response to GnRH testing (see Fig. 5–2) should distinguish this entity from CPP.[26] Ultrasound shows a prepubertal uterus and ovaries. However, differentiation may sometimes be difficult, and some individuals appear to have a slowly progressive or attenuated form of CPP, suggesting partial activation or incomplete suppression of the HPO axis.[27]

Longitudinal follow-up should distinguish premature thelarche from CPP and usually demonstrates regression of the breast tissue over 2 to 4 years.[28] Consequently, no therapy is indicated. Normal puberty subsequently occurs at an appropriate age, with attainment of normal adult height and development of normal reproductive capacity.[29]

Premature Pubarche

Premature pubarche is the early development of pubic hair. The normal minimum age is 8 years, although pubarche may occur several months earlier in black girls and usually occurs just before or synchronous with thelarche. Premature pubarche is understood to result from early maturation of the normal pubertal adrenal androgen secretory mechanism (adrenarche). With adrenarche, there is increased production and secretion of the adrenal androgens, dehydroepiandrosterone (DHEA), dehydroepiandrosterone sulfate (DHEAS), and androstenedione (AND). DHEA and AND are relatively weak androgens but may be peripherally converted to testosterone. Although pubarche may be the first manifestation of adrenarche to be noted, other signs (adult-type body odor, axillary hair, acne, and oily hair and skin) may sometimes precede pubarche.

Thus, premature pubarche is evidence of premature adrenarche without other evidence of activation of the HPO axis. Breast development is absent, although slightly accelerated growth velocity, tall stature, and advanced skeletal maturation may be present. Gonadotropin responses to GnRH are prepubertal. Whereas some individuals have elevated basal adrenal hormone levels, responses to adreno-corticotropic hormone (ACTH) stimulation tests show no evidence of defects in steroidogenesis.[30] There may be minimal to moderate progression of the pubic hair over time.[31] Normal puberty occurs subsequently at an appropriate age, and adult height is not compromised. No intervention is necessary apart from continued clinical observation.

Premature adrenarche is a diagnosis of exclusion, and disorders inducing sexual precocity and excessive androgen production should be eliminated from the differential diagnosis. Isosexual precocity will become apparent because of its progressive nature. A diagnostic difficulty may arise if excessive androgens beyond early pubertal levels are present. Although virilizing adrenal and ovarian tumors (discussed later) present with conspicuous, progressive evidence of hyperandrogenism, mild errors in steroidogenesis may present with more mild symptoms and signs of androgen excess.[32]

Congenital Adrenal Hyperplasia

Children with milder forms of congenital adrenal hyperplasia may have a clinical picture that is indistinguishable from those with simple premature adrenarche.[33] Basal levels of adrenal intermediate metabolites (DHEA or DHEAS, AND, 17-hydroxyprogesterone, and 17-hydroxypregnenolone) should be measured. If levels are elevated beyond those of early puberty, ACTH stimulation testing may be indicated to distinguish children with premature adrenarche from those with mild errors in steroidogenesis.[34] However, even though basal levels are not elevated, if androgenization is excessive (i.e., beyond that expected for early puberty) or if growth rate, height, or bone age is advanced, an ACTH stimulation test may be indicated to differentiate errors of steroidogenesis from simple premature adrenarche.[33, 34]

To perform an ACTH stimulation test, a pharmacologic dose (0.25 mg) of synthetic ACTH (cosyntropin [Cortrosyn]) is administered after a basal blood sample is obtained. An additional sample is obtained 30 or 60 minutes after cosyntropin is administered. Basal levels, incremental elevations (the difference between the stimulated and basal levels), and hormone ratios provide important information for the interpretation of ACTH stimulation tests. Specific steroids to be measured will be discussed subsequently.

Levels or responses slightly above the normal range do not in themselves constitute evidence of mild virilizing adrenal hyperplasia. This diagnosis should be restricted to those patients with clear evidence of hyperandrogenism. In addition, therapy for these disorders should generally be restricted to patients with excessive androgenization or frank virilization, with significantly advanced skeletal maturation, or with androgen levels greater than the upper limit for normal adult females.

The virilizing forms of congenital adrenal hyperplasia include decreased activity of the enzymes 21-hydroxylase, 11β-hydroxylase, and 3β-hydroxysteroid dehydrogenase. In these autosomal recessive disorders, increased ACTH secretion to maintain adequate cortisol production results in overproduction of adrenal androgens. In each of these forms, there is a spectrum of deficient enzyme activity ranging from profoundly decreased to slightly impaired. The milder forms of these steroidogenic defects can present with prepubertal or pubertal virilization (premature pubic or axillary hair, acne, adult-type body odor, excessive growth or bone age maturation, clitoromegaly, hirsutism, and oligomenorrhea).[35]

Elevated plasma levels of 17-hydroxyprogesterone, AND, and DHEA are characteristic of 21-hydroxylase deficiency. Obligate heterozygotes have increased incremental 17-hydroxyprogesterone elevations following ACTH stimulation. The diagnosis of 21-hydroxylase deficiency should not be made based on responses to ACTH stimulation unless clinical and laboratory data corroborate such a diagnosis.

Similar criteria should be applied for the diagnosis of 11β-hydroxylase deficiency; an increased incremental response of 11-deoxycortisol compared to normals alone is insufficient to make this diagnosis. The diagnosis of 3β-hydroxysteroid dehydrogenase deficiency is even more difficult; because there is considerable variation even among normal individuals, the ACTH stimulation data should include increases in both 17-hydroxypregnenolone and DHEA responses plus an increased stimulated ratio of 17-hydroxypregnenolone to 17-hydroxyprogesterone. These findings, together with clinical and laboratory evidence of hyperandrogenism, should be present to establish this diagnosis.

The diagnosis of mild congenital adrenal hyperplasia is frequently not possible at the time of initial presentation and may require observation and testing over time. Glucocorticoid therapy should not be initiated unless the manifestations are severe enough to justify the possible consequences of such therapy (i.e., adrenal suppression, the need for supplemental therapy with stress, required monitoring of the adequacy of therapy, and the risk of excessive glucocorticoid effects).

Steroid-Producing Tumors

In contrast to the mild adrenal hyperplasias, adrenocortical and androgen-secreting ovarian tumors present with noticeable and progressive evidence of androgen excess. Such androgenic tumors are more common in girls.[36] Increased muscle mass, early or excessive pubic hair, genital enlargement, and hypertension may be present. DHEAS, DHEA, and testosterone levels are elevated. Although elevated serum cortisol levels and urinary cortisol excretion may be present, the typical features of glucocorticoid excess, short stature, growth deceleration, and delayed skeletal maturation may be masked by the hyperandrogenism.[37]

Adrenal tumors are generally autonomously functioning and are not suppressed after dexamethasone administration. Useful imaging techniques are sonography, CT, and MRI. Clinical features, imaging studies, and even histologic findings may not distinguish adenoma from carcinoma because pleomorphism and capsular invasion have been noted in tumors with clinically benign behavior.[38] Pulmonary metastases may already exist at the time of presentation and should be sought in cases of malignancy. Surgical resection of the adrenal tumor is the treatment of choice in both benign and malignant disease and requires perioperative and postoperative glucocorticoid replacement. In patients with multiple metastases, treatment with the adrenolytic agent o, p'-dihydroxydinaphthyl disulfide (o, p'-DDD) or mitotane may be beneficial in lowering hormone secretion and ameliorating symptoms of the tumor.[38] Survival may be prolonged by therapy, and initiation of therapy in the immediate postoperative period is suggested. Nonetheless, patient prognosis remains poor. Other agents reported to be variably helpful in the management of this disease are spironolactone, ketoconazole, and RU-486.

Virilizing ovarian tumors, arrhenoblastomas, or lipoid cell tumors may present in preadolescence. A palpable mass may or may not be present. Both testosterone and AND levels may be elevated, but DHEA and DHEAS levels are not elevated. Serum gonadotropin concentrations are at prepubertal levels. Urinary 17-ketosteroids may or may not be elevated. Elevated urinary 17-ketosteroids do not eliminate the possibility of an ovarian source. Androgen-secreting tumors of the ovary may frequently be small and difficult to visualize by ultrasound, CT, or MRI.

Premature Menarche

Premature menarche (vaginal bleeding) normally may occur in the immediate neonatal period as a result of postnatal estrogen withdrawal. Otherwise, vaginal bleeding in the absence of other signs of puberty in prepubertal girls is uncommon. Nonendocrine causes such as vulvovaginitis, trauma, a foreign body, or child abuse may be associated with a bloody, foul vaginal discharge and must be excluded from the differential diagnosis. Bleeding from the urinary tract should also be excluded. Genital tumors such as rhabdomyosarcoma (botryoid sarcoma), endodermal carcinoma, mesonephric carcinoma, and clear-cell carcinoma may manifest with isolated vaginal bleeding.[39] In one study of 52 patients with isolated vaginal bleeding, 28 had local lesions (11 were malignant genital tract tumors), three had granulosa cell tumors, and six had isolated menses.[40]

Spontaneous regression of an ovarian cyst may induce isolated vaginal bleeding. Hypothyroidism can also cause vaginal bleeding without other evidence of pubertal development. In hypothyroid patients, skeletal maturation is generally delayed.[41, 42] McCune-Albright syndrome, a condition characterized by the development and regression of estrogen-producing ovarian cysts, may be associated with isolated vaginal bleeding.[43] Typically, although ovarian cysts may be visualized, uterine size is prepubertal. Gonadotropin levels are prepubertal, whereas estradiol levels are variable. Skeletal maturation is generally not advanced.[44]

The goal of evaluation of patients with isolated vaginal bleeding is to exclude serious causes of the bleeding. This requires a thorough physical examination, including (unless the cause is apparent) a pelvic examination, which may require anesthesia. Cultures for sexually transmitted diseases should be obtained. A pelvic ultrasound, bone age radiograph, and determination of gonadotropin and estradiol levels may be indicated to differentiate CPP from PPP. There do not appear to be long-term consequences of premature menarche for subsequent puberty and fertility.[45]

Evaluation of the Patient With Sexual Precocity

When evaluating the patient who presents with signs of precocity, the age at onset and the duration and progression of signs and symptoms are important historical information. Breast development is at least Tanner stage II with the areolae having a broadened, darkened, "stimulated" appearance. Genital changes may include fullness of the labia and pink dulling of the vaginal mucosa, reflecting estrogen-induced thickening of the vaginal mucosa. Increased vaginal leukorrhea may be found. Dark, coarse pubic hair—true sexual hair in contrast to the fine hair present during childhood—may be present. Additional androgen-dependent findings include acne and adult-type body odor. In girls, enhancement of general growth is coincident with the onset of estrogen-stimulated changes, and accelerated growth velocity, tall stature for age, and advanced skeletal maturation may be found.

The differentiation of CPP from PPP necessitates demonstration of pubertal gonadotropin secretion. The diagnostic evaluation required to document early pubertal development and differentiate central from peripheral causes is outlined in Table 5–2. Findings in the patient history consistent with a central cause include previous CNS trauma or infection, symptoms of an associated neurologic or neuroendocrine dysfunction, or a family history of early puberty. Exposure to exogenous hormones is indicative of a peripheral cause.

Physical findings suggestive of synchronous normal puberty are consistent with central precocity but do not rule out a peripheral cause. Particular attention should be paid to the neurologic examination and to any signs of neuroendocrine or endocrine dysfunction. Evidence of hypothyroidism, hyperadrenalism, or significant virilization implies a peripheral cause.

Useful laboratory studies include determinations of serum LH, FSH, estradiol, DHEA or DHEAS, TSH, thyroxine (T_4), and human chorionic gonadotropin (hCG) levels. DHEA or DHEAS levels may indicate adrenarche and, if markedly elevated, suggest an adrenal origin of PPP. Abnormal results on thyroid function tests and elevated hCG levels suggest the rare forms of nonpituitary gonadotropin-stimulated early puberty associated with chronic primary hypothyroidism and gonadotropin-secreting tumors.

Basal gonadotropin and estrogen levels may be similar in prepubertal and early pubertal

TABLE 5–2 ••• PHYSICAL FINDINGS AND LABORATORY RESULTS IN PRECOCIOUS PUBERTY

History and Physical Findings	Central Precocious Puberty	Peripheral Precocious Puberty	Premature Thelarche	Premature Adrenarche
Breast Tanner stage	II or greater	II or greater	II or greater	I
Pubic hair stage	I or greater	I or greater	I	II or greater
Stature for age	Tall	Tall	Normal or slight ↑	Normal or slight ↑
Growth rate	Accelerated	Accelerated	Normal or slight ↑	Normal or slight ↑
Adult-type body odor	Present	Generally absent	Absent	Absent
Laboratory studies				
LH and FSH*	Pubertal	Prepubertal	Prepubertal	Prepubertal
LH:FSH ratio	>1	<1	<1	<1
Estradiol*	Pubertal	Prepubertal†	Prepubertal	Prepubertal
DHEAS	Prepubertal	Prepubertal‡	Prepubertal	Pubertal
GnRH stimulation*	Pubertal	Prepubertal or suppressed	Prepubertal	Prepubertal
Skeletal age	Advanced	Advanced	Normal or slight ↑	Normal or slight ↑
Pelvic ultrasound	Pubertal ovaries	Prepubertal, adrenal tumor or ovarian tumor	Not indicated	Not indicated
MRI of CNS	Helpful§	Not indicated	Not indicated	Not indicated

*Levels vary depending on specific assay and range of prepubertal and pubertal values overlap.
†May be elevated with ovarian tumor.
‡May be elevated with adrenal tumor.
§May demonstrate specific cause.
↑, Increased; CNS, central nervous system; DHEAS, dehydroepiandrosterone sulfate; FSH, follicle-stimulating hormone; GnRH, gonadotropin-releasing hormone; LH, luteinizing hormone; MRI, magnetic resonance imaging.

subjects and may therefore fail to differentiate CPP from PPP. Because the pituitary gonadotropin response to GnRH increases with the onset of puberty, a clearly pubertal response of gonadotropins during GnRH testing best differentiates CPP from PPP. Gonadorelin hydrochloride (Factrel 100 μg) is administered by intravenous bolus, with blood samples obtained before administration and at 15- to 30-minute intervals for 1.5 to 2 hours after administration. A minimal increase in LH from low basal levels with a more pronounced FSH increase generally characterizes a prepubertal response. A robust LH increase, often overshadowing the FSH increase, is typical of a pubertal response. Accurate interpretation of GnRH stimulation test results requires the establishment of normal ranges for the populations being studied and for the particular assay method used.

Gonadotropins may be measured by radioimmunoassay (RIA), immunoradiometric assay (IRMA), enzyme-linked immunosorbent assay (ELISA), fluoroimmunometric assay (FIA), and chemiluminometricimmunoassay (CLIA). The gonadotropin standards for earlier radioimmunoassays contained free α and β subunits as well as altered gonadotropin structures and other pituitary hormones. The newer assays are more specific, often using two monoclonal antibodies directed toward different portions of the hormone molecule.[46]

Increased sleep-enhanced gonadotropin secretion (see Fig. 5–1) is one of the first manifestations of the onset of puberty.[47] However, nocturnal gonadotropin sampling to demonstrate this is cumbersome, is expensive, and risks a false-negative result if the patient is not acclimated to the testing environment.

All patients should undergo a baseline skeletal age radiograph, which reflects the degree of excessive hormone stimulation. Bone age radiographs help estimate additional growth potential and gauge pubertal progression. A CT or MRI scan of the hypothalamic-pituitary region should be considered in all cases of suspected central precocity to exclude a structural abnormality; it should also be considered in suspected PPP of uncertain origin.

Abdominopelvic ultrasonography may be obtained to document ovarian, uterine, and adrenal size and symmetry. A vaginal smear is a quick and simple bioassay used to determine the current level of estrogen stimulation, particularly when estradiol levels are prepubertal. Estrogen exposure of the prepubertal vaginal mucosa increases the number of cornified cells with small pyknotic nuclei. The results are expressed as a percentage of basal cells (deeply staining round or oval basal cells), intermediate cells (transitional cells), and superficial cells (flattened, poorly stained squamous cells). The greater the percentage of superficial cells, the greater the estrogen effect.

Treatment of Central Precocious Puberty

The treatment of choice for central sexual precocity is a gonadotropin-releasing hormone analogue (GnRHa). Analogues of GnRH are modifications of the native hormone, primarily at position six and at the carboxy-terminal end, that have greater resistance to degradation and increased affinity for the pituitary GnRH receptor.[48] Competitive inhibition by GnRHa induces downregulation of receptor function and gonadotropin secretion, resulting in temporary, reversible inhibition of the HPO axis as reflected by minimal or no response to GnRH stimulation (see Fig. 5–2) and regression of the manifestations of puberty.[49]

Treatment of individuals with CPP by GnRHa decreases gonadotropins and sex steroids to prepubertal or hypogonadal levels, which is followed by stabilization or regression of secondary sexual characteristics.[50, 51] Depending on the bone age at onset of therapy, growth velocity (Fig. 5–6) and skeletal maturation rates are slowed. If treatment is begun while bone age is still prepubertal, maturation proceeds appropriately for age, whereas adequate treatment begun during pubertal bone age decelerates maturation rate. The analogues either preserve or improve predicted height (see Fig. 5–6), unless bone age is so advanced that further growth is precluded. Recent evidence suggests that the benefit of GnRHa in reducing growth parameters is independent of changes in GH or IGF-I levels, although long-term suppression may induce a decline in GH secretion, but not IGF-I levels.[52, 53]

Treatment is continued until puberty is appropriate based on age, emotional maturity, height, and height potential. Resumption of puberty occurs after discontinuation of GnRHa therapy. Random and GnRH-stimulated gonadotropin and sex steroid levels return to or beyond pretreatment levels within a few months after stopping treatment.[54] Ovu-

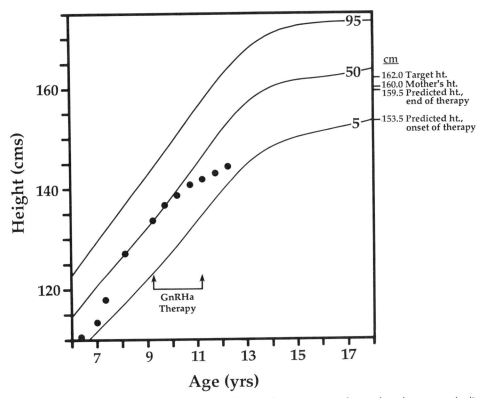

FIGURE 5–6 ••• Height according to age for a patient with central precocious puberty plotted on a standardized growth curve for females. Height was at the tenth percentile for age before the onset of puberty at age 7 years; thereafter the growth rate accelerated until GnRH analogue therapy was begun. Although growth rate and bone maturation rate slowed during therapy height remained appropriate for skeletal age, and projected height increased. Target height for females is mean parental height minus 5 cm.

latory menstrual cycles develop after discontinuation of GnRHa treatment.[54]

Children who develop sexual precocity secondary to a CNS lesion or its treatment, particularly those who receive CNS radiotherapy for malignancy, should be assessed and followed for GH deficiency. The diagnosis may not be readily apparent, because the accelerated growth velocity resulting from precocity may mask the evidence of GH deficiency. Growth velocity and IGF-I levels are greater in GH-deficient patients with sexual precocity than in those with isolated GH deficiency.[55] With initiation of GnRHa therapy, growth rates drop precipitously. Treatment with both GH and GnRHa is indicated for these patients.

If GnRHa cannot be used to treat central precocious puberty, medroxyprogesterone therapy may be used. With this treatment, progression of puberty and menses may be suppressed. Importantly, however, no effect on growth velocity, skeletal maturation, or adult height has been clearly demonstrated.[56]

Because precocious pseudopuberty is gonadotropin independent, GnRH analogues are not effective in its treatment. Choice of the appropriate therapy is based on the underlying disorder. Occasionally, GnRH analogues are useful adjunctive therapy when the underlying disorder has also caused premature maturation of the HPG axis.

Psychosocial Consequences of Precocity

Children with precocious puberty are often noticeably taller and more developed at the time of diagnosis and may therefore appear older than their peers. Parents, teachers, and others in authority may respond negatively to this age-appearance disparity and thereby increase the risk of adjustment reactions. These difficulties may be manifested as behavioral problems, especially withdrawal, depression, or aggression.[57] The effects of the stress of a chronic condition and the need for medication, frequent medical attention, and numerous physical examinations on the patient and her immediate family also contribute to the psychosocial aspects of CPP. Nevertheless, most girls with CPP do well psychologically. Concern is frequently expressed about the early initiation of heterosexual activity in such girls, but little evidence exists to support this concern. Appropriate sex education is recommended, with particular emphasis on avoiding being victimized by sexual abuse, as advanced sexual maturity combined with childlike responses to expressions of caring may make these children more at risk.

DELAYED PUBERTY

Delayed puberty is defined as the failure to exhibit the physical signs of puberty within the expected time period for puberty in normal children. Lack of evidence of the onset of puberty and failure of normal progression of puberty each constitutes pubertal delay. For boys, lack of testicular enlargement by 14 years of age is considered delayed puberty. For girls, delayed puberty means the absence of thelarche by 13 years and of menarche by 16 years. Using a 99% confidence interval (2.57 S.D.), 0.62% of normal females are, by inference, delayed in their development when compared with others in their age group. However, boys present with delayed puberty more often than girls. Lack of growth and development are the most common presentation in boys and are often recognized in relation to performance in sports and smaller stature. Girls most frequently present with questions related to sexual development (specifically, delayed menarche).

Pubertal delay may simply be a lag in the timing of normal pubertal development, a retardation of the reactivation of the HPG axis. Conversely, underlying abnormalities may include failure of hypothalamic activity, failure of pituitary transmission of the hypothalamic signal, or inability of the gonad to respond appropriately to this signal; all of these may present as delayed pubertal development.

Thus, the three major diagnostic categories of pubertal delay are (1) hypergonadotropic hypogonadism or gonadal failure; (2) hypogonadotropic hypogonadism; and (3) physiologic or constitutional delay (Table 5–3). Serious systemic illness, malnutrition, and untreated endocrine diseases may reversibly delay puberty. This discussion pertains to patients who are otherwise disease-free or whose illness is adequately treated.

Hypergonadotropic Hypogonadism

Hypergonadotropism occurs with primary gonadal failure. The most common cause of primary amenorrhea associated with primary gonadal failure is Turner syndrome. The classic findings of Turner syndrome (Fig. 5–7) are short stature and primary hypogonadism associated with a 45,X karyotype. However, clinical features and karyotype vary. Mosaic karyotypes and structural abnormalities of the X chromosome occur. Turner syndrome may manifest at birth with low birth weight and lymphedema, in childhood with short stature, or in adolescence with short stature and delayed puberty/primary amenorrhea. Additional clinical features include low posterior hairline, webbed neck, cubitus valgus, short fourth metacarpal, high arched palate, congenital heart disease, and renal abnormalities. There is an associated increased frequency of autoimmune disorders. During infancy and after age 7 to 8 years, gonadotropin levels, especially FSH, are elevated.[58] Turner syndrome and its variants are discussed in greater detail in Chapter 6.

Individuals with mixed gonadal dysgenesis may have somatic features typical of Turner syndrome, especially short stature. The most common karyotype is 45,X/46,XY. The external and internal genitalia reflect the extent of testosterone exposure in utero and thus may be female, ambiguous, or male. The gonads may vary from symmetric streak ovaries or dysgenetic testes to asymmetric gonads with a streak ovary on one side and a dysgenetic testis on the opposite side. The presence of the Y chromosome increases the chance of gonadal tumors, especially gonadoblastoma. Virilization may occur at puberty, and therefore, such gonads should be removed before puberty. Estrogen replacement will be required to induce puberty. The occurrence of spontaneous breast development suggests an estrogen-secreting gonadoblastoma. When the physical finding of ambiguous genitalia leads to the diagnosis of mixed gonadal dysgenesis, the decision regarding gender assignment or sex of rearing should be based on the potential for

TABLE 5–3 ••• ORIGINS OF DELAYED PUBERTY

I. Delayed puberty—no signs of pubertal development
  A. Hypergonadotropic hypogonadism
    1. Autoimmune oophoritis
    2. Galactosemia
    3. Gonadal agenesis (XX or XY)
    4. Gonadal dysgenesis, mixed
    5. "Resistant ovaries" syndrome
    6. Secondary to destruction of ovaries
      a. Chemotherapy
      b. Infection
      c. Irradiation
      d. Surgery
      e. Bilateral torsion
      f. Trauma
      g. Sickle cell disease
      h. Errors in steroidogenesis
        i. $P-450_{c17}$
        ii. $P-450_{scc}$
        iii. 17-Ketosteroid reductase
  B. Hypogonadotropism
    1. Permanent hypothalamic-pituitary defects
      a. Autoimmune disease
      b. Craniopharyngioma
      c. Granulomatous disease
      d. Hypothalamic tumors
      e. Idiopathic hypopituitarism
      f. Female Kallmann's syndrome
      g. Pituitary tumor
      h. Septo-optic dysplasia
      i. Syndromes
        i. Laurence-Moon-Biedl
        ii. Prader-Willi
      j. Secondary to
        i. Irradiation
        ii. Surgery

    2. Immature or reversible hypogonadotropism
      a. Anorexia nervosa
      b. Chronic illness
        i. Inflammatory bowel disease
        ii. Sickle cell disease
        iii. Cystic fibrosis
        iv. Rheumatoid arthritis
      c. Constitutional delay of puberty
      d. Endocrinopathies
        i. Cushing's syndrome
        ii. Diabetes mellitus
        iii. Growth hormone deficiency
        iv. Hyperprolactinemia
        v. Hypothyroidism
II. Breast development with primary amenorrhea
  A. Hypergonadotropic
    1. Androgen-insensitivity syndrome
  B. Normal or low gonadotropins
    1. Anatomic
      a. Imperforate hymen
      b. Mayer-Rokitansky-Küster-Hauser syndrome
    2. Pituitary
      a. Hyperprolactinemia
      b. Hypothyroidism
      c. Cushing's disease
III. Delayed puberty with virilization
  A. 5α-Reductase deficiency
  B. Congenital adrenal hyperplasia
  C. Virilizing tumors
  D. Mixed gonadal dysgenesis
  E. 17-Ketosteroid reductase

the external genitalia to fulfill a male or female sexual role in later life.

Normal or tall stature and hypergonadotropic hypogonadism are observed in pure gonadal dysgenesis. Characteristics associated with 46,XX gonadal dysgenesis are delayed puberty, bilateral streak gonads, and normal female internal genitalia. With 46,XY gonadal dysgenesis, delayed puberty may occur in its complete form, whereas ambiguous internal and external genitalia may be noted in incomplete 46,XY gonadal dysgenesis.

Prepubertal or pubertal gonadal injury may result in hypergonadotropic hypogonadism. However, the ovary is less vulnerable than the testis to most toxins. Chemotherapy for malignancies or immunologic disorders may damage gonads; nitrogen mustard compounds are particularly toxic in this regard. The degree of injury is greater when chemotherapy occurs during rather than before puberty.[59] Pelvic irradiation may also affect reproductive function, yet many girls treated for acute lymphocytic leukemia appear to retain ovarian function.[60]

Autoimmune oophoritis can occur in type I autoimmune polyglandular syndrome, which is characterized by hypoparathyroidism, Addison's disease, vitiligo, hypothyroidism, and pernicious anemia. Galactosemia is also associated with ovarian failure. *Resistant ovary syndrome* is the term applied to the state of anovulation in the presence of elevated gonadotropin levels and numerous primordial follicles on ovarian biopsy that fail to respond appropriately to endogenous or exogenous gonadotropins. The mechanism of this disorder is unclear but may involve deficient gonadotropin receptor function. However, the syndrome remains controversial, with many of the patients progressing to true premature ovarian failure, and therefore, for some patients the resistance may simply reflect a stage along the path to ovarian failure.

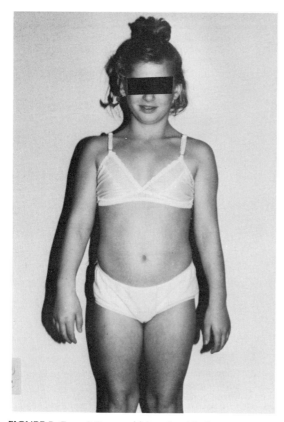

FIGURE 5–7 ••• A 9-year-old female with short stature and a karyotype of 45,X (Turner syndrome with minimal stigmata). Elevated gonadotropin levels indicated ovarian failure. This patient was treated with growth hormone to stimulate linear growth before institution of sex steroid replacement therapy.

Hypogonadotropic Hypogonadism

Congenital

Isolated gonadotropin deficiency (IGD), or idiopathic hypogonadotropic hypogonadism (IHH), is the most common form of hypogonadotropic hypogonadism. It is estimated to occur in only 1 in 50,000 women, a rate that is one fifth that seen in males.[61] Sporadic forms of this syndrome are most common, while autosomal recessive, autosomal dominant, and X-linked modes of inheritance have been described in males. The GnRH gene appears to be normal in these patients.[62]

A less common form of GnRH deficiency is Kallmann's syndrome, in which gonadotropin deficiency is associated with anosmia resulting from hypoplasia of the olfactory lobes, which may be demonstrable on CT or MRI scan.

This specific association of GnRH deficiency and anosmia is attributed to failure of migration of GnRH neurons from the forebrain during fetal differentiation.[63] The frequent association with microgenitalia is consistent with the concept that Kallmann's syndrome is the result of a developmental anomaly of pituitary differentiation. Using FIA, LH and FSH levels in patients with Kallmann's syndrome are reported to be indistinguishable from those in prepubertal children, whereas nocturnal augmentation of gonadotropin secretion has not been demonstrated in patients with Kallmann's syndrome.[46]

Not all patients with hypogonadotropic hypogonadism have Kallmann's syndrome. Low-frequency and low-amplitude pulses are found in many individuals with IHH who do not have Kallmann's syndrome, as well as in those with constitutional delayed puberty (discussed later). Indeed, in males with IHH, clear nocturnal enhancement of LH pulsatility is apparent in IHH associated with initiated but arrested puberty.[64] Hence, Kallmann's syndrome is a more profound form of IHH, usually associated with flat pulse studies and lack of gonadotropin response to GnRH stimulation testing (Fig. 5–8). Therefore, unless there is strong evidence that Kallmann's syndrome is present, pulse studies have limited usefulness in the differentiation or prognostication of pubertal delay in terms of IHH.

Acquired

Hypogonadotropic hypogonadism may also occur in association with other anterior pituitary hormone deficiencies. These congenital or acquired disorders may predominantly affect the hypothalamus, the pituitary, or both. Congenital hypopituitarism may be associated with structural abnormalities: midline facial defects, septo-optic dysplasia, and ectopic location of the posterior pituitary.[65] Most commonly, GH deficiency is the associated endocrine defect. Structural abnormalities of the hypothalamus may include craniopharyngiomas, hamartomas, gliomas, and hypothalamic cysts. Histiocytosis X, sarcoidosis, and radiation therapy are acquired causes of hypopituitarism. Granulomatous infiltrates may interfere with GnRH, LH, and FSH release. The coexistence of more than one tropic hormone deficiency, except in idiopathic hypopituitarism diagnosed in early childhood, strongly suggests an anatomic lesion. Diabetes insipidus or hyperpro-

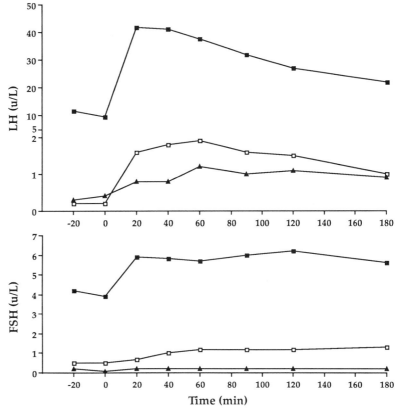

FIGURE 5–8 ••• Gonadotropin responses to GnRH stimulation testing in patients suspected to have hypogonadotropism. ■, A normal pubertal response in a 13-year-old female patient with growth hormone deficiency secondary to an eosinophilic granuloma who subsequently had normal spontaneous pubertal development. □, Lack of response in a 15-year-old female without pubertal development who had a brother with Kallmann's syndrome; this patient had the same diagnosis. ▲, Lack of response in a 14-year-old female with a history of a craniopharyngioma and panhypopituitarism. Height at various ages for these patients is plotted in Figure 5–9.

lactinemia in association with pubertal delay is particularly suggestive of a central lesion.

Prolactinomas may present with either delayed puberty or arrested pubertal development and with primary or secondary amenorrhea.[66, 67] Galactorrhea is not a constant finding. Gonadotropin levels are usually low. Clinically, some patients resemble those with anorexia nervosa because of poor appetite, weight loss, and delayed pubertal progression. Although most prolactinomas are responsive to bromocriptine therapy, transsphenoidal surgery or pituitary irradiation may occasionally be necessary.[68, 69]

Hemochromatosis leading to pituitary infiltration, whether idiopathic or secondary (such as occurs in sickle cell disease or thalassemia), may also result in gonadotropin deficiency because of the preferential affinity of iron for the gonadotrophs. Affected individuals may have delayed puberty.[70] Reversal of the pituitary gonadotropin deficiency and recovery of reproductive function may follow aggressive phlebotomy and chelation therapy in the idiopathic and familial forms of the disease.[71] Pituitary gonadotropin deficiency may occur in a similar fashion in Wilson's disease.

Functional

Anorexia nervosa is associated with delayed puberty, slowing of normal pubertal progression, and primary or secondary amenorrhea. Delayed puberty may also be observed in athletes and in individuals with chronic illnesses.[72] Failure to supply the requisite increased caloric intake for normal accelerated pubertal growth may frequently contribute to physiologic delay.[73] Frequently, in participants in certain sports (e.g., ballet, gymnastics, or track), pubertal delay may involve strenuous exercise, stress-related and intentional caloric restriction, or even an eating disorder. The chronic illnesses frequently associated with delayed puberty (i.e., inflammatory bowel disease, cystic fibrosis, chronic renal disease, and poorly controlled diabetes mellitus) are characterized by undernutrition. Serum gonadotropin levels are low, reflecting the absence or altered frequency of the normal GnRH pulsatile pattern.[74]

It is unclear whether these heterogeneous causes of functional hypogonadotropic hypogonadism share a common pathophysiologic mechanism. Altered neuroendocrine dynamics are described in functional hypothalamic amenorrhea.[75] Hypercortisolism and blunted cortisol responses to corticotropin-releasing hormone (CRH) have been detected in women with hypothalamic amenorrhea, suggesting involvement of the hypothalamic-pituitary-adrenal axis.[76] Pubertal hormonal secretion and menstrual periods usually occur after correction of the energy imbalance and weight gain.[77] Conversely, progressive exercise and caloric output have been shown to predictably and progressively attenuate HPO function.[78]

Hypothyroidism decreases growth velocity and slows skeletal maturation. Cold intolerance, constipation, and dry skin are suggestive of hypothyroidism. On physical examination, mild obesity for height; goiter; sluggishness; delayed reflexes; and cool, dry skin may be noted. Hypothyroidism delays maturation and thus, when present during childhood, may interfere in the pubertal process. Onset during or after pubertal development is associated with menstrual disorders, primary or secondary amenorrhea, and menometrorrhagia. Hypothyroidism during childhood may result in a height deficit.[79] Cushing's syndrome, although rare in childhood, may manifest with moon face, centripetal obesity, myopathy, striae, ecchymoses, hypertension, and hypercortisolemia in association with amenorrhea and low gonadotropin levels.

Several syndromes are characterized by hypogonadotropic hypogonadism. The Laurence-Moon-Biedl syndrome involves retinitis pigmentosa, polydactyly, obesity, mental retardation, and hypogonadism. Typical signs of the Bardet-Biedl subgroup of this syndrome are retinal dystrophy, dystrophic extremities (polydactyly, syndactyly, brachydactyly), obesity, and renal disease. Hypogonadism is more common in males. Although hypogonadism can occur in females, hirsutism and elevated LH levels appear to be more common.[80]

Short stature, hypotonia, and obesity are features of the Prader-Willi syndrome. Cryptorchidism, microphallus, and hypogonadotropic hypogonadism may occur. A deletion at the q11-13 region on chromosome 15 has been found in many patients.[81] Other unusual syndromes such as Alström's, Rud's, and Bloom's syndromes may also be associated with pubertal delay. Fröhlich's syndrome is simply the association of obesity and hypothalamic hypogonadism, not a separate entity in this spectrum of disorders.

Constitutional Delay of Growth and Development

The onset of puberty correlates better with skeletal maturity than chronologic age, a fact that may be particularly helpful in evaluating patients with constitutional delay of puberty. Other family members, such as the parents, may have had similarly delayed pubertal development. Children with constitutional delay are otherwise healthy but commonly have short stature. Their growth velocity during childhood is normal to low normal, with a more pronounced deceleration in growth velocity than usual just before the onset of puberty.

The diagnosis of constitutional delay is a diagnosis of exclusion. Commonly, there is already some physical evidence of the onset of puberty at presentation. To confirm the diagnosis, a short period of follow-up may be all that is required.

Therapy may be indicated when a diagnosis of constitutional delay is strongly suspected but unconfirmed, especially if delay is marked or psychosocial stress is intense. Therapy may be begun with low-dosage estrogen, with cyclical progestin added after 6 to 12 months, depending on the progress of physical development or when breakthrough bleeding occurs. Therapy for a tentative diagnosis of constitutional delay is usually reassessed after 3 to 6 months by interrupting treatment to determine if pubertal hormonal activity has commenced.

Other Causes of Delayed Puberty

Defects of Steroidogenesis

Decreased activity of steroidogenic enzymes can cause delayed puberty. Deficiency of 17α-hydroxylase/17,20-lyase (desmolase) (P-450$_{c17}$) affects both the adrenal and the gonad. This single enzyme, whose gene is located on chromosome 10, catalyzes both activities. Affected individuals are unable to synthesize sex steroid hormones, whether androgens or estrogens, and are therefore hypergonadotropic. Affected individuals with 46,XX karyotype have normal female external and internal genitalia with delayed puberty. Individuals with 46,XY karyotype have female or ambiguous external genitalia and absence of the uterus. Hypertension is often detected. Patients in both groups have elevated gonadotropin, 11-deoxycorticosterone, and corticosterone levels with low androgen, estrogen, and cortisol levels. Nucleotide duplications and point mutations of the gene in affected individuals have been reported.[82, 83] Both glucocorticoid and estrogen replacement are required.

Another cause of sexual ambiguity and delayed puberty is 17-ketosteroid reductase deficiency, a defect of testosterone biosynthesis. Impaired conversion of androstenedione to testosterone results in male pseudohermaphroditism. At birth, the external genitalia are female or ambiguous, and testes are usually palpable in the inguinal canal. The presence of müllerian inhibitory hormone (MIH) leads to regression of the müllerian structures such that there is often only a blind vaginal pouch. At puberty, androstenedione and estrone levels are elevated, and therefore both feminization and virilization may occur to varying degrees. In genetic females, hyperandrogenism may induce clitoromegaly, hirsutism, and amenorrhea.[84] Gonadotropin levels are generally, but not always, elevated. An elevated androstenedione-to-testosterone ratio is found following hCG administration.

Defects of Androgen Activity

Complete testicular feminization occurs as the result of an androgen receptor defect and is characterized by a female phenotype with primary amenorrhea, a short vagina, absent uterus, and absent sexual hair in the presence of an XY karyotype. Less commonly, an incomplete defect may occur with greater degrees of androgenization and virilization of the external genitalia. The functional testes, often detected as labial masses or inguinal hernias, induce müllerian regression in utero but fail to stimulate appropriate wolffian development. In adolescence, serum gonadotropin and testosterone levels are normal or somewhat elevated. Increased production, peripheral conversion, and unopposed action of estrogen may contribute to the feminization at puberty. There is an increased incidence of gonadal tumors in androgen insensitivity, and therefore orchidectomy is recommended, usually in the second decade of life after spontaneous pubertal development has occurred. Partial forms of androgen receptor insensitivity syndromes may manifest at birth with varying degrees of sexual ambiguity and later, at puberty, with varying degrees of virilization.

Sharing certain clinical features with the androgen insensitivity syndromes is the syndrome of 5α-reductase deficiency, the enzyme that catalyzes the conversion of testosterone to dihydrotestosterone. Defective enzyme activity in utero results in poor virilization of the genital tubercle and limited development of the penile urethra and fusion of the labioscrotal folds, a form of pseudohermaphroditism previously known as *pseudovaginal perineoscrotal hypospadias*. The presence of a normal testis secreting MIH in utero induces regression of müllerian structures. At puberty, further virilization of the external genitalia occurs as a result of increased testosterone secretion, with sufficient phallic growth for a male sexual role in some individuals. Peripheral effects of testosterone on muscle mass and linear growth are also seen at puberty in these patients. Severe hypospadias may not be an absolute barrier to fertility, but frequently the vasa deferentia may be incomplete and result in azoospermia. Normal to high serum testosterone levels are found with low dihydrotestosterone and mildly elevated or normal gonadotropin levels, whereas decreased conversion of testosterone to dihydrotestosterone occurs in cultured skin fibroblasts. Inheritance is sex-linked recessive, and the disorder is more common in certain ethnic groups.[85]

Delayed Menarche

Menarche may be delayed in the presence of normal secondary sexual development and may be related to anatomic obstruction of the outflow tract or to abnormalities of ovarian or adrenal steroidogenesis, commonly characterized by hyperandrogenism.

Anatomic Causes

Anatomic causes of primary amenorrhea should be excluded in the girl with full secondary sexual characteristics. Menarche, as mentioned earlier, occurs at a mean age of 12.5 years and at a time when breast and pubic hair development have reached Tanner stage IV. Failure of initiation of menses at a bone age of 13 or with the above degree of pubertal development should stimulate an evaluation for an anatomic cause of the delayed menarche.

Mayer-Rokitansky-Küster-Hauser syndrome is vaginal agenesis with or without uterine agenesis. It occurs in 1 in every 4000 to 10,000 female births. Remnants of müllerian structures may be palpable on rectoabdominal examination as a midline band of tissue. MRI and ultrasonography are useful diagnostic modalities.[86] Cyclic abdominal pain occurs in those patients in whom a partial endometrial cavity is present.[87] Severe unrecognized mittelschmerz may also occur and manifest as a possible "acute abdomen." Renal abnormalities, especially ectopic kidneys or unilateral renal agenesis, occur in approximately one third of such patients. Skeletal anomalies, especially spinal malformations, are also common and are often discovered serendipitously on radiologic studies. Adequate vaginal development for sexual function may occasionally be present, but more commonly, a vaginal dilator, with or without vaginoplasty, is usually necessary to achieve full sexual ability.[88] The patient's motivation is critical to the success of therapy.

An imperforate hymen is an easily determined and correctable cause of primary amenorrhea in the pubertal female with normal secondary sexual characteristics. Endocrine testing shows a normal female ovulatory profile, and ultrasound studies demonstrate normal müllerian structures.

Functional Causes

Primary or secondary amenorrhea may occur in association with hyperandrogenism, particularly with the more severe forms. Acne, hirsutism, and clitoromegaly are clinical manifestations of androgen excess. Increased androgen production may occur primarily through the adrenal gland or the ovary or secondarily through peripheral conversion of weakly androgenic precursors. Biochemical confirmation of hyperandrogenism should be obtained before an extensive diagnostic evaluation.

Hyperandrogenism of Ovarian Origin. Polycystic ovarian syndrome (PCOS) is a spectrum of disorders primarily characterized by oligomenorrhea and hyperandrogenism and ranging in severity from milder forms to the classic syndrome described by Stein and Leventhal.[88a] PCOS may also manifest as primary or secondary amenorrhea. The precise origin of this disorder is not apparent, and indeed, there may be several possible pathogenetic mechanisms, all of which induce elevated ovarian androgen levels with subsequent chronic anovulation. Increased activity of 17α-hydroxylase/17,20-lyase (P-450$_{c17}$) has been suggested as one cause of PCOS.[89] Another postulated mechanism involves altered central gonadotropin regulation with an increased LH-to-FSH ratio, leading to increased ovarian androgen production and suppression of folliculogenesis. Testing with ACTH or GnRH analogue may be necessary to distinguish chronic anovulatory syndromes from mild congenital adrenal hyperplasias, particularly where DHEAS and basal 17-hydroxyprogesterone levels are mildly elevated. Minor elevations of serum prolactin may be found in some patients with PCOS. Low-dose combination oral contraceptives offer a number of therapeutic advantages in PCOS: regulation of menstrual function, suppression of the ovarian androgen production, increased sex hormone–binding globulin production with reduction of free androgen levels, and often improvement of the other manifestations of hyperandrogenism such as acne and hirsutism.

Hyperandrogenism of Adrenal Origin. Mild congenital adrenal hyperplasias may manifest in the peripubertal period with premature adrenarche and hirsutism. Such disorders include decreased 21-hydroxylase activity (P-450$_{c21}$), decreased 11β-hydroxylase activity (P-450$_{c11}$), and decreased 3β-hydroxysteroid dehydrogenase activity. Deficiency of the 21-hydroxylase enzyme is by far the most common form of virilizing adrenal hyperplasia, occurring in 1 in every 5000 to 15,000 newborns, accounting for approximately 90% of cases.[90] The incidence of the nonclassic or late-onset form of the disorder is unknown, but the carrier state has been estimated to occur in as many as 1 in 50; both homozygotes and heterozygotes may present with peripubertal and postpubertal symptoms of hyperandrogenism.[91] Measurement of basal and stimulated adrenal steroid intermediate hormone levels after pharmacologic ACTH stimulation is necessary to confirm the diagnosis.[92] Both 11β-hydroxylase and 3β-hydroxysteroid dehydrogenase deficiency are less frequent causes of virilizing congenital adrenal hyperplasia and even less frequent but reported causes of peripubertal onset of signs of hyperandrogenism.[93, 94] Adrenal suppression using low-dose synthetic or semisynthetic glucocorticoid preparations results in lower androgen levels and regular menses.

Evaluation of the Patient with Delayed Puberty

The sequence for evaluation is determined by the patient history and physical examination (Table 5–4). Thorough questioning regarding past medical illnesses is important to assess for chronic conditions. A history of CNS, ocular, olfactory, pelvic, gonadal, and genital abnormalities should be obtained. Age of onset of pubertal development in both parents and siblings should be elicited. Linear growth for age should be carefully plotted (Fig. 5–9).

Height, weight, and the presence or absence of any evidence of pubertal development should be noted. Physical findings consistent with estrogen and androgen effects should be noted. Longitudinal growth data may be very helpful in the evaluation of pubertal delay. For example, a short girl with delayed puberty requires a determination of karyotype to exclude Turner syndrome in addition to an evaluation for endocrine disorders (e.g., growth hormone deficiency, thyroid hormone deficiency, or hypercortisolism). The presence of breast development and primary amenorrhea suggests testicular feminization as well as Mayer-Rokitansky-Küster-Hauser syndrome. In contrast, primary amenorrhea and hirsutism are more suggestive of hyperandrogenism.

Useful laboratory studies include determinations of LH, FSH, prolactin, DHEAS, and estradiol levels. Hypothyroidism should be excluded with measurements of T_4 and TSH levels. Bone age radiographs can be used to document degree of delay, monitor subsequent development, and provide an estimate of adult height. Elevated gonadotropin levels confirm a diagnosis of gonadal failure unless puberty is so delayed that the bone age is less than 10 to 11 years. A progesterone withdrawal test may be helpful in primary amenorrhea to assess estrogenization of the uterus and patency of the uterovaginal outflow tract. After ensuring that the patient is not pregnant, oral progesterone (10 mg daily) can be administered for 10 days. Withdrawal bleeding generally occurs within 72 hours of completing the progesterone treatment.

Differentiation of constitutional delay from hypogonadotropic hypogonadism is often difficult unless coincident disorders make hypothalamic-pituitary dysfunction probable. Low gonadotropin levels are present in both constitutional delay and permanent hypogonadotropic hypogonadism. Adrenal androgen serum levels indicate evidence of adrenarche and usually correlate with pubertal development. Therefore, prepubertal androgen levels are the usual finding in constitutional delay, whereas pubertal androgen levels in the absence of evidence of puberty may be more consistent with hypogonadotropic hypogonadism.

Responses to GnRH stimulation in both constitutional delay and hypogonadotropic hypogonadism are similar and not of prognostic value in cases of constitutional delay. Responses to GnRH may be useful in differentiating gonadotropin sufficiency from gonadotropin insufficiency in patients with other known pituitary disease or evidence of Kallmann's syndrome (see Fig. 5–8). No single blood test, imaging technique, or stimulation study distinguishes between these two entities. The variability of gonadotropin pulse patterns in individuals with pubertal delay and those with hypogonadotropic hypogonadism limits the utility of these studies. Even the apparent lack of pubertal sleep-enhanced increased gonadotropin secretion and poor synchronization of LH and FSH pulses in hypogonadotropic hypogonadal individuals may fail to differentiate the two conditions.[46] Longitudinal observation over time remains the best means to distinguish between these diagnoses.

Treatment of Delayed Puberty

For induction of the secondary sexual changes of puberty in girls, estrogen replacement therapy may be given as ethinyl estradiol (5 to 10 mg daily), conjugated equine estrogens (Premarin) (0.3 mg daily), or transdermal 17β-estradiol (Estraderm 0.025 mg). Because of first-pass hepatic effects, oral agents are associated with greater levels of sex hormone and other carrier proteins and renin substrate. High-density lipoprotein cholesterol levels are also greater.[95] Transdermal systems provide the added advantage of measurable blood levels of estradiol, and have been successfully utilized in hypogonadal girls.[96, 97] After 12 to 18 months of unopposed estrogen therapy or after vaginal bleeding occurs, a progestin should be added; for long-term replacement programs, the estrogen may be increased. Oral progestin, usually medroxyprogesterone acetate (Provera) 5 or 10 mg daily, can be added to the estrogen regimen in a sequential fashion. The patient may be given oral contraceptive therapy, particularly if she is sexually active,

TABLE 5–4 ••• FINDINGS IN DELAYED PUBERTY

Diagnosis	Breast	Sexual Hair	Stature	BA	LH	FSH	Estrogens	Androgens	Pelvic
Hypergonadotropic									
Turner syndrome	A	±	↓↓	↓	↑↑	↑↑	↓	N or ↓	Streak
Mixed gonadal dysgenesis	A	±	N or ↓	N or ↓	↑	↑	↓	N, ↓, or ↑	Streak
Pure gonadal dysgenesis	A	±	↑	N or ↓	↑	↑	↓	N, ↓, or ↑	Streak
Primary ovarian failure	A	±	N	N or ↓	↑	↑	↓	N or ↓	Variable
Hypogonadotropic									
Constitutional delay	A	A	N or ↓	↓	↓	↓	↓	↓	Normal
Female Kallmann's syndrome	A	A	N or ↑	↓	↓	↓	↓	↓	Normal
Miscellaneous									
Chronic disease	±	±	N or ↓	N or ↓	↓	↓	↓	↓	Normal
Anorexia nervosa	±	±	N	N or ↓	↓	↓	↓	N	Normal
Hypothyroidism	±	±	N or ↓	↓	↓	↓	↓	N	Normal
Cushing's syndrome	±	± or ↑	N or ↓	↓	↓	↓	↓	N or ↑	Normal
Virilizing errors in steroidogenesis	±	↑	N or ↑	↑	↓	↓	↓	↑	N/cyst
Androgen insensitivity	P	↓	N or ↑	N	↑	↓	↓	↑	No uterus
Mayer-Rokitansky-Küster-Hauser syndrome	P	P	N	N	N	N	N	N	Abnormal

±, Absent or present; ↓, decreased; ↑, increased; A, absent; cyst, polycystic ovaries; N, normal; P, present; streak, streak gonad.

72

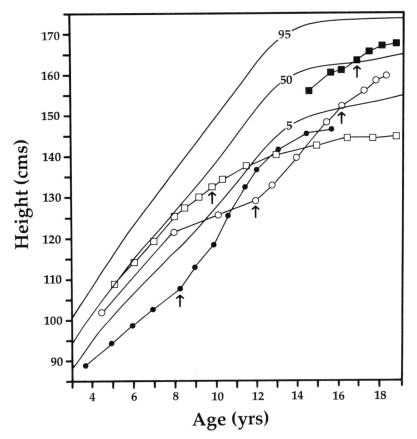

FIGURE 5–9 ••• Height according to age for four females who presented with delayed puberty. □, A patient with panhypopituitarism and severe mental deficit secondary to the presence and treatment of an astrocytoma. Diagnosis was made and the tumor treated at the point designated by the arrow. Because of mental deficit, the parents elected not to treat with growth hormone or pubertal hormones. Note the extreme short stature. ○, A girl with growth hormone and gonadotropin deficiency secondary to a craniopharyngioma in whom growth hormone therapy was begun at age 12 (*arrow*) and sex steroid therapy at age 16 (*arrow*). Note acceptable adult height. ●, A patient with growth hormone deficiency in whom growth hormone therapy was begun at age 8 years and who subsequently had spontaneous pubertal development. ■, A patient with Kallmann's syndrome first treated with sex steroids at age 17 years. Note normal stature for age.

although this approach to estrogen replacement therapy is less physiologic. Replacement treatment is also indicated to reduce the risk of osteoporosis.[98]

Height for age and growth potential, as projected by height, chronologic age, and skeletal age, should be major considerations in the timing and intensity of sex steroid therapy, particularly if treatment with other growth-promoting hormones is indicated (see Fig. 5–9). Untimely treatment or large dosages may disproportionately accelerate skeletal maturation and further shorten adult height.

Although this text focuses primarily on girls, similar considerations apply to boys. Intramuscular testosterone enanthate or testosterone cypionate can be used to induce pubertal development. Initial dosage is 50 to 100 mg administered monthly.

When constitutional delay cannot be clearly differentiated from hypogonadotropic hypogonadism, a course of hormone replacement therapy to induce secondary sexual characteristics, followed by a period of observation off therapy, may be beneficial for psychosocial reasons.

Psychosocial Aspects of Delayed Puberty

Significant delay in pubertal development may be associated with poor self-esteem and reduced academic performance and socialization with peers. Parents' and teachers' attitudes are partly determined by the physical maturity of the adolescent, and therefore, the difficulties of the adolescent may be compounded, particularly when short stature is associated, and lead to prolonged dependency on parents.[99]

References

1. Weitzman EB, Boyar RM, Kapen S, Hellman L. The relationship of sleep and sleep stages to neuroendocrine secretion and biological rhythms in man. Recent Prog Horm Res 1975; 31:399.
2. Mauras N, Rogol AD, Veldhuis JD. Specific, time-dependent actions of low-dose ethinyl estradiol administration on the episodic release of growth hormone, follicle-stimulating hormone, and luteinizing hormone in prepubertal girls with Turner's syndrome. J Clin Endocrinol Metab 1989; 69:1053.

3. Rappaport R, Prevot C, Brauner R. Somatomedin-C and growth in children with precocious puberty: A study of the effect of the level of growth hormone secretion. J Clin Endocrinol Metab 1987; 65:1112.

4. Hopwood NJ, Kelch RP, Helder LJ. Familial precocious puberty in a brother and sister. Am J Dis Child 1981; 135:78.

5. Ruvalcaba RHA. Isosexual precocious puberty. Am J Dis Child 1985; 139:1179.

6. Starceski PJ, Lee PA, Albright AL, Migeon CJ. Hypothalamic hamartomas and sexual precocity. Evaluation of treatment options. Am J Dis Child 1990; 144:225.

7. Zúñiga OF, Tanner SM, Wild WO, Mosier D Jr. Hamartoma of CNS associated with precocious puberty. Am J Dis Child 1983; 137:127.

8. Price RA, Lee PA, Albright AL, et al. Treatment of sexual precocity by removal of a luteinizing hormone-releasing hormone secreting hamartoma. JAMA 1984; 251:2247.

9. Cacciari E, Fréjaville E, Cicognani A, et al. How many cases of true precocious puberty in girls are idiopathic? J Pediatr 1983; 102:357.

10. Sigurjonsdottir TJ, Hayles AB. Precocious puberty—a report of 96 cases. Am J Dis Child 1968; 115:309.

11. Laue L, Comite F, Hench K, et al. Precocious puberty associated with neurofibromatosis and optic gliomas. Am J Dis Child 1985; 139:1097.

12. Rappaport R, Brauner R. Growth and endocrine disorders secondary to cranial irradiation. Pediatr Res 1989; 25:561.

13. Huseman CA, Kelch RP, Hopwood NJ, Zipf WB. Sexual precocity in association with septo-optic dysplasia and hypothalamic hypopituitarism. J Pediatr 1978; 92:748.

14. Penny R, Olambiwonnu NO, Frasier SD. Precocious puberty following treatment in a six-year-old male with congenital adrenal hyperplasia: Studies of serum luteinizing hormone (LH), serum follicle-stimulating hormone (FSH) and plasma testosterone. J Clin Endocrinol Metab 1973; 36:920.

15. Towne BH, Mahour GH, Woolley MM, Issacs H Jr. Ovarian cysts and tumors in infancy and childhood. J Pediatr Surg 1975; 10:311.

16. Raafat F, Rylance G. Juvenile granulosa cell tumor. Pediatr Pathol 1990; 10:617.

17. Lacson G, Gillis DA, Shawwa A. Malignant mixed germ cell–sex cord–stromal tumors of the ovary associated with isosexual precocious puberty. Cancer 1988; 61:2122.

18. Lightner ES, Kelch RP. Treatment of precocious pseudopuberty associated with ovarian cysts. Am J Dis Child 1984; 138:126.

19. Fleischer AC, Shawker TH. The role of sonography in pediatric gynecology. Clin Obstet Gynecol 1987; 30:735.

20. Foster CM, Ross JL, Shawker T, et al. Absence of pubertal gonadotropin secretion in girls with McCune-Albright syndrome. J Clin Endocrinol Metab 1984; 58:1161.

21. Lee PA, Van Dop C, Migeon CJ. McCune-Albright syndrome—long term follow up. JAMA 1986; 256:2980.

22. Weinstein LS, Shenker A, Gejman PV, et al. Activating mutations of the stimulatory G protein in the McCune-Albright syndrome. N Engl J Med 1991; 325:1688.

23. Levine MA. The McCune-Albright syndrome. The whys and wherefores of abnormal signal transduction. N Engl J Med 1991; 325:1738.

24. Comite F, Schiebinger RJ, Albertson BD, et al. Isosexual precocious pseudopuberty secondary to a feminizing adrenal tumor. J Clin Endocrinol Metab 1984; 58:435.

25. Wang C, Zhong CQ, Leung A, Low LCK. Serum bioactive follicle-stimulating hormone levels in girls with precocious sexual development. J Clin Endocrinol Metab 1990; 70:615.

26. Pescovitz OH, Hench KD, Barnes KM, et al. Premature thelarche and central precocious puberty: The relationship between clinical presentation and the gonadotropin response to luteinizing hormone-releasing hormone. J Clin Endocrinol Metab 1988; 67:474.

27. Fontoura M, Brauner R, Prevot C, Rappaport R. Precocious puberty in girls: early diagnosis of a slowly progressing variant. Arch Dis Child 1989; 64:1170.

28. Mills JL, Stolley PD, Davies J, Moshang T Jr. Premature thelarche—natural history and etiologic investigation. Am J Dis Child 1981; 135:743.

29. Van Winter JT, Noller KL, Zimmerman D, Melton LJ III. Natural history of premature thelarche in Olmsted County, Minnesota, 1940 to 1984. J Pediatr 1990; 116:278.

30. Korth-Schutz S, Levine LS, New MI. Serum androgens in normal prepubertal and pubertal children and in children with precocious adrenarche. J Clin Endocrinol Metab 1976; 42:117.

31. Kaplowitz PB, Cockrell JL, Young RB. Premature adrenarche: Clinical and diagnostic features. Clin Pediatr 1986; 25:28.

32. Siegel SF, Finegold DN, Lanes R, Lee PA. ACTH stimulation tests and plasma dehydroepiandrosterone sulfate levels in women with hirsutism. N Engl J Med 1990; 323:849.

33. Siegel SF, Finegold DN, Urban MD, et al. Premature pubarche: Etiologic heterogeneity. J Clin Endocrinol Metab 1992; 74:239.

34. Temeck JW, Pang S, Nelson C, New MI. Genetic defects of steroidogenesis in premature pubarche. J Clin Endocrinol Metab 1987; 64:609.

35. Siegel SF, Lee PA. Adrenal cortex and medulla. In: Hung W (ed). Clinical Pediatric Endocrinology. St Louis: Mosby-Year Book, 1992, p 179.

36. Daneman A, Chan HSL, Martin DJ. Adrenal carcinoma and adenoma in childhood: A review of 17 patients. Pediatr Radiol 1983; 13:11.

37. Lee PDK, Winter RJ, Green OC. Virilizing adrenocortical tumors in childhood: Eight cases and a review of the literature. Pediatrics 1985; 76:437.

38. Daneman A. Adrenal neoplasms in children. Semin Roentgenol 1988; 3:205.

39. Cowan BD, Morrison JC. Management of abnormal genital bleeding in girls and women. N Engl J Med 1991; 324:1710.

40. Hill NCW, Oppenheimer LW, Morton KE. The aetiology of vaginal bleeding in children. A 20 year review. Br J Obstet Gynecol 1989; 96:467.

41. Piziak VK, Hahn HB Jr. Isolated menarche in juvenile hypothyroidism. Clin Pediatr 1984; 23:177.

42. Schwarz HP, Duck SC, Johnson DA. Isolated precocious menstruation in primary hypothyroidism. Adolesc Pediatr Gynecol 1991; 4:33.

43. Jaffe SB, Jewelewicz R. Dysfunctional uterine bleeding in the pediatric and adolescent patient. Adolesc Pediatr Gynecol 1991; 4:62.

44. Blanco-Garcia M, Evain-Brion D, Roger M, Job JC. Isolated menses in prepubertal girls. Pediatrics 1985; 76:43.

45. Muram D, Dewhurst J, Grant DB. Premature men-

arche: A follow-up study. Arch Dis Child 1983; 58:142.

46. Wu FCW, Butler GE, Kelnar CJH, et al. Patterns of pulsatile luteinizing hormone and follicle-stimulating hormone secretion in prepubertal (midchildhood) boys and girls and patients with idiopathic hypogonadotropic hypogonadism (Kallman's syndrome): A study using an ultrasensitive time-resolved immunofluorometric assay. J Clin Endocrinol Metab 1991; 72:1229.

47. Boyar R, Finkelstein J, Roffwarg H, et al. Synchronization of augmented luteinizing hormone with sleep during puberty. N Engl J Med 1972; 287:582.

48. Conn PM, Crowley WF Jr. Gonadotropin-releasing hormone and its analogues. N Engl J Med 1991; 324:93.

49. Crowley WF Jr, Comite F, Vale W, et al. Therapeutic use of pituitary desensitization with a long-acting LHRH agonist: A potential new treatment for idiopathic precocious puberty. J Clin Endocrinol Metab 1981; 52:370.

50. Lee PA, Page JG. The Leuprolide Study Group. Effects of leuprolide in the treatment of central precocious puberty. J Pediatr 1989; 114:321.

51. Manasco PK, Pescovitz OH, Hill SC, et al. Six-year results of luteinizing hormone releasing hormone (LHRH) agonist treatment in children with LHRH-dependent precocious puberty. J Pediatr 1989; 115:105.

52. Sklar CA, Rothenburg S, Blumberg B, et al. Suppression of the pituitary-gonadal axis in children with central precocious puberty: Effects on growth, growth hormone, insulin-like growth factor-1, and prolactin secretion. J Clin Endocrinol Metab 1991; 73:734.

53. DiMartino-Nardi J, Wu R, Fishman K, Saenger P. The efficacy of long-acting analogue of luteinizing hormone-releasing hormone on growth hormone secretory dynamics in children with precocious puberty. J Clin Endocrinol Metab 1991; 73:902.

54. Manasco PK, Pescovitz OH, Feuillan PP, et al. Resumption of puberty after long term luteinizing hormone-releasing hormone agonist treatment of central precocious puberty. J Clin Endocrinol Metab 1988; 67:368.

55. Cara JF, Burstein S, Cuttler L, et al. Growth hormone deficiency impedes the rise in plasma insulin-like growth factor I levels associated with precocious puberty. J Pediatr 1989; 115:64.

56. Lee PA. Medroxyprogesterone therapy for sexual precocity in girls. Am J Dis Child 1981; 135:443.

57. Sonis WA, Comite F, Blue J, et al. Behavior problems and social competence in girls with true precocious puberty. J Pediatr 1985; 106:156.

58. Conte FA, Grumbach MM, Kaplan SL. A diphasic pattern of gonadotropin secretion in patients with the syndrome of gonadal dysgenesis. J Clin Endocrinol Metab 1975; 40:670.

59. Rivkees SA, Crawford JD. The relationship of gonadal activity and chemotherapy-induced gonadal damage. JAMA 1988; 259:2123.

60. Poplack DG. Acute lymphoblastic leukemia. In: Pizzo PA, Poplack DG (eds). Principles and Practice of Pediatric Oncology. Philadelphia: JB Lippincott, 1989, p 323.

61. Jones JR, Kemmann E. Olfacto-genital dysplasia in the female. Obstet Gynecol Ann 1976; 5:443.

62. Weiss J, Crowley WF Jr, Jameson JL. Normal structure of the gonadotropin-releasing hormone (GnRH) gene in patients with GnRH deficiency and idiopathic hypogonadotropic hypogonadism. J Clin Endocrinol Metab 1989; 69:299.

63. Schwanzel-Fukada M, Bick D, Pfaff DW. Luteinizing hormone-releasing hormone (LHRH) cells do not migrate normally in an inherited hypogonadal (Kallmann) syndrome. Mol Brain Res 1989; 6:311.

64. Spratt DI, Carr DB, Merriam GR, et al. The spectrum of abnormal patterns of gonadotropin-releasing hormone secretion in men with idiopathic hypogonadotropic hypogonadism: Clinical and laboratory correlations. J Clin Endocrinol Metab 1987; 64:283.

65. Root AW. Magnetic resonance imaging in hypopituitarism. J Clin Endocrinol Metab 1991; 72:10.

66. Sadeghi-Nejad A, Wolfsdorf JI, Biller BJ, et al. Hyperprolactinemia causing primary amenorrhea. J Pediatr 1981; 99:802.

67. Huseman CA, Rizk G, Hahn F. Long term bromocriptine treatment for prolactin-secreting macroadenoma. Am J Dis Child 1986; 140:1216.

68. Cheyne KL, Lightner ES, Comerci GD. Bromocriptine-unresponsive prolactin macroadenoma in a prepubertal female. J Adolesc Health Care 1988; 9:331.

69. Howlett TA, Wass JAH, Grossman A, et al. Prolactinomas presenting as primary amenorrhea and delayed or arrested puberty: Response to medical therapy. Clin Endocrinol 1989; 30:131.

70. De Sanctis V, Vullo C, Katz M, et al. Gonadal function in patients with β thalassaemia major. J Clin Pathol 1988; 41:133.

71. Kelly TM, Edwards CQ, Meikle AW, Kushner JP. Hypogonadism in hemochromatosis: Reversal with iron depletion. Ann Intern Med 1984; 101:629.

72. Mansfield MJ, Emans SJ. Anorexia nervosa, athletics, and amenorrhea. Pediatr Clin North Am 1989; 36:533.

73. Pugliese MT, Lifshitz F, Grad G, et al. Fear of obesity. A cause of short stature and delayed puberty. N Engl J Med 1983; 309:513.

74. Veldhuis JD, Evans WS, Demers LM, et al. Altered neuroendocrine regulation of gonadotropin secretion in women distance runners. J Clin Endocrinol Metab 1985; 61:557.

75. Berga SL, Mortola JF, Girton L, et al. Neuroendocrine aberrations in women with functional hypothalamic amenorrhea. J Clin Endocrinol Metab 1989; 68:301.

76. Biller BMK, Federoff HJ, Koenig JI, Klibanski A. Abnormal cortisol secretion and responses to corticotropin-releasing hormone in women with hypothalamic amenorrhea. J Clin Endocrinol Metab 1990; 70:311.

77. Kriepe RE, Churchill BH, Strauss J. Long-term outcome of adolescents with anorexia nervosa. Am J Dis Child 1989; 143:1322.

78. Bullen BA, Skrinar GS, Beitins IZ, et al. Induction of menstrual disorders by strenuous exercise in untrained women. N Engl J Med 1985; 312:1349.

79. Pantsiotou S, Stanhope R, Uruena M, et al. Growth prognosis and growth after menarche in primary hypothyroidism. Arch Dis Child 1991; 66:838.

80. Green JS, Parfrey PS, Harnett JD, et al. The cardinal manifestations of Bardet-Biedl syndrome, a form of Laurence-Moon-Biedl syndrome. N Engl J Med 1989; 321:1002.

81. Jones KL. Prader-Willi syndrome. In: Smith's Recognizable Patterns of Human Malformation. 4th ed. Philadelphia: WB Saunders, 1988, p 170.

82. Winter JSD, Couch RM, Muller J, et al. Combined 17-hydroxylase and 17,20-desmolase deficiencies: Evidence for synthesis of a defective cytochrome $P450_{c17}$. J Clin Endocrinol Metab 1989; 68:309.

83. Winter JSD. Clinical, biochemical, and molecular aspects of 17-hydroxylase deficiency. Endocr Res 1991; 17:53.

84. Pang S, Softness B, Sweeney WJ III, New MI. Hirsutism, polycystic ovarian disease, and ovarian 17-ketosteroid reductase deficiency. N Engl J Med 1987; 316:1295.

85. Imperato-McGinley J, Guerrero L, Gautier T, Peterson RE. Steroid 5α-reductase deficiency in man: An inherited form of male pseudohermaphroditism. Science 1974; 186:1213.

86. Hugosson C, Jorulf H, Bakri Y. MRI in distal vaginal atresia. Pediatr Radiol 1991; 21:281.

87. Griffin JE, Edwards C, Madden JD, et al. Congenital absence of the vagina—the Mayer-Rokitansky-Kuster-Hauser syndrome. Ann Intern Med 1976; 85:224.

88. Ellis CEG, Dewhurst J. A simplified approach to management of congenital absence of the vagina and uterus. Pediatr Adolesc Gynecol 1984; 2:25.

88a. Stein IF, Levanthal ML. Amenorrhea associated with bilateral polycystic ovaries. Am J Obstet Gynecol 1935; 29:181.

89. Rosenfield RL, Barnes RB, Cara JF, et al. Dysregulation of cytochrome P450c17α as the cause of polycystic ovary syndrome. Fertil Steril 1990; 53:785.

90. Pang S, Wallace MA, Hofman L, et al. Worldwide experience in newborn screening for classical congenital adrenal hyperplasia due to 21-hydroxylase deficiency. Pediatrics 1988; 81:866.

91. Miller WL, Morel Y. Molecular genetics of 21-hydroxylase deficiency. Annu Rev Genet 1989; 23:371.

92. White PC, New MI, Dupont B. Congenital adrenal hyperplasia. Part 1. N Engl J Med 1987; 316:1519.

93. Zachmann P, Tassinari D, Prader A. Clinical and biochemical variability of congenital adrenal hyperplasia due to 11β-hydroxylase deficiency. A study of 25 cases. J Clin Endocrinol Metab 1983; 56:222.

94. Pang S, Lerner AJ, Stoner E. Late-onset adrenal steroid 3β-hydroxysteroid dehydrogenase deficiency. I. A cause of hirsutism in pubertal and postpubertal women. J Clin Endocrinol Metab 1985; 60:428.

95. Powers MS, Schenkel L, Darley PE, et al. Pharmacokinetics and pharmacodynamics of transdermal dosage forms of 17β-estradiol: Comparison with conventional oral estrogens used for hormone replacement. Am J Obstet Gynecol 1985; 152:1099.

96. Chetkowski RJ, Meldrum DR, Steingold KA, et al. Biologic effects of transdermal estradiol. N Engl J Med 1986; 314:1615.

97. Illig R, DeCampo C, Lang-Muritano MR, et al. A physiological mode of puberty induction in hypogonadal girls by low dose transdermal 17β-oestradiol. Eur J Pediatr 1990; 150:86.

98. Emans SJ, Grace E, Hoffer FA, et al. Estrogen deficiency in adolescents and young adults: Impact on bone mineral content and effects of estrogen replacement therapy. Obstet Gynecol 1990; 76:585.

99. Mazur T, Clopper RR. Pubertal disorders—psychology and clinical management. Endocrinol Metab Clin North Am 1991; 20:211.

CHAPTER 6

◯◯◯ Disorders of Abnormal Sexual Differentiation

JOE LEIGH SIMPSON

Abnormalities of sexual differentiation usually become evident either at birth or at the expected time of puberty. Thus, the pediatric endocrinologist and adolescent gynecologist are integral parts of the diagnostic and management team. This chapter systematically surveys the major forms of abnormal sexual differentiation; more detailed genetic considerations are provided elsewhere.[1–4]

FETAL GONADS AND GENITAL DIFFERENTIATION

Primordial germ cells, which originate in the endoderm of the yolk sac during the eighth week of embryonic life, migrate to the genital ridge to form the indifferent gonad. The 46,XY and 46,XX gonads are indistinguishable at this stage. Indifferent gonads develop into testes if the embryo (or, more specifically, the gonadal stroma) is 46,XY. This process begins about 43 days after conception. The testes are morphologically identifiable 7 to 8 weeks after conception (9 to 10 gestational or menstrual weeks).[5]

Analysis of patients with structural abnormalities of the Y chromosome has localized the region responsible for testicular determinant(s) to the short arm of the Y.[6] However, the manner in which the Y causes testicular differentiation is still not clear. H-Y antigen[7] is no longer considered obligatory for testicular differentiation, although it may play a pivotal role in spermatogenesis.[8] For several years a 160-kb sequence coding for a DNA zinc-binding protein called *zinc finger Y* (ZFY) was considered the gene product of a unique Y testicular determinant.[9] However, more recently exceptions have invalidated this claim.[10] Whether the Y truly has a unique DNA sequence coding for a structural testis-determining factor (TDF) was even doubted. Indeed, other mechanisms of sex determination can be hypothesized (e.g., presence or absence of gonadal determinants on the X and the Y, differing in number between sexes solely as a result of X inactivation occurring in females but not males).[11, 12] The existence of autosomal loci integral for normal testicular differentiation is consistent with this idea.[1, 2] However, a very attractive gene involved in the process of sexual differentiation is the sex-determining region Y (SRY), particularly its highly conserved DNA-binding motif. Located near the pseudoautosomal boundary (Fig. 6–1), SRY has proved to be present in XX males (even those lacking ZFY) and absent in certain XY-females.[13] In addition, point mutations (e.g., frame shift mutation) have been found in patients with XY gonadal dysgenesis.[14, 15]

Sertoli cells are the first cells to become evident in testicular differentiation. These cells organize the surrounding cells into tubules. Both Leydig cells[16] and Sertoli cells[17] function in dissociation from testicular morphogenesis,

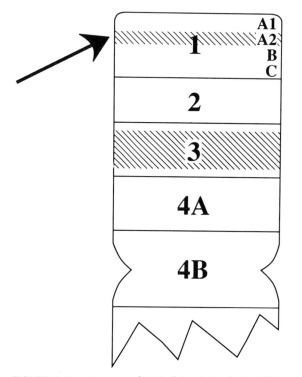

FIGURE 6–1 •• Location of testis-determining factor (TDF) and other loci on the Y chromosome. The region of Yp that contains TDF is interval 1 (Vergnaud et al.), as originally defined by DNA sequence DXYS5. Page et al. further subdivided region 1 into subintervals, one of which (1A2) is believed to contain TDF. (From Page DC, Mosher R, Simpson EM, et al. The sex-determining region of the human Y chromosome encodes a finger protein. Cell 1987:51:1091.)

which is consistent with their earlier directed gonadal development. These two cells secrete hormones that direct subsequent male differentiation (Fig. 6–2).

Fetal Leydig cells produce an androgen, probably testosterone, that stabilizes the wolffian ducts and permits differentiation of vasa deferentia, epididymides, and seminal vesicles. In the anlagen of the external genitalia, testosterone is converted to dihydrotestosterone (DHT) by the enzyme 5α-reductase. DHT, a more potent androgen, induces masculinization of the external genitalia. These actions can be mimicked by the administration of testosterone to female or castrated male embryos, as demonstrated clinically by the existence of female pseudohermaphroditism.[18] Fetal Sertoli cells produce a different hormone, a glycoprotein believed to diffuse locally to cause regression of müllerian derivatives (uterus and fallopian tubes). The gene for antimüllerian hormone (AMH) has been isolated and localized to chromosome 19.[19] Although this explanation of embryology is traditionally accepted, the situation may be more complex. The probability exists that AMH has other functions, as demonstrated by experiments in transgenic mice. When AMH is chronically expressed in XX mice, oocytes fail to persist, and tubule-like structures develop in gonads.[20]

In the absence of AMH and testosterone, internal genitalia develop along female lines (Fig. 6–3). Müllerian ducts develop into the uterus and fallopian tubes; wolffian ducts regress. External genitalia also develop along female lines. It was first shown decades ago in rabbits[21] that these changes also occur in 46,XX and castrated 46,XY human embryos.

In the absence of a Y chromosome, the indifferent gonad develops into an ovary. Transformation into fetal ovaries begins at 50 to 55 days of embryonic development. Initial ovarian differentiation may or may not require genes analogous to those on the Y chromosome. Actually, oocytes differentiate in 45,X embryos,[5, 22] only to undergo atresia at a rate more rapid than that expected in normal 46,XX embryos. Determinants for ovarian maintenance can be localized to specific regions of the X.[1, 2, 13, 23, 24] In addition, autosomal genes must also remain intact for successful oogenesis.

Independent of gonadal differentiation are ductal and external genital development, processes that depend on the presence or absence of certain hormones. Again, pivotal to the process is the development of the fetal testes, which then secrete two hormones (see Fig. 6–2). Fetal Leydig cells produce testosterone. Testosterone stabilizes the wolffian ducts, thereby permitting differentiation of vasa deferentia, epididymides, and seminal vesicles. After conversion by 5α-reductase to dihydrotestosterone, the previously indifferent external genitalia become virilized.[25] Fetal Sertoli cells produce a second compound, AMH, a glycoprotein that, as stated earlier, diffuses locally to cause regression of müllerian derivatives (uterus and fallopian tubes).[19, 26] In the absence of testosterone and AMH, external genitalia develop in female fashion. The müllerian ducts form the uterus and fallopian tubes, and wolffian ducts regress. Such changes occur in normal 46,XX embryos as well as in 46,XY embryos castrated before testicular differentiation.

Late genital and ductal differentiation is also governed by genetic processes, as evidenced by various genetic syndromes.[1, 3] However, the precise nature of the genes is uncertain. In

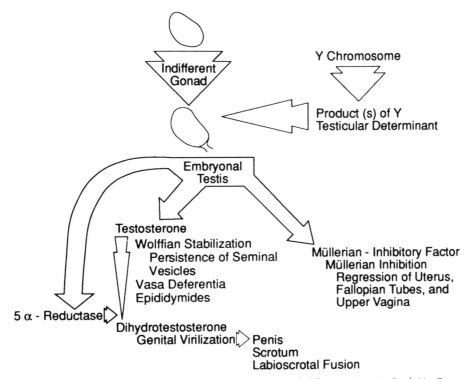

FIGURE 6–2 ••• Male embryology. (From Simpson JL. Genetics of sexual differentiation. In: Rock JA, Carpenter SE (eds). Pediatric and Adolescent Gynecology. New York: Raven Press, 1992.)

females, polygenic/multifactorial factors appear operative in müllerian aplasia and incomplete müllerian fusion, implying that normal müllerian differentiation is similarly governed.[3] Moreover, mendelian mutations are responsible for syndromes in which incomplete müllerian fusion and other uterine anomalies occur.[3] It may thus be assumed that autosomal genes must remain intact for normal genital differentiation. In males, similar conclusions are probably valid for genital and ductal development.

OVARIAN DYSGENESIS

Individuals with ovarian dysgenesis have absent or deficient numbers of oocytes, often resulting in so-called streak gonads. Many different chromosomal complements have been associated with gonadal dysgenesis, only a few of which will be discussed here. Forms associated with a normal chromosomal complement (XX and XY gonadal dysgenesis) also exist.

The term most frequently applied to gonadal dysgenesis is *Turner syndrome,* a term that unfortunately connotes different features to different investigators. In this chapter the term *gonadal dysgenesis* will be used for any individual with streak gonads; in contrast, the term *Turner stigmata* will be used for those with short stature and certain other somatic anomalies. In itself, the term *Turner stigmata* does not imply the presence of streak gonads.

Monosomy X (45,X)

Gonads

In most 45,X adults with gonadal dysgenesis, the normal gonad is replaced by a white fibrous streak, 2 to 3 cm long and about 0.5 cm wide, located in the position ordinarily occupied by the ovary (Fig. 6–4). A streak gonad is characterized histologically by interlacing waves of dense fibrous stroma that is indistinguishable from normal ovarian stroma (Fig. 6–5). Although oocytes are usually completely absent in 45,X adults, germ cells are present in 45,X embryos.[5] Thus, the pathogenesis of germ cell failure is increased atresia, not failure of germ cell formation and migration into the fetal ovary.

Although streak gonads are usually present

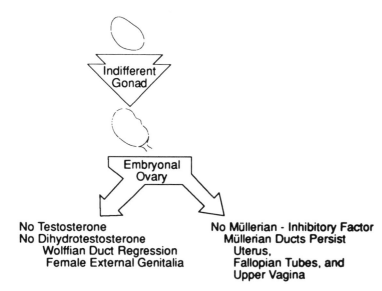

No Testosterone
No Dihydrotestosterone
Wolffian Duct Regression
Female External Genitalia

No Müllerian - Inhibitory Factor
Müllerian Ducts Persist
Uterus,
Fallopian Tubes, and
Upper Vagina

FIGURE 6–3 ••• Female embryology. (From Simpson JL. Genetics of sexual differentiation. In: Rock JA, Carpenter SE (eds). Pediatric and Adolescent Gynecology. New York: Raven Press, 1992.)

in 45,X individuals, about 3% of affected adults menstruate spontaneously at least twice, and 5% show breast development. Fertile patients have even been reported. Undetected 46,XX cells should be suspected in menstruating 45,X patients; however, it is plausible that a few 45,X individuals could be fertile, inasmuch as germ cells are present in 45,X embryos. The rare offspring of 45,X women are probably not at increased risk for chromosomal abnormalities,[27] although this has been disputed.[27, 28] However, menstruation and fertility occur so rarely that 45,X patients should be counseled to anticipate primary amenorrhea and sterility. Hormone therapy (estrogen and cyclic progestogens) can lead to normal uterine size, and 45,X women can carry pregnancies achieved through donor oocytes (in vitro fertilization or gamete intrafallopian transfer [GIFT]). Pregnancy is also feasible with donor embryos obtained by uterine lavage.

In untreated women, lack of normal ovarian development predictably leads to deficient secretion of sex steroids. Estrogen and androgen levels are decreased; follicle-stimulating hormone (FSH) and luteinizing hormone (LH) levels are increased. Estrogen-dependent processes show the predictable effects of hormonal deficiency. Breasts contain little parenchymal tissue, and the areolar tissue is only slightly

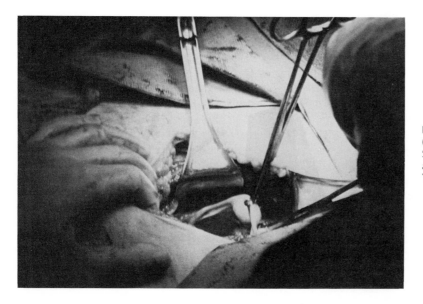

FIGURE 6–4 ••• A streak gonad. (From Simpson JL. Disorders of Sexual Differentiation: Etiology and Clinical Delineation. New York: Academic Press, 1976.)

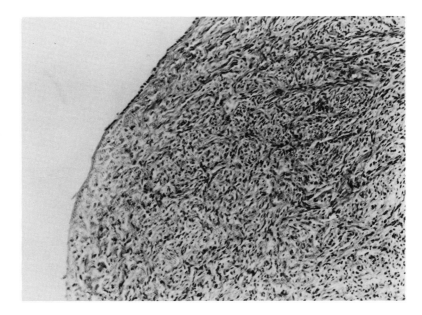

FIGURE 6–5 ••• Histologic appearance of streak gonad showing lack of oocytes. (From Simpson JL. Disorders of Sexual Differentiation: Etiology and Clinical Delineation. New York: Academic Press, 1976. Courtesy of Dr. Robert W. Wahl.)

darker than the surrounding skin (Fig. 6–6); the well-differentiated external genitalia, vagina, and müllerian derivatives remain small. At puberty, pubic and axillary hair fail to develop in normal quantity.

Somatic Anomalies and Growth Development

45,X individuals not only are short (less than 4 feet, 10 inches), but also often exhibit many features of Turner stigmata (Table 6–1). None of these features is pathognomonic, but in aggregate they form a characteristic spectrum that is more likely to occur in individuals with a 45,X complement than in individuals with most other sex chromosomal abnormalities. Renal, vertebral, cardiac, and auditory morphology and function should therefore be assessed routinely.

Individuals with a 45,X karyotype have decreased birth weight.[29] Total body length at birth is sometimes less than normal, but often is close to the 50th percentile. However, height velocity before puberty generally lies in the 10th to 15th percentile,[30] and the mean height of 45,X adults (≥16 years old) lies between 141 and 146 cm.[31–33]

Various treatments for short stature in 45,X patients (growth hormone, anabolic steroids, and low-dose estrogen) have been proposed. These are discussed in Chapter 3. Growth hormone abnormalities have long been proposed, but their existence is controversial.[34]

Treatment regimens appear to provide ostensible benefit, especially in the first few years of therapy. However, the efficacy of growth hormone or other treatment is yet to be determined. Observations that epiphyses in patients with a 45,X complement are structurally abnormal suggest that Turner syndrome can be considered a malformation syndrome. Not only are long bones abnormal, but so are the teeth[35] and skull.[36] Thus, individuals with a 45,X karyotype might be said to have a skeletal dysplasia.[37]

Intelligence

Most 45,X patients have normal intelligence, but any 45,X patient has a slightly higher probability of being retarded than a 46,XX individual.[31] Performance intelligence quotient (IQ) is lower than verbal IQ, with the latter similar to that in 46,XX matched controls.[38] 45,X individuals also have a cognitive defect characterized by poor spatial processing skills (space-form blindness). Predictable psychosocial deficits occur, primarily involving immaturity and social relationships.[39]

45,X/46,XX and 45,X/47,XXX Mosaicism

In general, individuals with 45,X/46,XX show fewer anomalies than do 45,X individu-

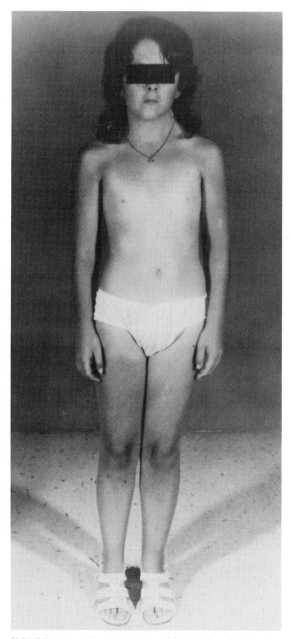

FIGURE 6–6 ••• Seventeen-year-old 45,X female showing sexual infantilism, webbing of the neck, low nuchal hair line, and pigmented nevi. (From Sutton E. Introduction to Human Genetics. 2nd ed. New York: Holt, Rinehart & Winston, 1975.)

than 152 cm.[31] Somatic anomalies are less likely to occur in 45,X/46,XX than in 45,X individuals.

Detected far less often, 45,X/47,XXX individuals are phenotypically similar to 45,X/

als. Twelve percent of 45,X/46,XX individuals menstruate, compared with only 3% of 45,X individuals.[31] Of 45,X/46,XX individuals, 18% experience breast development, compared with 5% of 45,X individuals. Mean adult height is greater in 45,X/46,XX than in 45,X individuals; more mosaic (25%) than nonmosaic (5%) patients reach adult heights greater

TABLE 6–1 ••• SOMATIC FEATURES ASSOCIATED WITH 45,X CHROMOSOMAL COMPLEMENT

Growth
  Decreased birth weight
  Decreased adult height (141–146 cm)
Intellectual function
  Verbal IQ > performance IQ
  Cognitive deficits (space-form blindness)
  Immature personality, probably secondary to short
    stature
Craniofacial
  Premature fusion (spheno-occipital and other sutures),
    producing brachycephaly
  Abnormal pinnae
  Retruded mandible
  Epicanthal folds (25%)
  High-arched palate (36%)
  Abnormal dentition
  Visual anomalies, usually strabismus (22%)
  Auditory deficits (sensorineural or secondary to middle
    ear infections)
Neck
  Pterygium coli (46%)
  Short, broad neck (74%)
  Low nuchal hair (71%)
Chest
  Rectangular contour (shield chest) (53%)
  Apparent widely spaced nipples
  Tapered lateral ends of clavicle
Cardiovascular
  Coarctation of aorta or ventricular septal defect (10%
    to 16%)
Renal (38%)
  Horseshoe kidneys
  Unilateral renal aplasia
  Duplication ureters
Gastrointestinal
  Telangiectasias
Skin and lymphatics
  Pigmented nevi (63%)
  Lymphedema (38%) resulting from hypoplasia of
    superficial vessels
Nails
  Hypoplasia and malformation (66%)
Skeletal
  Cubitus valgus (54%)
  Radial tilt of articular surface of trochlear
  Clinodactyly of fifth digit
  Short metacarpals, usually fourth metacarpal (48%)
  Decreased carpal arch (mean angle, 117 degrees)
  Deformities of medial tibial condyle
Dermatoglyphics
  Increased total digital ridge count
  Increased distance between palmar triradii a and b
  Distal axial triradius in position t'

Modified from Simpson JL. Disorders of Sexual Differentiation: Etiology and Clinical Delineation. New York: Academic Press, 1976.

46,XX individuals. Furthermore, 45,X/46,XY individuals may also show bilateral streak gonads; however, they more often show either a unilateral streak gonad and a contralateral dysgenetic testis (mixed gonadal dysgenesis) or bilateral testes. This is discussed in the section on male pseudohermaphroditism.

Deletions of the X Short Arm

The most common break point for a terminal deletion of the X short arm is band Xp11 (Fig. 6–7). In 46,X,del(X)(p11), only the proximal portion of the Xp remains; the distal (telomeric) regions are lost. The break point may also occur at Xp21 or Xp22, and interstitial deletions have been reported. Of 24 reported del(X)p(11.2→11.4) individuals, 13 individuals (54.2%) menstruated spontaneously; however, menstruation was rarely normal.[12, 24] Functional ovarian tissue thus persists more often in these del(Xp) individuals than in 45,X individuals. In fact, individuals with more distal deletions (i.e., del(X)(p21)) usually menstruate spontaneously, although approximately half are infertile (secondary amenorrhea). Thus, the terminal portion of Xp[X(pter→p21)] plays some role in ovarian

development, in contrast to previous beliefs that it was unimportant.[40]

Figure 6–8 shows heights of women with short-arm chromosome deletions. Statural determinants can be localized to Xp21→Xpter, because del(X)(p21) women are short even if they display normal ovarian function.[12, 40] Thus, regions on Xp responsible for ovarian and statural determinants must be distinct.[1, 2, 12, 23, 24, 40]

Isochromosome for the X Long Arm

Division of the centromere in the transverse rather than the longitudinal plane results in an isochromosome, a metacentric chromosome consisting of isologous arms. Both arms are structurally identical and contain the same genes. An isochromosome for the X long arm (i(Xq)) differs from a terminal deletion of Xp in that not just the terminal portion, but all of the Xp is deleted. An isochromosome for the X long arm is the most common X structural abnormality, but coexisting 45,X lines (mosaicism) are common.

Almost all reported 46,X,i(Xq) patients show streak gonads. Short stature and Turner stigmata are common as well.[31] Occasional

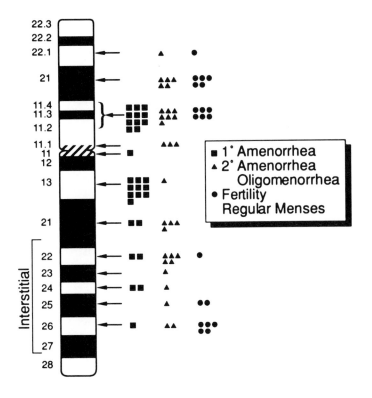

FIGURE 6–7 ••• Schematic diagram of the X chromosome, showing ovarian function as a function of terminal deletion. The bracketed area to the left connotes the interstitial deletion. (From Simpson JL. Localizing ovarian determinants through phenotypic-karyotypic deductions. Progress and pitfalls. In: Rosenfeld RG, Grumbach MM (eds). Turner Syndrome. New York: Marcel Dekker, 1988, pp 65–77.)

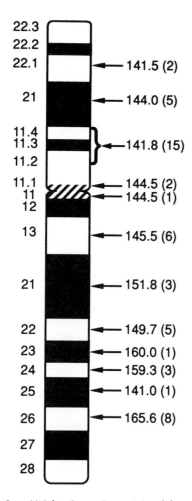

FIGURE 6–8 ••• Heights (in centimeters) in adults reported to have terminal deletions at various regions of chromosome X. Samples were restricted to adults (patients older than 15 years) in whom mosaicism was excluded. The numbers in parentheses indicate the numbers of cases. (From Simpson JL. Localizing ovarian determinants through phenotypic-karyotypic deductions: Progress and pitfalls. In: Rosenfeld RG, Grumbach MM (eds). Turner syndrome. New York: Marcel Dekker, 1988.)

46,X,i(Xq) individuals experience menstruation, but surveys support findings consistent with the rarity of menstruation.[31] The almost complete lack of gonadal development in 46,X,i(Xq) individuals contrasts with that in 46,X,del(Xp11) individuals, about half of whom menstruate or demonstrate breast development. This difference could be explained if gonadal determinants exist at several different locations on Xp. If so, a locus on Xp might be deficient in i(Xq), yet retained in del(X)(p11).

The mean height of nonmosaic 46,X,i(Xq) patients is 136 cm.[31] Somatic anomalies of

Turner stigmata occur about as frequently in 46,X,i(Xq) as in 45,X individuals, and the spectrum of anomalies associated with the two complements is similar.

Deletions of the X Long Arm

In nonmosaic deletions of the X long arm (see Fig. 6–7),[12, 23] many different break points have been reported. However, region Xq13 or Xq21 is probably the single most important region for ovarian maintenance deletions. Deletions originating at Xq13 are usually associated with primary amenorrhea, lack of breast development, and complete ovarian failure. Deletions involving region Xq25→27 are less deleterious, and affected individuals usually show only premature ovarian failure.[23, 41–43] Figure 6–8 suggests that the effect of distal Xq deletions on height may also be less deleterious than the effect of more proximal deletions.

Isochromosome of X Short Arm

In the past certain individuals were believed to have a 46,X,i(Xp) complement. Such women were said to show primary amenorrhea, and were usually normal in stature. The consensus now appears to be that i(Xp) probably does not exist or is very rare. Rather, the karyotype is now presumed to be del(X) (q22 or 24).

Other X Abnormalities

Many other X abnormalities have been reported. Centric fragments, dicentric fragments, and ring X chromosome are mitotically unstable rearrangements frequently associated with monosomic lines. The latter may be responsible for gonadal dysgenesis rather than the structurally abnormal X. However, it is not the rearrangement per se but rather the deficient loci that are responsible for associated abnormalities. Translocations between an autosome and an X chromosome may be associated with ovarian dysgenesis. Those involving the X long arm are especially likely to cause ovarian failure. X/autosome translocations may lead to familial gonadal dysgenesis.[40, 44]

Abnormalities of the Y Chromosome

The initial step in localizing the TDF occurred in the 1960s when 46,X,i(Yq) individuals were observed to be female in appearance.[45] It was because 46,X,i(Yq) individuals lacked Yp that TDF—and, later, SRY—could be localized to the Y short arm.[46.]

XX Gonadal Dysgenesis

Gonadal dysgenesis that is histologically similar to that detected in individuals with an abnormal sex chromosomal complement has been observed repeatedly in 46,XX individuals in whom mosaicism is reasonably excluded. The term *XX gonadal dysgenesis* is applied to these individuals.[47–49]

External genitalia and streak gonads of affected individuals are indistinguishable from those of individuals who have gonadal dysgenesis as a result of an abnormal chromosomal complement. Likewise, endocrine findings (elevated FSH and LH levels) and lack of secondary sexual development are similar to those in other individuals with streak gonads. Most individuals with XX gonadal dysgenesis are normal in stature (mean height, 165 cm).[48] Somatic features of Turner stigmata are usually absent.

XX gonadal dysgenesis is inherited in autosomal recessive fashion. Of gynecologic interest are families in which affected siblings demonstrated slightly different phenotypes: one with streak gonads, and another with primary amenorrhea and extreme ovarian hypoplasia (i.e., presence of a few oocytes).[48, 50, 51] This suggests that the mutant gene responsible for XX gonadal dysgenesis does not necessarily always cause complete ovarian failure. It follows that the mutation may also be responsible for sporadic cases of premature ovarian failure.

XX gonadal dysgenesis may occur as an isolated defect, or it may coexist with patterns of somatic anomalies. The combination of XX gonadal dysgenesis and neurosensory deafness (Perrault's syndrome) is accepted as a separate entity.[52–54] Other possible distinct syndromes include XX gonadal dysgenesis and myopathy[55]; XX gonadal dysgenesis and cerebellar ataxia[56]; and XX gonadal dysgenesis, microcephaly, and arachnodactyly.[57]

Gonadal dysgenesis in 46,XX individuals may also result from nongenetic causes (phenocopies). Plausible mechanisms include infections (e.g., mumps), infarctions, infiltrative processes (e.g., tuberculosis, neoplasia), and autoimmune phenomena.[58] Sometimes familial

aggregates are observed, illustrating that familial and genetic are not synonymous.[59]

XY Gonadal Dysgenesis

Gonadal dysgenesis may occur in individuals with apparently normal male (46,XY) chromosomal complements. The pathogenesis is readily explained by loss of testicular tissue before 7 to 8 weeks of embryogenesis. This would produce a female phenotype, as shown in castration experiments performed decades ago by Jost.[60] However, in some cases the gonads of these individuals are known to have been ovaries during embryologic development.[61]

Individuals with XY gonadal dysgenesis show female external genitalia, a uterus, and fallopian tubes. At puberty, secondary sexual development fails to occur. Height is normal, and somatic anomalies are usually absent. However, a relationship exists between XY gonadal dysgenesis and renal failure of uncertain pathogenesis.[27, 62, 63]

Approximately 20% to 30% of XY gonadal dysgenesis patients develop a dysgerminoma or gonadoblastoma.[64] Often the neoplasia arises in the first or second decade of life. About two thirds of XY gonadal dysgenesis individuals are H-Y antigen positive, and such individuals are far more likely to develop neoplasia than H-Y antigen–negative individuals.[7] Because of the relatively high probability of undergoing neoplastic transformation, gonads should be extirpated from all individuals with XY gonadal dysgenesis. The uterus and fallopian tubes should not be removed, even though it is technically easier to remove these organs than to extirpate only the streaks. Retention of the uterus allows pregnancy through donor oocytes or donor embryos, as mentioned for 45,X gonadal dysgenesis.

Genetic heterogeneity exists with respect to XY gonadal dysgenesis. At least one form segregates in the fashion expected of an X-linked recessive disorder.[48, 65] Neoplasia and H-Y positivity have been observed in some X-linked kindreds.[66] An autosomal recessive form of XY gonadal dysgenesis may or may not also exist,[65] and it is clear that cases that are clinically indistinguishable from the X-linked form can result from deletion of TDF from Yp.[67, 68] Specifically, deletion or point mutations within SRY may be involved.[15]

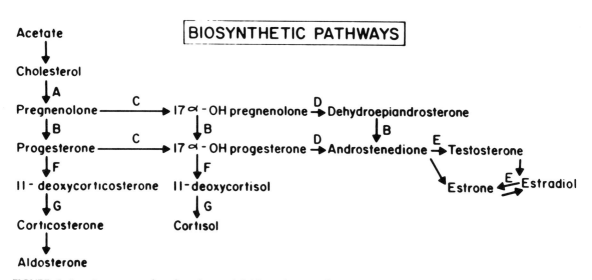

FIGURE 6–9 ••• Important adrenal and gonadal biosynthetic pathways. Letters designate enzymes required for the appropriate conversions. A, 20α-hydroxylase, and 20,22-desmolase; B, 3β-ol-dehydrogenase; C, 17α-hydroxylase; D, 17,20-desmolase; E, 17-ketosteroid reductase; F, 21-hydroxylase; G, 11β-hydroxylase. (From Simpson JL. Disorders of Sexual Differentiation: Etiology and Clinical Delineation. New York: Academic Press, 1976.)

However, relatively few cases appear to result from deletions of Yp.[69]

At least three syndromes have XY gonadal dysgenesis as one of their components: XY gonadal dysgenesis and campomelic dwarfism,[70, 71] XY gonadal dysgenesis and ectodermal anomalies,[72] and genitopalatocardiac (Gardner-Silengo-Wachtel) syndrome.[73]

Germ Cell Failure in Both Sexes

In each of five sibships reported in the literature, male and female siblings have each shown germinal cell failure. Affected females demonstrated streak gonads, whereas affected males demonstrated germ cell aplasia (Sertoli cell–only syndrome or del Castillo phenotype). In two families, the parents were consanguineous, and no somatic anomalies coexisted.[74, 75] In three other families, seemingly unique patterns of somatic anomalies suggested the existence of distinct entities. Hamet et al.[76] reported germ cell failure, hypertension, and deafness; Al-Awadi et al.[77] reported germ cell failure and alopecia; Mikati et al.[78] reported germ cell failure, microcephaly, short stature, and minor anomalies.

These families are biologically important in demonstrating that several different autosomal genes are capable of affecting germ cell development in both sexes. Presumably the genes act at a site common to early germ cell development.

FEMALE PSEUDOHERMAPHRODITISM

Female pseudohermaphrodites are 46,XX individuals whose external genitalia fail to develop as expected for normal females; the causes may be genetic or teratogenic. Usually anomalies are limited to the external genitalia, but in a few cases abnormalities of the embryonic hindgut, cloacal membrane, or urogenital membrane coexist.

Congenital Adrenal Hyperplasia

Syndromes of congenital adrenal hyperplasia, the most common cause of genital ambiguity, result from deficiencies of the various enzymes required for steroid biosynthesis (Fig. 6–9). Deficiencies of 21-hydroxylase, 11β-hydroxylase, and 3β-ol-dehydrogenase produce female pseudohermaphroditism. The common pathogenesis involves decreased production of adrenal cortisol, which regulates secretion of adrenocorticotropic hormone (ACTH) through a negative feedback inhibition mechanism. If cortisol production is decreased, ACTH secretion is not inhibited. Elevated

ACTH levels lead to increased quantities of steroid precursors, from which androgens can be synthesized. Because the fetal adrenal gland begins to function during the third month of embryogenesis, excessive production of adrenal androgens will virilize the external genitalia. Müllerian and gonadal development remain unaffected because neither is androgen dependent.

The syndromes of adrenal hyperplasia represent the most common causes of genital ambiguity. They must be excluded immediately when assessing an individual with genital ambiguity, because cortisol and corticosterone deficiencies result in sodium wasting.

Even if cortisol administration is begun immediately following birth, patients with adrenal hyperplasia usually only attain heights between the third and fifteenth percentiles.[79] If cortisol is not administered, affected individuals initially experience increased growth during early childhood, but premature epiphyseal closure leads to decreased final adult height.

Deficiency of 21-Hydroxylase

The gene for 21-hydroxylase is encoded by a gene on chromosome 6. If this gene is deficient, this P-450 enzyme fails to convert 17α-hydroxyprogesterone to 11-deoxycortisol (see Fig. 6–9). Deficiency of 21-hydroxylase is the most common cause of genital ambiguity. Cortisol and deoxycortisol levels are decreased; levels of 17α-hydroxyprogesterone (17α-OHP), androstenedione, estrone, and testosterone are increased. Increased levels of 17α-OHP, both in serum (affected neonate) and amniotic fluid (affected fetus), serve as the basis for diagnosis.

Females deficient for 21- or 11β-hydroxylase show clitoral hypertrophy, labioscrotal fusion, and displacement of the urethral orifice to a location more nearly approximating that of a normal male. The extent of virilization may vary among individuals with the same type of enzyme deficiency. Wolffian derivatives (vasa deferentia, seminal vesicles, epididymides) are rarely present, probably because fetal adrenal function begins too late in embryogenesis to stabilize the wolffian ducts. Müllerian derivatives develop normally, as would be expected in the absence of AMH. Ovaries, likewise, develop normally. Scrotal and areolar hyperpigmentation may occur, presumably because ACTH has melanocyte-stimulating properties. Moreover, there probably exists increased synthesis of proopiomelanocortin (POMC), the parent hormone of both melanocyte-stimulating hormone (MSH) and ACTH. In fact, hyperpigmentation suggests the diagnosis of 21- or 11β-hydroxylase deficiencies in males whose genitalia are normal at birth. If not ascertained at birth, the condition may pass undetected until the child is 2 years of age or older, when genital enlargement, pubic hair, and increased height are noted. If the sex of rearing is established by 18 months and genital reconstruction accomplished at 2 to 4 years of age, the child should be unequivocally female in psychosexual development.

Sodium wasting may or may not occur in 21-hydroxylase. In the form of 21-hydroxylase deficiency not associated with sodium wasting (non–sodium-wasting 21-hydroxylase deficiency), it is assumed that increased secretion of ACTH results in levels of aldosterone and cortisol sufficient to prevent sodium wasting.

As will be discussed in detail in Chapter 7, mineralocorticoid and sodium chloride must be administered to correct hyperkalemia and restore the fluid-electrolyte balance. If the condition goes untreated, hyponatremia, hyperkalemia, dehydration, and death may occur. Long-term replacement with sodium-retaining hormone (e.g., fluorinated hydrocortisone) is necessary if sodium wastage occurs. Cortisol administration must be continued into adulthood, although after infancy requirements per unit weight may diminish.

21-Hydroxylase deficiency is an autosomal recessive trait closely linked to human leukocyte antigen (HLA) on chromosome 6. This linkage facilitates heterozygote identification and antenatal diagnosis.

Deficiency of 11β-Hydroxylase

Less common than 21-hydroxylase deficiency, 11β-hydroxylase deficiency is inherited in autosomal recessive fashion. This disorder is characterized by decreased conversion of 11-deoxycortisol to cortisol. Deoxycortisol, deoxycorticosterone, and testosterone are increased, and therefore the major metabolite of 11-deoxycortisol, tetrahydrocortisol, is increased.

Because deoxycortisol and deoxycorticosterone are potent sodium-retaining hormones, increased levels may lead to hypervolemia and, hence, hypertension. Patients with 11β-hydroxylase deficiency thus manifest not only the genital virilization characteristic of 21-hydroxylase deficiency, but also hypertension. Except rarely, early sodium wasting does not usually occur. The gene for 11β-hydroxylase is located on chromosome 8.[80]

Deficiency of 3β-ol-Dehydrogenase

If 3β-ol-dehydrogenase (see Fig. 6–9) is deficient, the principal androgen synthesized is dehydroepiandrosterone (DHEA). This relatively weak androgen cannot be converted to either androstenedione or testosterone. Females with 3β-ol-dehydrogenase deficiency are thus less virilized than females with 21- or 11β-hydroxylase deficiencies. On the other hand, DHEA is such a weak androgen that males with 3β-ol-dehydrogenase deficiency fail to masculinize completely (male pseudohermaphroditism). 3β-ol-dehydrogenase deficiency is therefore the only form of adrenal hyperplasia in which both males and females show genital ambiguity. 3β-ol-dehydrogenase activity reaches its maximum capacity earlier in embryonic testes (third month) than in embryonic adrenals and ovaries (fourth month). Otherwise, one might expect the external genitalia to be identical in affected males and affected females.

Complete deficiency of 3β-ol-dehydrogenase results in severe sodium wasting secondary to deficiency of sodium-retaining hormones. Sodium wasting is often so pronounced that affected infants die precipitously. However, less severe deficiencies are compatible with long-term survival, and increasing numbers of cases are currently being detected in older infants.[81] The trait is inherited in an autosomal recessive fashion and is best diagnosed on the basis of levels of DHEA and other intermediate steroids measured in serum before and after ACTH stimulation.[81] The gene is located on chromosome 1.

Deficiency of 17α-Hydroxylase

If 17α-hydroxylase is deficient, pregnenolone cannot be converted to 17α-hydroxypregnenolone. If the defect is complete, then cortisol, androstenedione, testosterone, and estrogens cannot be synthesized; however, 11-deoxycorticosterone and corticosterone can be synthesized. As ACTH secretion compensatorily increases, 11-deoxycorticosterone and corticosterone increase. This results in hypernatremia, hypokalemia, hypervolemia, and hypertension. Aldosterone levels are decreased, presumably because hypervolemia suppresses the renin-angiotensin system. The gene controlling 17α-hydroxylase has been localized to chromosome 10, which has also been shown to be responsible for the subsequent conversion to 17,20-desmolase. The two enzyme deficiencies may occur together or separately.

Females with 17α-hydroxylase deficiency have normal external genitalia, but at puberty they fail to undergo normal secondary sexual development (primary amenorrhea). Their oocytes appear incapable of reaching a diameter >2.5 mm.[82] Affected males usually have genital ambiguity (male pseudohermaphroditism). 17α-hydroxylase deficiency is assumed to be an autosomal recessive trait.

Teratogenic Female Pseudohermaphroditism

Female pseudohermaphroditism can result from administration of androgens or certain progestins during pregnancy. Currently these forms of female pseudohermaphroditism are rare, but they are still important because they are preventable. Administration of testosterone and other androgens to pregnant women may masculinize their female offspring, producing phallic enlargement, labioscrotal fusion, displacement of the urogenital sinus invagination, and wolffian duct development. Again, excessive androgen production does not affect müllerian differentiation or ovarian differentiation.

The phenomenon of androgen-induced female pseudohermaphroditism in humans was more common several decades ago, when women were more frequently treated during pregnancy with high doses of synthetic progestins. Virilized female offspring often resulted.[18, 83] Currently administration of progestins during pregnancy is rarely indicated.[84]

Some hormones are more likely than others to produce clinical manifestations of female pseudohermaphroditism.[6, 18] Testosterone, ethinyl testosterone, norethindrone acetate, norethindrone, and danocrine are proven teratogens. Norethynodrel, medroxyprogesterone, and 17α-OH-progesterone caproate have rarely been implicated.

To interfere with genital differentiation, a teratogen must also be present during organogenesis. Before that time, no organ-specific structure can be affected. In humans the genital tubercle first becomes evident at about 5 weeks of embryogenesis (7 weeks gestation). If an androgenic teratogen is administered prior to 12 weeks of gestation, labioscrotal fusion may occur. After 12 weeks, an androgenic teratogen may cause clitoral enlargement but not labioscrotal fusion.

Frequently cited as a cause for masculinizing female fetuses, androgen-secreting tumors in pregnant women are actually a very rare cause of female pseudohermaphroditism. Fetal masculinization has been reported in pregnancies associated with Sertoli cell tumors (arrhenoblastoma), Leydig cell tumors, luteomas of pregnancy, and certain adenocarcinomas that metastasize to the ovary (e.g., Krukenberg's tumor). However, patients with preexisting androgen-secreting tumors rarely become pregnant. In 1973 Verhoeven et al[85] found only 45 reports in which virilizing tumors were associated with pregnancy. Among the offspring were 18 females whose external genitalia were described; nine had clitoral or labial hypertrophy, but only one had labioscrotal fusion.

Marked clitoral enlargement of unexplained origin sometimes results from hemangiomas, neurofibromas, or tumors. Occasionally, the enlargement appears idiopathic.

Other Forms of Female Pseudohermaphroditism

The literature contains reports of two siblings with clitoral hypertrophy, a single perineal orifice leading anteriorly to a urethra and posteriorly to a vagina, and numerous skeletal anomalies (hypoplasia of the mandible and maxilla, brachycephaly, narrow vertebral bodies, relatively long slender bones, dislocation or fusion of the radial heads leading to abnormal-appearing elbows, coxa valga, and phalangeal fusion of several toes).[86, 87] Müllerian derivatives and ovaries were normal. Both siblings developed breasts and pubic hair but failed to menstruate. Because their parents were consanguineous, autosomal recessive inheritance seems probable.

Female pseudohermaphroditism of unknown origin can also be associated with one or more of the following anomalies: absence or duplication of the uterus; renal absence, duplication, or hydronephrosis; and imperforate anus.[88] Short stature, mental retardation, deafness, ear and nasal malformation, and a blindly ending colon are less often associated; the ovaries are usually normal.

Genital abnormalities may also result from maldevelopment of the genital tubercle, cloacal membrane, urogenital membrane, or the entire hind end of the embryo (i.e., caudal regression syndrome). In some of these malformations the external genitalia may be so abnormal that the sex of rearing is in doubt. These rare disorders, discussed elsewhere in detail,[6] include exstrophy of the bladder, exstrophy of the cloaca, and sirenomelia.

MALE PSEUDOHERMAPHRODITISM

Male pseudohermaphrodites are individuals with a Y chromosome whose external genitalia fail to develop as expected for normal males. Some authors apply the term only to those whose external genitalia are ambiguous enough to confuse the sex of rearing; however, applying the term more liberally seems more useful clinically. Cytogenetic forms of male pseudohermaphroditism (45,X/46,XY and variants) are also discussed here to contrast their phenotype with those of genetic male pseudohermaphroditism.

Cytogenetic Forms

45,X/46,XY individuals have both a 45,X cell line and at least one cell line containing a Y chromosome. They may manifest a variety of phenotypes, ranging from almost normal males with cryptorchidism or penile hypospadias to females indistinguishable from those with 45,X Turner syndrome.[6, 89, 90] Different phenotypes presumably reflect different tissue distributions of the various cell lines. Not infrequently, a structurally abnormal Y chromosome is present.

45,X/46,XY individuals may be grouped clinically into one of three categories: unambiguous female external genitalia, ambiguous external genitalia (i.e., the sex of rearing is in doubt), or nearly normal male external genitalia.

Unambiguous Female External Genitalia

These 45,X/46,XY individuals may have Turner stigmata and thus be clinically indistinguishable from 45,X individuals. Such individuals usually are normal in stature and show no somatic anomalies. As in other types of gonadal dysgenesis, the external genitalia, vagina, and müllerian derivatives remain unstimulated because of the lack of sex steroids. Breasts fail to develop, and little pubic or axillary hair develops. If breast development occurs in a 45,X/46,XY individual, an estrogen-secreting tumor such as a gonadoblastoma or dysgerminoma should be suspected.[91] Occasionally virilization is claimed to result from gonadotropin stimulation of streak gonads.[92]

Although the streak gonads of 45,X/46,XY individuals are usually histologically indistinguishable from the streak gonads of individuals with 45,X gonadal dysgenesis, gonadoblastomas or dysgerminomas develop in about 15% to 20% of 45,X/46,XY individuals.[64] Neoplasia may develop in the first or second decade of life. Despite the possibility that loss of a region (locus) on Yq may confer a protective effect with respect to neoplasia,[93] we recommend gonadal extirpation for all 45,X/46,XY individuals having female external genitalia. The uterus should not be removed because of the possibility of pregnancy through donor oocytes or donor embryos.

Ambiguous External Genitalia

The term *asymmetric* or *mixed gonadal dysgenesis* is applied to individuals with one streak gonad and one dysgenetic testis. Such individuals usually have ambiguous external genitalia and a 45,X/46,XY complement. Occasionally only 45,X or only 46,XY cells are demonstrable. Many investigators believe that the phenotype is invariably associated with 45,X/46,XY mosaicism. Nonmosaic cases most likely reflect the inability to sample appropriate tissues.

An important clinical observation is that 45,X/46,XY individuals with ambiguous external genitalia usually have müllerian derivatives (e.g., a uterus). The presence of a uterus is diagnostically helpful, because that organ is absent in almost all genetic (mendelian) forms of male pseudohermaphroditism (discussed elsewhere in this section). If an individual has ambiguous external genitalia, bilateral testes, and a uterus, it is therefore reasonable to infer that such an individual has 45,X/46,XY mosaicism, regardless of whether both lines can be demonstrated cytogenetically. Occasionally the uterus is rudimentary, or a fallopian tube may fail to develop ipsilateral to a testis.

Nearly Normal Male External Genitalia

45,X/46,XY mosaicism may be detected in individuals with nearly normal male external genitalia. In fact, this phenotype may be the single most common form, based on the fact that 45,X/46,XY fetuses ascertained at amniocentesis usually (90%) have a normal male phenotype.[94] The observation that neonates with genital ambiguity seem more common reflects biases of selection. In addition, 45,X/46,XY individuals having almost normal male external genitalia do not seem to develop neoplasia as often as 45,X/46,XY individuals with female or frankly ambiguous genitalia.[64] Gonadal extirpation is thus probably not necessary if a male sex of rearing is chosen, provided gonads can be assessed periodically within the scrotum (i.e., through ultrasound and palpation).[64]

Disorders With Multiple Malformation Patterns

Genital ambiguity may occur in individuals with multiple malformation patterns. The coexistence of genital ambiguity with the Meckel-Gruber syndrome, the Smith-Lemli-Opitz type I syndrome, the brachio-skeletal-genital syndrome,[95] and the esophageal-facial-genital syndrome[96] has long been recognized. These disorders are inherited in an autosomal recessive or X-linked recessive fashion. Descriptions are provided in standard textbooks of dysmorphia.[97, 98]

Several recently recognized disorders are of special interest to the pediatric gynecologist. *Drash's syndrome* is the term currently applied to individuals with Wilms' tumor, aniridia, and male pseudohermaphroditism.[99, 100] Because Wilms' tumor is associated with deletion of chromosome 11p13, its association with Drash's syndrome has been interpreted as localization of an autosomal region integral for male development. Smith-Lemli-Opitz syndrome type II is an autosomal recessive condition in which 46,XY individuals show not only genital abnormalities, but also female external genitalia (sex reversal).[101] In the genitopalatocardiac (Gardner-Silengo-Wachtel) syndrome, 46,XY individuals show phenotypic variability, not only in external genitalia, but also in the gonads[73]; complete sex reversal can even occur in 46,XY individuals who have ovaries. Implications of these syndromes for sex-determining mechanisms are discussed by Simpson.[102]

Deficiencies in Testosterone Biosynthesis

Male pseudohermaphroditism may result from deficiencies of 17α-hydroxylase, 3β-ol-dehydrogenase, 17-ketosteroid reductase, 17,20-desmolase or one of the enzymes required to convert cholesterol to pregnenolone (congenital adrenal lipoid hyperplasia) (see Fig. 6–9). Deficiencies of 21- or 11β-hydroxylase, the most common causes of female pseudohermaphroditism, do not cause male pseudohermaphroditism.

An enzyme deficiency should be suspected if levels of testosterone or its metabolites are decreased. Although diagnosis of the conditions discussed below is not difficult in older children, detection may be difficult during infancy, because neonatal testosterone levels are normally low. Provocative tests (i.e., human chorionic gonadotropin [hCG]) are usually recommended to facilitate diagnosis.

Congenital Adrenal Lipoid Hyperplasia

In congenital adrenal lipoid hyperplasia, male pseudohermaphrodites show ambiguous or female-like external genitalia, severe sodium wasting, and adrenals characterized by foamy-appearing cells filled with cholesterol. Approximately 30 cases have been described.[103, 104] Accumulation of cholesterol has long indicated that this compound cannot be converted to pregnenolone (see Fig. 6–9). The cytochrome P-450 enzyme responsible for this defect is side chain cleavage (scc). This enzyme is required to convert cholesterol to pregnenolone via 20α-hydroxylase, 20,22-desmolase, and 22α-hydroxylase. Inheritance is presumed to be autosomal recessive on the basis of increased parental consanguinity. The gene is located on chromosome 15.

3β-ol-Dehydrogenase Deficiency

Deficiency of 3β-ol-dehydrogenase, also an autosomal recessive disorder, results in decreased synthesis of both androgens and estrogens (see Fig. 6–9). Perrone et al.[105] collected 27 cases in males. The major androgen produced is DHEA, which is a weaker androgen than testosterone and cannot adequately virilize the male fetus. Diagnosis is usually established on the basis of serum DNA before and after ACTH stimulation. In addition to genital abnormalities, 3β-ol-dehydrogenase deficiency is often associated with severe sodium wasting, because aldosterone and cortisol are decreased.

The incompletely developed external genitalia of males with 3β-ol-dehydrogenase deficiency are clinically similar to the external genitalia of most other male pseudohermaphrodites (i.e., small phallus, urethral opening proximal on the penis, and incomplete labioscrotal fusion). Testes and wolffian ducts differentiate normally. Given the fact that affected females (46,XX) also show genital ambiguity, 3β-ol-dehydrogenase is the only enzyme that, when deficient, produces male pseudohermaphroditism in males and female pseudohermaphroditism in females.

17α-Hydroxylase Deficiency

Males deficient in 17α-hydroxylase usually show ambiguous external genitalia; however, wolffian duct development and testicular development are normal. Severely affected males may even show female external genitalia.[106] Although affected females (46,XX) show hypertension, males deficient in 17α-hydroxylase usually display normal blood pressure. Inheritance is autosomal recessive.

17,20-Desmolase Deficiency

Zachmann et al.[107] reported a family in which two maternal cousins had genital ambiguity, bilateral testes, and no müllerian derivatives. A maternal "aunt" was said to have abnormal external genitalia and bilateral testes. The deficient enzyme was deduced to be 17,20-desmolase on the basis of both cousins showing low plasma testosterone and DHEA levels, despite normal urinary excretion of pregnanediol, pregnanetriol, and 17-hydroxycorticoids. In testicular tissue, testosterone could be synthesized from androstenedione or DHEA, excluding 17-ketosteroid reductase deficiency (see below) but suggesting 17,20-desmolase deficiency. That a single enzyme appears to be able to serve both 17α-hydroxylase and 17,20-desmolase function further produces genetic and nosologic confusion.[108]

Deficiency of 17-Ketosteroid Reductase

The inability of the testes to convert androstenedione to testosterone is the result of deficiency of 17-ketosteroid reductase (see Fig. 6–9). Approximately 25 cases have been reported.[109] Plasma testosterone levels are usually decreased, and androstenedione and DHEA levels are increased. Affected males show ambiguous external genitalia, bilateral testes, and no müllerian derivatives. Breast development may or may not be present and apparently is dependent on the estrogen-to-testosterone ratio.[110] Pubertal virilization is greater than in some other enzyme deficiencies, with gynecomastia sometimes not even evident.[111] In one remarkable case, the sex of rearing of an affected individual was changed from female to male after puberty.[110] This disorder can be either autosomal recessive or X-linked recessive.

Complete Androgen Insensitivity (Complete Testicular Feminization)

In complete androgen insensitivity (complete testicular feminization), 46,XY individuals show bilateral testes, female external genitalia, a blindly ending vagina, and no müllerian derivatives (Fig. 6–10). These findings are entirely predictable, given the underlying pathogenesis of the inability to respond to testosterone. However, AMH is synthesized as in the normal testis; the body responds normally to AMH, and for this reason no uterus is present. Affected individuals experience breast development and pubertal feminization.

Despite pubertal feminization, some individuals with androgen insensitivity show clitoral enlargement and labioscrotal fusion; the term *incomplete (partial) androgen insensitivity (incomplete testicular feminization)* is applied to these patients. Both complete and incomplete (partial) androgen insensitivity are inherited in an X-linked recessive fashion. Not only are the two disorders genetically distinct, but heterogeneity exists for each. Both complete androgen insensitivity and its incomplete counterpart result from mutations in the androgen receptor gene localized to region Xq.

As adults, individuals with the complete form of androgen insensitivity may be quite

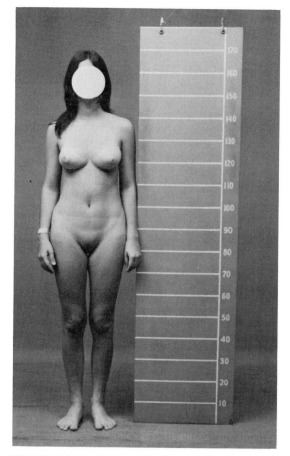

FIGURE 6–10 ••• Photograph of patient with complete testicular feminization. (From Simpson JL. Disorders of Sexual Differentiation: Etiology and Clinical Delineation. New York: Academic Press, 1976. Courtesy of Dr. Charles Hammond.)

attractive and show excellent breast development. However, most are similar in appearance to unaffected females in the general population. Breasts contain normal ductal and glandular tissue, but the areolae are often pale and underdeveloped. Pubic hair and axillary hair (terminal) are usually sparse (vellus hair is present), but scalp hair is normal. The vagina terminates blindly. Sometimes vaginal length is shorter than usual, presumably because müllerian ducts fail to contribute to formation of the vagina. Occasionally, the vagina is only 1 to 2 cm long or is represented merely by a dimple. Surgery or dilatation may then be necessary to create a neovagina, but this is relatively uncommon.

Neither a uterus nor fallopian tubes are ordinarily present. Occasionally there may be fibromuscular remnants, rudimentary fallopian

Exons, Binding Domains of the hAR

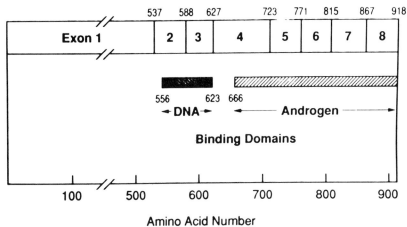

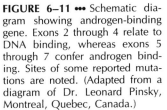

FIGURE 6–11 ••• Schematic diagram showing androgen-binding gene. Exons 2 through 4 relate to DNA binding, whereas exons 5 through 7 confer androgen binding. Sites of some reported mutations are noted. (Adapted from a diagram of Dr. Leonard Pinsky, Montreal, Quebec, Canada.)

tubes, or, rarely, even a uterus.[112] In fact, müllerian aplasia is approximately twice as common as complete androgen insensitivity.[6]

The testes are usually normal in size. They may be located in the abdomen, inguinal canal, labia, or anywhere along the path of embryonic testicular descent. If located in the inguinal canal, the testes may produce inguinal hernias. One half of all individuals with testicular feminization develop inguinal hernias. It is therefore worthwhile to determine the cytogenetic status of prepubertal girls with inguinal hernias, although most will prove to be 46,XX. Height is slightly increased when compared with normal women, but unremarkable when compared with 46,XY males.

The frequency of gonadal neoplasia is increased, but the exact magnitude is uncertain. The actual risk, once considered relatively high,[113] is probably no greater than 5%.[64, 83] The risk of malignancy is clearly low before 25 to 30 years of age and increases thereafter. Benign tubular adenomas (Pick's adenomas) are especially common in postpubertal patients, probably as a result of increased secretion of LH. Although orchiectomy is eventually necessary, it is acceptable to leave the testes in place until after spontaneous pubertal feminization. However, if a herniorrhaphy proves necessary before puberty, most surgeons perform the orchiectomy at the same time. There may also be some psychological benefit in prepubertal orchiectomies.

Genetic heterogeneity clearly exists. In 60% to 70% of cases, androgen receptors are not present (i.e., the patient is receptor negative).

In 30% to 40%, receptors are present (i.e., receptor positive), and in these, a defect at a more distal step in androgen action must be postulated. Receptor-positive and receptor-negative cases are clinically indistinguishable. Enormous progress has been made by applying molecular genetic technology to receptor-negative androgen insensitivity. A number of different mutations have been uncovered. Most lie in the androgen-binding domain (exons 5, 6, and 7) (Fig. 6–11).[114]

Incomplete or Partial Androgen Sensitivity (Incomplete Testicular Feminization and Reifenstein's Syndrome)

At puberty in certain 46,XY individuals, feminization (i.e., breast development) occurs despite the fact that the external genitalia are characterized by phallic enlargement and partial labioscrotal fusion (Fig. 6–12). Such individuals are said to have incomplete or partial androgen insensitivity (incomplete testicular feminization). Incomplete and complete androgen insensitivity share many features: bilateral testes with Leydig cell hyperplasia, no müllerian derivatives, pubertal breast development, lack of pubertal virilization, normal (male) plasma testosterone, and failure to respond to androgen.[115] The pathogenesis of partial androgen insensitivity may involve decreased numbers or qualitative defects of androgen receptors.[116–118] As noted earlier, mo-

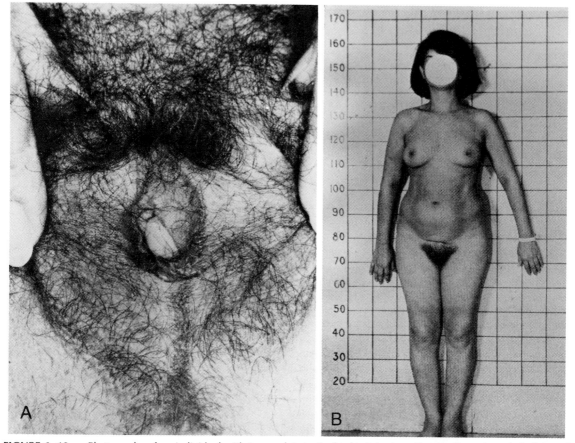

FIGURE 6–12 ••• Photographs of an individual with incomplete testicular feminization. Despite the enlarged phallus and labioscrotal fusion (*A*), breast development occurred at puberty (*B*). (From Park IJ, Jones HW. Familial male hermaphroditism with ambiguous external genitalia. Am J Obstet Gynecol 1970; 108:1197.)

lecular analysis has revealed several different mutations in the androgen-binding domains (exons 5, 6, and 7). At present, no correlation has been proved between the exon involved and phenotype.

Finally, it is worth recounting for nosologic reasons that incomplete (partial) androgen insensitivity is an X-linked recessive condition that encompasses several entities historically considered separate (i.e., Lubs' syndrome, Gilbert-Dreyfus syndrome, and Reifenstein's syndrome). In 1974 Wilson et al.[119] demonstrated occurrence in a single kindred of both the Reifenstein phenotype and the incomplete androgen insensitivity phenotype as traditionally defined. In 1984 the same group confirmed partial androgen receptor deficiency in two individuals with the Lubs' syndrome phenotype.[120] Thus the traditional separation between Reifenstein's syndrome, Lubs' syndrome, and incomplete androgen insensitivity

as defined earlier was not valid. These three disorders merely represent different spectrums of a single X-linked recessive disorder, here called *incomplete (partial) androgen insensitivity*. Individuals characterized by female genitalia and failure of posterior labioscrotal fusion may also fit into this spectrum, although those who apply a separate appellation would disagree. Genetic heterogeneity may still exist, but its basis should not be considered to consist merely of differences in clinical appearance.

The obvious clinical significance of incomplete (partial) androgen insensitivity is that this disorder must be excluded before a male sex of rearing can be assigned. The presence of androgen receptors and demonstration of a response to exogenous androgen excludes the condition; the converse, especially demonstration of a molecular defect in the androgen receptor gene, verifies the diagnosis.

5α-Reductase Deficiency (Pseudovaginal Perineoscrotal Hypospadias)

For decades it has been recognized that some genetic males show ambiguous external genitalia at birth, but at puberty undergo virilization like normal males. They experience phallic enlargement, increased facial hair, muscular hypertrophy, and voice deepening, but no breast development. Their external genitalia consist of a phallus that resembles a clitoris more than a penis, a perineal urethral orifice, and usually a separate, blindly ending, perineal orifice that resembles a vagina (pseudovagina). The testes are relatively normal in size and secrete testosterone in normal amounts.

In 1971, this trait, then called *pseudovaginal perineoscrotal hypospadias* (PPSH), was shown to be inherited in an autosomal recessive fashion.[121, 122] The disorder was later shown to result from deficiency of the enzyme 5α-reductase.[123–125] This enzyme converts testosterone to dihydrotestosterone (DHT). The fact that intracellular 5α-reductase deficiency results in the PPSH phenotype is consistent with observations that virilization of the external genitalia during embryogenesis requires dihydrotestosterone; wolffian differentiation requires only testosterone. Pubertal virilization also can be accomplished by testosterone alone.

5α-Reductase deficiency is an autosomal recessive disorder.[123] Diagnosis is most easily made on the basis of an elevated testosterone-to-DHT ratio following administration of hCG or testosterone propionate.[126] The ratio of the respective urinary metabolites of testosterone and DHT (i.e., etiocholanolone and androsterone) is also elevated. In infants, baseline levels of testosterone and DHT are so low that distinguishing normal from affected individuals may be difficult. Imperato-McGinley et al.[127] suggest an elevated urinary tetrahydrocortisol–to–5α-tetrahydrocortisol ratio as the basis for diagnosis; this is determined by gas chromatography or mass spectrometry.

Agonadia (Testicular Regression Syndrome)

In agonadia, gonads are absent, external genitalia are abnormal, and all but rudimentary müllerian or wolffian derivatives are absent. External genitalia usually consist of a phallus about the size of a clitoris, underdeveloped labia majora, and nearly complete fusion of the labioscrotal folds. A persistent urogenital sinus is often present. By definition, gonads are undetectable. Neither normal müllerian derivatives nor normal wolffian derivatives are ordinarily present; however, rudimentary structures may be present along the lateral pelvic wall. Somatic anomalies (craniofacial or vertebral anomalies or mental retardation) may coexist.[128]

The pathogenesis of agonadia must take into account not only the absence of gonads, but also abnormal external genitalia and the absence of internal ducts. Two explanations seem plausible:

1. Fetal testes functioned long enough to inhibit müllerian development, but not long enough to allow complete male differentiation (hence the appellation *testicular regression syndrome* preferred by some).

2. Alternatively, gonadal, ductal, and genital systems all could have developed abnormally as a result of either defective primordium, defective connective tissue, orteratogenic action.

The occasional coexistence of somatic anomalies is most consistent with the second hypothesis.

Among the approximately 30 reported cases are several sibships of affected males.[129] Autosomal recessive inheritance seems likely, but X-linked recessive inheritance cannot be excluded.

Leydig Cell Agenesis

46,XY patients showing complete absence of Leydig cells[130, 131] have female external genitalia, no uterus, and bilateral testes devoid of Leydig cells. Epididymides and vasa deferentia are present, and LH levels are elevated. Affected siblings have been reported,[132, 133] and parental consanguinity has been observed.[134] Thus, autosomal recessive inheritance is plausible.

TRUE HERMAPHRODITISM

True hermaphrodites have both ovarian and testicular tissue. They may have a separate ovary and a separate testis, or, more often, one or more ovotestes. Most true hermaphrodites (60%) have a 46,XX chromosomal complement; however, others have 46,XX/46,XY, 46,XY,46,XX/47,XXY, or other complements.[135] Although phenotype may depend on karyotype,[135, 136] it is preferable here to generalize about the phenotype of all true hermaphrodites.

Phenotype

If no intervention occurs, about two thirds of true hermaphrodites are raised as males. However, their external genitalia are usually ambiguous or predominantly female. Breast development usually occurs at puberty even with predominantly male external genitalia.

Gonadal tissue may be located in the ovarian, inguinal, or labioscrotal regions. A testis or an ovotestis is more likely to be present on the right than on the left. Spermatozoa are rarely present[137]; however, apparently normal oocytes are often present, even in ovotestes (Fig. 6–13). Several 46,XX true hermaphrodites have become pregnant,[138, 139] usually, but not always, after removal of testicular tissue.

The greater the proportion of testicular tissue in an ovotestis, the greater the likelihood of gonadal descent. In 80% of ovotestes, testicular and ovarian components are juxtaposed

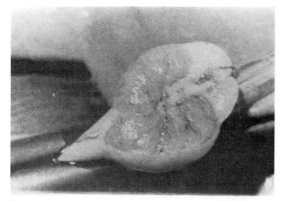

FIGURE 6–13 ••• A bisected ovotestis from a patient of Van Niekerk. The patient had a 46,XX complement. The ratio of ovarian to testicular tissue is about 1:4; ovarian tissue is present in the upper right. The testicular portion appeared yellowish brown, whereas the ovarian portion was white, although, in this photograph, color differentiation cannot be appreciated. The ovarian portion was firmer than the testicular portion. In 80% of ovotestes, just as in this patient, ovarian and testicular tissues are arranged end to end. (From Van Niekerk WA. True Hermaphoditism. New York: Harper & Row, 1974.)

end to end.[140] An ovotestis can thus be detected by inspection or by palpation, because testicular tissue is softer and darker than ovarian tissue. Ultrasound evaluation may also be useful. Accurate identification is particularly necessary if the inappropriate portion of an ovotestis is to be extirpated.

A uterus is usually present, although sometimes it is bicornuate or unicornuate. Absence of a uterine horn usually indicates an ipsilateral testis or ovotestis. The fimbriated end of the fallopian tube may be occluded ipsilateral to an ovotestis, and squamous metaplasia of the endocervix may occur.[140] Menstruation is not uncommon and is occasionally manifested as cyclic hematuria.[141]

Diagnosis is usually made only after excluding male and female pseudohermaphroditism. If a female sex of rearing is chosen, extensive surgery may or may not be necessary. If a male sex of rearing is chosen, genital reconstruction and selective gonadal extirpation are invariably indicated. Both gonadal neoplasia and breast carcinoma have been reported.[91, 135]

Etiology

True hermaphroditism is heterogeneous in origin. 46,XX/46,XY true hermaphroditism is caused by chimerism, which is the presence of two or more cell lines, each derived from different zygotes, in a single individual. Most 46,XY cases are unrecognized chimeras.[135] However, chimerism is not considered the explanation for 46,XX true hermaphrodites. Possible explanations for the presence of testes in those individuals who ostensibly lack a Y include (1) translocation of TDF, presumably SRY, from the Y to an X, (2) translocation of TDF from the Y to an autosome, (3) undetected mosaicism or chimerism, and (4) autosomal sex-reversal genes.

Although H-Y antigen is present in almost all 46,XX true hermaphrodites,[7] 46,XX true hermaphrodites fail to show DNA sequences from their father's Y that are presumed to contain TDF.[142] Detection of the DNA sequence of SRY in a 46,XX true hermaphrodite and a 46,XX male sibling gave a strong clue that Y/X translocation is involved.[15] However, more consistent with mendelian factors are sibships with XX true hermaphroditism.[135] The occurrence of 46,XX males and 46,XX true hermaphrodites in the same kindred has also been reported. The 46,XX males in these kindreds usually show genital ambiguity, unlike the typical 46,XX male. Interestingly, familial true hermaphroditism is more likely to be characterized by bilateral ovotestes and uterine absence than the nonfamilial type[135]; bilateral consistency favors a central basis for gonadal perturbation, as opposed to chimerism. It can thus be postulated that perturbation (derepression) of an ordinarily dormant autosomal gene induces inappropriate (testicular) gonadal development in 46,XX individuals. This argument has been developed elsewhere in more detail.[12, 23, 24]

HYPOGONADOTROPIC HYPOGONADISM

Isolated Gonadotropin Deficiency

Deficiency of the gonadotropins FSH and LH without deficiencies of other pituitary tropic hormones and without associated somatic anomalies is a rare cause of hypogonadism. Affected females have primary amenorrhea and lack secondary sexual development. Affected males fail to undergo normal secondary sexual development and thus usually consult a physician because of a small penis, small testes, high-pitched voice, and scanty beard growth. External genitalia are small yet well differentiated. Testes are characterized by decreased Leydig cells and retarded spermatogenesis. Ovaries show numerous primordial follicles but no oocytes. If somatic anomalies are present, a disorder other than isolated gonadotropin deficiency should be considered.

Pathogenesis could theoretically involve abnormalities of either the hypothalamus or the pituitary. In mice a similar disorder results from deficiency of gonadotropin-releasing hormone (GnRH). Existence of familial aggregates[143–149] suggest that isolated gonadotropin deficiency is inherited in autosomal recessive fashion. This mode of inheritance alone serves to distinguish this condition from Kallmann's syndrome.

Kallmann's Syndrome

Individuals with Kallmann's syndrome have not only isolated gonadotropin deficiency, but also decreased or absent olfaction (anosmia or hyposmia) secondary to aplasia of the olfactory

bulbs. Unilateral renal agenesis, cleft palate, and other somatic anomalies may also occur. This disorder is the most common cause of hypogonadotropic hypogonadism.[150]

Because Kallmann's syndrome was once believed to occur only in males, it was thought to be inherited in an X-linked recessive fashion. It is now apparent that females may also be affected, although hyposmia occurs less often than in males. Male-to-male transmission has been observed, thereby excluding X-linked inheritance. The mutant gene is inherited in autosomal dominant fashion, with variable expression.

Isolated LH Deficiency

Males with normal or nearly normal spermatogenesis who fail to undergo normal sexual development are said to be "fertile eunuchs." LH secretion is deficient. Affected individuals have high-pitched voices, poor muscle development, and scanty beard growth. Their testes have normal numbers of germ cells but practically no Leydig cells. Sperm counts are usually normal. Administration of hCG and testosterone has resulted in well-documented cases of paternity. Most cases are sporadic.

Isolated FSH Deficiency

Rabin and coworkers[151] and Bell et al.[152] reported a woman with primary amenorrhea and no secondary sex characteristics who appeared to have isolated FSH deficiency. Her ovaries were small. Numerous primordial follicles were present, but mature oocytes were not. FSH was undetectable (<3 mIU/ml), whereas LH was markedly elevated (40 to 90 mIU/ml). Given the current belief that only a single GnRH exists, the pathogenesis would seem more likely to involve the pituitary than the hypothalamus.

Pituitary Dwarfism

Deficiency of two or more pituitary tropic hormones, including gonadotropins, is a well-known cause of dwarfism. Hypopituitary dwarfs deficient in growth hormone (GH) may also be deficient in thyroid-stimulating hormone (TSH), ACTH, or FSH and LH. Hypopituitary hypogonadotropic hypogonadism is thus diagnosed easily on the basis of associated growth retardation, hypothyroidism, and hypoadrenalism. Causes include autosomal recessive gene, X-linked recessive gene, infection, or neoplasia involving the pituitary or hypothalamus.

DISORDERS OF GENITAL DUCTS

Transverse Vaginal Septa

Transverse vaginal septa are usually located near the junction of the upper and middle third of the vagina, but they may also be located more inferiorly. Other pelvic structures are usually normal, although occasionally the uterus is bicornuate. Transverse vaginal septa presumably result from failure of urogenital sinus derivatives and müllerian duct derivatives to fuse or canalize. An autosomal recessive gene is responsible for some cases, at least in Amish individuals.[153] Some patients with transverse vaginal septa also have polydactyly, and in these cases the term *McKusick-Kaufman* (or *Kaufman-McKusick) syndrome* is often applied. These cases may or may not be etiologically distinct from those without polydactyly. Clinical management is considered in Chapter 7.

Müllerian Aplasia

Aplasia of the müllerian ducts leads to absence of the uterine corpus, the uterine cervix, and the upper portion of the vagina.[6, 154] A 1- to 2-cm vagina is present, presumably derived exclusively from invagination of the urogenital sinus. Except for primary amenorrhea, secondary sexual development is normal. Some investigators call this condition *Mayer-Rokitansky-Küster-Hauser syndrome,* especially if rudimentary bands persist.

Renal anomalies are detected in about 40% of individuals with müllerian aplasia.[6, 154, 155] Pelvic kidney, renal ectopia, and unilateral renal aplasia are most common. Parenthetically, some investigators believe that a mutant dominant gene causes an entity characterized by renal dysplasia and müllerian aplasia.[156]

Siblings with müllerian aplasia have been reported on several occasions.[155] Shokeir[157] reported several kindreds in which the condition

appeared to be inherited in sex-limited autosomal dominant fashion; however, in a study of 24 probands, Carson et al.[155] found no affected siblings (0/30), paternal aunts (0/31), or maternal aunts (0/41). With the possible exception of the Canadian population studied by Shokeir,[157] the few reported familial aggregates seem most consistent with polygenic/multifactorial inheritance.

Cramer and coworkers[158] found galactose-1-phosphatidyl transferase deficiency or variants in two unrelated individuals with müllerian aplasia. This enzyme is known to be necessary for oogenesis,[159, 160] but germ cell differentiation need not, and usually does not, parallel ductal differentiation. Moreover, a relationship would be surprising, because galactosemic females usually have a normal uterus. The most common cause of congenital absence of the vagina and uterus, müllerian aplasia, and its surgical management are considered in Chapter 33.

Persistence of Müllerian Derivatives in Otherwise Normal Males

The uterus and fallopian tubes (müllerian derivatives) may persist in ostensibly normal males. The external genitalia, wolffian (mesonephric) derivatives, and testes develop as expected; virilization occurs at puberty. However, infertility is common, and about 5% of reported individuals develop a seminoma or other germ cell tumor. The disorder is sometimes ascertained because the uterus and fallopian tubes prolapse into an inguinal hernia (hence the term *uterine hernia inguinalis*).

Multiple affected siblings and concordant monozygotic twins have been reported.[30] In one family, maternal half-siblings were affected,[161] suggesting X-linked recessive inheritance. Another case consistent with that mode of transmission was reported by Naguib et al.[162] Failure of müllerian duct regression theoretically could result from either end-organ (uterus) insensitivity to AMH or from failure of Sertoli cells to synthesize or secrete AMH. If the origin truly is an X-linked recessive gene, the pathogenesis would not seem likely to involve the structural locus for AMH, because that gene has been localized to chromosome 19.[19] Instead, a receptor abnormality might be more plausible. However, Harbison et al.[163] reported an affected child in whom AMH was documented to be absent, not reduced. This suggested an abnormality of the AMH gene. Indeed, Knebelmann et al.[164] found an inappropriate stop codon involving AMH in an affected patient.

Incomplete Müllerian Fusion

During embryogenesis the müllerian ducts are originally paired organs. Fusion and canalization subsequently produce the upper vagina, uterus, and fallopian tubes. Failure of fusion results in two hemiuteri, each associated with no more than one fallopian tube. By contrast, in true müllerian duplication, each hemiuterus has two tubes. Thus, the common clinical term *double uterus* is a misnomer when applied to incomplete müllerian fusion. Clinical management is discussed in Chapter 33.

Familial aggregates of incomplete müllerian fusion are not rare. There are reports of multiple affected siblings, as well as an affected mother and daughter.[165] A proper genetic study would be difficult, as it would require invasive procedures to assess gynecologic status in relatives. One formal study found a low (1/37, or 2.7%) recurrence risk in female siblings,[166] consistent with polygenic/multifactorial inheritance.

Incomplete müllerian fusion may also be one component of a genetically determined malformation syndrome.[165] Meckel's syndrome, Fraser's syndrome, and Rudiger's syndrome are examples. Especially common is the hand-foot-uterus syndrome, an autosomal dominant disorder in which affected females have a bicornuate uterus and characteristic malformations of the hands and feet. The skeletal anomalies are frequently unappreciated by primary care physicians, and for this reason the condition is probably underdiagnosed.

References

1. Simpson JL. Human disorders of sex differentiation and the genetic control of sex differentiation. In: Pasqualini JR, Scholler R (eds). Hormones and Fetal Pathophysiology. New York: Marcel Dekker, 1992, pp 171–201.
2. Simpson JL. Genetic control of ovarian development. In: Boutaleb Y, Gzouli A (eds). Recent Developments in Fertility and Sterility Series. Vol 6: New Concepts in Reproduction. Lancaster, United Kingdom: Parthenon Publishing, 1992, pp 11–24.
3. Simpson JL, Golbus MS. Genetics in Obstetrics and Gynecology. 2nd ed. Philadelphia: WB Saunders, 1992.
4. Simpson JL. Genetics of sexual differentiation. In: Rock JA, Carpenter SE (eds). Pediatric and Adolescent Gynecology. New York: Raven Press, 1992, pp 1–37.
5. Jirasek J. Principles of reproductive embryology. In: Simpson JL (ed). Disorders of Sexual Differentiation. New York: Academic Press, 1976, p 51.
6. Simpson JL. Disorders of Sexual Differentiation: Etiology and Clinical Delineation. New York: Academic Press, 1976.
7. Wachtel SS. H-Y Antigen and the Biology of Sex Determination. New York: Grune & Stratton, 1983.
8. Simpson E, McLaren A, Chandler P, et al. Expression of H-Y antigen by female mice carrying SXR. Transplantation 1984; 37:1721.
9. Page DC. Hypothesis: A Y-chromosome gene causes gonadoblastoma in poorly dysgenetic gonads. Development (S) 1987; 101:151.
10. Palmer MS, Sinclair AH, Berta P. Genetic evidence that ZFY is not the testis determining factor. Nature 1989; 342:937.
11. Chandra HS. Is human X chromosome inactivation a sex determining device? Proc Natl Acad Sci USA 1985; 82:6947.
12. Simpson JL. Phenotypic-karyotypic correlations of gonadal determinants: Current status and relationship to molecular studies. In: Sperling K, Vogel F (eds). Human Genetics. Proceedings 7th International Congress Human Genetics (Berlin, 1986). Heidelberg: Springer-Verlag, 1987, p 224.
13. Sinclair AH, Berta P, Palmer MS, et al. A gene from the human sex-determining region encodes a protein with homology to a conserved DNA-binding motif. Nature 1990; 346:240.
14. Berta R, Hawkins JR, Sinclair AH, et al. Genetic evidence equating SRY and the testis-determining factor. Nature 1990; 348:448.
15. Jager RJ, Anvret M, Hall K, et al. A human XY female with a frame shift mutation in the candidate testis-determining-gene SRY. Nature 1990; 348:452.
16. Patsavoudi E, Magre S, Castinior M, et al. Dissociation between testicular morphogenesis and functional differentiation of Leydig cells. J Endocrinol 1985; 105:235.
17. Magre S, Jost A. Dissociation between testicular organogenesis and endocrine cytodifferentiation of Sertoli cells. Proc Natl Acad Sci USA 1984; 81:7831.
18. Carson SA, Simpson JL. Virilization of female fetuses following maternal ingestion of progestional and androgenic steroids. In: Mahesh VB, Greenblatt RB (eds). Hirsutism and Virilization. Littleton, MA: PSG Publishing, 1984, p 177.
19. Cohen-Haguenauer O, Picard JY, Mattei MG. Mapping of the gene for anti-müllerian hormone to the short arm of human chromosome 19. Cytogenet Cell Genet 1987; 44:2.
20. Behringer RR, Cate RL, Froekick GJ, et al. Abnormal sexual development in transgenic mice chronically expressing Müllerian inhibiting substance. Nature 1990; 345:167–170.
21. Jost A. Recerches sur la differenciation sexuelle de l'embryon de lapin II. Action des androgenes de syntheses sur l'histogenese genitale. Arch Anat Micor Morph Exper 1947; 36:242.
22. Singh PR, Carr DH. The anatomy and histology of XO human embryos and fetuses. Anat Rec 1966; 155:369.

23. Simpson JL. Genetic control of sexual development. In: Ratnam SS, Teoh SE, Anandakumar C (eds). Advances in Fertility and Sterility: Releasing Hormones and Genetics and Immunology in Human Reproduction. Vol 3. Proceedings 12th World Congress on Fertility and Sterility (Singapore, 1986). Lancaster, UK: Parthenon Press, 1987, p 165.

24. Simpson JL. Genetics of sex determination. In: Iizuka R, Seem K, Ohno T (eds). Human Reproduction—Current Status, Future Prospect. Proceedings of VIth World Congress on Human Reproduction (Toyko, 1987). The Netherlands: Elsevier, 1988, p 19.

25. Siiteri PK, Wilson JD. Testosterone formation and metabolism during male sexual differentiation in the human embryo. J Clin Endocrinol Metab 1974; 38:113.

26. Cates RL, Mattaliano RJ, Hession C, et al. Isolation of the bovine and human genes for Mullerian inhibiting substance and expression of the human gene in animal cells. Cell 1986; 45:685.

27. Simpson JL. Pregnancies in women with chromosomal abnormalities. In: Schulman JD, Simpson JL (eds). Genetic Diseases in Pregnancy. Academic Press, New York: 1981, p 440.

28. Dewhurst J. Fertility in 47,XXX and 45,X patients. J Med Genet 1978; 15:132.

29. Chen ATL. The effects of chromosome abnormalities on birth weight in man. I. Sex chromosome disorders. Hum Hered 1971; 21:543.

30. Brook CGD, Wagner H, Zachmann M, et al. Familial occurrence of persistent Mullerian structures in otherwise normal males. Br Med J 1973; 1:771.

31. Simpson JL. Gonadal dysgenesis and abnormalities of the human sex chromosomes: Current status of phenotypic-karyotypic correlations. Birth Defects 1975; 11(4):23.

32. Ranke MB, Pfluger H, Rosendahl W, et al. Turner's syndrome spontaneous growth in 150 cases and review of the literature. Eur J Pediatr 1983; 181:141.

33. Simpson JL. Localizing ovarian determinants through phenotypic-karyotypic deductions: Progress and pitfalls. In: Rosenfeld RG, Grumbach MM (eds). Turner Syndrome. New York: Marcel Dekker, 1988, pp 65–77.

34. Ranke MB, Blum WF, Hang F, et al. Growth hormone, somatomedin levels and growth regulation in Turner's syndrome. Acta Endocrinol (Copenh) 116, 1987.

35. Filippson R, Lindsten J, Almqvist S. Time of eruption of the permanent teeth cephalometric and tooth measurement and sulphation factor activities in 45 patients with Turner syndrome with different types of X chromosome aberration. Acta Endocrinol (Copenh) 1965; 48:91.

36. Lindsten J, Fraccaro M. Turner's syndrome. In: Rashad MN, Morton WRN (eds). Genital Anomalies. Springfield, IL: Charles C Thomas, 1969, p 396.

37. Lubin MB, Gruber HE, Rimoin DL, et al. Skeletal abnormalities in the Turner syndrome. In: Rosenfeld RG, Grumbach MM (eds). Turner Syndrome. New York: Marcel Dekker, 1990, p 281.

38. McCauley E, Kay T, Ito I, et al. The Turner syndrome: Cognitive defects, affective discrimination and behavior problems. Child Dev 1987; 58:464.

39. McCauley E, Sybert VP, Ehrhardt A. Psychological adjustments of adult women with Turner syndrome. Clin Genet 1986; 29:284.

40. Fraccaro M, Tiepolo L, Zuffardio-Chiumello G, et al. Familial XX true hermaphroditism and H-Y antigen. Hum Genet 1979; 48:45.

41. Krauss CM, Turkray RN, Atkins L, et al. Familial premature ovarian failure due to interstitial deletion of the long arm of the X chromosome. N Engl J Med 1987; 317:125.

42. Fitch N, de Saint VJ, Richer CL, et al. Premature menopause due to small deletion in long arm of the X chromosome: A report of three cases and a review. Am J Obstet Gynecol 1982; 142:968.

43. Tharapel AT, Anderson KP, Simpson JL, et al. Are all "terminal" Zq deletions interstitial? Reevaluation of a detected X-chromosome in a proband and her mother by Southern blotting and FISH analyses. Am J Hum Genet: In press.

44. Davis JR, Heine MW, Graap RF, et al. X-short arm deletion gonadal dysgenesis in two siblings. Clin Genet 1976; 10:202.

45. Jacobs PA, Ross A. Structural abnormalities of the Y chromosome in man. Nature 1966; 210:352.

46. Page DC, Mosher R, Simpson EM, et al. The sex-determining region of the human Y chromosome encodes a finger protein. Cell 1987; 51:1091.

47. Simpson JL, Christakos AC, Horwith M, et al. Gonadal dysgenesis associated with apparently chromosomal complements. Birth Defects 1971; 7(6):215.

48. Simpson JL. Gonadal dysgenesis and sex chromosome abnormalities. Phenotypic/karyotypic correlations. In: Vallet HL, Porter IH (eds). Genetic Mechanisms of Sexual Development. New York: Academic Press, 1979, p 365.

49. Simpson JL. Gonadal dysgenesis XX type. In: Buyse ML (ed). Birth Defects Encyclopedia. Cambridge, MA: Blackwell Scientific Publishers, 1990, p 805.

50. Boczkowski K. Pure gonadal dysgenesis and ovarian dysplasia in sisters. Am J Obstet Gynecol 1970; 106:626.

51. Portuondo JA, Neyro JL, Benito JA, et al. Familial 46,XX gonadal dysgenesis. Int J Fertil 1987; 32:56.

52. Christakos AC, Simpson JL, Younger JB, et al. Gonadal dysgenesis as an autosomal recessive condition. Am J Obstet Gynecol 1969; 104:1027.

53. Pallister PD, Opitz JM. The Perrault syndrome: Autosomal recessive ovarian dysgenesis with facultative, non sex-limited sensorineural deafness. Am J Med Genet 1979; 4:239.

54. McCarthy DJ, Opitz JM. Perrault syndrome in sisters. Am J Med Genet 1985; 22:629.

55. Lundberg PO. Hereditary myopathy, oliophrenia, cataract, skeletal abnormalities and hypergonadotrophic hypogonadism: A new syndrome. Eur Neurol 1973; 10:261.

56. Skre H, Bassoe HH, Berg K, et al. Cerebellar ataxia and hypergonadism in the two kindreds. Chance occurrence, pleiobokism or linkage? Clin Genet 1976; 9:234.

57. Maximilian C, Ionescu B, Bucur A. Deux soeurs avec dysgenesie gonadique majeure, hypotrophic staturale, microcephalie, arachnodactylie et caryotype 46,XX. J Genet Hum 1970; 18:365.

58. Verp MS. Environmental causes of ovarian failure. Semin Reprod Endocrinol 1983; 1:101.

59. Aleem FA. Familial 46,XX gonadal dysgenesis. Fertil Steril 1981; 35:317.

60. Jost A. Problems of fetal endocrinology. The gonadal and hypophyseal hormones. Recent Prog Horm Res 1953; 8:379.

61. Cussen LK, McMahon R. Germ cells and ova in dysgenetic gonads of a 46,XY female dizygote twin. Arch Dis Child 1979; 133:373.

62. Simpson JL, Chaganti RSK, Mouradian J, et al. Chronic renal disease myotonic dystrophy, and gonadoblastoma in an individual with XY gonadal dysgenesis. J Med Genet 1982; 19:73.

63. Haning RV Jr, Chesney RW, Moorthy AV, et al. A syndrome of chronic renal failure and XY gonadal dysgenesis in young phenotypic females without genital ambiguity. Am J Kidney Dis 1985; 6:40.

64. Simpson JL, Photopulos G. The relationship of neoplasia to disorders of abnormal sexual differentiation. Birth Defects 1976; 12(1):15.

65. Simpson JL, Blagowidow N, Martin AO. XY gonadal dysgenesis: Genetic heterogeneity based upon clinical observations. H-Y antigen status and segregation analysis. Hum Genet 1981; 58:91.

66. Mann JR, Corkery JJ, Fisher HJW, et al. The X-linked recessive form of XY gonadal dysgenesis with high incidence of gonadal cell tumours: Clinical and genetic studies. J Med Genet 1983; 20:264.

67. Disteche CM, Casanova M, Saal H, et al. Small deletions of the short arm of the Y chromosome in the 46,XY female. Proc Natl Acad Sci USA 1986; 83:7841.

68. Page DC. Sex reversal: Deletion mapping the male determining function of the Y chromosome. Cold Spring Harbor Symp Quant Biol 1986; 51:229.

69. Piunik S, Wachtel SS, Woods D, et al. Mutations in the conserved domain of SRY are uncommon in XY gonadal dysgenesis. Hum Genet. In Press.

70. Bricarelli FD, Fraccaro M, Lindsten J, et al. Sex-reversed XY females with campomelic dysplasia are H-Y negative. Hum Genet 1981; 57:15.

71. Puck SM, Haseltine FP, Francke U. Absence of H-Y antigen in an XY female with campomelic dysplasia. Hum Genet 1981; 57:23.

72. Brosnan PC, Lewandowski RC, Toguri AG, et al. A familial syndrome of the 46,XY gonadal dysgenesis with anomalies of ectodermal and mesodermal structures. J Pediatr 1981; 97:586.

73. Greenberg F, Gresik MW, Carpenter RJ, et al. The Gardner-Silengo-Wachtel or Genito-Palato-Cardiac syndrome: Male pseudohermaphroditism with micrognathia, cleft palate, and conotruncal cardiac defects. Am J Med Genet 1987; 26:59.

74. Smith A, Fraser IS, Noel M. Three siblings with premature gonadal failure. Fertil Steril 1979; 32:528.

75. Granat M, Amar A, Mor-Yosef S, et al. Familial gonadal germinative failure: Endocrine and human leukocyte antigen studies. Fertil Steril 1983; 40:215.

76. Hamet P, Kuchel O, Nowacynski JM, et al. Hypertension with adrenal genital, renal defects, and deafness. Arch Intern Med 1973; 131:563.

77. Al-Awadi SA, Farag, FI, Teebie AS, et al. Primary hypergonadism and partial alopecia in three sibs with Mullerian hypoplasia in the affected females. Am J Med Genet 1985; 22:619.

78. Mikati MA, Samir SN, Sahil IF. Microcephaly, hypergonadotropic hypogonadism, short stature and minor anomalies. A new syndrome. Am J Med Genet 1985; 22:599.

79. Riddick DH, Hammond CB. Long-term steroid therapy in patients with adrenogenital syndrome. Obstet Gynecol 1975; 45:15.

80. Mornet E, White PC. Analysis of genes encoding steroid 11-betahydroxylase. Abstract. Cytogenet Cell Genet 1989; 51:1047.

81. Bongiovanni AM. Further studies of congenital adrenal hyperplasia due to 3β-hydroxysteroid dehydrogenase deficiency. In: Vallet HL, Porter IH (eds).

Genetic Mechanisms of Sexual Development. New York: Academic Press, 1979, p 189.

82. Araki S, Chikazawa K, Sekisuchi I, et al. Arrest of follicular development in a patient with 17 alpha-hydroxylase deficiency: Folliculogenesis in association with a lack of estrogen synthesis in the ovaries. Fertil Steril 1987; 47:169.

83. Grumbach MM, Ducharme JR, Moloshak RE. On fetal masculinizing action of certain oral progestins. J Clin Endocrinol Metab 1959; 19:1369.

84. Simpson JL, Carson SA. Genetic and nongenetic causes of spontaneous abortion. In: Sciarra JJ (ed). Gynecology and Obstetrics. Vol 5. Philadelphia: JB Lippincott, 1991.

85. Verhoeven ATM, Mastboom JL, Van Leusden HAIM, et al. Virilization in pregnancy coexisting with an (ovarian) mucinous cystadenoma: A case report and review of virilizing ovarian tumors in pregnancy. Obstet Gynecol Surv 1973; 28:597.

86. Jones HW, Park IJ. A classification of special problems in sex differentiation. Birth Defects 1971; 7(6):113.

87. Park IJ, Jones HW, Melham RE. Nonadrenal familial female hermaphroditism. Am J Obstet Gynecol 1971; 112:930.

88. Lubinsky MS. Female pseudohermapahroditism and associated anomalies. Am J Med Genet 1980; 6:123.

89. McDonough PG, Tho PT. The spectrum of 45X/46,XY gonadal dysgenesis and its implications (a study of 19 patients). Pediatr Adolesc Gynecol 1983; 1:1.

90. Rosenberg C, Frota-Pessoa O, Vianna-Morgante AM, et al. Phenotypic spectrum of 45,X/46,XY individuals. Am J Med Genet 1987; 27:553.

91. Verp MS, Simpson JL. Abnormal sexual differentiation and neoplasia. Cancer Genet Cytogenet 1987; 25:191.

92. Boscze P, Szamel I, Molnar F, Laszlo J. Non-neoplastic gonadal testosterone secretion as a cause of vaginal cell maturation in streak gonad syndrome. Gynecol Invest 1986; 22:153.

93. Lukusa T, Fryns JP, Van den Berge H. Gonadoblastoma and Y-chromosome fluorescence. Clin Genet 1986; 29:311.

94. Hsu LYF. Prenatal diagnosis of chromosome abnormalities through amniocentesis. In: Milunsky A (ed). Genetic Disorders and the Fetus. 3rd ed. Baltimore: Johns Hopkins Press, 1986, p 155.

95. Elshay AI, Waters WR. The brachio-skeleto-genital syndrome. Plast Reconstr Surg 1971; 48:542.

96. Opitz JM, Howe JJ. The Meckel syndrome (dysencephalic splanchnocystica, the Gruber syndrome). Birth Defects 1969; 5(2):167.

97. Jones KL. Smith's Recognizable Patterns of Human Malformation. 4th ed. Philadelphia: WB Saunders, 1988.

98. Buyse ML. Birth Defects Encyclopedia. Edinburgh: Blackwell Scientific, 1990.

99. Eddy AA, Mauer M. Pseudohermaphroditism, glomerulopathy and Wilms tumor (Drash syndrome): Frequency in end-stage renal failure. J Pediatr 1985; 106:584.

100. Habib R, Loirat C, Gubler MC, et al. The nephropathy associated with male pseudohermaphroditism and Wilms' tumor (Drash syndrome): A distinctive glomerular lesion—report of 10 cases. Clin Nephrol 1985; 24:269.

101. Curry CRJ, Carey JC, Holland JS, et al. Smith-Lemli-Opitz syndrome-type II: Multiple congenital

anomalies with male pseudohermaphroditism and frequent early lethality. Am J Med Genet 1987; 26:45.

102. Simpson JL. Genetic heterogeneity in XY sex-reversal: Potential pitfalls in isolating the Testes-Determining-Factor: TDF. In: Wachtel SS (ed). Evolutionary Mechanisms in Sex Determination. Baton Rouge, LA: CRC Press, 1989, p 265.

103. Frydman M, Kauschansky A, Zamir R, et al. Familial lipoid adrenal hyperplasia: Genetic marker data and an approach to prenatal diagnosis. Am J Med Genet 1986; 25:319.

104. Chung BC, Matteson KJ, Voutilainen R, et al. Human cholesterol side-chain cleavage enzyme P450scc:cDNA cloning assignment of the gene to chromosome 15 and expression in the placenta. Proc Natl Acad Sci USA 1986; 83:8962.

105. Perrone L, Criscuolo T, Sinisi AA. Male pseudohermaphroditism due to 3β-hydroxysteroid dehydrogenase-isomerase deficiency associated with atrial septal defect. Acta Endocrinol (Copenh) 1985; 110:532.

106. Heremans GFP, Moolenaar AJ, Van Gelderen HM. Female phenotype in a male child due to 17α-hydroxylase deficiency. Arch Dis Child 1976; 51:721.

107. Zachmann M, Vollmin JA, Hamilton W, et al. Steroid 17,20-desmolase deficiency: A new cause of male pseudohermaphroditism. Clin Endocrinol 1972; 1:369.

108. Nebert DW, Nelson DR, Adesnik M, et al. The P-450 superfamily: Updated listing of all genes and recommended nomenclature for the chromosomal loci. DNA 1989; 8:1.

109. Balducci R, Toscano V, Wright F, et al. Familial male pseudohermaphroditism with gynaecomastia due to 17β-hydroxysteroid dehydrogenase deficiency. A report of 3 cases. Clin Endocrinol (Oxf) 1985; 23:439.

110. Imperato-McGinley J, Peterson RE, Stoller R, et al. Male pseudohermaphroditism secondary to a 17α-hydroxysteroid dehydrogenase deficiency: Gender role with puberty. J Clin Endocrinol Metab 1979; 49:391.

111. Caufriez A. Male pseudohermaphroditism due to 17-ketoreductase deficiency: Report of a case without gynecomastia and without vaginal pouch. Am J Obstet Gynecol 1986; 154:148.

112. Ulloa-Aguirre A, Mendez PJ, Chavez A, et al. Incomplete regression of Mullerian ducts in the androgen insensitivity syndrome. Fertil Steril 1990; 53:1024.

113. Morris JM, Mahesh VB. Further observations on the syndrome "testicular feminization." Am J Obstet Gynecol 1963; 87:731.

114. Prior L, Bordet S, Trifèro MA, et al. Replacement of arginine 773 by cysteine or histidine in the human androgen receptor causes complete androgen insensitivity with different receptor phenotypes. Am J Hum Genet 1992; 51:143.

115. Park IJ, Jones HW. Familial male hermaphroditism with ambiguous external genitalia. Am J Obstet Gynecol 1970; 108:1197.

116. Griffin JE, Punyashthiki K, Wilson JD. Dihydrotestosterone binding by culture human fibroblasts. Comparison of cells from control subjects and from patients with hereditary pseudohermaphroditism due to androgen resistance. J Clin Invest 1976; 57:1342.

117. Pinksy L, Kaufman M. Genetics of steroid receptors and their disorders. Adv Hum Genet 1985; 16:299.

118. Pinsky L, Kaufman M, Levitzsky LL. Partial androgen resistance due to a distinctive qualitative defect of the androgen receptor. Am J Med Genet 1987; 27:459.

119. Wilson JD, Harrod MJ, Goldstein JL, et al. Familial incomplete male pseudohermaphroditism type I. N Engl J Med 1974; 290:940.

120. Wilson JD, Harrod MJ, Goldstein JL, et al. Familial incomplete male pseudohermaphroditism. N Engl J Med 1984; 290:1097.

121. Simpson JL, New M, Peterson RE, et al. Pseudovaginal perineoscrotal hypospadias (PPSH) in sibs. Birth Defects 1971; 7(6):140.

122. Opitz JM, Simpson JL, Sarto GE, et al. Pseudovaginal perineoscrotal hypospadias. Clin Genet 1971; 3:1.

123. Imperato-McGinley J, Guerrero L, Gauiter T, Peterson RE. Steroid 5α-reductase deficiency: An inherited form of male pseudohermaphroditism. Science 1974; 186:1213.

124. Walsh C, Madden JD, Harrod MJ, et al. Familial incomplete male pseudohermaphroditism, type 2. N Engl J Med 1974; 291:944.

125. Peterson RE, Imperato-McGinley J, Gautier T, et al. Male pseudohermaphroditism due to steroid 5α-reductase deficiency. Am J Med 1977; 62:170.

126. Green S, Zachmann M, Mannella B. Comparison of two tests to recognize or exclude 5α-reductase deficiency in prepubertal children. Acta Endocrinol (Copenh) 1987; 114:113.

127. Imperato-McGinley J, Gautier T, Pichardo M, Shackleton C. The diagnosis of 5 alpha-reductase in infancy. J Clin Endocrinol Metab 1986; 63:1313.

128. Sarto GE, Opitz JM. The XY gonadal agenesis syndrome. J Med Genet 1973; 10:288.

129. de Grouchy J, Gompel A, Salmon-Bernard Y. Embryonic testicular regression syndrome and severe mental retardation in sibs. Ann Genet 1985; 28:154.

130. Brown DM, Markland C, Dehner LP. Leydig cell hypoplasia: A case of male pseudohermaphroditism. J Clin Endocrinol Metab 1976; 46:1.

131. Lee PA, Rock JA, Brown TR, et al. Leydig cell hypofunction resulting in male pseudohermaphroditism. Fertil Steril 1981; 37:675.

132. Perez-Palacios G, Scaglia HE, Kofman-Afaro S. Inherited male pseudohermaphroditism due to gonadotrophin unresponsiveness. Acta Endocrinol (Copenh) 1982; 98:148.

133. Saldanha PH, Arnhold IJP, Mendonca BB, et al. A clinico-genetic investigation of Leydig cell hypoplasia. Am J Med Genet 1987; 26:337.

134. Schwartz M, Imperato-McGinley J, Peterson RE, et al. Male pseudohermaphroditism secondary to an abnormality in Leydig cell differentiation. J Clin Endocrinol Metab 1981; 53:123.

135. Simpson JL. True hermaphroditism. Etiology and phenotypic considerations. Birth Defects 1978; 14(6C):9–15.

136. Van Niekerk WA, Retief AE. The gonads of human true hermaphrodites. Hum Genet 1981; 58:117.

137. Aaronsen I. True hermaphroditism. A review of 41 cases with observations on testicular histology and function. Br J Urol 1985; 57:775.

138. Tegenkamp TR, Brazzell JW, Tegenkamp I, et al. Pregnancy without benefit of reconstructive surgery in a bisexually active true hermaphrodite. Am J Obstet Gynecol 1979; 135:427.

139. Minowada S, Fukutani K, Hara M, et al. Childbirth in a true hermaphrodite. Eur Urol 1984; 10:414.

140. Van Niekerk WA. True Hermaphroditism. New York: Harper & Row, 1974.

141. Raspa RW, Subramanian AP, Romas NA. True hermaphroditism presents as intermittent hematuria and groin pain. Urology 1986; 28:133.

142. Ramsay M, Bernstein R, Zwane E, et al. XX true hermaphroditism in South African blacks: An enigma of primary sexual differentiation. Am J Hum Genet 1988; 43:4.

143. LeMarquand HS. Congenital hypogonadotropic hypogonadism in 5 members of a family, 3 brothers and 2 sisters. Proc R Soc Med 1954; 47:422.

144. Ewer RW. Familial monotropic pituitary gonadotropin insufficiency. J Clin Endocrinol 1968; 28:783.

145. Faiman C, Hoffman DL, Ryan RJ, Albert A. The 'fertile eunuch' syndrome: Demonstration of isolated luteinizing hormone deficiency by radioimmunoassay technique. Mayo Clin Proc 1968; 43:661.

146. Santen RJ, Paulsen CA. Hypogonadotrophic eunuchoidism: Gonadal responsiveness to exogenous gonadotropins. J Clin Endocrinol Metab 1973; 36:55.

147. Boyar RM, Wu RHK, Kapen S, Hellman L, Weitzman ED, Finkelstein JW. Clinical and laboratory heterogeneity in idiopathic hypogonadotrophic hypogonadism. J Clin Endocrinol Metab 1976; 43:1268.

148. Betend B, Lebacq E, David L. Familial idiopathic hypogonadotrophic hypogonadism. Acta Endocrinol (Copenh) 1977; 84:246.

149. Toledo SP, Arnhold IJ, Luthold W, et al. Leydig cell hypoplasia determining familial hypergonadotropic hypogonadism. Prog Clin Biol Res 1983; 200:311.

150. Santen RJ, Paulsen CA. Hypogonadotrophic eunuchoidism. I. Clinical study of the mode of inheritance. J Clin Endocrinol Metab 1973; 36:47.

151. Rabin D, Spitz I, Bercovici B, et al. Isolated deficiency of follicle-stimulating hormone. N Engl J Med 1972; 289:1313.

152. Bell J, Benveniste R, Spitz I, Rabinowitz D. Isolated deficiency of follicle-stimulating hormone. Further studies. J Clin Endocrinol Metab 1975; 40:790.

153. McKusick VA, Weilbaecher RG, Gregg CW. Recessive inheritance of a congenital malformation syndrome. JAMA 1968; 204:113.

154. Griffin JE, Edwards C, Madden JD, et al. Congenital absence of the vagina. The Mayer-Rokitansky-Küster-Hauser syndrome. Ann Intern Med 1976; 85:224.

155. Carson SA, Simpson JL, Malinak LR, et al. Heritable aspects of uterine anomalies. II. Genetic analysis of Mullerian aplasia. Fertil Steril 1983; 34:86.

156. Opitz JM. Vaginal atresia (von Mayer-Rokitansky-Küster or MRK anomaly) in hereditary renal adysplasia (HRP). Am J Med Genet 1987; 26:873.

157. Shokeir MHK. Aplasia of the Mullerian system: Evidence for probable sex-limited autosomal dominant inheritance. Birth Defects 1978; 14(6C):147.

158. Cramer DW, Ravnikar VA, Craighill M, et al. Mullerian aplasia associated with maternal deficiency of galactose-1-phosphate uridyl transferase. Fertil Steril 1987; 47:930.

159. Kaufman F, Kogut MD, Donnell GN, et al. Ovarian failure in galactosemia. Lancet 1979; 2:737.

160. Hoefnagel D, Wurster-Hill D, Child EL. Ovarian failure in galactosemia. Lancet 1979; 2:1197.

161. Sloan WR, Walsh PC. Familial persistent Mullerian duct syndrome. J Urol 1976; 115:459.

162. Naguib KK, Teebi AS, Farag TI, et al. Familial uterine hernia syndrome: Report of an Arab family of four affected males. Am J Med Genet 1989; 33:180.

163. Harbison MD, Magid ML, Josso N, et al. Antimullerian hormone in three intersex conditions. Ann Genet 1991; 34:226.

164. Knebelmann B, Baussin L, Guerrier D, et al. Antimullerian hormones: A nonsense mutation associated with persistent mullerian duct syndrome. Proc Natl Acad Sci USA 1991; 88:3367.

165. Verp MS, Simpson JL, Elias S, et al. Heritable aspects of uterine anomalies. I. Three familial aggregates with Mullerian fusion anomalies. Fertil Steril 1983; 34:80.

166. Elias S, Simpson JL, Carson SA, et al. Genetic studies in incomplete Mullerian fusion. Obstet Gynecol 1984; 63:276.

○○○

CHAPTER 7

Abnormal Sexual Differentiation and Hypogonadism: Management and Therapy

SELMA F. SIEGEL

SARAH BERGA

PETER A. LEE

Sexual differentiation, or the development of internal and external genitalia, is a complex process dependent on a normal chromosomal constitution in the presence of a gender-appropriate hormonal milieu. Genetic sex, determined at fertilization, directs the differentiation of the bipotential structures, which are composed of analogous cell types: germ cells; granulosa-Sertoli cells; and theca-Leydig cells.[1] When the chromosomes are 46,XY, the bipotential gonad differentiates into a testis by 6 to 7 weeks of gestation. When the chromosomes are 46,XX, ovarian differentiation occurs later, at 9 to 10 weeks of gestation.

Testis-determining factors have been localized to the short arm of the Y chromosome. Through analysis of the genomes of XX males and XY individuals, a 35-kilobase conserved region of the Y chromosome has been identified as sex-determining region Y (SRY). The protein encoded by this gene is homologous to others with DNA-binding function.[2] De novo point mutations within this region have been described in seven 46,XY females;[3, 4] but in three cases the identical mutations were shared

with their fertile fathers, implying that additional genes may be involved in the process of sexual differentiation.[4]

Pseudoautosomal regions occur on the X and Y chromosomes. These regions are distal segments of the short arms of the X and Y chromosomes that are highly homologous (Fig. 7–1). These regions appear to escape X chromosome inactivation such that gene dosage is equivalent.[5] Indeed, MIC2, which encodes a cell surface antigen and is located within the pseudoautosomal region, is expressed from both X chromosomes in normal females.[6] The SRY gene is located adjacent to the pseudoautosomal region. Divergent evolution of homologous ancestral chromosomes is speculated to have led to localization of the male sex-determining "factors" to the Y chromosome, with development of this pseudoautosomal region allowing pairing of the X and Y chromosomes during meiosis.[7]

While genetic sex influences gonadal differentiation, external genital development is dependent on the intercellular signaling systems of testosterone metabolism and the androgen

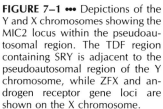
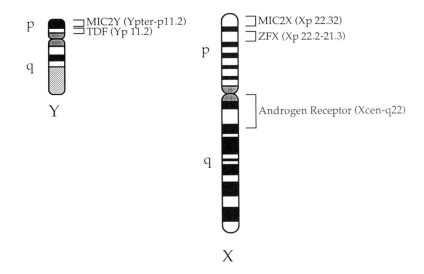

FIGURE 7–1 ••• Depictions of the Y and X chromosomes showing the MIC2 locus within the pseudoautosomal region. The TDF region containing SRY is adjacent to the pseudoautosomal region of the Y chromosome, while ZFX and androgen receptor gene loci are shown on the X chromosome.

receptor. In the presence of testosterone and dihydrotestosterone, male external genital development is induced. In the absence of effective androgen stimulation, the "default" developmental program is female.

Genital ambiguity indicates an abnormality in sexual differentiation. Disordered gonadal differentiation can be secondary to aneuploidy or abnormalities of all or part of the sex chromosomes. Abnormal hormonal milieu can affect genital structure development. For example, increased androgen levels during gestation of a female fetus will induce virilization of the external genitalia. In contrast, decreased androgen levels or impaired androgen action interferes with the development of the external genitalia of a male fetus.

CHROMOSOMAL DISORDERS

Turner Syndrome

In 1930, Ullrich reported a syndrome that was further characterized by Henry Turner in 1938 as including short stature, lack of pubertal development, webbed neck, low posterior hairline, and cubitus valgus (Fig. 7–2).[8] Subsequently, this clinical phenotype was determined to be associated with X chromosome monosomy.[9] Mosaic karyotypes can occur with a spectrum of phenotypic abnormalities; the incidence is 1 in 2500 to 3000 female births. Diagnosis is usually made at birth as a result of typical dysmorphic features (Table 7–1) or in early adolescence as a result of short stature and delayed puberty.[10]

Short stature, or a mean adult height of approximately 143 cm, is a characteristic feature of Turner syndrome.[11] The etiology of the short stature is unclear. Intrauterine growth retardation with low birth weight is common.

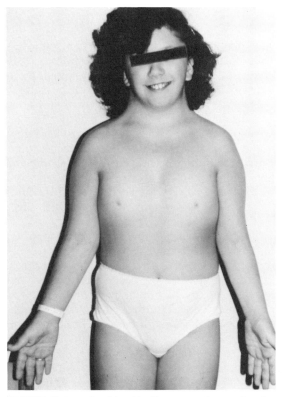

FIGURE 7–2 ••• A girl with Turner syndrome showing cubitus valgus (wide carrying angle), neck webbing, and widely spaced nipples.

TABLE 7–1 ••• FEATURES OF TURNER SYNDROME

Short stature
Skeletal abnormalities
    Shortening of the fourth metacarpal
    Widening head of the distal phalanges
    Madelung's deformity
    Cubitus valgus
    Schmorl's nodes
    Scheuermann's disease
    Osteoporosis
Chronic otitis media
    Cholesteatoma
Cardiac abnormalities
    Coarctation of the aorta
    Bicuspid aortic valves
    Partial anomalous venous return
    Hypertension
Lymphatic abnormalities
    Cystic hygroma
    Puffy hands and feet
Renal anomalies
    Horseshoe kidney
    Duplicated collecting systems
    Malrotation
    Abnormalities of the renal vascular system
Inflammatory bowel disease
Endocrine abnormalities
    Hypothyroidism
    Carbohydrate intolerance
    Hypergonadotropic hypogonadism
    Infertility

The majority of girls with Turner syndrome have normal growth hormone responses (>10 ng/ml) to pharmacologic and physiologic evaluations of growth hormone secretory status.[12] During the prepubertal years, growth hormone and insulin-like growth factor I (IGF I) levels are comparable to those in normal children. Mean 24-hour growth hormone concentrations were similar in girls with Turner syndrome and normal individuals prior to 9 years of age, but were lower in girls with Turner syndrome after 9 years of age when compared with age-matched normal girls.[13, 14]

Skeletal abnormalities are often recognized in Turner syndrome (Table 7–2). Shortening of the fourth metacarpal secondary to premature epiphyseal fusion occurs frequently, but this also occurs in pseudohypoparathyroidism, pseudopseudohypoparathyroidism, brachycephaly E syndrome, and basal cell nevus syndrome. Shortening of the fourth metatarsal may also occur. The "drumstick" appearance of the distal phalanges is due to widening of the head of the distal phalanges. When impaired distal radial growth and premature fusion of the distal radial growth plate occur in association with shortening of the ulna, Ma-

delung's deformity of the wrist develops. Cubitus valgus, or an increased carrying angle of the elbow, is common. Characteristic knee findings include projection and enlargement of the metaphyseal portion of the medial aspect of the tibial condyle, which is associated with enlargement of the medial femoral condyle.[15]

In the spine, abnormalities of the cartilaginous end plates (Schmorl's nodes) and of the epiphyseal rings (Scheuermann's disease) may be found. Typically, Scheuermann's disease is not associated with significant pain. Scoliosis occurs but is generally not severe or progressive. This is perhaps due to the lack of a normal pubertal growth spurt.

Osteoporosis has been recognized as a component of Turner syndrome for many years.[16] No consistent differences have been detected on histologic examination between bone obtained from Turner syndrome patients and that obtained from normal individuals. Bone density (gm/cm) and bone mineral content (gm/cm^2) are decreased when compared with chronologic or skeletal age, but not when compared with height age.[17] Despite a theoretical risk of increased fractures, they are usually not a major problem for girls with Turner syndrome. Physical activity and hormone replacement therapy correlate with skeletal mineralization in adult women with Turner syndrome.[18]

TABLE 7–2 ••• TREATMENT ASPECTS OF TURNER SYNDROME

Short stature
    Growth hormone treatment*
Skeletal abnormalities
    Observe for scoliosis and osteoporosis
    Prevention of osteoporosis is another justification for
        hormonal replacement therapy
Chronic otitis media
    Antibiotic therapy as needed
    Tympanotomy tubes
    Observe for cholesteatoma
Cardiac abnormalities
    Echocardiogram
    Appropriate therapy for any intrinsic cardiac lesions
    Subacute bacterial endocarditis prophylaxis
    Monitor blood pressure
Renal anomalies
    Renal ultrasound
Endocrine abnormalities
    Monitor thyroid function studies
    Document hypergonadotropic state
    Hormonal replacement therapy to initiate and
        maintain secondary sexual development

*Should be considered on an individual basis.

Facial features include high arched palate, micrognathia, and downward droop of the lateral corners of the eyes. Chronic or recurrent otitis media persisting into adolescence and hearing loss are associated with Turner syndrome.[19] In 2 of 22 patients, a cholesteatoma sac was identified.[20] Hence, significant morbidity may result from the otologic manifestations of Turner syndrome.

Because abnormalities of the left side of the heart are associated with Turner syndrome, patients benefit from a cardiac evaluation that includes echocardiography. The characteristic anomalies are coarctation of the aorta and bicuspid aortic valves.[21] A pathogenetic relationship may exist among prenatal lymphatic obstruction, webbing of the neck, nuchal cystic hygroma, and left-sided congenital heart disease.[22, 23] Partial anomalous venous return has been reported in patients with Turner syndrome. Severe congenital heart disease appears to be more common in those with the 45,X karyotype than in those with mosaic karyotypes.[24] Aortic dissection with pathologic evidence of cystic medial necrosis is a potentially catastrophic complication.[25] Reevaluation in adolescence and young adulthood is recommended because of this devastating but treatable complication. Patients with recognized valvular abnormalities should receive standard subacute bacterial endocarditis (SBE) prophylaxis.

Renal anomalies, especially horseshoe kidney, duplicated collecting systems, malrotation, or abnormalities of the renal vascular system, are associated with Turner syndrome.[26] Because urinary tract infections, with secondary effects on renal function, may occur, patients should undergo a renal imaging study. Renal ultrasound is usually an adequate screening measure.[27] Hypertension may develop because of coarctation of the aorta, renal disease, or idiopathic hypertension. The increased blood pressure may be difficult to control.

Affected individuals often have increased numbers of nevi. Many patients have a tendency to form keloids. This tendency is important when considering surgery, especially cosmetic surgery.

Both Crohn's disease and ulcerative colitis occur with increased frequency in patients with Turner syndrome.[28] These inflammatory bowel diseases may further reduce growth velocity.[29]

Carbohydrate intolerance has also been recognized to occur in Turner syndrome. While fasting glucose levels are generally normal, oral glucose tolerance testing revealed higher glucose and insulin levels in 16 of 41 girls studied.[30]

Differential Diagnosis

Short stature and delayed puberty are the most frequent presenting complaints for girls with Turner syndrome. Subnormal growth velocity may also be the initial symptom of hypothyroidism, hypercortisolism, growth hormone deficiency, chronic renal disease, or inflammatory bowel disease. In addition, there is an increased incidence of some of these disorders in Turner syndrome. Short stature may also be attributed to familial short stature. Girls who present in early adolescence are short for chronologic age and for corrected midparental height with a height standard deviation score more than two standard deviations below the mean for age or corrected midparental height.[10] Hence, all short girls should be evaluated for the possibility of Turner syndrome.

The diagnosis of Turner syndrome is based on chromosomal analysis. Peripheral blood lymphocyte analysis is usually sufficient, but in some mosaic patients, analysis of fibroblasts from skin biopsy is necessary. Buccal smears do not provide adequate information. Despite attempts to localize the chromosomal determinant of ovarian failure and short stature, it appears that there are loci on both the short and long arms for ovarian maintenance and stature.[31] In infancy and beginning in late childhood, gonadotropin levels are elevated because of the lack of negative feedback within the hypothalamic-pituitary-gonadal axis.[32]

Girls with Noonan's syndrome may have physical stigmata reminiscent of Turner syndrome (e.g., short stature, webbed neck, cubitus valgus, and midfacial hypoplasia). However, right-sided congenital heart disease and a greater incidence of developmental delay are associated with Noonan's syndrome. Typically, girls with Noonan's syndrome have a normal karyotype.[33]

Treatment

The effects of treatment with steroid hormones and growth hormone on growth velocity and adult height have been investigated (see

Table 7–2). Early studies were inconclusive because of small numbers of patients, inconsistent hormone dosages, and brief periods of longitudinal observation.

A pair-matched study of oxandrolone (0.1 mg/kg/day for 1 year) showed improved growth velocity and adult height.[34] However, potential problems with oxandrolone—accelerated skeletal maturation, clitoromegaly, acne, deepening of the voice, and hirsutism—have limited its usefulness.

Low doses of estradiol promote growth, while higher doses are inhibitory. Estrogens may enhance growth hormone secretion and have a direct effect on bone growth. However, premature pubertal development and accelerated skeletal maturation may occur with estradiol treatment.[35]

During 1 year of therapy, human growth hormone increased the mean growth velocity from 3.2 ± 0.8 cm/yr to 5.9 ± 1.4 cm/yr.[36] With the increased availability of recombinant growth hormone, its use, either alone or in combination with sex steroids, has been evaluated in Turner syndrome. Comparison of oxandrolone therapy alone (0.125 mg/kg/day), growth hormone therapy alone (0.375 mg/kg/week), and combination therapy showed annual growth velocities of 7.6 ± 1.5, 6.6 ± 1.2, and 9.8 ± 1.4 cm/yr, respectively, compared with the control growth velocity of 3.8 ± 1.1 cm/yr.[37] The oxandrolone dosage was decreased to 0.0625 mg/kg/day in later years of this study because of the occurrence of excessive virilizing side effects. Analysis after 3 years of this multicenter study showed greater height increment without excessive advancement of skeletal maturation in patients treated with growth hormone, either alone or in combination with oxandrolone.[38]

With the use of recombinant growth hormone therapy, short-term growth velocity may be improved in individual patients with Turner syndrome (Fig. 7–3).[39, 40] The improvement in growth velocity tends to vary among patients and is modest compared with the response of growth hormone–deficient individuals. However, preliminary results suggest that adult height may be increased by growth hormone therapy. This may also permit the initiation of feminizing doses of estrogens at a more appropriate chronologic age. The precise mechanism of growth hormone action in Turner syndrome is not well defined. Plasma IGF I, serum procollagen III N-terminal peptide (a parameter of collagen metabolism), and osteocalcin

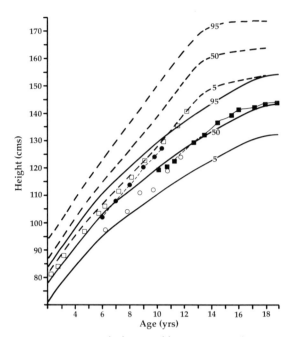

FIGURE 7–3 ••• Height for age of four patients with Turner syndrome plotted on a grid showing the 5th, 50th, and 95th percentile for heights for age from the National Center for Health Statistics *(dashed lines)* and for untreated patients with Turner syndrome *(solid lines)*. The open circles (○) depict the heights at various ages for a patient with spontaneous ovarian function who was not treated for short stature. The solid circles (●) represent heights for a patient during GH therapy. The open squares (□) show the heights for age of a patient with relatively good stature and growth rate who had spontaneous pubertal development. The solid squares (■) show heights for a patient when untreated *(unconnected squares)*, during hGH therapy *(dashed line)*, and while receiving estrogen therapy *(solid line)*. (Adapted from Lyon AJ, Preece MA, Grant DB. Growth curves for girls with Turner syndrome. Arch Dis Child 1985; 60:932–935.)

(a parameter of bone metabolism) levels were increased by growth hormone administration.[41]

Oxandrolone alone or with growth hormone resulted in impaired glucose tolerance associated with insulin resistance; fasting glucose levels and glycosylated hemoglobin levels remained within the normal range.[42] Hyperinsulinemia, noted before growth hormone treatment using the hyperglycemic glucose-clamp technique, markedly increased after growth hormone therapy in seven girls with Turner syndrome.[43] The acute and chronic clinical consequences of impaired glucose tolerance and hyperinsulinemia are uncertain. While hyperinsulinism may facilitate the effects of growth hormone and anabolic steroids on linear growth, it may also contribute to hypertension, atherosclerosis, and cardiomegaly.[43, 44]

Psychosocial and Educational Aspects of Turner Syndrome

Comprehensive education of the patient and her family is a major goal of treatment.[45] Indeed, surveys of affected middle-aged women indicate the need to fully inform these girls and their families about Turner syndrome.[46] Telling a young girl that nothing is wrong when she visits a "special" doctor on a regular basis doesn't fool her. Such denial may only convince her that she has a terrible disease. This inconsistency may intensify the negative impact that short stature and delayed puberty have already made on her self-esteem. Diagnosis at the time of puberty is not optimal for the use of growth hormone therapy or for patient–parent education.

Earlier literature implied that girls with Turner syndrome are "retarded." Because the verbal intelligence and school performance of affected girls are comparable to those of unaffected sisters, it is crucial that this inaccurate information be dealt with promptly.[47] However, when considered as a group, there is an increased incidence of impaired spatial skills. Geometry and hand-eye coordination require this cognitive skill and may be more difficult for some girls with Turner syndrome. Additional tasks that require spatial abilities include estimating distances of objects, traveling through unfamiliar areas, and playing sports with fast-moving balls.[48] Overall, educational and vocational achievement are congruent with innate intellectual abilities, while social adjustment tends to be more mediocre.[49]

Situations that "set up" failure are best avoided. For example, it may be helpful for families to be aware that the cubitus valgus and wrist deformity may make playing the violin difficult. Parents, educators, and physicians should focus on positive attributes. These girls should be encouraged to participate in sports in which stature is not important (e.g., ice skating, diving, or swimming). Stores catering to petite sizes provide sophisticated clothing for the adolescent or adult woman with Turner syndrome.

Delaying the induction of puberty to maximize growth potential may have adverse effects on the patient's self-esteem, as one affected individual eloquently stated:

Without breasts and other secondary sexual development, the boys did not "notice" me in usual junior-high-school fashion. Perhaps I would not have worried so much about that, for I sensed that I was not ready for predating boy-girl relationships, had it not also tended to isolate me from girlfriends. Few of them were dating regularly, but all were claiming boyfriends and sharing their interests in dating in intimate sessions. Because they, too, responded to my youthful appearance, I was largely excluded from much of the normal friendships and socialization of early adolescence. I was confused and angry.[50]

Reproductive issues should be put in a positive perspective: the girl will most likely have her family by adoption. As discussed later in this chapter, donor oocytes and techniques for in vitro fertilization have expanded the reproductive options for hypogonadal women.

Gonadal Dysgenesis

The term *gonadal dysgenesis* is used for conditions in which gonadal differentiation is aberrant. Histologic examination reveals streak ovaries and dysgenetic testicular tissue. Gonadal dysgenesis is further subclassified as either "mixed" or "pure." Currently, patients are classified by phenotypic appearance and gonadal histology. As the mechanism of sexual differentiation is elucidated through the tools of molecular biology, a more precise classification of affected individuals may emerge.

Mixed gonadal dysgenesis is defined as streak gonads with dysgenetic testicular elements. Patients may be recognized at birth because of ambiguous genitalia. The spectrum of external genital appearance extends from phenotypic female to phenotypic male.[51, 52] Affected individuals can show many phenotypic similarities to those with Turner syndrome, including short stature, renal anomalies, webbed neck, and low posterior hairline. Karyotypes are usually 45,X/46,XY, but additional mosaic karyotypes (i.e., 45,X/46,XX/46,XY) may occur. One analysis of prenatally diagnosed cases revealed that many 45,X/46,XY fetuses have normal male external genitalia without correlation between the percent mosaicism and the occurrence of genital or gonadal abnormalities.[53] While there is often a streak gonad on one side and a dysgenetic testis on the other side (Fig. 7–4), the spectrum of gonadal differentiation extends from bilateral streak gonads to bilateral dysgenetic testes.[54]

The degree of masculinization reflects testicular function. Individuals with dysgenetic testes often have deficient müllerian inhibitory

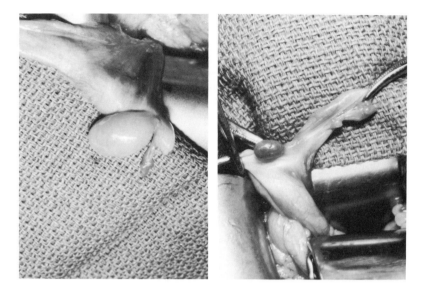

FIGURE 7–4 ••• Internal reproductive structures of a patient with mixed gonadal dysgenesis. The photo on the left shows a testis, while the photo on the right depicts a uterus, uterine tube, and streak gonad.

hormone secretion in utero, resulting in regression of wolffian structures and the presence of fallopian tubes and uterus. Asymmetry of internal and external genital structures, frequently found in this disorder, is a valuable physical finding in the evaluation of individuals with ambiguous genitalia. Importantly, at puberty there may be sufficient testosterone secretion from the dysgenetic testis to induce significant virilization.

The risk for gonadoblastoma is increased in the presence of dysgenetic testicular elements.[55] Although such tumors are more frequent during late adolescence and the early adult years, they have also been reported in infancy.[56] A gonadoblastoma is composed of admixed nests of germ cells and sex cord cells.[57] Calcification may occur. It has been suggested that gonadoblastomas are carcinomas in situ from which invasive germ cell tumors, seminoma, embryonal carcinoma, teratoma, choriocarcinoma, and dysgerminoma may evolve.[58, 59] Gonadectomy is generally curative for gonadoblastoma. However, additional treatment may be indicated if invasive elements are present.[60]

Pure gonadal dysgenesis may occur with either a 46,XX or a 46,XY karyotype. The eponym *Swyer's syndrome* refers to individuals with female phenotypic appearance and 46,XY karyotype. These patients usually are diagnosed in adolescence when they present with delayed puberty or primary amenorrhea. Typical findings include normal or tall stature and bilateral streak gonads with fibrous tissue. X-linked recessive or male-limited autosomal dominant inheritance has been reported for the familial forms. Sporadic forms also occur. Aberrant testicular differentiation in utero leads to impaired müllerian inhibitory hormone secretion and decreased testosterone production. This results in preservation of müllerian structures and regression of wolffian structures.

Deletions of Y chromosomal material have been described.[61] In some 46,XY females, the sex-determining region of the Y chromosome has been lost.[62, 63] Mutations in the SRY gene have been reported in 46,XY females.[3, 64] From the gonadal histology of individuals with pure gonadal dysgenesis, complete failure of testicular differentiation, leading to ovarian development with secondary degeneration because of the lack of a second X chromosome, may be hypothesized.[65]

Affected individuals also have an increased risk of gonadal tumors, primarily gonadoblastoma, although dysgerminoma may also occur. Malignant degeneration of the germ cell elements of a gonadoblastoma may occur, resulting in metastatic disease. Indeed, the presence of breast development often signifies the presence of a gonadal tumor with increased estrogen secretion.[66]

Pure gonadal dysgenesis with a 46,XX karyotype is also characterized by delayed puberty with poor breast development, sparse sexual hair, and primary amenorrhea.[67] The typical clinical phenotype is normal to tall stature without stigmata of Turner syndrome. Familial forms show autosomal recessive inheritance.

True hermaphroditism, by definition, is the simultaneous occurrence of ovarian tissue with follicles and testicular tissue with tubules. The gonads can be ovary, testis, or ovotestis. Most commonly, there is an ovary on one side and an ovotestis on the other side.[68] The majority of such individuals have a 46,XX karyotype. The phenotypic appearance ranges from phenotypic female to genital ambiguity. Hypospadias, undescended testes, and inguinal hernias are common. A gonad or uterus is often found within the hernia sac. Because gonadal function varies considerably among affected individuals, ovulation and fertility may be possible. Sufficient testosterone production for pubertal virilization may occur, but azoospermia is typical. Heterosexual development (virilization in affected phenotypic females and gynecomastia in affected phenotypic males) is not uncommon.

HORMONAL DISORDERS

Disorders of Cortisol Biosynthesis

In the congenital adrenal hyperplasias, inadequate cortisol synthesis caused by decreased steroidogenic enzyme activity results in increased ACTH secretion. Distinctive biochemical patterns of abnormal hormone secretion by the adrenal gland occur depending on which specific enzyme activity is affected (Table 7–3). The resulting hormonal milieu leads to characteristic phenotypic findings.

Decreased 21-Hydroxylase Activity

Decreased 21-hydroxylase activity is the most common form of the congenital adrenal hyperplasias, with a reported incidence of 1 in 5000 to 1 in 15,000.[69–71] The enzyme, 21-hydroxylase or cytochrome $P-450_{c21}$, converts 17-hydroxyprogesterone to 11-deoxycortisol and progesterone to deoxycorticosterone. The clinical spectrum of this disorder ranges from severely affected individuals with genital ambiguity and salt loss to clinically asymptomatic individuals.[72]

In affected 46,XX fetuses, the inadequate cortisol secretion leads to increased ACTH secretion, resulting in increased adrenal androgen secretion. These weaker androgenic hormones, dehydroepiandrosterone (DHEA) and androstenedione, undergo extraadrenal conversion to testosterone and induce virilization of the fetus, resulting in genital ambiguity (Fig. 7–5). Varying degrees of masculinization of the external genitalia occur, ranging from significant genital ambiguity to posterior labial fusion in the absence of clitoromegaly.[73, 74] Most importantly, no matter how well developed the scrotum and phallus appear, the external genitalia appear to be symmetric, and there are no palpable gonads. Such infants have normal functional ovaries and normally developed müllerian structures because of the absence of müllerian inhibitory hormone. Similar physical findings may be present when maternal hyperandrogenism, such as that caused by androgen-secreting tumors, occurs.

Affected 46,XY fetuses appear normal at

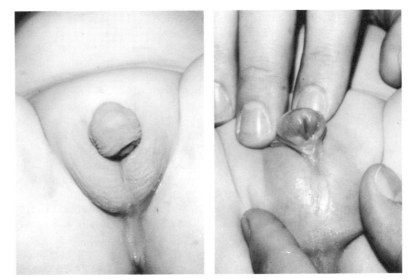

FIGURE 7–5 ••• Masculinization of the external genitalia of a female infant with clitoromegaly and labioscrotal fusion. The urethral opening is on the ventral side of the clitoris, not at the base on the left at the end of the glans.

TABLE 7–3 ••• ENZYME DEFECTS IN STEROIDOGENESIS

| Enzyme | Karyotype | Differs Between Sexes | |
		Prenatal	Puberty
21-hydroxylase			
Severe	46,XX	Virilization	Premature pubarche
Moderate		± Virilization	Hirsutism
Mild		Normal	Clitoromegaly
Severe	46,XY	Normal	Premature
Moderate		Normal	Pubarche
Mild		Normal	Normal
11β-hydroxylase			
Severe	46,XX	Virilization	Premature pubarche
Mild, Moderate		± Virilization	Hirsutism
Severe	46,XY	Normal	Premature pubarche
Mild, Moderate		Normal	± Childhood virilization
3β-hydroxydehydrogenase			
Severe	46,XX	Virilization	Premature pubarche
Mild, Moderate		± Virilization	Hirsutism
Severe	46,XY	↓ Masculinization	± Virilization
Mild, Moderate		± ↓ Masculinization	± Premature pubarche
17α-hydroxylase/17,20-lyase	46,XX	Normal	Delayed/absent
	46,XY	↓ Masculinization	Delayed/absent
Cholesterol desmolase	46,XX	Normal	Delayed/absent
	46,XY	↓ Masculinization	Delayed/absent
5α-reductase†	46,XY	↓ Masculinization	Virilization
17-ketosteroid reductase	46,XX	Normal	Virilization
	46,XY	↓ Masculinization	Virilization

*May present with salt loss in infancy.
†Affects males only.
↑, Increased; ↓, decreased; +, present; −, absent; DHEA, dehydroepiandrosterone; N, normal.

birth. If mineralocorticoid deficiency is present, the affected male generally presents within the first 3 weeks of life with weight loss and dehydration secondary to salt loss.

The molecular genetics of 21-hydroxylase deficiency have been well characterized. The gene encoding for 21-hydroxylase is located within the class III region of the major histocompatibility complex on the short arm of chromosome 6.[75] Two 21-hydroxylase loci, a functional gene (CYP21) and a pseudogene (CYP21P), are arranged in a tandem duplication pattern with C4A and C4B, which encode serologically and functionally distinct proteins for the fourth component of serum complement.[76] At least three deleterious mutations are recognized in the pseudogene that prevent encoding a functional protein.[77] Through the use of restriction fragment length polymorphisms and DNA sequencing, specific mutations have been recognized in individuals with

decreased 21-hydroxylase activity.[78–80] Approximately 25% of severely affected individuals have a 30-kb deletion extending from the 5' portion of the pseudogene through C4B into the functional gene. Gene conversions occur in which the structure of the functional gene is "converted" to that of the pseudogene.[81]

Diagnostic findings include elevated urinary 17-ketosteroid secretion. Plasma 17-hydroxyprogesterone levels are elevated and are often greater than 10,000 ng/dl in the neonatal period. Mildly affected individuals and heterozygotes have elevated 17-hydroxyprogesterone responses following ACTH administration (0.25 mg cosyntropin [intravenous or intramuscular], with samples at 0 and 30 or 60 minutes). Prenatal diagnosis is possible in affected families. This can be done through comparison of conventional human leukocyte antigen (HLA) typing to determine which haplotype carries the affected allele. Analysis of

TABLE 7–3 ••• ENZYME DEFECTS IN STEROIDOGENESIS *Continued*

			For Both Sexes				
			Plasma Concentration				
Salt Loss	Hypertension	Principal Elevated Steroid(s)	17-Hydroxy-progesterone	DHEA	Andro-stenedione	Testosterone	Renin
+	−	17-Hydroxyprogesterone	↑↑↑	↑, N	↑↑	↑	↑↑
−	−		↑↑	↑, N	↑↑	↑	N, ↑
−	−		↑	N, ↑	↑	N, ↑	N
−*	+	Desoxycortisol	↑	↑, N	↑↑	↑	↓, N
−	+,−		↑, N	↑, N	↑	↑, N	↓, N
+	−	17-Hydroxypregnenolone, DHEA	↓	↑↑	N, ↑	N	↑
−	−		↓	↑	N, ↑	N	N
−	+, −	Progesterone	↓, N	↓	↓	↓	↓, N
−	+, −						
+	−	Cholesterol	↓	↓	↓	↓	↑
−	−	Testosterone	↑, N	↑, N	↑	↑	N
−	−	Androstenedione	↑	↑	↑↑	↓	N
−	−						

the DNA pattern of the proband and families is the most accurate method. Chorionic villus sampling and amniocentesis can be utilized. However, virilization of the external genitalia begins before such laboratory results are available. Hence, maternal treatment with dexamethasone from the time of the first missed menstrual period can decrease the magnitude of virilization of the external genitalia.[82] If the fetus is male or unaffected, then dexamethasone may be discontinued. Limitations of prenatal therapy include undetermined effects of dexamethasone treatment; all at-risk pregnancies must be treated, and a proband must be previously identified.[83]

Decreased Activity of 11β-Hydroxylase

Decreased activity of 11β-hydroxylase, cytochrome P-450$_{c11}$, can manifest similar ambiguity of the external genitalia of a 46,XX fetus. 11β-Hydroxylase converts 11-deoxycortisol to cortisol and deoxycorticosterone to corticosterone.[84] While this form of congenital adrenal hyperplasia is characterized by hypertension, salt loss may occur in the neonatal period or in treated patients with adrenal suppression.[85] Levels of 11-deoxycortisol and deoxycorticosterone are elevated. Heterozygotes have variable responses following adrenocorticotropic hormone (ACTH) stimulation tests.[86]

Decreased Activity of 3β-Hydroxysteroid Dehydrogenase

Decreased activity of 3β-hydroxysteroid dehydrogenase causes ambiguous genitalia in both sexes. This enzyme catalyzes the conversion of pregnenolone to progesterone and 17-hydroxypregnenolone to 17-hydroxyprogesterone. In the 46,XX fetus, this results in increased DHEA secretion, which causes masculinization of the external genitalia. In contrast, in the 46,XY fetus, there is inadequate testosterone synthesis for normal development of the external genitalia.[87] Mineralocorticoid and glucocorticoid deficiencies also occur. Diagnostic findings include elevated levels of 17-hydroxypregnenolone and DHEA, with an increased 17-hydroxypregnenolone–to–17-hydroxyprogesterone ratio and an increased DHEA-to-androstenedione ratio.

Decreased Activity of 17α-Hydroxylase/17,20 Lyase

The enzyme 17α-hydroxylase/17,20 lyase is a single enzyme, P-450$_{c17}$, which converts pregnenolone to 17-hydroxypregnenolone and 17-hydroxypregnenolone to DHEA.[88] Decreased activity of this enzyme interferes with glucocorticoid and sex steroid synthesis.[89] However, clinical findings of hypocortisolism are uncommon, despite impaired glucocorticoid production.[90] The hypothesis that there are two differentially regulated enzyme sites is clinically correlated in that some patients appear to have more significant impairment of one enzyme activity.[91] An affected XX fetus will have normal female genitalia, while an affected XY fetus may have genital ambiguity secondary to inadequate testosterone production. Because of the presence of müllerian inhibitory hormone, müllerian structures are absent in XY fetuses. Genetic females present with delayed puberty, including absence of breast tissue, absence of sexual hair, primary amenorrhea, and elevated gonadotropin levels. The magnitude of hypertension and hypokalemia, attributed to increased deoxycorticosterone and corticosterone secretion, is variable. Mutations in the structural P-450$_{c17}$ gene have been identified in affected individuals.[92–94]

Decreased Activity of Cholesterol Desmolase

Cholesterol desmolase (P-450$_{scc}$) is the enzyme that converts cholesterol to pregnenolone. Deficiency of this enzyme impairs synthesis of glucocorticoids, mineralocorticoids, and sex steroids. Affected 46,XX fetuses have normal female external genitalia, while 46,XY fetuses are undervirilized. Histologic examination of the adrenals and testes has revealed lipid-laden cells.

Treatment

Treatment of glucocorticoid and mineralocorticoid deficiency disorders requires physiologic replacement. Such therapy decreases the excessive adrenal androgen secretion. In children, oral hydrocortisone is the most commonly used glucocorticoid, because it provides the best approximation of physiologic dosage. The goal of therapy is adequate adrenal suppression to prevent continued virilization and accelerated skeletal maturation while avoiding oversuppression characterized by subnormal growth velocity. Physiologic replacement therapy is based on daily cortisol production rates of 7 to 12 mg/m^2/day in children and adults.[95, 96] For most patients, an oral cortisol dosage of between 12 and 20 mg/m^2/day is sufficient for normal growth and development. Adequacy of replacement therapy can be assessed by the lack of progressive virilization, growth velocity, skeletal maturation, serum adrenal androgen levels, and urinary 17-ketosteroid excretion.

The usual mineralocorticoid replacement regimen consists of oral fludrocortisone (Florinef). The typical dose is 0.1 mg administered as a daily single dose. Neonates and infants may require as much as 0.2 to 0.3 mg daily because of greater aldosterone production rates during infancy. In the older child, a dietary history regarding salt intake provides a clinical parameter of the sufficiency of the mineralocorticoid replacement regimen. Plasma renin levels furnish another index of the adequacy of mineralocorticoid replacement therapy. However, plasma renin levels do not indicate whether dosage is excessive.

Increased glucocorticoid dosage is necessary at times of physiologic stress (e.g., fever [>101°F], persistent vomiting, significant trauma, and surgical procedures). Two to three times the usual daily glucocorticoid dose is generally adequate, but higher doses may be necessary for surgical procedures. All families should have injectable hydrocortisone (Solu-Cortef) available for emergencies. Recommended dosage is 50 mg in children under 4 years of age and 100 mg for all others. During surgical procedures, hydrocortisone can be administered by continuous intravenous infusion with the usual intravenous fluids. Because of the short half-life of intravenous hydrocortisone, administration must be continuous. When oral mineralocorticoid replacement is not tolerated, intravenous normal saline may be necessary, because parenteral deoxycorticosterone acetate is generally unavailable. Individuals with 11β-hydroxylase deficiency who are on suppressive glucocorticoid therapy may require mineralocorticoid replacement when under stress.

Disorders of Testosterone Biosynthesis

Male sexual differentiation is dependent on sufficient local concentrations of testosterone and dihydrotestosterone to maintain the wolffian ducts. Steroid biosynthesis utilizes a common pathway in both the adrenal gland and the testis. In addition to decreased activity of 17α-hydroxylase/17,20-lyase, reduced activity of either 5α-reductase or 17-ketosteroid reductase impairs testosterone synthesis. In these disorders, absence of müllerian-derived structures with underdevelopment of wolffian structures is typical as a result of normal müllerian inhibitory hormone secretion in utero. Varying degrees of genital ambiguity occur in the 46,XY fetus depending on the magnitude of the impaired enzyme activity.

Decreased activity of 5α-reductase disrupts normal male external genital development, leading to pseudovaginal perineoscrotal hypospadias. There is usually a blind vaginal pouch with a urogenital sinus and clitoral-like phallus. Structures derived from wolffian ducts are present. At puberty, virilization occurs, with deepening of the voice and phallic growth. However, facial hair is often sparse, and male-pattern baldness is uncommon. Impaired spermatogenesis is often present.[97]

Clusters of this autosomal recessive disorder have been reported in socially isolated populations with considerable consanguinity in the Dominican Republic, Turkey, and New Guinea.[98–100] While the initial sex of rearing may be female, the psychosexual orientation has been described to become masculine as the affected individual virilizes with the onset of puberty. In the Dominican Republic, affected individuals are known as "guevedoces," or "penis at 12."[98] In these populations, cultural expectations influence the psychosexual identity and self-esteem of the male pseudohermaphrodites.[101] Familiarization with Western culture may modify the particular societal beliefs.

The increased testosterone-to-dihydrotestosterone ratio is amplified following human chorionic gonadotropin (hCG) stimulation.[102] Urinary metabolites show increased etiocholanolone-to-androsterone and tetrahydrocortisol-to–5α-tetrahydrocortisol ratios. Specific enzyme activity can be assayed in genital skin fibroblasts. Gonadotropin levels are normal to slightly increased. Deletion of the gene encoding the 5α-reductase isoenzyme in genital skin has been reported in two related individuals with 5α-reductase deficiency.[103]

The enzyme, 17-ketosteroid reductase, converts androstenedione to testosterone and estrone to estradiol. With decreased 17-ketosteroid reductase activity, external genitalia are feminine or ambiguous with a blind vaginal pouch. Puberty is characterized by clitoral enlargement, deepening of the voice, and male-pattern sexual hair, because androstenedione undergoes peripheral tissue conversion to testosterone.[104] Gynecomastia may occur. Like in individuals with 5α-reductase deficiency, a change in gender identity from female to male may occur at puberty.

There is a clustering of affected individuals within an inbred Arab population of the Gaza strip.[105] Because the majority of reported cases involve 46,XY individuals, there appears to be an ascertainment bias in this presumably autosomal recessive disorder. Investigation of a 46,XX individual who had hirsutism, secondary amenorrhea, and polycystic ovaries revealed biochemical evidence consistent with decreased 17-ketosteroid reductase deficiency.[106] After hCG stimulation, the androstenedione-to-testosterone ratio is increased in affected individuals. When diagnosed in infancy, the clinical response to testosterone can be assessed so that male sex of rearing can be assigned.[107]

Disorders of Androgen Action

The androgen insensitivity syndromes refer to complete or partial resistance to androgen action at the receptor or postreceptor level. In the 46,XY fetus with complete androgen insensitivity, the inability of the target cell to respond to androgen stimulation results in impaired stabilization of the wolffian ducts, while normal müllerian inhibitory hormone secretion by the testes leads to regression of the müllerian ducts. Hence, affected 46,XY fetuses have phenotypically normal female external genitalia and absence of internal genital ducts. Such individuals may present with labial masses, inguinal hernias, or primary amenorrhea. The vagina is short and blind or absent. The testes may be intraabdominal, within the inguinal canal, or within the labia majora. At puberty, the loss of negative gonadotropin feedback leads to increased luteinizing hormone (LH) secretion with subsequent increased testosterone production. Increased conversion of testosterone to estradiol frequently induces spontaneous breast development. Axillary and pubic hair is sparse. In infants, adolescents, and adults, LH levels are elevated, while follicle-stimulating hormone (FSH) levels may be normal or elevated.

In partial androgen insensitivity syndromes, a degree of androgen responsiveness is present. Such individuals may present with ambiguous genitalia or peripubertal virilization. Reifenstein, Gilbert-Dreyfus, and Lubs are eponyms for partial androgen insensitivity syndromes. Although the spectrum of phenotypic findings may vary widely within a single family, these syndromes are all secondary to mutations in the androgen receptor gene.[108]

At a target cell, testosterone diffuses into the cell, where it binds directly to the intranuclear androgen receptor or undergoes conversion to dihydrotestosterone by the enzyme 5α-reductase, which then binds to the androgen receptor (Fig. 7–6). Ligand binding induces allosteric activation of the receptor, which then binds to specific steroid response elements (SREs) in DNA. The formation of stable hormone-receptor-SRE complexes results in changes in DNA transcription.[109]

The gene encoding the androgen receptor is localized to the Xq11-Xq12 region of the long arm of the X chromosome.[110, 111] The androgen receptor, analogous to other steroid/thyroid hormone/retinoic acid receptors, is characterized by a DNA-binding domain, hormone-binding domain, and a variable N-terminal region that modulates gene expression (Fig. 7–7). The two zinc finger motifs, located within the DNA-binding domain, are believed to stabilize the binding of the receptor-ligand complex to the SRE in DNA.[112]

Abnormalities of the androgen receptor have been categorized as receptor negative, in which androgen binding is absent in cultured genital fibroblasts, or as receptor positive, in which androgen binding is present. Although gene deletions have been described, point mutations of the androgen receptor gene are much more common.[108, 113] The effects of identified point mutations include premature termination of translation, resulting in a truncated defective receptor protein; altered half-life of the ligand-receptor complex; and impaired ligand-receptor complex interaction with the SRE.[114–117]

"Vanishing Testes" Syndrome

Individuals with bilateral congenital anorchia but well-developed male external genitalia are considered to have the "vanishing testes" syndrome. Such individuals had testes that secreted adequate testosterone at the appro-

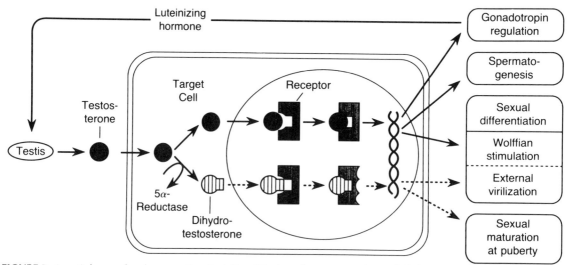

FIGURE 7–6 ••• Scheme of androgen action depicting diffusion of testosterone intracellularly to bind the androgen receptor or be converted to dihydrotestosterone (DHT), which in turn binds the receptor. Androgen actions are mediated by testosterone or DHT. (From Griffin JE. Androgen resistance—the clinical and molecular spectrum. Reprinted by permission of The New England Journal of Medicine 326; 612, 1992.)

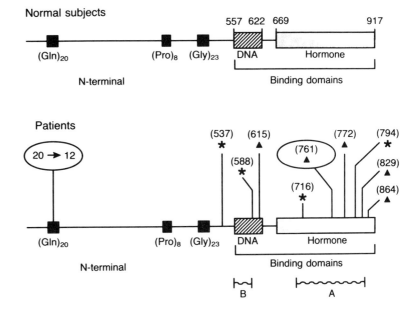

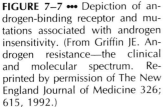

FIGURE 7–7 ••• Depiction of androgen-binding receptor and mutations associated with androgen insensitivity. (From Griffin JE. Androgen resistance—the clinical and molecular spectrum. Reprinted by permission of The New England Journal of Medicine 326; 615, 1992.)

priate time of gestation to induce male sexual differentiation. However, testicular regression, perhaps because of inadequate vascular supply, may have occurred. Affected individuals have no significant testosterone response to hCG injections.

Persistent Müllerian Duct Syndrome

Persistent müllerian duct syndrome represents an abnormality in müllerian inhibitory hormone secretion or action. Normal male external genitalia with cryptorchidism is typical. Derivatives of müllerian structures are usually located within an inguinal hernia. Both testes have been found within the hernia sac with the müllerian structures on one side or embedded in the round ligaments in an ovarian position. Müllerian inhibitory hormone–positive and –negative forms have both been reported.[118] A nonsense mutation in the gene encoding müllerian inhibitory hormone has been described.[119]

MANAGEMENT: SEX OF REARING

After an infant's first cry in the delivery room, the child's gender is announced. The occurrence of genital ambiguity—with its med-

ical, sexual, psychosocial, and genetic implications—disrupts this expected sequence of events. While genital ambiguity represents a developmental aberration to the clinician, it is a social *emergency* for the anxious parents and extended family. Compounding the difficulties are cultural attitudes on sexual dimorphism, preexisting expectations regarding the child's sex, and feelings of guilt for having a child with a birth defect, especially a defect that is very emotionally charged.[120]

It is helpful to tell the parents that their child's genitalia were incompletely formed. This incomplete development represents a birth defect that could be equated to a defect such as a cleft palate. Explanations of normal fetal sexual differentiation, with emphasis on the bipotentiality of genital structures, can help parents understand what has happened, as well as the rationale for specific diagnostic procedures. Demonstration of the specific abnormalities on physical examination can also be beneficial for the parents. Importantly, the infant should be referred to as "your baby" or "your child" rather than "it," "he," or "she." Naming and birth registration should be postponed until the diagnostic evaluation has enabled selection of the most appropriate sex of rearing.

Determinants for sex of rearing for the 46,XY infant include the extent of erectile tissue, the magnitude of reconstructive surgery for male or female sex of rearing, the prognosis for spontaneous pubertal development, and the risk for gonadal neoplasms. Consideration of these factors in relation to the family's cultural attitudes should lead to an individualized decision.

The first step of the diagnostic evaluation is a thorough physical examination (Fig. 7–8). Relevant features are palpable gonads, symmetry of structures, extent of phallic development, presence of other anomalies, and the status of müllerian structures. These physical features describe the fetal hormonal milieu and do not identify the genetic sex. A family history to ascertain other possibly affected individuals is important.

Additional diagnostic studies include a karyotype study to determine genetic sex and imaging studies to ascertain the status of the müllerian structures. Although basal steroid hormone levels may be diagnostic, stimulation with ACTH or hCG may be necessary to discriminate defects in steroidogenesis. For example, an elevated basal 17-hydroxyprogesterone level in a 46,XX infant with ambiguous genitalia and without palpable gonads confirms the diagnosis of 21-hydroxylase deficiency and necessitates lifelong glucocorticoid replacement therapy. In contrast, an hCG stimulation test may be necessary to diagnose 17-ketosteroid reductase deficiency or 5α-reductase deficiency in a 46,XY infant with genital ambiguity and palpable gonads. Gonadotropin, glucose, and electrolyte levels should be deter-

mined, in addition to 17-hydroxypregnenolone, 17-hydroxyprogesterone, 11-deoxycortisol, DHEA, androstenedione, testosterone, and dihydrotestosterone levels. Simultaneous occurrence of hyponatremia and hyperkalemia confirms mineralocorticoid deficiency. Importantly, although gonadal histology confirms the diagnosis of true hermaphroditism, it may not accurately determine the specific pathophysiology in a patient with ambiguous genitalia.[121]

Androgen insensitivity syndromes are characterized by elevated LH and testosterone levels in the neonatal period.[122] When the diagnosis of partial androgen insensitivity is suspected in a newborn with genital ambiguity, palpable gonads, and a typical hormonal profile, the response to exogenous androgen stimulation can be determined to help with the decision regarding sex of rearing. The amount of phallic growth following one or more monthly testosterone injections (e.g., 25 mg testosterone enanthate for 1 to 3 months) provides a clinical assessment of androgen sensitivity. The clinical and biochemical responses (penile growth and testosterone production) to hCG can also be assessed. If the response is judged to be satisfactory to provide an adequate penis, male sex of rearing is appropriate. For infants with partial androgen insensitivity and poor responses to exogenous androgen stimulation, female sex of rearing is indicated.

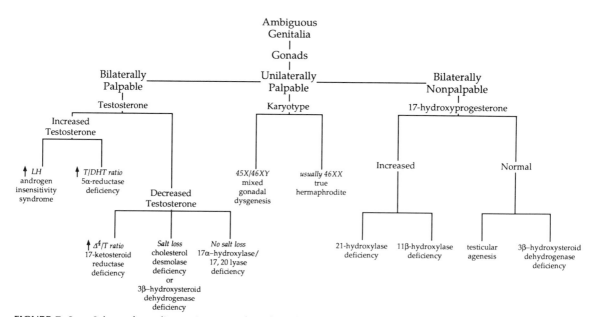

FIGURE 7–8 ••• Schema for a diagnostic approach to the infant presenting with ambiguous genitalia. Possible diagnoses are suggested using the presence of palpable gonads and indicated diagnostic tests.

The demonstration of absent androgen binding in genital skin fibroblasts confirms receptor-negative androgen insensitivity syndromes. The diagnosis of receptor-positive androgen insensitivity syndromes, either complete or partial, may be confirmed by ascertainment of the specific molecular defect in the androgen receptor. These results may not be available for timely gender assignment.

As soon as the etiology of the genital ambiguity has been reasonably classified, the decision regarding sex of rearing must be made. Because a decision regarding sex of rearing should be made promptly, a precise diagnosis may not be available. The predominant issue is the potential for achievement of satisfactory adult sexual function. Additional important concerns are the prospects for fertility and appropriate gonadal steroidogenesis. In the 46,XX infant with 21-hydroxylase deficiency, female sex of rearing with genital reconstructive surgery is clearly appropriate, as these infants have the potential for normal female pubertal development and reproductive abilities if maintained on glucocorticoid therapy. Clitoral reduction and perineal reconstruction are generally performed in early infancy. Vaginoplasty, frequently requiring dilatation, is often delayed until adolescence. In contrast, the 46,XY infant with partial androgen insensitivity who has a minimal response to exogenous testosterone would be best raised as a female.

Once the sex of rearing is determined, gender identity should be unequivocal. The infant is either a boy or a girl. Issues relating to genital appearance, sexual functioning, and potential for fertility should be addressed. Genetic implications such as the risk of recurrence need to be discussed with the family.

Diagnosis of complete androgen insensitivity syndromes, true hermaphroditism, and 17α-hydroxylase/17,20-lyase deficiency may be delayed beyond the neonatal period, because such infants typically have normal female external genitalia and are assigned to female sex of rearing at birth. Labial masses, bilateral inguinal hernias, or delayed puberty bring these individuals to medical attention. Because gender identity is generally well established, the goal of medication intervention is to support the chosen identity.

HORMONE REPLACEMENT IN HYPOGONADAL FEMALES

Customarily, sex hormone replacement is recommended in the female with hypogonad-ism. However, if short stature, especially in association with Turner syndrome, is present, the possible benefits of growth hormone therapy should be considered before instituting sex hormone replacement, because epiphyseal maturation may diminish the potential for additional linear growth.[123–127]

One potential exception, however, is the girl or woman with functional hypothalamic amenorrhea, oligomenorrhea, or polymenorrhea as a result of life-style factors such as excessive exercise, performance pressures, depression, and/or eating disorders. In these circumstances, the hypogonadism is theoretically reversible, and behavior management can be attempted initially.[128] Discussion of the potential complications of chronic hypoestrogenism and the possibility of "weak bones" may facilitate behavior modification, especially in athletes.[129]

Estrogen therapy is used to initiate or promote pubertal development of secondary sexual characteristics and organs, particularly the breast, vagina, and uterus. Current evidence suggests that estrogen therapy may increase bone mass and provide cardioprotection, including induction of beneficial alterations in the lipoprotein profile.[130–133] The potential psychological impact of estrogens is not well understood, but mood lability or increased libido may result.[134, 135]

When a uterus is present, progestins are employed to protect against the eventual induction of endometrial hyperplasia or carcinoma by unopposed estrogen treatment.[136, 137] Progestins may affect other processes (e.g., bone density, mood, libido, breast maturation, and cardiovascular function), but the overall risk-to-benefit ratio is poorly understood at present.[135, 138–141] There are no conclusive data regarding the role of progestin therapy in the patient lacking a uterus.

Estrogens and progestins can be administered in a variety of regimens. The three major types of estrogen preparations (Table 7–4)[142–144] are (1) physiologic preparations such as 17β-estradiol, (2) synthetic preparations such as ethinyl estradiol, and (3) conjugated natural estrogens such as Premarin. Ethinyl estradiol (EE) is a more potent estrogen than estradiol, even when EE is delivered vaginally.[145, 146] The transdermal 17β-estradiol patch has largely supplanted the need to employ vaginal, injectable, or implantable estrogen preparations.[142] When compared with orally administered estrogen preparations, the transdermal estradiol patch delivers estradiol in a more physiologic pattern with fewer peaks and troughs in the

TABLE 7–4 ••• COMMON COMMERCIALLY AVAILABLE ESTROGEN PREPARATIONS

	Route	Doses
Estradiol	Oral	1, 2* mg
Estradiol	Transdermal	0.05,* 0.10 mg
Ethinyl estradiol	Oral	0.005, 0.010, 0.020* mg
Estropipate (Estrone)	Oral	0.625, 1.25,* 2.5, 5 mg
Conjugated equine estrogens	Oral	0.3, 0.625,* 0.9, 1.25, 2.5 mg

*Minimum dose thought to be effective to prevent osteoporosis.[142–144]

serum concentrations and thus avoids the effects that oral agents have on the liver.[147] The use of the transdermal estradiol patch preserves the physiologic 1:1 estrone-to-estradiol ratio achieved by the ovary. This ratio is elevated greatly by the use of oral preparations, even oral estradiol, because the liver metabolizes and converts orally administered estrogens before their distribution in the circulation.[148] Because transdermal estradiol appears to provide efficacious prophylaxis against osteoporosis and induction of beneficial lipoprotein profiles in postmenopausal women, it is an alternative to oral preparations in the young hypogonadal woman.[143, 149–152] The serum concentrations achieved by the patch can be readily determined and the dose adjusted, if necessary. While many adolescents prefer the transdermal patches to oral medication, some are bothered by local skin irritation secondary to the adhesive and the visible sign of "being different."[129]

Progesterone can be administered orally, rectally, or vaginally; a transdermal preparation is not currently available.[153, 154] Prolonged progesterone administration by vaginal or rectal routes is inconvenient. Progestins differ with regard to their androgenicity and their impact on the endometrium and lipoproteins, but at present there is no clear advantage of one oral progestin over another.[138, 155–158]

With regard to the timing of the initiation of replacement therapy, it should be realized that young adolescents aspire to be like their friends. Failure to develop secondary sexual characteristics and the absence of the "landmark event" of menarche may make affected girls feel different, with secondary effects on self-esteem.[159] Hence, the decision to initiate replacement therapy should be personalized with consideration to the underlying diagnosis (i.e., need for growth hormone treatment) and individual psychosocial outlook. Low-dose estrogen therapy can be initiated with gradual

dosage increase to maximize long-bone growth and lessen the nausea, breast tenderness, and other potential negative side effects that may compromise compliance.[35, 160–162] In this setting, the initiation of progestins can be delayed for several months. Breast development can be induced with 5 to 10 μg ethinyl estradiol daily, 0.3 mg Premarin daily, or transdermal estradiol patches (0.05/mg) biweekly. Once vaginal bleeding occurs or there has been 6 to 12 months of unopposed estrogen treatment, cyclic estrogen-progestin therapy can then be initiated.

Cyclic estrogen-progestin regimens include continuation of the current estrogen treatment (oral or transdermal estrogen) with the addition of 5 to 10 mg medroxyprogesterone (Provera) for 12 to 14 days of each month or oral contraceptives with 20 to 35 μg ethinyl estradiol. The advantage of oral contraceptives is the simplicity of taking one pill per day, but this is more expensive than therapy with separate oral estrogen and progestin preparations. With cyclic menses, the dose of progestin necessary to fully transform the endometrium from proliferative to secretory can be titrated. To simplify this approach, the estrogen preparation is given daily, and the progestin is prescribed for 12 to 14 days, frequently beginning with the first calendar day of the month. If the dose of progestin is adequate, menses should occur on day 11.[163] The patient can be instructed to record the first day of bleeding on a calendar and to continue progestin therapy for 12 to 14 days, even if bleeding occurs. Simple inspection of the calendar will allow the physician to determine whether the dose should be adjusted. If bleeding occurs on or before day 10, then the daily progestin dose can be increased. Extrapolating from data regarding postmenopausal women, it may not be necessary to discontinue estrogen administration for 5 to 7 days each month after completion of the cyclic progestin exposure; this break may induce hot flashes or withdrawal headaches in sensitive individuals.

Side effects may limit compliance. For example, a 14-year-old girl with gonadal dysgenesis who is 61 inches tall and weighs 100 pounds may be "overdosed" by a standard low-dose oral contraceptive preparation containing 35 μg of ethinyl estradiol.[164] Protracted breast tenderness generally improves by decreasing the daily estrogen dose. However, if monotherapy is desired, an oral contraceptive containing 20 μg of ethinyl estradiol and 1 mg of norethindrone (Loestrin 1/20) might be a better choice. If amenorrhea is desired, this combination pill could be administered in a continuous fashion.[165] Most women exposed to a regimen of continuous estrogen and progestin will become amenorrheic after 3 to 9 months. Endometrial biopsies after 9 months of continuous daily oral administration of conjugated equine estrogens (0.625 mg) and medroxyprogesterone acetate (2.5 mg), revealed an inactive endometrium.[166] While there may be no firm evidence to suggest that menses are a physiologic or medical necessity, cyclic menses are regarded as a symbol of a normal female.[158, 166]

Because continuous low-dose transdermal estradiol would likely not prevent ovulation, pregnancy could result without the patient or physician recognizing it acutely because of the preceding amenorrhea. In instances in which pregnancy may be possible, oral contraceptives could be used to provide hormone replacement and contraception simultaneously.

In general, the clinician who is managing hormone replacement therapy should be familiar with a variety of oral contraceptive preparations (e.g., the transdermal estradiol patch; oral estrogen preparations, including conjugated equine estrogens, estradiol, and estrone; and the available progestin preparations) (see Tables 7–2 and 7–3). The clinician should also note, that while the literature initially favored the concept that the cardioprotective benefits of a given hormonal preparation could be assessed by its effects on the lipoprotein profile, new evidence suggests that estrogens and progestins may be cardioprotective even when the lipoprotein profile is altered by progestins at levels that were previously assumed to be deleterious.[167–170] Thus, at the present time, the benefits of estrogen replacement appear to clearly outweigh the risks in most circumstances, even when progestins are employed.

FERTILITY IN HYPOGONADAL FEMALES

The development of techniques for in vitro fertilization has expanded the reproductive options of women with irreversible hypogonadism. Currently, the minimum requirement for becoming pregnant is the presence of a uterus and the willingness to receive donor oocytes.[171] Donor oocytes can be obtained from anonymous volunteers undergoing elective tubal ligation, women undergoing assisted reproductive techniques, and relatives or anonymous volunteers who are willing to undergo controlled ovarian hyperstimulation and retrieval.[172] The relative merits of each of these approaches to obtaining donor oocytes is beyond the scope of this chapter, and all approaches may not be available at every medical center.

To initiate a pregnancy, donor oocytes are inseminated in vitro with the partner's sperm. If fertilization occurs, the woman with hypogonadism undergoes an embryo transfer (ET), in which a small catheter containing one or more embryos is passed transcervically into the fundus of the uterus. The procedure for embryo transfer generally takes less than 5 minutes. The pregnancy rate when three or more embryos are transferred generally exceeds 25% (with a subsequent 20% to 25% miscarriage rate).[173, 174] Because the transfer procedure itself involves minimal surgical risk, the potential problem for the patient is exposure to infectious agents via the receipt of donor oocytes. However, donors generally are screened according to defined criteria, including, but not limited to, a thorough family history and serologic testing for the human immunodeficiency virus (HIV).[175, 176] Unless the donors must be reimbursed for the cost of ovarian stimulation and oocyte retrieval, the majority of the cost of the procedure involves the laboratory charges associated with the handling of gametes and embryo culture.

If the recipient is functionally agonadal, synchronization of donor and recipient cycles is straightforward.[177, 178] Recipients, who should already be receiving hormone replacement therapy, are instructed to continue or begin oral or transdermal estradiol and discontinue all progestin therapy a minimum of 2 weeks before the expected time of oocyte retrieval. To induce a secretory transformation of the endometrium and prepare it for implantation, progesterone administration can begin either at the time the donor receives hCG to initiate the process of ovulation (with retrieval in 36 hours) or at the time of the donor oocyte retrieval.[178] The advantage of this second plan is that progesterone is not begun unless a sufficient quantity of oocytes is available for donation. If progesterone is withheld in the event of insufficient oocytes, the proposed recipient does not have to wait another cycle to receive the next available donor oocytes.

Embryo transfer with donor oocytes and the partner's sperm provides a realistic alternative to adoption. Although it is not possible to match phenotypic characteristics and blood group in oocyte donation as closely as in sperm donation, the prospective parents may be spared the potential legal entanglements of adoption. The prospective mother is able to experience gestation; to control exposure of the fetus to tobacco, alcohol, and illegal drugs; and to breast-feed the infant postpartum. Experiencing pregnancy and childbirth may enhance the self-esteem of these women, who frequently doubt their femininity.

References

1. Ohno S. Overview and summary of Y chromosome/XY antigen/organogenesis. In: Rosenfeld RG, Grumbach MM (eds). Turner Syndrome. New York: Marcel Dekker, 1990, pp 57–63.
2. Sinclair AH, Berta P, Palmer MS, et al. A gene from the human sex-determining region encodes a protein with homology to a conserved DNA-binding motif. Nature 1990; 346:240.
3. Berta P, Hawkins JR, Sinclair AH, et al. Genetic evidence equating SRY and the testis-determining factor. Nature 1990; 348:448–450.
4. Harley VR, Jackson DI, Hextall PJ, et al. DNA binding activity of recombinant SRY from normal males and XY females. Science 1992; 255:453.
5. Simmler M-C, Rouyer F, Vergnaud G, et al. Pseudoautosomal DNA sequences in the pairing region of the human sex chromosomes. Nature 1985; 317:692–7.
6. Goodfellow PJ, Darling SM, Thomas NS, Goodfellow PN. A pseudoautosomal gene in man. Science 1986; 234:740–743.
7. Shapiro LJ. X and Y chromosome organization. The pseudoautosomal region. In: Rosenfeld RG, Grumbach MM (eds). Turner Syndrome. New York: Marcel Dekker, 1990, pp 3–11.
8. Turner HH. A syndrome of infantilism, congenital webbed neck, and cubitus valgus. Endocrinology 1938; 23:566–578.
9. Ford CE, Jones KW, Polani PE, et al. A sex chromosome anomaly in a case of gonadal dysgenesis (Turner's syndrome). Lancet 1959; 1:711.
10. Massa GG, Vanderschueren-Lodeweyckx M. Age and height at diagnosis in Turner syndrome: Influence of parental height. Pediatrics 1991; 88:1148–1152.
11. Lyon AJ, Preece MA, Grant DB. Growth curves for girls with Turner syndrome. Arch Dis Child 1985; 60:932–935.
12. Ranke MB, Blum WF, Haug F, et al. Growth hormone, somatomedin levels and growth regulation in Turner's syndrome. Acta Endocrinol 1987; 116:305–313.
13. Ross JL, Long LM, Loriaux DL, Cutler GB Jr. Growth hormone secretory dynamics in Turner syndrome. J Pediatr 1985; 106:202–206.
14. Albertsson-Wikland K, Rosberg S. Dynamics of growth hormone secretion in girls with Turner syndrome. In: Rosenfeld RG, Grumbach MM (eds). Turner Syndrome. New York: Marcel Dekker, 1990, pp 233–246.
15. Beals RK. Orthopedic aspects of the XO (Turner's) syndrome. Clin Orthop 1973; 97:19–30.
16. Brown DM, Jowsey J, Bradford DS. Osteoporosis in ovarian dysgenesis. J Pediatr 1974; 84:816–820.
17. Ross JL, Long LM, Feuillan P, et al. Normal bone density of the wrist and spine and increased wrist fractures in girls with Turner's syndrome. J Clin Endocrinol Metab 1991; 73:355–359.
18. Naerra RW, Brixen K, Hansen RM, et al. Skeletal size and bone mineral content in Turner's syndrome: relation to karyotype, estrogen treatment, physical fitness, and bone turnover. Calcif Tissue Int 1991; 49:77–83.
19. Watkin PM. Otological disease in Turner's syndrome. J Laryngol Otol 1989; 103:731–738.
20. Sculerati N, Ledesma-Medina J, Finegold DN, Stool SE. Otitis media and hearing loss in Turner syndrome. Arch Otolaryngol Head Neck Surg 1990; 116:704–707.
21. Miller MJ, Geffner ME, Lippe BM, et al. Echocardiography reveals a high incidence of bicuspid aortic valve in Turner syndrome. J Pediatr 1983; 102:47–50.
22. Clark EB. Neck web and congenital heart defects: A pathogenic association in 45 XO Turner syndrome. Teratology 1984; 29:355–361.
23. Lacro RV, Jones KL, Benirschke K. Coarctation of the aorta in Turner syndrome: A pathologic study of fetuses with nuchal cystic hygromas, hydrops fetalis, and female genitalia. Pediatrics 1988; 81:445–451.
24. Mazzanti L, Prandstraller D, Tassinari D, et al. Heart disease in Turner's syndrome. Helv Paediatr Acta 1988; 43:25–21.
25. Lin AE, Lippe BM, Geffner ME, et al. Aortic dilation, dissection, and rupture in patients with Turner syndrome. J Pediatr 1986; 109:820–826.
26. Matthies F, Maciarmid WD, Rallison ML, Tyler FH. Renal anomalies in Turner's syndrome. Clin Pediatr 1971; 10:561–565.
27. Lippe B, Geffner ME, Dietrich RB, et al. Renal malformations in patients with Turner syndrome: Imaging in 141 patients. Pediatrics 1988; 82:852–856.
28. Arulanantham K, Kramer MS, Gryboski JD. The association of inflammatory bowel disease and X chromosomal abnormality. Pediatrics 1980; 66:63–67.
29. Manzione NC, Kram M, Kram E, Das KM. Turner's syndrome and inflammatory bowel disease: A case report with immunologic studies. Am J Gastroenterol 1988; 83:1294–1297.
30. Polychronakos C, Letarte J, Collu R, Ducharme JR. Carbohydrate intolerance in children and adolescents with Turner syndrome. J Pediatr 1980; 96:1009–1014.
31. Simpson JL. Localizing ovarian determinants

through phenotypic-karyotypic deductions. Progress and pitfalls. In: Rosenfeld RG, Grumbach MM (eds). Turner Syndrome. New York: Marcel Dekker, 1990, pp 65–77.

32. Conte FA, Grumbach MM, Kaplan SA, et al. A diphasic pattern of gonadotropin secretion in patients with the syndrome of gonadal dysgenesis. J Clin Endocrinol Metab 1975; 40:670.

33. Mendez HMM, Opitz JM. Noonan syndrome: A review. Am J Med Genet 1985; 21:493–506.

34. Joss E, Zuppinger K. Oxandrolone in girls with Turner's syndrome—a pair-matched controlled study up to final height. Acta Paediatr Scand 1984; 73:674–679.

35. Martínez A, Heinrich JJ, Domené H, et al. Growth in Turner's syndrome: Long term treatment with low dose estradiol. J Clin Endocrinol Metab 1987; 65:253–257.

36. Raiti S, Moore WV, Van Vliet G, Kaplan SL. Growth-stimulating effects of human growth hormone therapy in patients with Turner syndrome. J Pediatr 1986; 109:944–949.

37. Rosenfeld RG, Hintz RL, Johanson AJ, et al. Three-year results of a randomized prospective trial of methionyl human growth hormone and oxandrolone in Turner syndrome. J Pediatr 1988; 113:393–400.

38. Rosenfeld RG, Hintz RL. Growth hormone therapy in Turner syndrome. In: Rosenfeld RG, Grumbach MM (eds). Turner Syndrome. New York: Marcel Dekker, 1990, pp 393–404.

39. Wilton P. Growth hormone treatment in girls with Turner's syndrome. Acta Paediatr Scand 1987; 76:193–200.

40. Takano K, Shizume K, Hibi I, et al. Clinical trials of human growth hormone therapy in Turner syndrome in Japan. In: Rosenfeld RG, Grumbach MM (eds). Turner Syndrome. New York: Marcel Dekker, 1990, pp 421–431.

41. Bergmann P, Valsamis J, Van Perborgh J, et al. Comparative study of the changes in insulin-like growth factor-I, procollagen-III N-terminal extension peptide, bone gla-protein, and bone mineral content in children with Turner's syndrome treated with recombinant growth hormone. J Clin Endocrinol Metab 1990; 71:1461–1467.

42. Wilson DM, Frane JW, Sherman B, et al. Carbohydrate and lipid metabolism in Turner syndrome: Effect of therapy with growth hormone, oxandrolone, and a combination of both. J Pediatr 1988; 112:210–217.

43. Caprio S, Boulware SD, Press M, et al. Effect of growth hormone treatment on hyperinsulinemia associated with Turner syndrome. J Pediatr 1992; 120:238–243.

44. Amiel A, Caprio S, Sherwin RS, et al. Insulin resistance of puberty: A defect restricted to peripheral glucose metabolism. J Clin Endocrinol Metab 1991; 72:277–282.

45. Nielsen J. What more can be done for girls and women with Turner's syndrome and their parents? Acta Pediatr Scand (Suppl) 1989; 356:93.

46. Sylvén L, Hagenfeldt K, Bröndum-Nielsen K, von Schoultz B. Middle-aged women with Turner's syndrome. Medical status, hormonal treatment and social life. Acta Endocrinol 1991; 125:359–365.

47. Nielsen J. Mental aspects of Turner syndrome and the importance of information and Turner contact groups. In: Rosenfeld RG, Grumbach MM (eds). Turner Syndrome. New York: Marcel Dekker, 1990, pp 451–467.

48. Berch DB. Psychological aspects of Turner syndrome. Adolesc Pediatr Gynecol 1989; 2:175.

49. Aran O, Galatzer A, Kauli R, et al. Social, educational and vocational status of 48 young adult females with gonadal dysgenesis. Clin Endocrinol 1991; 36:405–410.

50. Orten JL. Coming up short: The physical, cognitive, and social effects of Turner's syndrome. Health Social Work 1990; 15:100–106.

51. Aranoff GS, Morishima A. XO/XY mosaicism in delayed puberty. J Adolesc Health Care 1988; 9:501.

52. Wallace TM, Levin HS. Mixed gonadal dysgenesis. Arch Pathol Lab Med 1990; 114:679–688.

53. Chang HJ, Clark RD, Bachman H. The phenotype of 45,X/46,XY mosaicism: An analysis of 92 prenatally diagnosed cases. Am J Hum Genet 1990; 46:156–167.

54. Roach DJ, Tho SPT, Plouffe L, McDonough PG. Asymmetric gonadal dysgenesis in a 46,XY individual. Adolesc Pediatr Gynecol 1988; 1:129.

55. Müller J, Skakkebaek NE. Gonadal malignancy in individuals with sex chromosome anomalies. Birth Defects 1991; 26:247–255.

56. Olsen MM, Caldamone AA, Jackson CL, Zinn A. Gonadoblastoma in infancy: Indications for early gonadectomy in 46XY gonadal dysgenesis. J Pediatr Surg 1988; 23:270.

57. Rutgers JL. Advances in the pathology of intersex conditions. Hum Pathol 1991; 22:884–891.

58. Sully RE. Gonadoblastoma. A review of 73 cases. Cancer 1970; 25:1340.

59. Müller J, Skakkebaek NE, Ritzén M, et al. Carcinoma in situ of the testis in children with 45,X/46,XY gonadal dysgenesis. J Pediatr 1985; 106:431.

60. Chapman WHH, Plymyer MR, Dresner ML. Gonadoblastoma in an anatomically normal man: A case report and literature review. J Urol 1990; 144:1472.

61. Disteche CM, Casanova M, Saal H, et al. Small deletions of the short arm of the Y chromosome in 46,XY females. Proc Natl Acad Sci 1986; 83:7841.

62. Levilliers J, Quack B, Weissenbach J, Petit C. Exchange of terminal portions of X- and Y-chromosomal short arms in human XY females. Proc Natl Acad Sci 1989; 86:2296–2300.

63. Page DC, Fisher EMC, McGillivray B, Brown LG. Additional deletions in sex-determining region of human Y chromosome resolves paradox of X,t(Y;22) female. Nature 1990; 346:279–281.

64. Jäger RJ, Anvret M, Hall K, Scherer G. A human XY female with a frame shift mutation in the candidate testis-determining gene SRY. Nature 1990; 348:452.

65. Berkovitz GD, Fechner PY, Zacur HW, et al. Clinical and pathologic spectrum of 46,XY gonadal dysgenesis: Its relevance to the understanding of sex differentiation. Medicine (Baltimore) 1991; 70:375–383.

66. Scully RE. Gonadal pathology of genetically determined diseases. In: Kraus FT, Damjanov I, Kaufman N (eds). Pathology of Reproductive Failure. Baltimore: Williams & Wilkins, 1991, pp 257–285.

67. de S Nazareth HR, Farah LMS, Cunha AJB, Vieira FJPB. Pure gonadal dysgenesis (type XX). Hum Genet 1977; 37:117–120.

68. Ramsay M, Bernstein R, Zwane E, et al. XX true hermaphroditism in Southern African Blacks: An enigma of primary sexual differentiation. Am J Hum Genet 1988; 43:4.

69. Pang S, Wallace MA, Hofman L, et al. Worldwide experience in newborn screening for classical congenital adrenal hyperplasia due to 21-hydroxylase deficiency. Pediatrics 1988; 81:866.

70. Speiser PW, Dupont B, Rubenstein P, et al. High frequency of nonclassical steroid 21-hydroxylase deficiency. Am J Hum Genet 1985; 37:650–667.

71. Thilen A, Larsson A. Congenital adrenal hyperplasia in Sweden 1969–1986. Acta Pediatr Scand 1990; 79:168–175.

72. Morel Y, Miller WL. Clinical and molecular genetics of congenital adrenal hyperplasia due to 21-hydroxylase deficiency. In: Harris H, Hirschhorn K (eds). Advances in Human Genetics. New York: Plenum Press, 1991, pp 1–68.

73. Wolff PB, Wilbois RP, Weldon VV, et al. Posterior fusion without clitoromegaly in a female with partial 21-hydroxylase deficiency. J Pediatr 1977; 91:951.

74. Marshall WN, Lightner ES. Congenital adrenal hyperplasia presenting with labial fusion without clitoromegaly. Pediatrics 1980; 66:312.

75. Dupont B, Oberfield SE, Smithwick ER, et al. Close genetic linkage between HLA and congenital adrenal hyperplasia (21-hydroxylase deficiency). Lancet 1977; 2:1309.

76. Yu CY, Campbell RD, Porter RR. A structural model for the location of the Rodgers and the Chiodo antigenic determinants and their correlation with the human complement component C4A/C4B isotypes. Immunogenetics 1988; 27:399–405.

77. White PC, New MI, Dupont B. Structure of human steroid 21-hydroxylase genes. Proc Natl Acad Sci 1986; 83:5111–5115.

78. Morel Y, Andre J, Uring-Lambert B, et al. Rearrangements and point mutations of P450c21 genes are distinguished by five restriction endonuclease haplotypes identified by a new probing strategy in 57 families with congenital adrenal hyperplasia. J Clin Invest 1989; 83:527.

79. Mornet E, Crete P, Kutenn F, et al. Distribution of deletions and seven point mutations on CYP21B genes in three clinical forms of steroid 21-hydroxylase deficiency. Am J Hum Genet 1991; 48:79.

80. Strachan T, White PC. Molecular pathology of steroid 21-hydroxylase deficiency. J Steroid Biochem Mol Biol 1991; 40:537.

81. Higashi Y, Tanae A, Inoue H, et al. Aberrant splicing and missense mutations cause steroid 21-hydroxylase [P-450(C21)] deficiency in humans: possible gene conversion products. Proc Natl Acad Sci 1988; 85:7486–7490.

82. Speiser PW, Laforgia N, Kato K, et al. First trimester prenatal treatment and molecular genetic diagnosis of congenital adrenal hyperplasia (21-hydroxylase deficiency). J Clin Endocrinol Metab 1990; 70:838.

83. Migeon CJ. Comments about the need for prenatal treatment of congenital adrenal hyperplasia due to 21-hydroxylase deficiency. Editorial. J Clin Endocrinol Metab 1990; 70:836.

84. Yanagibashi K, Haniu M, Shively JE, et al. The synthesis of aldosterone by the adrenal cortex. J Biol Chem 1986; 261:3556–3562.

85. Zadik Z, Kahana L, Kaufman H, et al. Salt loss in hypertensive form of congenital adrenal hyperplasia (11β-hydroxylation deficiency). J Clin Endocrinol Metab 1984; 58:384.

86. Pang S, Levine LS, Lorenzen F, et al. Hormonal studies in obligate heterozygotes and siblings of patients with 11β-hydroxylase deficiency congenital adrenal hyperplasia. J Clin Endocrinol Metab 1980; 50:586–589.

87. Cara JF, Moshang T Jr, Bongiovanni AM, et al. Elevated 17-hydroxyprogesterone and testosterone in a newborn with 3-beta-hydroxysteroid dehydrogenase deficiency. N Engl J Med 1985; 313:618.

88. Zuber MX, Simpson ER, Waterman MR. Expression of bovine 17α-hydroxylase cytochrome P450 cDNA in nonsteroidogenic (COS 1) cells. Science 1986; 234:1258.

89. Biglieri EG, Herron MA, Brust N. 17α-hydroxylase deficiency in men. J Clin Invest 1966; 45:1946.

90. Yanase T, Simpson ER, Waterman MR. 17α-hydroxylase/17,20-lyase deficiency: From clinical investigation to molecular definition. Endocr Rev 1991; 12:91–108.

91. Goebelsmann U, Zachmann M, Davajan V, et al. Male pseudohermaphroditism consistent with 17,20-desmolase deficiency. Gynecol Invest 1976; 7:138–156.

92. Yanase T, Kagimoto M, Matsui N, et al. Combined 17α-hydroxylase/17,20-lyase deficiency due to a stop codon in the N-terminal region of 17α-hydroxylase cytochrome P450. Mol Cell Endocrinol 1988; 59:249.

93. Kagimoto K, Waterman MR, Kagimoto M, et al. Identification of a common molecular basis for combined 17α-hydroxylase/17,20-lyase deficiency in two Mennonite families. Hum Genet 1989; 82:285.

94. Yanase T, Sanders D, Shibata A, et al. Combined 17α-hydroxylase/17,20 lyase deficiency due to a 7 base pair duplication in the N-terminal region of the cytochrome P450c17α (CYP17) gene. J Clin Endocrinol Metab 1990; 70:1325.

95. Kenny FM, Preeyasombat C, Migeon CJ. Cortisol production rate II. Normal infants, children, and adults. Pediatrics 1966; 37:34.

96. Linder BL, Esteban NV, Yergey AL, et al. Cortisol production rate in childhood and adolescence. J Pediatr 1990; 117:892–896.

97. Johnson L, George FW, Neaves WB, et al. Characterization of the testicular abnormality in 5α-reductase deficiency. J Clin Endocrinol Metab 1986; 63:1091–1099.

98. Imperato-McGinley J, Guerrero L, Gautier T, Peterson RE. Steroid 5α-reductase deficiency in man: An inherited form of male pseudohermaphroditism. Science 1974; 186:1213–1215.

99. Akgun S, Ertel NH, Imperato-McGinley J, et al. Familial male pseudohermaphroditism due to 5-alpha-reductase deficiency in a Turkish village. Am J Med 1986; 81:267–274.

100. Imperato-McGinley J, Miller M, Wilson JD, et al. A cluster of male pseudohermaphrodites with 5α-reductase deficiency in Papua New Guinea. Clin Endocrinol 1991; 34:293–298.

101. Herdt GH, Davidson J. The Sambia "Turnim-Man": Sociocultural and clinical aspects of gender formation in male pseudohermaphrodites with 5-alpha-reductase deficiency in Papua New Guinea. Arch Sex Behav 1988; 17:33–56.

102. Imperato-McGinley J, Gautier T, Pichardo M, Shackleton C. The diagnosis of 5α-reductase deficiency in infancy. J Clin Endocrinol Metab 1986; 63:1313–1318.

103. Andersson S, Berman DM, Jenkins EP, Russell DW. Deletion of steroid 5α-reductase gene in male pseudohermaphroditism. Nature 1991; 354:159–161.

104. Millán M, Audí L, Martinez-Mora J, et al. 17-ketosteroid reductase deficiency in an adult patient without gynecomastia but with female psychosexual orientation. Acta Endocrinol 1983; 102:633–640.

105. Eckstein B, Cohen S, Farkas A, Rosler A. The nature of the defect in familial male pseudohermaphroditism in Arabs of Gaza. J Clin Endocrinol Metab 1989; 68:477–485.

106. Pang S, Softness B, Sweeney WJ III, New MI. Hirsutism, polycystic ovarian disease, and ovarian 17-ketosteroid reductase deficiency. N Engl J Med 1987; 316:1295–1301.

107. Gross DJ, Landau H, Kohn G, et al. Male pseudohermaphroditism due to 17β-hydroxysteroid dehydrogenase deficiency: Gender reassignment in early infancy. Acta Endocrinol 1986; 112:238–246.

108. Griffin JE. Androgen resistance—the clinical and molecular spectrum. N Engl J Med 1992; 326:611–618.

109. O'Malley B. The steroid receptor superfamily: More excitement predicted for the future. Mol Endocrinol 1990; 4:363–369.

110. Brown CJ, Goss SJ, Lubahn DB, et al. Androgen receptor locus on the human X chromosome: Regional localization to Xq11-12 and description of a DNA polymorphism. Am J Hum Genet 1989; 44:264–269.

111. Imperato-McGinley J, Ip NY, Gautier T, et al. DNA linkage analysis and studies of the androgen receptor gene in a large kindred with complete androgen insensitivity. Am J Med Genet 1990; 36:104–108.

112. Evans RM, Hollenberg SM. Zinc fingers: Guilt by association. Cell 1988; 52:1–3.

113. Quigley CA, Friedman KJ, Johnson A, et al. Complete deletion of the androgen receptor gene: Definition of the null phenotype of the androgen insensitivity syndrome and determination of carrier status. J Clin Endocrinol Metab 1992; 74:927–933.

114. Marcelli M, Tilley WD, Wilson CM, et al. Definition of the human androgen receptor gene structure permits the identification of mutations that cause androgen resistance: Premature termination of the receptor protein at amino acid residue 588 causes complete androgen resistance. Mol Endocrinol 1990; 4:1105–1116.

115. Ris-Stalpers C, Trifiro MA, Kuiper GGJM, et al. Substitution of aspartic acid-686 by histidine or asparagine in the human androgen receptor leads to a functionally inactive protein with altered hormone-binding characteristics. Mol Endocrinol 1991; 5:1562–1569.

116. Marcelli M, Zoppi S, Grino PB, et al. A mutation in the DNA-binding domain of the androgen receptor gene causes complete testicular feminization in a patient with receptor-positive androgen resistance. J Clin Invest 1991; 87:1123–1126.

117. Zoppi S, Marcelli M, Deslypere J-P, et al. Amino acid substitutions in the DNA-binding domain of the human androgen receptor are a frequent cause of receptor-binding positive androgen resistance. Mol Endocrinol 1992; 6:409–415.

118. Guerrier D, Tran D, Vanderwinden JM, et al. The persistent müllerian duct syndrome: A molecular approach. J Clin Endocrinol Metab 1989; 68:46–52.

119. Knebelmann B, Boussin L, Guerrier D, et al. Anti-müllerian hormone Bruxelles: A nonsense mutation associated with the persistent müllerian duct syndrome. Proc Natl Acad Sci 1991; 88:3767–3771.

120. Baker SW. Psychological management of intersex children. Pediatr Adolesc Endocrinol 1981; 8:261–269.

121. Bale PM, Howard NJ, Wright JE. Male pseudohermaphroditism in XY children with female phenotype. Pediatr Pathol 1992; 12:29–49.

122. Lee PA, Brown TR, LaTorre HA. Diagnosis of the partial androgen insensitivity syndrome during infancy. JAMA 1986; 255:2207–2209.

123. Linder BL, Cassorla F. Short stature: Etiology, diagnosis and treatment. JAMA 1988; 260:3171–3175.

124. Frasier SD, Lippe BM. Clinical review 11: The rational use of growth hormone during childhood. J Clin Endocrinol Metab 1990; 71:269–273.

125. Crawford JD. Treatment of tall girls with estrogen. Pediatrics 1978; 62:1189–1195.

126. Boepple PA, Mansfield MJ, Link K, et al. Impact of sex steroid and their suppression on skeletal growth and maturation. Am J Physiol 1988; 255:E559–E566.

127. Bourguignon J-P. Linear growth as a function of age at onset of puberty and sex steroid dosage: Therapeutic implications. Endocr Rev 1988; 9:467–488.

128. Berga SL, Girton LG. The psychoneuroendocrinology of functional hypothalamic amenorrhea. Psychiatr Clin North Am 1989; 12:105–116.

129. Emans SJ, Goldstein DP. Pediatric and Adolescent Gynecology. 3rd ed. Boston: Little, Brown, 1990, pp 176–182.

130. Bush TL, Barrett-Connor E, Cowan LD, et al. Cardiovascular mortality and noncontraceptive use of estrogen in women: Results from the Lipid Research Clinics Program Follow-up Study. Circulation 1987; 75:1102–1109.

131. Stampfer MJ, Colditz GA, Willett WC, et al. Postmenopausal estrogen therapy and cardiovascular disease. N Engl J Med 1991; 325:756–762.

132. Ross RK, Paganini-Hill A, Mack TM, Henderson BE. Cardiovascular benefits of estrogen replacement therapy. Am J Obstet Gynecol 1989; 160:1301–1306.

133. Thorneycroft IH. The role of estrogen replacement therapy in the prevention of osteoporosis. Am J Obstet Gynecol 1989; 160:1306–1310.

134. Warren MP, Brooks-Gunn J. Mood and behavior at adolescence: Evidence for hormonal factors. J Clin Endocrinol Metab 1989; 69:77–83.

135. Sherwin BB. The impact of different doses of estrogen and progestin on mood and sexual behavior in postmenopausal women. J Clin Endocrinol Metab 1991; 72:336–343.

136. Nachtigall LE, Nachtigall RH, Nachtigall RD, Beckman EF. Estrogen replacement therapy. II. A prospective study in the relationship to carcinoma and cardiovascular and metabolic problems. Obstet Gynecol 1979; 54:74–79.

137. Whitehead MI, Townsend PT, Pryse-Davies J, et al. Effects of estrogens and progestins on the biochemistry and morphology of the postmenopausal endometrium. N Engl J Med 1981; 305:1599–1605.

138. Hirvonen E, Malkonen M, Manninen V. Effects of different progestogens on lipoproteins during postmenopausal replacement therapy. N Engl J Med 1981; 304:560–563.

139. Mandel FP, Davidson BJ, Erlik Y, Judd HL, Meldrum DR. Effects of progestins on bone metabolism in postmenopausal women. J Reprod Med 1982; 27:511–514.

140. Dennerstein L, Burrows G. Psychological effects of progestogens in the post-menopausal years. Maturitas 1986; 8:101–106.

141. Henderson BE, Ross RK, Lobo RA, et al. Re-evaluating the role of progestogen therapy after the menopause. Fertil Steril 1988; 49(suppl):9S–15S.

142. Miller-Bass K, Adashi EY. Current status and future prospects of transdermal estrogen replacement therapy. Fertil Steril 1990; 53:961–974.

143. Stevenson JC, Cust MP, Gangar KF, et al. Effects of transdermal versus oral hormone replacement therapy on bone density in spine and proximal femur in postmenopausal women. Lancet 1990; 335:265–269.

144. Horsman A, Jones M, Francis R, Nordin C. The effect of estrogen dose on postmenopausal bone loss. N Engl J Med 1983; 309:1405–1407.

145. Mashchak CA, Lobo RA, Dozono-Takano R, et al. Comparison of pharmacodynamic properties of various estrogen formulations. Am J Obstet Gynecol 1982; 144:511–518.

146. Goebelsmann U, Mashchak CA, Mishell DR Jr. Comparison of hepatic impact of oral and vaginal administration of ethinyl estradiol. Am J Obstet Gynecol 1985; 151:868–877.

147. Powers MS, Schenkel L, Darley PE, et al. Pharmacokinetics and pharmacodynamics of transdermal dosage forms of 17β-estradiol: Comparison with conventional oral estrogens used for hormone replacement. Am J Obstet Gynecol 1985; 152:1099–1106.

148. Steingold KA, Matt DW, DeZiegler D, et al. Comparison of transdermal to oral estradiol administration on hormonal and hepatic parameters in women with premature ovarian failure. J Clin Endocrinol Metab 1991; 73:275–280.

149. Riis BJ, Thomsen K, Strom V, Christiansen C. The effect of percutaneous estradiol and natural progesterone on postmenopausal bone loss. Am J Obstet Gynecol 1987; 156:61–65.

150. Stanczyk FZ, Shoupe D, Nunez V, et al. A randomized comparison of nonoral estradiol delivery in postmenopausal women. Am J Obstet Gynecol 1988; 159:1540–1546.

151. Jensen J, Riis BJ, Strom V, et al. Long-term effects of percutaneous estrogens and oral progesterone on serum lipoproteins in postmenopausal women. Am J Obstet Gynecol 1987; 156:66–71.

152. Moorjani S, Dupont A, Labrie F, et al. Changes in plasma lipoprotein and apolipoprotein composition in relation to oral versus percutaneous administration of estrogen alone or in cyclic association with utrogestan in menopausal women. J Clin Endocrinol Metab 1991; 73:373–379.

153. Padwick MB, Endacott J, Matson C, Whitehead MI. Absorption and metabolism of oral progesterone when administered twice daily. Fertil Steril 1986; 46:402–407.

154. Nillius SJ, Johansson EDB. Plasma levels of progesterone after vaginal, rectal, or intramuscular administration of progesterone. Am J Obstet Gynecol 1971; 110:470–477.

155. Lobo RA. The androgenicity of progestational agents. Int J Fertil 1988; 33(suppl):6–12.

156. King RJB, Whitehead MI. Assessment of the potency of orally administered progestins in women. Fertil Steril 1986; 46:1062–1066.

157. Christiansen C, Riis BJ. 17β-estradiol and continuous norethisterone: A unique treatment for established osteoporosis in elderly women. J Clin Endocrinol Metab 1990; 71:836–841.

158. Jensen J, Riis BJ, Strom V, Christiansen C. Continuous oestrogen-progestogen treatment and serum lipoproteins in postmenopausal women. Br J Obstet Gynaecol 1987; 94:130–135.

159. Tesch L-G. Turner syndrome: A personal perspective. Adolesc Pediatr Gynecol 1989; 2:186–188.

160. Ross JL, Cassorla FG, Skerda MC, et al. A preliminary study of the effect of estrogen dose on growth in Turner's syndrome. N Engl J Med 1983; 309:1104–1106.

161. Attie KM, Ramirez NR, Conte FA, et al. The pubertal growth spurt in eight patients with true precocious puberty and growth hormone deficiency: Evidence for a direct role of sex steroids. J Clin Endocrinol Metab 1990; 71:975–983.

162. Ho KY, Evans WS, Blizzard RM, et al. Effects of sex and age on the 24-hour profile of growth hormone secretion in man: Importance of endogenous estradiol concentrations. J Clin Endocrinol Metab 1987; 64:51–58.

163. Padwick ML, Pryse-Davies J, Whitehead MI. A simple method for determining the optimal dosage of progestin in postmenopausal women receiving estrogens. N Engl J Med 1986; 315:930–934.

164. Goldzieher JW, Brody SA. Pharmacokinetics of ethinyl estradiol and mestranol. Am J Obstet Gynecol 1990; 163:2114–2119.

165. Williams SR, Frenchek B, Speroff T, Speroff L. A study of combined continuous ethinyl estradiol and norethindrone acetate for postmenopausal hormone replacement. Am J Obstet Gynecol 1990; 162:438–446.

166. Hammarback S, Backstrom T, Holst J, et al. Cyclical mood changes as in the premenstrual tension syndrome during sequential estrogen-Progestagen postmenopausal replacement therapy. Acta Obstet Gynecol Scand 1985; 64:393–397.

167. Clarkson TB, Adams MR, Kaplan JR, et al. From menarche to menopause: Coronary artery atherosclerosis and protection in cynomolgus monkeys. Am J Obstet Gynecol 1989; 160:1280–1285.

168. Mishell DR Jr. Symposium: Optimizing contraceptive decisions: Clinical implications of the triphasic randomized clinical trial. Correcting misconceptions about oral contraceptives. Am J Obstet Gynecol 1989; 161:1385–1389.

169. Clarkson TB, Shively CA, Morgan TM, et al. Oral contraceptives and coronary artery atherosclerosis of cynomolgus monkeys. Obstet Gynecol 1990; 75:217–222.

170. Adams MR, Clarkson TB, Koritnik DR, Nash HA. Contraceptive steroids and coronary artery atherosclerosis in cynomolgus macaques. Fertil Steril 1987; 47:1010–1018.

171. Mahlstedt PP, Greenfeld DA. Assisted reproductive technology with donor gametes: The need for patient preparation. Fertil Steril 1989; 52:908–914.

172. Frydman R, Bydlowski M, Letur-Konirsch H, et al. A protocol for satisfying the ethical issues raised by oocyte donation: The free, anonymous, and fertile donors. Fertil Steril 1990; 53:666–672.

173. Serhal PF, Craft IL. Oocyte donation in 61 patients. Lancet 1989; I:1185–1187.

174. Sauer MV, Paulson RJ, Lobo RA. A preliminary report on oocyte donation extending reproductive potential to women over 40. N Engl J Med 1990; 323:1157–1160.

175. The American Fertility Society. New guidelines for

the use of semen donor insemination: 1990. Fertil Steril 1990; 53(suppl):1S–13S.

176. The American Fertility Society. Revised minimum standards for in vitro fertilization, gamete intrafallopian transfer, and related procedures. Fertil Steril 1990; 53:225–226.

177. Navot D, Laufer N, Kopolovic J, et al. Artificially induced endometrial cycles and establishment of pregnancies in the absence of ovaries. N Engl J Med 1986; 314:806–811.

178. Navot D, Bergh PA, Williams M, et al. An insight into early reproductive processes through the in vivo model of ovum donation. J Clin Endocrinol Metab 1991; 72:408–414.

CHAPTER 8

○○○ # Nutrition, Growth, and Development

GILBERT B. FORBES

The importance of proper nutrition cannot be overstated, as ultimately the functioning of all physicochemical processes is dependent on an adequate supply of dietary nutrients. Although there is some latitude in the amounts needed, a minimum requirement for each nutrient does exist, and excessive amounts of some nutrients can be harmful. The body can function for a time without food, albeit at less than full capacity, but a more or less continuous supply of nutrients is needed to provide those ingredients that cannot be manufactured within: essential amino acids, vitamins, minerals, and energy. In some respects human beings are more at risk than other mammals, some of whom can synthesize certain vitamins or, with the help of intestinal bacteria, can thrive without a dietary supply of essential amino acids. Hibernating animals conserve energy by reducing metabolic rate.

Growth is one of the prime indicators of nutritional adequacy; indeed, growth rate can serve as a bioassay of nutritional status. For many years this has been the standard practice of nutritionists, who have used the growth rate of animals to test the adequacy of various diets. For instance, the observation many years ago that highly purified diets did not provide normal growth in rats led to a search for missing ingredients, resulting in the discovery of some vitamins. The biologic value of various dietary proteins was also established using this technique.

Growth requires energy plus an adequate supply of all essential nutrients; hence, there is no single dietary "growth factor." The effect of a deficiency of one essential nutrient, or of dietary energy, cannot be rectified by giving an excess of the others. In children in underdeveloped areas of the world, growth faltering is known to occur with diets low in vitamin A, zinc, vitamin D, or protein as well as with diets low in dietary energy. Even chloride deficiency can cause growth failure. However, diets in developed countries usually provide sufficient essential nutrients because of the wide variety of foods available, the plentiful supplies of milk, and the fact that a number of foods are fortified with vitamins and minerals. The one exception is iron, for it is known that some adolescents are deficient in this element. Thus, in growth-deficient individuals, the energy content of the diet is most frequently at fault.

Figure 8–1 illustrates the importance of growth rate as an indicator of nutrient deficiency (in this case, vitamin A). Growth rate is exceeded in sensitivity only by female reproductive performance, and thus it will reflect milder deficiency states than can be detected by other techniques.[1]

The great sensitivity of the growth rate to a reduction in energy intake means that growth per se is an integral, inescapable part of adolescent life. Insufficient food has a negative impact on the entire adolescent functional unit (i.e., metabolic rate, activity level, physical performance, and sexual maturation), as well as on growth rate. If energy intake is inade-

The research was supported by National Institutes of Health grant HD18454.

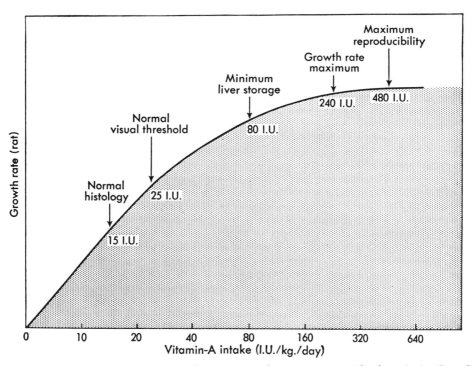

FIGURE 8–1 ••• Growth rate of rats as a function of vitamin A intake—comparison with other criteria. (From Bessey OA. Evaluation of nutritive status by chemical and other methods. In: Scheinberg IH [ed]. Infant Metabolism. New York: Macmillan, 1956.)

quate, growth will suffer along with other bodily functions.

The growing body also responds to energy surfeit. Deliberate overfeeding of adults and adolescents results in weight gain. About two thirds of this gain is fat, and about one third is lean; of interest is the finding that the weight increment per unit of excess food consumed is the same for women as it is for men.[2] Obese children, who can achieve such a state only via a positive energy balance, are apt to be taller and to have a larger lean weight and larger bones than their thinner peers. Longitudinal studies of children who became obese during childhood show that most of them had had an increase in height percentile status once they had become obese; this change in height status occurred either coincident with the increase in weight or sometime thereafter, but never before.[3]

The plane of nutrition also has an effect on sexual maturation. Girls who have an early menarche tend to be heavier and taller at menarche than their premenarchal age-matched peers, and those with a late menarche tend to be lighter than their postmenarchal age-matched peers, though stature is comparable.

Thus, early maturers have an elevated body mass index (BMI) (weight/height[2]), and late maturers have a smaller BMI than their age-matched peers. A plot of the data provided by Zacharias et al.[4] shows a progressive fall in BMI with age at menarche, in distinct contrast to the progressive increase in BMI that occurs normally at this time of life (Fig. 8–2). However, it should be noted that there is wide variation in menarchal weight; of the 600 subjects studied by Zacharias et al., the heaviest girl was 2½ times the weight of the lightest girl at time of menarche; the coefficient of variation was 15%. Using data from several surveys, Garn and LaVelle[5] have documented the fact that a body weight of less than the proclaimed "critical value" of 47 kg is not necessarily an impediment to menarche or conception.

Two lines of evidence support the concept that nutrition has an effect on sexual maturation in humans. As noted earlier, obese girls tend to have an early menarche, and Stark et al.[6] have shown that early-maturing girls are already overweight by the age of 7 years. Girls living in underdeveloped countries tend to have a later menarche. Thus, overnutrition

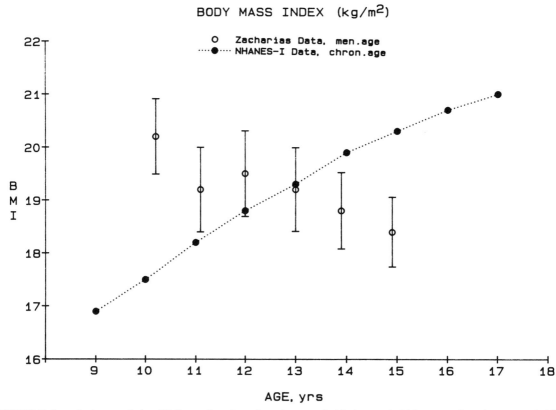

BODY MASS INDEX (kg/m²)

FIGURE 8–2 ••• Body mass index (BMI) as a function of age in normal girls (● . . .●). 50th percentile values compiled by Cronk and Roche[16] from data obtained during the National Health and Nutrition Survey. Vertical bars show means and standard errors of BMI at menarche for girls of different menarchal age. (Data from Zacharias L, Rand WM, Wurtman RJ. A prospective study of sexual development and growth in American girls: The statistics of menarche. Obstet Gynecol Surv 1976; 31:325.)

speeds up the maturation process, and undernutrition slows it. Of interest is the demonstration of compromised ovarian function in young women who undergo small degrees of weight reduction.[7]

Underfed animals experience delayed puberty. Young female rats who are underfed have reduced levels of pituitary gonadotropin-releasing hormone (GnRH), as well as fewer GnRH receptors, so that gonadotropin production and/or release is subnormal, and vaginal opening does not occur. This situation is promptly reversed by adequate food: normal hormonal function is restored, and sexual maturation takes place.[8]

It has been demonstrated that undernutrition diminishes the production of somatomedins, important facilitators of growth, produced in the liver by the action of growth hormone. Reduced plasma levels of somatomedins have been recorded in infants with kwashiorkor, and even brief periods of undernutrition in adults result in a striking reduction

in plasma levels of somatomedins, which are promptly restored by adequate food intake.[9] Deliberate overfeeding is accompanied by a small increase in levels of somatomedins.[10] Thus, nutrition can influence hormones as well as somatic growth.

Several changes have occurred in the growth of children and adolescents since the nineteenth century. Secular increases in height and weight have been noted in all industrialized societies for which reliable data exist. Female adolescents are taller and heavier than their age-matched peers of a century ago, and puberty (as judged by menarchal age) is occurring at an earlier age. These changes accompanied the rise of modern nutritional science, and most observers favor the hypothesis that improved nutrition is responsible for such changes. However, two additional factors may have played a role: the decline in chronic infection, and the phenomenon of hybrid vigor.

All of the preceding information must be

viewed in the context of heredity. At all ages past infancy there is a reasonable correlation between the heights of children and the heights of their parents. Studies of twins and adoptees show that inheritance is a major factor influencing weight, stature, BMI, lean weight, and body fat.[11, 12]

ASSESSMENT OF GROWTH IN HEIGHT AND WEIGHT

The most commonly used height and weight charts are those based on data collected by the National Committee on Health Statistics on thousands of white children in the United States (Fig. 8–3). Percentile plots are preferred over means and standard deviations, because frequency distributions are often skewed. Although black children and adolescents tend to be a bit taller and Hispanics and Orientals somewhat shorter than whites, these charts have proven satisfactory.* Every effort should be made to make an accurate measurement of height and weight and to record age to the nearest month. The best instrument for measuring height is the Holtain stadiometer,† which consists of a fixed vertical member attached to the wall on which rides a movable headboard maintained in a horizontal position, a direct reading dial, and a footboard with a heel plate. Unfortunately, however, this instrument is expensive. A satisfactory substitute is a meter stick attached to the wall next to a bare floor, with a movable headboard positioned perpendicular to the wall. The sliding-stick devices attached to platform scales are not accurate and should not be used (see Fig. 2–5).

The subject must remove his or her shoes and stand erect next to the measuring device in the nonlordotic position, with the eyes and ears forming a horizontal plane; some observers prefer to give a gentle upward tug on the chin. It should be remembered that people are often 1 to 2 cm shorter in the late afternoon than in the early morning. Weight should be determined with the subject dressed in light indoor clothing and the shoes removed.

Older children and adolescents may want to know how tall they will be when fully grown; this is especially true of undergrown boys and tall girls. There are two common techniques for making such estimates. The simplest is to average the parents' heights, and then add 6.5 cm for boys and subtract 6.5 cm for girls. Another method is to obtain a roentgenogram of the wrist and enter bone age and present stature into the prediction tables provided by Bayley and Pinneau.[14]

CHANGES IN BODY COMPOSITION DURING GROWTH

A number of organ systems comprise body weight. Modern technology has made it possible to estimate several components of the body in a relatively nontraumatic manner. The growth of these components during adolescence differs somewhat from the growth of the body as a whole.

Methods for Estimating Body Composition

The weight of body fluids (plasma volume, total red cell mass, extracellular fluid volume, total body water) is estimated by the principle of isotopic dilution.

Lean body mass (LBM) (or, as some prefer, fat-free mass) can be estimated in several ways, based on the fact that neither electrolytes nor water are bound by neutral fat, and by the fact that LBM has a different density than fat. Hence, a measurement of total body water or total body potassium can yield an estimate of LBM; body fat is weight minus LBM. Measurement of body density yields an estimate of the percentage of body fat and LBM. Urine creatinine excretion is used as an index of muscle mass.

Estimates of skeletal mass are made from the size and density of various bones, using the degree of attenuation of monoenergetic gamma rays; this is referred to as *single-* or *dual-photon absorptiometry*. The cross-sectional area of the second metacarpal cortex, as read from a plain radiograph, has also been used for this purpose. Computed tomography (CT) and magnetic resonance imaging (MRI) can define the size and shape of various organs, as well as determine muscle mass and body fat.

---

*Tanner and Davies[13] have devised some charts that portray height velocity as a function of age for average adolescents, and for early and late maturers. These charts are available from Serono Laboratories, Inc., 280 Pond St., Randolph, MA 02368.

†Holtain Ltd., Crosswell, Crymmych, Pembrokeshire, U.K.

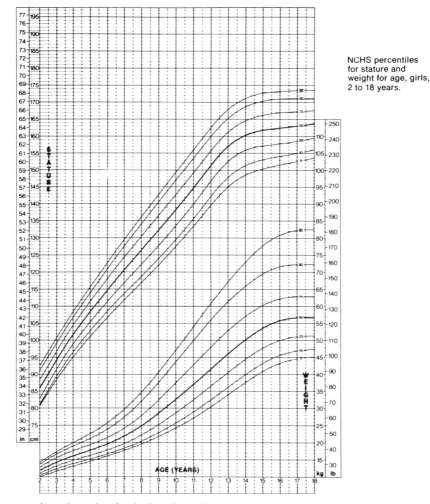

NCHS percentiles for stature and weight for age, girls, 2 to 18 years.

FIGURE 8–3 ••• Height and weight of girls, based on data from the National Center for Health Statistics. (From Moore WH, Jeffries JE. In: Johnson TR, Moore WM, Jeffries JE (eds). Children are Different. Columbus, OH: Ross Laboratories, 1978. Used and reprinted with permission of Ross Laboratories, Columbus, OH 43216, from NCHS Growth Charts, © 1982, Ross Laboratories.)

Two new techniques are currently being studied. Total body conductivity and bioimpedance are used to estimate lean weight. The former measures the perturbation of an electromagnetic field produced by the presence of the subject; the latter measures the resistance to a weak alternating current passed between the hand and the foot.

Most of these techniques are more suitable for the research laboratory; some require expensive instrumentation, and some involve radiation exposure. Details can be found in work reported by Forbes.[2]

Although it does not carry a high degree of precision, anthropometry provides an inexpensive and easily used technique for estimating body fat. The two most commonly used techniques are the measurement of skinfold (actually fatfold) thickness, and various body circumferences.

Because human skin is only 0.5 to 2 mm thick, the subcutaneous fat layer contributes the bulk of the skinfold thickness. The measurement is made by grasping the skin plus subcutaneous tissue between the thumb and forefinger, shaking it gently to exclude underlying muscle, and stretching it just far enough to permit the jaws of a spring-actuated caliper to pinch the tissue. Because the jaws of the caliper compress the tissue, the caliper reading diminishes for a few seconds, and then the dial is read.

The most frequent site of measurement is over the triceps muscle at a point halfway between the shoulder and elbow; other sites are over the biceps, at the inferior tip of the scapula, and at the iliac crest. Individuals with moderately firm subcutaneous tissue and those with very firm tissue that is not easily deformable present something of a problem. In individuals who have recently lost weight, the subcutaneous tissue is often flabby; in the very obese, the tissue thickness may exceed the maximum jaw width (40 mm) of the caliper.

The ratio of abdomen circumference to hip circumference can be used as an index of body fat distribution. There is some evidence to suggest that adults with high ratios have large accumulations of intraabdominal fat and are somewhat more prone to cardiovascular disease and stroke. Forbes[15] has described the changes in this ratio during the adolescent and adult years in normal individuals. It is noteworthy that sex differences first appear during adolescence, with girls having a lower ratio than boys.

The cross-sectional area of arm muscle and bone and of fat can be calculated from measurements of arm circumference and skinfold thickness* (many authors use the term *arm muscle area*, which is incorrect). Although this technique yields reliable results in thin individuals, it may overestimate arm muscle and bone area and thereby underestimate arm fat area in obese individuals.

Finally, it should not be forgotten that the use of relative weight—either percentage weight for height or BMI—while far from perfect, can be useful in evaluating large numbers of individuals. Those with high values almost always have increased body fat, especially girls and women. A nomogram for determining BMI from weight and height is shown in Figure 8–4. This index is age dependent, as shown in Figure 8–2, which depicts the 50th percentile for white children and adolescents who participated in the 1971–1974 National Health and Nutrition Survey.[5] Values for adolescent black females tend to be a little higher (by 1% to 4%) than those for whites. Values for Dutch children and for French children are comparable to those shown in the figure.

Table 8–1 lists the various percentile values for girls as compiled by Cronk and Roche.[16] It is evident that the distributions at all ages

---

*Arm muscle + bone area is $(C - \pi SF)^2/4$, and arm fat area is $\frac{SF}{4}(2C - \pi SF)$, where C is arm circumference and SF is skinfold thickness.

shown are strongly skewed toward higher values. In evaluating data on BMI, it should be kept in mind that body weight is the sum of lean and fat; hence, individuals with a large body frame may have a generous BMI without excess body fat.

Subcutaneous Fat

As stated earlier, the region over the triceps muscle is the most commonly used site for measuring the thickness of skin plus subcutaneous tissue. Measurements at other sites usually yield different values, indicating that the subcutaneous fat mantle does not have a uniform thickness; indeed, CT scans and MRI studies show that a large fraction of total subcutaneous fat in women is located in the hips and thighs. However, the triceps site is easily accessible, and the triceps skinfold thickness does bear a relationship to total body fat content.

Figure 8–5 shows the changes in triceps skinfold thickness during adolescence in white girls who participated in the 1971–1974 National Health and Nutrition Survey. It is apparent that the frequency distributions are strongly skewed toward higher values.

Menarche is an event of considerable physiologic as well as hormonal significance. It has been known for many years that the peak of the height velocity curve occurs just before menarche and that there is a temporal association with changes in basal oxygen consumption, pulse rate, and blood pressure. In addition, data show that the perimenarchal years are accompanied by an array of changes in body composition, skeletal size, distribution of body fat, muscle strength, and urinary hydroxyproline excretion. Indeed, the increase in LBM at this time of life is fully as great as the increase in body fat.[17]

Lean Body Mass and Body Fat

Figure 8–6 shows the time course for body weight, LBM, and body fat (average values) for boys and girls. The developing sex difference in LBM during adolescence is clearly evident; by the end of the second decade of life, the male LBM is roughly equal to female body weight; the male-to-female ratio for LBM is about 1.44:1, in contrast to 1.25:1 for body weight. This is one reason boys are stronger

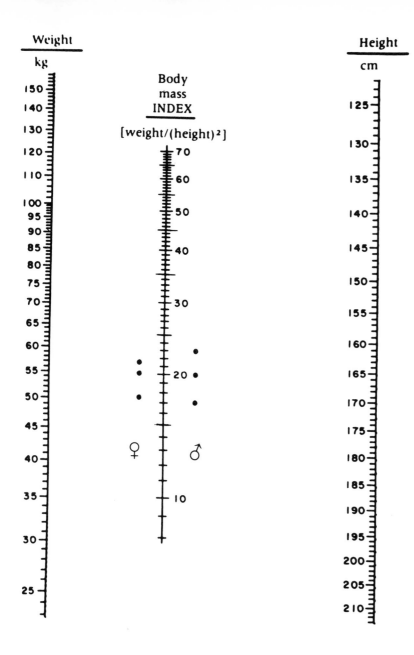

FIGURE 8–4 ●●● By laying a straight edge connecting weight and height, the BMI can be read. The three dots on the left side of the BMI line represent 50th percentile values for females age 20 (*top*), 15 (*middle*), and 10 years (*bottom*); those on the right side are for males of similar age.

TABLE 8–1 ●●● BODY MASS INDEX (kg/m²) FOR GIRLS

Age (yr)	Percentile						
	5th	*10th*	*25th*	*50th*	*75th*	*90th*	*95th*
6	12.8	13.5	14.0	15.0	16.0	16.9	17.3
7	13.1	13.8	14.5	15.6	16.8	18.4	19.2
8	13.5	14.2	15.1	16.2	17.7	19.9	21.1
9	13.9	14.6	15.6	16.9	18.7	21.3	23.0
10	14.4	15.1	16.2	17.5	19.6	22.7	24.8
11	14.9	15.5	16.7	18.2	20.4	23.8	26.3
12	15.3	16.0	17.3	18.8	21.2	24.8	27.7
13	15.8	16.4	17.8	19.3	21.9	25.6	28.8
14	16.2	16.8	18.2	19.9	22.5	26.1	29.6
15	16.6	17.2	18.6	20.3	23.0	26.5	30.2
16	16.9	17.5	18.9	20.7	23.5	26.7	30.6
17	17.1	17.8	19.2	21.0	23.8	26.9	30.9
18–20	17.6	18.4	19.7	21.6	24.3	27.2	31.2
21–23	17.7	18.5	19.8	21.8	24.4	27.7	31.5

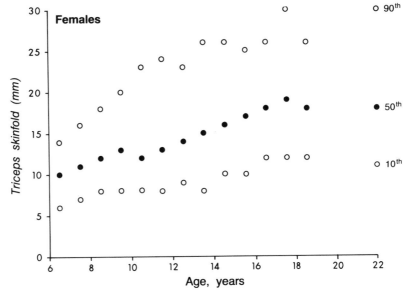

FIGURE 8–5 ••• Triceps skinfold thickness for females—90th, 50th, and 10th percentiles. (Data from Cronk CE, Roche AF. Race- and sex-specific reference data for triceps and subscapular skinfolds and weight/stature[2]. Am J Clin Nutr 1982; 35:351.)

than girls and have a greater energy requirement.

LBM has physiologic and nutritional importance. It constitutes the active metabolic mass of the body, as body fat is relatively inert. There is little or no sex difference in basal metabolic rate when LBM is used as a reference point; total energy expenditure, blood volume, and maximum oxygen consumption are all functions of LBM. Accretion rates of various body constituents are more closely related to LBM than to weight with its variable component of fat.

LBM is a function of height at all ages, and

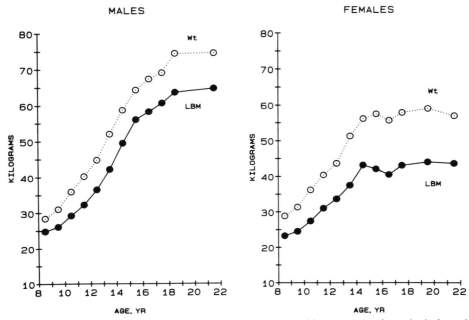

FIGURE 8–6 ••• Growth of weight and lean body mass (LBM) for girls and boys (mean values); body fat is the difference between weight and LBM. Data based on potassium 40 counting in 551 white females and 559 white males. (From McAnarney ER, Krrepe RE, Orr DP, Comerci GD. Textbook of Adolescent Medicine. Philadelphia: WB Saunders, 1992.)

TABLE 8–2 ••• BODY MEASUREMENTS AND CONSTITUENTS AT SELECTED AGES

	Age 10 (M/F)	Age 20 (M/F)	Daily Accretion av Entire Decade (M/F)
Body weight (kg)*	33/34	71/57	
Lean body mass (kg)*	27/26	62/43	
Total body nitrogen (gm)†	840/780	1980/1290	0.31/0.14
Total body calcium (gm)‡	330/290	1100/710§	0.21/0.12
Total body iron (mg) ‖	1480/1430	3560/2270	0.57/0.23
Blood volume (ml) ‖	2450/2400	5350/3950	
Arm muscle + bone area (cm²)¶	24.4/22.6	59.0/34.0	
Urine creatinine (mg/24 hr)	730/700	1990/1300	
Metacarpal cortex (cm²)#	0.27/0.26	0.56/0.42	

*Author's data (Fig. 8–6).

†To convert to grams of protein, multiply by 6.25.

‡Data from Christian et al. (1975), extrapolated from photon density measurements of forearm bones; referenced in Forbes GB. Human Body Composition: Growth, Aging, Nutrition, and Activity. New York: Springer-Verlag, 1987.

§Values obtained by neutron activation (S. Cohn et al., 1971, 1980) are 1100 gm for males and 830 gm for females; referenced in Forbes GB. Human Body Composition: Growth, Aging, Nutrition, and Activity. New York: Springer-Verlag, 1987.

‖ Data compiled by Hawkins (1964); referenced in Forbes GB. Human Body Composition: Growth, Aging, Nutrition, and Activity. New York: Springer-Verlag, 1987.

¶Midarm cross-sectional area, calculated from skinfold thickness and arm circumference. Data compiled by Frisancho (1981); referenced in Forbes GB. Human Body Composition: Growth, Aging, Nutrition, and Activity. New York: Springer-Verlag, 1987.

#Midshaft cross-sectional area, second metacarpal. Data from Garn et al. (1976); referenced in Forbes GB. Human Body Composition: Growth, Aging, Nutrition, and Activity. New York: Springer-Verlag, 1987.

the same is true for total body calcium in adults; hence, tall children should have an athletic advantage over those who are shorter. The variability in LBM for subjects of a given age and sex is less than that for weight, and thus body fat variability accounts for a large proportion of the variation in body weight.

Table 8–2 lists average values of a number of body measurements and body constituents for 10-year-olds and 20-year-olds, together with estimates of daily accretion rates for nitrogen, calcium, and iron over the entire decade. At the peak of the adolescent growth spurt, these accretion values will be two to three times greater. At the beginning of the decade there is little, if any, sex difference for any of these values, but it can be seen that the accretion rates (i.e., the amounts added to the body as a result of growth) are considerably greater in boys. By age 20 years, the male-to-female ratios for the various measurements are in the range of 1.3:1 to 1.7:1, in contrast to a weight ratio of only 1.25:1 and a height ratio of 1.08:1. On average, boys acquire about twice as much nitrogen, calcium, and iron and much more muscle mass, as reflected by arm muscle plus bone cross-sectional area and the daily excretion of creatinine. It should be remembered that these are accretion rates, not dietary requirements, which must take into consideration gastrointestinal absorption and urinary, fecal, and cutaneous losses.

COMPOSITION OF WEIGHT GAIN AND WEIGHT LOSS

Generally speaking, a significant loss of weight, which is the result of nutritional deficit, involves both LBM and fat. The relative contribution of these two body components to the total weight loss depends on the initial body fat content and on the magnitude of the energy deficit. Thin individuals tend to lose relatively more lean tissue, and obese people lose relatively more fat.[18] Very low energy diets result in considerable erosion of the LBM, despite adequate protein intake, whereas diets providing more than 1000 kcal/day are less hazardous in this respect. Exercise tends to mitigate the effect of low energy intakes, but only to a degree; a weight loss of more than a few kilograms will still be accompanied by some loss of LBM. Careful studies have shown that an energy deficit, the result of exercise, produces about the same degree of weight loss and negative nitrogen balance as a comparable deficit from eating less food. Athletes should be told to eat properly, and girls who aspire to a very thin figure run the risk of subnormal lean weight and thinner bones.

Weight gain, the result of nutritional surfeit, also involves both LBM and fat. The fact that obese individuals usually have a somewhat larger LBM than thin individuals favors the hypothesis that obesity is indeed a nutritional disease, the result of a positive energy balance. There is even some evidence for increased skeletal size and slightly higher blood hemoglobin levels. Indeed, obese individuals need to eat more than thin individuals to stay in energy balance: data on free-living adults and adolescents engaged in light physical activity show that an extra 16 to 20 kcal/day are needed for each additional kilogram of body weight.[2, 19] Data from dietary histories that purport to show otherwise must be regarded with great skepticism.

There are two exceptions to the general rule that LBM and fat increase and decrease together. The first relates to the effect of anabolic agents: androgenic-anabolic steroids given in significant amounts and for long enough periods cause an increase in LBM (including muscle) and a decrease in body fat; the same is true of human growth hormone. This is the reason athletes take steroids and risk undesirable side effects in an effort to augment athletic performance. The second exception is the Prader-Willi syndrome, in which LBM is decreased in the presence of an excess of body fat.[20] Body composition changes in these patients mimic those seen in animals with experimental hypothalamic obesity.

Exercise

A regular program of exercise over a period of several weeks can produce a modest increase (1 to 3 kg) in LBM and a decrease in body fat. However, a weight loss of more than a few kilograms will usually cause some loss of LBM even with adequate exercise.[21] Excessive exercise can lead to fatigue and even some loss of appetite; the latter, of course, will lead to weight loss.

The fact that the dominant arm of professional tennis players has larger muscle and bone mass testifies to the phenomenon of local muscle hypertrophy in response to vigorous use over prolonged periods. The large muscle bulk of some body builders is sometimes hailed as a result of exercise and muscle training, but without special tests to measure serum testosterone and gonadotropins, it is difficult to exclude the effects of unreported use of androgenic-anabolic steroids. Certainly the generous deltoid muscles of some runners may provide circumstantial evidence of steroid use.

Many athletes, boys and girls alike, have a larger LBM and less body fat than nonathletes. It is not known whether this is the result of training or is principally hereditary. As noted earlier, a generous intake of food can augment the LBM, but body fat increases at the same time.

Successful athletes constitute a special group. A study of female participants in the 1972 and 1976 Olympic Games showed that almost all of the finalists in the various events were taller than the average for American women age 18 to 24 years (exceptions were gymnasts, coxswains, and participants in equestrian jumping); the mean difference was 7 cm. However, with the exception of discus throwers and shot putters, average BMI values were close to the 50th percentiles shown in Table 8–1 and Figure 8–2.[22] This must mean that the smaller body fat burden of the female athlete is counterbalanced by a somewhat larger LBM.

Special Situations

Nutrition is a most important determinant of growth.[23] Suboptimal nutrition slows the rate of growth and sexual maturation, and excess calories speed up both processes. It has been established that significant changes in body weight incident to nutritional factors involve both the lean and the fat components of the body: both components decrease with undernutrition and increase with overnutrition.

Adolescents vary considerably in body size. All other things being equal, larger teenagers need more to eat than those who are small. Basal metabolic rate is known to be a function of body size when expressed in absolute terms (i.e., kilocalories per unit time). Studies of adolescent girls using advanced techniques have shown that total energy expenditure is related to body size; the slope of the regression line for adolescent girls is 20 kcal/day per kilogram body weight.[19] Obviously, obese girls must eat more than their thin peers to maintain their greater body weight.

There are three situations in adolescence for which nutritional surveillance and advice are particularly important.

The first is pregnancy, which involves rapid weight gain, almost all of it in the second and third trimesters. The average gain is 75 gm/day; assuming an energy expenditure of 8 kcal/gm, the extra energy need is about 600 kcal daily, or about 25% of the average nonpregnant female intake. Extra iron and calcium are needed to support the increased maternal blood volume and the demands of the fetal skeleton. Underweight and poorly nourished girls deserve special consideration.

Second, athletes have a higher energy expenditure than the average adolescent and therefore need more food if they are not to lose weight. With the possible exception of iron, there is no need for extra nutrients other than calories. Hot weather increases the need for water and, if sweating is profuse and prolonged, for salt.

The third group are those who partake of fad diets, which may be deficient in one or more essential nutrients. Growth faltering can occur with diets low in cholesterol and saturated fat if attention is not given to energy intake.

A word should be said regarding the nutritional benefits of exercise. Exercise demands more food but not necessarily more essential nutrients; assuming a well-balanced diet, the result will be a higher intake of such nutrients and thus less likelihood of a specific deficiency. Support for the long-term benefits comes from a study showing that even modest exercise programs can reduce the risk of non–insulin-dependent diabetes mellitus.[24]

References

1. Bessey OA. Evaluation of nutritive status by chemical and other methods. In: Scheinberg IH (ed). Infant Metabolism. New York: Macmillan, 1956, p 284.
2. Forbes GB. Human Body Composition: Growth, Aging, Nutrition, and Activity. New York: Springer-Verlag, 1987.
3. Forbes GB. Nutrition and growth. J Pediatr 1977; 91:40.
4. Zacharias L, Rand WM, Wurtman RJ. A prospective study of sexual development and growth in American girls: The statistics of menarche. Obstet Gynecol Surv 1976; 31:325.
5. Garn SM, LaVelle M. Reproductive histories of low-weight girls and women. Am J Clin Nutr 1983; 37:862.
6. Stark O, Peckham CS, Moynihan C. Weight and age at menarche. Arch Dis Child 1989; 64:383.
7. Lager C, Ellison PT. Effect of moderate weight loss on ovarian function assessed by salivary progesterone measurements. Am J Hum Biol 1990; 2:303.
8. Delemarre-van de Waal HA, Plant TM, van Rees GB, et al (eds). Control of the Onset of Puberty. III. New York: Excerpta Medica, 1989.
9. Clemmons DR, Klibanski A, Underwood LE, et al. Reduction of plasma immunoactive somatomedin-C during fasting in humans. J Clin Endocrinol Metab 1981; 53:1247.
10. Forbes GB, Brown MR, Welle SL, Underwood LE. Hormonal response to overfeeding. Am J Clin Nutr 1989; 49:608.
11. Bouchard C, Savard R, Despres J-P, et al. Body composition in adopted and biological siblings. Hum Biol 1985; 57:61.
12. Stunkard AJ, Sorensen TIA, Hanis C, et al. An adoption study of human obesity. N Engl J Med 1986; 314:193.
13. Tanner JM, Davies PSW. Clinical longitudinal standards for height and height velocity for North American children. J Pediatr 1985; 107:317.
14. Bayley N, Pinneau SR. Tables for predicting adult height from skeletal age: Revised for use with the Gruelich-Pyle hand standards. J Pediatr 1952; 40:432.
15. Forbes GB. The abdomen:hip ratio. Normative data and observations on selected patients. Int J Obes 1990; 14:149.
16. Cronk CE, Roche AF. Race- and sex-specific reference data for triceps and subscapular skinfolds and weight/stature^2. Am J Clin Nutr 1982; 35:351.
17. Forbes GB. Body size and composition of perimenarchal girls. Am J Dis Child 1992; 146:63.
18. Forbes GB. Lean body mass–body fat interrelationships in humans. Nutr Rev 1987; 45:225.
19. Bandini LG, Schoeller DA, Dietz WH. Energy expenditure in obese and nonobese adolescents. Pediatr Res 1990; 27:198.
20. Schoeller DA, Levitsky LL, Bandini LG, et al. Energy expenditure and body composition in Prader-Willi syndrome. Metabolism 1988; 37:115.
21. Forbes GB. Exercise and body composition. J Appl Physiol 1991; 70(3):994.
22. Khosla T. Sport for tall. Br Med J 1983; 287:736.
23. Phillips LS. Nutrition, metabolism, and growth. In: Daughaday WH (ed). Endocrine Control of Growth. New York: Elsevier, 1981.
24. Helmsick SP, Ragland DR, Leung RW, Paffenbarger RS. Physical activity and reduced occurrence of non-insulin-dependent diabetes mellitus. N Engl J Med 1991; 325:147.

CHAPTER 9

Effects of the Thyroid on Gonadal and Reproductive Function

THOMAS P. FOLEY, Jr.

The interrelationships between the hypothalamic-pituitary-gonadal (HPG) axis and thyroid function have been known for nearly two centuries. The alterations in thyroid function tests in pregnancy and in women receiving oral contraceptives are familiar to physicians even though errors in interpretation occur not infrequently. Specific thyroid diseases alter normal reproductive function, particularly in females, at puberty and during adult life.[1, 2] The most common causes of acquired abnormalities of thyroid function in areas of the world in which dietary iodine is sufficient are autoimmune thyroid disease (ATD), Graves' disease, and autoimmune (Hashimoto's) thyroiditis. Autoimmune diseases, including ATD, are much more common in adolescent and adult women than in men.[3]

HYPOTHALAMIC-PITUITARY-THYROID REGULATION: THYROID HORMONE

Metabolism and Action

The regulation of thyroid hormone secretion and action is less complex than that of the HPG system, particularly in females (Fig. 9–1). There are two sources for the iodothyronines in serum:

1. Thyroxine (T_4) and, in much smaller amounts, the triiodothyronines (T_3 and reverse T_3) are synthesized and secreted directly by the thyroid gland.

2. The monodeiodination of T_4 generates the most potent of the iodothyronines—3,3′,5-l-triiodothyronine (T_3)—and the biologically inactive stereoisomer—reverse T_3 (rT_3, known chemically as 3,3′,5′-l-triiodothyronine).[4] These hormones exist in the circulation and are predominantly bound to three distinct proteins: thyroxine-binding globulin (TBG), transthyretin, and albumin. TBG has the greatest binding affinity for the iodothyronines, and albumin has the greatest binding capacity. However, the biologically active hormones that mediate the action of thyroid hormones at the cellular level exist in the unbound, or free, form. The concentrations of free T_4 and free T_3 directly correlate with the biologic status of thyroid hormone function and can be directly measured using methods that are generally available in commercial laboratories.[5]

Thyroid-stimulating hormone (TSH), a pituitary glycoprotein, regulates thyroid hormone synthesis and secretion and, in part, thyroid glandular growth.[6] In addition, thyroid

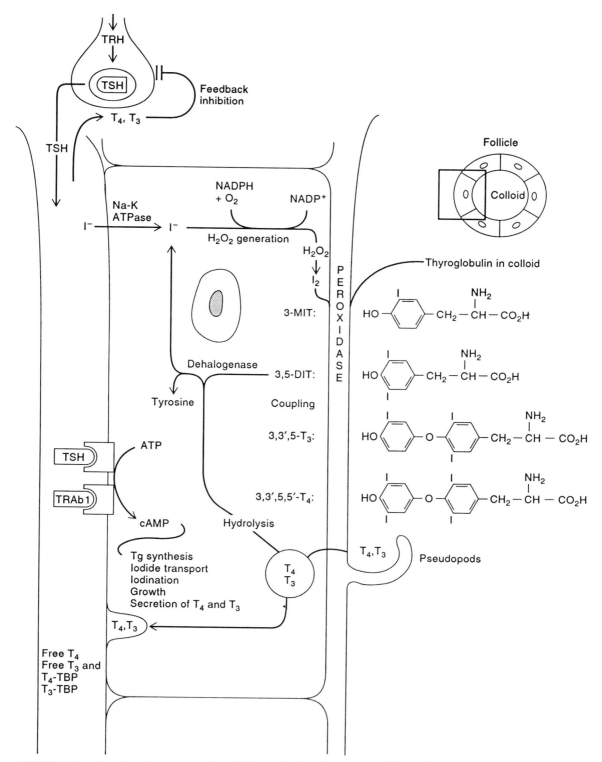

FIGURE 9–1 ••• A schematic representation of the synthesis and secretion of thyroid hormones by the thyroid gland. Dietary sources of iodide are absorbed into the circulation, concentrated by the thyroid, and immediately oxidized to iodine and incorporated into tyrosyl residues on thyroglobulin; mono- and diiodotyrosyl residues are coupled to form tetraiodothyronine (T_4) or triiodothyronine (T_3); T_4 and T_3 are released by proteolysis and secreted into the circulation on stimulation by thyroid-stimulating hormone (TSH).

growth probably is controlled by local growth factors such as insulin-like growth factor I (IGF I) and epidermal growth factor (EGF).[5] The synthesis and release of TSH is regulated in part by stimulation of the hypothalamic hormone, thyrotropin-releasing hormone (TRH), and in part by the pituitary intracellular concentration of T_3. The latter is derived from circulating free T_3 concentrations and by the intrapituitary conversion of T_4 to T_3. This enzymatic reaction is very important in the regulation of TSH synthesis and release. When the availability of T_4 for conversion to T_3 is decreased within the pituitary gland, TSH synthesis and secretion increase in an effort to restore free T_4 concentrations to normal.[7] Therefore, T_4 concentrations are very important in the regulation of TSH secretion, even though their biologic potency at the cellular level is minimal compared with that of T_3. The earliest sign of thyroid gland failure is a decrease in T_4 secretion. Initially, however, the concentration of circulating free T_4 usually remains within the normal range. The decrease in free T_4 concentration is recognized by the pituitary, and the first detectable abnormality in thyroid function in response to thyroid gland failure is an increase in pituitary TSH content and release into the circulation to increase the concentration of TSH in serum.

The gonadotropins—follicle-stimulating hormone (FSH), luteinizing hormone (LH), TSH, and human chorionic gonadotropin (hCG)—are glycoproteins that share identical α subunits within a species.[6] The β subunits mediate the biologic response only when the α and β subunits are combined to form the intact hormone and when posttranslational glycosylation is completed. There are sequence homologies between the β subunits of TSH, LH, and hCG such that these hormones, when present in high concentrations, may display the biologic properties of their related glycoproteins. These activities may be important as partial explanations for increased thyroid gland function in the presence of increased concentrations of hCG and the precocious onset of puberty that is observed in children with severe primary hypothyroidism, or myxedema.

The deiodination of T_4 to T_3 and rT_3 in peripheral tissues is regulated by the nutritional and metabolic needs of the organism and may be altered in certain pathophysiologic conditions (see Fig. 9–1).[4] During nutritional deprivation, particularly when carbohydrate intake is reduced, there is preferential deiodination of T_4 to rT_3. Similarly, during acute severe illnesses, there is preferential deiodination of T_4 to rT_3; this is known as the nonthyroidal illness (NTI) syndrome, or the euthyroid sick syndrome. In addition, there may be a decrease in total T_4, but free T_4 levels remain normal to high normal when measured by definitive methods such as equilibrium or direct dialysis. Maintenance of high-normal free T_4 concentrations in the NTI syndrome is the likely mechanism whereby TSH secretion remains in the normal range even in the presence of a low T_3 concentration. These metabolic alterations are thought to be a mechanism in which the organism adapts to a decreasing need for a highly catabolic hormone (T_3) by producing the biologically inactive stereoisomer, rT_3. Therefore, when a patient with the NTI syndrome is tested, the results include a low total T_3, an elevated rT_3, a normal or decreased total T_4, a normal or high-normal free T_4, and a normal, measurable TSH. In advanced severe stages of the NTI syndrome, free T_4 concentrations may decline, even though serum TSH values remain normal or low, suggesting that a state of hypothalamic hypothyroidism had developed.

The metabolic effects of thyroid hormone are mediated by T_3 at the cellular level.[8] This action is very similar to that of the steroid hormones in that T_3 binds to a thyroid hormone response element that is bound to the DNA receptor that controls transcription and translation and thereby regulates protein synthesis. There is also evidence to suggest that T_3 may directly stimulate oxidative phosphorylation in the mitochondria, an action that may be separate and distinct from its effect on protein synthesis.

There are important physiologic and pathophysiologic relationships between thyroid function and gonadal function.[1, 2] The concentration of estrogen in serum during pregnancy and during oral contraceptive therapy stimulates hepatic synthesis and secretion of TBG. This estrogen effect will alter thyroid function tests but will not change the thyroid status of the patient. In the presence of an increased concentration of TBG, there will be an increase in total T_4, normal levels of free T_4, and normal levels of TSH. When indirect measurements of free T_4 are made using the resin uptake test with radiolabeled T_3 (RT_3U) in the presence of estrogen, the effect of increased TBG will be to increase the total T_4 and decrease the RT_3U. The estimated free thyroxine (EFT) or free T_4 index (FTI) is calculated by the product of the total T_4 and RT_3U.

The high T_4 and low RT_3U values will give a product that is normal, reflecting a normal free T_4 concentration in this circumstance.

When patients are born with an absent or very low level of TBG, the total T_4 is low, the RT_3U is elevated, and the product, FTI, is normal. Because familial TBG deficiency usually is inherited as an X-linked trait, the female is the heterozygote and has mildly decreased or intermediately low levels of total T_4. When the RT_3U test is performed, the value is increased, and the calculated FTI is normal. This disorder is relatively common and may lead to inappropriate treatment with T_4 when women are tested for thyroid hormone abnormalities during an infertility evaluation.

There are other medications that either alter the binding of thyroid hormones to thyroid hormone–binding proteins or interfere with binding (Table 9–1). Anabolic steroids and androgens decrease TBG synthesis, secretion,

and serum concentrations. Certain anticonvulsant medications, particularly phenytoin, (Dilantin), compete with T_4 for binding to TBG. Thyroid function tests will show normal TBG levels and decreased total T_4 values, and in some instances there are artifactual abnormalities in the RT_3U test. In these cases, direct measurement of free T_4 using the equilibrium or direct dialysis methods may be the only reliable way to assess the free T_4 concentration and differentiate alterations in T_4 binding from hypothalamic or pituitary hypothyroidism.[9] These methods are available from commercial laboratories with expertise in endocrine testing and are important to use when there are discrepancies in the expected results of thyroid function tests, or when certain therapeutic or clinical conditions are present. Such conditions include the NTI syndrome, when alterations in thyroid function may result in an incorrect diagnosis of hypothalamic or pituitary hypo- or hyperthyroidism.

There are other tests of thyroid function whose results differ between men and women and are altered during contraceptive therapy or pregnancy.[1, 2] TSH and prolactin responses to TRH are greater in women than in men. This effect is particularly evident when estrogen concentrations in preovulatory women are increased compared with women in the luteal phase of the cycle or with men. During pregnancy, associated changes in thyroid function include increases in thyroid size, in total production of thyroid hormone, in secretory activity of the thyroid by histologic evaluation, and in the uptake of radioactive iodine.

TABLE 9–1 ••• CLINICAL CONDITIONS AND PHARMACEUTICAL AGENTS THAT INTERFERE WITH IODOTHYRONINE BINDING TO THYROID-BINDING PROTEINS

Decreased thyroxine-binding globulin (TBG) concentration
  Active acromegaly
  Androgenic steroids
  Medications: L-asparaginase
  Familial TBG deficiency
  Glucocorticoids
  Nephrotic syndrome
  Severe illness
  Thyrotoxicosis
Inhibitors of binding
  Medications
    5-Fluorouracil
    Halofenate
    Mitotane
    Phenylbutazone
    Phenytoin
    Salicylate
Increased TBG concentrations
  Acute intermittent porphyria
  Medications
    Clofibrate
    Diacetylmorphine hydrochloride (heroin)
    Methadone
    Perphenazine
  Estrogens (endogenous and exogenous)
    Contraceptives
    Neonatal estrogen
    Pregnancy
  Familial TBG excess
  Hepatitis (infectious and chronic active)
  Hypothyroidism
Familial abnormalities of albumin and transthyretin
Iodothyronine antibodies (anti-T_4 and anti-T_3)

Thyrotoxicosis and the Reproductive System

There is a long history of the association of thyrotoxicosis and abnormalities in HPG regulation. The first report of thyrotoxicosis, by Parry in 1825, described menstrual abnormalities in two women as follows:

She nursed for a year the child of her first lying-in, during which time she did not menstruate. Subsequently to that period she had five times miscarried; and for the last four months her menses had been irregular as to intervals, and defective in quantity and colour.[10]

This woman had been seen in 1786 with tachycardia, exophthalmos, and goiter. In another case the description read, "menses, since the commencement of the malady, defective." In 1940, von Basedow reported the occurrence of amenorrhea as a common symptom in postmenarchal women.[11]

Menarche may occur at an earlier than normal age if hyperthyroidism develops in prepubertal girls, presumably as a result of the effects of excessive thyroid hormones on mild advancement of skeletal maturation, which is an indication of an advance in biologic maturation.[1] However, the onset of menses may be delayed in prepubertal thyrotoxic girls, an effect that is analogous to amenorrhea in adult women. Oligomenorrhea, anovulation, and menometrorrhagia also have been reported, although the last condition is seen more commonly in association with hypothyroidism. These changes would be expected to return to normal when euthyroidism is achieved during therapy.[1]

Pathogenesis

Autoimmune thyrotoxicosis (Graves' disease or Parry's disease) is the most common cause of thyrotoxicosis (Table 9–2). The disease is caused by an abnormality in the immune system that results in the production of an immunoglobulin G (IgG), usually subclass 1, that stimulates the TSH receptor.[12] Thyroid hormones do not modulate the stimulatory response of the thyroid to these antibodies, known as TSH receptor antibodies (TRAb), and an unregulated excessive secretion of T_4 and T_3 causes most of the clinical symptoms of the disease. These symptoms are found in any disease associated with thyrotoxicosis and are not specific for Graves' disease. However, specific antibodies, either the same antibody clone or an antibody distinct from the thyroid-stimulating antibody, are reported to cause the exophthalmos and other eye signs in autoimmune thyrotoxicosis.[13] Exophthalmos is a clinical sign specifically associated with Graves' disease, and its presence is diagnostic.

The other causes of thyrotoxicosis are very uncommon or rare during adolescence and include the unusual cases of TSH-mediated hyperthyroidism from either pituitary TSH-secreting adenomas or the syndrome of pituitary resistance to thyroid hormone; ingestion of excessive amounts of thyroid hormones; toxic thyroiditis from the release of preformed thyroid hormones after a viral (subacute thyroiditis) or autoimmune (Hashimoto's disease) insult to the thyroid; autonomous hyperfunction of the thyroid either from a thyroid adenoma, the McCune-Albright syndrome or, very rarely, thyroid carcinoma; iodide-induced hyperthyroidism (Jodbasedow's disease); and tumor-secreting thyroid stimulators that are rarely seen in women with hydatidiform mole and choriocarcinoma.[14] In these last diseases, high levels of hCG stimulate the thyroid to increase the secretion of thyroid hormones and cause hyperthyroidism.

Clinical Symptoms and Signs

During childhood and adolescence, the symptoms and signs of thyrotoxicosis are sim-

TABLE 9–2 ••• ETIOLOGY AND PATHOGENESIS OF JUVENILE HYPERTHYROIDISM AND HYPOTHYROIDISM

Juvenile Hyperthyroidism	Juvenile Hypothyroidism
Autoimmune (Graves' disease)	Chronic autoimmune thyroiditis
Autonomous hyperfunctioning nodular disease	Lymphocytic thyroiditis with thyromegaly
Toxic adenoma	Hashimoto's thyroiditis (struma lymphomatosa) with
McCune-Albright syndrome	thyromegaly
Hyperfunctioning thyroid carcinoma (rare)	Fibrous variant with atrophy
TSH-mediated hyperthyroidism	Congenital hypothyroidism, late-onset, mild disease
TSH-secreting pituitary adenoma	Ectopic thyroid dysgenesis
Pituitary resistance to thyroid hormone	Dyshormonogenesis
Toxic thyroiditis	Peripheral resistance to thyroid hormone
Thyrotoxic phase of subacute thyroiditis	Endemic goiter
Thyrotoxic presentation of autoimmune thyroiditis	Iodine deficiency
Ingestion of thyroid hormone	Environmental goitrogen
Iodide-induced hyperthyroidism (Jodbasedow's	Drug-induced
disease)	Lithium
Tumor-secreting thyroid stimulators (rare)	Antithyroid drugs
Hydatidiform mole	Iodide excess in association with other thyroid disease
Choriocarcinoma	Thyroid irradiation
	Thyroidectomy

ilar to those in adults (Table 9–3). Children and adolescents often experience deteriorating academic performance; abnormal sleeping habits (enuresis, difficulty falling asleep, and restlessness during sleep); and the expected symptoms of muscle weakness, fatigue, heat intolerance, excessive perspiration, increased appetite with loss in weight or stable weight, nervousness, irritability, and emotional lability. Thyromegaly is almost always present in the child and young adult when hyperthyroidism (excess thyroid hormone secretion from the thyroid gland) is the cause of thyrotoxicosis. Except when a thyroid nodule secretes thyroid hormone, the gland is diffusely enlarged, soft to firm, nontender, smooth, and usually symmetrically enlarged (Fig. 9–2).[14] Tachycardia with an increased pulse pressure is expected; proptosis from exophthalmos usually is mild to moderate in severity during childhood and adolescence and occurs less often and is less severe than in adults (see Fig. 9–2). Other eye signs seen in children and adolescents are generally limited to stare, eyelid lag, and retraction, although periorbital edema and conjunctival injection and edema are occasionally observed.

Diagnostic Evaluation

The patient presenting with the classic symptoms and signs of Graves' disease—diffuse thyromegaly, exophthalmos, and tachycardia—requires minimal diagnostic procedures before therapy.[14] Thyroid function tests should include measurement of serum free T_4 and TSH using a sensitive assay that discriminates

TABLE 9–3 ••• THYROTOXICOSIS

Clinical Symptoms and Signs	Initial Clinical Evaluation
Thyromegaly	T_3, T_4, free T_4, TSH
Tachycardia	Complete blood cell and
Nervousness and	differential counts
insomnia	TRAb
Increased pulse pressure	Radionuclide image *only* in
and palpitations	presence of nodule(s)
Proptosis	Radioiodide uptake *only*
Increased appetite, often	when diagnosis and origin
with weight loss	are uncertain
Tremor, restlessness	
Heat intolerance	
Deteriorating school	
performance	
Enuresis	

TRAb, TSH receptor antibody.

normal from low values, a complete blood cell count with differential, and preferably (although not required) measurement of TRAb by a TSH-receptor–binding inhibitory immunoglobulin (TBII) method to document an autoimmune origin (see Table 9–3).

When the origin of thyrotoxicosis is less certain, other diagnostic tests may be necessary to exclude other causes of thyrotoxicosis.[15] Such tests include measurement of serum T_3 whenever a thyroid nodule is present or free T_4 is normal or only slightly elevated; measurement of radioiodide uptake at 4 to 6 hours and 24 hours after the tracer dose to differentiate hyperthyroid from nonhyperthyroid causes of thyrotoxicosis; a thyroid radiograph if there is nodular thyroid disease; and a pituitary magnetic resonance imaging (MRI) scan and determination of serum α subunit if the serum TSH is inappropriately normal or elevated in the presence of elevated concentrations of free T_4 and T_3.[16]

Thyroglobulin and thyroperoxidase antibody titers in serum may be useful to determine the presence of autoimmune thyroiditis (Hashimoto's disease), either as the cause of transient, toxic thyroiditis with thyrotoxicosis or as a coexisting disease with autoimmune thyrotoxicosis (Graves' disease).

Management

The initial therapy for thyrotoxicosis is directed toward control of the exaggerated adrenergic responsiveness that occurs in moderate and severe thyrotoxicosis and the excessive thyroid hormone secretion or release.[15, 17] Usually symptoms can be controlled by β-adrenergic blocking agents such as propranolol in doses for adolescents as low as 10 to 20 mg every 6 to 8 hours, assuming no contraindications for their use (e.g., asthma or congestive heart failure). After 2 to 3 weeks, as euthyroidism develops in response to antithyroid therapy, the dose of propranolol can be tapered and discontinued over 1 or 2 weeks.[18]

Antithyroid medications—methimazole (MTZ) and propylthiouracil (PTU)—are prescribed in three divided doses totaling 0.5 to 1.0 mg/kg/day for MTZ or 5 to 10 mg/kg/day for PTU.[15, 19] Once euthyroidism is achieved, the maintenance dose of MTZ and possibly of PTU can be prescribed once daily[20, 21]; PTU may need to be continued in either two or three divided doses. When the thyroid is blocked and the total and free T_4 and T_3 values

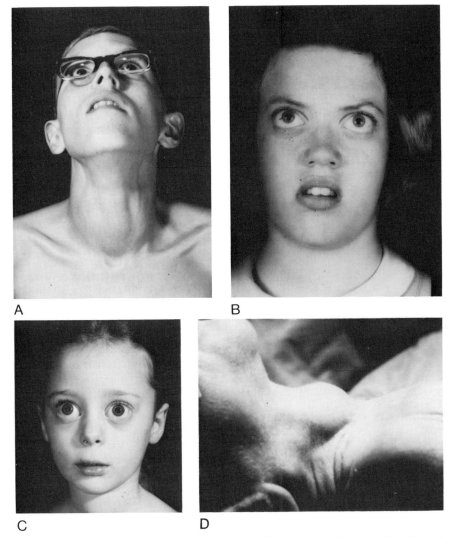

FIGURE 9–2 ••• Patients with autoimmune thyrotoxicosis (Graves' disease). *A,* Adolescent with diffuse thyromegaly. *B,* Adolescent with exophthalmos and diffuse thyromegaly. *C,* Young girl with exophthalmos and diffuse thyromegaly. *D,* Neonate with diffuse thyromegaly secondary to congenital transient Graves' disease. (Courtesy of the Endocrine Clinic, Children's Hospital of Pittsburgh, PA.)

decrease into the hypothyroid range, the serum TSH may remain suppressed below normal levels for several weeks as a result of the effect of prolonged hypothalamic-pituitary suppression from chronically elevated T_4 and T_3 concentrations. Once serum TSH values become elevated, there are two options for maintenance therapy: (1) the addition of T_4 in a once daily dose of 1 μg/kg while maintaining the blocking doses of the antithyroid drug (known as combined therapy); or (2) a stepwise decrement in the antithyroid dose.[15] The advantage of combined therapy is the need for less frequent patient monitoring to ensure the op-

timal dose for the antithyroid medication and the ability to suppress thyroid gland function and expression of the antigen, the TSH receptor. Continuation of T_4 therapy after remission and discontinuation of antithyroid therapy has been reported to reduce the risk of subsequent relapse of thyrotoxicosis in adults.[22]

The most effective and safest mode of definitive therapy for autoimmune thyrotoxicosis is radioiodide ablation.[15, 23, 24] Permanent hypothyroidism requiring T_4 replacement therapy is the goal of radioiodide therapy and often is the preferred initial treatment for adults, particularly in North America. If thyroid tissue is ablated rather than partially damaged, the risk for benign or malignant tumors of the thyroid has not been reported to differ from that in the general population; this therapy is acceptable for both adolescents and adults.[24] There is very limited experience with radioiodide ablative therapy in young children, even though the risk for thyroid tumors theoretically would be low if the gland is completely destroyed. Because radioiodine readily crosses the placenta and will ablate the fetal thyroid after 11 to 12 weeks of gestation, it is contraindicated during pregnancy. A screening test for pregnancy is mandatory before radioiodine therapy is initiated in female patients between the time of menarche and menopause.[25]

The current indications for surgical therapy for thyrotoxicosis are limited.[17] The presence of a toxic thyroid nodule and a nodule within the thyroid gland of patients with Graves' disease, which may be indicative of thyroid carcinoma, is an indication for definitive surgical therapy. Subtotal thyroidectomy may be indicated for treatment of Graves' disease during pregnancy when antithyroid drugs, given in lower doses to present low risk to the fetus, are not successful in maintaining mild hyperthyroidism or euthyroidism. Definitive surgical therapy is also indicated in the patient in whom one or two courses of radioiodide therapy have failed or there are other contraindications for radioiodide exposure.

Hypothyroidism and the Reproductive System

Hypothyroidism may have a profound effect on growth and sexual maturation of children and adolescents.[26] In severe primary hypothyroidism, there may be complete cessation of growth and a profound delay in skeletal maturation. In most cases, pituitary or hypothalamic hypothyroidism is associated with other pituitary hormone deficiencies and causes deceleration in growth, particularly when associated with growth hormone deficiency. However, even in panhypopituitarism, some growth is observed.

Hypothyroidism that occurs during the prepubertal years usually causes delay in the onset of puberty; when it develops during puberty, it causes a cessation in sexual maturation.[27] Hypothyroidism—whether primary, pituitary (secondary), or hypothalamic (tertiary)—is an important cause of delayed puberty, is associated with a deceleration in growth, and is reversed with thyroxine therapy. An enlarged sella turcica may be found in patients with primary hypothyroidism as a result of the hyperplasia of thyrotrophs in response to the marked increase in TSH secretion. This abnormality usually is differentiated by MRI from hypothalamic and pituitary tumors, which cause deficiencies in the secretion of TRH and/or TSH.

Infrequently, hypothyroidism that develops during childhood may be associated with isosexual precocity and precocious menstruation in females[28, 29] and with testicular enlargement in males.[30] Gonadal stimulation from pubertal levels of gonadotropins is evidenced by breast development in girls and testicular enlargement in boys. However, there is no evidence for precocious adrenarche, as pubic and axillary hair are absent. The hypothesis to explain sexual precocity is based on the common α subunits; partial sequence homology of the β subunits and weak cross-reacting bioactivity of the pituitary glycoproteins (LH, FSH, TSH, and hCG); and the stimulation of gonadotropin secretion, in the presence of a very active hypothalamic-pituitary system, for the secretion of TSH.[29, 30]

Causes of Hypothyroidism: Primary, Pituitary, and Hypothalamic

The most common cause of acquired primary hypothyroidism is chronic autoimmune thyroiditis.[26] There are three common variants: lymphocytic thyroiditis of childhood and adolescence with thyromegaly, but usually not severe hypothyroidism; Hashimoto's thyroiditis with thyromegaly, also known as struma lymphomatosa; and a chronic fibrous variant.[26, 31] These diseases present with growth deceleration and/or thyromegaly.

Other causes of primary hypothyroidism include late-onset, mild, congenital hypothyroidism; sporadic thyroid dysgenesis with ectopic tissue; familial thyroid dyshormonogenesis with thyromegaly; or the very rare disease known as peripheral resistance to thyroid hormone.[27] Nearly all cases of congenital primary hypothyroidism are detected by newborn screening programs and rarely present during childhood except when screening is not available or is inadequate or when the condition is missed by the screening program. The most common cause of primary hypothyroidism is endemic goiter and cretinism caused by iodine deficiency and/or environmental goitrogens. With the increased use of ionizing radiation in the treatment of cervical, cranial, and thyroid tumors, there are an increasing number of patients with radiation-induced primary hypothyroidism. During the early recovery phase of toxic thyroiditis from subacute or viral thyroiditis, primary hypothyroidism is present for a transient interval of several weeks until the thyroid gland recovers. Certain medications are known to block either thyroid hormone synthesis (propylthiouracil, methimazole) and thyroid hormone release (iodides, lithium) and cause primary hypothyroidism usually with goiter.[27]

The pituitary and hypothalamic forms of hypothyroidism usually are caused by space-occupying lesions in and between the hypothalamus and pituitary or by the effects of radiation therapy for tumors in this region.[32] Isolated TRH or TSH deficiency has been reported as both a familial and a sporadic disease.[33] Other causes, usually occurring in association with other pituitary hormone deficiencies, include congenital midline malformations of the central nervous system, trauma, infections and inflammatory processes.

Clinical Symptoms and Signs

During childhood and adolescence, the most characteristic clinical presenting signs of hypothyroidism are deceleration of growth, thyromegaly, and abnormal sexual development (see Chapter 3).[26] Nonspecific symptoms such as lethargy, easy fatiguability, weight gain (although usually not obesity), weakness, cold intolerance, constipation, and dry skin may be present (Table 9–4). Because these symptoms develop very gradually, the child or parent often is not aware of them until thyroxine therapy is initiated and the symptoms recede. Other signs include delayed dental maturation and tooth eruption, coarse hair and hair loss, galactorrhea, and a sallow appearance of the skin (Fig. 9–3). These symptoms and signs are seen infrequently in hypothalamic and pituitary hypothyroidism because of the mild degree of hypothyroidism.[32, 33]

Diagnostic Evaluation

The diagnosis of primary hypothyroidism is confirmed by the elevation of serum TSH, usually a value greater than 20 mU/L.[26] Patients with growth deceleration and the symp-

TABLE 9–4 ••• HYPOTHYROIDISM

Clinical Symptoms and Signs	Initial Clinical Evaluation
Deceleration of linear growth	Growth curve
	TSH
Delayed skeletal maturation	T_4, free T_4
Delayed pubertal development; rarely, precocious puberty	Bone age
	Thyroid antibodies: TpAb, TgAb, TRAb, TRBAb
Delayed dental development and tooth eruption	
	Radioiodide uptake *only* when diagnosis and origin are uncertain
Myopathy, weakness, fatigue, muscular hypertrophy	
Pale, dry, sallow skin	
Galactorrhea	
Constipation	
Cold intolerance	
Pseudotumor cerebri	

TgAb, Thyroglobulin antibody; TpAb, thyroperoxidase (thyroid microsomal) antibody; TRAb, TSH receptor antibody; TRBAb, TSH receptor blocking antibody.

toms and signs of hypothyroidism will have very low levels of T_4 and free T_4, but serum T_3 values may remain within the normal range until these patients develop the classic presentation of myxedema. The diagnosis of autoimmune thyroiditis can be established by the presence of thyroid antibodies (thyroglobulin and thyroid peroxidase), also known as microsomal antibodies, or TSH receptor–blocking antibodies in serum. Pituitary and hypothalamic hypothyroidism are confirmed by a low free T_4 level with a normal, undetectable, or, on rare occasions in hypothalamic hypothyroidism, mildly elevated serum TSH level that is less than 20 mU/L.[34] The latter occurs because the biologic activity of TSH is impaired in hypothalamic hypothyroidism as a result of reduced or abnormal glycosylation of the molecule; however, TSH can be measured by immunoassays, because the antibodies in the assay are directed against the peptide portion of the molecule that is secreted in response to the low circulating free T_4 values.[35] No other evaluation or tests are usually required for diagnosis.

Management

Hypothyroidism is one of the easiest diseases to manage, and the cost of therapy is low.[26] The pure synthetic preparations of levothyroxine should be used, particularly in children. In older children and adolescents, a dosage of 1 to 3 µg/kg/day (approximately 100 µg/M²/day) generally renders the patient clinically and

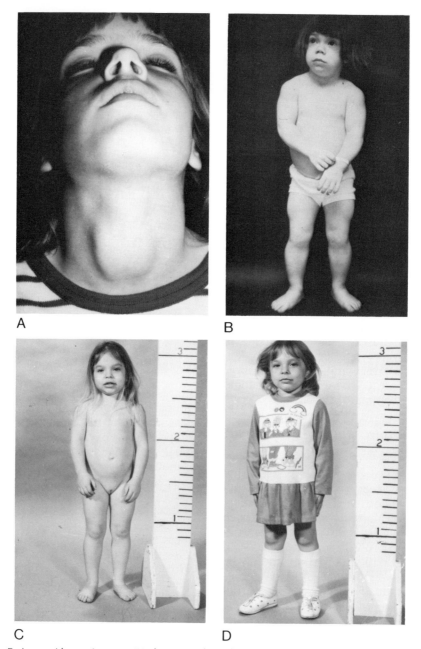

FIGURE 9–3 ••• Patients with autoimmune (Hashimoto's) thyroiditis. *A,* Young adolescent with diffuse thyromegaly and the right lobe larger than the left. *B,* Young boy with primary hypothyroidism and the Kocher-Debré-Sémélaigne syndrome (muscular hypertrophy in chronic primary juvenile hypothyroidism). *C,* Young girl with advanced primary hypothyroidism, growth retardation, and myxedema secondary to the fibrous variant of autoimmune (Hashimoto's) thyroiditis. *D,* Young girl in C after 2 months of levothyroxine therapy. (Courtesy of the Endocrine Clinic, Children's Hospital of Pittsburgh, PA.)

biochemically euthyroid. To avoid interference in absorption by certain foods, thyroxine should be taken at least 30 minutes before a meal or at bedtime.[27] If the patient forgets a dose, a double dose should be taken the next day. Once normal levels of serum T_4 and TSH are achieved, thyroid function tests need only be monitored annually, unless patient compliance or the reliability of thyroxine preparations is of concern.

CLINICAL PRESENTATIONS AND THE ROLE OF THYROID HORMONES IN PATHOGENESIS

Pubertal Delay. In the evaluation of the child with pubertal delay, both primary hypothyroidism and hypothalamic-pituitary disease with or without hypothyroidism must be excluded. For the diagnosis of autoimmune thyroiditis with primary hypothyroidism, serum TSH (elevated), free T_4 (low) and thyroperoxidase and thyroglobulin antibodies (positive in titers greater than 1:4 in children and 1:100 in young adults) are the initial and often definitive diagnostic indicators. An elevated TSH level without an abnormally low T_4 level is considered compensated primary hypothyroidism and would not be expected to account for pubertal delay. Because hypothalamic-pituitary hypothyroidism after age 8 years is nearly always associated with other hypothalamic or pituitary hormone abnormalities, pubertal delay in such cases is associated with gonadotropin deficiency. Confirmation of the diagnosis of hypothalamic or pituitary hypothyroidism requires a low serum free T_4 level, (preferably determined using a definitive test such as direct or equilibrium dialysis)[9] and a low, normal, or mildly elevated TSH level (not greater than 20 mU/L).[34] An MRI scan of the hypothalamic-pituitary area is necessary to distinguish a space-occupying lesion from idiopathic hypothalamic-pituitary hypothyroidism.[32] A TRH test is required to differentiate hypothalamic from primary pituitary disease as a cause of central hypothyroidism.[32, 35] The failure to demonstrate a rise in TSH following TRH in the presence of low free T_4 would support the diagnosis of primary pituitary TSH deficiency. In such cases the prolactin (PRL) response to TRH would be normal or exaggerated unless there was complete destruction of the pituitary gland, in which case there would be no TSH or PRL response.

Precocious Puberty. Early onset of breast development or testicular enlargement without adrenarche is a rare presentation of advanced primary hypothyroidism. The usual cause is autoimmune thyroiditis, but it may also be caused by any disease associated with primary hypothyroidism of chronic duration, usually with symptoms and signs of myxedema and onset during childhood. The initial thyroid evaluation is the same as that described for primary hypothyroidism and pubertal delay (i.e., measurement of serum TSH, free T_4, and thyroid antibodies).

Hyperprolactinemia. Primary and hypothalamic hypothyroidism can both be associated with hyperprolactinemia, and pubertal or adult patients may present with amenorrhea and galactorrhea. In early stages of disease with mild hypothyroidism, the basal PRL level may be normal, but the PRL response to TRH may be exaggerated, as with the TSH response. Young adults presenting either with an unexplained elevated PRL level or galactorrhea should be screened for hypothyroidism (i.e., with measurement of serum TSH and free T_4).

Growth Aberrations. Mild accelerations in growth may occur with thyrotoxicosis, but such patients will have obvious clinical disease by the time growth acceleration is observed. In hypothyroidism, however, the first and only sign of the disease may be a deceleration in growth velocity. These patients must be screened for hypothyroidism.

Rapid Pubertal Advance During Treatment of Hypothyroidism. Patients with chronic primary hypothyroidism associated with growth deceleration and retarded skeletal maturation who present during late childhood or early adolescence may experience both rapid growth acceleration and pubertal advance when euthyroidism is restored with appropriate doses of thyroxine.[36] The onset of puberty may occur before growth has caught up to the growth percentile achieved before the development of hypothyroidism. Furthermore, because the pubertal response may progress more rapidly than the growth response, the patient may reach adult height with epiphyseal fusion before catch-up growth is completed and thereby not attain the genetically predetermined height, known as the target height.[36] This problem is demonstrated in Figure 3–3. The patient grew at the 50th percentile before hypothyroidism developed at age 6 years; however, after therapy and completion of pubertal development, the patient's height was only at the 25th percentile. Short adult stature is more likely to occur in children with hypothyroidism of greater severity and duration who begin treatment in the early teenage years.

References

1. Longcope C. The Male and Female Reproductive Systems in Thyrotoxicosis. In: Braverman LE, Utiger

RD (eds). Werner and Ingbar's The Thyroid. 6th ed. Philadelphia: JB Lippincott Co., 1991, pp 828–835.

2. Longcope C. The Male and Female Reproductive Systems in Hypothyroidism. In: Braverman LE, Utiger RD (eds). Werner and Ingbar's The Thyroid. 6th ed. Philadelphia: JB Lippincott, 1991, pp 1052–1055.

3. Foley TP Jr. Acute, subacute and chronic thyroiditis. In: Kaplan SA (ed). Clinical Pediatric and Adolescent Endocrinology. Philadelphia: WB Saunders, 1982, pp 96–109.

4. Kohrle J, Hesch D, Leonard JL. Intracellular pathways of iodothyronine metabolism. In: Braverman LE, Utiger RD (eds). Werner and Ingbar's The Thyroid. 6th ed. Philadelphia: JB Lippincott, 1991, pp 144–189.

5. Dumont JE, Vassart G, Refetoff S. Thyroid disorders. In: Scriver CR, Beaudet AL, Sly WS, et al (eds). The Metabolic Basis of Inherited Disease. 6th ed. New York: McGraw-Hill, 1989, p 1843.

6. Scanlon MF. Neuroendocrine Control of Thyrotropin Secretion. In: Braverman LE, Utiger RD (eds). Werner and Ingbar's The Thyroid. 6th ed. Philadelphia: JB Lippincott, 1991, p 230–256.

7. Larsen PR, Silva JE, Kaplan MM. Relationships between circulating and intracellular thyroid hormones: Physiological and clinical implications. Endocr Rev 1981; 2:87–102.

8. Oppenheimer JH, Schwartz HL, Mariash CN, et al. Advances in our understanding of thyroid hormone action at the cellular level. Endocr Rev 1987; 8:288.

9. Nelson JC, Tomei RT. Direct determination of free thyroxine in undiluted serum by equilibrium dialysis/radioimmunoassay. Clin Chem 1988; 34:1737–1744.

10. Parry CH. Collections from the unpublished medical writings of the late Caleb Hillier Parry. Elements of Pathology and Therapeutics, 1825; 2:111–128.

11. von Basedow CA. Exophthalmos durch Hypertrophie des Zellgewebes in der Augenhöhle. Wochenschr Heilk 1840; 6:197–204, 220–228.

12. Weetman AP, Yateman ME, Ealey PA, et al. Thyroid-stimulating antibody activity between different immunoglobulin G subclasses. J Clin Invest 1990; 86:723–727.

13. Hiromatsu Y, Fukazawa H, Wall JR. Cytotoxic mechanisms in autoimmune thyroid disorders and thyroid-associated ophthalmopathy. Endocrinol Metab Clin North Am 1987; 16:269–286.

14. Foley TP. Thyrotoxicosis in childhood. Pediatr Ann 1992; 21:43–49.

15. Dallas JS, Foley TP. Hyperthyroidism. In: Lifshitz F (ed). Pediatric Endocrinology: A Clinical Guide. New York: Marcel Dekker, 1990, pp 483–500.

16. Weintraub BD, Gershengorn MC, Kourides IA, et al. Inappropriate secretion of thyroid stimulating hormone. Ann Intern Med 1981; 95:339.

17. Solomon B, Glinoer D, Lagasse R, Wartofsky L. Current trends in the management of Graves' disease. J Clin Endocrinol Metab 1990; 70:1518–1524.

18. Levey GS. The heart and hyperthyroidism. Use of beta-adrenergic blocking drugs. Med Clin North Am 1975; 59:1193–1201.

19. Cooper DS. Antithyroid drugs. N Engl J Med 1984; 311:1353.

20. Jansson R, Dahlberg PA, Johansson H, Lindström B. Intrathyroidal concentrations of methimazole in patients with Graves' disease. J Clin Endocrinol Metab 1983; 57:129–132.

21. Okuno A, Yano K, Inyaku F, et al. Pharmacokinetics of methimazole in children and adolescents with Graves' disease. Studies on plasma and intrathyroidal concentrations. Acta Endocrinol (Copenh) 1987; 115:112–118.

22. Hashizume K, Ichikawa K, Sakurai A, et al. Administration of thyroxine in treated Graves' disease. N Engl J Med 1991; 324:947–953.

23. Becker DV. The role of radioiodine treatment in childhood hyperthyroidism. J Nucl Med 1979; 20:890–894.

24. Levy WJ, Schumacher OP, Gupta M. Treatment of childhood Graves' disease. Cleve Clin J Med 1988; 55:373–382.

25. Stoffer SS, Hamburger JI. Inadvertent ^{131}I therapy for hyperthyroidism in the first trimester of pregnancy. J Nucl Med 1976; 17:146–149.

26. LaFranchi S. Thyroiditis and acquired hypothyroidism. Pediatr Ann 1992; 21:29–39.

27. Dallas JS, Foley TP Jr. Hypothyroidism. In: Lifshitz F (ed). Pediatric Endocrinology: A Clinical Guide. New York: Marcel Dekker, 1990, pp 469–481.

28. Hubble D. Endocrine relations. Lancet 1955; 1:1.

29. Van Wyk J, Grumbach MM. Syndrome of precocious menstruation and galactorrhea in juvenile hypothyroidism: An example of hormonal overlap pituitary feedback. J Pediatr 1960; 57:416.

30. Franks RC, Stempfel RS. Juvenile hypothyroidism and precocious testicular maturation. J Clin Endocrinol Metab 1963; 23:805.

31. Foley TP, Schubert WK, Marnell RT, McAdams AJ. Chronic lymphocytic thyroiditis and juvenile myxedema in uniovular twins. J Pediatr 1968; 72:201–207.

32. Arslanian S, Foley TP Jr, Lee PA. Endocrine and systemic manifestations of brain tumors in children. In: Deutsch M (ed). Management of Childhood Brain Tumors. Boston: Kluwer Academic, 1990, pp 137–173.

33. Foley TP Jr. Congenital hypopituitarism. In: Dussault JH, Walker PA (eds). Congenital Hypothyroidism. New York: Marcel Dekker, 1983, pp 331–348.

34. Illig R, Krawczynska H, Torresani T, Prader A. Elevated plasma TSH and hypothyroidism in children with hypothalamic hypopituitarism. J Clin Endocrinol Metab 1975; 41:722–728.

35. Pinchera A, Martino E, Faglia G. Central hypothyroidism. In: Braverman LE, Utiger RD (eds). Werner and Ingbar's The Thyroid. 6th ed. Philadelphia: JB Lippincott, 1991, pp 968–984.

36. Rivkees SA, Bode HH, Crawford JD. Long-term growth in juvenile acquired hypothyroidism: The failure to achieve normal adult stature. N Engl J Med 1988; 318:599–602.

CHAPTER 10

Molecular Biology and Genetic Aspects

LEE P. SHULMAN
STEPHEN S. WACHTEL

The clinical applications of molecular biology have increased considerably since the 1980s. Genetics is no longer the domain of geneticists alone; molecular methods have become important diagnostic tools in most clinical specialties, including diverse ones such as infectious disease, pathology, and clinical immunology. These methods have enabled more accurate diagnosis and have improved the delineation of disease and the monitoring of treatment modalities. In addition, molecular biology has entered the arena of adolescent and pediatric gynecology. Health care professionals providing gynecologic care to adolescent and pediatric patients should be aware of the molecular techniques applicable to the diagnosis and management of problems they are likely to encounter.

The molecular methods currently available to clinicians include identification of specific DNA sequences by Southern blotting and hybridization, DNA sequence analysis, genetic fingerprinting, and amplification of specific DNA sequences by polymerase chain reaction. This chapter discusses these methods and reviews their application to two problems frequently encountered in the adolescent and pediatric population: sexual assault and abnormal sexual development. A comprehensive description of laboratory methodology is beyond the scope of this chapter, and interested readers are encouraged to review the technical literature referenced throughout the text.

MOLECULAR BIOLOGY: RECOMBINANT DNA METHODS

Restriction Enzymes

The fleas we know have other fleas,
Upon their backs to bite 'em,
And these in turn have other fleas,
And so ad infinitum.

The validity of this little rhyme has yet to be ascertained, but we do know that bacterial cells are hosts for viruses known as *bacteriophages* or simply *phages*—minute particles existing in the mysterious and obscure reaches between the realms of life and nonlife.

Regardless of whether they are alive, bacterial viruses are parasites of the bacterial cell. In general, the individual phage particle consists of a duplex molecule of DNA surrounded by a protein coat. The phage attaches to the cell wall of the bacterium and injects its DNA into the cell. As a consequence of that injection, the protein- and DNA-synthesizing programs of the bacterial cell are subverted: viral proteins and DNA chains, not chains of the bacterium, are produced. These components are assembled into new virus particles inside the bacterium so that the infected cell becomes little more than a shell containing a hundred or so viruses. The cell virtually explodes, thereby releasing the nascent viruses into the surrounding milieu.

Students of medicine know that the entire life cycle of a virus lasts about 20 minutes and that billions of viruses can be produced within a couple of hours, given the proper host and environment. However, bacterial cells are not without their defenses; among the proteins produced by bacteria are enzymes that cut viral DNA into harmless pieces. These enzymes recognize very short base sequences that are common in viral DNA but rare in bacterial DNA. An example is *Eco*RI (for *Escherichia coli* restriction enzyme one), which cuts DNA wherever it encounters the following sequence:

— GAATTC —
— CTTAAG —

The cut is made as follows:

— G • AATTC —
— CTTAA • G —

Bacterial enzymes that cut DNA in this way are called *restriction enzymes* because they restrict the ability of viruses to infect and reproduce. Many different restriction enzymes have been identified in a variety of bacteria. The sequence of bases that the restriction enzyme cuts is called a *restriction site* or *recognition sequence*. The fragments resulting from digestion of DNA with a particular restriction enzyme are called *restriction fragments*.

Restriction enzymes are valuable tools for molecular biology because they allow geneticists to dissect, analyze, and restructure DNA in a predictable and controlled fashion. For example, by using several alternative restriction enzymes with a given sample of DNA, it is possible to produce a *restriction map* showing a linear sequence of restriction sites and restriction fragments in the sample under study. (Differences in restriction maps among individuals are called *restriction fragment length polymorphisms*, or RFLPs.) As another example, geneticists can use restriction enzymes to remove a sequence of bases from between two restriction sites in one piece of DNA and insert it into another piece of DNA that contains the same restriction sites. The product of this kind of manipulation is called *recombinant DNA*.

The techniques of recombinant DNA allow human DNA sequences to be placed into bacterial (plasmid) or viral DNA. This enables large-scale replication of the human sequences; when the bacterial or viral DNA is replicated, the human DNA also is replicated. Given the short life cycle of bacteria and bacterial viruses, it is thus possible to generate millions of copies of a desired sequence. This is called *cloning*. The target DNA can be removed from the recombinant molecule by applying the same restriction enzyme used to insert it. Cloning allows comprehensive analysis of DNA—determination of the exact sequence of nucleotide bases, for example, and thereby elucidation of the precise order of amino acids in the corresponding protein.[1]

Probes

The human genome contains about 3×10^9 base pairs (bp) of DNA. Hence, the DNA in a single gene (usually about 300 to 2000 bp) represents only a tiny fraction of the total. To identify a particular gene, a specific *probe*—a sequence of DNA able to react with the target sequence—is required. The probe may correspond to the entire gene or to sequences within the gene.

One way to obtain a probe is to identify a target messenger RNA (mRNA) by separation from newly synthesized protein, for example, and to synthesize DNA by use of the mRNA as a template. The enzyme that catalyzes this reaction is called *reverse transcriptase*. The initial product of the reaction is a hybrid molecule consisting of one strand of mRNA and one strand of complementary DNA (cDNA). When the reaction is complete, the mRNA is degraded with alkali, and the single-stranded cDNA is converted, by use of the enzyme *DNA polymerase*, into double-stranded cDNA. The double-stranded cDNA can be cloned and used as a probe.[2]

There are alternative ways to develop probes. For instance, enriched populations of Y chromosomes or any other chromosomes can be obtained by flow cytometry. If the Y chromosomal DNA is digested with restriction enzymes, the result is a series of Y-specific DNA fragments. Some of these can be used as probes to evaluate children with ambiguous genitalia, as the presence of a Y chromosome or portion thereof may be responsible for some cases of sexual ambiguity in children. In addition, Y-specific probes are valuable for evaluating XX males. Because sex reversal in XX males usually is due to Y-X crossovers involving transfer of the testis-determining gene (*TDF*), and because Y-X crossovers may involve more or less Y material, those probes that are closer to *TDF* would be expected in a greater proportion of XX males than would those that are more distal. This has enabled construction of maps depicting the relative positions of a number of Y probes and has led to the discovery of the zinc finger Y (*ZFY*) gene, an early candidate for the human *TDF*, and, more recently, to the discovery of sex-determining region (*SRY*) gene, the prime candidate.

Identification of Specific Sequences

Southern Blotting

For the sake of illustration, say that a young woman presenting with amenorrhea, eunuchoid habitus, and short stature is found to have a karyotype of 46,X + marker. The marker chromosome is small and could represent part of the short arm of either the X or the Y. Keeping in mind that females possessing Y fragments have an increased risk of gonadal malignancy,[3] we wish to determine the nature of the marker chromosome. Let us assume that we have a probe—call it Y-1—representing a DNA segment proximal to the Y centromere. By the following method, called *Southern blotting* after its inventor,[4] we can then determine whether the marker is Y derived.

A sample of DNA is first extracted from the patient's blood. The DNA is then fractionated by digestion with restriction enzyme. Say that the *Eco*RI restriction enzyme is used. Wherever the enzyme encounters its recognition site (—GAATTC—), it will cut (—G / AATTC—), and the result will be a series of fragments of varying sizes. Next the DNA fragments are placed in a gel matrix and exposed to an electric field, in which they migrate according to size; the smaller fragments migrate faster than the larger fragments. The fragments can accordingly be classified by the number of DNA base pairs that they contain. It is convenient to describe the size of such fragments in terms of the thousands of base pairs. These are referred to as *kilobases* (kb). A particular fragment might contain 5.5 kb, for instance, or 6.8 kb.

When the migration (*electrophoresis*) is completed, the DNA fragments are denatured and transferred (*blotted*) onto a nitrocellulose or nylon matrix and thereby immobilized. By this method, the DNA fragments can be removed from the gel and transferred in exactly the same positions that they occupied in the gel.

Copies of the probe, Y-1, are placed onto the filter under conditions that favor *hybridization*, the reaction of sequences in the probe with complementary sequences in the target DNA, which is denatured before transfer (so probe and target DNA both are single stranded). The hybridization reaction is visualized by the use of radiolabeled or chemiluminescent probes. The result is a band or series of bands on the filter or photographic plate, identifying the fragment to which the probe has bound. The size of the fragment is determined by comparing the position of the band with markers of known size (Fig. 10–1).

In the test being described, DNA from the patient would be compared with samples of DNA from normal male and female controls. Given that the probe is specific to the Y chromosome, we would expect at least a single hybridization band in the male DNA and absence of that band in the female DNA. Presence of the band in the patient would signal the presence of at least that part of the Y chromosome corresponding to the probe. By use of alternative probes from across the Y, one could determine the approximate amount of Y material in the marker chromosome.

When a probe represents part or all of a specific gene, it is possible to determine whether that gene is present in a genome. In certain cases, by the application of small (*oligonucleotide*) probes, geneticists can use Southern blotting techniques to identify particular mutations within genes.

Northern Blotting

The Northern blotting technique is essentially similar to the technique described for Southern blotting, except that mRNA rather than DNA is probed. As a result, the geneticist obtains a measure of transcription (expression) of the target gene. Say, for example, that a gene has been identified as a candidate for *TDF*. By Northern blotting it may be ascer-

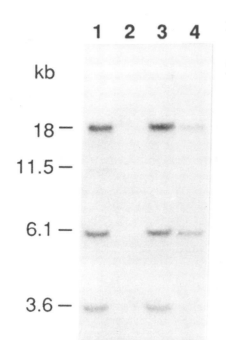

FIGURE 10–1 ••• Southern blot. Autoradiograph of genomic DNA hybridized with radioactive phosphorus (^{32}P)—labeled probe pT5.1.1.PH, which identifies Y chromosome–specific sequences in the mouse. Lanes contain mouse DNA as follows: 1, normal XY male; 2, normal XX female; 3, sex-reversed XX male with Y-X crossover; 4, sex-reversed XX male carrying deleted Y-X crossover. The sizes of the fragments identified by the probe can be estimated by comparison with the kilobase (kb) markers at left. (From Mitchell MJ, Bishop CE. A structural analysis of the Sxr region of the mouse Y chromosome. Genomics 1992; 12:26.)

tained whether the gene is transcribed in testis, male lung, or kidney, and it may be shown whether the gene is transcribed in the gonadal ridge at about the time of testicular differentiation. That is precisely how Northern blotting was used to evaluate the candidacy of the *SRY* gene, currently accepted as *TDF*. An RNA transcript hybridizing with the *SRY* probe (pY53.3) was identified in testis but not in male lung or kidney,[5] and a corresponding transcript was identified in the gonadal ridge of the fetal mouse, just before emergence of the seminiferous tubules.[6]

Dot Blots and Slot Blots

Methods exist for rapid screening of desired sequences in DNA and RNA. The samples to be analyzed are first digested and denatured, as in Southern or Northern blotting. However, the extracted DNA or RNA is then applied directly to nitrocellulose or another matrix without electrophoresis. By application of a particular probe, one can then determine whether the corresponding sequence is present in the sample, without reference to the size of the fragments that may be recognized by the probe. (This information is lacking in the absence of electrophoresis.) The difference between slot blots and dot blots lies in the shape of the recess or template in the apparatus used to capture the DNA or RNA under study. The slot is a thin rectangle, whereas the dot is a small circle. In both cases, the formats facilitate consistent loading of samples. The amount of sample hybridizing with a particular probe can be quantified by densitometry.

Stringency

Stringency refers to the conditions of the hybridization reaction that determine the stability of the resulting DNA duplex. A stringency of 80% means that 80% of the base pairs in a duplex are matched. It is possible to vary the stringency of hybridization, in Southern blots for example, by changing the temperature and salt concentration when the filter is washed. At higher stringency (i.e., higher temperature, lower salt concentration), a greater degree of base pair matching is required between probe and target DNA for hybridization to occur (that is, in order for the probe to recognize the target sequence). By varying the temperature and salt concentration, the geneticist can apply the probe to the identification of sequences related to, but not identical with, the target sequence.

Consider this example. The gene for the platelet-activating factor receptor (PAFR) has been cloned recently in guinea pig DNA, but the corresponding human gene has not been cloned. Given the likelihood of strong evolutionary conservation (PAFR belongs to the G protein–coupled receptor superfamily), the guinea pig probe might be used to isolate a corresponding human sequence by screening a human cDNA library at reduced stringencies. Fragments with which the probe hybridizes could then be cloned and the desired human sequence identified by testing for function or by partial sequence analysis (see next section).

DNA Sequencing

It may be said that the chief goal of genetics is to determine the nucleotide sequence of genes, for this would allow comparison of normal (wild type) and mutant genes, and thus correlation of discrete lesions (nucleotide base substitutions, deletions, etc.), with particular disorders. In fact, current methods enable the geneticist to routinely decipher the sequence of a gene or a particular DNA fragment. Two methods in particular have been employed in this regard: the method of Maxam and Gilbert,[7] which involves chemical modification and cleavage of specific nucleotides, followed by electrophoresis of the resulting fragments in high-resolution acrylamide gels; and the dideoxy chain termination method of Sanger et al.,[8] which involves synthesis of small fragments of DNA in a way that curtails elongation of each fragment at a position corresponding to a particular base; this is also followed by electrophoresis in acrylamide. The method of Sanger et al.,[8] which is perhaps the more widely used, is reviewed.

First, a series of 2', 3'-dideoxynucleotides, representing each of the four bases (ddATP, ddTTP, ddCTP, ddGTP), is prepared. Because each of these bases possesses a normal 5'-triphosphate, each can be taken up into the growing DNA chain by DNA polymerase. However, once it is incorporated, a dideoxynucleotide (ddNTP) blocks chain growth because it will not form a bond with the deoxynucleotide (dNTP) next in line; elongation of that fragment is terminated. For sequencing, four polymerase reactions are performed, each involving one of the four nucleotide bases, which has been labeled. When the ddNTPs are mixed with "normal" bases (dNTPs) in the correct ratio, some of the polymerizing reactions are terminated, while most others continue. The result is a series of DNA fragments, each one a single base longer than the preceding one, and each terminating at a particular base (A,T,C,G). The fragments are then separated by electrophoresis in an acrylamide gel. The pattern of migration, which corresponds exactly to the particular sequence of nucleotides in the segment of DNA under study, is visualized by autoradiography or chemiluminescence (Fig. 10–2). With this method it is possible to determine the sequence of about 250 to 300 bases at a time. For large segments, 250 to 300 bp are read in alternative fragments, and the

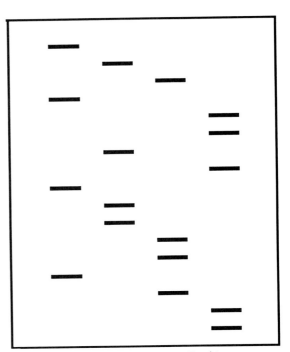

FIGURE 10–2 ••• DNA sequencing. Graphic representation of autoradiograph depicting nucleotide bands in a sequencing gel. The order of nucleotides in the segment analyzed is C-C-A-T-A-A-G-G-T-C-G-C-C-T-A-G-T.

overlapping sequences are combined to give the complete sequence.

DNA Fingerprinting

The human genome contains long repetitive DNA sequences known as *satellites*, so called because they are representative of small shoulders, or "satellites," off the main peak in cesium chloride density ultracentrifugation profiles of DNA (Fig. 10–3). Satellite DNA occurs typically in the heterochromatic regions of the chromosomes, which are usually genetically inert; the DNA in these regions is sometimes called "junk DNA." Within these regions, the G:C and A:T base pairs are distributed unequally, and thus satellite DNA has a density that is different from the density of the main body of DNA.

A number of polymorphic "minisatellites" have been identified in human DNA. These consist of tandem repeats of a core sequence containing, say, from 10 to 15 bp, as in the (AGGGCTGGAGG)n sequence described by

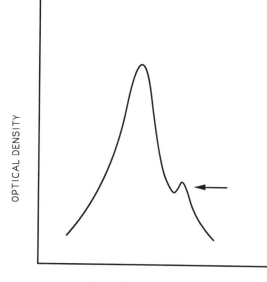

OPTICAL DENSITY

◄—— BUOYANT DENSITY

FIGURE 10–3 ••• Satellite DNA. The buoyant density of double-stranded DNA—a function of G-C content—may be determined by centrifugation through a cesium chloride density gradient. The main peak depicted in the figure includes 90% of the DNA in the genome. This is centered around a value of 1.70 gm/cm⁻³ corresponding to an average G-C content of 42%, which is typical of mammals. The small peak at the right (*arrow*) represents 10% of the genome. This is a satellite DNA with a G-C content of 30% and a buoyant density of 1.69 gm/cm⁻³. Satellites may have densities that are larger or smaller than those represented by the main peak.

Jeffreys et al.[9] This particular type of satellite DNA is also known as *variable numbers of tandem repeats* (VNTRs), as these repeated sequences are characterized by hypervariable numbers of these sequences throughout the genome. The great variability in the number of repeated sequences is probably generated by unequal crossing over, thereby yielding a composite of specific VNTRs that differs from individual to individual—in other words, a *DNA fingerprint*. Southern blotting and hybridization with probes comprising multiple repeats of the core sequence can be used to detect several distinct sequences simultaneously, thereby enabling identification of individuals for family, demographic, and linkage studies. Evidently these sequences are inherited in mendelian fashion; they exhibit germline and somatic stability.

DNA fingerprinting has been used to identify individuals and to determine genetic relationships in many species, including dogs, cats, house sparrows, lesser snow geese, and various

sea turtles and whales. An example of DNA fingerprinting in the sea turtle is given in Figure 10–4. In humans, DNA fingerprinting is used in paternity testing and forensic medicine. In an immigration case in England, DNA fingerprinting enabled positive identification of a Ghanian boy desiring to live with his mother.[10]

Despite this, the validity of DNA fingerprint analysis has been questioned, particularly in criminal cases involving sexual assault. The major problem is that the methods for identification of DNA samples may yield inconclusive or even spurious data. In an editorial on the subject of genetic fingerprinting, Lander[11] pointed out that artifacts can be generated with the use of forensic DNA samples, which are likely to be degraded or contaminated. In citing the paper by Budowle et al.,[12] Lander noted that when fresh DNA from the victim's blood was compared with forensic samples from the vaginal epithelium in 111 cases of rape, corresponding fragments differed by as much as 5% ± 1.5% (S.D.) molecular weight, and forensic samples exhibited a tendency to migrate faster during electrophoresis than did freshly extracted samples. In addition, he noted that little has been published concerning laboratory-to-laboratory variation in fingerprint analysis (or even variation within the same laboratory), and that the problem of "bandshifting" resulting from contamination, degradation, or differences in sample concentration remains to be solved.

Polymerase Chain Reaction

The ability to amplify a particular segment of DNA—to produce billions or even trillions of copies of a single DNA molecule—has sparked a revolution in molecular biology. DNA amplification by polymerase chain reaction (PCR) was first described by Saiki et al.[13] The method has since found a broad spectrum of applications in medicine, genetics, and evolutionary biology.[14]

The PCR consists of three basic steps: denaturation of double-stranded DNA, attachment of oligonucleotide primers that delineate a target sequence, and synthesis of new DNA corresponding to the target sequence. Usually each step is carried out at a particular temperature; for example, denaturation from 94°C to 98°C, primer attachment ("annealing") from 37°C to 65°C, and replication at 72°C. The target sequence is amplified by running the

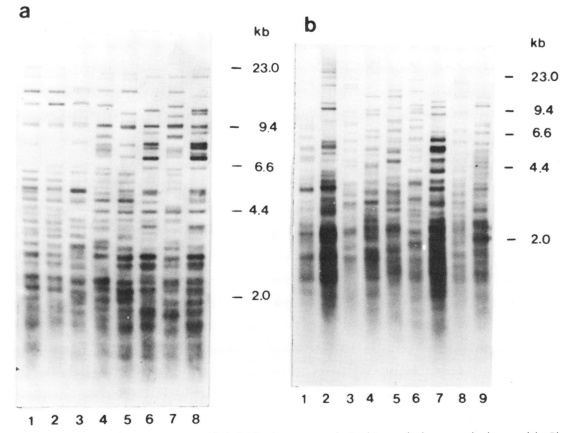

FIGURE 10–4 ••• DNA fingerprinting. Variable hybridization patterns obtained in two freshwater turtles by use of the Bkm probe (GATA) after digestion of DNA with the restriction enzyme BstN1: *A, Trionyx spiniferous* (spiny soft shell); *B, Trachemys scripta* (red-eared slider). Each of the numbered lanes contains the "fingerprint" of a particular animal. The size of the individual fragments (or bands) can be approximated by reference to the kb markers to the right of each Southern blot. (From Demas S, Wachtel S. DNA fingerprinting in reptiles: Bkm hybridization patterns in Crocodilia and Chelonia. Genome 1991; 34:472.)

PCR through several (say, from 20 to 40) cycles; this results in an exponential increase in the number of target sequences, because the products generated in cycle *n* can serve as templates in the next cycle ($n + 1$).

Although large fragments of DNA can be amplified in the PCR, many reactions are limited to segments of about 400 bp or less. As an example, say that we wish to amplify a 300-bp segment within a particular gene. We must have the nucleotide sequences of the regions immediately flanking the target sequence. Then we can produce the oligonucleotide primers that will delineate the sequence to be amplified. The primers are single-stranded DNA molecules of about 18 to 24 bases in length. Once annealed to the target sequence, they serve in initiating replication and in controlling the direction of synthesis (Fig. 10–5). The reaction is catalyzed by the heat-stable enzyme *Taq* polymerase, obtained from the thermophilic bacterium, *Thermus aquaticus*. Use of *Taq* polymerase enables the entire reaction to be carried out in a single tube in a temperature-cycling apparatus.

The potential applications of PCR are numerous. The following are a sample:

1. *Diagnosis:* In the aforementioned female patient with the 46,X, + mar karyotype, the origin of the marker chromosome was identified by Southern blotting. This could be done more easily using PCR with oligonucleotide primers delineating Y chromosome–specific sequences. As another example, the products of PCR amplification can be tested for single base changes with oligonucleotide *probes*, as in the original report by Saiki et al.,[13] in which the authors describe a method for diagnosis of sickle cell anemia by detection of polymorphism within the β-globin gene.

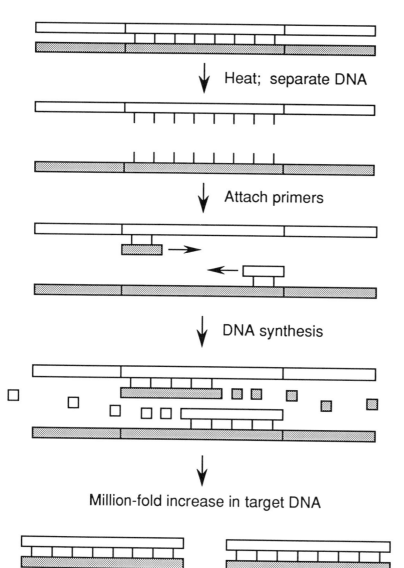

Heat; separate DNA

Attach primers

DNA synthesis

Million-fold increase in target DNA

FIGURE 10–5 ••• Polymerase chain reaction (PCR). The weak bonds that unite the individual DNA strands are broken by heating, and the strands are separated. Then the single-stranded primers are attached. The primers delineate the sequence to be replicated and determine the orientation of DNA synthesis. Replication is accomplished in the presence of heat-resistant Taq polymerase; the small squares represent the incoming nucleotides. The process may be repeated through numerous cycles, generating millions or billions of copies of a desired sequence. See text for a detailed description.

2. *Oncology:* Mutations within the *ras* oncogene, common in certain tumors, can likewise be diagnosed by PCR in combination with short DNA probes used to hybridize with the amplified fragments.

3. *Forensics:* PCR has enabled evaluation of minute quantities of degraded DNA in samples that could not be used for standard DNA fingerprint analysis. The alternative method, involving Southern blotting, calls for greater quantities of intact high-molecular-weight DNA than are needed in PCR.

4. *Evolutionary biology:* One of the more fascinating applications of PCR is in the study of DNA from extinct species such as the wooly mammoth and quagga, an African equine resembling the zebra. There is one case involving amplification of sequences from the brain of a 7500-year old mummy.

5. *Genetics:* By reverse transcription, it is also possible to amplify DNA from mRNA templates. This enables study not only of the presence of a gene, but also of its expression.

For a more detailed description of the applications of PCR, see Erlich.[14]

Contamination. Anyone who has used PCR is familiar with the problem of contamination. Because billions of copies of a sequence can be produced from a single template, it is necessary to ensure that contaminating templates are not present in the reaction mixture. Given that templates can be provided by a single foreign cell, or even a single molecule, the risk of contamination is significant, and the use of sterile reagents and utensils and containment facilities is advisable. Several methods are under development to eliminate or reduce contamination, especially methods to control the potential for carryover of PCR product from one reaction to another.

FORENSIC APPLICATIONS OF RECOMBINANT DNA TECHNOLOGY: SEXUAL ASSAULT

The methods described here have generated considerable enthusiasm in forensic medicine; as noted earlier, recombinant DNA techniques can provide data concerning the identification of individuals and can be applied to the analysis of tissue specimens not previously amenable to forensic analysis. DNA analysis is currently widely used to determine parentage; to identify people *physically* involved in homicide, sexual assault, and other crimes; and to identify the victims of kidnapping, murder, or natural disasters. DNA methodology does not necessarily require fresh blood or tissue samples for analysis, but can be applied to the analysis of blood or tissue samples exposed to the environment for varying periods of time.

Pediatric and adolescent gynecologists are frequently called on to assess the young victims of sexual assault. In addition to the gynecologist's central role in the emotional and physical care of these victims of sexual assault, he or she must also assist government authorities in identifying the responsible parties. Thus, pediatric and adolescent gynecologists must be aware of the methods currently used for inclusion or exclusion of sexual assault suspects. This section reviews the application of recombinant DNA techniques to the evaluation of sexual assault, as well as the applications and limitations of such technologies in various legal jurisdictions.

Forensic DNA Fingerprinting. DNA fingerprinting, or DNA profiling, can be used to identify the source of seminal fluid or other tissues recovered from sexual assault victims. This technology can also be utilized to detect more than one assailant. In addition, if the sexual assault occurred soon after consensual sexual intercourse with a different partner, DNA profiling can effectively differentiate the tissue of a husband or boyfriend from that of an assailant. Despite the power of DNA fingerprinting in identifying sexual assailants, there are limitations to the data produced by such analyses, with problems ranging from improper preparation of specimens to inaccurate interpretation of data.[15] These problems have limited the universal acceptance of DNA fingerprinting in cases of sexual assault.[16]

DNA Extraction. DNA for forensic analysis can be obtained from any nucleated cell. However, the quality of analysis directly correlates with the quality of the specimen from which the DNA was extracted. Extraction of high-quality DNA is related to the size and age of the specimen and the environmental conditions in which the specimen was found and eventually stored.[17] For example, a 72-hour-old dried semen specimen will not usually yield the same quality DNA as a specimen obtained from the vagina 6 hours after ejaculation. A general rule is that a specimen recently produced and not exposed to extreme heat or cold will yield higher quality DNA than an older specimen exposed to the environment. However, universal standards regarding tissue volume and environmental conditions have yet to be determined.

DNA Storage and Transport. Despite the desirability of immediate extraction of DNA from a specimen at a crime scene, this is not always possible. Appropriate conditions for storage of various tissues amenable to forensic DNA analysis are given in Table 10–1. Determination of which storage condition to use

TABLE 10–1 ••• STORAGE OF TISSUE OR EXTRACTED DNA

	Storage Requirements
Unextracted tissue	Room temperature
	4°C
	−25°C to 195°C
	Fixed in alcohol or saline
Extracted DNA	Room temperature
	4°C
	Chloroform (5 μl/ml)
	Frozen (kept indefinitely)
Tissue lysate	Unextracted tissue placed in a solution containing 100 mmol *tris*-HCl, 40 mmol ethylenediaminetetra-acetic acid, 0.2% sodium dodecyl sulfate (pH, 8.0)

depends on the specific tissue, the type of analysis to be performed, and the amount of time that the sample or extracted DNA will be stored or transported.

DNA is relatively stable and, once extracted, can be shipped at room temperature or kept indefinitely if frozen. However, repetitive freezing and thawing will result in degradation and are not recommended. DNA can also be stored in chloroform (optimal concentration: 5 μl/ml) for long periods of time.

VNTRs. The specific method used to identify individuals involved in sexual assault will depend on the quality and quantity of specimen available and the type of information desired. For cases in which a recently ejaculated seminal specimen is recovered, DNA fingerprinting utilizing probes of VNTRs is widely used. VNTRs are characterized by repetitive sequences found in specific regions of the human genome and are polymorphic in different individuals (i.e., the number and location of these sequences differ from person to person).[18-21] Thus, analysis of VNTRs in DNA extracted from seminal fluid recovered from the vagina of assault victims can be used to differentiate the victim's own DNA and the DNA of consensual sexual partners from that of the purported sexual assailant.

Once it is extracted from the seminal specimen, the DNA is exposed to restriction enzymes, subjected to gel electrophoresis, and blotted onto a nitrocellulose filter (see "Molecular Biology: Recombinant DNA Methods"). Hybridization using either multilocus or single-locus VNTRs probes may then be performed; the decision as to which probes to use is based on the type of information required. Multilocus VNTR probes produce a complex banding pattern (see Fig. 10–4) for each individual and are used for paternity determination and to resolve questions of relatedness. Single-locus probes produce a maximum of two bands, representing the two alleles at a given genetic locus. Several single-locus probe analyses can be performed to provide data concerning several genetic loci and can usually include or exclude a sexual assailant suspect. The sensitivity and specificity of VNTR analysis depend on the clarity of the DNA banding pattern, which is directly related to the quality of the DNA and to the quality control program implemented by the individual laboratory.[16]

Single-Locus Polymorphism. Unfortunately, recently ejaculated seminal specimens are not always recoverable from the crime scene. In some cases, victims do not obtain medical treatment for several days after the assault; in other cases, the assailant does not ejaculate within the vagina or does not ejaculate at all. In these cases, degraded seminal specimens, fingernail scrapings, or hair samples may provide the only DNA recoverable from the assailant; the amount of such DNA is usually small and not amenable to either multilocus or single-locus VNTR probe analysis. For these cases, single-locus polymorphism probes can be used to exclude sexual assailant suspects.[22]

Single-locus polymorphism probes identify deletions, additions, or inversions at specific sites within the genome, the presence or absence of which may differ among individuals.[23] Such probes may be applied to small or degraded DNA specimens; Southern blot and dot blot techniques may both be used in the analyses. The dot blot technique, which is similar to Southern blotting but without the electrophoresis, is especially appealing, because it depends simply on hybridization of the probe and a DNA sample and does not involve electrophoresis. Thus, dot blots provide data in a more timely fashion and are less costly than Southern blots. Despite the advantages of single-locus polymorphism probe analysis, the technique is not very specific and may require multiple probes to include or exclude suspects.[22]

Statistical Analysis. The prime question addressed by molecular methods in cases of sexual assault cases is whether the DNA obtained at the crime scene is the same as a suspect's DNA. Statistical analysis is used to estimate the probability that DNA obtained at the crime scene is that of a particular suspect. The analyst must take into account not only the frequency in the general population of the studied alleles, but also the probability that the alleles analyzed are sufficient to include or exclude suspects. Selection of specific statistical methods thus depends on the data available and the information desired. A review of statistical tests used in forensic medicine is found in Kirby.[16]

Legal Considerations. Despite the relatively wide acceptance of DNA analysis by civil and criminal courts, the limitations previously mentioned have served to prevent universal admissibility of molecular results into criminal and civil legal proceedings. DNA forensic technology is relatively new,[9] and for this reason the data generated by DNA techniques are considered novel and not always accepted as evidence. Novel scientific data, if it is to be admitted as evidence in a court of law, usually must pass two "tests": the Frye test and the relevancy test. The Frye test[24] is based on the case *Frye v. United States*,[25] in which the District of Columbia Court of Appeals ruled that ". . . the thing from which the deduction is made must be sufficiently established to have gained general acceptance in the particular field to which it belongs." The Frye test thus is meant to ensure that only data resulting from reliable scientific tests can be admitted as evidence. Once data from a novel scientific diagnostic test are admitted as evidence in a certain legal jurisdiction, similar data can be admitted in the future *in that specific legal jurisdiction* without the need to further demonstrate the reliability of the method. Without universal standards and guidelines, data from DNA analyses resulting from different DNA techniques or performed in different laboratories may be required to "pass" another Frye test within a certain legal jurisdiction that may have already admitted, as evidence, similar DNA analyses performed in a different laboratory.

The relevancy test asserts that novel scientific data are similar to other expert testimony,[26] allowing the data to be admitted but also ". . . attacked by cross-examination and refutation."[27] The relevancy approach neither accepts nor refutes the Frye test, but instead permits judges more latitude in accepting such evidence. The relevancy approach has been promulgated by some Federal jurisdictions; the Third Circuit Court of Appeals has held that ". . . some scientific evidence can assist the trier of fact in reaching an accurate determination of facts in issue even though the principles underlying the evidence have not become generally accepted in the field to which they belong." Such rulings permit parties to attempt refutation of the findings of DNA analysis based on demonstration of one or several of the aforementioned limitations.

As more legal jurisdictions accept molecular methods as commonplace, data generated by DNA analysis will be more easily utilized in criminal and civil cases. However, data generated by DNA analyses may not be considered "relevant" if discrepancies in the analysis or its interpretation are demonstrated in court. Only strict, universal quality control standards for all aspects of DNA analysis,[17] as are currently in place for forensic blood protein tests, will serve to ensure that information generated by DNA analysis will truly be representative of the individuals involved and thus properly utilized to assess innocence or guilt.

MOLECULAR TECHNIQUES IN THE STUDY OF SEXUAL DIFFERENTIATION

Pediatric and adolescent gynecologists are frequently called on to evaluate abnormal sexual differentiation or genital tract abnormalities. Although normal sexual and genital tract differentiation involves complex interaction among genetic, hormonal, and environmental factors, genetic factors have begun to play an increasing role in the diagnosis of abnormal sexual and genital tract differentiation. This section reviews genetic aspects of normal sexual differentiation and discusses the genetics of normal and abnormal development of the female reproductive tract.

Normal Sex Differentiation

It is well known that the Y chromosome determines sex (the embryo becomes a male in the presence of the Y and a female in its absence), but it is not known how this is accomplished. In recent years, several Y-situated genes and sequences have been candidates for *TDF*. These include the *HYS* gene, which governs expression of the serologic H-Y ("male") antigen; the Bkm minisatellite, a tetranucleotide originally recovered from the sex-determining W chromosome of the banded krait (a snake); the *ZFY* gene, which encodes a zinc finger protein; and the *SRY* gene, which encodes a protein with a conservative DNA binding motif.

Among these sequences,[28] the *SRY* gene seems to be the most likely candidate for several reasons. It is highly conservative. *SRY*-like sequences are found in a broad spectrum of vertebrate species, including representatives of five major classes.[5, 29] The *SRY* gene contains a conservative motif of 80 amino acids, with "striking" homology to part of the Mc mating-type protein of the fission yeast, *Schizosaccharomyces pombe*, and to a DNA binding motif found in the nuclear high-mobility-group proteins, HMG1 and HMG2. The mouse homologue (written *Sry*) is located in the smallest region of the mouse Y chromosome known to induce the testis and is deleted in a line of XY females. It is expressed in the gonadal ridge of the mouse embryo at precisely the time of testicular development, and its transcription is curtailed after formation of the seminiferous tubules. It is expressed in the somatic cells of the gonad and not in the germ cells (presence of germ cells is not a prerequisite for testicular differentiation). Finally, microinsertion of a 14-kb segment of DNA containing *Sry* evoked development of testes in at least some transgenic XX mice.[30]

Further evidence of a testis-inducing role of *SRY* is provided in cases of sex reversal in the human. For example, the *SRY* gene is found in most XX males (indicating that XX sex reversal is, in general, secondary to Y-X crossover of the testis-determining locus), and mutations within *SRY* have been discovered in certain women with XY gonadal dysgenesis, characterized by failure of testicular differentiation, presence of streak gonads, and primary amenorrhea.

Some XX males do not possess *SRY*, and most women with XY gonadal dysgenesis appear to have *SRY* genes indistinguishable from those in normal males, at least with respect to the conservative region. These findings, together with other data that will be summarized here, provide evidence of the role of other genes in testicular organogenesis and some insights into the nature of primary (gonadal) sex differentiation. Thus, absence of *SRY* in certain XX males[31] argues for unregulated expression of "downstream" X-linked or autosomal testis-determining genes, and the presence of apparently intact *SRY* genes in (most) women with XY gonadal dysgenesis argues for mutation in those same genes. Indeed, X-linked and autosomal transmission is indicated in familial cases of XY gonadal dysgenesis, and X-chromosomal rearrangements have been correlated with failure of testicular development in those with Gardner-Silengo-Wachtel (genito-palato-cardiac) syndrome.

Autosomal Genes in XY Gonadal Dysgenesis. According to the scheme advanced by Wolf et al.,[32] the structural genes for testicular differentiation are on an autosome, repressed by genes in the noninactivated part of the X and derepressed by a gene on the Y. It follows that some forms of XY gonadal dysgenesis are a result of failure of the autosomal genes and are transmitted as autosomal recessive traits. After excluding kindreds with likely X-linked inheritance, Simpson et al.[33] evaluated segregation ratios in 24 families. Among these were 12 families with a single case of XY gonadal

dysgenesis, six with two cases, and six with three cases. Although X-linked recessive and male-limited autosomal dominant transmission could not be ruled out, the frequency of affected relatives was not different from the frequency that would be expected if the condition were inherited as an autosomal recessive trait limited to XY embryos. Moreover, autosomal genes would seem likely in the etiology of XY gonadal dysgenesis, as the majority of cases seem to arise sporadically.

X-linked Genes in XY Gonadal Dysgenesis. Several cases of XY gonadal dysgenesis can be attributed directly to failure of X-linked genes. Among the familial cases surveyed by Simpson et al.,[33] X-linked recessive inheritance was demonstrated in four.[34] The last family was described in Mann et al.[35] This included three affected sisters, an affected maternal second cousin, and a maternal aunt. The maternal grandmother of the affected siblings had a sister who was infertile and presumed to be an XY female. The maternal great-grandmother had three infertile sisters, each presumed to be an affected XY female.

As noted earlier, rearrangements of the X chromosome have been detected in cases of the Gardner-Silengo-Wachtel syndrome, which involves sex reversal in XY female infants with multiple congenital abnormalities.[36] For example, Bernstein and coworkers[37] described an anomalous additional band in the short arm of the X chromosome in a profoundly retarded girl with somatic features, including ventricular septal defect, cleft palate, and asymmetric skull and facies. The karyotype was 46,Xp+Y, representing a duplication of part of the short arm [46,dup(X)(p21pter)Y]. When the child died at 5 years of age, necropsy disclosed hypoplastic uterus and tubes. Ovaries could not be detected macroscopically, but histologic examination of the uterine adnexa revealed a small focus of ovarian stroma with scattered degenerative follicles. There was no sign of testicular architecture. The external genitalia were those of a normal female. When amniocentesis revealed the abnormal 46,Xp+Y karyotype in fetal cells during a later pregnancy, the parents elected to abort the fetus at 20 weeks of gestation. The fetus was a phenotypic female exhibiting the various abnormalities extant in the proband, but in this case, the gonads were normal ovaries with numerous follicles and germ cells. Similar findings including the duplicated X chromosome have been reported by Stern et al.[38] in a single infant and by Scherer et al.[39] in sisters, and we are currently studying another case in collaboration with Arn (unpublished). These findings point to a function of the X chromosome in development of the testis. When this is blocked by duplication of a region within the X short arm, the result is an XY ovary, which degenerates at or around the time of birth.

Genetics of Testicular Differentiation. In aggregate, the data that we have reviewed indicate the existence of at least three genes in a differentiative pathway culminating in organization of the fetal testis. One of the genes would be situated on the Y chromosome, one on the X, and one on an autosome. A simple scheme would have the primary switch on the Y chromosome. This gene (*SRY*) would encode a protein that binds to and activates another gene or group of genes. Failure or deletion of any of these genes would result in the formation of an XY ovary that would degenerate, being replaced by a streak gonad (XY gonadal dysgenesis). Translocation of the Y gene to an X, or activation of the downstream autosomal or X-linked genes in the absence of the Y, would result in an XX male.

Ovarian Genes. It seems reasonable to assume that ovarian differentiation is likewise under genetic control, but the genes responsible for development of the female gonad have not been identified. Human embryos with the 45,X karyotype (indicating loss of the second sex chromosome) develop the characteristic features of Turner syndrome: short stature, epicanthal folds, high-arched palate, low nuchal hair line, webbed neck, shieldlike chest, coarctation of the aorta, and ventricular septal defect. As in 46,XY gonadal dysgenesis, the gonads initially develop as ovaries but, in the absence of the second X chromosome, degenerate and are replaced at around the time of birth or shortly thereafter by streak gonads, which are endocrinologically inert. This indicates occurrence of X-linked genes that are critical for the maintenance of the ovary.[40]

In addition to X-linked genes, certain autosomal genes are required for maintenance of the ovary, because autosomal inheritance is indicated in certain forms of gonadal dysgenesis occurring in females with a "normal" 46,XX karyotype. In some families one sibling may exhibit gonadal dysgenesis, whereas another may exhibit primary amenorrhea with extreme ovarian hypoplasia. In other cases, XX gonadal dysgenesis may occur in those with severe somatic anomalies. An example is Perrault's syndrome, in which XX gonadal

dysgenesis and neurosensory deafness are combined.[40]

Genetic Contributions to Normal and Abnormal Female Genital Tract Development

Normal development of the female reproductive tract involving proper differentiation of the müllerian ducts and the urogenital sinus depends on complex interaction among genetic, hormonal, and environmental factors. Perturbation of this interaction can result in a wide spectrum of genital tract abnormalities, including imperforate hymen, vaginal septa, vaginal atresia, incomplete müllerian fusion, and müllerian aplasia, which may be isolated or associated with other anomalies. Moreover, several mendelian disorders include abnormalities of the female reproductive tract as a component of their phenotypic expression.

In pediatric and adolescent patients, müllerian tract abnormalities may result in gynecologic problems requiring assessment, diagnosis, and appropriate treatment. Here we review the genetic factors contributing to müllerian or wolffian duct anomalies in young girls; diagnosis and management of müllerian duct abnormalities are reviewed in Chapter 6.

Embryology

There are two primordial genital duct systems in all embryos: the wolffian, or *mesonephric*, ducts and the müllerian, or *paramesonephric*, ducts. One duct system persists in each sex, and one regresses. The wolffian ducts drain the mesonephric kidneys, which disappear at 11 to 12 weeks of fetal development. In XY embryos, under the influence of androgens secreted by the newly differentiated testes, the wolffian ducts form the epididymis, ductus deferens, and ejaculatory duct.[41] In the absence of androgens, or in androgen-insensitive embryos, the wolffian ducts fail to differentiate and then regress, leaving behind only small remnants. Unlike müllerian duct regression, which requires müllerian inhibiting substance (MIS), wolffian duct regression does not require the presence of a specific substance but instead occurs in the absence of androgens.

The müllerian ducts develop as invaginations on the lateral surface of the wolffian ducts. The superior portions of the müllerian ducts remain separate and eventually form the fallopian tubes. The inferior portions become the Y-shaped uterovaginal primordium, consisting of a uterine segment and a vaginal segment.[42]

The external genitalia arise from a common, undifferentiated primordium. At 4 weeks of fetal development, a genital tubercle with lateral labioscrotal and urogenital folds appears at the cranial end of the cloacal membrane. The genital tubercle elongates to become a phallus that is equally long in males and females. In the absence of dihydrotestosterone (DHT), a 5α-reductase metabolite of testosterone, growth of the phallus slows considerably, and the genital tubercle forms the clitoris, the urogenital folds do not fuse (they form the labia minora[43]), and the labioscrotal folds become the labia majora. The vaginal vestibule, into which the urethra, vagina, and vestibular ducts open, arises from the cavernous tissue derived from walls of the urogenital sinus.[42]

Clinical Presentations and Evaluation

The discovery of genital abnormalities causes significant psychological and emotional duress for girls and their families. Such discoveries lead to in-depth diagnostic testing, and symptomatic abnormalities frequently are treated by surgical repair. Although most female genital abnormalities occur sporadically, an important part of the diagnostic evaluation of affected girls and women should be a detailed family history, as familial clustering of a particular abnormality or associated abnormalities is useful in formulating a correct diagnosis and in assessing the risk for other family members and offspring of affected individuals.

Most patients with müllerian and urogenital sinus anomalies undergo normal secondary sexual development and present with amenorrhea or abnormal menses. This is because müllerian and urogenital anomalies are end-organ abnormalities and therefore not often associated with mutations of the primary sex-determining genes. Hence, these patients usually have normal levels of sex steroids and regulatory hormones. However, genital tract abnormalities occurring as a result of sex chromosome abnormalities may be associated with gonadal dysgenesis.

Most forms of isolated müllerian duct and urogenital sinus abnormalities are inherited in polygenic/multifactorial fashion. (Mendelian forms of isolated müllerian duct abnormalities are discussed later.) In addition, some müllerian duct abnormalities may be a component of a mendelian multiple malformation syndrome.

Specific Female Genital Tract Abnormalities

Fusion of the Labia Minora. In girls, agglutination of the labia minora usually follows genital infection or trauma resulting from sexual abuse. Congenital fusion of the labia minora is a rare occurrence that has been reported in siblings and in several families.[44, 45]

Imperforate Hymen. The hymen usually ruptures spontaneously during the prenatal period, permitting outflow of mucus during the prepubescent period and menstruum at menarche. If the hymen is imperforate, accumulation of mucus (hydrocolpos) or blood (hematocolpos) within the vagina or blood within the uterus (hematometra) occurs. Although cases affecting siblings have been described,[46] most cases are isolated events.

Transverse Vaginal Septa. Transverse vaginal septa are believed to arise from a failure in fusion and/or canalization of the urogenital sinus and müllerian duct derivatives. Two observations support this statement: (1) septa usually occur at predicted sites of fusion of the müllerian and urogenital sinus derivatives, and (2) cranial surfaces of septa are lined with columnar (müllerian) epithelium, whereas caudal surfaces are lined with squamous (urogenital sinus) epithelium.[47] Although transverse vaginal septa usually occur sporadically, McKusick et al.[48] have described an autosomal recessive disorder (MIM#46000*) occurring in the Amish population in which affected females have transverse vaginal septa in addition to ophthalmologic (congenital cataracts) and orthopedic abnormalities (severe scoliosis, unilateral absence of the leg). Kaufman et al.[49] reported another autosomal recessive disorder (MIM#236700) in which affected patients have not only transverse vaginal septa, but also congenital heart disease and postaxial polydactyly; this disorder has not been reported among the Amish.

Longitudinal Vaginal Septa. Vaginal septa

---

*MIM# refers to the reference number describing the appropriate Mendelian disorder found in McKusick VL. Mendelian Inheritance in Man. Baltimore, MD: Johns Hopkins University Press, 1991.

also occur in the longitudinal axis in either a coronal or a sagittal orientation. Unlike transverse septa, longitudinal septa probably do not arise from fusion or canalization abnormalities but instead arise from abnormal mesodermal proliferation or persistence of epithelium during canalization.[47] As with transverse septa, most longitudinal septa occur sporadically in the population. However, Edwards and Gale[50] have described an autosomal dominant syndrome (MIM#114150) characterized by longitudinal vaginal septa, urinary tract anomalies, and hand abnormalities (camptobrachydactyly). Johanson and Blizzard[51] described an autosomal recessive disorder (MIM#243800) characterized by longitudinal vaginal septa, aplastic nasal ala, microcephaly, deafness, hypothyroidism, skeletal dysplasia, and gastrointestinal malabsorption.

Vaginal Atresia. Vaginal atresia occurs when the urogenital sinus fails to contribute to the inferior portion of the vagina. The lower portion of the vagina is thus replaced by fibrous tissue, above which well-developed müllerian structures are usually found. As with both types of vaginal septa, most cases occur sporadically. Nonetheless, vaginal atresia may be part of an autosomal recessive syndrome (MIM#267400) consisting of renal, genital, and middle ear anomalies. Winter et al.[52] and Turner[53] described families in which female siblings exhibited vaginal atresia, anomalies of the ossicles of the middle ear, and varying degrees of renal dysgenesis.

Müllerian Aplasia. Müllerian aplasia, often called Mayer-Rokitansky-Küster-Hauser syndrome, is the congenital absence or hypoplasia of the fallopian tubes, uterine corpus, uterine cervix, and proximal portion of the vagina.[54-57] Müllerian aplasia must be distinguished from vaginal atresia, a condition in which the distal vagina is replaced by fibrous tissue but with normal müllerian structures

superior to the vaginal aplasia (Fig. 10–6). Because ovarian function is usually unaffected, patients with müllerian aplasia undergo normal secondary sexual development but lack uterine enlargement and menarche. The blind-ending vagina is shortened (1 to 2 cm) and is derived totally from invagination of the urogenital sinus.[47] In addition to the abnormalities in the müllerian duct derivatives, a high percentage of patients with müllerian aplasia exhibit urologic and skeletal abnormalities. Duncan et al.[58] suggested that the aforementioned müllerian, renal, and cervicospinal abnormalities be grouped in a distinctive, nonrandom association known as müllerian-renal-cervicospinal (MURCS).

Most patients with müllerian aplasia have a 46,XX karyotype, but some patients exhibit sex chromosome mosaicism (45,X/46,XX; 46,XX/47,XXX)[59] or deletions in the short arm of a G group autosome.[60] Although familial aggregates of müllerian aplasia have been well documented,[61, 62] the mode of inheritance is still unclear. Lischke et al.[63] reviewed three families in which monozygotic twins were discordant, making an autosomal recessive mode of inheritance unlikely. Shokeir[64] proposed a sex-limited (female) autosomal dominant mode of inheritance based on his study of 16 families in Saskatchewan. However, Carson et al.[65] found no other affected relatives among the families of 23 probands, suggesting multifactorial/polygenic inheritance. These discrepant results could be explained by genetic heterogeneity; that is, expression of different genes could result in similar phenotypes. The MURCS anomalad usually occurs sporadically. Greene et al.[66] reported a family in which several female members were diagnosed as having the MURCS anomalad.

Incomplete Müllerian Fusion. Incomplete müllerian fusion results in a spectrum of anomalies that include unicornuate uterus, arcuate

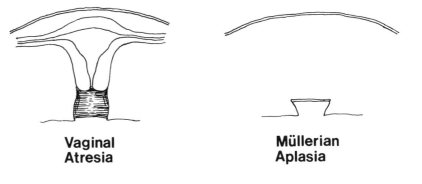

FIGURE 10–6 ••• Müllerian aplasia. Diagrammatic comparison of vaginal atresia and müllerian aplasia. Vaginal abnormality is a cardinal feature of both disorders. (From Shulman LP, Elias S. Developmental abnormalities of the female reproductive tract: Pathogenesis and nosology. Adolesc Pediatr Gynecol 1988; 1:230.)

Vaginal Atresia

Müllerian Aplasia

uterus, subseptate uterus, septate uterus, uterus bicornis unicollis (bicornuate uterus), uterus bicornis bicollis, and didelphic uterus (completely separate hemiuteri, each of which leads to a separate cervix and vagina) (Fig. 10–7). Most retrospective surveys estimate the prevalence of incomplete fusion at around 0.1%,[67, 68] but obstetricians who have explored uteri immediately after delivery have reported a prevalence of 2% to 3%.[69, 70] In the latter studies, a relatively high percentage of affected patients exhibited an arcuate or subseptate uterus, anomalies that are often difficult to detect except in the immediate postpartum period.

Although familial aggregates of incomplete müllerian fusion have been described,[71] the only formal genetic analysis was reported by Elias et al.,[72] who sought to determine the frequency with which symptomatic müllerian fusion anomalies occurred in relatives of a small but genetically unbiased sample of 24 probands. Only one of 37 (2.7%) female siblings older than 16 years appeared to have a symptomatic uterine anomaly; none of 24 mothers, 45 maternal aunts, or 50 paternal aunts were affected. This low frequency of affected relatives is more consistent with a polygenic/multifactorial etiology than with other genetic etiologies.

Incomplete müllerian fusion may also occur as a component of a multiple malformation syndrome. Fraser's syndrome (MIM#219000) is an autosomal recessive disorder characterized by cryptophthalmos, middle and outer ear malformations, hypertelorism, laryngeal stenosis, and syndactyly; affected females may also have a bicornuate uterus.[73] The hand-foot-genital (HFG) syndrome (MIM#140000) is an autosomal dominant disorder in which patients exhibit skeletal abnormalities of the hands and feet (small feet, short great toes, abnormal thumbs, clinodactyly); hypospadias and displaced urethral meatus in affected males; and incomplete müllerian fusion anomalies, urinary incontinence, and malposition of ureteral orifices in affected females.[74] As with other dominantly inherited disorders, HFG syndrome demonstrates considerable variation in expression among affected family members.

Persistence of Müllerian Structures in Males. Persistence of the uterus and fallopian tubes in males is a result of absence or mutation of the müllerian-inhibiting substance or its receptor. Affected males usually present with inguinal hernias, cryptorchidism, and/or infertility. Diagnosis is frequently made at the time of surgical intervention when rudimentary or developed müllerian duct derivatives are discovered. Nilson[75] reported the first case in 1939; familial aggregates were subsequently reported.[76, 77] Study of the familial aggregates

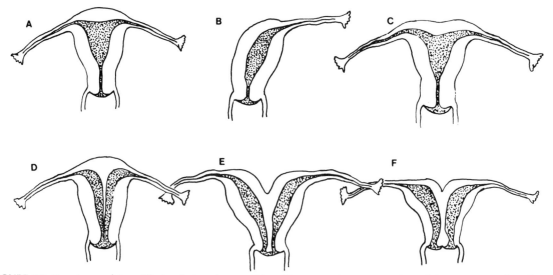

FIGURE 10–7 ••• Incomplete müllerian fusion abnormalities. Diagrammatic representation of the spectrum of müllerian fusion anomalies. *A*, Normal uterus; *B*, uterus unicornis (unicornuate uterus); *C*, uterus arcuatus (arcuate uterus) *D*, uterus septus (septate uterus); *E*, uterus bicornis unicollis (bicornuate uterus); *F*, uterus didelphys (didelphic uterus). (From Shulman LP, Elias S. Developmental abnormalities of the female reproductive tract: Pathogenesis and nosology. Adolesc Pediatr Gynecol 1988; 1:230.)

revealed a recessive mode of inheritance, although it is not clear whether the inheritance is autosomal or X linked (see Table 10–1).[78]

References

1. Watson JD, Tooze J, Kurtz DT. Recombinant DNA. New York: WH Freeman and Co, 1983.
2. Berger SL, Kimmel AR. Guide to Molecular Cloning Techniques. New York: Academic Press, 1987.
3. Simpson JL. Disorders of Sexual Differentiation: Etiology and Clinical Delineation. New York: Academic Press, 1976.
4. Southern EM. Detection of specific sequences among DNA fragments separated by gel electrophoresis. J Molec Biol 1975; 98:503.
5. Sinclair AH, Berta P, Palmer MS, et al. A gene from the human sex-determining region encodes a protein with homology to a conserved DNA-binding motif. Nature 1990; 346:244.
6. Koopman P, Münsterberg A, Blanche C, et al. Expression of a candidate sex-determining gene during mouse testis differentiation. Nature 1990; 348:450.
7. Maxam A, Gilbert W. A new method for sequencing DNA. Proc Natl Acad Sci USA 1977; 74:560.
8. Sanger F, Nicklen S, Coulson AR. DNA sequencing with chain-terminating inhibitors. Proc Natl Acad Sci USA 1977; 74:5463.
9. Jeffreys AJ, Brookfield JFY, Semenoff R. Positive identification of an immigration test-case using human DNA fingerprints. Nature 1985; 317:818.
10. Jeffreys AJ, Wilson V, Thein SL. Individual-specific "fingerprints" of human DNA. Nature 1985; 316:76.
11. Lander ES. Research on DNA typing catching-up with courtroom application. Invited editorial. Am J Hum Genet 1991; 48:819.
12. Budowle B, Giusti AM, Waye JS, et al. Fixed-bin analysis for statistical evaluation of continuous distributions of allelic data from VNTR loci for use in forensic comparisons. Am J Hum Genet 1991; 48:841.
13. Saiki RK, Scharf S, Faloona F, et al. Enzymatic amplification of β-globin sequences and restriction site analysis for diagnosis of sickle cell anemia. Science 1985; 37:170.
14. Erlich HA. PCR Technology. Principles and Applications for DNA Amplification. New York: Stockton Press, 1989.
15. King M-C. An application of DNA sequencing to a human rights problem. In Friedmann T (ed). Molecular Genetic Medicine. New York: Academic Press, 1991, pp 117–134.
16. Kirby LT. DNA Fingerprinting: An Introduction. New York: Stockton Press, 1990.
17. Mudd JL, Hartmann JM, Kuo MC, et al. Guidelines for a quality assurance program for DNA restriction fragment length polymorphism analysis. Crime Lab Digest 1991; 16:41.
18. Chandley AC, Mitchell AR. Hypervariable minisatellite regions are sites for crossing-over at meiosis in man. Cytogenet Cell Genet 1988; 48:152.
19. Jeffreys AJ. Highly variable minisatellites and DNA fingerprints. Biochem Soc Trans 1987; 15:309.
20. Jeffreys AJ, Royle NJ, Wilson V, et al. Spontaneous mutation rates to new length alleles at tandem-repetitive hypervariable loci in human DNA. Nature 1988; 332:278.
21. Royle NJ, Clarkson RE, Wong Z, et al. Clustering of hypervariable minisatellites in the proterminal regions of human autosomes. Genomics 1988; 3:352.
22. Zumwalt RE. Application of molecular techniques to forensic pathology. In: Fenoglio-Preiser CM, Willman CL (eds). Molecular Diagnostics in Pathology. Baltimore: Williams & Wilkins, 1991; pp 339–354.
23. Schumm JW, Knowlton R, Braman J, et al. Identification of more than 500 RFLPs by screening random genomic clones. Am J Hum Genet 1988; 42:143.
24. Levin R. DNA typing on the witness stand. Science 1989; 244:1033.
25. *Frye v. United States*, 293 F 1013 (DC Cir 1923).
26. Comment. DNA identification tests and the courts. 63 Wash L Rev 1988; 903, 905, no 2.
27. *United States v. Baller*, 519 F 2d463, 466 (4th Cir, 1975).
28. Wachtel SS, Wachtel G, Nakamura D. Sexual differentiation. In: Pang PKT, Schreibman MP (eds). Vertebrate Endocrinology: Fundamentals and Biomedical Implications. Vol 4. Part B. San Diego: Academic Press, 1991, pp 149–180.
29. Tiersch TR, Mitchell MJ, Wachtel SS. Studies on the phylogenetic conservation of the *SRY* gene. Hum Genet 1991; 87:571.
30. Koopman P, Gubbay J, Vivian N, et al. Male development of chromosomally female mice transgenic for *Sry*. Nature 1991; 351:117.
31. Ferguson-Smith MA, North MA, Affara NA, et al. The secret of sex. Lancet 1990; 336:809.
32. Wolf U, Fraccaro M, Mayerová A, et al. A gene controlling H-Y antigen on the X chromosome. Hum Genet 1980; 54:149.
33. Simpson JL, Blagadowidow N, Martin AO. XY gonadal dysgenesis: Genetic heterogeneity based upon clinical observations, H-Y antigen status and segregation analysis. Hum Genet 1981; 58:91.
34. Wachtel SS. Genetics of XY gonadal dysgenesis. In: Wachtel SS, Simpson JL (eds). Molecular Genetics of Sex Determination. San Diego: Academic Press, in press.
35. Mann JL, Corkery JJ, Fisher HJW, et al. The X-linked recessive form of XY gonadal dysgenesis with a high incidence of gonadal germ cell tumors: Clinical and genetic studies. J Med Genet 1983; 20:264.
36. Greenberg F, Greesick MV, Carpenter RJ, et al. The Gardner-Silengo-Wachtel syndrome: Male pseudohermaphroditism with micrognathia, cleft palate, and cono-truncal cardiac defect. Am J Hum Genet 1987; 26:59.
37. Bernstein R, Koo GC, Wachtel SS. Abnormality of the X chromosome in human 46,XY female siblings with dysgenetic ovaries. Science 1980; 207:768.
38. Stern HJ, Garrity AM, Saal HM, et al. Duplication of Xp21 and sex reversal: Insight into the mechanism of sex determination. Am J Hum Genet 1990; 47(suppl):A41.
39. Scherer G, Schempp W, Baccichetti C, et al. Duplication of an Xp segment that includes the ZFX locus causes sex inversion in man. Hum Genet 1989; 81:291.
40. Neely EK, Rosenfeld RG. Phenotypic correlations of X chromosome loss. In: Wachtel SS, Simpson JL (eds). Molecular Genetics of Sex Determination. San Diego: Academic Press, in press.
41. Gyllensten L. Contributions to embryology of the urinary bladder: Development of definitive relationships between openings of the wolffian ducts and the ureters. Acta Anat 1949; 7:305.
42. Bulmer D. The development of the human vagina. J Anat 1957; 91:490.

43. Jirasek JE. Atlas of Human Prenatal Morphogenesis. Boston: Martinus-Nijhoff, 1983, pp 64–68.

44. Sueriro MB, Piloto R. Aderencia incompleta dos pequinos labios com caracter familiar. Gaz Med Port 1963; 16:513.

45. Willman SP, Carr BR, Klein VR. Familial fusion of the labia minora. Abstract. Proc Greenwood Genet Center 1988; 7:140.

46. Mcllroy DM, Ward IV. Three cases of imperforate hymen occurring in one family. Proc R Soc Med 1930; 23:633.

47. Simpson JL. Gynecologic disorders. In: King RA, Rotter JI, Motulsky AG (eds). The Genetic Basis of Common Disease. Oxford, England: Oxford University Press, 1992, 564–576.

48. McCusick VA, Weilbaecher RG, Gragg GW. Recessive inheritance of a congenital malformation syndrome. JAMA 1968; 204:111.

49. Kaufman RL, Hartmann AF, McAlister WH. Family studies in congenital heart disease. II. A syndrome of hydrometrocolpos, postaxial polydactyly and congenital heart disease. Birth Defects 1972; VIII:85.

50. Edwards JA, Gale RP. Camptobrachydactyly: A new autosomal dominant trait with two probable homozygotes. Am J Hum Genet 1972; 24:464.

51. Johanson A, Blizzard R. A syndrome of congenital aplasia of the alae nasi, deafness, hypothyroidism, dwarfism, absent permanent teeth and malabsorption. J Pediatr 1971; 79:982.

52. Winter JSD, Kohn G, Mcllman WJ, et al. A familial syndrome of renal, genital and middle ear anomalies. J Pediatr 1968; 72:88.

53. Turner G. A second family with renal, vaginal and middle ear anomalies. J Pediatr 1970; 76:641.

54. Mayer G. Über Verdoppelungen des Uterus und ihre Arten, nebst Bemerkungen über Hasenscharte und Wolfsrachen. J Chir Auger 1829; 13:525.

55. Küster H. Uterus bipartitus solidus rudimentarius cum vagina solida. Z Geburtshilfe Gyn 1910; 67:692.

56. Rokitansky H. Über die sogenannten Verdoppelungen des Uterus. Med Jb Öst Staat 1938; 26:39.

57. Hauser GA, Schreiner WE. Das Mayer-Rokitansky-Küster syndrome. Schweiz Med Wochenschr 1961; 91:381.

58. Duncan PA, Shapiro LR, Klein RM. The MURCS association. Am J Obstet Gynecol 1987; 156:1554.

59. Stott RB, Cameron JS, Ogg CS, et al. XO/XX mosaicism in the Rokitansky-Küster-Hauser syndrome. Lancet 1971; ii:1380.

60. Linquette M, Gasnault JP, Dupont-Lecompte J, et al. Le syndrome de Rokitansky-Küster-Hauser et les syndromes voisins d'aplasie uterovaginale. Rev Fr Endocrinol Clin 1962; 9:41.

61. Anger D, Hemet J, Ensel J. Forme familial du syndrome de Rokitansky-Kuster-Hauser. Bull Fed Gynecol Obstet Franc 1966; 18:229.

62. Jones HW, Mermut S. Familial occurrence of congenital absence of the vagina. Am J Obstet Gynecol 1972; 114:1100.

63. Lischke JH, Curtis CH, Lamb EJ, et al. Discordance of vaginal agenesis in monozygotic twins. Obstet Gynecol 1973; 41:920.

64. Shokeir MHK. Aplasia of the müllerian system: Evidence for probable sex-limited autosomal dominant inheritance. Birth Defects 1978; XIV(6C):147.

65. Carson SA, Simpson JL, Malinak LR, et al. Heritable aspects of uterine anomalies. II. Genetic analysis of müllerian aplasia. Fertil Steril 1983; 40:86.

66. Greene RA, Bloch MJ, Huff DS, et al. MURCS association with additional congenital anomalies. Hum Pathol 1986; 17:88.

67. Simpson JL. Genetic aspects of gynecologic disorders occurring in 46,XX individuals. Clin Obstet Gynecol 1972; 15:157.

68. Semens JP. Congenital anomalies of female genital tract. Functional classification based on review of 56 personal cases and 500 reported cases. Obstet Gynecol 1962; 68:371.

69. Hay D. Uterus unicollis and its relationship to pregnancy. J Obstet Gynecol Br Emp 1961; 82:330.

70. Greiss FC, Manzy CH. Genital anomalies in women. An evaluation of diagnosis, incidence and obstetric performance. Am J Obstet Gynecol 1961; 82:330.

71. Verp MS, Simpson JL, Elias S, et al. Heritable aspects of uterine anomalies. I. Three familial aggregates with müllerian fusion anomalies. Fertil Steril 1983; 40:80.

72. Elias S, Simpson JL, Carson SA, et al. Genetic studies in incomplete müllerian fusion. Obstet Gynecol 1984; 63:276.

73. Fraser GR. Our genetical "load." A review of some aspects of genetical variation. Ann Hum Genet 1962; 25:387.

74. Elias S, Simpson JL, Feingold M, et al. The hand-foot-uterus syndrome: A rare autosomal dominant disorder. Fertil Steril 1978; 9:239.

75. Nilson O. Hernia uteri inguinalis beim manne. Acta Chir Scand 1939; 83:231.

76. Sloan WR, Walsh CR. Familial persistent müllerian duct syndrome. J Urol 1976; 115:459.

77. Brook CGD, Wagner H, Zachmann M, et al. Familial occurrence of persistent müllerian structures in otherwise normal males. Br Med J 1973; 1:771.

78. Imperato-McGinley J, Peterson RE. Male pseudohermaphroditism: The complexities of male phenotypic development. Am J Med 1976; 61:251.

79. Mitchell MJ, Bishop CE. A structural analysis of the Sxr region of the mouse Y chromosome. Genomics 1992; 12:26.

80. Demas S, Wachtel S. DNA fingerprinting in reptiles: Bkm hybridization patterns in *Crocodilia* and *Chelonia*. Genome 1991; 34:472.

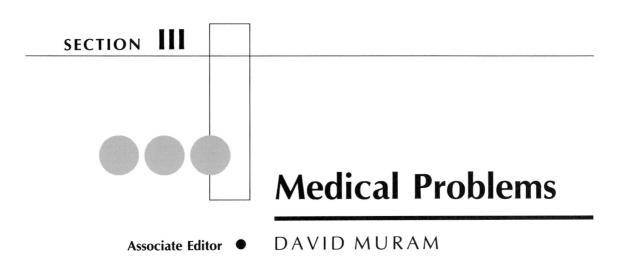

Medical Problems

Associate Editor ● DAVID MURAM

CHAPTER 11

Genital Examination of Prepubertal and Peripubertal Females

SUSAN F. POKORNY

The information in this chapter will not be optimally used if the physician cannot adequately examine the child's reproductive organs, but the physician examining a young child should keep in mind that experiences related to the genitourinary and rectal area play a key role in psychological development. Thus the physician should consider the appropriateness of the examination in terms of both the timing and the type of information needed from the examination. The full pelvic examination sequence as applied to the reproductive-age woman is never used in a prepubertal child, but there is no physical reason why, with proper physician skill and patient preparation, a speculum examination cannot be performed on a virginal adolescent.

APPROPRIATENESS OF THE EXAMINATION

Educational Examinations

Prevailing thought in American culture is that the female genital system should be kept out of sight and out of mind until some "magic moment" when a woman should be knowl-edgeable about "womanly things."[1] This does not allow children to develop the cognitive skills necessary to acknowledge early signs or symptoms of genital disorders, nor does it help children ward off the coercive, clandestine advances of sexual molesters or abusers. With this in mind, it seems appropriate that all pediatric primary care providers should include a detailed educational genital examination with each annual physical examination.

The child should be allowed to leave the undergarments on until time for the genital examination, as this symbolically tells the child that the genitals are a special area of the body. When it comes time for the genital examination, the physician might say something like, "Now I'm going to check a special part of your body to see that everything is growing well." The examination can then be carried out as described later in this chapter and information obtained from the examination shared with both the child and parent. Because children and young adolescents are concrete thinkers, it is during the course of the examination per se that the most meaningful information can be imparted.

During or immediately after the examination, it is important that the physician point out to the child that the examination was sanctioned by the parent or guardian who was present. The physician might use this moment to explain to the child that no one else should attempt to examine or touch her genital area, and if this happens, she should inform the parent or guardian. As already stated, children are concrete thinkers and need this type of explicit instruction.[2]

By addressing issues referable to the genital area in an open and comfortable fashion, very often the physician is also providing the parent with vocabulary and communication skills that will sustain future parent-child dialogues pertaining to the child's reproductive system.

Diagnostic Examinations

When a child is brought for a specific genital complaint, the physician starts with a patient history and then follows with a physical examination. Because genital symptoms are frequently presented in colloquialisms and anatomically incorrect terms, the physician will have to rely most heavily on the physical examination for the diagnosis of most pediatric gynecologic disorders.

The physician planning a diagnostic genital examination must look for features in the history that will dictate what information should be obtained from the examination and the sequence in which such information is to be obtained. For example, not every 4-year-old girl with vaginal discharge will need to undergo a vaginoscopy, but many will, particularly if the discharge is copious, bloody, or persistent. On the other hand, there is no reason to put a 4-year-old child with lichen sclerosus through a vaginal examination when the diagnosis can be made using external procedures.

Genital examination of the prepubertal child relies on obtaining patient compliance by promising to do her no physical harm. Occasionally there is not enough time for the physician to develop a rapport with the child and thereby develop her trust for compliance. For example, in cases of a penetrating perineal injury or a recent sexual assault, it is imperative that an examination be performed immediately, regardless of the child's compliance. In these situations, the physician should consider the appropriateness of an examination under anesthesia or heavy sedation.

On the other hand, if the genital complaint is chronic or the injury clearly superficial, then the physician can consider allowing a diagnostic examination to evolve over several sessions (i.e., sequential examinations).

The timing between sequential examinations will also be dictated by certain aspects of the history. A history of bleeding at any time during the course of the illness that cannot be explained on the first examination will dictate a more urgent follow-up visit for further studies.[3] On the other hand, the spacing of follow-up examinations for chronic vulvitis might be more leisurely, allowing time for removal of environmental contact irritants and for therapeutic trials of medications, etc.

Because children have a low level of circulating sex steroid hormones compared with reproductive-age women, it is important to remember that the vast majority of pediatric gynecology complaints will be in reference to growth, inflammation, lesions, or reactions of the skin and mucosa of the external genitalia or, to a lesser degree, of the mucosa of the vaginal canal. The cervix, uterus, and fallopian tubes are so hormonally inert and undeveloped that they are typically evaluated only when a neoplasm grows to a pathologically obvious size; colposcopy of the cervix and hysterosalpingograms cannot be performed in children because of the small size of these structures. The ovaries likewise are not routinely evaluated unless signs and symptoms of a neoplastic or endocrine disorder are apparent.

The physician must decide which cases warrant only an external examination and which cases require visualization of the vaginal canal. If there is a history of bleeding and no cause has been found, or there is persistent or recurrent infection, then vaginoscopy is mandatory to rule out a foreign object or neoplasm.

PERFORMING AN ADEQUATE GENITAL EXAMINATION

Getting the Child to Comply

Giving the child a sense of control over the examination and making a commitment to not cause discomfort during the examination sets the stage to obtain maximal information and to give age-appropriate educational guidance (Table 11–1).

If the child is being seen because of a genital complaint, it is advisable to have some idea as to the area of the family's concern before

TABLE 11–1 •• SUGGESTIONS FOR GENITAL EXAMINATIONS OF YOUNG CHILDREN AND ADOLESCENTS

Obtain the patient's cooperation
  This is necessary for teachable moments and for adequate examinations.
Get the patient to comply
  She must have control over the examination.
  She must be promised no physical pain.
  Define the information that is to be obtained.
Special aspects of the prepubertal female's examination
  Inform the child that the genital examination is sanctioned.
  Involve the child with a hand-held mirror and magnification device.
  Position the child with the feet in the stirrups, with the feet on the examiner's lap, or sitting on the parent's lap drape the child's legs over the parent's thighs.
  Attempt both the supine and knee-chest positions.
  Be knowledgeable about the various spread methods to see the vestibule.
  There is only a limited need to use instruments.
Special aspects of the peripubertal genital examination
  Understand the impact of estrogen.
  Use extinction of stimuli phenomenon.
  Choose the proper speculum width after the introitus is evaluated.

contact with the patient. If too much time is spent verbally obtaining all the historical details of the complaint, the child will become restless and anxious. This history can be obtained most expeditiously by use of a questionnaire before the patient's contact with the physician. This questionnaire should include the following: the length of time the problem has existed; the pivotal issues, signs, or symptoms; the presence or absence of common environmental irritants; past treatments and diagnoses; skin and/or allergic conditions of the patient and/or family members; and recently prescribed medications not related to the complaint, particularly antibiotics. Occasionally the physician will have to address past traumatic genital events in the child's history to clarify a confusing array of symptoms and concerns. By keeping an open, nonjudgmental approach to eliciting these concerns, caretaker practices that might be contributing to the child's signs and symptoms will be detected.[4]

The questionnaire allows the physician to move more rapidly to the examination itself and to concentrate on developing a rapport with the child. The patient is much more likely to comply with the examination when the physician is able to succinctly explain to the child why the examination needs to be done and that the examination will not hurt her. A simple way of doing this is to say something like, "I understand your mother has some worries about your girl parts. Why don't we just look and I'll tell you what I see."

Compliance for a genital examination in a premenarchal child is greatly facilitated by the use of a hand-held mirror. The mirror can be held by the patient, a nurse, or the patient's parent so that the patient can see her external genitalia at the same time that the examination is being performed.

The patient can be shown the mirror and how it will facilitate visualization of her genitalia before removing her clothing. While the patient is sitting on the edge of the examination table or on her parent's lap, the physician or nurse can demonstrate how the patient can see her shoes or feet with the use of the mirror. Once the patient knows how to do this, it is simple to slightly adjust the mirror so that she can see her external genital area. This can be described as a "trick" to look around corners.

Once the child knows how the mirror will allow her to observe the examination, it is easy to get her to remove her clothing. A comment from the examiner about not being able to see through underpants is usually an adequate clue, and the patient will typically quickly remove her underclothing so that the examination can proceed.

Videocolposcopy is a technique advocated by some clinicians that also allows the patient and parent to visualize the external genitalia. Proponents of this technique believe it reduces anxiety for the patient.

At the time the child is removing her underclothing, she should be offered a drape. Most young children will not request a drape and will not know how to use it without instructions. Nevertheless, by draping the child's lower body for the genital examination, the physician is again indicating to the child that the genital area is a special part of the body, and that the physician has respect for any modesty the patient might have. The physician does not want to be so casual about the examination that the child might stop in the waiting room to show everyone else the parts of her anatomy that the physician has just shown her. The use of drapes symbolizes to the child that the physician-directed genital examination is a special situation.

Positioning the Child for the Examination

The ideal position for good visualization of the child's external genitalia is the supine position with the buttocks on the end of a gyne-cologic examination table. Her head should be elevated so that constant communication with the examiner, who is positioned at the end of the table, is maintained. The examiner should be comfortably seated and have an adequate light source. The child's feet can be placed in the gynecologic table stirrups or in the exam-iner's lap.

The child can also sit on her parent's lap with her legs spread open and draped across the parent's thighs. Ideally, the parent should sit, semireclined, on the end of the gynecologic table, with both feet in the stirrups. There are several advantages to this position: the parent can hold the mirror so that both he or she and the child can see the child's external genital area; the parent's arms enwrap and reassure the child; and the elevated position of the child makes the examination much easier.

After as much visual information as possible has been obtained from the supine frog-legged position, the child should be encouraged to assume the prone knee-chest position, prefer-ably with her back slightly swayed. Although this is a more anxiety-provoking position and

the child cannot watch the examination with the hand-held mirror, by retracting the peri-neal tissues laterally and superiorly, a different and sometimes more thorough examination of the hymen can be accomplished (Figs. 11–1, 11–2). The main advantage to this position, if the child cooperates and relaxes her abdominal muscles, is that more of the vaginal canal can be visualized than in the supine frog-legged position. Occasionally, with a well-focused light and if there is minimal discharge or in-flammation, the cervix can be identified at the vaginal apex.

The Noncompliant Child

Occasionally a child will have been so trau-matized by previous examinations or by sexual abuse that even though all of these steps are followed, the child will not allow an external genital examination. At this point, if the ex-aminer makes a particularly strong appeal to the child's "need to know that everything down there is okay," it is surprising how many will eventually comply with the examination.

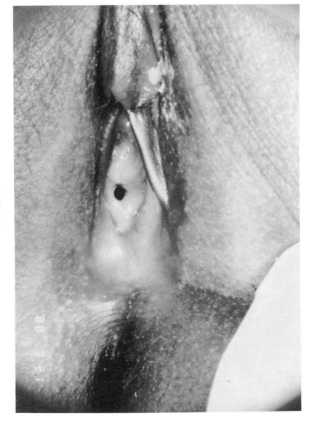

FIGURE 11–1 ••• Appearance of normal external geni-talia of a prepubertal female in the supine position using the lateral spread technique. (From Pokorny SF. Pediatric gynecology. In: Stenchever MA [ed]. Office Gynecology. St. Louis: Mosby–Year Book, 1992, pp 106–135.)

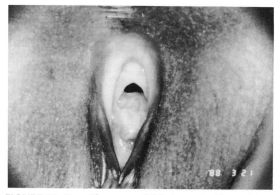

FIGURE 11–2 ••• The same child shown in Figure 11–1, but in the knee-chest position. (From Pokorny SF. Pediatric gynecology. In: Stenchever MA [ed]. Office Gynecology. St. Louis: Mosby–Year Book, 1992, pp 106–135.)

If the examiner has the impression that a child who has been previously traumatized is being manipulative, the child should be told that she can leave but cannot be assured that everything is okay. The examiner might even leave the room to go see other patients, giving the victimized child time to reconsider and allow the examination. As stated earlier, invariably these children will position themselves to allow an external examination. If a child is extremely frightened, she should be allowed to use her own hands to spread the labia laterally so that the vaginal introitus can be visualized.

To force a genital examination on any child is symbolically saying that older and stronger individuals have the right to access that part of her body. With the current concern about sexual abuse of children, this is not the message that should be given. An examination forced on a previously traumatized child might cause further psychological harm. Furthermore, no matter how many individuals are restraining the child, the examination will be inadequate, as the perineum must be somewhat relaxed for adequate visualization of the hymen.

Sedation of the anxious, fearful child for a genital examination frequently fails to be adequate or requires a degree of sedation dangerous for most outpatient settings. Like a forced examination, an examination with inadequate sedation symbolizes to the child that older, stronger individuals have the right to access the child's genital area without her permission, and any educable moments are missed. If a pathologic condition is strongly expected, an examination under anesthesia is usually warranted. If a pathologic condition is unlikely or of minimal clinical consequence, it is advisable to continue to work sequentially with the patient on an outpatient basis until an adequate examination can be performed.

Clearly, a noncompliant child taxes the patience of the examiner and everyone else involved. Nevertheless, the cultural message given and the long-term therapeutic benefits obtained from allowing the child to control the pace of the examination process will far outweigh the information obtained from a forced genital examination.

Magnification and Documentation

The physician should not begin a genital examination of a prepubertal child without having available some means to magnify the tissue. The genital structures are small, and minute details derived from the examination are frequently needed for a correct diagnosis and for therapeutic intervention. An otoscope with the truncated ear canal piece removed, a hand-held map-reading magnifying glass, operative microscopic eye loops, a dermatology circular magnifying light, a colposcope, and a cervicoscope have all been used as magnifying instruments. The cost of the instrument, its ease of use and mobility, and the setting for its use must all be considered. The colposcope and cervicoscope have photographic capabilities that aid in documentation of structures and lesions not afforded by the other instruments, but they are expensive and cumbersome to use.

The advantages of magnification and the discipline required to document what is noted improve the visual acumen of the examiner. Physicians should approach the examination with the idea that they will be seeing normal genital structures that have the potential for individual, physiologic, and acquired variations.

All adequate genital examinations of the prepubertal child should be documented in the child's medical record by a detailed, labeled sketch of the external genitalia (Figs. 11–3, 11–4). This detailed sketch becomes part of a database from which future genital complaints for that child can be interpreted.

A simple way to sketch findings is to start with a diamond-shaped space representing the vestibule of a child in the supine position; the

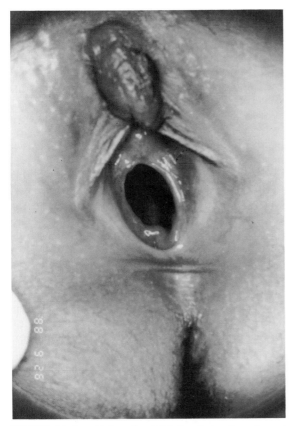

FIGURE 11–3 ••• Vulva of a child showing a disruption of the hymen's posterior rim at the 6 o'clock position, associated with a small bump at the 7 o'clock position.

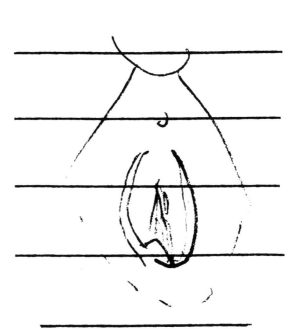

FIGURE 11–4 ••• Example of how the vulva of a prepubertal child can be sketched in the medical record for documentation of minute details. This is a sketch from the medical record of the child in Figure 11–3.

clitoris would be positioned at 12 o'clock, the patient's left side at 3 o'clock, the posterior fourchette at 6 o'clock, and the patient's right side at 9 o'clock. The urethra and vaginal opening can be placed within the diamond space and lesions or other details properly placed.

This explicit detailed documentation of findings is extremely important for the very young preverbal child and for the mentally or verbally handicapped child who cannot, should there ever be a need, make an "outcry" about sexual abuse. A baseline documentation of genital findings at a given point in time is invaluable should a future examination produce evidence of unexplained genital trauma.

Visualizing the Vestibule

The small structures of the vestibule cannot usually be adequately evaluated unless the adjacent labia majora are spread laterally and posteriorly. By placing the index finger from each hand or the index and middle finger or thumb and index finger from one hand on both labia majora, lateral to the vestibule and slightly posterior to the vaginal orifice, the examiner can usually spread the tissues later-

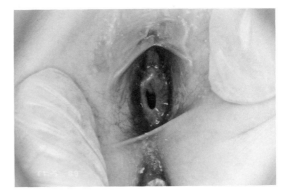

FIGURE 11–5 ••• Vulva of a 3-year-old child; note the denseness of capillaries on the vestibular sulcus. (Erythema of the atrophic mucosa can be confused with inflammation.) Also note the bands and crypts of the minor vestibular glands in the periurethral sulcus. (From Pokorny SF. Physical examination of the reproductive systems of female children and adolescents. Curr Probl Obstet Gynecol Fertil 1990; 13[5]:202–213.)

ally and posteriorly enough so that the vestibular structures can be adequately visualized. This is called the *supine lateral-spread method* (Fig. 11–5).

If this attempt is inadequate, each labium major should be gently grasped in the same location used for the two-fingered method described above, but using both hands. Gentle traction is placed on the labia, pulling toward the examiner as well as slightly posteriorly and laterally. While doing this, the examiner should continue to reassure the patient, being careful to not "pinch" the grasped labia. At the point of maximal traction, if the child is instructed to take a deep breath, the change in intraabdominal pressure so created will invariably allow the vestibular tissues to fan out so that the hymen and vaginal opening can be readily visualized. This is called the *supine lateral traction method*.

PHYSICAL FINDINGS

Anatomic Structures

The physical findings of the external genital examination should be recorded using standardized, anatomically correct terms (Fig. 11–6). The *vulva* encompasses the mons, the labia majora, and the vestibule; the *vestibule* is the externalized mucosal surface demarcated by the clitoris, the labia minora, Hart's line, and the posterior fourchette; the *perineal body* is the bridge of tissue between the vestibule and the rectum; the *perineum* encompasses all structures from the anterior mons or pubic symphysis, the lateral border of the labia majora or ischial tuberosities, and the posterior perirectal area or coccyx; *introitus* refers to a mouth or an opening.

The most obvious landmark of the perineum of the prepubertal female is the clitoris. Because of extreme variability in both clitoral size and the subcutaneous adipose tissue of the mons pubis, the clitoris can occasionally seem quite strikingly large.

Once the clitoral complex is identified, the next most prominent structures are the labia minora. These raised, thin mounds form the lateral anterior margins of the vestibule and course medially toward the midline to meet under the clitoral complex. A thin, sharp apex of the labia minora is compatible with the atrophic state of most prepubertal females.

The vestibule is lined with glabrous epithelium. The vestibular sulcus between the vaginal orifice and the posterior fourchette, the fossa navicularis, can be deep, forming a considerable pocket, or shallow and almost nonexistent

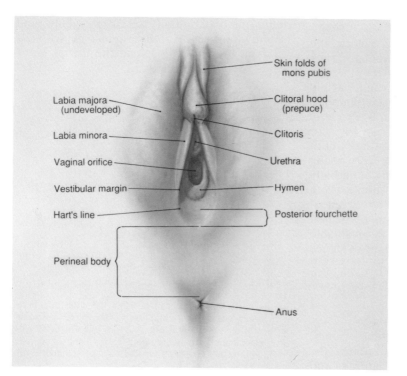

Labia majora (undeveloped)

Labia minora

Vaginal orifice

Vestibular margin

Hart's line

Perineal body

Skin folds of mons pubis

Clitoral hood (prepuce)

Clitoris

Urethra

Hymen

Posterior fourchette

Anus

FIGURE 11–6 ••• External genitalia of the prepubertal female. The goal of the external genital examination is to identify all of these structures.

as an entity. The fossa navicularis and the lateral vestibular sulci are extremely vascular; the density of capillaries in these areas makes them persistently erythematous.

The urethra is in the anterior vestibule. It might be a minute, pinpoint orifice; cleftlike; or surrounded by a marked and variable amount of mucosa; it can at times appear quite patulous. In the periurethral area, there are frequently noted bands of tissue or deep crypts. There is great variability in the appearance of these structures caused by the minor vestibular glands.

Posterior to the urethra, with the child in the dorsal supine position, is the opening into the vagina. The vaginal orifice or introitus is surrounded by a collar of tissue called the *hymen*. Lateral and circumferential to the vaginal orifice is a sulcus in the vestibule. Crypts occur in this sulcus and are quite variable in their appearance. Again, these are the minor vestibular glands; they are less apparent and not seen as frequently as in the periurethral area.

In cases of vulvovaginitis or marked estrogen depletion of the tissues, spreading the labial tissues laterally for visualization of the vestibular structures can inadvertently cause a fissure in the superficial tissue of the posterior fourchette. This heals rapidly with a warm tub bath and removal of irritants.

Estrogen Status

Understanding the estrogen status of the young female is essential to determine the manner in which the genital examination should be performed. This determination is also important in order to arrive at an appropriate diagnosis and a treatment plan. Although estrogen stimulation drops rapidly after birth with removal of the maternal circulation, for a variable period of time the newborn infant's gonadotropin levels remain elevated, and estrogen effect on the vulvar tissues persists well into the third year of life. Capillaries cannot be seen in the estrogenized mucosa, which has a moist, whitish-pink color.

From the toddler years until the peripubertal years of 9 or 10, estrogen effect is minimal, and the vulvovaginal mucosa is extremely thin and atrophic. "Road map" capillary beds should be visible. In areas where these capillaries are dense (i.e., the sulcus of the vestibule and very often the periurethral area), the tissue

is erythematous and can be confused with inflammation. In the situation in which inflammation is causing the erythema, there is a more generalized redness of the tissue, which is thickened and edematous, thereby obscuring the capillary beds so easily seen in the normal atrophic prepubertal mucosa.

The Hymen: Variations, Configurations, and Alterations

Most hymenal membranes have a distinct orifice. In some cases the orifice is so small as to justify the term *microperforation* (Fig. 11–7). Another, more common variation is the septated hymen (Fig. 11–8), in which there are two distinct orifices with an intervening bridge of tissue that usually runs in the anterior to posterior dimension but can also run horizontally or diagonally. It is important to distinguish a septated hymen, which has no association with upper reproductive tract müllerian duplication anomalies, from a longitudinally

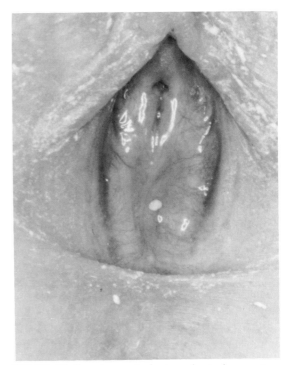

FIGURE 11–7 ••• A seemingly imperforate hymen in a prepubertal female. A small probe was passed into the vagina via a microperforate opening in the suburethral area. (From Pokorny SF, Pokorny WJ. Pediatric gynecology. In: Ashcraft KW, Holder TM [eds]. Pediatric Surgery. 2nd ed. Philadelphia: WB Saunders, 1993, p 975.)

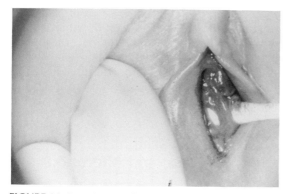

FIGURE 11-8 ••• Septated hymen with a probe demonstrating that this is not a duplicate vagina. (From Pokorny SF. Pediatric gynecology. In: Stenchever MA [ed]. Office Gynecology. St. Louis: Mosby–Year Book, 1992, pp 106–135.)

septated vagina, which has a high association with müllerian duplication anomalies.

It is not uncommon for a seemingly imperforate hymen to ultimately be discovered with sequential examinations to be a microperforate hymen. Gentle probing with a small catheter or feeding tube in the suburethral area will usually identify a passage into the vagina. This usually requires no surgical intervention, since drainage is not impeded, and under estrogen stimulation at the time of puberty, many of these microperforations enlarge.

When an imperforate hymen is detected at birth because of a small hydrocolpos that does not extend above the pelvic brim, a hymenotomy can be performed in the newborn nursery. The infant is stabilized in the dorsal lithotomy position by assistants, local anesthetic is applied, a cruciform incision is made in the bulging membrane, and the redundant margins are excised. Because of the extremely well estrogenized mucosa of the neonate, hemostasis is rarely a problem and can usually be managed by silver nitrate cauterization.

If a child is suspected of having an imperforate hymen (Fig. 11–9) and has no retention of secretions (i.e., a hydromucocolpos), which can be easily detected on rectal examination, surgery should be postponed until estrogen production is noted at puberty but before development of a significant hematocolpos.

Periurethral cysts in the neonate are frequently confused with a small hydromucocolpos and bulging imperforate hymen (Fig. 11–10). If the physician carefully probes in the suburethral area, the anteriorly placed vaginal introitus will be found. The probe or feeding tube can then be glided posteriorly past the cyst and into the vagina, proving the patency of the latter. The hymen may be stretched thin over the 2- to 4-cm yellowish suburethral cyst (Fig. 11–11). These cysts spontaneously resolve over the first month or so of life and do not require excision or drainage unless they become infected or symptomatic.

In reviews of 265 prepubertal hymens and 333 newborn hymens, Pokorny and Kozinetz[5] and Mor, Merlob, and Reisner[6] found a combined incidence of 3.8% and 3% for hymen variants (septations, microperforations, or imperforations), respectively.

Hymenal Configurations

In addition to the above congenital variants, the physician should be aware that the hymen of a prepubertal child has a wide range of variation in how it surrounds the vaginal orifice. These are termed *hymenal configurations* (Fig. 11–12).[7] If the hymen is thought of as a skirt or collar of tissue surrounding the mouth

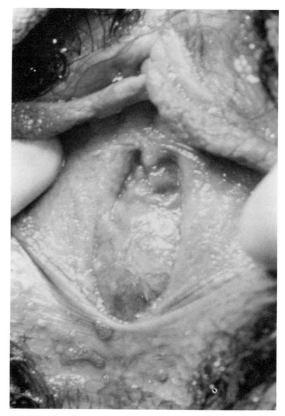

FIGURE 11-9 ••• A bulging imperforate hymen with a hematocolpos in a 13-year-old girl.

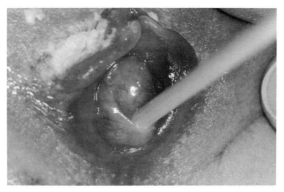

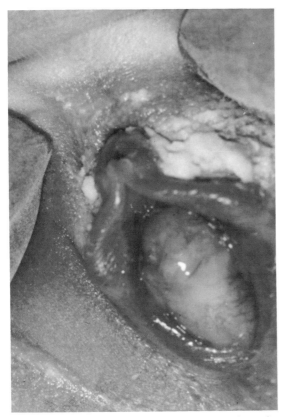

FIGURE 11–10 ••• A periurethral cyst in a newborn that gives the appearance of an imperforate hymen and a small hydromucocolpos. (From Pokorny SF. Pediatric gynecology. In: Stenchever MA [ed]. Office Gynecology. St. Louis: Mosby-Year Book, 1992, p 119.)

FIGURE 11–11 ••• Photograph of the same patient shown in Figure 11–10, illustrating that the hymen was stretched thin over the yellowish periurethral cyst, which spontaneously resolved over several months. (From Pokorny SF, Pokorny WJ. Pediatric gynecology. In: Ashcraft KW, Holder TM [eds]. Pediatric Surgery. 2nd ed. Philadelphia: WB Saunders, 1993, p 975.)

of the vagina, then the various configurations can be better conceptualized.

In most children, the hymenal collar completely surrounds the vaginal orifice. If the opening in the membrane is not centrally located, it is almost always anteriorly displaced toward the urethra. This type of hymen is considered to be *annular* or *circumferential* (see Fig. 11–5).[7–9]

If the orifice is placed so far anteriorly that there is no room for development of a hymenal rim in the suburethral area, there will be no

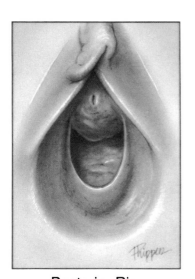

Posterior Rim

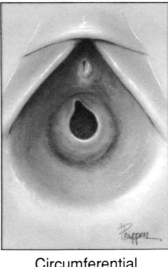

Circumferential Smooth Rim

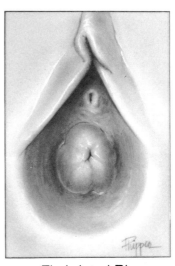

Fimbriated Rim

FIGURE 11–12 ••• Various hymen configurations. (From Pokorny SF. Configuration of the prepubertal hymen. Am J Obstet Gynecol 1987; 157:950–956.)

hymenal tissue from 10 o'clock or 11 o'clock clockwise to 1 or 2 o'clock. This hymenal configuration is called a *crescent* or a *posterior rim*.[7-9] Depending on how high the collar of tissue is, this might be a "high" (Fig. 11–13) or a "low" (Fig. 11–14) posterior rim.

In other children, the hymen seems to be more redundant and not infrequently has scallops on its free-standing margin. This configuration is definitely more common in the estrogenized state (Fig. 11–15), but aspects of this configuration, especially the scallops on the margins of a redundant hymen, occur in prepubertal children. This configuration has been called *fimbriated* or *denticular*.[7-9]

The hymenal orifice diameter can be influenced by the type of hymen configuration, by the method for spreading the vulvar tissues, and by the degree of perineal muscular relaxation at the time the diameter measurements are taken. Two other factors that influence orifice diameter, because they thicken the hymenal tissue and thereby make the orifice smaller, are inflammation and estrogenization of the tissue.

Occasionally a physician will examine a child who seems to have no hymenal tissue at all; if

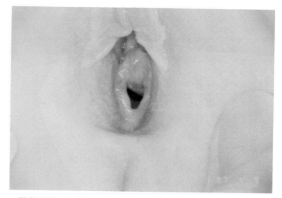

FIGURE 11–14 ••• Hymen with a low posterior rim.

any can be visualized, it is only in irregularly placed nubbins of tissue surrounding the mouth of the vagina (Fig. 11–16). All females are born with a hymen, and falls and severe blows to the adjacent perineal or vulvar tissues do not result in the finding of no hymenal tissue.[10] In adult patients, hymenal caruncles occur after the stretch trauma of vaginal childbirth. Similarly, hymenal remnants or caruncles are evidence of significant stretch trauma to the prepubertal child's vaginal introitus and

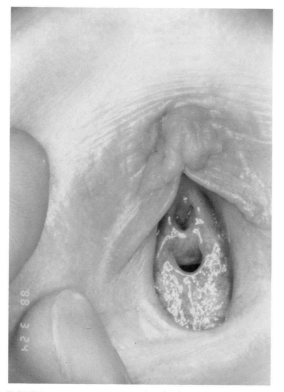

FIGURE 11–13 ••• Hymen with a high posterior rim. Note that there is no hymenal tissue in the suburethral area.

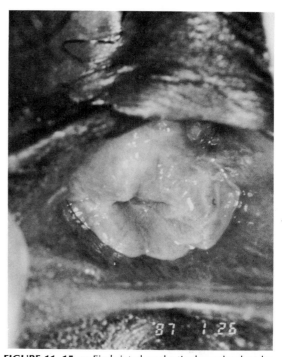

FIGURE 11–15 ••• Fimbriated or denticular redundant hymen with scallops along its rim. (From Pokorny SF. Configuration of the prepubertal hymen. Am J Obstet Gynecol 1987; 157:950–956.)

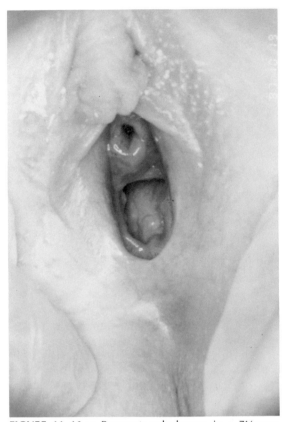

FIGURE 11–16 ••• Remnants-only hymen in a 7½-year-old girl several years after multiple episodes of penile–vaginal penetration. (From Pokorny SF. Pediatric vulvovaginitis. In: Kaufman R, Fredrich EG, Gardner HL [eds]. Benign Diseases of the Vulva and Vagina. Chicago: Year Book Medical, 1989, p 58.)

are the most consistent residual physical findings of severe childhood sexual abuse involving vaginal penetration. As such, hymenal caruncles in the prepubertal child should not be ignored by the clinician and should be reported to proper authorities for investigation of sexual abuse.

Evaluation of the prepubertal hymen should proceed in a stepwise fashion. Is this a hymen variant such as an imperforate, microperforate, or septated hymen? How is the hymen configured around the vaginal introitus (general variations)? Are there any breaks or bumps (minute variations)?

The greatest hymen contour variability will be noted in the suburethral area, but the majority of hymens will have a smooth free margin from 3 o'clock clockwise to 9 o'clock with no irregularities, mounds, or indentations. If such variations are noted, it is imperative that they be described in anatomically

descriptive terms, *not* action descriptive terms such as "ruptured," "virginal," or "marital" (Fig. 11–17).

Many annular hymens have a cleft or an indentation in the hymenal collar in the suburethral hymen from 10 o'clock clockwise to 2 o'clock (see Fig. 11–5). The crescent hymen not infrequently has symmetric scallops, flaps, or wings of tissue of the same color and thickness as the remainder of the hymen bilaterally on the hymen margins from 9 o'clock to 3 o'clock. The scallops that grace the free margins of the fimbriated hymen are noted to be uniform in their arrangement. These scallops occasionally form a "stellate" orifice, but because this term describes an orifice and not a hymen, its use should be discouraged. When evaluating these scalloped hymen contours, it is important to document the integrity of the hymenal tissue collar and to confirm that the scallop indentations do not represent breaks that extend through the collar of tissue down to the vaginal wall (Fig. 11–18).

Hymenal tags are not uncommon in new-

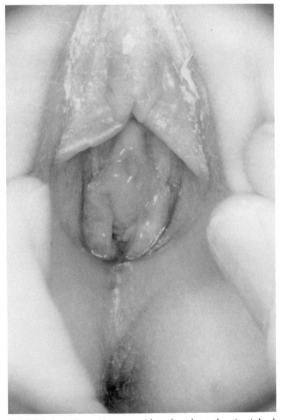

FIGURE 11–17 ••• Hymen with a break at the 6 o'clock position.

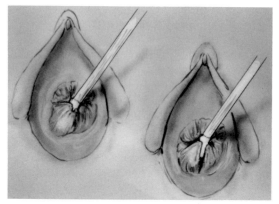

FIGURE 11–18 ••• Fimbriated redundant hymens occasionally need to be examined with a small probe or swab to determine whether an indentation extends to the base of the hymen collar. This figure shows a tear at the 6 o'clock position. (From Pokorny SF. Physical examination of the reproductive systems of female children and adolescents. Curr Probl Obstet Gynecol Fertil 1990; 13[5]:202–213.)

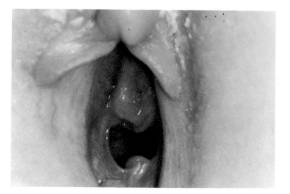

FIGURE 11–20 ••• Vestibule of a 5-year-old child. Note the patulous urethra. A biopsy of a mound of tissue on the hymen margin at the 6 o'clock position demonstrated fibroelastic tissue, compatible with hymenal septal remnant. (From Pokorny SF. Physical examination of the reproductive systems of female children and adolescents. Curr Probl Obstet Gynecol Fertil 1990; 13[5]:202–213.)

borns and seem to be related to estrogen stimulation. In the newborn these are isolated exophytic mucosal lesions of small dimensions (1 mm × 3 mm), and the majority resolve. Occasionally one will persist, most likely secondary to end-organ heightened sensitivity to low levels of estrogen. In the older child, these tags typically are isolated asymmetric mounds of tissue; their thickness and color resemble that of the hymen collar. Occasionally, they outgrow their blood supply, become more polypoid, and create an inflammatory and occasionally bloody discharge. When these latter alterations occur, it is difficult to distinguish the tags from a pedunculated friable condyloma acuminatum; in these cases excisional biopsy is warranted (Fig. 11–19).

Some mounds of tissue on the hymen margin at 6 o'clock most likely represent remnants of a septated hymen (Fig. 11–20). Other bumps on the hymen margin are thought to be acquired. Some are situated on the rim of the hymen on one side or the other, usually from 3 o'clock clockwise to 9 o'clock on the posterior hymenal margin, and, like the retracted septal remnant described earlier, are thicker than the hymen itself and in many cases are discolored (i.e., more erythematous than the hymen) (Fig. 11–21). Biopsies have proven that many of these consist of inflammatory granulation tissue or are histologically suggestive of human papillomavirus. It is unclear whether inflammation alone can cause these isolated hymenal bumps to form or a traumatic event must precede their development.[6]

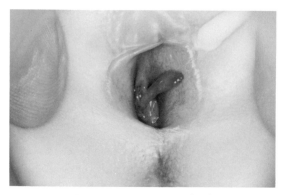

FIGURE 11–19 ••• Hymenal polyp.

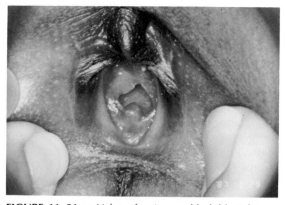

FIGURE 11–21 ••• Vulva of a 4-year-old child. A biopsy of a mound of erythematous tissue at the 6 o'clock position on hymen rim revealed chronic inflammation. (From Pokorny SF. Physical examination of the reproductive systems of female children and adolescents. Curr Probl Obstet Gynecol Fertil 1990; 13[5]:202–213.)

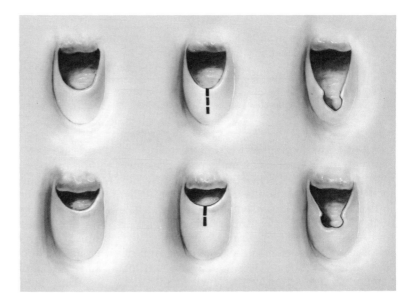

FIGURE 11–22 ••• Posterior rim breaks. (From Pokorny SF, Kozinetz CA. Configuration and other anatomic detail of the prepubertal hymen. Adolesc Pediatr Gynecol 1988; 1:99.)

Symmetric bumps on the hymen may represent retractions of a traumatic hymenal laceration at the 6 o'clock position (Figs. 11–22, 11–23). Interpretation of bumps and breaks on the hymen is controversial, but in a reported series of 265 prepubertal hymens, such bumps and breaks were three times more likely to be associated with sexual abuse than with other pediatric gynecologic conditions.[6]

INSTRUMENTATION OF THE VAGINA

Vaginal Aspirator

Although the estrogen effect on the mucosa of prepubertal children varies from child to child, the majority of children who are past the stage of toilet training have very atrophic genital mucosa. This atrophic mucosa is very sensitive to touch and can easily be lacerated by inflexible instruments. Furthermore, cotton-tipped swabs, which are often used to obtain secretions from the vagina, are abrasive and painful.

A soft rubber catheter is excellent for flushing the vagina with fluid, but is not ideal for obtaining undiluted vaginal secretions. Because the vagina is a closed space, when vaginal fluid is aspirated back into the catheter, invariably the catheter tip will be sucked against the vaginal wall, yielding a variable, but usually disappointingly small, amount of vaginal aspirant.

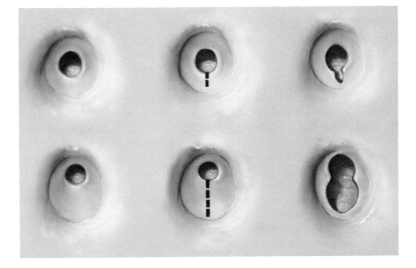

FIGURE 11–23 ••• Circumferential breaks. (From Pokorny SF, Kozinetz CA. Configuration and other anatomic detail of the prepubertal hymen. Adolesc Pediatr Gynecol 1988; 1:99.)

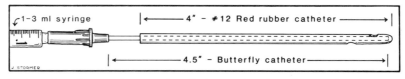

FIGURE 11–24 ••• Catheter-in-catheter aspirator used to obtain secretions from the prepubertal vagina. (From Pokorny SF, Stormer J. Atraumatic removal of secretions from the prepubertal vagina. Am J Obstet Gynecol 1987; 156[3]:581–582.)

An atraumatic method for obtaining vaginal aspirant fluid involves a makeshift catheter-within-a-catheter[11] (Fig. 11–24). Using aseptic technique, the proximal 4 inches of a butterfly intravenous tube is passed into the distal 4½ inches of a soft No. 12 urinary bladder catheter. A 1-ml tuberculin syringe with 0.5 to 1.0 ml of aspirating fluid is attached to the hub of the butterfly tubing. The entire amount of vaginal wash solution can be flushed into the vagina and aspirated back into the syringe; this can be done several times to obtain a good admixture of upper vaginal secretions. The aspirant can be used for wet mounts, Gram stains, cultures, and forensic material.

Because young children do not have a concept of the vaginal canal, it is frequently frightening for them to watch the catheter slide into the vaginal canal. Therefore, if at all possible they should not be encouraged to watch this procedure with the hand-held mirror.

Most children will comply with the above vaginal wash procedure if they are shown that no needles are attached to the catheter apparatus. Sometimes squirting a few drops of the flushing fluid onto their hand or allowing them to touch and feel a sample catheter reassures them. The procedure is performed with the child in the supine frog-legged position. The examiner should explain what will happen in terms the child can understand (e.g., he or she is going to wash the child's girl parts out, and the child will feel it, but it will not hurt). Then, using one hand to spread the labia so that the vaginal introitus is visualized, the catheter apparatus, held in the other hand, is quickly slipped at least 2 to 3 cm into the child's vagina. The examiner should brace his or her hand against the child's mons pubis or thigh so that if the child should move suddenly when the catheter is inserted into the vagina, the catheter will stay in place. Once the child is again assured that the catheter is not hurting her, the examiner can inject and aspirate the fluid in and out of the vagina a few times to get a good admixture of vaginal secretions,

aspirate the fluid back into the syringe, and then quickly remove the entire apparatus.

Topical anesthetics are occasionally helpful for pediatric gynecologic procedures (e.g., when the vaginal canal needs to be vigorously flushed to remove a foreign object, such as toilet paper wads, or vaginoscopy). Because local anesthetic might interfere with the results, it is not routinely used when vaginal aspirant is needed for cultures or forensic material.

Viscous xylocaine (2% jelly) can be applied with a cotton ball or dripped directly on the vestibule. After it has had time to take effect, a urinary bladder catheter is placed into the child's vagina. With her buttocks over the drain basin on the end of the gynecologic examination table, aseptic solution (e.g., bladder irrigant with povidone-iodine) is flushed into her vagina.

Other Instruments

To adequately visualize the vaginal canal of a prepubertal child, the instrument of choice must be narrow in diameter and have irrigating capabilities. Instillation of the irrigation fluid will expand the vaginal canal, as well as flush out discharge and debris, so that the entire vaginal canal and cervix can easily be visualized. Hysteroscopes and pediatric cystoscopes are ideal for this task.

All bivalved instruments, even nasal specula, cause damage to the atrophic tissues of the prepubertal child's vagina and rarely can be opened wide enough to provide the same degree of visualization as described earlier. The large otoscope and the Cameron-Myers vaginoscope, although the latter was designed specifically for children, also give inferior visualization of the vaginal canal when compared with the visualization provided by an endoscope and a fluid-expanded vaginal canal. Pediatric specula are a misnomer, as they are too short (<8 cm) to see the vaginal apex of a peripubertal child and too wide for the vaginal introitus of a small child, which they can severely traumatize.

Any inflexible instrument has the potential to injure an unanesthetized prepubertal child's vulva, should the child inadvertently move while the instrument is in the vagina. In situations in which the vaginal canal must be visualized and it is thought that the child will comply with the examination, the instrument of choice is a flexible fiberoptic endoscope with irrigating capabilities.

As described earlier, viscous xylocaine can be placed on the vestibule. The fiberoptic endoscope with infusing irrigating fluid can then be gently inserted into the vaginal canal. Once the scope is in the canal, the labial tissues can be gently squeezed together to allow the irrigating fluid to expand the vagina.

Ideally, for this procedure the child should sit, semireclined, with her buttocks slightly over the end of the gynecology table and her feet in the stirrups. The drain basin of the table should be positioned so that the irrigating fluid will drain into it.

Promising the child that she will also be allowed to look into the scope once the examiner is finished aids in obtaining patient compliance. Most fiberoptic scopes are long enough that the intravaginal aspect of the scope can be steadied and the eyepiece handed to the patient, allowing her to look also.

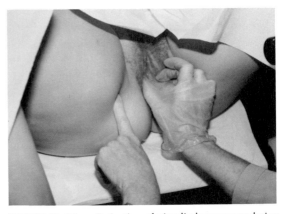

FIGURE 11–25 ••• Extinction of stimuli phenomenon being applied to obtain patient compliance for her first pelvic examination. Note the nonexamining finger being pressed into the patient's perineum in preparation for placement of the examiner's finger into the patient's vaginal introitus.

ulum blade width that will afford the most comfort *and* the best visibility.

Applying the "extinction of stimuli" phenomenon is valuable for a young female's first pelvic examination. This is a neurologic phenomenon whereby a primary distracting stimulus is used to lessen, defuse, and extinguish the intensity of the second stimulus. This consists of instructing the patient about sensations she will be experiencing as the examining index finger enters the vaginal introitus.

In essence, the examiner presses the nonexamining finger into the patient's perineum

SPECIAL ASPECTS OF THE PERIPUBERTAL GENITAL EXAMINATION

It is appropriate to consider the use of a speculum for genital examination of the estrogenized peripubertal female. Estrogen has a profound impact on the introital tissues, allowing a degree of pliability and distention not found in the nonestrogenized prepubertal state. The same speculum that can be used in a peripubertal girl would have lacerated her vulvar tissues just a year or so earlier.

The examiner should first attempt to place the examining index finger *through* the vaginal introitus before insertion of the speculum. There are several advantages to this practice: it allows detection of hymenal variants, it is necessary for teaching the patient to relax, and it allows the examiner to determine the spec-

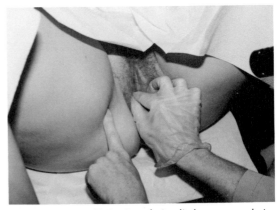

FIGURE 11–26 ••• Extinction of stimuli phenomenon being demonstrated for a patient's first pelvic examination. Note that the nonexamining finger continues to be pressed into the patient's perineum while the examiner's other index finger probes the patient's introitus.

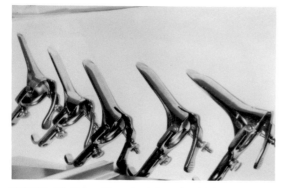

FIGURE 11–27 ••• The physician should have a broad spectrum of speculum widths (0.8 to 3.0 cm) to choose from when performing a girl's first pelvic examination. (From Pokorny SF. Physical examination of the reproductive systems of female children and adolescents. Curr Probl Obstet Gynecol Fertil 1990; 13[5]:202–213.)

close to the pantyline before touching the patient's introitus with the examining finger. The examination should not proceed until the patient acknowledges that the pressure sensation she is feeling is not painful; she should acknowledge an awareness of a pressure sensation (Fig. 11–25).

The patient is then forewarned that she will feel the same type of pressure sensation as the examining finger slowly enters the vaginal introitus. The more anxious the patient is and the tighter the introital tissues feel, the more the nonexamining, distracting finger should apply pressure to the perineum to defuse and extinguish the sensation the patient is experiencing at the introitus (Fig. 11–26).

Once the examining finger is worked through the introitus, it should remain there. At this point, the patient can be instructed how to relax the perineal body by allowing her knees to drop outward. Once this is accomplished the proper speculum width can easily be chosen (Fig. 11–27).

References

1. Cassell C. Swept Away. Why Women Fear Their Own Sexuality. New York: Simon and Schuster, 1984.
2. Jenny C, Sutherland SE, Sandahl BB. Developmental approach to preventing the sexual abuse of children. Pediatrics 1986; 78:1034.
3. Cowan BD, Morrison JC. Management of abnormal genital bleeding in girls and women. N Engl J Med 1991; 324(24):1710–1715.
4. Herman-Giddens ME, Berson NL. Harmful genital care practices in children. JAMA 1989; 261:577.
5. Pokorny SF, Kozinetz CA. Configuration and other anatomic details of the prepubertal hymen. Adolesc Pediatr Gynecol 1988; 1:97.
6. Mor N, Merlob P, Reisner SH. Types of hymen in the newborn infant. Eur J Obstet Gynecol Reprod Biol 1986; 22:225.
7. Pokorny, SF. Configuration of the prepubertal hymen. Am J Obstet Gynecol 1987; 157:950–956.
8. Emans SJ, Woods ER, Flagg NT, et al. Genital findings in sexually abused symptomatic and asymptomatic girls. Pediatrics 1987; 79:778.
9. Enos W, Conrath T, Byer J. Forensic evaluation of the sexually abused child. Pediatrics 1986; 78:385–398.
10. Pokorny SF, Pokorny WJ, Kramer W. Acute genital injury in the prepubertal female. Am J Obstet Gynecol 1992; 166(5):1461–1466.
11. Pokorny SF, Stormer J. Atraumatic removal of secretions from the prepubertal vagina. Am J Obstet Gynecol 1987; 156(3):581–582.

CHAPTER 12

Vulvovaginitis

FREDERICK J. RAU
CLAUDETTE E. JONES
DAVID MURAM

VULVOVAGINITIS IN CHILDREN

Vulvovaginal inflammation is the most common gynecologic complaint in the prepubertal female, accounting for 40% to 50% of visits to pediatric gynecology clinics.[1] There has been an increasing interest in the microbiology as well as the sequelae of vulvovaginitis. Various infectious agents initially affecting the lower genital tract may result in a serious health risk. For example, vulvovaginal infection caused by the human papillomavirus (HPV) is associated with an increased risk of neoplastic change.[2] In prepubertal children, the relative frequency of the various microbiologic organisms is different when compared with those seen in adolescent and adult women. In addition, the diagnosis of specific venereal diseases should prompt appropriate investigative steps by child protective service agencies.

Research on the clinical aspects of vulvovaginal infections is rapidly increasing. In children and adolescents especially, the presence of a genital infection, along with the implications of a possible sex-related infection, can be very significant for the patient and her caretaker. Thus, it is important for the clinician to have a rational and caring approach to patients with vulvovaginitis to improve patient education and thus increase compliance with the suggested therapy.[3]

Definition

Vulvovaginitis is defined as inflammation of the vulvar and vaginal tissues and may result from a wide variety of causes. Commonly, in prepubertal children with altered vaginal bacteriologic environments as a result of disturbed homeostasis, vulvitis occurs initially and may exist alone or involve the vagina.

Risk Factors

Prepubertal children are anatomically, physiologically, and behaviorally at relative risk for a number of varieties of vulvovaginitis. Recognized predisposing factors for the development of vulvovaginitis in prepubertal children are given in Table 12–1. Other potential risk factors for vulvovaginitis include obesity, systemic illness (e.g., diabetes mellitus), preexisting vulvar dermatoses, and altered immune status.

Symptoms and Signs

Acute vulvovaginitis may denude the vulvar and vaginal epithelium, resulting in symptoms related by the child or her caretaker. The patient is commonly brought to the clinician with complaints of discharge staining her un-

TABLE 12–1 ••• PREDISPOSING FACTORS FOR VULVOVAGINITIS IN PREPUBERTAL CHILDREN

Suboptimal perineal hygiene
Short distance between the vagina and anus
Small hymenal opening, obstructing egress of secretions
Lack of vulvar fat pads and pubic hair
Unestrogenized, atrophic vagina
pH of 6.5 to 7.5
Impaired local immune mechanisms

derclothing; at times blood stains are noted. This may be associated with genital discomfort, including pruritus, vulvar "burning," or stinging, especially on urination when the urine comes in contact with the irritated tissues (vulvar dysuria). The child may scratch the area, leading to excoriations and increased inflammatory reaction. Dysuria may lead to an erroneous diagnosis of a lower urinary tract infection, especially if a voided specimen is contaminated with vaginal secretions and contains white blood cells. If the parent examines the child's vulva, erythema, discharge, and an offensive odor may be noted. Young children usually cannot verbalize specific symptoms, and reliance on parental observations of irritability, rubbing, or scratching is required. The child may cry if the area is touched or may be noted to sit or walk in ways indicating genital discomfort.

Approach to Evaluation

The initial history taking of the patient and her caretaker should include pertinent questions communicated in terms appropriate for the age of the child. As is true for nearly all pediatric patients, a different approach from that used with adult women must be taken. In young patients, gaining the child's trust and occupying her attention with an interesting and nonthreatening conversation provides a great deal of assistance in minimizing the potential for a negative experience.

Commonly, the patient's parent(s) will relate part or all of the history, but the child should always be included in the initial interaction. The child may have received a variety of physician-prescribed or "home" remedies, most or all of which provided no therapeutic effect. The vulvar symptoms may well have resulted in sleepless nights for parent and child. Symptoms usually have been present for days, weeks, or months in an intermittent

pattern before a physician is consulted. As a result, the clinician may evaluate the patient when the parent has exhausted all other resources in caring for the child. Moreover, the parent may be concerned about other implications of genital disorders, including sexual abuse and sexually transmitted disease, poor hygiene, foreign bodies, cancer, or future reproduction.

History

The history should focus on those aspects of the symptoms that may be helpful at narrowing the possible etiologic factors. The duration, quantity, consistency, and color of the discharge should be noted. The presence of a new or offensive odor is usually indicative of anaerobic bacterial secretion products. Because the vulvar skin is delicate and has a thin epithelial cover, any cause of increased heat, moisture, vulvar friction, or bacteriologic contamination may incite vulvovaginitis. Behaviorally, inadequate hygiene along with incorrect urinary and bowel habits (e.g., back-to-front wiping after a bowel movement or urinating with the knees tightly closed), genital manipulation with contaminated hands, and minor trauma associated with outdoor play (i.e., sandbox vulvitis) may contribute to epithelial maceration and subsequent vulvovaginitis. Close-fitting and poorly absorbent clothing (e.g., leotards, tights, and one-piece sleepers) may predispose a child to develop inflammation. In younger children, the type of diapers used should be noted. Other areas of concern include recent systemic infection in the patient or family members (upper respiratory, gastrointestinal, or dermatologic), recent treatment with medication, bed wetting or soiling problems, bubblebath use, history of atopic dermatitis or other dermatoses, and nocturnal perianal pruritus. The possibility of childhood sexual abuse must be considered when evaluating children with vulvovaginitis.

Physical Examination

The clinical examination of children with vulvovaginitis is described in Chapter 11. The physician should be able to visualize the labia majora and minora, introitus and hymen, clitoris, urethra, anus, and the lower portion of the vagina. The frog-legged position with gentle lateral and downward retraction of the labia majora usually provides an adequate view

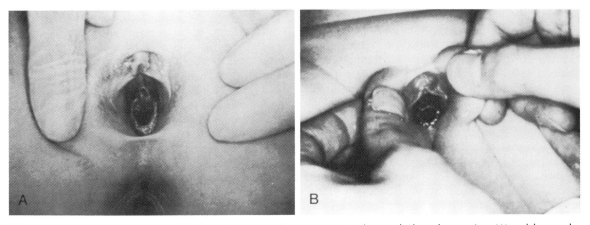

FIGURE 12–1 ••• Examination of the vulva, hymen, and anterior vagina by gentle lateral retraction *(A)* and by gentle gripping of the labia, pulling anteriorly *(B)*. (From Emans SJ, Goldstein DP. Office evaluation of the child and adolescent. In: Pediatric and Adolescent Gynecology. 3rd ed. Boston: Little, Brown and Company, copyright 1990, p 7. Reprinted with permission.)

(Fig. 12–1). Obtaining a sample of the discharge for microscopic examination and bacteriologic study is usually necessary at the time of visualization. This can be accomplished using a variety of nontraumatic methods. In children with nonrecurrent vulvovaginitis, vaginoscopy is not necessary if no bleeding is present and a foreign body is not suspected. Occasionally, an in-office vaginoscopic examination using a variety of appropriately sized instruments can be accomplished in a very cooperative patient. Emotional and physical trauma clearly must be avoided.

The findings at physical examination in children with vulvovaginitis are extremely variable (Table 12–2). Commonly, no discharge is seen, and there are no obvious signs of inflamma-tion. When present, the amount of vaginal discharge varies from minimal, dried secretions on the vulva to copious amounts identified at the vaginal introitus and on the underclothing. The color may vary from a clear or white mucoid discharge to any variety of yellow, green, or gray-brown. Evidence of suboptimal perineal hygiene is seen in some children, including debris within the intralabial sulci or stool contamination of the vulva. Vulvar erythema, edema, and excoriations are commonly seen. Injection of the superficial vessels of the vaginal introitus and vestibule may be increased. The hymen should be evaluated for its configuration and degree of inflammation. Signs of trauma such as scarring, tears, or loss of hymenal continuity can be seen in the setting

TABLE 12–2 ••• CLINICAL FEATURES OF VULVOVAGINITIS

	Candidiasis	**Gardnerella Vaginalis**	**Trichomoniasis**
Signs and symptoms	Pruritus Vulvovaginitis erythema White curdlike discharge	Vulvitis (rare) Gray-white "amine-like" discharge	Pruritus Vaginal erythema
Vaginal smear	Filaments and spores (10% potassium hydroxide)	Epithelial cells with bacteria "clue" cells Gram-negative rods Positive whiff test Fishy odor with potassium hydroxide	Motile, flagellated organisms (saline)
pH	Acidic with nitrazine paper	5.0 to 5.5	6.5 to 7.5
Treatment	Clotrimazole Miconazole Nystatin Gentian violet or boric acid	Metronidazole Ampicillin	Metronidazole

Douching is not usually recommended for the adolescent.
From Sanfilippo JS. Adolescent girls with vaginal discharge. Pediatr Ann 1986; 15(7):509–519.

of childhood sexual abuse. Gentle "gripping" of the labia majora and depression of the perineum assists in visualization of the distal vagina to detect discharge or foreign bodies lodged behind the hymen. The perineal skin and anus should always be examined and can demonstrate inflammation and/or excoriations or other signs of trauma. To test for pinworm infestation, a piece of clear tape is dabbed on the perineal skin and anus when the child awakens and the debris examined for the characteristic ova (Fig. 12–2). If indicated, a gentle rectoabdominal examination is usually well tolerated by children and is helpful in detecting a pelvic mass. Expressing remaining discharge, assessing rectal tone, and occasionally palpating a hard foreign body may also be necessary.

Examination of the vaginal secretions is of paramount importance if an accurate diagnosis is to be made. Various methods have been described for the atraumatic collection of vaginal secretions in prepubertal children. One method, described by Pokorny and Stormer, is the catheter-within-a-catheter technique.[4] This involves placing the plastic portion of a No. 14 or No. 16 intravenous catheter within

a shortened No. 12 plastic or rubber urinary catheter. A small syringe with 1 to 2 ml of bacteriostatic saline is attached to the hub. Standing at the side of the examining table, the clinician can gently but quickly place the red rubber catheter tip into the hymenal opening. The examiner can move the syringe within the barrel several times to distribute the saline and collect the vaginal secretions. The device is then removed and appropriate microscopic examination and cultures performed. Another method of collection of vaginal secretions in children includes instilling saline from a syringe into the vagina and collecting the fluid as it accumulates in the lower vagina and vestibule. Direct collection with saline-moistened urethral or regular cotton-tipped swabs or Calgiswabs has also been described. Microscopic examination of the discharge for mycotic organisms, white and red blood cells, estrogen effect on vaginal squamous epithelium, and parasitic ova, "clue" cells, or trichomonads should be performed. Appropriate bacteriologic assessment will confirm the diagnosis. However, if no clear signs of discharge or inflammation are noted on examination, vaginal cultures are unlikely to add clinically useful information.

Hormonal Alterations Associated with Vaginal Discharge

The presence of a noticeable vaginal discharge without symptoms or signs of vulvovaginal inflammation is a common presenting complaint. There are two points in the developmental timetable of genital maturation when this is likely to be seen as a normal physiologic process. In the neonatal period, a mucoid white discharge may be noted at the vaginal introitus. This is due to stimulation of the endocervical glands and transudation of vaginal fluid secondary to maternal estrogens. The discharge is composed of endocervical mucus and desquamated cervicovaginal epithelial cells. As estrogen levels fall, the discharge decreases but may be accompanied by a small amount of estrogen-withdrawal bleeding from the endometrium. Occasionally, minor degrees of breast development or hymenal estrogenization can be noted. These changes should gradually disappear by 6 weeks postnatally. The typical prepubertal appearance of the vulva, hymen, and vagina remains throughout childhood until ovarian estrogen production

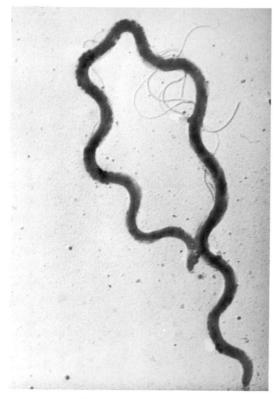

FIGURE 12–2 ••• Pinworms.

begins. Following thelarche, estrogen stimulation of endocervical mucus production and vaginal transudation and desquamation of cells produces a vaginal discharge. The secretion is mucoid and yellow-white in appearance, is nonirritating, and does not have a foul odor. The color may change to yellowish-brown after drying on the child's underclothing. Discharge secretion is associated with other estrogen-dependent changes, including labial enlargement, sebaceous gland stimulation, thickening and rugae formation of the vagina, hymenal thickening and redundancy, and increased uterine fundal growth in relation to the cervix. Patient and parental education and reassurance are helpful in this setting to prevent unnecessary overtreatment of presumed pathologic vulvovaginitis.

Etiology and Management of Vulvovaginitis

Specific Vaginitis

Microbiologic cultures of vaginal secretions in children presenting with vaginal symptoms have been studied by Paradise et al.[5] These investigators found that in 24 prepubertal patients without vaginal discharge, all had "normal" flora appropriate for their age group (i.e., lactobacilli, α-hemolytic streptococci, and diphtheroids). Additionally, other isolates were found in 10 of these 24 children. These included *Escherichia coli, Haemophilus influenzae* type B, and *Bacteroides* sp. No yeast species were cultured from any prepubertal patients presenting with or without vaginal discharge. Five patients, all with discharge on examination, had positive cultures for *Neisseria gonorrhoeae* or *Shigella sonnei*. To minimize potential contamination, Gerstner et al.[6] employed vaginoscopy while culturing symptomatic and asymptomatic prepubertal girls for aerobic and anaerobic organisms. The most common aerobic organisms found were *Staphylococcus epidermidis*, enterococci, and *E. coli*, which are representative of normal cutaneous and enteric flora. Predominant anaerobic organisms were *Peptococcus* sp., *Peptostreptococcus* sp., *Veillonella parvula*, eubacteria, *Propionibacterium* sp., and *Bacteroides* sp.

Although the array of organisms was similar in girls with and without symptoms and signs of vaginitis, there were a number of differences. Anaerobic organisms such as *Peptococcus* sp., *Peptostreptococcus* sp., *Bacteroides fragilis*, and *Clostridium perfringens* were isolated more frequently from patients exhibiting signs of vulvovaginitis.

Conversely, lactobacilli were significantly less common in symptomatic patients. *Candida albicans* was isolated in only 3.2% of asymptomatic children but was identified in 25% of symptomatic patients. Overall, there was a minor trend toward isolating aerobic organisms in children with vulvovaginitis. Thus, it appears that the microbiologic characteristics of children with symptomatic vulvovaginitis involve differences in quantity of the various organisms, in addition to an overpopulation of specific anaerobic species. In association with these changes, the population of lactobacilli is diminished, and *Candida* species may proliferate. The inciting factors and host response to these microbiologic alterations have yet to be clearly elucidated. It seems likely that children differ in their local immune response to a variety of organisms and their secretion products. This may partially account for the wide array of clinical manifestations and responses seen in childhood vulvovaginitis.

Nonspecific Vaginitis

The presenting symptoms of all patients are similar. Careful examination and the use of microscopy and microbiologic studies are helpful in planning appropriate therapy. However, the majority of vulvovaginal infections in children are caused by disturbed bacterial homeostasis, which is commonly related to inadequate fecal and urinary hygiene. This entity is termed *nonspecific vaginitis* and accounts for up to 70% of all pediatric vulvovaginitis cases. It is thought to involve subtle alterations in the local microbiologic flora and/or host defense and homeostatic mechanisms, leading to symptoms of vulvar and distal vaginal inflammation, vaginal discharge, and odor. The inflammation involves the introitus, hymen, and labial epithelium. The discharge can be scant or copious, is seen by the parent on the child's underclothing, and may be yellow-white, green, or tan. The odor is a source of great concern to the older child and parent. Vulvar skin changes such as excoriation resulting from scratching, erythema, edema, maceration, and denudation of epithelium may also be seen. Occasionally, the clinician may note no signs of inflammation, or only minimal erythema.

A saline wet mount reveals a mixture of white blood cells, bacteria, and other debris. Other findings, such as the presence of "clue" cells, trichomonads, and yeast species, should be noted but are rarely identified in a typical case. Vaginal cultures obtained using one of the methods previously discussed may assist the clinician in identifying a predominant or clearly pathologic organism. If no discharge is seen and the signs of vulvovaginal inflammation are minimal, the bacteriologic cultures are unlikely to be positive.

Based on available data, nonspecific vulvovaginitis may be viewed as a condition in which overpopulation of anaerobic, and likely aerobic, bacterial species are present. This may result from unknown inciting factors or may clearly be associated with inadequate perineal hygiene. The child's individual vulvovaginal local immune mechanisms respond in an idiosyncratic manner to produce a variety of signs and symptoms.

The mainstay of therapy consists of improved perineal hygiene. This improvement is necessary to decrease the contaminant bacterial population derived from the gastrointestinal tract. Sitz/tub baths twice a day for 30 minutes help eliminate irritating, bacteria-containing discharge from the vulvar structures. Nonirritating soap (e.g., glycerine-based or super-fatted soap) often is useful. Increased supervision at the time of urination or defecation to encourage adequate front-to-back wiping is encouraged. Permitting the child to go without underwear at home and the use of small amounts of baby powder on the vulva promote drying and decrease inflammation.

Objective data with respect to various therapeutic efforts in childhood vulvovaginitis are currently not available. Clinical experience has shown that local measures alone can produce improvement in most patients. However, if an abnormal population of bacteria is present, antimicrobial therapy would be expected to contribute to clinical improvement. Amoxicillin (20 to 40 mg/kg/day in three divided doses) is effective against a variety of potentially pathogenic organisms in patients with nonspecific vulvovaginitis. Amoxicillin–clavulanic acid (Augmentin) may provide improved coverage if anaerobic or β-lactamase–producing organisms are present. Local corticosteroid therapy (e.g., 1% hydrocortisone cream, betamethasone valerate) relieves vulvar symptoms such as itching, irritation, and erythema.

The clinician may request a follow-up visit. If the symptoms persist after approximately 2 weeks of therapy, reexamination should be performed and consideration given to vaginoscopy. This allows evaluation of the entire vagina, specifically looking for a nidus of infection (e.g., foreign body, neoplasm, or abnormal communication with the urinary or gastrointestinal tract). The clinician should communicate any laboratory results to the parent. Reassurance and a review of preventive methods are helpful.

Secondary Inoculation

Blood-borne inoculation of the vulva and vagina by organisms causing an infection elsewhere in the body and transmission by contaminated hands are other causes of vulvovaginitis in children. The child may present with signs and symptoms of discharge and vulvar inflammation. A history of another infection affecting the upper respiratory tract, pharynx, skin, and urinary or gastrointestinal tract or other sites may be present. Culture of the discharge or vaginal saline irrigation usually reveals the same organism thought to be responsible for the original infection. The symptoms and signs of secondary vulvovaginitis are similar to those previously described.

Planning therapy for this group of patients depends on defining the primary source of infection, obtaining culture results, and determining previous treatment. Good perineal hygiene and sitz baths as described earlier are important to provide relief from symptoms and prevent recurrence. Antibiotic therapy prescribed for the primary infection is likely to clear the vaginal infection as well. If the initial therapy has been completed and symptoms still persist, treatment with a second course of antibiotics is reasonable. The choice of agent depends on the previous treatment, response, and culture results. Topical corticosteroids can be effective in decreasing the inflammatory reaction. If persistent discharge or inflammation persists or recurs after a second course of therapy, vaginoscopy is then required.

Shigella Vulvovaginitis

Shigella vulvovaginitis is rare in children. It is commonly associated with a diarrheal illness in either the patient or a family member. Vaginal discharge is present, and blood may be seen in the discharge in up to 40% to 50% of cases. *Shigella flexneri* is the most common species (85%), with *S. sonnei* and *S. boydii*

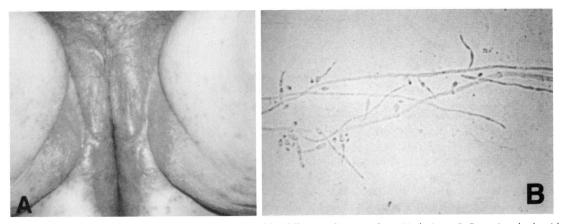

FIGURE 12–3 ••• *A*, Candida vulvovaginitis characterized by diffuse erythema and pruritic lesions. *B*, Potassium hydroxide (KOH) vaginal preparation. Note the hyphae and budding yeast. (From Sanfilippo JS. Adolescent girls with vaginal discharge. Pediatr Ann 1986; 15[7]:509.)

being much less common.[6] *Shigella* infestation of the vagina in association with a gastrointestinal infection substantiates the concept that the prepubertal vagina is susceptible to enteric pathogens. Treatment consists of systemic antibiotics to which the specific pathogen is susceptible. Topical therapy is not effective. Such treatment may not result in cure of the associated vaginitis, and additional therapy may be necessary.[7]

Sexually Transmitted Diseases

When a child is found to have a venereal disease, the origin of the inciting inoculation must be determined. Inherent in this evaluation is the possibility of abusive sexual contact. Certain specific vulvovaginitis entities are recognized as indicators of sexual abuse (e.g., gonorrhea or syphilis). Other sexually transmitted diseases may be acquired at birth when the infant passes through an infected birth canal. The various venereal diseases in children are discussed in greater detail in Chapter 20.

Candida Vulvovaginitis

Candida vulvovaginitis is common in adolescents and adults but appears to be somewhat less common in prepubertal children. However, data on the prevalence of *Candida* sp. in various populations of children with vulvovaginitis vary considerably. Paradise et al. evaluated 36 prepubertal girls with genital symptoms or signs of vulvovaginitis. No *Candida* sp. were isolated when vaginal cultures were obtained

in girls either with or without vaginal discharge.[5] Conversely, in another study vaginoscopic culture techniques were used in 31 asymptomatic and 36 symptomatic prepubertal girls. The investigators found that *Candida* was present in 3% of the asymptomatic children and 25% of the symptomatic girls.[6]

The child with candidal vulvovaginitis will complain of severe vulvar pruritus and secondary vulvar dysuria. There may be a small amount of white or yellow curdlike discharge. Examination reveals diffuse erythema and hyperemia of the vulva. Inflammation may extend inferiorly to the perianal region or laterally toward the inner thighs. Excoriation and desquamated areas are seen. White plaques or satellite *Candida* lesions may be identified. The dermatologic appearance can sometimes be confused with lichen sclerosus. The diagnosis is established by examination of the fungal hyphae and buds with a saline or potassium hydroxide wet mount (Fig. 12–3). A culture can be obtained if the diagnosis is in doubt.

Because candidal vulvovaginitis is less common in childhood, predisposing factors should be determined. Antibiotic therapy can alter the microbiologic flora of the prepubertal vagina predisposing to candida. Diabetes mellitus can also result in candidal infections and a glucose screening, and if necessary, glucose tolerance test may be appropriate especially with recurrent candidal infection. Transmission by close contact, bed clothes etc., appears to be less likely.

Treatment of candidal vulvovaginitis in children is limited by the difficulty in administering intravaginal topical therapy. Options include topical vulvar therapy with an antifungal cream (miconazole, buconazole, clotrimazole) complemented, if necessary, with a corticosteroid preparation. In resistant infections documented to be caused by *Candida*, intravaginal administration of antifungal cream can be performed in the office using a catheter-syringe method. Alternatively, 1 ml of nystatin liquid can be instilled intravaginally three times daily. Intravaginal tablets (clotrimazole) can be used in older prepubertal girls and adolescents. Gentian violet liquid is reserved for recalcitrant infections, as it stains clothing and tissues and may cause vulvar irritation. Oral nystatin for recurrent infections has not been well studied in children.

VULVOVAGINITIS IN ADOLESCENTS

Adolescence is often associated with unique gynecologic concerns. Pubertal hormonal changes promote an alteration of the vaginal flora from that of a child to that of an adult. As a result, infectious processes are different and more prevalent. It has been noted that the signs and symptoms of vulvovaginitis (e.g., vaginal discharge and pruritus) were second only to menstrual disorders as the presenting complaint in more than 2000 visits by adolescent females to a gynecology clinic.[2]

The sequelae of these infections include more serious disorders of the upper genital tract (e.g., salpingo-oophoritis with resultant infertility). Other concerns, including premature rupture of membranes and asymptomatic cervicitis, may be noted in this patient population. Finally, the epidemic of human papillomavirus (HPV) infections has been linked to an increased risk of developing cervical cancer.

Evaluation of an adolescent who presents with signs and symptoms of vulvovaginitis must take into consideration the pubertal status, current or recent sexual involvement (voluntary or associated with assault), and contraceptive method (if any), as these may affect management. The possibility of sexually transmitted infection is of significant concern to these patients, and thus the clinical setting provides the opportunity to educate the patient and facilitate compliance with recommended therapy. Sexual activity among adolescents predisposes them to exposure to a host of pathogens. Because sexually transmitted diseases are discussed in Chapter 21, the present discussion is limited to the evaluation and management of the common causes of vulvovaginitis in adolescents.

Definition and Risk Factors

Vulvar and vaginal inflammation may result from a wide variety of causes. In postpubertal adolescents, especially those who are sexually active, it usually begins as a primary vaginitis; the associated discharge may induce a secondary vulvitis. In many patients, it may be impossible to accurately identify the anatomic origin of the presenting symptoms, and additional history may be necessary to determine whether the upper genital tract is affected.

Hormonal Changes

After puberty, the vaginal ecosystem resembles that of the adult, with an epithelial lining, enzymes, substrates, microflora, and secretions. Vaginal secretions are composed of the products of vaginal transudation, endocervical mucus secretions, endometrial and tubal fluids, exfoliated cells, and fluid from sebaceous, sweat, and Bartholin's glands. The vaginal flora is dependent on pH and glycogen-glucose availability for bacterial metabolism. Under the influence of endogenous estrogens, the vaginal mucosa proliferates, thickens, and accumulates glycogen. Fermentation of glycogen results in a decrease in the pH to levels of 4.0 to 4.5. This environment favors acidogenic, glycogen-metabolizing bacteria, predominantly lactobacilli.[8] Other such bacteria include acidogenic corynebacteria, *Enterobacteriaceae* sp., and *Bacteroides fragilis*. Various staphylococci, streptococci, diphtheroids, *C. albicans*, and other species of anaerobic bacteria have also been noted.

Lactobacilli help control the vaginal microflora and maintain its steady state. Lactic acid, produced during lactobacillus metabolism as well as by vaginal epithelial cells, promotes a low vaginal pH. Lactobacilli continue to thrive in this environment. They also possess many antagonistic properties, and some strains produce metabolites (such as H_2O_2) that help to maintain this dominance.[9] Changes in pH or glycogen status affect the lactobacilli, thereby permitting other organisms to predominate. Antibiotics, douches, alkaline secretions during menses, alkaline soaps, and poorly controlled diabetes mellitus are among the more common causes of such changes in microflora. A variation in dominance and population levels of each bacterial species is noted throughout the cycle as the vaginal pH varies from neutral to acidic. Some researchers suggest that frequent and unprotected intercourse may also alter pH status because of the strongly alkaline nature of seminal fluid and vaginal lubricating secretions.[9]

Hormonal Alterations Producing Discharge. Six to 12 months before menarche, physiologic vaginal secretions may increase in production, resulting in a physiologic discharge (leukorrhea). In general this discharge is clear or yellow-white in appearance, mucoid in texture, and nonirritating. It is frequently copious, with no specific malodor. Staining of underclothing may result from the drying of secretions, with a resultant change to a yellow-brown color. Dried secretions may also cause vulvar pruritus, although the vulva is not inflamed.[10] Evaluation of the discharge by microscopy notes normal flora with an absence of leukocytes or pathogenic bacteria. The pH of the secretions is <4.5. Good perineal hygiene should be encouraged, and the patient should be reassured that this is not indicative of a disease.

Risk Factors for Vulvovaginitis

Sexual activity increases the risk of vulvovaginal infections and sexually transmitted diseases in adolescents. The use of oral contraceptives and douches, as well as the alteration of immune mechanisms caused by chemotherapeutic agents (antibiotics, etc.) or systemic illness (diabetes mellitus) potentially increase the risk of developing vulvovaginitis. Certain sexual practices; obesity; the wearing of tight, noncotton underclothing; and poor perineal hygiene may also play a role in the development of vulvovaginitis in the adolescent female. When evaluating young females with symptoms suggestive of vulvovaginitis, it is very helpful to identify these risk factors, as they may suggest the possible pathogen.

Clinical Features of Vulvovaginitis

The presenting symptoms may differ according to the organism. Once the normal vaginal flora is replaced by a pathogen, the vaginal mucosa becomes irritated and inflamed, often with a resulting increase in production of vaginal secretions and discharge and a change in odor or color. Adolescents with vulvovaginitis may note these changes. The color ranges from yellow or white to greenish-brown, especially if the discharge is associated with some bleeding. Pruritus and vulvar irritation symptoms are common. These include burning, dyspareunia, vulvar dysuria, or ill-defined discomfort of the genitalia. Pelvic pain, abnormal uterine bleeding, and other signs of pelvic inflammatory disease may be evident if an ascending infection is present.

Approach to the Adolescent Patient

Conveying the belief that her problem is significant helps greatly in establishing a trusting relationship with the adolescent patient. Confidentiality is of utmost importance to the adolescent, and reassurances as to the physician-patient relationship should be clearly stated. This is especially true when sexual activity is of concern. The clinician must also be aware that adolescents often use common gynecologic symptoms as a prelude to the discussion of more pressing concerns such as possible pregnancy, contraceptive needs, or fear of a sexually transmitted illness. Sensitive listening and "reading between the lines" must be practiced in this setting.

Patient History

It is important to note the characteristics of the discharge and associated vulvar inflammation. Additional information should include pubertal status, menstrual history, the use of menstrual hygiene products, and medications. Timing of the onset of symptoms with respect to the menstrual cycle, sexual activity, or the use of medications should also be noted. Inquiry should be made, if applicable, as to the number of sexual partners, any recent change in partners, a history of dyspareunia, dysuria or orogenital sexual activity.[11] Open-ended questions such as "Do you have a boyfriend?" and "Is it serious?" are useful in establishing communication early on. With time, more direct questions can be asked.

The presence of the parent or guardian usually limits discussion regarding sexuality. Talking with the adolescent in private leads to a more accurate history. In some cases, the vulvovaginal symptoms may cause embarrassment to the young teenager, who may have difficulty revealing pertinent historical data and may be very reluctant to be examined. Supportive and nonthreatening discussion is critically important.

Physical Examination

For the younger adolescent with vulvovaginitis, this will often be the first pelvic examination. This setting provides an excellent opportunity to discuss pubertal changes, reproductive health, and the importance of routine gynecologic care. Discussion and reassurance regarding the pelvic examination and its importance are extremely helpful in creating a positive experience. Adult stirrups may be successfully used for most teenage patients.

The initial phase of the genital examination consists of an inspection of the vulva for distribution of pubic hair and signs of inflammation or vulvar skin disease, discharge, or trauma. After emphasizing normal findings or confirming visualization of potentially abnormal areas, the labia are gently separated, and the hymen and vestibule are inspected. The degree of estrogenization and caliber of the orifice are noted.

Decisions about how the discharge is sampled and whether a speculum is used are based primarily on the degree of relaxation, the size of the hymenal opening, and previous sexual activity. If an adolescent is not sexually active and has a small hymenal orifice, vaginal cultures and/or saline and potassium hydroxide wet mounts can be obtained using an intravaginal saline-soaked, cotton-tipped swab without the use of a speculum. This may be especially appropriate if the girl has not used tampons in the past. If the patient has successfully used tampons, the Huffman-Graves speculum may be used to visualize the cervix and collect the appropriate specimens. In the sexually active adolescent, the cervix should be sampled for gonorrhea and chlamydia. A Pap smear is important in sexually active teenagers to screen for HPV or other manifestations of cervical inflammation or dysplasia. A rectoabdominal or vaginoabdominal examination is required to detect uterine or adnexal tenderness or, at times, the presence of a pelvic mass.

Etiology and Management

In adolescents, mixed infections are common. Evaluation of the discharge with respect to magnitude, color, character, odor, and pH is important. Microscopic evaluation of a wet-mount preparation is a significant part of the office evaluation. A specific culture may be required to determine whether a chlamydial or gonorrheal infection is present. The most common causes of vulvovaginitis are bacterial vaginosis, trichomoniasis, and candidiasis (see Table 12–2).

Bacterial Vaginosis

Overgrowth of aerobic and anaerobic vaginal bacterial flora upsets the normal lactobacillus predominance and results in bacterial vaginosis. This is the most common cause of vulvovaginitis during the reproductive age.[12] Bacterial vaginosis accounts for approximately one third of all of vulvovaginitidies in women.[13] It occurs when the normal flora is replaced by *Gardnerella vaginalis* (a gram-negative rod), *Mycoplasma hominis, Bacteroides* sp., or *Mobiluncus* sp. (a curved gram-negative rod).

Bacterial vaginosis is not presently considered a sexually transmitted disease, as its prevalence in sexually active as well as virginal females has been found to be similar.[14] However, many of the sexual partners of females with bacterial vaginosis have been found to be colonized with the same organism, and symptoms often follow unprotected intercourse. Some women may be more susceptible to acquiring bacterial vaginosis. Eschenbach et al. have observed that women with bacterial vaginosis lack the H_2O_2-producing strains of lactobacilli that usually inhibit the growth of the etiologic pathogens.[15]

Clinical Features. Although many women remain asymptomatic, the common presenting symptom of bacterial vaginosis is that of vaginal discharge with a foul odor. Often a thin, homogeneous, gray discharge with a "fishy" odor is noted. The organism, a surface parasite, is unable to invade the vaginal wall, and therefore, acute inflammatory reaction is rare. Bacterial vaginosis has been associated with upper genital tract disorders (e.g., endomyometritis, chorioamnionitis, and pelvic inflammatory disease). *Mobiluncus* sp. have been associated with vaginal bleeding.[16]

On examination, discharge is usually noted at the introitus and may also be found adherent to the vaginal walls. The mucosal surface often appears normal, without signs of acute inflammation. The vaginal pH is >4.5, and on mixture of the fluid with a 10% potassium hydroxide solution, a "fishy" odor may be noticed (the whiff test). Metabolism of *G. vaginalis* produces amines. This positive "whiff" test is caused by the alkalinization of amines produced by the organism. Microscopic evaluation of a saline wet-mount preparation shows stippled vaginal epithelial cells, the borders of which appear obscured by the adherent bacteria. This typical appearance is called the "clue" cell, and when 20% or more of the vaginal epithelial cells show these features, some investigators consider it to be diagnostic for bacterial vaginosis[17] (Fig. 12–4*A*). Few, if any, leukocytes are noted. The corkscrew movement pattern of the highly motile *Mobiluncus* bacterial rods may be another diagnostic feature seen on wet-mount slides[18] (Fig. 12–4*B*). A Gram stain of the vaginal fluid reveals mixed flora with relatively few lactobacilli.[6]

Routine cultures are generally not helpful, and the diagnosis of bacterial vaginosis is confirmed on the basis of the presence of the clinical and wet-mount observations outlined in Table 12–3.[19]

Treatment. The current treatment of bacterial vaginosis consists of an oral 7-day course of metronidazole (500 mg administered twice daily).[20] Using this regimen, an 80% to 90% cure rate has been reported. A single 2-gm dose has been suggested to improve patient compliance; however, it has been associated with a significant failure rate.[17] Clindamycin, either oral or intravaginal, is an alternative treatment regimen.[21] It is unclear whether an

TABLE 12–3 ••• CLINICAL AND WET-MOUNT CRITERIA IN BACTERIAL VAGINOSIS

A homogenous, adherent discharge
Positive whiff test
"Clue" cells
pH > 4.5

asymptomatic patient should be treated, although in light of the potential for an ascending infection, it may well be necessary to treat asymptomatic women. Sexual partners are often not treated unless recurrent bacterial vaginosis occurs.[22]

Trichomoniasis

Trichomonas vaginalis, a motile protozoan, is a common cause of vulvovaginitis in adolescent females, accounting for 15% to 20% of all cases of vulvovaginitis.[17] Although the organism is known to survive for several hours in wet towels or chlorinated water reservoirs,[23] it is transmitted primarily through sexual contact.

Clinical Features. The presenting complaint is usually a vaginal discharge. Because *T. vaginalis* also infects the urethra and Skene's glands, dysuria and vulvar pruritus are often present. Dyspareunia may be a rare symptom of trichomoniasis. The discharge ranges from scant to profuse; is usually malodorous; and may be yellow, green, or gray in appearance. The trichomonads produce carbon dioxide, which may cause the discharge to appear frothy.

On examination, vulvar and vaginal erythema are common. Punctate hemorrhages of

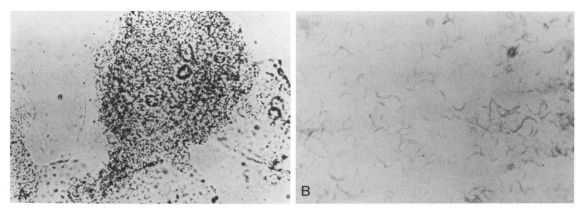

FIGURE 12–4 ••• *A,* Typical "clue" cell of bacterial vaginosis. Note *Gardnerella vaginalis* attached to vaginal epithelial cell. *B,* Typical "comma"-shaped cell seen in bacterial vaginosis caused by the curved rod–shaped *Mobiluncus* species. (From Mårdh P-A. The vaginal ecosystem. Am J Obstet Gynecol 1991; 165:1165–1166.)

the vagina and cervix ("strawberry cervix") are visibly noted in about 20% of cases.[11] Colposcopic evaluation may enhance detection of this abnormality in about 45% of cases.[17] Such cervical involvement may result in postcoital bleeding, which may alter the color of the discharge.

Growth of the organism is optimal at a pH of 5.5 to 6.0; the vaginal pH in patients with trichomoniasis is generally >5.0. Diagnosis is made on microscopic examination of the wet-mount preparation. Motile, flagellated tear-shaped organisms are seen (Fig. 12–5), although commonly a number of seemingly lifeless ones can be observed. Many leukocytes are also identified. Unlike in bacterial vaginosis, lactobacilli may be present. Occasionally, trichomonads are noted on routine urinalysis. The Pap smear detects the presence of trichomonads in about 60% of cases but is an unreliable test because of a high false-positive rate.[24] Gram stains are of little value.[17] Cultures are very sensitive but are rarely required to confirm the diagnosis.

Treatment. Treatment may consist of antibiotic therapy and local vulvar care. Systemic therapy is preferred to adequately treat the urethral and periurethral reservoirs. Metronidazole remains the medication of choice. The oral 7-day regimen of 250 mg three times per day has a cure rate of 95%;[25] the one-time dose of 2 gm has a cure rate of 88%.[17] Single-dose therapy facilitates patient compliance and can even be administered in an office setting. Sexual partners should be treated simultaneously with the single-dose regimen. Metronidazole-resistant strains have been identified,[26] and infections with such strains may require treatment with higher doses for longer periods of time or, alternatively, a combination of oral and vaginal therapy. Monif suggests habitual use of condoms and postcoital douching with an acid preparation solution as preventive therapy.[11]

Candidal Vulvovaginitis

Candidal vulvovaginitis is fairly common in adolescents. Although prevalence estimates for this group are not readily available, it probably accounts for about 25% of vulvovaginitidies among women. Asymptomatic colonization may be present in up to 20% of healthy women.[17]

C. albicans comprises between 85% and 90% of all yeast organisms isolated from the vagina.[17] Non–*C. albicans* species (e.g., *Candida tropicalis, Torulopsis glabrata* [also known as *Candida glabrata*], and *Candida parapsilosis*) are becoming more prevalent as the causative agent in vulvovaginitis. This increase probably reflects an increase in resistance of

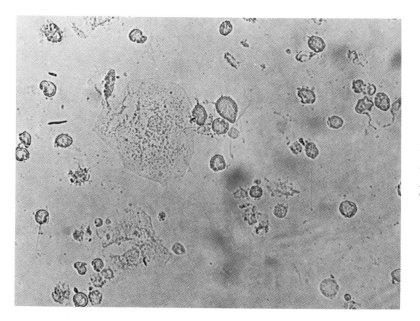

FIGURE 12–5 ••• A wet mount showing motile trichomonads in the center and nonviable forms mixed with white blood cells in the periphery. (From Friedrich EG Jr. Vulvar Disease. 2nd ed. Philadelphia: WB Saunders, 1983.)

these organisms to conventional antifungal therapy. This results in an increased prevalence of treatment failures and recurrent candidal infections.[27] Although penile colonization has been found in 20% of the male partners of women with recurrent candidal infections,[28] candidal vulvovaginitis is not considered a sexually transmitted disease.

Candidal infection often follows disturbances in the normal vaginal ecosystem (e.g., diabetes mellitus, pregnancy, the use of broad-spectrum antibiotics, or other immunosuppressive states). The clinical observation that candidal vulvovaginitis most frequently appears in the luteal phase of the menstrual cycle is supported by the idea that modulation of the immune system may be influenced by the hormonal status of women.[29] Combination oral contraceptives containing estrogen predispose patients to candidal vulvovaginitis in a similar manner. A recent course of antibiotics can alter the microbiologic flora of the pubertal vagina, making *Candida* more likely to overgrow. Diabetes mellitus can predispose the patient to candidal infections, and glucose screening up to and including a glucose tolerance test may be appropriate, although the latter has not been found to be cost effective on a routine screening basis.[17] Transmission by close contact (e.g., bed clothes) appears to be less likely. Increased body moisture associated with tight or restrictive clothing is a predisposing factor. Fashion consciousness among adolescents may increase the importance of this last factor as a cause for vulvovaginitis.

Clinical Features. The presenting complaint in candidal vulvovaginitis is usually severe vulvar pruritus. Secondary vulvar dysuria and dypareunia may also be present. There may be a small amount of white or yellow curdlike discharge that tends not to have an odor. The non–*C. albicans* species rarely cause dyspareunia or dysuria and therefore are associated with less discomfort than *C. albicans*.

Examination reveals diffuse erythema and hyperemia of the vulva. Inflammation may extend inferiorly to the perianal region or laterally toward the inner thighs. Excoriation and desquamated areas may be seen. White plaques or satellite candidal lesions may be identified. The dermatologic appearance can sometimes be confused with lichen sclerosus. The pH of the discharge is <4.5.

The diagnosis is made by examination of the fungal hyphae and buds with a saline or potassium hydroxide wet-mount preparation (Fig. 12–6). Leukocytes and epithelial cells are usually present. Hyphae and pseudohyphae are noted on Gram stain. Culture may be obtained if the diagnosis is in doubt.

Treatment. Predisposing factors should be assessed and, if possible, corrected. Control of serum glucose, use of oral contraceptives containing low-dose estrogen, discontinuation of the use of perfumed vaginal hygiene products, completion of antibiotic therapy or a change to cotton undergarments, preferably less tight fitting, may be necessary.

Intravaginal therapy with antimycotic preparations (creams, suppositories, or tablets) for 3 to 7 days is the standard regimen. Traditional therapy consists of any of the imidazoles (i.e., miconazole, buconazole, clotrimazole). Recent discovery of the triazoles (e.g., terconazole) provides for broad-spectrum coverage of *C. albicans* as well as non–*C. albicans* species.[27] In adolescent females, a shorter course of therapy promotes enhanced patient compliance, as deference to the desires of the sexual partner(s) may be a factor. Treatment of the male partner is not routinely recommended.

Recurrent Candidal Vulvovaginitis. Recurrent or chronic candidal vulvovaginitis has become a problem. Whether this clinical situation is due to the presence and persistence of vaginal yeast species or to incomplete therapy (associated with patient noncompliance) has been debated. More frequent use of broad-spectrum antibiotic therapy has also been implicated. Defective T-cell function in immu-

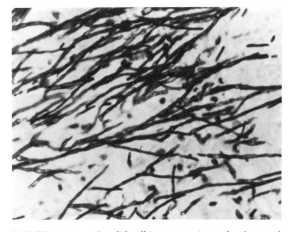

FIGURE 12–6 ••• *Candida albicans* growing as hyphae and pseudohyphae within infected tissue (× 320). (From Monif GRG. Infectious Disease in Obstetrics and Gynecology. Hagerstown, MD: Harper & Row, 1974.)

nodeficient states allows for persistence of the organisms.[30] Over-the-counter availability of imidazoles may allow for subsequent selection of non–*C. albicans* species. Use of the newer triazoles in initial therapy may prevent this situation. However, in cases of recurrence, prophylactic postmenstrual therapy with intravaginal clotrimazole (500 mg each month)[31] or suppressive therapy with low-dose oral ketoconazole (100 mg daily for 6 months)[17] have been found to be beneficial. Treatment of sexual partners has not been shown to be useful.

Unusual Causes of Vulvovaginitis

A foreign body within the vagina can produce persistent discharge with secondary vulvar irritation that will be unresponsive to medical therapy. In adolescents, the most common vaginal foreign body is a forgotten tampon, usually found high in the proximal vagina where it may have been "resting" for days or weeks. The discharge is usually dark brown, purulent, and malodorous. On removal of the tampon, symptoms abate. Vaginal ulcerations may appear if several weeks have elapsed before discovery and removal of the object.[23]

Chemical or allergic vulvovaginitis is more common in adolescents who use exogenous chemicals such as feminine hygiene sprays, douches, and deodorant tampons or creams, all of which may lead to vaginal irritation.[6] Severe vulvar pruritus, burning, and discomfort are common. It is important to obtain a thorough history of possible allergens or irritants so that the diagnosis of candidal vulvovaginitis is not established incorrectly.[17]

References

1. Grunberger W, Fisch LF. Pediatric gynecological outpatient department. A report on 600 patients. Wien Klin Wochenschr 1982; 94:614–618.
2. Schiffman MH. Recent progress in defining the epidemiology of human papillomavirus infection and cervical neoplasia. J National Cancer Institute 1992; 84(6):394–398.
3. Russo JF. The spectrum of outpatient adolescent gynecologic pathology. J Adolesc Health Care 1982; 3:126–127.
4. Pokorny SF, Stormer J. Atraumatic removal of secretions from the prepubertal vagina. Am J Obstet Gynecol 1987; 156:581–582.
5. Paradise JE, Compos JM, Friedman HM, Frishmuth G. Vulvovaginitis in premenarchal girls: Clinical features and diagnostic evaluation. Pediatrics 1982; 70:193–198.
6. Gerstner GJ, Grunberger W, Boschitsch E, Rotter M. Vaginal organisms in prepubertal children with children with and without vulvovaginitis. A vaginoscopic study. Arch Gynecol 1982; 231:247–252.
7. Murphy TV, Nelson JD. Shigella vaginitis: Report of a case and review of the literature. Pediatrics 1979; 63:511–515.
8. Friedrich EG. Vaginitis. Am J Obstet Gynecol 1985; 152:247–251.
9. Redondo-Lopez V, Cook RL, Sobel JD. Emerging role of lactobacilli in the control and maintenance of the vaginal bacterial microflora. Rev Infect Dis 1990; 12(5):856–872.
10. Sanfilippo JS. Adolescent girls with vaginal discharge. Pediatr Ann 1986; 15(7):509–519.
11. Monif GRG. Infectious Vulvovaginitis. Keystone Heights, Florida: Rose Printing, 1985.
12. Kent HL. Epidemiology of vaginitis. Am J Obstet Gynecol 1991; 165:1168–1176.
13. Sobel J. The diagnosis and management of bacterial vaginosis. STD Bull 1992; 11(3):3–11.
14. Bump RC, Bueshing WJ. Bacterial vaginosis in virginal and sexually active adolescent females: Evidence against exclusive sexual transmission. Am J Obstet Gynecol 1988; 158(4):935–939.
15. Eschenbach DA, Davick PR, Williams BL, et al. Prevalence of hydrogen peroxide-producing lactobacillus species in normal women and women with bacterial vaginosis. J Clin Microbiol 1989; 27(2):251–256.
16. Larsson PB, Bergman BB. Is there a causal connection between motile, curved rods, *Mobiluncus* species and bleeding complications? Am J Obstet Gynecol 1986; 154:107–108.
17. Sobel JD. Vaginal infections in adult women. Med Clin North Am 1990; 74(6):1573–1602.
18. Mårdh P-A. The vaginal ecosystem. Am J Obstet Gynecol 1991; 165:1163–1168.
19. Amsel R, Toten PA, Spiegel CA, et al. Nonspecific vaginitis: Diagnostic criteria and microbial and epidemiologic associations. Am J Med 1983; 74:14–22.
20. Centers for Disease Control. 1989 sexually transmitted diseases treatment guidelines. MMWR 1989; 38(no. S-8):36.
21. Hillier S, Krohn MA, Watts H, et al. Microbiologic efficacy of intravaginal clindamycin cream for the treatment of bacterial vaginosis. Obstet Gynecol 1990; 76(3):407–413.
22. Thomason JL, Gelbart SM, Scaglione NJ. Bacterial vaginosis: Current review with indications for asymptomatic therapy. Am J Obstet Gynecol 1991; 165:1210–1217.
23. Altchek A. Vulvovaginitis, vulvar skin disease, and pelvic inflammatory disease. Pediatr Clin North Am 1981; 28(2):397–431.
24. Krieger JN, Tam MR, Stevens CE, et al. Diagnosis of trichomoniasis: Comparison of conventional wet-mount examination with cytologic studies, cultures and monoclonal antibody staining of direct specimens. JAMA 1988; 259:1223–1227.
25. Lossick JG, Kent HL. Trichomoniasis: Trends in diagnosis and management. Am J Obstet Gynecol 1991; 165:1217–1222.
26. Grossman JH III, Galask PG. Persistent vaginitis caused by metronidazole-resistant trichomonas. Obstet Gynecol 1990; 76(3):521–522.

27. Horowitz BJ. Mycotic vulvovaginitis: A broad overview. Am J Obstet Gynecol 1991; 165:1188–1192.

28. Horowitz BJ, Edelstein SW, Lippman L. Sexual transmission of *Candida*. Obstet Gynecol 1987; 69:883–886.

29. Kalo-Klein A. *Candida albicans*: Cellular immune system interaction during different stages of the menstrual cycle. Am J Obstet Gynecol 1989; 161:1132–1136.

30. Ashman RB, Papadimitriou JM. What's new in the mechanisms of host resistance to Candida albicans infection? Pathol Res Pract 1990; 186:527–534.

31. Roth AC, Milsom I, Forrsman L, Wahlen P. Intermittent prophylactic treatment of recurrent vaginal candidiasis by postmenstrual application of a 500 mg clotrimazole vaginal tablet. Genitourin Med 1990; 66:357–360.

CHAPTER 13

Vulvar Disorders

C. MARJORIE RIDLEY

An effort to cover all dermatologic conditions of the vulva would require a complete textbook. This chapter will describe in sufficient detail common and uncommon conditions that are of considerable importance. Rarer entities of less general significance will be merely noted or referred to where relevant for differential diagnosis. There are a number of sources available for those seeking details of either dermatologic conditions in general or vulvar lesions in particular.[1, 2]

Specialists in many clinical disciplines may find disorders of the vulvar area somewhat unfamiliar. It is often difficult to appreciate normal limits, which vary with respect to the neonate, the child, and the adolescent; also, the child or parent may be reluctant to permit full examination. The appearance of lesions is modified by the warmth and moisture of the locality; bullae rupture, and scaling areas become moist and the surfaces readily become macerated. The dermatologist is aware that vaginal conditions may be relevant and that examination is best carried out by the gynecologist; however, pediatricians and gynecologists are frequently unacquainted with cutaneous lesions. There is a self-evident need for cooperation and for a common framework of morphologic description and classification (see Table 13–3).

Evaluation. Multispecialty clinics can be very useful for evaluation. The first essential point is an adequate examination. The easiest way to accomplish this is to have the child lying on her back with the legs abducted. The labia minora will spontaneously separate, and

the vestibule will be clearly visible. The perianal area can also be evaluated in this position; if not, the left lateral position or the knee-chest position may be used. Examination should be systematic, and it is often helpful to document findings with a diagram. In some circumstances, a photograph may be desirable (see Chapter 11). Very often there will be a need to examine the rest of the patient's body. When internal examination is indicated, examination with anesthesia may be required; in such a case, expressly designed instruments should be used. When infection is suspected, appropriate diagnostic tests should be obtained. In most vulvar abnormalities, diagnosis will be achieved by a combination of clinical examination of the vulva and appropriate testing for infection. There are many times when the diagnosis is uncertain, but the condition appears to be banal; sensible symptomatic management is then justifiable. However, it is vital in this situation to reevaluate the child until a firm diagnosis has been reached or until the signs have completely cleared.

Biopsy Procedure. There are times when biopsy is indicated, and in most cases this can be done on a simple outpatient basis with local anesthetic. A 2% lidocaine ointment or prilocaine/lidocaine (EMLA cream) is applied; natural occlusion by adduction of the thighs ensures absorption and numbing of the area in 10 to 15 minutes.[3] In children, the possibility of methemoglobinemia with the use of this local anesthetic has been raised.[4] Absorption through vulvar skin is usually quite rapid—the effect being obtained in 10 minutes rather than the hour or more required on keratinized skin; therefore, the amount of medication applied must be as small as possible. A 1% or 2% lidocaine solution then must be introduced; needle insertion will be pain free. A formal elliptical excision with suture placement may be difficult to achieve; in practice a punch biopsy (2, 3, or 4 mm) yields a good sample, is much quicker to obtain, and needs no suturing, with hemostasis achieved by pressure, cautery, or a silver nitrate stick. The specimen should be placed on a piece of blotting paper or card before it goes into permanent fixative; this procedure ensures that the pathologist will receive a specimen capable of being oriented for sectioning. Sometimes tissue is required for additional histologic and/or electron microscopy studies. Specimens should be taken from an area beside the lesion rather than from the lesion per se, rinsed in sterile saline or water, and placed in a special transport medium or snap frozen. A cooperative parent can be helpful in the procedure, but it is better kindly but firmly to exclude parents who are likely to be upset by the situation.

VULVAR DISORDERS IN THE NEONATE AND INFANT

Infants born prematurely tend to have immature skin that is imperfectly keratinized and easily damaged, losing heat and water readily.[5] The normal neonate has anatomically mature skin, but a number of functional deficiencies (e.g., insufficient eccrine sweating) commonly lead to skin changes. Excessive sebaceous gland secretion is also present, and the skin is susceptible to infection. Throughout life, the vulvar skin responds in a very different way physiologically from other areas of skin—for example, in absorption capacity, transepidermal water evaporation, water-holding capacity of the stratum corneum, susceptibility to irritant factors, and blood flow.[6] Bacterial counts are increased at the vulva compared with control sites.[7] Lesions readily become macerated or infected, with partial obliteration of typical features.

Hymenal Polyps. The gynecologic examination in the newborn may reveal a polypoid structure at the area of the introitus. This represents a thickening of the dorsal segment of the hymen manifested as a "rounded tag." Incidence is reported in 6% of newborn girls within the first 48 hours of life.[8] Treatment

usually involves observation, since the polypoid structure tends to diminish within several days as the "normal degree" of vulvar edema decreases (Fig. 13–1).

Perianal Dermatitis. Perianal dermatitis has been described in the newborn, especially when the infant was fed a formula based on cow's milk. The skin is red and eroded, and there may or may not be an associated diaper rash. Treatment consists of careful cleaning, bland lubricants, and protective agents (petroleum jelly).

Miliaria. Miliaria related to obstruction of the eccrine sweat duct is common in neonates and to some extent in infants, perhaps in relation to both immaturity of the duct and overheating. The diaper area is a common site (diaper dermatitis). *Miliaria crystallina* refers to obstruction in the stratum corneum and *miliaria rubra* to deeper obstruction. The latter is the form occurring in the diaper area as well as elsewhere in infants. Groups of papules and papulovesicles or pustules on a red background develop and last for a few days. Secondary infection may occur. The diagnosis must be differentiated from toxic erythema of the newborn; lesions in the latter are pustular and contain eosinophils.

Intertrigo. Intertrigo in the genitocrural area is common and develops in relation to friction, obesity, and moisture. Miliaria and secondary infection are often associated. The affected areas are red and macerated. Careful hygiene, together with bland emollients and perhaps a mild corticosteroid are effective in treatment.

Impetigo. Impetigo is also a risk in the first week of life. It is usually caused by *Staphylococcus aureus*, usually phage group II, especially type 71, which may be acquired from the mother, other relatives, or staff. Impetigo

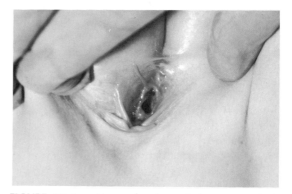

FIGURE 13–1 ⦁⦁⦁ Hymenal polyp noted on gynecologic examination of a newborn.

tends to affect the vulva and umbilical areas, causing lesions of blisters that later become crusted. Extensive spread and complications may ensue if treatment with antibiotics is not swift and adequate.

Diaper Dermatitis. Diaper dermatitis is a common problem occurring in the first 2 to 3 weeks of life. The most common form is an irritant dermatitis from friction and wetting, exacerbated by the effects of ammonia, urine of pH > 8, and secondary infection with *Candida* sp. or bacteria. The erythema may have a somewhat glazed appearance and tends to be marked around the edges (Fig. 13–2). Sometimes papules with eroded, shallow, ulcerated summits develop (Fig. 13–3). Although this usually clears uneventfully when the child is out of diapers, it may be part of an atopic dermatitis, so the prognosis is guarded.

Seborrheic Dermatitis Localized to the Vulva (Diaper Related). This is a condition probably not related to seborrheic dermatitis in later life (Fig. 13–4). It is often associated with lesions elsewhere, particularly on the scalp. The diaper area tends to be more diffusely red than in irritant type cases. The presence of lesions elsewhere can be helpful for diagnosis, but differentiation can be difficult in a child with an irritant type of diaper rash as well as atopic dermatitis with lesions elsewhere. Pruritus tends to be absent in the seborrheic type, and immunoglobulin E (IgE) levels are not elevated as in atopic dermatitis. However, some clinicians do not regard these two conditions as distinct.

Diaper Psoriasis. This is probably not a

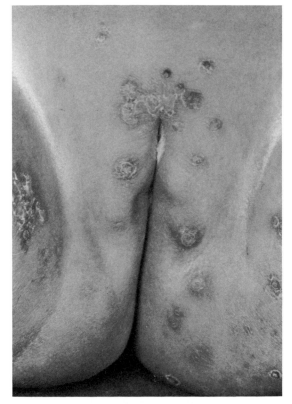

FIGURE 13–3 ••• Note diaper rash, with eroded papules. (From Ridley M, Oriel JD, Robinson AJ. A Colour Atlas of Diseases of the Vulva. London, Chapman and Hall, 1992.)

manifestation of psoriasis (Fig. 13–5), although it may be that in a minority of children with a psoriatic diathesis, true psoriasis is triggered by a diaper rash. The typical human leukocyte antigen (HLA) types associated with psoriasis are not associated with diaper psoriasis. The lesions are well defined and scaly, resembling psoriasis, and occur on the trunk

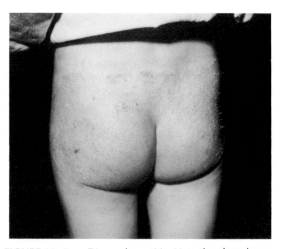

FIGURE 13–2 ••• Diaper dermatitis. Note the clear demarcation of the diaper area with the irritation.

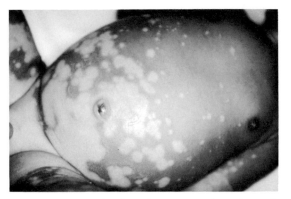

FIGURE 13–4 ••• Seborrheic dermatitis involving the trunk and vulvar area.

and limbs as well as at the diaper area. The differential diagnosis in all cases of diaper rash includes Langerhans' cell histiocytosis (histiocytosis X), acrodermatitis enteropathica, and congenital syphilis, all of which are rare.

TREATMENT OF DIAPER-RELATED PROBLEMS

In general, most types of diaper-related problems will respond to general measures such as keeping the area dry and open as much as possible and using bland emollients such as zinc and castor oil cream or aqueous cream, followed by a mild topical corticosteroid with or without antiseptic or antibiotics. Fluorinated corticosteroids may lead to local atrophy or even to wasting and absorption. One-way disposable diapers are often helpful, although concern has been expressed that dioxin used as a fabric whitener may be found in one layer of disposable diapers. When prevention of skin

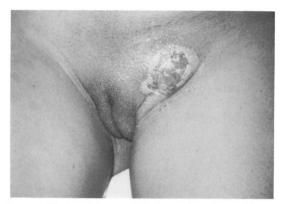

FIGURE 13–6 ••• Infantile gluteal granuloma located in the left inguinal area.

wetness is used as a test of diaper quality (measured on the forearm in adult subjects), super-absorbent disposable type diapers are the most effective, with other types being no better than cloth diapers.[9] If cloth diapers are used, a middle layer of a different nonwoven component is recommended. The frequency of diaper changes of any type is most important, as is careful rinsing and the avoidance of irritant or dangerous antiseptics.

Infantile Gluteal Granulomata. These are categorized by oval nodules with eroded surfaces on the buttocks, usually associated (although not exclusively) with a previously existing diaper rash (Fig. 13–6).[10] The diagnosis is confirmed histologically. Fluorinated topical corticosteroids and *Candida* organisms have been suspected as a cause but may not account for all cases. Treatment with a mild corticosteroid (0.5% to 1% hydrocortisone cream) with or without a topical antifungal (clotrimazole hydrocortisone ointment) leads to regression, although sometimes with scarring.

Labial Adhesions. Labial adhesions were present in 1.4% of infants in one reported series.[11] In another series of 50 children, the patients usually were affected before age 2, with none presenting before 2 months of age.[12] A survey of 5000 newborn females established that the condition was not found in the newborn and therefore does not appear to be analogous to the subpreputial adhesions in male newborns.

Although the etiology is unknown, estrogen deficiency has been postulated; inflammation also may be a factor. The labia minora become adherent either in part or totally. If incomplete, the fusion is usually posterior. In extreme cases, a tiny aperture situated just below the clitoris is the only patent area (Fig. 13–7).

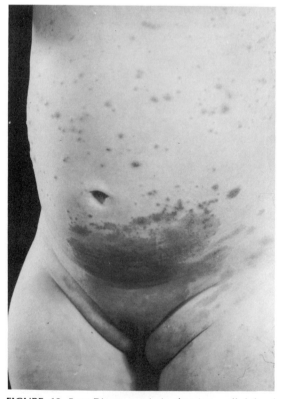

FIGURE 13–5 ••• Diaper psoriasis showing well-defined lesions of the diaper area of the trunk. (From Ridley M, Oriel JD, Robinson AJ. A Colour Atlas of Diseases of the vulva. London, Chapman and Hall, 1992.)

Occasionally the condition is confused with ambiguous genitalia, but the presence of a midline raphe is usually clear. Other important differential diagnoses include lichen sclerosus, where the picture is primarily one of obliteration of contours rather than simple fusion;[13] fusion as a result of inflammation following child sexual abuse; and, occasionally, rarer conditions such as childhood cicatricial pemphigoid. The condition may be asymptomatic, but dysuria, urine retention, and occasionally urinary tract infection may be present.[14] The labia can be separated by the mother, with or without the use of emollients or estrogen

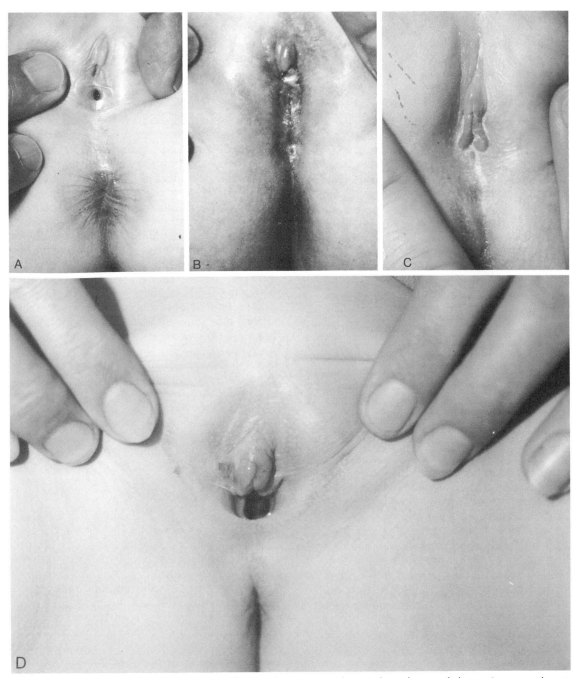

FIGURE 13–7 ••• Labial adhesions. *A–C,* Small vaginal opening with complete closure of the vagina secondary to adhesions. *D,* An intact hymen and introitus with lateral displacement of the adherent area.

cream, or separated under general anesthesia. The rationale for the use of estrogen is uncertain; side effects of systemic absorption of estrogen include pigmentation of the vulva and breast enlargement. There is some evidence that spontaneous resolution is quite common; in one series of 10 children with labial adhesions, five experienced regression in 6 months, nine in 12 months, and all 10 in 18 months, without recurrence.[15] In the presence of symptoms, however, separation is obviously advisable. Recurrences may be anticipated.

INFECTIONS AND INFESTATIONS

Sexually transmitted diseases and infective causes of vulvovaginitis are discussed in Chapters 20 and 21. This section discusses infestations and other infective conditions in children and adolescents, as well as lesions of human papillomavirus (HPV), herpes simplex virus (HSV), and molluscum contagiosum, in which the issue of sexual transmission is in question.

Enterobius **Infection.** *Enterobius* (threadworm, whipworm) infection is common. These worms live in the large bowel and travel out of the anus to lay eggs at night. Larvae hatch and reenter the canal, reactivating the cycle. Pruritus ani is the usual accompanying symptom. Sometimes the worms enter the vagina, and pruritus vulvae ensues. Cellophane tape swabs applied to the perianal area in the morning before washing or at bedtime is a convenient way to isolate the ova, which then can be identified under the microscope. Piperazine salts are the accepted treatment and should be administered to the patient and the family. Hygienic measures (i.e., hand washing and nail scrubbing after defecation and before meals) are very important in preventing reinfection. Occasionally, *Ascaris* and *Trichuris* have been found in children.

Candida **Infection.** *Candida* infection is a frequent factor in diaper rashes. Candidal vulvovaginitis is rare in children but less so in adolescents. Vulvar lesions may occur in chronic mucocutaneous candidiasis, a rare condition in which plaques of *Candida*-infected tissue are associated with immunosuppression.[16] Underlying factors (e.g., diabetes) should be determined. Treatment with an imidazole cream is usually effective except in cases of chronic mucocutaneous candidiasis.

Pityriasis Versicolor. This condition, caused by *Pityrosporon orbiculare*, manifests as scaly macules of the trunk in postpubertal patients, but lesions have been reported on the face and in the genital area in West Indian infants of African extraction.[17] The diagnosis is made easily by visualization of hyphae in spores in 10% potassium hydroxide. Treatment with topical imidazoles (e.g., clotrimazole) is effective.

Pyococcal Infection. Pyococcal infection may or may not be associated with poor hygiene. Staphylococci may cause impetigo and are also responsible for folliculitis in the pubic area in adolescence. Oral antibiotics may be required, or a topical antibiotic such as mupirocin may be used along with a general antiseptic such as povidone-iodine used as a skin wash. Staphylococcal infections of Bartholin's gland and duct are rare before adulthood. Streptococcal cellulitis tends to occur and recur in chronically edematous tissue. More common, however, is a streptococcal dermatitis without true cellulitis.[18] This is divided into three types: one in which the perianal skin is pink, moist, and tender; one in which it is reddened with fissures; and one in which it is beefy red with scaling and crusting. The source may be the gastrointestinal tract or contact with the fingers, throat, or skin. In all cases, β-hemolytic streptococci are involved. Such lesions may complicate underlying skin conditions; in practice, a common one is lichen sclerosus. Penicillin V or erythromycin is the usual treatment. Topical antiseptics such as povidone-iodine used as a wash are helpful in preventing recurrence.

Varicella Zoster. Varicella zoster may affect the vulva as part of the generalized rash. Herpes zoster is rare in children and adolescents, and thus genital involvement is very unlikely. Lesions of sacral nerve 3 (S-3) will lead to vulvar lesions.

HSV, HPV, and Molluscum Contagiosum. These three conditions are frequently encountered in the genital area but may or may not be sexually transmitted. They are considered in detail in Chapters 20 and 21.

HSV. HSV types 1 and 2 are involved in vulvar lesions. The types are not site specific, but type 2 is commonly responsible for genital lesions and type 1 for facial or oral lesions. The virus lies latent in the dorsal root ganglia and is periodically reactivated, causing outbreaks on the skin or mucosa. Papules become vesicles that in turn become eroded and crusted. Primary lesions tend to be more severe than recurrences. Precipitating factors for genital lesions include stress, intercourse, and menstruation. The cervix may be involved, and if sacral radiculitis is a feature, there may be urinary retention. Differential diagnosis includes any eroded or blistering lesions, as well as herpes zoster in segmental lesions; definitive diagnosis is made by culturing the virus or visualizing it by electron microscopy. Treatment with acyclovir orally for the primary attack, or as an ointment applied at the time of prodromal symptoms for the recurrent attack, reduces viral shedding and accelerates healing in the adolescent. In special circumstances, long-term acyclovir therapy can be considered. Nonsexual transmission of genital lesions is possible; however, the occurrence of such lesions in a child indicates a strong possibility of child sexual abuse.

HPV. There are many HPV serotypes; serotypes 6, 11, 16, and 18 usually are associated with anogenital lesions (Fig. 13–8); types 16 and 18 are particularly associated with malignant and premalignant lesions. The clinical manifestations are more florid and more resistant to treatment in the presence of immunosuppression and/or pregnancy. The differential diagnosis includes molluscum contagiosum, condyloma latum, and vulvar intraepithelial neoplasia. The presence of anogenital warts in children raises the possibility of child sexual abuse.[19–21] However, lesions may also be transmitted by casual domestic contact, including baths, fomites, sometimes from the patient's own hands, and vertically through maternal infection at the time of birth. Even when adequate typing of the HPV is achieved and it is known whether the responsible types are usually associated with genital or nongenital lesions, it is clear that typing does not prove the presence or absence of sexual transmission.[22] Treatment is as unsatisfactory as in adults, and early recourse to surgical treatment under general anesthesia is probably advisable.

Molluscum Contagiosum. There are two distinct virus types of molluscum contagiosum, but there appears to be no site specificity.[23] The lesions are firm papules with an umbilicated center from which whitish material extrudes, and there is rarely any diagnostic difficulty. Curetted material can be examined as a wet-mount film or sent for complete histologic examination if there is any doubt. Treatment by local destruction is effective but painful, a circumstance that becomes problematic for children. Children usually have extragenital lesions, but some have anogenital lesions; whether investigation into the possibility of child sexual abuse is instigated will depend on the circumstances. Adolescents may have sexually transmitted anogenital lesions.

SYSTEMIC DISEASE

Acrodermatitis Enteropathica. This rash is a consequence of zinc deficiency (Fig. 13–9). It can be inherited as a recessive characteristic leading to a defect of zinc absorption or acquired—for example, as a result of prematurity, drug effects (penicillamine therapy or chelating agents), or total parenteral nutrition. The histology is nonspecific. The lesions affect the face and anogenital area; they are bright red, often eroded, well defined, and resistant to conventional treatment for diaper rash or eczema. If treatment is long deferred, hair will

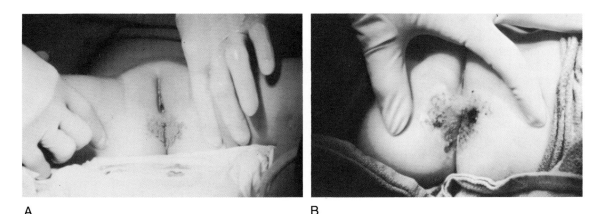

A   B

FIGURE 13–8 ••• *A,* A 24-month-old female with recurrent condylomata acuminata refractory to medical therapy. *B,* Same patient during intraoperative CO$_2$ laser treatment of the condylomata.

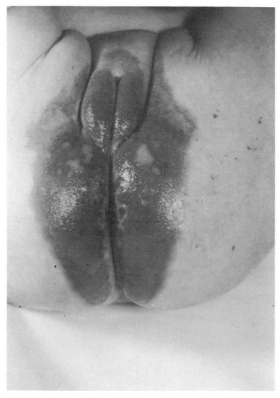

FIGURE 13–9 ••• Zinc deficiency. Note red, eroded areas. (From Ridley M, Oriel JD, Robinson AJ. A Colour Atlas of Diseases of the Vulva. London, Chapman and Hall, 1992.)

be lost. Serum zinc levels are usually low but can be unreliable, and clinical diagnosis is of paramount importance. Oral zinc treatment is effective, and such treatment is temporary or permanent according to etiology.

Crohn's Disease. Crohn's disease is a condition of unknown etiology that can affect both children and adolescents.[24] Histologic analysis of bowel lesions shows noncaseating epithelioid granulomata, but lesions outside the bowel may be either typical or nonspecific. Cutaneous signs, usually oral and genital, may predate bowel signs and symptoms. The labial and buccal mucosa may be thickened ("cobblestoning") (Fig. 13–10). The vulva shows edema and lymphangiectasia or sinuses, abscesses, and tags.[25] Treatment of the bowel lesions often alleviates the skin condition.

Langerhans' Cell Histiocytosis (Histiocytosis X). In the acute disseminated Letterer-Siwe form, the diaper area is the site of infection (Fig. 13–11). Histiocytosis X cells show Langerhans' granules on electron microscopy and are mixed with histiocytes, eosinophils, and giant cells. The diaper area as well as the trunk

and scalp are often involved. The lesions are firm, yellowish, and often purpuric papules. Systemic involvement is frequent, and the prognosis is variable. Differentiating the diagnosis from a diaper rash usually is not difficult if the condition is suspected; histologic analysis is diagnostic.

GENETIC DISORDERS

Darier's disease is inherited as a dominant characteristic. Its lesions begin in late childhood and gradually increase. The histologic analysis is diagnostic, with hyperkeratosis, parakeratosis, and acanthosis being identified. Acantholytic cells keratinize to form abnormal cells, the corps ronds. Wide areas of the body tend to be involved, with the skin flexures being especially vulnerable. Horny papules coalesce, becoming macerated and infected. Patients are prone to bacterial and viral infection, and the vulva appears to be a site of predilection for severe outbreaks. Topical treatment with mild corticosteroids, antibiotics, and antiseptics is somewhat efficacious. Severe cases can be improved dramatically with the use of oral etretinate (Tegison), but its side effects and teratogenic potential significantly limit its use.

DISORDERS OF HAIR

Folliculitis. After the development of pubic hair, folliculitis may arise, either spontaneously or as a result of shaving or the use of depilatory preparations. The papulopustules must be differentiated from molluscum contagiosum and the possibility of pediculosis excluded. Bathing with povidone-iodine solution once or twice a day, along with a course of oral antistaphylococcal antibiotics if the condition is severe, appears to be effective. It may be necessary to continue topical treatment if perineal involvement is noted.

Alopecia Areata. This is not uncommon in adolescents, and patches may affect the pubic area, usually in combination with lesions elsewhere. Histologic assessment in the early stage identifies lymphatic infiltration focused on the hair bulb. Later there is no inflammation, but the follicles appear smaller and higher in the dermis than is normal. The areas are round patches without apparent redness or scaling. It is doubtful whether topical corticosteroids

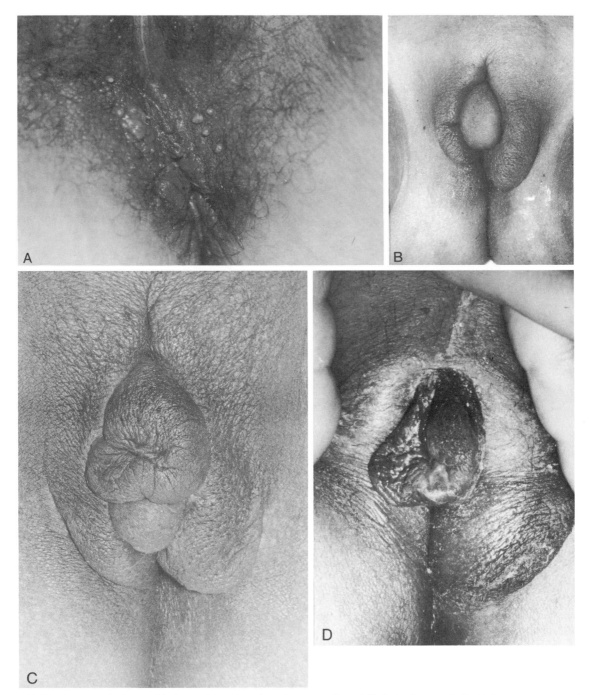

FIGURE 13–10 ••• *A*, Perianal lesions of lymphangiectasia, suggestive of Crohn's disease. *B–D*, Vulvar appearance of patients with Crohn's disease involving the vulva. (*A* from Ridley M, Oriel JD, Robinson AJ. A Colour Atlas of Diseases of the Vulva. London, Chapman and Hall, 1992.)

have more than placebo value, but patient prognosis usually is good.

Effects of Cytotoxic Drugs. Children on cytotoxic drugs may temporarily lose hair at all sites as a result of premature entry of anagen follicles into catagen.

DISORDERS OF PIGMENTATION

Hyperpigmentation

Acanthosis Nigricans. In childhood and adolescence, the appearance of this unusual pigmented condition in the inguinal areas and other flexures may accompany endocrinologic abnormalities or occur alone; there is no cause for concern about any associated malignancy as there is in adults. There is hyperkeratosis, acanthosis, and papillomatosis, and the skin is dark and thickened. The condition must be differentiated from the diffuse darkening in these areas common in obese patients, particularly dark-skinned individuals. Deposits of hemosiderin may be found in cases of lichen sclerosus. Other causes of hyperpigmentation include lentigines and moles.

Hypopigmentation

In dark-skinned individuals, hypopigmentation follows the lesions of pityriasis versicolor or any inflammatory condition (Fig. 13–12). *Vitiligo* is a complete loss of pigment (Fig. 13–13); melanocytes may be absent, reduced, or normal but nonfunctional. It may affect the genital area at any age. Segmental lesions are perhaps more common in children than the usual symmetric patchy loss. The pigment is unlikely to return. The differential diagnosis includes atrophy and pallor of lichen sclerosus, with which it may be significantly associated.

DISORDERS OF SWEAT GLANDS

Apocrine lesions do not develop before puberty. *Hidradenitis* is the most frequent and

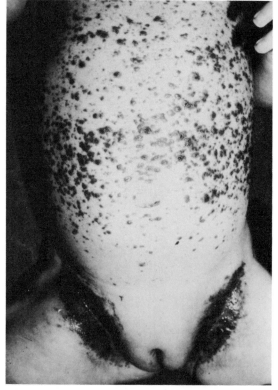

FIGURE 13–11 ••• Langerhans' cell histiocytosis, showing papules on the trunk and diaper area. (From Ridley M, Oriel JD, Robinson AJ. A Colour Atlas of Diseases of the Vulva. London, Chapman and Hall, 1992.)

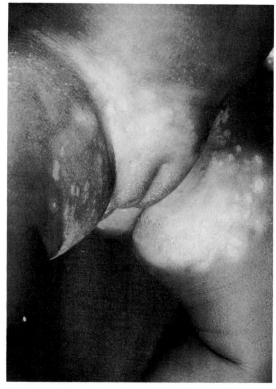

FIGURE 13–12 ••• Hypopigmentation in the diaper area after resolution of diaper rash in a dark-skinned child. (From Ridley CM. The Vulva. Edinburgh: Churchill Livingstone, 1988.)

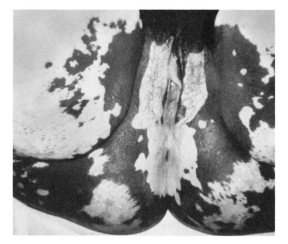

FIGURE 13–13 ••• Vitiligo. Note the depigmented areas of the vulva.

important condition. The breasts, axillae, and particularly the anogenital area are affected. The etiology is uncertain. Many of the changes seen are in the apocrine glands, but recent work suggests that apocrine gland involvement is secondary to a primary abnormality of follicular epithelium.[26] Painful reddened nodules develop into abscesses, often with sinuses and fistulae. In quiescent periods, small bridged scars with comedones remain. Severe examples involve the whole area in a painful, unsightly mass. Oral antibiotics, especially metronidazole, and topical antiseptics have a limited role. Isotretinoin (Accutane) appears to be of no value; etretinate (Tegison) is probably of little value and should not be used in patients of child-bearing years unless alternative therapies have been exhausted.[27] Antiandrogens have been helpful, but surgery is probably the best treatment available; either local excision of small areas or extensive surgical extirpation with grafting can be very successful. The differential diagnosis includes chronic infection such as granuloma inguinale and lymphogranuloma inguinale, but perhaps the most common condition to cause difficulty in the differential diagnosis is Crohn's disease.

BEHÇET'S SYNDROME AND OTHER ULCERATIVE CONDITIONS

A classification of two ulcerative lesions is presented in Table 13–1.

Behçet's Syndrome. A serious and rare multisystem disease of probable viral origin, Behçet's syndrome may have its onset in adolescence. The diagnosis should not be established hastily and often cannot be established with certainty until the events are clarified by the passage of time. Criteria have been established for diagnosis of this syndrome.[28]

Arthritic, neurologic, ocular, and mucocutaneous subgroups are described. The histology of the lesions is nonspecific or may show thrombosis of arterioles. Cutaneous lesions include erythema nodosum, pyoderma, and sterile pustules. Mucocutaneous lesions affect the eyes, mouth, and genitalia. Vulvar lesions are commonly on the labia minora and appear as painful, shallow, persistent ulcers, often leading to scar formation. The prognosis is variable depending on involvement of other systems.

Topical use of bland preparations, corticosteroids, and anesthetic agents (e.g., xylocaine jelly) along with systemic steroids may be useful. Colchicine has also proved beneficial.

Aphthous Ulcers. Of uncertain etiology, these often affect the mucosa of both the genitalia and the oral cavity and are divided into major and minor types (Fig. 13–14). Histologic analysis is nonspecific. Major aphthous ulcers are deep and painful and often leave scars; there may be a family history of aphthous ulceration. Oral thalidomide is effective but clearly not appropriate in children and adolescents. Topical steroid and tetracycline

TABLE 13–1 ••• ULCERATIVE LESIONS

Lesion	Etiology	Incidence	Family History	Other Sites Affected	Histology	Scarring
Behçet's syndrome	Unknown, possibly viral	Very rare	Negative	Mandatory for diagnosis	Nonspecific	Common
Aphthous ulceration	Unknown, some cases genetic	Rare but less so than Behçet's syndrome	Often positive	Mouth only	Nonspecific	Common

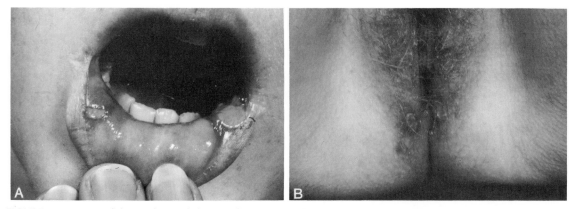

FIGURE 13–14 ••• Aphthous ulcers of the mouth *(A)* and vulvar area *(B)*. (From Ridley CM. The Vulva. Edinburgh: Churchill Livingstone, 1988.)

combinations in an appropriate base are helpful. Sometimes ulcers appear, without recurrence, in adolescents who manifest fever with or without other systemic disease (e.g., infectious mononucleosis); sometimes the lesion may be a specific manifestation of such a disease.[29]

BULLOUS DISEASES

A simplified classification of bullous disease is presented in Table 13–2.

Epidermolysis Bullosa. This genetically determined mucocutaneous bullous condition has many different forms that can be differentiated on clinical, genetic, and electron microscopic grounds (Fig. 13–15). Some forms affect mucous membranes, and depending on the level of bulla formation, there will be scarring. The latter is associated with a split below the lamina lucida, as opposed to within it. The labia and the vaginal walls may be fused and the vestibule narrowed. Anal scarring may lead to constipation. Genetic counseling is important.

Hailey-Hailey Disease. Also known as *benign familial chronic pemphigus*, this is a rare condition genetically determined as a dominant characteristic. Lesions appear in adolescence in the genital area and other flexures. They usually are considered to remain confined to the keratinized skin, but some reports suggest that the vagina may be involved.[30, 31] Histologic evaluation identifies dramatic acantholysis, and thus this can be easily confused with Darier's disease; the two conditions can probably coexist. Immunofluorescence is negative. The lesions are moist, red, and fissured,

with or without visible blistering. They are exacerbated by infection, whether fungal *(Candida)*, bacterial, or viral, and by allergic contact dermatitis. Topical corticosteroids and antibiotics suffice in mild cases, and long-term oral antibiotics are helpful. Other patients may need systemic steroids or even excision and grafting.

Stevens-Johnson Syndrome. This is a variant of erythema multiforme with mucosal involvement and is often precipitated by drugs or HSV. Bullae are subepidermal, characterized by vasculitic dermal changes and epidermal necrosis, and rupture to leave denuded painful areas. Acral target-like skin lesions may coexist, and there is usually considerable systemic disturbance. Scarring may remain, and introital adenosis has been reported to be a rare complication.[32, 33]

Toxic Epidermal Necrolysis (TEN). TEN is considered by some to be a severe variant of erythema multiforme, but most consider it a distinct disorder[34] precipitated by medications, but not HSV. It can occur at any age, even infancy. The epidermis is necrotic and detached from the dermis, which shows little change. The skin peels off over large areas, usually without the target lesions so typical of erythema multiforme. Mucosal areas are severely affected. The patient becomes very ill, with fever, pain, secondary infection, and multisystem involvement. Sequelae include scarring, especially ocular; the vagina may also be affected. Differential diagnosis of erythema multiforme and TEN includes toxic shock syndrome, which occurs in adolescence, usually in relation to use of a tampon; the distinction usually is not difficult.

TABLE 13–2 ••• BULLOUS DISEASES

Disease	Etiology	Site of Bullae	Immunofluorescence	Treatment
Epidermolysis bullosa	Genetic	Variable, depending on type	Negative	Symptomatic
Hailey-Hailey disease (Benign familial chronic pemphigus)	Genetic	Intraepidermal with acantholysis	Negative	Antibiotics Corticosteroids Occasionally excision and grafting
Stevens-Johnson syndrome	Unknown (sometimes drug or herpes simplex virus induced)	Subepidermal with epidermal necrosis Vasculitic changes in dermis	Negative	Symptomatic (intensive care) Not systemic steroids
Toxic epidermal necrolysis	Unknown (sometimes drug)	Subepidermal with marked epidermal necrosis	Negative	Symptomatic (intensive care) Not systemic steroids
Staphylococcal scalded skin syndrome	Infective (staphylococcal)	Intraepidermal	Negative	Antibiotics
Impetigo, bullous type	Staphylococcal	Intraepidermal	Negative	Antibiotics
Pemphigus vulgaris	Immunologic	Intraepidermal with acantholysis	IgG on intercellular substance of epidermis	Systemic steroids Immunosuppressants
Chronic bullous disease of childhood	Immunologic	Subepidermal	Linear IgA at basement membrane zone	Dapsone or sulfapyridine
Childhood cicatricial pemphigoid	Immunologic	Subepidermal with dermal fibrosis	Linear IgA at basement membrane zone	Dapsone or sulfapyridine
Bullous pemphigoid	Immunologic	Subepidermal	IgG at basement membrane zone	Dapsone or sulfapyridine Systemic steroids

Staphylococcal Scalded Skin Syndrome (SSSS). SSSS is a condition that results from staphylococcal toxins of noncutaneous origin and is more common in children than TEN is. The genital mucosa is not affected; the genitocrural area may be involved in the initial generalized faint rash that precedes peeling. If there is any doubt about the diagnosis, histologic assessment will make the differentiation, as splitting occurs at the level of the granular layer in this syndrome. For severe Stevens-Johnson syndromes and for TEN, hospitalization in an intensive care burn unit is recommended. Silver sulfadiazine cream, commonly used for burns, is avoided, however, as sulfonamides are a common cause of TEN. Systemic steroids are contraindicated. The mortality rate for those with TEN is as high as 30%.

Pemphigus Vulgaris. This is a rare condition in adults and very rare in children or adolescents. However, cases have been reported in association with a specific tumor.[35]

Chronic Bullous Disease of Childhood (CBDC). CBDC is the term that has supplanted the formerly used *juvenile dermatitis herpetiformis (DH)*. The blisters are subepidermal, but immunofluorescence demonstrates linear immunoglobulin A (IgA) at the base of the basement membrane zone (BMZ) rather than the familiar papillary granular pattern of DH; the clinical picture is distinctive (Fig. 13–16). In a published surgical review, the age of affected patients ranged from 6 months to 10 years.[35] Tense bullae develop on the trunk, especially in the genital area. Typically they are grouped to form a "cluster-of-jewels" pattern, or they may take on a circinate or polycyclic appearance. It has been shown that involvement of ocular, oral, genital, and nasal

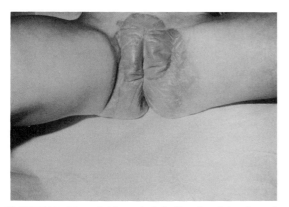

FIGURE 13–15 ••• Epidermolysis bullosa involving the vulvar area.

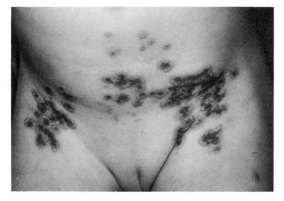

FIGURE 13–16 ••• Chronic bullous disease of childhood. Note the clustered lesions on the lower trunk. (From Ridley CM. The Vulva. Edinburgh: Churchill Livingstone, 1988.)

mucosa is common (64%), and ocular scarring may occur.[36] Patient prognosis is usually good, with the rash clearing within 2 years, but cases persisting into adult life have been described. Treatment with oral dapsone, sulfapyridine, or sulfamethoxypyridazine is effective; oral steroids have also been given, with uncertain benefit. Dapsone is usually less well tolerated in children than in adults, and sulfapyridine is most often the treatment of choice.

Childhood Cicatricial Pemphigoid (CCP). CCP was previously thought to be very rare in childhood, but an increasing number of cases are being reported.[36] The bullae are subepidermal and associated with dermal fibrosis. Immunofluorescence shows linear IgA at the BMZ. The bullae are usually widespread and mucosal involvement invariable. The lesions tend to persist into adult life, especially the mucosal component, and ocular scarring is a prominent feature; in one report describing four cases with onset between 2.5 and 10 years, the vulva was involved in two.[36] As in chronic bullous disease of childhood, the condition is responsive to dapsone and sulfapyridine. CBDC and CCP therefore show overlap with each other and with adult linear IgA disease. It has been suggested that CCP is a more severe form of chronic bullous disease of childhood.

Bullous Pemphigoid. Bullous pemphigoid, in which subepidermal bullae are associated with linear immunoglobulin G (IgG) at the BMZ with no scarring, tends to be a disease of the elderly, but well-authenticated cases have been reported in children and reviewed.[37]

Blisters associated with impetigo are noted elsewhere. Blisters may also be a manifestation of nonaccidental injury.

Psoriasis. Psoriasis often has a flexural component, and lesions of this type are seen sometimes in the anogenital area (Fig. 13–17). Histologic evaluation is rarely sought but will identify the typical parakeratosis, acanthosis, elongation of rete ridges, reduced granular layer, and perivascular dermal inflammation. Occasionally, collections of neutrophils are seen in the parakeratotic horny layer. The scaling is not obvious in the genital area, but the bright erythema and the sharp outline usually make diagnosis easy. There is often a fissure when the natal cleft is involved. The condition is chronic but usually can be managed well with topical corticosteroids and bland emollients. Tar and dithranol should be avoided.

Seborrheic Dermatitis. This condition demonstrates mild eczema on histologic examination and tends to occur in flexures. The lesions are less bright and well defined than those of psoriasis, but the two can be difficult to distinguish; indeed, they may coexist or change from one to the other from time to time in the same patient.

Eczema. Even if severe elsewhere, atopic eczema rarely affects the vulvar area in older children and adolescents, although, as has been noted, it may be associated with a diaper rash. Eczema in the anogenital area is more likely to be an irritant or allergic reaction complicating some other dermatologic condition. The histologic picture of eczema consists of spongiosis, acanthosis, and parakeratosis, along with inflammation in the dermis. With rubbing and scratching, the epidermis becomes more acanthotic (lichenification). Clinically, the picture is that of erythema with various degrees of erosion, excoriation, and thicken-

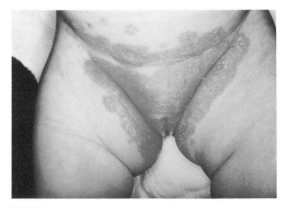

FIGURE 13–17 ••• Psoriasis involving the vulvovaginal area.

ing. With gross thickening, the skin color can become either a dull, earthy shade or quite pale, depending on the site and the degree of maceration. Treatment is with soothing preparations such as saline or potassium permanganate baths followed by corticosteroid cream; secondary infection also should be treated as necessary. While a stronger topical corticosteroid may be necessary initially, maintenance is often satisfactory with a milder one (i.e., hydrocortisone), coupled with an antibacterial and antifungal preparation such as miconazole. Management should include a review of the underlying condition. Contact dermatitis or irritant effects often arise from injudicious applications. The most common causes of allergic contact dermatitis in this area are preservatives, perfumes, and topical anesthetics or antihistamines. When allergy is suspected, patch testing should be carried out; the patient should be referred to a dermatologist for this procedure.

Lichen Simplex and Lichenification. *Lichen simplex* refers to thickening of the skin in response to itching, the skin originally being apparently normal; this is rare in children and adolescents. *Lichenification* is thickening in response to rubbing of the skin, which is originally abnormal because it is involved in psoriasis, eczema, or lichen sclerosus, for example. Histologically, the skin becomes hyperkeratotic and acanthotic with dermal inflammation. Clinically, it appears pale or earthy in color, and skin markings are increased. The condition will respond to bland applications and a topical corticosteroid until underlying factors causing the problem can be ascertained. These changes have been termed *hyperplastic dystrophy* in the past (Table 13–3).

Lichen Sclerosus. Lichen sclerosus (lichen sclerosus et atrophicus)[38] is a condition that affects all areas of the body in both sexes and at all ages; its etiology is unknown. It is significantly associated with autoimmune disease, but no differences can be demonstrated in the pattern and behavior of the condition regardless of whether this association is present (Fig. 13–18*A,B*).[39] Evidence linking it to certain HLA types is as yet uncertain;[40] a familial incidence, however, is well recognized and significant. Evidence regarding its pathogenesis remains to be fully demonstrated. There has been evidence in the past of a possible association with acid-fast bacilli. Attention has been focused more recently on the significance of *Borrelia burgdorferi*, but as yet no definite one- for-one correlation can be made.[41, 42]

The histologic appearance reveals a hyperkeratotic epidermis, later becoming atrophic, with acanthosis and follicular plugging. Typically there is an edematous hyalinized area in the dermis, often containing extravasated red cells with an underlying band of inflammatory cells. The elastic tissue subsequently tends to disappear. Probably as a reaction to irritation, there can be epithelial hyperplasia and increased keratinization, with strikingly pointed or forked rete ridges. Clinically, the lesions consist of ivory colored, flat-topped, polygonal papules, often coalescing into large plaques that may appear clinically atrophic (Fig. 13–18*C*). Purpuric speckling and frank ecchymosis are quite common, and the Koebner effect is well recognized. Lesions at the vulva affect the labia minora, the clitoris, and the surrounding tissue of the genitocrural folds, as well as the inner aspects of the labia majora once they have developed. There is a frequent figure-of-

TABLE 13–3 ••• THE INTERNATIONAL SOCIETY FOR THE STUDY OF VULVAR DISEASE AND THE INTERNATIONAL SOCIETY OF GYNECOLOGICAL PATHOLOGISTS (ISSVD AND ISGYP) CLASSIFICATION OF NON-NEOPLASTIC EPITHELIAL DISORDERS, VULVAR SKIN AND MUCOSA, 1987

1. Lichen sclerosus
2. Squamous cell hyperplasia (formerly called hyperplastic dystrophy)
3. Other dermatoses

Mixed epithelial disorders may occur. In such cases, it is recommended that both conditions be reported. For example: lichen sclerosus with associated squamous cell hyperplasia (formerly classified as mixed dystrophy) should be reported as lichen sclerosus and squamous cell hyperplasia. Squamous cell hyperplasia with associated vulvar intraepithelial neoplasia (formerly called hyperplastic dystrophy with atypia) should be diagnosed as vulvar intraepithelial neoplasia.

Squamous cell hyperplasia is used for those instances in which the hyperplasia is not attributable to another cause. Specific lesions or dermatoses involving the vulva (e.g., psoriasis, lichen planus, lichen simplex chronicus, *Candida* infection, condyloma acuminatum) may include squamous cell hyperplasia but should be diagnosed specifically and excluded from this category.

Adapted from Ridley CM, Frankman O, Jones ISC, et al. New nomenclature for vulvar disease. Report of the Committee on Terminology. Am J Obstet Gynecol 1989; 160:769. With permission of Mosby-Year Book, Inc.

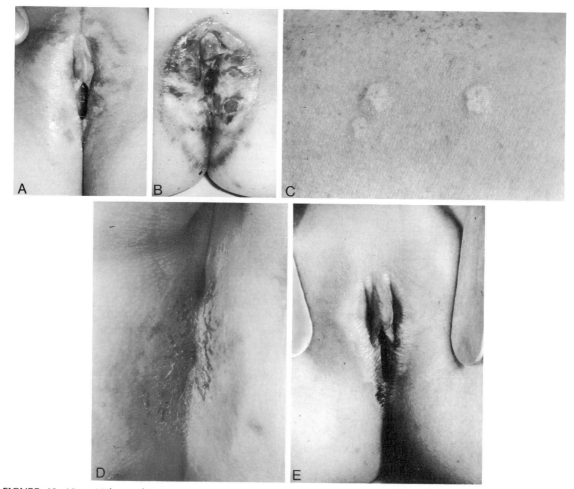

FIGURE 13–18 ••• Lichen sclerosus. *A,* Lichenified areas with associated white epithelium. *B,* Vulvar lesions with secondary ulcerations. *C,* Ivory papules on the trunk. *D,* Perianal secondary infection. *E,* Intense purpura that bleeds with minimal trauma.

eight pattern involving the anogenital area as a whole. Lesions are quite commonly found on the rest of the body (6% in one series[39]). The lesions may be symptomless or may lead to soreness and pruritus. Secondary infection is a common problem, and cutaneous lesions cause difficulty in passing urine or defecating. The clinical appearance, regardless of biopsy findings, is readily recognized by dermatologists but less often recognized by gynecologists and pediatricians.[43] Failure to diagnose this condition can lead to inappropriate treatment for constipation. Other differential diagnoses include vaginitis, suspected because of the general moistness of the area; intertrigo; threadworm infestation; and, most importantly, sexual abuse. Sexual abuse often is suspected because of the fragility of the area, the pres-

ence of secondary infection, and bleeding (Fig. 12–18*D,E*). The fusion and loss of tissue substance occurring in lichen sclerosus may be mistaken for labial adhesions of the type sometimes considered indicative of sexual abuse. It has been postulated that the trauma of sexual abuse could provoke lichen sclerosus, but the general opinion is that this is unlikely. Sexual abuse and lichen sclerosus can certainly coexist, however, and each clinical case must be investigated carefully on its own merit.

Management is with simple bland emollients and attention to hygiene, with topical antiseptics or antibiotics used as necessary. Mild or moderately potent topical corticosteroids are adequate to suppress any symptoms. Whether the use of a highly potent topical corticosteroid (clobetasol propionate 0.05%) would halt the process of the disease or reverse it and prevent distortion and loss of tissue in later life is uncertain. In treatment in adult patients, this may be the case; if loss of tissue appears to be very marked, use of such agents would, in children, be justifiable.

Prognosis. Published work has stressed that symptoms and signs tend to improve around the time of puberty.[2, 38, 43] What is not certain is whether the condition really does regress at that time or simply lessens in severity or clears for a time, only to return. Most reports are based on subjective evidence rather than on biopsy results or prolonged observation; a prospective study would be of great value. Parents should be assured that adequate treatment is likely to keep the condition well under control and that intercourse and pregnancy will be possible.

Cysts. Cysts are found in patients of any age, from infancy to adolescence. They are mucinous when in the vestibule and mesonephric when more lateral.[44] Sebaceous gland cysts, Bartholin's gland duct cysts, and epidermoid cysts are unlikely to occur before adult life.

Neoplasms. Any mass of the vulva, unless the clinical diagnosis is beyond doubt, should be excised or undergo biopsy.

Nonepithelial Neoplasms. These are very rare, whether benign or malignant, but can occur at any age.[45] A number of these tumors may affect the vagina in infants and young children and present as a vulvar mass.

Neurofibromatosis. Type II lesions appear in childhood or adolescence and may affect the vulva; isolated lesions also occur occasionally in patients with no evidence of generalized disease. They may consist of nodules or be more diffuse. Histologic examination identifies Schwann cells, collagen, and mucoid material or expanded nerve branches with collagen and Schwann cells (the plexiform pattern). Clitoral involvement in childhood is notoriously likely to lead to a mistaken diagnosis of ambiguous genitalia. Sometimes the condition is diagnosed in this way, offering the opportunity for appropriate genetic counseling.[46] It is likely that such lesions tend to be selectively reported, and the true incidence of neurofibromatosis of the vulva is not accurately known. Malignant change is possible but unusual.

Hemangioma. Some consider these lesions to be hamartomas rather than true neoplasms (Fig. 13–19). The one most commonly seen on the vulva is the cavernous hemangioma, or strawberry mark. Histologically, these are vas-

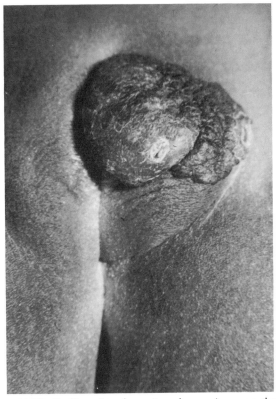

FIGURE 13–19 ••• Strawberry type hemangioma on the vulva.

cular channels lined with a single layer of endothelial cells. The lesion appears as a large vascular mass that may become ulcerated or secondarily infected. The prognosis is good, with the lesions gradually acquiring pale areas and becoming lax and shriveled. Ulceration is treated with topical antiseptics or antibiotics, and hemorrhage is rarely a problem except in the rare case of Kasabach-Merritt syndrome in which there is thrombocytopenia. In these cases, systemic steroids are required. Any unsightly remnants of a resolved hemangioma can be treated with plastic surgery.

Lymphangiomas. Lymphangiomas also occasionally affect the vulva. The histologic appearance is that of lymphatic spaces lined by endothelial cells and containing lymphocytes and erythrocytes. One type of lymphangioma presents as a soft mass, usually in the labia majora. The tiny frogspawn-like vesicles of lymphangioma circumscription may appear in young adults. The vesicles are sometimes dark and may mimic angiokeratomas, which are rarely seen before adulthood. Excision is not easy, as there is often communication with deep lymphatic vessels.

Lipomas. These can occur at any age, including childhood. They usually affect the labia majora and present no unusual features, consisting of mature fat cells and presenting as soft rounded masses.

Epithelial Tumors. The most common benign epithelial lesion in the young is the genital wart.[47]

Vulvar Intraepithelial Neoplasia. This condition is encountered in adolescents, increasingly so in more recent years. It presents in a clinically varied fashion, appearing as red, white, dark, or warty areas that are single or multiple. It is closely associated with HPV lesions and is considered in more detail in Chapter 38. At least three cases demonstrating similar changes have been reported in children.[48–50] One was in a 3-year-old girl, a victim of child sexual abuse; the lesion regressed after biopsy.[48] Another was in a male child aged 2; the lesion was found to contain HPV-16 and resolved spontaneously.[49] The third case was a lesion in a female child 2 years and 10 months of age who had no evidence of child sexual abuse; HPV-16 and HPV-18 were found, and the lesion responded to cryotherapy.[50]

Squamous Cell Carcinoma. This malignancy has been reported in adolescents but is extremely rare.

Melanocytic Lesions

Lentigo is not uncommon on the vulva. It occurs singly or affects large areas (lentiginosis), and the appearance of both is relatively unusual in children and adolescents. There are more melanocytes and increased pigmentation of the basal layer, with some melanophages in the underlying dermis. The lesions are brown and macular. An example of the LAMB syndrome (lentigines, atrial myxoma, mucocutaneous myxomas, blue nevi) has been reported in a girl of 13 years of age who had lentigines of the vulva.[51]

A *juvenile mole* (Spitz nevus) may occur on the vulva as a brown nodule. It is benign and has a distinctive histologic appearance, showing spindle and epithelioid nevus cells in the epidermis, sometimes with giant cells. The groups of cells are well demarcated. *Intradermal, compound,* and *junctional nevi* are quite commonly found at the vulva. In a series of 301 females (including an unspecified number of children) examined for vulvar nevi, although 10% had some pigmented lesions, only 2% had nevi; few patients were aware of having the lesions.[52] It has been noted that some unusual compound nevi in young women can be easily mistaken for malignant melanoma; nests of unusually shaped nevus cells are found in the epidermis, but they are benign.[53]

Malignant melanoma has been reported in a patient of 14 who also had lichen sclerosus.[54]

Adnexal Neoplasms

The only adnexal tumor in this class likely to be encountered in adolescents is the syringoma, a benign tumor of eccrine differentiation. The histologic appearance is that of comma-shaped ducts surrounded by fibrous tissue; the ducts are lined with epithelial cells. Many cases of vulvar lesions have been reported in young adults, usually in association with lesions elsewhere; they have also been reported in children.[55] The lesions are benign, small, skin-colored papules.

Bartholin's gland lesions are rare in childhood and adolescence, as are lesions of the urethra.

References

1. Champion RH, Burton JL, Ebring FJG (eds). Rook Wilkinson Ebring Textbook of Dermatology. 5th ed. London, Blackwell Scientific, 1992.
2. Ridley CM (ed). The Vulva. Edinburgh: Churchill Livingstone, 1988.
3. Byrne M. Topical anaesthesia with lidocaine prilocaine cream for vulval biopsy. Br J Obstet Gynaecol 1989; 96:497.
4. Frayling IM, Addison GM, Chattergee K, Meakin G. Methaemaglobinaemia in children treated with prilocaine-lignocaine cream. Br Med J 1990; 301:153.
5. Immature skin. Lancet 1989; ii(8672):1138.
6. Oriba HA, Elsner P, Maibach HI. Vulvar physiology. Semin Dermatol 1989; 8:2.
7. Aly R, Britz MB, Maibach HI. Quantitative microbiology of the vagina. Br J Dermatol 1979; 101:445.
8. Borglin NE, Selander P. Hymenal polyps in newborn infants. Acta Paediatr (Suppl) 1962; 135:28.
9. Wilson PA, Dallas MJ. Diaper performance: Maintenance of healthy skin. Pediatr Dermatol 1990; 7:179.
10. Bluestein J, Furner EB, Phillips D. Granuloma gluteale infantum: Case report and review of the literature. Pediatr Dermatol 1990; 7:196.
11. Christensen EH, Oster J. Adhesions of labia minora (synechia vulvae) in childhood. Acta Paediatr Scand 1971; 60:709.
12. Capraro VJ, Greenberg H. Adhesions of the labia minora: A study of 50 patients. Obstet Gynecol 1972; 39:65.
13. Muram D. Labial adhesions in sexually abused children. Correspondence. JAMA 1988; 259:352.
14. Finlay HVL. Adhesions of the labia minora in childhood. Proc R Soc Med 1965; 58:929.
15. Jenkinson SD, Mackinnon AE. Spontaneous separation of fused labia minora in prepubertal girls. Br Med J 1984; 289:160.
16. Odds FC, Candida and Candidosis. 2nd ed. London: Baillière Tindall, 1988.
17. Jelliffe DB, Jacobson FW. The clinical picture of tinea versicolor in negro infants. J Trop Med Hyg 1954; 57:290.

18. Krol AL. Perianal streptococcal dermatitis. Pediatr Dermatol 1990; 7:97.
19. Rock B, Naghashfar L, Barnett N, et al. Genital tract papillomavirus infection in children. Arch Dermatol 1986; 122:1129.
20. Oriel JD. Anogenital papillomavirus infection in children. Br Med J 1988; 296:1484.
21. Obalek S, Jablonska S, Pavre M, et al. Condylomata acuminata in children: Frequent association with human papillomaviruses responsible for cutaneous warts. J Am Acad Dermatol 1990; 23:205.
22. Padel AF, Venning VA, Evans MF, et al. Human papillomaviruses in anogenital warts in children: Typing by in situ hybridisation. Br Med J 1990; 300:1491.
23. Porter CD, Blake NW, Archard LC, et al. Molluscum contagiosum virus types in genital and non-genital lesions. Br J Dermatol 1989; 120:37.
24. Lally MR, Orenstein SR, Cohen BA. Crohn's disease of the vulva in an 8 year old girl. Pediatr Dermatol 1988; 5:103.
25. Handfield-Jones SE, Prendiville WJ, Norman S. Vulval lymphangiectasia. Genitourin Med 1989; 65:335.
26. Yu CCW, Cook MG. Hidradenitis suppurativa: A disease of follicular epithelium rather than apocrine glands. Br J Dermatol 1990; 122:763.
27. Mortimer PS, Dawber RPR, Gales MA, Moore RA. A double blind controlled cross-over trial of cyproterone acetate in females with hidradenitis suppurativa. Br J Dermatol 1986; 115:263.
28. Wechsler B, Davatchi F, Mizushima Y, et al. Criteria for diagnosis of Behcet's disease. Lancet 1990; 335:1078.
29. Portnoy J, Ahronheim GA, Ghibu F, et al. Recovery of Epstein-Barr virus from genital ulcers. N Engl J Med 1984; 311:966.
30. Vaclavinkova V, Neumann E. Vaginal involvement in familial benign chronic pemphigus (Morbus Hailey-Hailey). Acta Derm Venereol 1982; 62:80.
31. Brandrup F, Petri J, Algidius J. Acantholytic lesions in the vagina. Correspondence. Br J Dermatol 1990; 123:691.
32. Wilson EE, Malinak LR. Vulvovaginal sequelae of Stevens-Johnson syndrome and their management. Obstet Gynecol 1988; 71:478.
33. Bonafe JL, Thibaut I, Hoff J. Introital adenosis associated with the Stevens-Johnson syndrome. Clin Exp Dermatol 1990; 15:356.
34. Roujeau J-C, Chosidow O, Saiag P, Guillanme J-C. Toxic epidermal necrolysis (Lyell's syndrome). J Am Acad Dermatol 1990; 23:1039.
35. Coulson IH, Cook MG, Bruton J, Penfold C. Atypical pemphigus vulgaris associated with angio-follicular lymph node hyperplasia (Castleman's disease). Clin Exp Dermatol 1986; 11:656.
36. Wojnarowska F, Marsden RA, Bhogal B, Black MM. Chronic bullous disease of childhood, childhood cicatricial pemphigoid and linear IgA disease of adults. J Am Acad Dermatol 1988; 19:792.
37. Guenther LC, Shum D. Localized childhood vulvar pemphigoid. J Am Acad Dermatol 1990; 22:762.
38. Ridley CM. Lichen sclerosus et atrophicus. Semin Dermatol 1989; 8:54.
39. Meyrick Thomas RH, Ridley CM, McGibbon DH, Black MM. Lichen sclerosus et atrophicus and autoimmunity—a study of 350 women. Br J Dermatol 1988; 118:41.
40. Purcell KG, Spencer LV, Simpson PM, et al. HLA antigens in lichen sclerosus et atrophicus. Arch Dermatol 1990; 126:1043.
41. Orss SA, Sanchez JL, Taboas JO. Spirochetal forms in the dermal lesions of morphea and lichen sclerosus et atrophicus. Am J Dermatopathol 1990; 12:357.
42. Aberer E, Killegger H, Kristoferitsch W, Stanek G. Neuroborreliosis in morphea and lichen sclerosus et atrophicus. J Am Acad Dermatol 1988; 19:820.
43. Berth-Jones J, Graham-Brown RAC, Burns DA. Lichen sclerosus et atrophicus—a review of 15 cases in young girls. Clin Exp Dermatol 1991; 16:14.
44. Fox H, Buckley CH. Tumour-like lesions and cysts of the vulva. In: Ridley CM (ed). The Vulva. Edinburgh: Churchill Livingstone, 1988.
45. Fox H, Buckley CH. Non-epithelial and mixed tumours of the vulva. In: Ridley CM (ed). The Vulva. Edinburgh: Churchill Livingstone, 1988.
46. Friedrich EG, Wilkinson EJ. Vulvar surgery for neurofibromatosis. Obstet Gynecol 1985; 65:135.
47. Buckley CH, Fox H. Epithelial tumours of the vulva. In: Ridley CM (ed). The Vulva. Edinburgh: Churchill Livingstone, 1988.
48. Halasz C, Silvers D, Crum CP. Bowenoid papulosis in a 3-year-old girl. J Am Acad Dermatol 1986; 14:326.
49. Breneman DL, Lucky AW, Ostrow RS, et al. Bowenoid papulosis of the genitalia associated with human papillomavirus DNA type 16 in an infant with atropic dermatitis. Pediatr Dermatol 1985; 2:297.
50. Weitzner JM, Fields KW, Robinson MJ. Pediatric Bowenoid papulosis: Risks and management. Pediatr Dermatol 1989; 6:303.
51. Rhodes AR, Silverman RA, Harrist TJ, Perez-Atayde AR. Mucocutaneous lentigines cardiomuco-cutaneous myxomas and multiple blue nevi: The LAMB syndrome. J Am Acad Dermatol 1984; 10:72.
52. Rock B, Hood AF, Rock JA. Prospective study of vulvar nevi. J Am Acad Dermatol 1990; 22:104.
53. Friedman RJ, Ackerman AB. Difficulties in the histologic diagnosis of melanocytic nevi on the vulva of premenstrual women. In: Ackerman AB (ed.). Pathology of Malignant Melanoma. Chicago: Year Book Medical Publishers, 1981, p. 119.
54. Friedman RJ, Kopf AW, Jones WB. Malignant melanoma in association with lichen sclerosis on the vulva of a 14-year-old girl. Am J Dermatolpathol 1984; 6:253.
55. Scherbenske JM, Lupton GP, Hames WD, Kirkle DB. Vulvar syringomas occurring in a 9-year-old child. Correspondence. J Am Dermatol 1988; 19:575.

○○○

CHAPTER 14

Vaginal Bleeding in Childhood and Menstrual Disorders in Adolescence

DAVID MURAM
JOSEPH S. SANFILIPPO
S. PAIGE HERTWECK

Bleeding in an adolescent girl is of clinical significance when it is prolonged or when blood loss is excessive. In comparison, vaginal bleeding in early childhood, regardless of its duration and quantity, is always of clinical importance. Vaginal bleeding in children may be caused by local vulvar or vaginal lesions or may arise from the endometrium as a manifestation of precocious puberty. In adolescent girls, excessive or irregular bleeding from the vagina is one of the most common disorders of menstrual function. Most of these patients suffer from dysfunctional uterine bleeding. Determining the cause of vaginal bleeding in children and adolescents can indeed be a challenge to the clinician.

BLEEDING GENERATED BY VULVAR AND VAGINAL DISORDERS

A detailed history and careful inspection of the external genitalia will determine the cause of bleeding in many children with vulvar lesions. Vaginoscopy and examination under anesthesia are the mainstays of evaluation to exclude the presence of local vaginal lesions (e.g., tumors, foreign bodies). In infants and children, the hymenal orifice normally will admit a 0.5-cm vaginoscope. An instrument 0.8 cm in diameter can be used to examine most older premenarchal girls. Although some patients cooperate well in the office, many young patients are very apprehensive, and vaginoscopy often is best performed under general anesthesia.[1, 2] The more common vulvar and vaginal disorders that cause bleeding in children are listed in Table 14–1.

Vulvovaginitis

Vulvovaginitis is the most common gynecologic disorder in children. Young children are susceptible to infections because perineal hygiene is often less than adequate and contamination by stool and debris is common. In

TABLE 14–1 ••• VULVAR AND VAGINAL CAUSES OF BLEEDING IN CHILDREN

Vulvovaginitis
Foreign body
Trauma
Sarcoma botryoides
Adenocarcinoma of the cervix or vagina
Urethral prolapse
Vulvar skin disorders

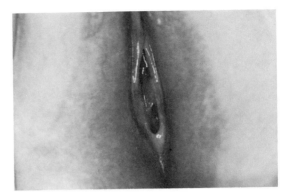

FIGURE 14–1 ••• Acute vulvovaginitis. Note the typical area of distribution.

addition, the vaginal mucosa is thin and atrophic and therefore less resistant to infections. The symptoms of vulvovaginitis vary from minor discomfort to relatively intense perineal pruritus or a sensation of burning accompanied by a foul-smelling discharge. The irritating discharge inflames the vulva and often causes the child to scratch the affected area to the point of bleeding. Acute vulvovaginitis may denude the thin vulvar or vaginal mucosa, but bleeding usually is minimal, and, as a rule, the discharge is little more than bloodstaining. Inspection of the vagina reveals an area of redness and soreness that may be minimal or may extend laterally to the thighs and posteriorly to the anus (Fig. 14–1). Vaginoscopy is necessary to exclude a foreign body or tumor in a girl with recurrent vaginal infections or a foul-smelling, bloody discharge.[2]

Wet-mount specimens and cultures often confirm the diagnosis.[2–4] In general, broad-spectrum antibiotics (e.g., ampicillin) are extremely useful. In all instances, proper instructions regarding vulvar hygiene should be given to both the parent and the child. When infection is severe and extensive mucosal damage is noted, a short course of topical estrogen cream (one fingertip applied twice daily for 7 to 10 days) is prescribed to promote healing of vulvar and vaginal tissues. When irritation is intense, ½% to 1% hydrocortisone cream may be necessary to alleviate the pruritus.

Foreign Bodies

Foreign bodies in the vagina induce an intense inflammatory reaction and result in a blood-stained, foul-smelling discharge (Figs. 14–2, 14–3). The child usually does not recall inserting the foreign object or will not admit to it. The most commonly found foreign bodies are rolled pieces of toilet paper that appear as amorphous conglomerates of grayish material. They are found most frequently on the poste-

rior vaginal wall (Fig. 14–4). Because many foreign bodies are not radiopaque, radiographs are of little value. Vaginoscopy is essential to remove objects situated in the vagina and to exclude other causes for the bleeding. A foreign body in the lower third of the vagina often can be removed by washing out the vagina with warm saline. Unfortunately, however, recurrences are quite common.[2, 3, 5]

Urethral Prolapse

Vulvar bleeding is occasionally the result of urethral prolapse (Fig. 14–5). The urethral mucosa protrudes through the meatus and forms a hemorrhagic, sensitive vulvar mass that bleeds quite easily.[6] Prolapse of the urethra is diagnosed when the urethral orifice is identified in the center of the mass, which is separate from the vagina. When the lesion is small and urination is unimpaired, a short

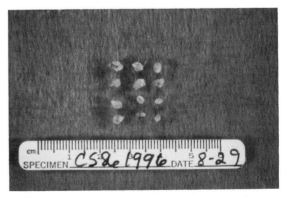

FIGURE 14–2 ••• Rolled toilet paper removed from a child's vagina.

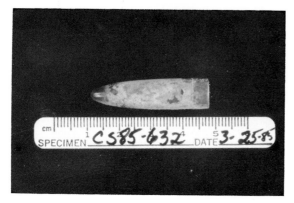

FIGURE 14–3 ••• Pen top removed from a 3½-year-old child.

course of therapy with estrogen cream is beneficial. Resection of the prolapsed tissue and insertion of an indwelling catheter for 24 hours may be necessary when urinary retention is present or if the lesion is large and necrotic.[2, 5, 7]

Lichen Sclerosus

Lichen sclerosus of the vulva is a hypertrophic dystrophy (Fig. 14–6). Although it

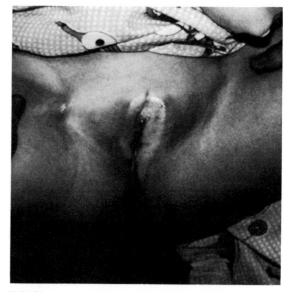

FIGURE 14–5 ••• Urethral prolapse in a 6-year-old child.

ordinarily affects postmenopausal women, it also occasionally affects young children. Symptoms consist of vulvar irritation, dysuria, and pruritus. Examination of the vulva reveals flat, ivory-colored papules that may coalesce into plaques. The clitoris, posterior fourchette, and anorectal area frequently are affected. The lesions do not extend laterally beyond the middle of the labia majora or spread into

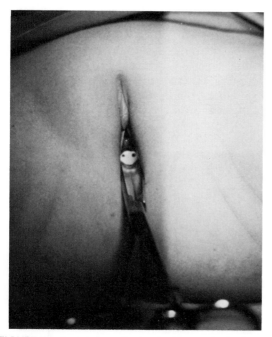

FIGURE 14–4 ••• A large foreign body seen in the lower vagina.

FIGURE 14–6 ••• Lichen sclerosus of the vulva in a 6-year-old child.

the vagina, and they tend to bruise easily, forming bloody blisters that become susceptible to secondary infections. Histologically, the skin shows flattening of the rete pegs, hyalinization of the subdermal tissues, and keratinization. Histologic confirmation is not usually indicated in children.

Treatment consists of improved local hygiene, reduction of trauma, and short-term use of steroid cream to alleviate the pruritus. Treatment may be repeated when exacerbations occur. Improvement in symptoms and appearance of the skin lesions following puberty has been described.[2, 3, 8] (See Chapter 13.)

Genital Trauma

The external genitalia of children, compared with those in adults, are not as well protected against injury. Fortunately, most of these injuries are minor. Commonly, the trauma is caused by a blunt blow to the vulva, although infrequently the injury results from a fall on a sharp object that may penetrate the perineal body or vagina. Although most injuries are accidental, there is a significant number of children whose genital tract injuries are caused by physical or sexual abuse. Therefore, it is extremely important for the examining physician to determine how the child sustained the injury. In the case of sexual abuse, the victimized child must be removed from an unsafe environment.[9]

A blunt injury may cause blood vessels beneath the perineal skin to rupture. Blood accumulates under the skin and forms a hematoma, producing a rounded, tense, and tender swelling, the size of which depends on the amount of bleeding (Fig. 14–7). A contusion to the vulva usually does not require treatment. A small vulvar hematoma often can be controlled by pressure with an ice pack, but a large hematoma, or one that continues to increase in size, should be incised, the clotted blood removed, and the bleeding points ligated. Use of prophylactic broad-spectrum antibiotics is advisable. The vulva should be kept clean and dry.[5]

Most vaginal injuries occur when an object penetrates the vagina through the hymenal opening. Hymenal injuries rarely involve the hymen alone. The thin vaginal mucosa often is lacerated along with the hymen. Usually there is very little bleeding from a hymenal

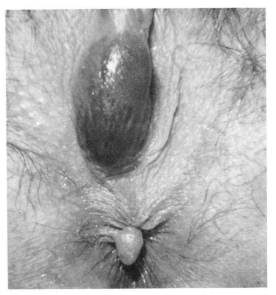

FIGURE 14–7 ••• Vulvar hematoma caused by a straddle injury.

injury, but any such bleeding is indicative of vaginal penetration, and thus the possibility of additional vaginal injuries exists. Consequently, a detailed examination is necessary to exclude injuries to the upper vagina. When a vaginal laceration extends to the vaginal vault, a laparotomy is indicated to exclude extension of the tear into the broad ligament or the peritoneal cavity. Bladder and bowel integrity must be confirmed by catheterization and rectal palpation.[2, 3, 10]

Genital Tumors

Benign tumors of the vulva, particularly hemangiomas, may cause vulvar bleeding. Capillary hemangiomas cause only minimal bleeding, if any (Fig. 14–8). They usually disappear as the child grows older and thus require no therapy except for reassurance to the parent. In contrast, cavernous hemangiomas are composed of vessels of considerable size, and injury to them may cause serious hemorrhage. Thus they are best treated surgically, either by excision or occlusion of the feeding vessels.[3]

Although uncommon, genital tumors must be considered whenever a girl is found to have a chronic genital ulcer, an atraumatic swelling of the external genitalia, tissue protruding from the vagina, or a foul-smelling, bloody discharge (Table 14–2). Embryonal carcinoma

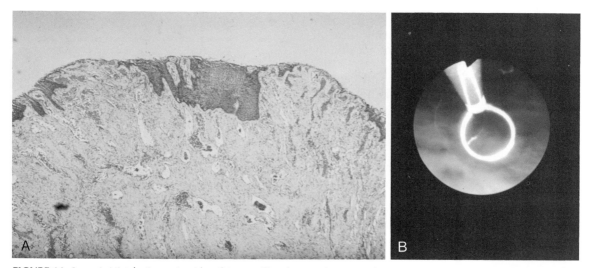

FIGURE 14–8 ••• *A,* Histologic section identifying capillary hemangioma noted in a 5-year-old child during vaginal biopsy. *B,* Cystoscopic view of a capillary hemangioma showing loop coagulation of bleeding areas of the bladder mucosa.

of the vagina, or rhabdomyosarcoma (sarcoma botryoides), is seen most commonly in children (Fig. 14–9). The tumors arise in the submucosal tissue and spread rapidly beneath an intact vaginal epithelium. The vaginal mucosa then bulges into a series of polypoid growths that may protrude through the vaginal orifice. The diagnosis is confirmed by histologic examination of a biopsy specimen. A combination chemotherapy regimen including vincristine, d-actinomycin, and cyclophosphamide has been employed with success.[11] If the tumor is amenable to surgical removal after chemotherapy, radical hysterectomy and vaginec-

tomy are performed, preserving the ovaries. Exenteration is not recommended. If the tumor is still unresectable after chemotherapy, radiotherapy is employed to assist in shrinking and controlling tumor growth[11] (see Chapter 38).

During childhood and early adolescence, three types of vaginal carcinoma may appear:

1. Endodermal carcinoma, which occurs most often in young children.

2. Mesonephric carcinoma, which arises in

TABLE 14–2 ••• PREOPERATIVE WORKUP FOR CHILDREN AND ADOLESCENTS WITH OVARIAN CANCER

Required:
   Complete blood cell counts
   Blood chemistry tests
   Liver function tests
   Urinalysis
   Tumor markers (i.e., α-fetoprotein, β–human
     chorionic gonadotropin, carcinoembryonic antigen)
   Chest radiograph
   Intravenous pyelogram
   Pelvic sonogram

Obtain when indicated:
   Gastrointestinal series
   Computed tomography scan
   Liver and brain scans
   Magnetic resonance imaging
   Hormone assays (i.e., serum androgens, serum
     estrogen)
   Lymphangiogram

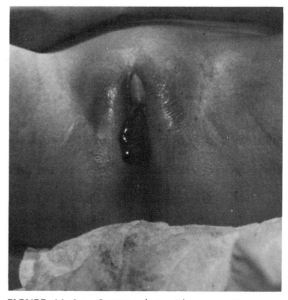

FIGURE 14–9 ••• Sarcoma botryoides presenting as a hemorrhagic growth extruding from the vagina.

a remnant of a mesonephric duct and occurs more often in girls 3 years of age or older.

3. Clear-cell adenocarcinoma, which is often associated with a history of antenatal exposure to diethylstilbestrol and is encountered most frequently in postmenarchal teenage girls.

The clinical features and treatment of these malignant lesions of the vagina and cervix are similar to those in adult women.

ENDOMETRIAL SHEDDING

Bleeding that arises from the endometrium per se usually represents endometrial shedding; in the pediatric age group it is often associated with sexual precocity. Precocious puberty is the onset of sexual maturation at any age that is >2 S.D. earlier than the norm. At present, the appearance of secondary sexual characteristics before 8 years of age or onset of menarche before age 10 is considered precocious.[12–14] Occasionally, for reasons that remain unclear, only one sign of pubertal development will be present (e.g., premature thelarche or premature menarche). This may be caused by a transient elevation in the circulating levels of estrogen or by extreme sensitivity of the target tissue to the very low, prepubertal level of sex hormones. However, such isolated development may be the first sign of precocious puberty, and therefore reevaluation at regular intervals is indicated. When endometrial shedding occurs, the following are recommended to determine the cause[15–19]:

1. Determination of blood estradiol levels or, as an alternative, cytologic evaluation of a vaginal smear (maturation index) to determine whether estrogen stimulation is present.

2. Gonadotropin-releasing hormone (GnRH) stimulation test to assess pubertal aberrancy.

3. Pelvic ultrasound and, if necessary, a computed tomographic (CT) scan of the abdomen and pelvis to exclude gonadal or adrenal neoplasm.

4. CT scan of the head to rule out central nervous system lesions.

The disorders responsible for endometrial shedding in children are listed in Table 14–3.

Physiologic Endometrial Shedding

During the first few weeks of life, the newborn female physiologically responds to the

TABLE 14–3 ••• CAUSES OF ENDOMETRIAL SHEDDING IN CHILDREN

Physiologic
  Neonatal withdrawal bleeding
Early sexual development (incomplete form)
  Premature menarche
Early sexual development (complete forms)
  Immature hypothalamic-pituitary-ovarian axis
    Exposure to estrogens
     In the food chain
     Through medications
    Endogenous estrogen production
     Functional ovarian cysts
     Ovarian neoplasms
     Other hormone-producing neoplasms
  Mature hypothalamic-pituitary-ovarian axis
    Idiopathic precocious puberty
    Central nervous system lesions
    McCune-Albright syndrome

stimulation of placentally acquired maternal estrogens. The effects may be seen for perhaps a month, but rarely longer. The most obvious effect—breast budding—occurs in nearly all infants born at term. Vaginal discharge is quite common, as the cervical glands secrete a considerable amount of mucus, which combines with exfoliated vaginal cells. Occasionally, after birth and with subsequent declining estrogen levels, the stimulated endometrial lining is shed and vaginal bleeding occurs. However, the bleeding ceases within the first 7 to 10 days of life. Further evaluation is required if bleeding is initiated or persists after 10 days of age.[2, 3, 5]

DYSFUNCTIONAL UTERINE BLEEDING

Dysfunctional uterine bleeding (DUB) is defined as excessive, prolonged, or unpatterned bleeding from the uterine endometrium that is unrelated to anatomic lesions of the uterus.[20] The most common cause of DUB is anovulation secondary to a disturbance of the normal hypothalamic-pituitary-ovarian axis. Anovulation accounts for more than 75% of all cases of DUB.[21] It has been advocated that DUB perhaps should be renamed "anovulatory uterine bleeding."

The normal menstrual cycle usually consists of a mean interval of 28 days with a mean duration of 4 days (±2 to 3 days).[22] Normal menstrual flow is approximately 30 ml/cycle,[23] with an upper normal limit of 60 to 80 ml.[24] Bleeding occurring at an interval of 21 days or less for >7 days duration of flow and/or 80 ml total volume is considered abnormal. Definitions of various menstrual abnormalities are listed in Table 14–4.

Approximately 10% to 15% of all gynecologic patients have DUB, but it is more commonly seen in the adolescent.[21] As stated earlier, the etiologic factors involve the slow maturation of the hypothalamic-pituitary-ovarian axis, especially for the first 18 months after menarche in the adolescent female, and thus cycles are usually anovulatory. Although menarche occurs, on the average, at 12.8 years of age in the United States, up to 5 years may be needed for regular ovulatory cycles to ensue.[25] McDonough and Ganett observed anovulation in 55% to 82% of cycles in adolescents between the time of menarche and 2 years after menarche, in 30% to 55% of the cycles from 2 to 4 years after menarche, and in up to 20% of cycles from 4 to 5 years after menarche.[26] Jones reported abnormal bleeding in more than 500 adolescent females who were followed for 5 years; 75% of these were anovulatory, thus indicating a relatively high association of anovulation with DUB in the adolescent patient.[27]

Normal ovulation involves a regular cyclic production, first of estradiol (initiating ovarian follicular growth and endometrial proliferation), and then of ovulation (producing a significant increase in progesterone, which stabilizes the endometrium). Without ovulation and subsequent progesterone production, a state of unopposed estrogen occurs. This causes dilation of the spiral arterial supply in the endometrium, with resultant endometrial growth and associated abnormal height without proper structural support, the result of which is spontaneous superficial breakage with random asynchronous bleeding.[23] Eventually, increased estrogen has a negative effect on the hypothalamus and pituitary gland, causing a decrease in GnRH, follicle-stimulating hormone (FSH), and luteinizing hormone (LH), as well as a decrease in estrogen. This results in vasoconstriction and collapse of a thickened hyperplastic endometrial lining, with heavy and often prolonged bleeding.[28]

Although anovulation is the most common finding associated with DUB, there are a number of ovulatory patients who have intermenstrual bleeding; the mechanism surrounding this particular disorder is uncertain. In addition, conditions involving prolonged progesterone excretion after ovulation as a result of a persistent corpus luteal cyst (Halban's syndrome) can result in 6 to 8 weeks of amenorrhea, followed by irregular menstrual flow.[29]

Diagnosis

DUB is a diagnosis of exclusion. Initial attempts at diagnosis of anovulation as the cause of irregular bleeding should be directed at eliminating the possibility of organic lesions in the reproductive tract and of coagulation disorders. Organic disorders that can cause symptoms resembling those of simple anovulatory bleeding include intrauterine benign neoplasms, reproductive tract malignancies, bleeding with early pregnancy (as in threatened abortion), ectopic pregnancy, and hydatidiform mole. Associated blood dyscrasias include thrombocytopenic purpura, von Willebrand's disease, platelet dysfunctions, and platelet storage pool diseases (Table 14–5).

Despite extensive possibilities, the usual diagnosis in an adolescent patient remains anovulation. As previously stated, the most common cause of anovulation in the adolescent is immaturity of the hypothalamic-pituitary-ovarian axis. However, any hypothalamic dysfunction associated with stress, exercise or weight loss, or systemic disease also can affect ovulation. In particular, congenital adrenal hyperplasia, Cushing's syndrome, hepatic dysfunction, adrenal insufficiency, and thyroid dysfunction can interfere with the process.[20] In some cases, the interaction is not well understood, but the hormonal derangement associated with adrenal dysfunction interacts with the central regulating mechanisms of ovulation, and it is thought that thyroid abnormalities and liver dysfunction result in a derangement of the metabolic clearance rate of estrogen.[21]

TABLE 14–4 ••• MENSTRUAL ABNORMALITIES

Polymenorrhea: Frequent irregular bleeding at less than 18-day intervals.
Oligomenorrhea: Infrequent irregular bleeding at intervals of more than 45 days.
Metrorrhagia: Intermenstrual bleeding between regular periods.
Menorrhagia: Excessive uterine bleeding occurring regularly (synonymous with the term *hypermenorrhea*).
Hypomenorrhea: Decreased menstrual flow at regular intervals.
Menometrorrhagia: Frequent, irregular, excessive, and prolonged uterine bleeding.

TABLE 14–5 ••• DIFFERENTIAL DIAGNOSIS OF DYSFUNCTIONAL UTERINE BLEEDING

Pregnancy complications
  Abortion
  Ectopic pregnancy
  Trophoblastic disease
Benign and malignant neoplasms of the genital tract
  Cervical polyp
  Vaginal adenosis
  Vaginal carcinoma
  Cervical carcinoma
  Granulosa–theca cell tumors
  Endometriosis
  Leiomyoma
Genital tract infection
  Vaginitis
  Cervicitis
  Vaginal foreign body
  Intrauterine contraceptive device
  Salpingo-oophoritis
Endocrinopathies
  Polycystic ovarian disease
  Hyperprolactinemia
  Hypothyroidism
  Hyperthyroidism
Administration of drugs or hormones
Trauma
Coagulation disorders
  Idiopathic thrombocytopenic purpura
  Von Willebrand's disease
Chronic systemic illness
  Liver cirrhosis
  Renal failure

TABLE 14–6 ••• EVALUATION OF PATIENTS WITH SUSPECTED COAGULOPATHY

Blood tests
  Complete blood cell count
  Blood smear
  Platelet count
  Prothrombin time
  Partial thromboplastin time
Other
  Bleeding time

the hemostasis achieved in a bleeding menstrual endometrium, and therefore deficiencies in these constituents, as seen in thrombocytopenia and von Willebrand's disease, cause the associated increased blood loss with menses.[23] Similarly, there have been case reports of menorrhagia in individuals with platelet storage pool disease, a defect causing inability of platelet aggregation (Table 14–6).[31]

Evaluation

An evaluation for abnormal bleeding is initiated with a detailed gynecologic history, which should include age at menarche, frequency and duration of menses, and last and previous menstrual periods, as well as a sexual history. Medications also should be carefully recorded, as they, too, can play an integral role in associated anovulatory bleeding. Medications that tend to increase the cytochrome P-450 mechanism in the liver (e.g., seizure medications) also increase the metabolism of steroid hormones and thus may result in DUB. A careful systems review should be obtained, with particular emphasis on evaluation of bleeding disorders (easy bruisability, epistaxis, gingival bleeding) and endocrinologic disorders (hirsutism, galactorrhea, thyroid dysfunction). The physical examination provides an opportunity to assess Tanner staging and signs of endocrine abnormalities. A pelvic examination must determine the possibility of pregnancy, the presence of a foreign body, or an anatomic source of the bleeding.

Essential laboratory tests (Table 14–7) include a complete blood cell count with platelet evaluation, a blood smear, a serum pregnancy test, and a coagulation profile, including prothrombin time and partial thromboplastin time. In severe cases, a von Willebrand factor assessment and a binding time should be ordered. These coagulation tests should be com-

The second most common cause of abnormal uterine bleeding in the adolescent is a coagulopathy.[30] Claessens and Cowell, in a 9-year review, examined all admissions for acute menorrhagia at Children's Hospital and determined that 19% were the result of primary coagulation disorders.[30] These disorders included idiopathic thrombocytopenic purpura, von Willebrand's disease, Glanzmann's disease (a primary qualitative platelet defect), Fanconi's anemia, and thalassemia major. The patients in this study who presented with acute menorrhagia at menarche included 45 with a coagulation disorder, illustrating the importance of excluding a hematologic problem whenever menorrhagia occurs at menarche.[30] An underlying coagulation disorder can be noted in one out of four girls with severe menorrhagia (especially if the hemoglobin concentration is <10 gm/100 ml) and in one of two adolescents presenting at the time of menarche.[30] Of those patients with bleeding dyscrasias, 10% present with cyclic hypermenorrhea. The most common hematologic disorder in the adolescent is thrombocytopenic purpura.[25] Platelets and fibrin play a direct part in

TABLE 14–7 ••• EVALUATION OF PATIENTS WITH DYSFUNCTIONAL UTERINE BLEEDING

Blood tests
   Complete blood cell count
   Pregnancy test
   Prolactin
   Thyroid function tests (in selected cases only)
Urinalysis
Other
   Cervical smear
   Vaginal smear for maturation index

pleted before transfusion or hormonal treatment. Endocrinologic evaluation should be complemented by thyroid function studies. Usually, thyroxin (T_4) and thyroid-stimulating hormone (TSH) levels are sufficient. Because hyperprolactinemia can interfere centrally, causing menstrual dysfunction, serum prolactin levels also should be determined.

Treatment

Management of DUB in large part depends on the presenting signs and symptoms, examination findings, and the hemoglobin/hematocrit level (Table 14–8). Irregular vaginal bleeding may be controlled with oral contraceptives. In general, a 35-μg preparation is adequate. For the short-term, it may be necessary to

TABLE 14–8 ••• MANAGEMENT OF DYSFUNCTIONAL UTERINE BLEEDING

Hemoglobin > 12 gm/100 ml
   Reassurance
   Menstrual calendar
   Iron supplements
   Periodic reevaluation
Hemoglobin 10–12 gm/100 ml
   Reassurance and explanation
   Menstrual calendar
   Iron supplements
   Cyclic progestin therapy or oral contraceptives
   Reevaluation in 6 mo
Hemoglobin < 10 gm/100 ml
   No active bleeding
      Explanation
      Transfusion/iron supplements
      Oral contraceptives
      Reevaluation in 6–12 mo
   Acute hemorrhage
      Transfusion
      Fluid replacement therapy
      Hormonal hemostasis (intravenous conjugated estrogen)
      Intensive progestin therapy
      D & C when hormonal hemostasis fails
      Oral contraceptives for 6–12 mo

increase the dose of ethinyl estradiol to 50 μg if the original dose is ineffective. Oral contraceptives reduce menstrual blood flow by at least 60% in patients with a normal uterus.[32] Failure to control hypermenorrhea with cyclic estrogen-progestin therapy implies the possibility of an anatomic cause such as a myoma, polyp, or bleeding diathesis.

In anovulatory bleeding, it is feasible to substitute only the missing progestin. Progesterones and progestins are antiestrogenic when given in pharmacologic doses.[33] Progesterone induces the enzyme 17-hydroxysteroid dehydrogenase in endometrial cells. This enzyme complex converts estradiol to estrone. Progestins diminish the estrogenic effect on target cells by inhibiting augmentation of estrogen cytosol receptors, which ordinarily modulate estrogen action. These influences account for the antimitotic antigrowth impact of progestins on the endometrium.[33] In the treatment of oligomenorrhea, withdrawal flow can be initiated by a progestational agent such as medroxyprogesterone acetate (10 mg daily for 10 days/month). If this regimen fails to induce bleeding, further evaluation is necessary. In the treatment of menometrorrhagia or polymenorrhea, progestins are prescribed for 10 to 14 days to induce stromal stability, which is followed by a withdrawal flow.

During an acute anovulatory bleeding episode, the bleeding may be controlled with a 50-μg estrogen-progestin oral contraceptive. Therapy consists of one pill taken four times daily for 1 to 5 days. If this dosage does not cause the menstrual flow to cease, a diagnosis other than anovulation must be considered, including the presence of myomas or polyps. If the flow diminishes significantly or abates predictably, the oral contraceptive should be tapered down to once per day for the remainder of the 21-day cycle, after which withdrawal flow occurs.

Intermittent vaginal bleeding frequently is associated with lower circulating estrogen levels and resultant breakthrough bleeding. Progestins do not control this type of bleeding. Such bleeding is common in the adolescent patient in whom there has been prolonged anovulation leading to persistent desquamation and leaving little residual endometrial tissue. Therefore, estrogen therapy must be administered before progestin therapy. In cases of acute or heavy uterine bleeding, intravenous conjugated estrogens (15 to 25 mg) may be administered and repeated in 6 to 12 hours.[34] After the bleeding ceases, the patient may be placed either on cyclic combination estrogen-progestin oral contraceptives or on cyclic progestins. For patients in whom the bleeding is less dramatic, estrogen-containing oral contraceptives or oral conjugated estrogens (1.25 mg orally for 7 to 10 days) may be prescribed.

Physicians frequently encounter irregular bleeding in patients on long-standing oral contraceptive therapy or on medroxyprogesterone acetate (Depo-Provera). Irregular bleeding occurs in the first part of the cycle and may be secondary to decreased estrogen input, resulting in an unstable, atrophic endometrial lining. This irregular bleeding also occurs in 25% of patients on medroxyprogesterone for similar reasons. Cyclic estrogen in the form of conjugated estrogens (2.5 mg daily for 7 days during the cycle) should control this problem.

Antiprostaglandins act on the endometrial vasculature. The concentrations of prostaglandins E (PGE) and $F_{2\alpha}$ ($PGF_{2\alpha}$) increase progressively in the endometrium during the menstrual cycle. The prostaglandin synthetase inhibitors appear to decrease menstrual blood loss.[35] This may result from altering the balance between the platelet-proaggregating vasoconstrictor thromboxane (both A_2 and B_2) and the antiaggregating vasodilator prostacyclin. Whatever the exact mechanism, prostaglandin inhibitors diminish menstrual blood loss in adolescents, as well as the bleeding associated with chronic endomyometritis (as, for example, with intrauterine contraceptive device use). These compounds may be prescribed in conjunction with cyclic hormonal therapy. Commonly, they are initiated at the first sign of menses or with the first cramping episode at the time of menses and continued throughout the menstrual cycle.

Failure to respond to medical therapy usually occurs when progestins are used to control bleeding in patients with hypoestrogenic or desquamated endometrium. Dilation and curettage (D & C) is the last line of therapy in anovulatory irregular bleeding in the adolescent and is rarely necessary except in the patient with a known bleeding diathesis. In such patients, bleeding should be controlled immediately using D & C, after which appropriate medical therapy should begin. If bleeding persists, the physician should suspect an anatomic abnormality not identified during the D & C. Further diagnostic evaluation (e.g., hysteroscopy) should be considered.

In rare situations in which hormonal therapy is contraindicated or bleeding is excessive and uncontrollable, the use of gonadotropin-releasing hormone analogues (GnRHag) have been recommended, not only to decrease menorrhagia, but also to produce amenorrhea.[30, 36] McLauchlen et al. reported that, after 12 weeks of intranasal GnRHag (buserelin) treatment in four patients with menorrhagia, total menstrual blood loss decreased significantly by the second and third posttreatment cycle.[36]

The long-term prognosis for adolescents with irregular bleeding can be described as guarded at best. About 5% continue to have severe episodes of anovulatory bleeding and merit endocrinologic evaluation.[37] The importance of continued follow-up is illustrated by the results of a 25-year prospective evaluation of adolescents with DUB.[37] Of 291 patients, 60% continued bleeding for 2 years after initial onset. Persistent problems were noted in 50% of patients after 4 years and in 30% after 10 years.[37] Except in patients with blood dyscrasias, patients who had normal menses before irregular bleeding have a more favorable prognosis.

References

1. Emans SJH, Goldstein DP. Pediatric and Adolescent Gynecology. 3rd ed. Boston: Little, Brown, 1990.
2. Muram D. Pediatric and adolescent gynecology. In: Pernol ML, Benson RC (eds). Current Gynecologic and Obstetric Diagnosis and Treatment. Norwalk, CT: Appleton & Lange, 1991, pp 629–656.
3. Huffman JW, Dewhurst CJ, Capraro VJ. The Gynecology of Childhood and Adolescence. 2nd ed. Philadelphia: WB Saunders, 1981.
4. Huffman JW. Premenarchal vulvovaginitis. Clin Obstet Gynecol 1977; 20:581.
5. Muram D, Massouda D. Vaginal bleeding in children. Contemp Obstet Gynecol 1985; 27:41–52.
6. Capraro VJ, Bayonet-Rivera NP, Magosas I. Vulvar tumor in children due to prolapse of urethral mucosa. Am J Obstet Gynecol 1970; 108:572.
7. Mercer LJ, Mueller CM, Hajj SN. Medical treatment of urethral prolapse. Adolesc Pediatr Gynecol 1988; 1:182–184.
8. Dewhurst J. Lichen sclerosus of the vulva in childhood. Pediatr Adolesc Gynecol 1983; 1:149.
9. Muram D. Detecting and managing sexual abuse in children. Contemp Obstet Gynecol 1988; 31:34–48.
10. Muram D. Genital tract trauma in pre-pubertal children. Pediatr Ann 1986; 15:616–620.
11. Dewhurst J. Botryoid sarcoma of the cervix and vagina in children. In: Studd J (ed). Progress in Obstetrics and Gynecology. 3rd ed. Edinburgh: Churchill Livingstone, 1983, pp 151–157.
12. Dewhurst CJ. Practical Pediatric and Adolescent Gynecology. New York: Marcel Dekker, 1980.
13. Dewhurst Sir J. Female Puberty and Its Abnormalities. Edinburgh: Churchill Livingstone, 1984.
14. Zacharias L, Rand WM, Wurtman RJ. A prospective study of sexual development and growth in American

girls: The statistics of menarche. Obstet Gynecol Surv 1976; 31:325.

15. Grant DB. Vaginal bleeding in childhood. Pediatr Adolesc Gynecol 1983; 1:173.

16. Grant DB. Variations in the clinical and endocrine patterns of female precocious puberty. In: Cacciari E, Prader A (eds). Pathophysiology of Puberty. London: Academic Press, 1980.

17. Dickerman Z, Prager-Lewis R, Laron Z. Response of plasma LH and FSH to synthetic LH-RH in children at various pubertal stages. Am J Dis Child 1976; 130:634.

18. Andreotti RF, Zusmer NR, Sheldon JJ, Ames M. Ultrasound and magnetic resonance imaging of pelvic masses. Surg Gynecol Obstet 1988; 166:327–332.

19. Council on Scientific Affairs: Magnetic resonance imaging of the abdomen and pelvis. JAMA 1989; 261:420–433.

20. American College of Obstetricians and Gynecologists. Dysfunctional uterine bleeding. ACOG Technical Bulletin no. 134; Washington, D.C., 1985.

21. Sanfilippo J, Yussman M. Gynecologic problems of adolescence. In: Lavery J, Sanfilippo J (eds). Pediatric and Adolescent Obstetrics and Gynecology. New York: Springer-Verlag, 1985, p 61.

22. Mishell D. Abnormal uterine bleeding. In: Droegemueller W, Herbst AL, Mishell DR, Stenchever MA (eds). Comprehensive Gynecology. St Louis: CV Mosby, 1987, p 953.

23. Speroff L, Glass R, Kase N. Dysfunctional uterine bleeding. In: Clinical Gynecologic Endocrinology and Infertility. 4th ed. Baltimore: Williams & Wilkins, 1989, p 265.

24. Hallberg L, Hogdahl AM, Nilsson L, Ribrybo G. Menstrual blood loss—a population study: Variations at different ages and attempts to define normality. Acta Obstet Gynecol Scand 1966; 45:320.

25. Gidwani GP. Vaginal bleeding in adolescents. J Reprod Med 1984; 29:419.

26. McDonough PG, Ganett P. Dysfunctional uterine bleeding in the adolescent. In: Barrom BN, Belisle BS (eds). Adolescent Gynecology and Sexuality. New York: Masson, 1982.

27. Jones GS. Endocrine problems in the adolescent. Md State Med J 1967; 16:45.

28. Spellacy WN. Abnormal bleeding. Clin Obstet Gynecol 1983; 26:702.

29. Dunnihoo D. Abnormal uterine bleeding. In: Fundamentals of Gynecology and Obstetrics. Philadelphia: JB Lippincott, 1990, p. 543.

30. Claessens EA, Cowell CA. Acute adolescent menorrhagia. Am J Obstet Gynecol 1981; 139:277.

31. Walker RW, Gustavson LP. Platelet storage pool disease in women. J Adolesc Healthcare 1983; 3:264.

32. Nilsson L, Ribrybo G. Treatment of menorrhagia. Am J Obstet Gynecol 1971; 110:712.

33. Gurpide E, Gusberg SB, Tseng L. Estradiol binding and metabolism in human endometrial hyperplasia and adenocarcinoma. J Steroid Biochem 1976; 7:891.

34. DeVore GR, Owens O, Kase N. Use of intravenous Premarin in the treatment of dysfunctional uterine bleeding—double-blind, randomized control study. Obstet Gynecol 1982; 59:285.

35. Anderson AB, Haynes PJ, Guillebaud J, et al. Reduction of menstrual blood loss by prostaglandin-synthetase inhibitors. Lancet 1976; 1:774.

36. McLauchlen RI, Healy DL, Burger HG. Clinical aspects of LH/RH analogs in gynecology: A review. Br J Obstet Gynecol 1986; 93:431.

37. Southam AL, Richart RM. The prognosis for adolescents with menstrual abnormalities. Am J Obstet Gynecol 1966; 94:637.

CHAPTER 15

Dysmenorrhea and Pelvic Pain

GITA P. GIDWANI

MARSHA KAY

Pelvic pain is a frequent complaint in pediatric and adolescent females. This chapter discusses the causes of acute and chronic pelvic pain, as well as management of the patient with pelvic pain and dsymenorrhea.

The differential diagnosis of pelvic pain can be a clinical challenge. Stress and the coping mechanisms of the young adult and her family may exacerbate the intensity of the symptoms. In patients with recurrent abdominal pain who have a negative clinical evaluation, an acute surgical emergency may arise, and the health care team must be able to ask appropriate questions to determine the source of the pain.

ACUTE PELVIC PAIN

The causes of acute pelvic pain are outlined in Table 15–1. Gynecologic causes may be associated with the complications of intrauterine or tubal pregnancy; torsion, rupture, or hemorrhage of an ovarian cyst; or infection of pelvic organs (e.g., postabortal endometritis or acute pelvic inflammatory disease). Any adolescent or premenarchal female with acute pelvic pain must undergo a pelvic or rectal examination when acute pelvic pain is present; otherwise, a number of diagnostic possibilities may be missed.

Nongynecologic causes (e.g., appendicitis, volvulus of the bowel, intestinal obstruction, perforation of the bowel, mesenteric adenitis) will produce acute peritoneal irritation and may require immediate surgical intervention. Urinary tract lesions—acute cystitis, acute pyelonephritis, or a ureteral calculus—may present with acute pain. Rarer causes of acute pelvic pain include bone and joint infections

TABLE 15–1 ••• CAUSES OF ACUTE PELVIC PAIN IN ADOLESCENT FEMALES

Gynecologic causes
  Pregnancy complications (e.g., incomplete or threatened abortion, tubal pregnancy)
  Infections (e.g., postabortal endometritis or acute pelvic inflammatory disease)
  Ovarian cyst—rupture, torsion, or hemorrhage
  Obstructive anomalies of the müllerian duct system (e.g., hematocolpos, complete transverse vaginal septum)
Nongynecologic causes
  Gastrointestinal causes
    Acute appendicitis
    Volvulus
    Meckel's diverticulitis
    Intestinal obstruction
    Mesenteric adenitis
    Regional enteritis
    Ulcerative colitis
    Pancreatitis
  Urinary tract causes
    Acute cystitis
    Acute pyelonephritis
    Ureteral calculus
  Other causes
    Bone and joint infections of the sacrum, ileum, or hip
    Slipped femoral epiphysis
    Intraabdominal abscess

of the sacrum, ileum, or hip; a slipped femoral epiphysis; or an intraabdominal abscess.

An adequate history must be taken for any young female who presents in the office or emergency department with acute pelvic pain. Many times such patients are too frightened to provide a history of sexual activity or of missed or abnormal periods, especially if these questions are asked in the presence of an anxious parent. Measurement of vital signs, an abdominal examination to identify signs of peritoneal irritation or to rule out a palpable mass or tenderness, and a pelvic examination must be performed. In prepubertal patients or in patients in whom sexual activity has not occurred, a rectal examination may suffice.

Narrow vaginal speculums (e.g., small Pedersen) must be available for examination of young girls. Cultures for gonococcal and chlamydial organisms are obtained when necessary. The size of the uterus, the presence or absence of tenderness of the cervix and adnexa, and the presence or absence of an adnexal mass all provide support for the diagnosis.

The basic laboratory work must include a pregnancy test, complete blood cell count, urinalysis (with cultures if indicated), and determination of the erythrocyte sedimentation rate. A pelvic ultrasound may be useful to identify free fluid in the cul-de-sac, suspected pregnancy, or a leaking, torsed, or hemorrhagic ovarian cyst.

Management will depend on how definitive the clinical diagnosis is from the clinical examination. If the diagnosis is not clear, surgical intervention is necessary. Laparoscopy is increasingly being used for treatment of ectopic pregnancy and hemoperitoneum secondary to a ruptured corpus luteum cyst. Some acute conditions (e.g., urinary tract infection, pelvic inflammatory disease, gastroenteritis, and mesenteric adenitis) are treated medically. Further tests (e.g., a urogram) may be necessary to diagnose urinary calculi.

Patients in whom the diagnosis is not clear present a clinical dilemma. Examples include patients with clinical evidence suggestive of pelvic inflammatory disease but who are not responding to the appropriate antibiotic therapy and in whom cultures are negative; patients with a ruptured ovarian cyst or incomplete torsion of an ovarian cyst; and patients with questionable appendicitis. In these patients, according to Goldstein,[1] laparoscopic examination and definitive treatment prevent long periods of inpatient observation and pain

and also avoid surgical catastrophes (e.g., a ruptured ectopic pregnancy or a ruptured appendix). The patient can also be discharged quickly after the laparoscopy and can resume scholastic and athletic activities within 48 to 72 hours.

According to data from Boston Children's Hospital collected between 1980 and 1986, 47% of 121 laparoscopy patients had some complications related to ovarian cysts, 11% had appendicitis, and in 17%, no abnormality was found.[2]

Whitworth et al.,[3] in a study of female patients, suggested that a diagnostic laparoscopy should be considered for young women with suspected appendicitis, even when classic signs and symptoms are present. The surgical risk involved in laparoscopy with general anesthesia is low. As such surgical procedures become more common, endoscopic appendectomy may indeed become the procedure of choice, even in acute cases.

RECURRENT ABDOMINAL PAIN

Recurrent abdominal pain (RAP) is defined as lower abdominal pain of at least 3 months' duration that has disrupted both school and social life and is not relieved by a non-narcotic analgesic. The patient has usually been evaluated in the emergency department or physician's office at least three times with no definitive diagnosis.

In 1959, Apley and Naish reported that 10% to 15% of pediatric and adolescent females presented with recurrent abdominal pain,[4] but they were able to identify an organic origin of the pain in only 1 of 20 patients. Since 1959, advances in endoscopy have aided in determining an organic cause in a significant percentage of patients. Apley noted that an organic cause must be ruled out before the patient can be considered "functional." Obviously not all patients will fit into the "organic" or "psychogenic" category; some are best managed by reassurance and the use of other available consultants, as necessary.

CHRONIC PELVIC PAIN

Chronic pelvic pain (CPP) in adult gynecologic patients has been similarly defined as noncyclical pelvic pain of greater than 6 months duration that is not relieved by non-

TABLE 15–2 ••• CAUSES OF RECURRENT ABDOMINAL PAIN IN ADOLESCENT FEMALES

Gynecologic causes
   Dysmenorrhea
   Mittelschmerz
   Pelvic inflammatory disease
   Endometriosis
   Müllerian obstructive anomalies
   Ovarian cysts
Nongynecologic causes
   Lactose malabsorption
   Chronic constipation
   Giardiasis
   Crohn's disease
   Irritable bowel syndrome
   Unusual causes
      Meckel's diverticulum
      Midgut malrotation
      Schönlein-Henoch purpura
      Acute intermittent porphyria
      Ureteropelvic junction obstruction
   Abdominal wall trigger points
   Psychogenic causes

narcotic analgesics. CPP is a very nonspecific term that includes pain associated with laparoscopically evident abnormalities (e.g., endometriosis), nongynecologic somatic pathologic abnormalities (e.g., irritable bowel syndrome), and nonsomatic "psychogenic" disorders. In adult patients, CPP accounts for a significant number of laparoscopies and hysterectomies. The direct and indirect costs of this syndrome have been estimated to be $2 billion annually.[5] Aggressive management of RAP in the female adolescent can prevent her from becoming an adult with CPP.

More than 100 entities can present with abdominal pain. The more common conditions are listed in Table 15–2.

DYSMENORRHEA

The literal translation of the term *dysmenorrhea* means "difficult menstrual flow." Primary dysmenorrhea is painful menstruation in the absence of gross pathologic conditions of the pelvic organs. Secondary dysmenorrhea denotes painful menstrual periods in the presence of gross pathologic conditions of the pelvic organs (e.g., endometriosis, salpingitis, or congenital anomalies of the müllerian system).

Incidence

Andersch and Milsom[6] noted that dysmenorrhea was reported by 72% of 19-year-old women from an urban Swedish population. The scoring system used for dysmenorrhea is shown in Table 15–3 and may be of assistance in planning additional questionnaire studies. Table 15–4 shows the prevalence and severity of dysmenorrhea in Andersch and Milsom's population sample.[6] It can be noted that 15.4% of the responders said that their menstrual cycle limited daily activity; however, 27.6% had no dysmenorrhea. There was a significant correlation between the severity of dysmenorrhea, the duration of menstruation, and the quantity of menstrual flow as assessed by the respondents. There was no significant difference in the prevalence and severity of dysmenorrhea between nulliparous women and women in whom pregnancy had been terminated by induced or spontaneous abortion. The prevalence and severity of dysmenorrhea in parous women were significantly lower. This study also noted that a total of 50.9% of the respondents had missed time from work or school as a result of dysmenorrhea.[6]

Only 31% of these women had been evaluated by a physician for dysmenorrhea. The authors believed that failure to report dysmenorrhea to a physician was a result of women's acceptance of dysmenorrhea as normal or their belief that treatment was not available.

Another epidemiologic study of dysmenorrhea was completed by Klein and Litt.[7] This consisted of a survey of a representative cross section of a "national probability sample" based on a study of 22 million, noninstitutionalized adolescents aged 12 to 17 years. The data were collected between 1966 and 1970 by the National Center for Health Statistics. Of the approximately 7000 adolescents surveyed, 2699 were menarchal. The prevalence of dysmenorrhea was striking: 59.7% reported discomfort or pain in connection with menstrual periods. Of those reporting pain, 14% described it as severe, 37% as moderate, and 49% as mild. The prevalence of dysmenorrhea increased with chronologic age, from 39% for 12-year-olds to 72% for 17-year-olds. Dysmenorrhea also increased with sexual maturity, from 38% of those at Tanner stage III to 66% at Tanner stage V, and from 31% at gynecologic age 1 to 78% at gynecologic age 5.

Of the total sample, 14% frequently missed school because of menstrual pain, and of those with severe dysmenorrhea, 50% reported missing school. Although black adolescents reported no increased incidence of dysmenorrhea, they were absent from school more frequently than whites because of dysmenor-

TABLE 15–3 ••• VERBAL MULTIDIMENSIONAL SCORING SYSTEM FOR ASSESSMENT OF DYSMENORRHEA

Grade	Working Ability	Systemic Symptoms	Analgesics
Grade 0: Menstruation is not painful, and daily activity is unaffected.	Unaffected	None	Not required
Grade 1: Menstruation is painful but seldom inhibits normal activity; analgesics are seldom required; mild pain.	Rarely affected	None	Rarely required
Grade 2: Daily activity affected; analgesics required and give sufficient relief so that absence from work or school is unusual; moderate pain.	Moderately affected	Few	Required
Grade 3: Activity clearly inhibited; poor effect of analgesics; vegetative symptoms (e.g., headache, fatigue, nausea, vomiting, and diarrhea); severe pain.	Clearly inhibited	Apparent	Poor effect

From Andersch B, Milsom I. An epidemiologic study of young women with dysmenorrhea. Am J Obstet Gynecol 1982; 144:655.

rhea, even when socioeconomic status was taken into account. Only 14.5% of the adolescents with dysmenorrhea had ever sought help for this problem. Interestingly, 30% of parents were not aware of their daughter's dysmenorrhea.

In Widholm and Kanter's study, the frequency of dysmenorrhea in Finnish adolescents aged 13 to 20 years ranged from 36% to 56%, with an overall school absence rate of 23.4%.[8] Thus, it is apparent from American, Swedish, and Finnish studies that a significant number of adolescents suffer from dysmenorrhea and many do not consult a health care provider. The reason for this can probably be understood by an historical review of dysmenorrhea.[9]

History and Pathogenesis

The discovery of prostaglandins by Pickles,[10] as well as intrauterine studies by Ackerland et al.,[11] proved that menstrual pain was not a myth, but a condition that could be treated with specific agents—namely, nonsteroidal anti-inflammatory drugs (NSAIDs).[12]

Prostaglandins and Their Pharmacology

The precursor for the synthesis of prostaglandins is arachidonic acid, an essential fatty acid that is derived from dietary sources and is stored primarily in cell plasma membranes. Any type of thermal, mechanical, or chemical stimulus is thought to cause the release of arachidonic acid from the depots, leading to the synthesis of prostaglandins. In the uterus, these prostaglandins are formed by two different enzyme systems: the cyclooxygenase pathway, which results in formation of prostaglandins, and the lipoxygenase pathway, which produces a series of monohydroxy acids and leukotriene products (Fig. 15–1).[13]

The cyclooxygenase pathway of arachidonic acid metabolism has been well studied. This pathway produces the classic prostaglandins—PGE_2, PGD_2, and $PGF_{2\alpha}$—as well as thromboxanes and prostacyclin. All of these products have potent and diverse physiologic activities, many of which are opposing (e.g., vasoconstriction vs. vasodilation and smooth muscle contraction vs. relaxation). It is the cyclooxygenase enzyme system that becomes compromised when patients are treated with NSAIDs.

The second pathway by which arachidonic

TABLE 15–4 ••• DYSMENORRHEA PREVALENCE AND SEVERITY

	Number of Patients	Percentage
Grade 0	162	27.6
Grade 1	201	34.3
Grade 2	133	22.7
Grade 3	90	15.4

From Andersch B, Milsom I. An epidemiologic study of young women with dysmenorrhea. Am J Obstet Gynecol 1982; 144:655.

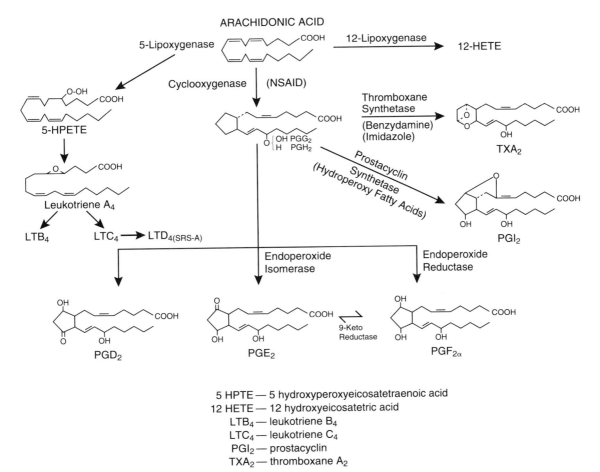

FIGURE 15–1 ••• Metabolism of arachidonic acid. (From Dawood MY, McGuire JL, Demers LM [eds]. Premenstrual Syndrome and Dysmenorrhea. Munich: Urban & Schwarzenberg, 1985. © 1985, Williams & Wilkins Co., Baltimore.)

acid is converted to prostaglandins is the lipoxygenase pathway. In this synthetic process, the leukotrienes, extremely potent smooth muscle–stimulating substances, are the end product. Several forms of lipoxygenase systems exist in cells. The 5-lipoxygenase and 12-lipoxygenase compounds are the two most prevalent in tissues and cells and catalyze the oxidation of arachidonic acid to one of two monohydric acids: 5-hydroperoxyeicosatetraenoic acid (5-HPETE) or 12-hydroperoxyeicosatetraenoic acid (12-HPETE). 5-HPETE ultimately gives rise to the leukotrienes, which can affect uterine activity. Currently it is believed that in the 30% to 40% of patients with dysmenorrhea who do not respond to cyclooxygenase inhibitors, the contribution of the lipoxygenase pathway may produce the symptoms of dysmenorrhea.

It is important to note that prostaglandins are not stored, and their de novo synthesis is

the reason they are found in tissues and biologic fluids when menstruation starts. These substances are rapidly bioinactivated, and the enzymes involved in the biodegradation of $PGF_{2\alpha}$ and PGE_2 are widely distributed throughout the body.[14–16] A major increase in prostaglandin release generally occurs within the first 36 to 48 hours of the onset of menses; as illustrated in Figure 15–2, this increase in uterine prostaglandins coincides with the loss of hormonal support of the endometrial lining. The source of prostaglandins is believed to be the human endometrium, which can synthesize both $PGF_{2\alpha}$ and PGE_2.[14–16]

Diagnosis

Primary Dysmenorrhea

It is imperative to differentiate primary from secondary dysmenorrhea. Primary dysmenor-

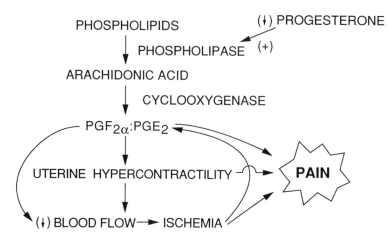

FIGURE 15–2 •• Prostaglandins in dysmenorrhea. (From Dawood MY, McGuire JL, Demers LM [eds]. Premenstrual Syndrome and Dysmenorrhea. Munich: Urban & Schwarzenberg, 1985. © 1985, Williams & Wilkins Co., Baltimore.)

rhea has characteristic features that must be obtained in the history. Primary dysmenorrhea occurs 6 to 12 months after menarche, when ovulatory cycles have been established. The onset of symptoms dates back to menarche or shortly thereafter. Patients who present with what seems to be primary dysmenorrhea but in whom the onset of symptoms occurred later in life usually have an organic cause (e.g., endometriosis [secondary dysmenorrhea]). The duration of dysmenorrhea is usually 48 to 72 hours. The pain begins characteristically with or after the beginning of the menstrual flow. If it starts before the period begins, it usually occurs several hours before the onset of menstrual flow. Dysmenorrhea that starts 2 or 3 days before the period is not primary dysmenorrhea and usually has an organic cause.[13]

The pain is typically described as crampy, spasmodic, labor-like, and localized over the lower abdomen and the suprapubic region. It sometimes may be described as a dull ache or a stabbing feeling. The pelvic examination is normal. A rectal examination, which can be performed with ease even in a tense, nervous adolescent, is an integral part of the evaluation, as abnormalities of the müllerian system will be easily missed without this examination. Thus, primary dysmenorrhea must be differentiated from all other causes of secondary dysmenorrhea.

Secondary Dysmenorrhea

The causes of secondary dysmenorrhea are shown in Table 15–5. This type of dysmenorrhea usually occurs a few years after menarche. The pain may start 1 or 2 days before menses, and the pelvic examination may reveal a num-

ber of signs (e.g., nulligravid retroverted uterus, adnexal tenderness, or an ovarian cyst).[14] A family history of endometriosis must alert the physician to the possibility of endometriosis in a teenager.[15] A past history of pelvic inflammatory disease (PID) or the use of any type of intrauterine device should indicate a probable diagnosis of secondary dysmenorrhea. Dyspareunia, infertility, dysmenorrhea, or heavy menstrual periods suggest organic disease.[16] Adequate laboratory tests, an abdominopelvic sonogram, and cultures from the cervix must be performed. Definitive diagnosis can almost always be established with diagnostic laparoscopy.[17]

Treatment

The general measures include reassurance and educational counseling. Mild analgesics and a simple explanation to allay anxiety after an adequate evaluation will help the patient cope with mild symptoms. Narcotic analgesics should not be routinely prescribed because of the high risk of abuse.

TABLE 15–5 •• CAUSES OF SECONDARY DYSMENORRHEA

Endometriosis
Pelvic inflammatory disease
Adenomyosis
Uterine polyps, uterine myomas
Congenital obstructive müllerian malformations
Cervical stricture or stenosis
Ovarian cysts
Pelvic adhesions

TABLE 15–6 ••• PROSTAGLANDIN SYNTHETASE
INHIBITORS

Carboxylic acids (type I)
  Salicylic acid esters (e.g., aspirin, Diflunisal
    [Dolobid])
  Acetic acids (e.g., indomethacin [Indocin],
    sulindac [Clinoril], tolmetin [Tolectin],
    diclofenac [Voltaren])
  Propionic acids (e.g., ibuprofen [Motrin, Advil,
    Nuprin, Rufin], feroprofen [Nalfon], naproxen
    [Naprosyn], naproxen sodium [Anaprox],
    ketoprofen [Orudis], suprofen [Suprol],
    flurbiprofen [Ansaid])
  Fenamic acids (e.g., mefenamic acid [Ponstel],
    meclofenamate [Meclomen], tolfenamic acid,
    flufenamic acid)

Enolic acids (type II)
  Pyrazolones (e.g., phenylbutazone [Butazolidin])
  Oxicans (e.g., piroxicam [Feldene])

NSAIDs

Prostaglandin synthetase inhibitors have had a profound impact on the treatment of primary dysmenorrhea.[18] They are considered NSAIDS in large part because they reduce the edema and erythema associated with inflammation. They are potent antipyretic agents, act as antithrombotic agents (i.e., inhibit the production of prostaglandins, which mediate the aggregatory response of these blood elements), and are extremely potent analgesic agents.[19] The two classes—carboxylic acids (type I) and enolic acids (type II)—are shown in Table 15–6. The type I prostaglandin synthetase inhibitors inhibit cyclooxygenase enzymes and therefore block the conversion of arachidonic acid to cyclic endoperoxides. Type II inhibitors tend to decrease isomerase and reductase enzyme activity and therefore prevent the conversion of cyclic endoperoxide to prostaglandins. Because cyclic endoperoxides are more potent than prostaglandins in their uterotonic effects, it is preferable to use type I inhibitors in the treatment of dysmenorrhea.

The doses of various NSAIDs are included in Table 15–7, and their side effects are shown in Table 15–8. Although all NSAIDs have the common property of inhibiting prostaglandin synthesis, a given NSAID may have different enzymatic activity associated with different tissue sources and for this reason may exhibit varying pharmacologic properties in the laboratory and in clinical practice. Thus, aspirin is a good antipyretic but lacks effective antiinflammatory action and may increase menstrual flow; therefore, it is less often used in the treatment of dysmenorrhea. The varying se-

verity of side effects of these drugs also determines their frequency of use. For example, indomethacin provides excellent relief of pain but has a number of side effects and thus is not commonly prescribed.

Ibuprofen and naproxen have been widely used in clinical practice.[20, 21] A trial of mefenamic acid (Ponstel) is useful when propionic acids are ineffective. Fenamates are potent inhibitors of prostaglandins and can antagonize the action of already-synthesized prostaglandins.[22] NSAIDs have definite advantages over oral contraceptives, as they are administered for only 2 or 3 days. Their success has confirmed the role of prostaglandins as the major factor in the etiology of dysmenorrhea. In the adolescent patient, a trial of 6 months, with necessary changes in dose and compound, usually proves effective.

NSAIDs reduce not only uterine hypercontractility, but also other side effects of dysmenorrhea (e.g., dizziness, nausea, and vomiting). The high rate of success with NSAIDs has made them the first line of treatment in the therapy of dysmenorrhea. However, there is a persistent, low treatment failure rate with NSAIDs in some patients, suggesting that there may be other mediators (e.g., leukotrienes) involved in this disorder.

Oral Contraceptives

Oral contraceptives have been known to prevent menstrual cramps. In an adolescent who is sexually active, an oral contraceptive will have the dual function of preventing pregnancy and treating dysmenorrhea. In clinical practice, a trial period of 2 to 3 months of oral contraceptives for the control of dysmenorrhea will demonstrate whether the patient is going to respond. If the patient does not respond to the use of NSAIDs or oral contraceptives, then an aggressive evaluation, including a diagnostic laparoscopy, should be performed to rule out an organic cause.[14]

Other Treatment Measures

After an anomaly has been ruled out by the use of laparoscopy, other methods are available for the control of dysmenorrhea. Transcutaneous electrical nerve stimulation (TENS) was used in 32 female patients for two cycles and provided excellent relief in 42.4%.[23] Acupuncture has also been found to be successful in managing the pain of primary dysmenorrhea; in a study of 43 patients, 90.9% showed improvement after acupuncture treatment.[24]

TABLE 15–7 ••• CLINICAL TRIALS OF NSAIDs IN DYSMENORRHEA

Class	Number of Patients	Regimen	Pain Relief (% of Patients)
Salicylates			
Aspirin	92 (1978–1980)	500–650 mg qid	Slight to no effect
Acetic acids			
Indomethacin	278 (1975–1979)	25–50 mg tid	71–100
Declofenac sodium	35 (1981)	25 mg tid	69
Propionic acids			
Naproxen (NA†)	224 (1977–1983)	200–285 mg qid	61–90
Ibuprofen	245 (1974–1983)	400 mg tid	56–100
Ketoprofen	23 (1979)	50 mg tid	90
Suprofen	610 (1983)	200 mg qid	63–84
Fenamates			
Flufenamic acid	90 (1974–1979)	125–200 mg tid	77–100
Mefenamic acid	138 (1977–1983)	250–500 mg tid	59–95
Meclofenamate	18	Single dose	71
Butaphenenes			
Phenylbutazone		NA	NA
Oxyphenbutazone		NA	NA
Oxicans			
Piroxicam (Feldene)	68	20–40 mg	90

NA, No information available.
Modified from Dawood MY, McGuire JL, Demers LM (eds). Premenstrual Syndrome and Dysmenorrhea. Munich: Urban & Schwarzenberg, 1985. © 1985, Williams & Wilkins Co., Baltimore.

Calcium channel blockers (e.g., nifedipine and flunarizine) have been shown to reduce intrauterine pressure and are effective in dysmenorrheic patients.[25] However, other symptoms (i.e., nausea, vomiting, and diarrhea) were not relieved, suggesting that the effect of the medication was restricted to smooth muscle relaxation. The side effects associated with calcium channel blockers were severe, and therefore these agents have limited clinical utility. Further research to develop lipoxygenase inhibitors and leukotriene antagonists, in combination with cyclooxygenase inhibitors, may increase the success rate of medical therapy to 100%.

Treatment Considerations

Durant et al.[26] found that girls with increased life crisis events experienced greater severity of symptoms during the first month of therapy for dysmenorrhea when compared with the

TABLE 15–8 ••• SIDE EFFECTS OF NONSTEROIDAL ANTIINFLAMMATORY DRUGS

Gastrointestinal
Indigestion
Nausea
Constipation
Vomiting
Diarrhea

Central nervous system
Headache
Dizziness
Vision and hearing disturbances
Irritability
Drowsiness

Other
Allergic reactions (e.g., skin rash)
Bronchospasm
Hematologic disease
Renal dysfunction (e.g., fluid retention)

Modified from Dawood MY, McGuire JL, Demers LM (eds). Premenstrual Syndrome and Dysmenorrhea. Munich: Urban & Schwarzenberg, 1985. © 1985, Williams & Wilkins Co., Baltimore.

control population. As therapy was continued, however, life stresses ceased to have a significant influence on the severity of dysmenorrhea. Clinicians should encourage patients to eat an adequate diet, decrease caffeine and chocolate intake, exercise regularly, and seek professional help for unusual stresses in their lives. However, it is important to understand that having control over pain enables the teenager to deal more easily with other stresses. Thus, a very aggressive treatment approach for the control of dysmenorrhea is paramount.

Because primary dysmenorrhea is a cyclic phenomenon, treatment is necessary during each menstrual cycle. Indeed, as soon as treatment is discontinued, a number of these patients experience recurrence of symptoms.

DIAGNOSIS AND TREATMENT OF OTHER CAUSES OF PELVIC PAIN

Gynecologic Causes of Pelvic Pain

Mittelschmerz

Mittelschmerz is characterized by pain at the time of ovulation. The pain may be described as severe, as colicky, or as a dull ache and may be accompanied by a clear discharge or sometimes even bleeding. Pain usually lasts for 6 to 7 hours but may persist for as long as 48 to 72 hours. This condition can be very easily diagnosed by recording the dates of pain along with the dates of menstruation, or even by keeping a formal basal body temperature chart to demonstrate that the pain is cyclic and related to ovulation. Spillage of fluid from the ruptured ovarian follicle may be seen on ultrasound. The use of NSAIDs, or sometimes simply acetaminophen or another analgesic, will sufficiently relieve symptoms in most cases.

Pelvic Inflammatory Disease

PID has been noted with increasing frequency in the young population. Gonococcal and chlamydial organisms are primarily responsible. The clinician must have high index of suspicion for this entity so that appropriate cultures can be obtained from the cervix in adolescents with lower abdominal pain, vaginal discharge, and dysuria.

Kleinhaus et al.[27] performed diagnostic laparoscopy in 50 girls aged 12 to 15 years to evaluate abdominal pain that was severe enough to warrant hospitalization. Twenty-three (46%) had had previous episodes of salpingitis but had negative cultures at the time of admission; 18 (36%) had no significant past medical history and totally normal physical findings. Laparoscopy established the diagnosis of PID in 28 of these patients; in the 32 patients in whom a specific preoperative diagnosis of PID was considered, laparoscopy proved to be incorrect in 15. Symptoms were relieved in all patients in whom laparoscopy resulted in a specific treatment, and there was no mortality or morbidity.

Adolescents with RAP and in whom PID is suspected must receive a laparoscopic examination of the pelvis in either of the following clinical situations:

1. Diagnosis of recurrent PID established without positive cervical cultures or other objective signs and symptoms.
2. Aggressive treatment for culture-proven PID for 4 to 7 days but continued significant pelvic pain and symptoms.

Jacobsen and Westrom objectively measured the accuracy of clinical diagnosis of pelvic pain and found that when laparoscopy was used, the positive predictive value for salpingitis was 70%.[28] Sellers et al.[29] demonstrated that the routine use of diagnostic laparoscopy was a valuable supplement to evaluation when negative cultures were obtained by endometrial and fimbrial minibiopsy. Thus, laparoscopy is of definite benefit to accurately diagnose PID.

Because the cost of undiagnosed PID, which results in subsequent infertility, may be particularly high in the adolescent patient, the cost and risk-to-benefit ratio of the laparoscopic procedure must be weighed when considering this surgical procedure in adolescents. Conversely, adolescents should not be diagnosed with "chronic PID" without adequate documentation. This subject is further discussed in Chapter 41.

Endometriosis

Endometriosis in the adolescent was not well known before the publishing of articles in the late 1970s.[16, 17] Adolescent endometriosis has been described by the authors previously.[14]

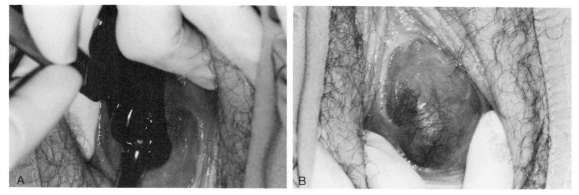

FIGURE 15–3 ••• *A*, Hematocolpos in a 12-year-old white female who presented with abdominal pain. She had been seen by her pediatrician five times, 3 to 4 weeks apart, with no major physical findings on abdominal examination. This time an abdominal mass was palpated, and a pelvic examination revealed a bulging membrane with no hymenal opening. Incision and drainage of 600 ml of thick, tarry blood was done in surgery, with disappearance of the mass (*B*).

This entity as a cause of chronic pelvic pain is discussed in Chapter 41.

Müllerian Obstructive Anomalies

Müllerian obstructive anomalies may be missed for a long time in an adolescent complaining of acute or chronic recurrent pain (Figs. 15–3 and 15–4). The obstructive anomalies may be missed unless one does a pelvic examination to rule out such anomalies. Goldstein et al.[16] showed that müllerian anomalies had been missed for a long time in patients with chronic pelvic pain, and these anomalies were discovered only on a laparoscopic examination. See Chapter 41 for further discussion of these patients.

Ovarian Cysts

Ovaries with multifollicular cysts measuring 3 to 4 cm are common in adolescent patients. They are caused by a burst of gonadotropins at the level of the "gonadostat"; such gonadotropins frequently have not become cyclic, as in the adult. A number of these young patients present with persistent discomfort and large, tender multifollicular ovaries, whereas other patients are totally asymptomatic. Occasionally, acute rupture or complete or partial torsion of a cyst may occur. Usually these patients can be managed using reassurance and observation consisting of several ultrasounds; a few may require judicious use of antiprostaglandins or oral contraceptives to relieve discomfort. If at all possible laparotomy with cystectomy for functional cysts must be avoided, as this will give rise to pelvic adhesions (see Chapter 41).

Nongynecologic Causes of Pelvic Pain

Gastrointestinal and urologic sources of chronic abdominal pain may be difficult to distinguish from those of gynecologic origin.

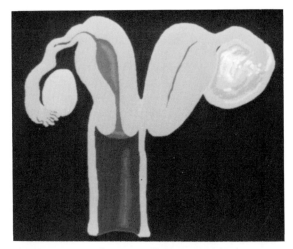

FIGURE 15–4 ••• Illustration of the reproductive tract in a 15-year-old white female who had severe, incapacitating dysmenorrhea since menarche at age 12 years. She had a difficult psychosocial history and had been seen for psychological counseling after her dysmenorrhea did not respond to antiprostaglandins and oral contraceptives. She was referred to a gynecologist by the counselor. An ultrasound revealed a didelphic uterus with noncanalization of the hemiuterus. The patient had a hemihysterectomy, as she had developed hematometra and hematosalpinx in the obstructed uterus.

Recurrent abdominal pain is thought to affect at least 10% of school age children, but only 10% of these cases are reported to physicians.[30] Several studies have shown a female predominance.[31]

Nonorganic pain is usually periumbilical and is characterized by a family medical history of functional gastrointestinal problems. The length and severity of attacks are often not helpful in elucidating the cause.[31] Differentiating between gastrointestinal and gynecologic origins of chronic abdominal pain is particularly difficult in an adolescent female.

Lactose Malabsorption

One common cause of gastrointestinal pain is lactose malabsorption.[32] This disorder affects between 5% and 20% of the population and is increased in certain ethnic or national groups, including blacks and Italians. Lactose malabsorption is characterized by abdominal pain, excess flatus, diarrhea, and bloating. Most patients seem to benefit from lactose withdrawal from their diet. This benefit, however, is not limited to those who are lactose malabsorbers; patients who are lactose absorbers also seem to benefit from lactose withdrawal. Lactose absorption is best evaluated by a breath hydrogen test. After a standard oral lactose load (usually 2 gm/kg, to a maximum of 50 gm), serial analyses of breath hydrogen samples are performed. An increase of more than 10, and especially of more than 20 parts per million (ppm) from the baseline, confirms lactose malabsorption and suggests that a dietary trial of lactose withdrawal may be warranted.[32] If lactose malabsorption is not indicated by the results of this test, a second confirmatory test, a lactulose tolerance test, is performed. Lactulose is a nonabsorbable disaccharide, and after administration of a standard lactulose load, breath hydrogen analysis should reveal an increase of at least 10 to 20 ppm. This test is used to detect individuals who cannot produce significant amounts of hydrogen in the colon and hence do not excrete it in their breath, and thereby it helps to eliminate false-negative results. It confirms that a negative breath hydrogen test indeed represents normal lactose absorption.

Chronic Constipation

A second cause of chronic abdominal pain that is often confused with pain of gynecologic origin is chronic constipation. The true incidence of this disorder is difficult to elucidate, although a significant number of individuals are affected. Chronic constipation may be determined by a history of infrequent bowel movements or of straining with bowel movements. Some younger children also develop overflow incontinence with chronic constipation, and a history of fecal soiling should be elicited as part of the history. This diagnosis can often be established on physical examination. Important confirmatory tests include rectal motility to evaluate the degree of distention in the rectum and to rule out a diagnosis of Hirschsprung's disease. Rectal motility may also be the initial step in the use of biofeedback therapy to assist these patients in overcoming their abdominal pain. Some authors have noted a decrease in the frequency of attacks of recurrent abdominal pain with the addition of dietary fiber; the mechanism is thought to be an alteration in chronic transit time.[33]

Irregular bowel habits may be a component of some gynecologic disorders including endometriosis, and the presence of constipation does not exclude other intraabdominal or intrapelvic abnormality.[34]

Giardiasis

The incidence of both symptomatic and asymptomatic *Giardia* infection is highly variable. It may represent a significant pathogen in young children, especially those who attend day-care centers.[35] Other individuals at risk include family members of children attending day-care facilities, travelers, refugees, swimmers in contaminated water, campers, and individuals who are immunodeficient.[36] The clinical presentation is highly variable and may be characterized by acute enteritis or a persistent and relapsing diarrhea. The patient may also have abdominal distention, nonspecific cramping, flatulence, and failure to thrive. Occasionally, patients will develop urticaria or bronchospasm related to *Giardia*.[36] The diagnosis is best established by serial stool cultures obtained on three separate occasions with examination for ova and parasites. A small-bowel biopsy may also be required for diagnosis. Individuals who have contact with contaminated water should be considered at risk for this disorder. Treatment is with quinacrine, metronidazole, or furazolidone. Treatment may be repeated if necessary.

Crohn's Disease

Crohn's disease is a serious cause of abdominal pain that may be missed without serial follow-up of patients, as evidenced by long-term studies performed at the Mayo Clinic.[37] On retrospective review of an outpatient population evaluated between 1950 and 1973, researchers found that the mean age at onset of symptoms of Crohn's disease was 11.6 years. However, there was a mean diagnostic delay of 9.5 months.[37] Although Crohn's disease is characterized by abdominal pain, diarrhea, weight loss, anorexia, fever, impaired growth, and joint symptoms, up to 7% of patients may present with isolated abdominal pain. Others may present with amenorrhea. Failure to gain weight appropriately on a height-to-weight basis and poor progression through the Tanner stages are clinical evidence suggestive of Crohn's disease. Many patients have a family history of either ulcerative colitis or Crohn's disease, especially in first-degree relatives, as has been demonstrated in studies from the Cleveland Clinic Foundation.[38]

The presence of Crohn's disease may be suggested by abnormal results on screening laboratory tests, including a complete blood cell count and erythrocyte sedimentation rate. A rectal examination should be performed to check for occult blood in every patient with recurrent abdominal pain. Many patients undergo surgery for abdominal pain and cramps before the correct diagnosis of Crohn's disease is made.

Irritable Bowel Syndrome

Irritable bowel syndrome may be a cause of recurrent abdominal pain in the older adolescent or young adult. It is especially prevalent in patients who present for gynecologic evaluation.[39] Patients characteristically have an altered bowel habit alternating between constipation and diarrhea. Dietary therapy that includes additional fiber may provide symptomatic relief in these patients. It is important to establish that the abdominal distention is not related to menses and that the pain is long-standing. Irritable bowel syndrome must be excluded if there is any evidence of blood on examination, if the patient has undergone previous bowel resection, or if a diagnosable organic disease is found.

Esophagitis, Gastritis, and Duodenitis

In the past, these conditions were often unable to be diagnosed using standard gastrointestinal radiographs. However, the development of fiberoptic endoscopy and its subsequent application to pediatrics have enabled diagnosis of these problems in children and adolescents. Tam and Saing[40] retrospectively reviewed 533 endoscopies performed in children over a 13-year period; in 34%, the indication was abdominal pain. They found that 22% of the patients had esophagitis, gastritis, duodenitis, or ulcerative disease. There was no endoscopy-related mortality in this series,[41] and difficulty in establishing a diagnosis occurred in only two infants with tracheoesophageal fistula. In children, unlike in adults, historical findings alone may not suggest this diagnosis because of the child's inability to localize the abdominal pain or determine precipitating or exacerbating factors. Tam et al.[41] reviewed their 18-year experience with peptic ulcer disease, predominantly chronic duodenal ulcers, in children. Forty-six percent of their patients had a history of epigastric pain, and of these, only 43% (one fourth of the total patients) had typical "ulcer pain." In fact, the location of the pain may lead to diagnostic errors. Five children with perforated duodenal ulcers presented with right lower quadrant pain and were thought preoperatively to have appendicitis.[41]

The development of endoscopy has led to a high accuracy rate in establishing the appropriate diagnosis in patients with abdominal pain. Nord et al.[42] did a retrospective review of children ultimately noted to have peptic ulcer disease. In patients who underwent upper gastrointestinal (UGI) series before endoscopy, 50% of gastric ulcers and 11% of duodenal ulcers were not detected. However, endoscopy provided an accurate diagnosis in 97% of these patients. In one patient with a duodenal ulcer, the endoscope could not be passed to visualize the ulcer because of a deformed duodenal bulb; that ulcer was diagnosed by UGI study.

Although its pathologic role in the development of gastritis is controversial, some authors believe *Helicobacter pylori* to be a pathogen in children with recurrent abdominal pain. Bujanover et al.[43] retrospectively studied 14 children who underwent endoscopy for recurrent abdominal pain. Antral biopsies, Giemsa staining, and urease testing were performed in all patients. In 6 of the 14, endoscopically obtained stains were positive for *Helicobacter* gastritis. Two of the six also had duodenitis. After 10 days of amoxicillin therapy and 6 weeks of bismuth subsalicylate therapy, the abdominal pain resolved in all six, and they remained symptom free for a follow-up period of 6 months.

Uncommon Nongynecologic Causes of Abdominal Pain

Many uncommon causes of chronic or recurrent abdominal pain may mimic pain of gynecologic origin. These include both anatomic and nonanatomic abnormalities.

Meckel's Diverticulum. This is the most frequent congenital anomaly of the intestinal tract, occurring in 0.3% to 3% of the population. Patients with complications related to a Meckel's diverticulum are usually very young (i.e., less than 2 years). Approximately 55% of patients with Meckel's diverticulum have an abnormal mucosa within the diverticulum, with gastric mucosa found in 80% to 85%.[36]

Complications of a Meckel's diverticulum include bleeding, which can be diagnosed using a technetium scan with pentagastrin stimulation; obstruction caused by intussusception or volvulus; diverticulitis; or perforation. Pain may be secondary to ulceration of the normal intestine adjacent to the diverticulum. This cause of abdominal pain occasionally has an acute onset. A large number of patients with a Meckel's diverticulum are asymptomatic, and the condition is discovered at autopsy.

Midgut Malrotation. Another unusual cause of abdominal pain that may present with chronic cramping is midgut malrotation.[44] In a retrospective review at Texas Children's Hospital, of 16 children older than 6 weeks of age who were operated on for midgut malrotation, the mean patient age was 4 years, with an age range of up to 15 years. Approximately half of these patients presented with chronic abdominal pain or vomiting. Another clue to the presence of malrotation was visible peristalsis. The pain was characteristically intermittent, and symptoms had been present for a mean duration of 6 months. Symptoms were often related to partial duodenal obstruction with the presence of Ladd's bands, and symptoms resolved postoperatively. Appropriate evaluation of these patients includes a UGI series with small-bowel follow-through.

Schönlein-Henoch Purpura. This disease is characterized by purpura, arthritis, and abdominal pain with or without glomerulonephritis.[45] Abdominal pain is present in two thirds of patients and may be severe or colicky. Up to 10% of patients may undergo exploratory laparotomy before the diagnosis is established. Fifty percent of patients have heme-positive stools, and 30% have melanotic stools. The abdominal pain of Schönlein-Henoch purpura may develop before the characteristic rash. This disease may also be complicated by intussusception or massive gastrointestinal bleeding, and early diagnosis is imperative. Older children seem to have an increased severity of the disease when compared with toddlers. Abdominal radiographs may reveal the characteristic thumbprinting, scalloping patterns. Corticosteroids have been prescribed for this disorder, with mixed results.[46]

Acute Intermittent Porphyria. This is an autosomal dominant disorder with an increased incidence in females. The onset characteristically is in late puberty or early adulthood; it is caused by diminished uroporphyrin synthetase activity. Precipitating factors, which may be found in 75% of patients, include the use of barbituates or sulfonamides, premenstrual segment of the cycle, infection, fasting, and alcohol consumption.

Acute intermittent porphyria is characterized by recurrent attacks of neurologic, abdominal, and psychologic symptoms. The attacks may last several days, with intervening asymptomatic periods. Patients also experience constipation and associated vomiting. In some, a history of pain or paresthesias in the extremities may be elicited, and up to 20% of patients may have tonic-clonic seizures related to this disorder. If the disorder goes undiagnosed, death may occur from respiratory paralysis or cardiac arrhythmia secondary to "sympathetic overdrive." Therapy consists of avoidance of precipitating factors. A correct diagnosis is important to reduce long-term morbidity.[47]

Abdominal Epilepsy. Some authors have described abdominal epilepsy as a very rare cause of recurrent abdominal pain. The pain is characteristically paroxysmal, abrupt in onset, located in the mid to upper abdomen, and associated with autonomic phenomena and mental status changes.[48] Patients have postictal symptoms after the attack and then are able to resume normal activity. The characteristic electroencephalogram finding is a spike wave pattern with a temporal lobe focus. The existence of this disorder is controversial, and its actual prevalence in pediatric patients is difficult to determine. A response to anticonvulsant medication is required for the diagnosis to be considered correct.[49]

Ureteropelvic Junction Obstruction. Although this is an uncommon cause of recurrent abdominal pain, occurring in fewer than 1% of patients evaluated for this disorder, abdominal pain as an isolated finding is not an uncommon presentation and may occur in up to 70% of patients older than 1 year. The abdominal pain is nonspecific and may radiate to the groin, upper quadrants, and flanks. Only a small percentage of patients have gross hematuria associated with this disorder. The problem is usually unilateral, with the left side affected more often than the right. However, in up to 20% of patients, the condition is bilateral, and the diagnosis of ureteropelvic junction obstruction on the opposite side may occur later than on the first. The condition is caused by intrinsic anomalies at the ureteropelvic junction, including adherent vessels, fibrous bands, and kinks. The diagnosis is readily established with an intravenous pyelogram, and a high index of suspicion is required.[50]

Psychogenic Disorders. There is preliminary evidence to suggest that recurrent and chronic abdominal pain may also be the result of a psychogenic disorder and may represent an altered response to the normal everyday stresses of life. Some studies have found that children with recurrent abdominal pain are likely to have a history of manifesting stress as gastrointestinal disorders (e.g., preschool stomachaches).[51] However, there is no evidence to suggest an increased incidence of psychosis in these children or a disrupted social environment. However, these patients do have a high incidence of a family history of functional gastrointestinal disorders.

ABDOMINAL WALL TRIGGER POINTS

Slocumb,[52] in a study of 122 chronic pelvic pain patients, found that the single most common area of pain is the abdominal wall. Needle localization was used to identify sources of pain in the fat and fascial planes above the aponeurosis in these patients. The tender points generated the majority of pain experienced in 90% of his series of patients. Tension of the rectus muscle, produced either by ele-

vating both legs or by lifting the head and shoulder, exacerbated the abdominal wall pain, because the tender points were pressed against the firm rectus muscles.[53]

Diagnosis and treatment of focal tender points in the abdominal wall by infiltration of local anesthetic (e.g., 1% procaine or 0.25% bupivacaine) has been shown to block this pain. Slocumb found that pain relief lasted for days or months, beyond the duration of the local anesthetic. This therapeutic modality has also been combined with the use of antidepressants and nonsteroidal antiinflammatory agents, as well as psychologic counseling whenever necessary.

During the examination the physician should try to elicit any abdominal trigger points in patients with chronic pain. The workup of patients with chronic pain can be accomplished in a stepwise fashion.

Patient History

One should begin by asking the patient to describe the pain, localizing it, and then soliciting information regarding factors that aggravate pain. If the pain is related to endometriosis, a cluster of symptoms, at least in the early stages, seem to occur around the menstrual cycle or at the time of ovulation.

A careful history of bowel function will elucidate irritable bowel symptoms. Manning et al.[54] administered a questionnaire listing 156 different symptoms, to 109 selected patients. Four symptoms—distention, relief of pain with bowel movement, loose and frequent bowel movements with onset of pain and mucus, and a sense of incomplete evacuation—were commonly seen in patients with irritable bowel. A guaiac test is recommended, and if the sedimentation rate is increased, the possibility of inflammatory bowel disease (e.g., Crohn's disease) must be kept in mind. The physician should note the presence of hard stool at the time of physical examination. This helps in counseling the patient regarding constipation as a possible cause of pain.

The physician should also try to elicit any history of bulimia and anorexia nervosa. The patient with anorexia nervosa can easily be diagnosed if she is at least 25% below her expected body weight, has an intense fear of gaining weight and a distorted body image, and has missed at least three consecutive menstrual periods. The patient with bulimia, on the other hand, may be very outgoing, sociable, sexually active, have normal periods, and be very secretive about her symptoms of binging. Associated findings include recurrent bouts of depression, low self-esteem, and substance abuse. The binging and purging puts these patients at risk for chronic constipation and laxative dependence, dental erosion and caries, and esophageal irritation along with electrolyte imbalance.

Denial of symptoms by the patient and sometimes by the family is characteristic. Again, diagnosis can only be established if the physician suspects an eating disorder and tries to obtain a history, which may not be available until the second or third visit.

It is also important to elicit any history of lactose intolerance, constipation, drinking of large amounts of carbonated drinks or iced tea, or gum chewing. A musculoskeletal examination, which may involve a straight leg–raising test and compression of different trigger points, must also be done.

Most importantly in the evaluation of chronic abdominal or pelvic pain, the workup must proceed in a stepwise and directed manner. Initial screening examinations should include a complete blood cell count with differential, determination of erythrocyte sedimentation rate, liver function tests, urinalysis with culture, amylase determination, plain film abdominal radiograph, stool cultures for ova and parasites, stool guaiac test, measurements of height and weight recorded on growth charts, and gynecologic examination. Secondary evaluation may include breath hydrogen tests, determination of lead levels, lipoprotein electrophoresis, porphyrin determinations, intravenous pyelography, UGI series with small-bowel follow-through, and barium enema.

An ultrasound of the pelvis is very commonly used in the evaluation of these patients. Ultrasound will ordinarily identify any major müllerian abnormalities but will not reveal endometriosis or PID unless these are accompanied by a large ovarian abscess or endometrioma. On the other hand, an ovarian cyst 1 to 2 cm in diameter in such a patient can lead to the belief that the cyst is causing the pain. However, the cyst may not account for the symptoms. It is therefore important that physicians be selective with respect to appropriate diagnostic testing. Laparoscopic examination and other gastrointestinal endoscopy are necessary in a number of these patients.

Management

Often these patients are angry and frustrated, because they have seen many physicians, have had numerous tests, and usually have missed a considerable amount of scholastic and extracurricular activities. Parents and teachers can become overprotective. Generally physicians should avoid recommending tutoring at home or giving special permits (e.g., notes to excuse the patient from physical fitness activities). It is best to complete the evaluation as quickly as possible and, as stated earlier, in a stepwise fashion. The physician must place the adolescent in proper perspective with respect to emotional development as related to her chronologic age. For example, a 16-year-old who is dependent on her mother will need to be followed until late adolescence.

Every attempt must be made to rule out organic causes by using noninvasive tests and, if necessary, by endoscopic examination of the gastrointestinal tract and liberal use of the laparoscope.

An adolescent should never be told, "The pain is in your head" or "You'll grow out of it" and then referred for psychiatric evaluation when the condition has an organic cause. Similarly, when a history of sexual or physical abuse is obtained or a triggering event (e.g., the death of a parent or friend) is noted, a search still must be undertaken to rule out organic causes that may have been causing the pain. After the workup has been completed, patients can be managed according to the specific cause.

Depression in the adolescent can also be associated with abdominal pain. Formal psychiatric treatment with antidepressants may be necessary. Depending on the diagnosis, methods of pain reduction may include biofeedback, stress management, and self-hypnosis. These modalities are used effectively by neurologists and other specialists to manage chronic degenerative disease of the back and migraine headaches. A psychogenic cause of abdominal pain is truly a diagnosis of exclusion.

Long-term follow-up and availability of the physician for any type of emergency situation is a necessity in the management of patients with abdominal pain. The goal of the health care team is to diagnose the cause of pain and allow the adolescent to resume normal activity. Recurrent pelvic pain is a pervasive problem in pediatric and adolescent patients and requires aggressive evaluation, often with a multidisciplinary approach, to arrive at the correct diagnosis and appropriate treatment.

References

1. Goldstein DP. Acute and chronic pelvic pain. Pediatr Clin North Am 1989; 36:573.
2. Emans SJ, Goldstein DP. Pelvic pain, dysmenorrhea, and the premenstrual syndrome. In: Emans SJ, Goldstein DP (eds). Pediatric and Adolescent Gynecology. 3rd ed. Boston: Little, Brown, 1989, p 273.
3. Whitworth CM, Whitworth PW, Sanfilippo J, Polk HC. Value of diagnostic laparoscopy in young women with possible appendicitis. Surg Gynecol Obstet 1988; 167(3):187–190.
4. Apley J, Naish N. Recurrent abdominal pain: A field survey of disease in childhood. Arch Dis Child 1958; 33:165.
5. Reiter RC. Chronic pelvic pain. In: Pitkin RM, Scott JR (eds). Clinical Obstetrics and Gynecology. Philadelphia: JB Lippincott, 1990, p 117.
6. Andersch B, Milsom I. An epidemiologic study of young women with dysmenorrhea. Am J Obstet Gynecol 1982; 144:655.
7. Klein J, Litt J. Epidemiology of adolescent dysmenorrhea. Pediatrics 1981; 68(5):661.
8. Widholm O, Kanter RC. Menstrual patterns of adolescent girls according to the chronological and gynecological ages. Acta Obstet Gynecol Scand 1971; 50(suppl 14):30.
9. Gidwani G. Dysmenorrhea—myths and facts. Cleve Clin Q 1983; 50:567.
10. Pickles VR. Prostaglandins and dysmenorrhea—historical survey. Acta Obstet Gynecol Scand 1979; 87(suppl 58):7.
11. Ackerland M, Anderson KF, Ingemarsson I. Effects of terbutaline on myometrial activity, uterine blood flow and lower abdominal pain in women with primary dysmenorrhea. Br J Obstet Gynecol 1976; 38:673–678.
12. Schwartz A, Zor U, Lindner HR, Naor S. Primary dysmenorrhea alleviation by an inhibitor or prostaglandin synthesis and action. Obstet Gynecol 1974; 44:709–712.
13. Dawood MY, McGuire JL, Demers LM (eds). Premenstrual Syndrome and Dysmenorrhea. Baltimore-Munich: Urban & Schwarzenberg, 1985.
14. Gidwani GP. Treating endometriosis in the adolescent. Contemp OB/GYN 1989; 33(4):75.
15. Malinak LR, Buttram VC, Jr, Elias S, et al. Heritable aspects of endometriosis. Am J Obstet Gynecol 1980; 137:332–337.
16. Goldstein DP, deCholnoky C, Leventhal JM, Emans S. New insights into the old problem of chronic pelvic pain. J Pediatr Surg 1979; 14:675–680.
17. Chatman DL, Ward AB. Endometriosis in adolescents. J Reprod Med 1982; 27:156–160.
18. Jacobsen J, Cavalli-Bjorkman K, Lundstrom V, et al. Prostaglandin synthetase inhibitors and dysmenorrhea—a survey and personal clinical experience. Acta Obstet Gynecol Scand 1979; 87(suppl 1):73.
19. Dawood MY. Dysmenorrhea and prostaglandins: Pharmacological and therapeutic considerations. Drugs 1981; 22:42.
20. Chan WY, Fuchs F, Powell AM. Effects of naproxen sodium on menstrual prostaglandins and primary dysmenorrhea. Obstet Gynecol 1983; 61:285.
21. Jacobsen J, Lundstrom V, Nilsson B. Naproxen in treatment of OC resistant primary dysmenorrhea. Acta Obstet Gynecol Scand [Suppl] 1983; 113:87.
22. Smith RP, Powell JR. Simultaneous objective and subjective evaluation of meclofenamate sodium in the treatment of primary dysmenorrhea. Am J Obstet Gynecol 1987; 157(3):611.
23. Dawood MY, Ramos J. Transcutaneous electrical nerve stimulation (TENS) for the treatment of primary dysmenorrhea—a randomized crossover comparison with placebo, TENS and ibuprofen. Obstet Gynecol 1990; 75(4):656–660.
24. Helms JM. Acupuncture for the management of primary dysmenorrhea. Obstet Gynecol 1987; 69(1):51–56.
25. Pasquale SA, Rathauser R, Dolese HM. A double blind placebo controlled study comparing three single dose regimens of piroxicam with ibuprofen in patients with primary dysmenorrhea. Am J Med 1988; 84(5A):30.
26. Durant RH, Jay MS, Shoffith T. Factors influencing adolescents for dysmenorrhea. Am J Dis Child 1985; 139:489.
27. Kleinhaus S, Hein K, Sheran M. Laparoscopy for diagnosis and treatment of abdominal pain in adolescent girls. Arch Surg 1977; 112:1178–1179.
28. Jacobsen L, Westrom L. Objectivized diagnosis of acute pelvic inflammatory disease. Am J Obstet Gynecol 1969; 105:1088.
29. Sellers J, Mahony J, Goldsmith C, et al. The accuracy of clinical findings and laparoscopy in pelvic inflammatory disease. Am J Obstet Gynecol 1991; 164:113–120.
30. Pineiro-Carrero V, Andres J, Davis R, et al. Abnormal gastroduodenal motility in children with recurrent functional abdominal pain. J Pediatr 1988; 113:820–825.
31. Poole S. Recurrent abdominal pain in childhood and adolescence. Am Fam Physician 1984; 30:131–137.
32. Blumenthal I, Kelleher J, Littlewood J. Recurrent abdominal pain and lactose intolerance in childhood. Br Med J 1981; 282:2013–2014.
33. Feldman W, McGrath P, Hodgson C, et al. The use of dietary fiber in the management of simple childhood idiopathic recurrent abdominal pain. Am J Dis Child 1985; 139:1216–1218.
34. Gidwani G. Endometriosis more common than you think. Contemp Pediatr 1989; 6:99–110.
35. Ish-Horowicz M, Korman S, Shapiro M, et al. Asymptomatic giardiasis in children. Pediatr Infect Dis J 1989; 8:773–779.
36. Korman S, Deckelbaum R. Giardiasis in children—diagnosis and treatment. Resident Staff Physician 1989; 35:61–65.
37. Castile R, Telander R, Cooney D, et al. Crohn's disease in children: Assessment of the progression of disease, growth and prognosis. J Pediatr Surg 1980; 15:462–469.
38. Farmer RG, Michener WM, Mortimer EA. Studies of family history among patients with inflammatory bowel disease. Clin Gastroenterol 1980; 9:271–277.
39. Hogston P. Irritable bowel syndrome as a cause of chronic pain in women attending a gynecology clinic. Br Med J 1987; 284:934–935.
40. Tam P, Saing H. Pediatric upper gastrointestinal endoscopy: A 13 year experience. J Pediatr Surg 1989; 24:443–447.

41. Tam P, Saing H, Lav J. Diagnosis of peptic ulcer in children: The past and present. J Pediatr Surg 1986; 21:15–16.

42. Nord K, Rossi T, Lehenthal E. Peptic ulcer in children. Am J Gastroenterol 1981; 75:153–157.

43. Bujanover Y, Konikoff F, Baratz M. Nodular gastritis and helicobacter pylori. J Pediatr Gastroenterol Nutr 1990; 11:41–44.

44. Brandt M, Pokorny W, McGill C, et al. Late presentation of mid gut malrotation in children. Am J Surg 1985; 150:767–771.

45. Goldman L, Lindenberg R. Henoch-Schoenlein purpura. Am J Gastroenterol 1981; 75:357–360.

46. Rosenblum N, Winter H. Steroid effects in the course of abdominal pain in children with Henoch-Schoenlein purpura. Pediatrics 1987; 79:1018–1021.

47. Pattison C, Haynes I. Acute intermittent porphyria. Practitioner 1984; 22:420–421.

48. Peppercorn M, Herzog A. The spectrum of abdominal epilepsy in adults. Am J Gastroenterol 1989; 84:1294–1296.

49. Singhi P, Kaur S. Abdominal epilepsy misdiagnosed as psychogenic pain. Postgrad Med J 1988; 64:281.

50. Byrne W, Arnold W, Stannard M, et al. Ureteropelvic junction obstruction presenting with recurrent abdominal pain—a diagnosis by ultrasound. Pediatrics 1985; 76:934–937.

51. McGrath P, Goodman J, Firestone P, et al. Recurrent abdominal pain: A psychogenic disorder? Arch Dis Child 1983; 58:888–890.

52. Slocumb JC. Neurologic factors in chronic pelvic pain: Trigger points and abdominal pelvic pain syndrome. Am J Obstet Gynecol 1984; 149:536.

53. Thomson WH, Dawes RF, Couter SS. Abdominal wall tenderness: A useful sign in chronic abdominal pain. Br J Surg 1991; 78(2):223–225.

54. Manning AP, Thompson WG, Heaton KW, Morris AF. Towards positive diagnosis of irritable bowel. Br Med J 1978; 11:653–654.

CHAPTER 16

Androgens and the Adolescent Girl

JOSÉ F. CARA

ROBERT L. ROSENFIELD

Androgen excess during childhood and adolescence produces a variety of clinical signs and symptoms that must be appropriately recognized, evaluated, and treated. Hyperandrogenism must be considered in any female with premature development of pubic hair, premature or excessive development of acne, menstrual irregularity (whether it be oligomenorrhea or dysfunctional uterine bleeding), or obesity. The most common cause of hyperandrogenism presenting in a teenage girl is the syndrome of polycystic ovaries (PCO). However, the differential diagnosis includes "exaggerated adrenarche," late-onset congenital adrenal hyperplasia, intersexuality, virilizing tumors, Cushing's syndrome, hyperprolactinemia, acromegaly, and abnormalities of cortisol metabolism. This chapter will discuss current concepts of androgen physiology, advances in understanding the etiology of hyperandrogenic disorders, and recommendations for diagnosis and treatment of hyperandrogenism in childhood and adolescence.

ANDROGEN PHYSIOLOGY AND PATHOPHYSIOLOGY

Androgen Biosynthesis

Steroid hormone biosynthesis involves the sequential enzymatic processing of cholesterol to form one of five possible end products: progestins, mineralocorticoids, glucocorticoids, androgens, and estrogens (Fig. 16–1).[1] Although only the adrenal cortex and gonads secrete steroids, other tissues (including liver, adipose tissue, and skin) contain enzymes that allow for the further processing of steroids synthesized within the adrenal gland and gonads.[2–4] Although steroid hormone biosynthesis requires many steps, there are only a relatively small number of enzymes in the steroid biosynthetic cascade, many of which can perform more than one sequential reaction. These enzymes have been purified and cloned, and most have been determined to be members of the cytochrome P-450 group of oxidases localized within the mitochondria or endoplasmic reticulum of steroidogenic tissues.[1] Like other P-450 enzymes, these require the presence of flavoproteins (such as adrenodoxin, adrenodoxin reductase, or cytochrome P-450 reductase) for the transport of electrons to and from their respective substrates. Others, including Δ^5-isomerase-3β-hydroxysteroid dehydrogenase (3β-HSD) and 17-ketosteroid oxidoreductase, are non–P-450 steroidogenic enzymes located within the membranes of the endoplasmic reticulum.

As with other steroid hormones, the first step in the biosynthesis of androgens begins with side chain cleavage of cholesterol to pregnenolone by P-450$_{scc}$ (Figs. 16–1, 16–2), an enzyme mediating the three chemical reactions involved in side chain cleavage. This is a tropic hormone–dependent step and is rate limiting

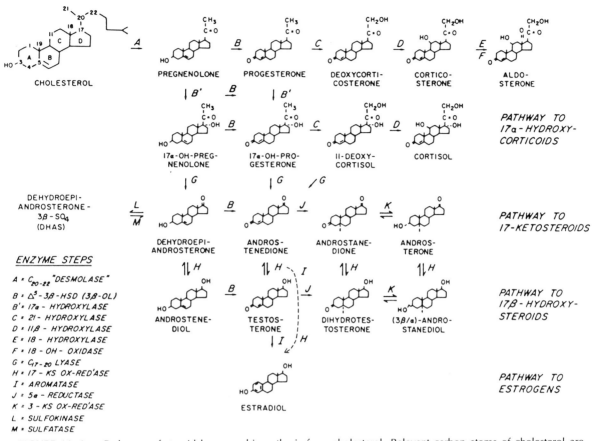

FIGURE 16–1 ••• Pathways of steroid hormone biosynthesis from cholesterol. Relevant carbon atoms of cholesterol are designated by conventional numbers; rings are designated by letters. The flow of hormonogenesis is generally downward and to the right. The first line shows the pathway to progestins and mineralocorticoids, the second line the pathway to glucocorticoids, the third line the pathway to 17-ketosteroids, and the fourth line to androgens. The bottom and dotted lines indicate the pathways to estrogen (the long dotted line involves the 17-keto-estrogen, estrone [not shown] as an intermediate). The terms *desmolase* and *lyase* are often used interchangeably, as are the terms *hydroxysteroid dehydrogenase* and *ketosteroid (oxido) reductase*. HSD, Hydroxysteroid dehydrogenase; KS, ketosteroid; OH, hydroxy. (From Rosenfield RL. The ovary and female sexual maturation. In: Kaplan SA [ed]. Clinical Pediatric Endocrinology. 2nd ed. Philadelphia: WB Saunders, 1989, p 259.)

for the secretion of all steroid hormones.[1] P-450$_{c17}$, which possesses both 17α-hydroxylase and 17,20-lyase (desmolase) activities, is a key enzyme that is also dependent on tropic hormones and is rate limiting for the formation of its products.[1, 5] In the adrenal cortex, it controls a branch point of steroid hormone biosynthesis because of its ability to direct formation of either glucocorticoids or sex steroids. In the case of androgen biosynthesis, P-450$_{c17}$ mediates conversion of pregnenolone by a two-step chemical reaction involving 17α-hydroxylation (to 17-hydroxypregnenolone) followed by 17,20-lyase activity (to dehydroepiandrosterone (DHEA).[3] Alternatively, pregnenolone may first be converted to progesterone by 3β-HSD before being 17α-hydroxylated to form

17-hydroxyprogesterone by P-450$_{c17}$. 17-Hydroxyprogesterone is the key precursor for both glucocorticoids and, via 17,20-lyase activity, androstenedione.[1, 6–9]

DHEA and androstenedione are 17-ketosteroids synthesized by both the adrenal glands and the gonads. They have important functions as prohormones, because they can be converted in peripheral tissues to form testosterone and other androgens.[2, 8] Furthermore, in the gonads, androstenedione is the major precursor for both testosterone and estrogen synthesis; it is converted by the enzyme 17-ketosteroid oxidoreductase to form testosterone or is aromatized by P-450$_{arom}$ to form estrogen.[10]

In women, the ovaries and adrenal glands normally contribute about equally to testoster-

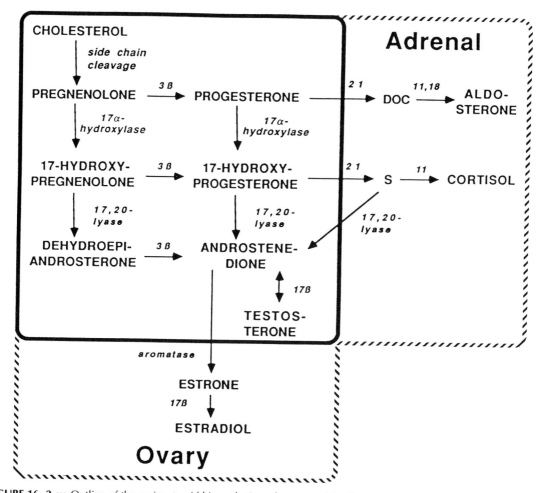

FIGURE 16–2 ••• Outline of the major steroid biosynthetic pathways used by the gonads and the adrenal glands. The area enclosed by the solid line contains the core steroidogenic pathway used by both the ovaries and the adrenal glands. The areas enclosed by the dotted lines contain the steroidogenic pathways utilized specifically by the ovaries and adrenal glands, as indicated. The Δ^5 path is in the left column; the Δ^4 path is in the right column. Both sets of glands have some 5α-reductase activity and thus secrete small amounts of dihydrotestosterone (not shown). DOC, deoxycorticosterone; S, 11-deoxycortisol. The steroidogenic enzymes are italicized: *3β*, 3β-hydroxysteroid dehydrogenase; *21*, 21-hydroxylase; *11,18*, 11β-hydroxylase/18-hydroxylase-dehydrogenase; *17β*, 17β-hydroxysteroid dehydrogenase. (Modified from Ehrmann DA, Rosenfield RL. An endocrinologic approach to the patient with hirsutism. J Clin Endocrinol Metab 1990; 71:1–4. © 1990, by The Endocrine Society.)

one production.[8, 11] Approximately half of the total testosterone originates from direct secretion, and the other half is derived from peripheral conversion of secreted 17-ketosteroids. The major clinically important site of this peripheral conversion is the liver, but nonsplanchnic tissues also contribute.

Regulation of Androgen Secretion

Androgens are secreted by both the adrenal glands and the ovaries in response to their respective tropic hormones, adrenocorticotropic hormone (ACTH) and luteinizing hormone (LH).[1, 6, 9] Because androgens are, in a sense, by-products of estradiol and cortisol secretion by the ovary and adrenal gland, respectively, androgen levels in females are not under specific hormonal control; there is no sensitive negative feedback control by the pituitary gland as there is in the case of cortisol and estradiol secretion.

Adrenal Gland

Adrenal 17-ketosteroid secretion gradually begins during mid childhood as a result of adrenarche, an incomplete aspect of puberty in which maturational changes in adrenal steroid hormone synthesis make the adrenal cortex capable of secreting androgenic precursors.[10, 12] Although young children secrete as much cortisol in proportion to body size as adults, they form virtually no 17-ketosteroids.[6, 8, 13] During adrenarche, there is a change in the pattern of the adrenal secretory response to ACTH, with striking increases in 17-hydroxypregnenolone and DHEA production (Fig. 16–3).[13] As a result, DHEA sulfate (DHEAS, the sulfated derivative of DHEA) increases markedly at adrenarche, becoming the predominant androgen secreted by the adrenal gland (Fig. 16–4).[8, 13, 14]

The exact cause of the maturational changes underlying adrenarche is not clear. Both in vivo and in vitro data indicate that there are maturational increases in the 17-hydroxylase

and 17,20-lyase activities of $P-450_{c17}$ responsible for adrenal androgen production.[1, 13, 15, 16] These adrenarchal changes seem to be related in part to the development of the zona reticularis of the adrenal cortex, an adrenal zone that produces large amounts of DHEA and DHEAS.[15, 17–19] This zone has been postulated to originate from cells of the fetal adrenocortical zone that have failed to undergo involution. Its development as a continuous zone begins at about 6 years of age and correlates with the increasing DHEAS production.[19]

The nature of the factor or factors responsible for bringing about the adrenarchal change within the adrenal gland has been the subject of considerable controversy. A pituitary source of the putative adrenarche factor has been postulated,[20] and several substances have been implicated as being the pituitary hormone responsible for bringing about the adrenarchal

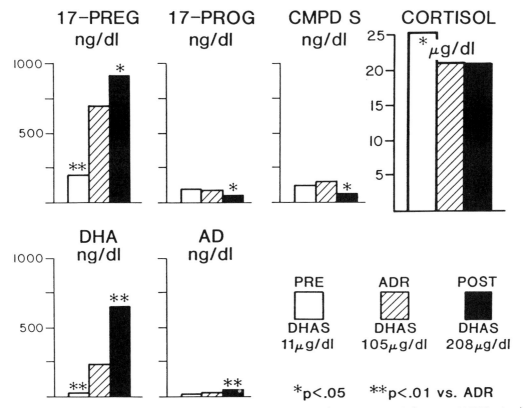

FIGURE 16–3 ••• Changing pattern of adrenal steroidogenic response to adrenocorticotropic hormone (ACTH) stimulation with maturation. Shown are the plasma steroid levels 30 minutes after a 10 μg/m² intravenous bolus of ACTH in prepubertal children (PRE), children with precocious adrenarche (ADR), and follicular phase adult females (ADULT). The layout is organized according to the biosynthetic pathway (see Figs. 16–1 and 16–2). Note that children with precocious adrenarche have 17-hydroxypregnenolone (17-PREG) and dehydroepiandrosterone (DHA) responses that are intermediate between those of prepubertal children and adults. AD, Androstenedione; CMPD S, 11-deoxycortisol; 17-PROG, 17-hydroxyprogesterone. (From Rosenfield RL. The ovary and female sexual maturation. In: Kaplan SA [ed]. Clinical Pediatric Endocrinology. 2nd ed. Philadelphia: WB Saunders, 1989, p 259.)

PLASMA DHAS IN RELATION TO MATURATIONAL STAGE

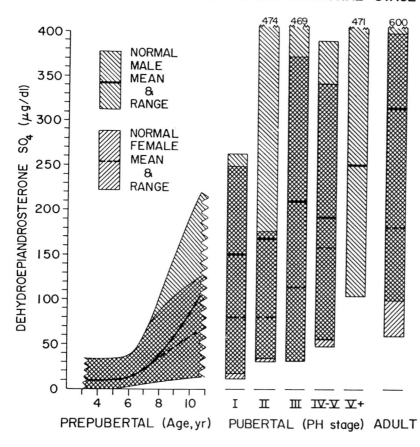

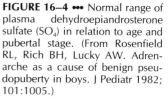

FIGURE 16–4 ••• Normal range of plasma dehydroepiandrosterone sulfate (SO_4) in relation to age and pubertal stage. (From Rosenfield RL, Rich BH, Lucky AW. Adrenarche as a cause of benign pseudopuberty in boys. J Pediatr 1982; 101:1005.)

change; these include cortical androgen-stimulating hormone and proopiomelanocortin-related peptides.[12, 20, 21] The fact that adrenarche represents a change in the steroidogenic response pattern of the adrenal gland to ACTH suggests that potential adrenarche factor(s) may control the growth and differentiation of the zona reticularis or regulate steroidogenic enzyme activity, especially the 17,20-lyase activity of P-450$_{c17}$.[6, 7, 13, 21, 22] Intraadrenal factors, such as estradiol, have also been postulated as potential adrenarchal factors, and they may function as modulators of adrenal steroidogenic enzyme activity.

In most individuals, adrenarchal androgen production becomes clinically apparent (as pubarche, the appearance of pubic hair) at about the same time as does true pubertal development (also called gonadarche). However, because the control mechanisms responsible for initiating adrenarche are different from those responsible for initiating puberty, adrenarche is sometimes not chronologically related to

true puberty. Adrenarche and gonadarche are dissociated in a variety of clinical conditions, including idiopathic premature puberty, gonadal dysgenesis, isolated gonadotropin deficiency, and constitutional delay of puberty.[14, 23] Whereas neither adrenal androgens nor corticoids are stimulated by gonadotropins,[24] DHEAS production is depressed moderately in hypogonadism, for reasons that are not clear.[25]

Ovary

The combined action of LH on theca-interstitial cells and of follicle-stimulating hormone (FSH) on ovarian granulosa cells is necessary for the development and maintenance of normal ovarian function. In the two-cell–two-gonadotropin theory of ovarian steroidogenesis (Fig. 16–5), androgenic precursors (especially androstenedione) produced by theca-interstitial (thecal) cells under LH stimulation are aromatized to estrogen by FSH-stimulated gran-

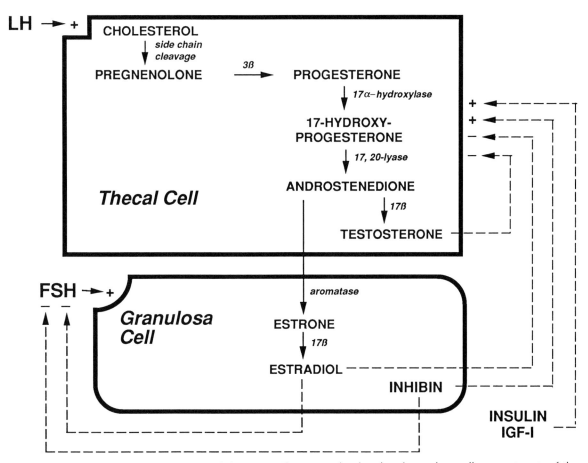

FIGURE 16–5 ••• Functional organization of the ovary. Shown are the thecal and granulosa cell compartments of the ovary with representative endocrine, paracrine, and autocrine factors that either stimulate (+) or inhibit (−) ovarian P-450$_{c17}$ activities. 3β, 3β-Hydroxysteroid dehydrogenase; 17β, 17β-hydroxysteroid dehydrogenase. (From Ehrmann D, Rosenfield RL, Barnes RB, et al. Detection of functional ovarian hyperandrogenism in women. N Engl J Med 1992; 327:157. Reprinted with permission of The New England Journal of Medicine.)

ulosa cell aromatase activity.[9, 26–28] Estrogens, acting in concert with FSH and LH, induce granulosa cell growth and follicular maturation.[27, 28] Androgens, in turn, through their atretogenic effect, limit the number of follicles that are allowed to mature and so may be involved in the selection of a single follicle for ovulation.[27–29] As the dominant follicle emerges, increased amounts of both androstenedione and estradiol are secreted, with the ratio favoring estradiol in healthy follicles.

Ovarian androgen production depends on LH stimulation of the thecal cell compartment of the ovary. The binding of LH to the LH receptor of these cells, a member of the G protein–coupled receptor family, increases intracellular adenylate cyclase, stimulating the activity of P-450$_{scc}$ and P-450$_{c17}$.[30] Thecal cell androstenedione production is thus directly

increased by LH. Because of the pubertal increase in LH secretion, ovarian androgen and estrogen secretion increases during puberty. However, the normal female pattern of gonadotropin response to gonadotropin-releasing hormone (GnRH) is one of relatively low LH and relatively high FSH,[24] thereby favoring estradiol secretion.

Androgens can be viewed as a necessary evil in the ovary. On one hand, they are obligate intermediates in the biosynthesis of estradiol (see Fig. 16–5).[9, 28] On the other hand, intraovarian androgens induce premature atresia of developing follicles.[31, 32] Atretic follicles are predominantly androgenic, as they are relatively deficient in aromatase activity.[9, 28, 33] Consequently, androgen-induced follicular atresia seems to result in further androgen production, producing a vicious cycle of hyperandrogenism. Therefore, it seems critical for the function of the ovary that intraovarian androgen concentration be kept to a minimum. It is not known how ovarian androgen secretion is minimized while the formation of estrogen is optimized, but because there is no long-loop feedback (via the pituitary) for specifically regulating ovarian androgen secretion, another mechanism must exist. It has been postulated that androgen excess is normally prevented primarily by the down-regulation process whereby excessive or protracted LH stimulation leads to intraovarian desensitization of the responses to LH at the level of P-450$_{c17}$.[6, 7]

A number of hormones and growth factors appear to be involved in the intraovarian modulation of steroidogenic responsiveness to LH (see Fig. 16–5). It is likely that estrogen inhibits this response by a short-loop (paracrine) negative feedback mechanism.[6, 7] Androgens, on the other hand, may well be inhibitory as the result of an autocrine mechanism.[7] These inhibiting modulators seem to be counterbalanced by hormones and growth factors that amplify 17α-hydroxylase and 17,20-lyase activities, including insulin, insulin-like growth factor I (IGF I), and inhibin,[34–36] among others.[9, 28]

Blood Levels and Transport of Androgens

The total plasma concentrations of androgens and intermediates in their biosynthesis are shown in Table 16–1.[8] Whereas plasma DHEAS levels normally reflect adrenal androgen production, plasma testosterone and androstenedione levels mirror both ovarian and adrenal androgen secretion.[8] Plasma 17-hydroxyprogesterone, like plasma testosterone and androstenedione, may arise from either the adrenal glands or ovaries. Of the circulating androgens, testosterone is the most important biologically and clinically because of its relatively high plasma concentration and potency at the target organ level.

More than 96% of the plasma testosterone and structurally related 17β-hydroxysteroids circulate in plasma bound to carrier proteins, with only a small fraction remaining free.[37, 38] Sex hormone–binding globulin (SHBG) and albumin are the principal sex steroid–binding proteins in plasma. Although there has been interest in the possibility that albumin-bound testosterone is bioactive, most evidence suggests that only the free steroid intermediate is

bioavailable.[39, 40] Because of SHBG's high binding affinity, SHBG concentration is the major determinant of the fraction of 17β-hydroxysteroids binding to plasma albumin and of the fraction remaining free and biologically active in blood.

SHBG is a glycoprotein synthesized in the liver.[38, 41] Isoelectric focusing studies have shown heterogeneity of the circulating forms, but the clinical significance of this finding is not known. SHBG is structurally homologous to a noncirculating androgen-binding protein synthesized in the Sertoli cells of the testis.[41] Its synthesis is modulated by a number of physiologic and pathologic states that ultimately affect its plasma concentration: SHBG levels are increased by estrogens and thyroid hormone excess and decreased by androgen, glucocorticoid, growth hormone and insulin.[38, 42] Because SHBG levels are often decreased in hyperandrogenic states and obesity, serum free testosterone levels are often elevated in women whose total testosterone levels are normal. Consequently, the plasma free testosterone concentration is elevated in women with hirsutism or acne more often than is the plasma total testosterone concentration, reflecting the truly elevated plasma concentration of bioavailable androgen.[43]

Mechanisms of Androgen Action

Testosterone exerts its biologic actions by binding to the androgen receptor of target tissues (Fig. 16–6). However, the biologic activity of testosterone depends in large part on its previous conversion to dihydrotestosterone (DHT), which has greater biologic potency than testosterone because of its higher affinity for and slower dissociation from the androgen receptor.[44]

The conversion of testosterone to DHT is mediated by the 5α-reductase activity of target tissues and liver.[45, 46] In skin, 5α-reductase activity resides primarily in sebaceous and sweat glands, as well as the dermis, rather than in hair per se. Plasma 3α-androstanediol glucuronide, a metabolite of DHT, has been touted as a marker of hypersensitivity of the hair follicle to androgen.[46] However, the extent to which this metabolite arises from hepatic or skin 5α-reductase activity is controversial.[46, 47] The conversion of testosterone and other precursors to DHT determines, to a significant

TABLE 16–1 ••• TYPICAL NORMAL RANGES FOR PLASMA ANDROGENS AND INTERMEDIATES*

	17-Hydroxy-pregnenolone (ng/dl)	17-Hydroxy-progesterone (ng/dl)	11-Deoxy-cortisol (ng/dl)	Cortisol (µg/dl)	DHEA (ng/dl)	Andro-stenedione (ng/dl)	Testosterone (ng/dl)
Prepubertal, 2–8 yr	<25–235	<25–65	<25–160	5–25	<25–120	<25–50	<15
Adrenarchal†	<25–355	<25–95	<25–120	5–25	100–420	30–75	10–45
Adult female	40–360	30–130‡	30–220	5–25	100–1000	55–200	20–75

*Normal range may differ slightly among laboratories.
†Children with premature adrenarche.
‡17-Hydroxyprogesterone increases in the preovulatory phase to peak as high as 360 ng/L in the luteal phase of the cycle.
From Rosenfield RL. Hyperandrogenism in peripubertal girls. Pediatr Clin North Am 1990; 37:1333.

extent, the expression of androgen action at the level of the pilosebaceous unit.[48, 49]

The androgen receptor has been cloned and the gene determined to be located on the X chromosome near the centromere between Xq13 and Xp11.[44] Together with the corticoid, estrogen, progesterone, and thyroid hormone receptor, as well as the v-*erb* A oncogene product, it forms part of a superfamily of nuclear receptors with homologous structures and similar modes of action.[50, 51] Androgen binding to the androgen receptor in the nucleus leads to an activated ligand-receptor complex that binds to acceptor sites on nuclear DNA,

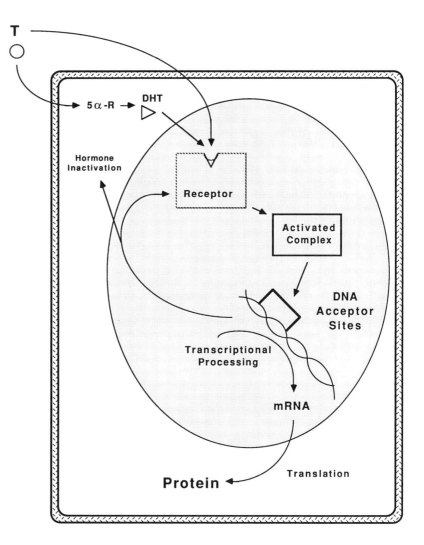

FIGURE 16–6 ••• Mechanism of action of testosterone on target cells. Testosterone (T) binds to its intracellular receptor directly or after its previous conversion to dihydrotestosterone (DHT). The resulting activated receptor complex binds to DNA acceptor sites, stimulating transcription and translation of specific genes. 5α-R, 5α-Reductase.

stimulating transcription of target genes and leading to increased protein synthesis. As expected in androgen target tissues, androgen receptors have been demonstrated in the pilosebaceous unit.[52] Studies have shown that genetic mutations in the androgen receptor can lead to quantitative or qualitative abnormalities in androgen receptor function, producing the various syndromes of androgen resistance.[53]

Cutaneous Manifestations of Androgen Excess

The cutaneous manifestations of androgen excess include hirsutism, acne, and balding.[54] However, these manifestations of hyperandrogenism are variably expressed; some patients have hirsutism or acne alone, others have both, still others have neither, or balding can be the sole symptom. Hyperandrogenemia should be suspected if there is premature development of pubic hair (before 8.5 years of age in girls) or hirsutism. It should also be considered if inflammatory acne appears before feminization at puberty, if acne is moderately severe during puberty, or if mild acne is persistent through the teenage years (Table 16–2).

Hair can be categorized as vellus hair or terminal hair.[22, 45] Vellus hair is fine, soft, and not pigmented, while terminal hair is long, coarse, and pigmented. Virtually all hair follicles are associated with sebaceous glands to form pilosebaceous units (PSUs). The growth of the hair follicle of PSUs is controlled by an as-yet-uncharacterized induction factor elaborated by the dermal papilla. In target areas,

androgens cause the prepubertal PSU to differentiate into either a sexual hair follicle (in which the vellus hair transforms into a terminal hair) or a sebaceous follicle (in which the sebaceous component proliferates and the hair remains vellus). Androgens are thus necessary for sexual hair and sebaceous gland development. Antiandrogens reverse this process, causing PSUs to revert to the prepubertal state.[45, 55] Male-pattern sexual hair development (for example, mustache and beard) occurs in sites where relatively high levels of androgen are necessary for PSU differentiation. The greater density of terminal hairs in the androgen-sensitive areas of men than in women is accounted for by a greater proportion of PSUs with terminal rather than vellus hairs. Male-pattern baldness is largely the result of conversion of terminal hair to vellus follicles.[45]

Hirsutism is defined as excessive male-pattern hair growth in women.[22] Hirsutism must be distinguished from hypertrichosis, which is the proper term to describe the excessive growth of androgen-independent hair, which is vellus, prominent in nonsexual areas, and most commonly familial or caused by metabolic disorders (e.g., thyroid disturbances, anorexia nervosa) or medications (e.g., phenytoin, minoxidil, or cyclosporine). In white women, hirsutism can be defined as a total score of 8 or more on the scale of Ferriman and Gallwey (Fig. 16–7). Thus, it is normal for women to have a few sexual hairs in "male" areas (e.g., mustache and beard).

An increase in plasma free testosterone concentration is responsible for half of the cases of mild hirsutism and a third of the cases of persistent mild acne in adolescents.[54] Moderately severe hirsutism or cystic acne is even more likely to be hyperandrogenic.[54, 56] However, it must be noted that sexual hair and sebaceous gland development seem to depend as much on the factors determining sensitivity of the PSUs to androgens as they depend on the plasma androgen level itself. At one end of the normal spectrum are women whose PSUs seem hypersensitive to normal blood free androgen levels; this seems to account for "idiopathic" hirsutism and acne. At the other end of the spectrum are women whose PSUs are relatively insensitive to androgen; this seems to account for "cryptic" hyperandrogenemia (hyperandrogenism without skin manifestations).

TABLE 16–2 ••• CLINICAL SCORING SYSTEM FOR ACNE VULGARIS*

Score	Class	Lesions
	Microcomedones	Comedones, <2 mm diameter
1	Minor	Comedones, 2 mm or greater (<10)
2	Mild	Comedones (10–20; pustular or nonpustular)
3	Moderate	Comedones (>20) or pustules (<20)
4	Severe	Pustules (>20)
5	Cystic	Inflammatory lesions >5 mm

*Face and trunk may be graded separately.
From Rosenfield RL. Hyperandrogenism in peripubertal girls. Pediatr Clin North Am 1990; 37:1333.

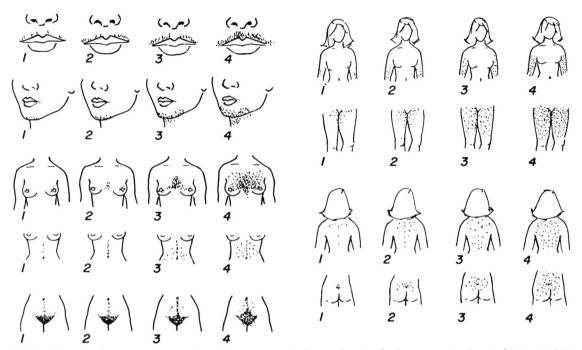

FIGURE 16–7 ••• Hirsutism scoring scale of Ferriman and Gallwey. The nine body areas possessing androgen-sensitive pilosebaceous units are graded from 0 (no terminal hair) to 4 (frankly virile) and totaled. (From Ehrmann DA, Rosenfield RL. An endocrinologic approach to the patient with hirsutism. J Clin Endocrinol Metab 1990; 71:1–4. © 1990, by The Endocrine Society.)

HYPERANDROGENIC DISORDERS

Androgen excess arises from abnormal adrenal or ovarian function in most cases, but occasionally from abnormalities in the peripheral formation of androgens. Functional abnormalities (Table 16–3) are much more common than neoplasms.

Adrenal Disorders

Premature Adrenarche

Normally, the first manifestation of the adrenarchal or gonadarchal increases in androgen production is pubarche, the appearance of pubic hair. Presexual pubic hair (Tanner II) appears in girls at 11.2 ± 1.1 (mean ± S.D.) years of age and sexual pubic hairs (Tanner III) appear at 11.9 ± 1.1 years of age.[8] Premature pubarche in girls refers to the appearance of sexual pubic hair before 8.5 years of age.

Premature pubarche is usually the result of premature adrenarche.[8, 14] That is, most children with the precocious onset of pubic hair

have undergone early maturation of adrenal androgen secretion. In others, less commonly, premature pubarche represents inordinate sensitivity of sexual hair follicles to normal adrenal androgen levels. The best hormonal indicator

TABLE 16–3 ••• CAUSES OF FUNCTIONAL HYPERANDROGENISM

Functional adrenal hyperandrogenism
  Premature adrenarche
  Exaggerated adrenarche/dysregulation
  Congenital adrenal hyperplasia
  Cushing's disease
  Hyperprolactinemia
  Abnormal cortisol action or metabolism
Functional gonadal hyperandrogenism
  Functional ovarian hyperandrogenism
  (polycystic ovarian syndrome)
    Increased intraovarian androgen
      Extraovarian hyperandrogenemia
      Dysregulation of P-450$_{c17}$
        LH elevation
        Hyperinsulinemia
        IGF-I excess
    Ovarian steroidogenic defects
    Increased follicular atresia
    Insulin resistance
  Hermaphroditism
Peripheral androgen overproduction
  Obesity
  Other

of adrenarche is a plasma DHEAS level of more than 40 μg/dl (see Fig. 16–3). In children with premature adrenarche, plasma testosterone levels also rise into the mid-pubertal range. Clinically, the androgen excess is so subtle that the only other sign of increased androgen production may be a few microcomedones. Typically, there is no other evidence of virilization: no clitoromegaly, no growth spurt, and no discordant advancement in bone age.[14] In more than 90% of children with premature adrenarche, the responses of steroid intermediates to ACTH are in between the prepubertal and adult range (see Fig. 16–3; Table 16–4).

The distinction of premature adrenarche from mild virilizing congenital adrenal hyperplasia (CAH) has been a matter of considerable controversy. In some clinics, as many as 40% of children presenting with premature pubarche have been diagnosed as having non-classic CAH caused by 21-hydroxylase deficiency.[57] This high incidence is clearly skewed by the presence in these clinics of patients from ethnic groups with a high incidence of CAH (e.g., Ashkenazi Jews and Hispanics).[58] However, much of the dispute centers around the distinction of mild 3β-HSD deficiency from premature adrenarche based on the responses of steroid intermediates to ACTH stimulation. Some investigators have designated Δ⁵-steroid responses greater than those of Tanner stage II–III controls as indicating 3β-HSD deficiency, thus concluding that 3β-HSD deficiency is a common cause of premature adrenarche.[57] However, the interpretation of several authors[13, 14, 59–62] is that this designation is inappropriate, because adrenarchal androgen production increases rapidly, approximately doubling, between stage II of puberty and adulthood, and because there is considerable variability in the overall response of the adrenarchal adrenal to ACTH stimulation (see Fig. 16–3 and Table 16–4). The diagnosis of 3β-HSD should be made only if the responses to ACTH of the Δ⁵-steroids (namely, 17-hydroxypregnenolone and DHEA) are greater than those of normal *adults*.[63] As additional criteria for this diagnosis, there should be a subnormal rise in Δ⁴-steroids (17-hydroxyprogesterone and androstenedione) accompanied by an inordinate advancement of bone age. Table 16–4 shows the typical ranges of steroid intermediate responses to ACTH in normal and prematurely adrenarchal subjects.

Exaggerated Adrenarche

Adrenal hyperandrogenism resulting from "exaggerated adrenarche" is the most common single cause of adrenal hyperandrogenism presenting in the perimenarchal period.[6, 7] This designation stems from the observation that fully one half of women with 17-ketosteroid hyperresponsiveness to ACTH have a pattern of steroid intermediates that resembles an exaggeration of adrenarche.[64] Typically, they have androstenedione hyperresponsiveness to ACTH, together with moderately excessive 17-hydroxypregnenolone and/or DHEA responses.

Some investigators have considered such patients to have mild 3β-HSD deficiency or, alternatively, symptomatic heterozygosity for 21-hydroxylase deficiency. The first appears unlikely, because GnRH agonist testing in half the cases of exaggerated adrenarche shows a pattern of ovarian steroid response that is different from that encountered in 3β-HSD deficiency.[24, 65] In addition, many patients who have been assigned a diagnosis of mild 3β-HSD deficiency have greater than average androstenedione responses to ACTH stimulation, which suggests that they, too, have exaggerated adrenarche rather than 3β-HSD deficiency. Symptomatic heterozygosity for 21-hydroxylase deficiency, on the other hand, is often suspected because a slightly elevated 17-

TABLE 16–4 ••• TYPICAL NORMAL RANGE OF STEROID LEVELS POST-ACTH*

	17-Hydroxy-pregnenolone (ng/dl)	17-Hydroxy-progesterone (ng/dl)	11-Deoxy-cortisol (ng/dl)	Cortisol (μg/dl)	DHEA (ng/dl)	Andro-stenedione (ng/dl)
Prepubertal, 2 yr	130–340	80–180	<25–350	13–50	45–120	<25–80
Adrenarchal†	240–1100	40–190	40–300	13–50	285–495	55–140
Adult female	150–1070	35–130‡	40–200	13–50	225–1470	55–185

*30 min post-ACTH 10 μg/m² as intravenous bolus. Values 60 min after 250 μg ACTH are similar.
†Children with typical premature adrenarche.
‡17-Hydroxyprogesterone increases in the preovulatory phase to peak as high as 360 ng/dl in the luteal phase of the cycle.
From Rosenfield RL. Hyperandrogenism in peripubertal girls. Pediatr Clin North Am 1990; 37:1333.

hydroxyprogesterone response is often found in women with an otherwise typical exaggerated adrenarche steroid pattern. However, the ratio of Δ^5 to Δ^4 steroid levels in response to ACTH seems to distinguish these women from carriers of 21-hydroxylase deficiency.[6]

The cause of exaggerated adrenarche is unknown. It may represent hyperplasia of the zona reticularis or, alternatively, it may be caused by abnormal regulation (dysregulation) of adrenal P-450$_{c17}$ activity of the same sort that seems to coexist in half of the cases of functional ovarian hyperandrogenism.[6, 7, 64, 65] Whether it is related to premature adrenarche is unknown. Although the menstrual cycle is usually normal in those women with isolated exaggerated adrenarche, some would consider this an adrenal variant of the PCO syndrome[66, 67] (see "PCO Syndrome").

Congenital Adrenal Hyperplasia

CAH results from an autosomal recessive defect in the activity of any one of the steroidogenic enzymes necessary for the synthesis of corticosteroid hormones by the adrenal gland (see Figs. 16–1 and 16–2).[68, 69] Because of the enzyme defect, the adrenal gland cannot efficiently secrete glucocorticoids (especially cortisol) or mineralocorticoids (primarily aldosterone). This nonsecretion causes a lack of negative feedback inhibition of ACTH or of renin-angiotensin secretion, respectively, which markedly increases the secretion of these trophic hormones and leads to compensatory hyperplasia of the adrenal cortex. The result is defective synthesis of the end product and accumulation of steroid precursors immediately before the enzyme defect.

Each enzyme deficiency leads to a characteristic clinical syndrome and biochemical abnormality, depending on which of the adrenal end products is deficient and which precursors accumulate. The clinical presentation also depends on the severity of the enzyme deficiency. Generally, if the enzyme deficiency is severe, adrenal insufficiency and salt wasting present early in the neonatal period and may be associated with accumulation of androgenic precursors, which leads to virilization of female infants and sexual ambiguity. However, when the enzyme deficiency is mild, secretion of end product is sometimes restored to normal, but only at the expense of the accumulation of precursors before the defective enzyme step. In these cases, the disorder may not become

clinically apparent until childhood or adolescence, when the individual presents with variable signs of virilization as a result of excessive androgen accumulation.

Several clinical syndromes resulting from deficient adrenal enzyme activity have been described; these include sex hormone deficiency CAH, isolated mineralocorticoid deficiency CAH, and virilizing CAH.[68–71] Related steroidogenic disorders of the testes that do not affect adrenal corticosteroid secretion cause male pseudohermaphroditism with ambiguous genitalia characterized by pseudovaginal perineoscrotal hypospadias.

Sex hormone deficiency CAH is the result of P-450$_{scc}$ deficiency or a deficiency of the 17α-hydroxylase and/or 17,20-lyase activities of P-450$_{c17}$. In these disorders, severe deficiency causes sexual ambiguity in males and sexual infantilism in females. P-450$_{scc}$ deficiency causes lipoid adrenal hyperplasia, a defect that leads to deficient mineralocorticoid, glucocorticoid, and sex steroid synthesis. Complete P-450$_{c17}$ deficiency is associated with excessive mineralocorticoid production and hypertension and deficient glucocorticoid synthesis and sex steroid production. A variant of P-450$_{c17}$ deficiency is isolated 17,20-lyase deficiency, characterized by normal glucocorticoid and mineralocorticoid function but deficient synthesis of C-19 steroids (including testosterone and estradiol).

Mineralocorticoid deficiency CAH results from 18-hydroxylase or 18-hydroxysteroid dehydrogenase deficiencies, which result in deficient aldosterone synthesis.[72] Glucocorticoid and sex steroid production are unaffected, resulting in clinical syndromes characterized by isolated salt wasting without genital ambiguity, hyperandrogenism, or cortisol deficiency.

Virilizing CAH occurs as the result of 3β-HSD, 11β-hydroxylase, or 21-hydroxylase deficiency. In virilizing CAH, inefficient cortisol synthesis is associated with the accumulation of androgenic precursors, which produce excessive virilization of female infants with genital ambiguity in the neonatal period or hyperandrogenism later in childhood. These disorders are classically associated with altered mineralocorticoid production, mineralocorticoid deficiency with salt wasting (in the case of 3β-HSD and 21-hydroxylase deficiency), and salt retention with hypertension in the case of 11β-hydroxylase deficiency.

Severe 3β-HSD deficiency leads to defective cortisol and mineralocorticoid synthesis, with adrenal insufficiency presenting in the neonatal period. Because of deficient synthesis of Δ^4-steroids (including androgens), affected male infants classically have insufficient virilization with sexual ambiguity. Affected female infants, on the other hand, are often virilized because of the very high levels of the weakly androgenic DHEA and its more androgenic metabolites.[73] When the enzyme deficiency is mild, virilization later in childhood or adolescence may be the first sign of the accumulation of these androgenic precursors.[63, 74] The controversy regarding the distinction of mild 3β-HSD deficiency from simple premature adrenarche was previously discussed in the section, "Premature Adrenarche."

11β-hydroxylase deficiency classically presents with genital ambiguity in the female and subsequent incomplete sexual precocity in association with hypertension. Atypical cases with late-onset hirsutism without hypertension have been reported.[75]

Virilizing CAH Caused by 21-Hydroxylase Deficiency. Whereas most of the enzyme deficiencies resulting in the various clinical CAH syndromes described earlier are rare, 21-hydroxylase deficiency is a common inherited condition that can lead to excessive virilization either early in life or later in childhood and adolescence. It has an overall incidence in the general population of about 1 in 12,000. Several distinct clinical syndromes have been described; these are the result of a spectrum of variations in the severity of the enzyme defect.[68–71] "Classic" 21-hydroxylase deficiency is the result of a severe enzyme deficiency that presents in the neonatal period with variable signs and symptoms of excessive virilization and adrenal insufficiency. It leads to ambiguous genital development in female infants and can be associated with mineralocorticoid deficiency (salt-wasting CAH) or, in many cases, with normal mineralocorticoid function (simple virilizing CAH). Because the genital development of males is not affected, males will usually present with either adrenal insufficiency and salt wasting shortly after birth (when associated with mineralocorticoid deficiency) or with signs of androgen excess later in childhood (in simple virilizing CAH).

CAH can also be "nonclassic" in its presentation, manifesting in its "late onset" form as premature pubarche or presenting with perior postpubertal onset of hirsutism, acne, or amenorrhea. Such nonclassic cases account for about 1% to 5% of cases of adult hirsutism.[7] Additional cases are entirely cryptic, manifest-ing as isolated biochemical disorders with no clinical abnormalities. These late-onset forms of 21-hydroxylase deficiency CAH have been shown to be due to distinct 21-hydroxylase mutations that cause only mild enzyme deficiencies.[76]

As previously mentioned, there is considerable controversy about the frequency with which late-onset 21-hydroxylase deficiency results in premature pubarche in childhood. Although some clinicians believe that late-onset CAH is a frequent cause of precocious pubarche in children, this frequency is probably because there is a high prevalence of late-onset CAH in certain ethnic populations. Regardless, it is clear that late-onset CAH is an important cause of hyperandrogenism in childhood and adolescence that needs to be appropriately recognized and treated. Fortunately, CAH can be easily separated from premature adrenarche based on the steroidogenic profiles after acute ACTH stimulation (see later discussion).

Studies of the molecular biology of 21-hydroxylase deficiency have provided important tools for the diagnosis of this condition. The gene for 21-hydroxylase (P-450$_{c21}$) is located on chromosome 6 and is closely linked to the human major histocompatibility complex (MHC) or human leukocyte antigen (HLA), residing between HLA-B and HLA-DR.[1, 68, 69] The linkage between HLA and 21-hydroxylase thus allows for the detection of individuals who have the genetic abnormality, provided the HLA haplotypes of the individual and index case are known. For example, a child possessing HLA haplotypes identical to the index case can be predicted to be affected, one who shares one haplotype can be predicted to be a heterozygote, and one sharing no haplotype can be said to be unaffected. Additionally, prenatal diagnosis is possible in affected families, allowing for potential in utero therapies to prevent the genital abnormalities present in severely affected individuals.[77, 78]

Using HLA typing and ACTH response patterns, New and colleagues have developed normative data that have greatly aided the diagnosis of the different 21-hydroxylase deficiency syndromes (Fig. 16–8).[76] These investigators have shown that the rapid 17-hydroxyprogesterone response to an intravenous bolus of ACTH distinguishes both mild and classic virilizing CAH better than baseline steroid levels. The degree of clinical severity is correlated with the degree of 21-hydroxylase deficiency elucidated by the ACTH test. Impor-

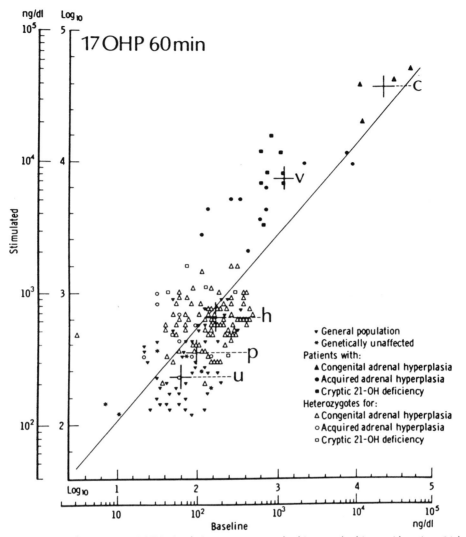

FIGURE 16–8 ••• Patterns of response to ACTH stimulation among normal subjects and subjects with various 21-hydroxylase deficiency syndromes. The graph shows the baseline and ACTH-stimulated levels of 17-hydroxyprogesterone in unaffected individuals (u), the general population (p), heterozygotes for 21-hydroxylase deficiency (h), nonclassical variants homozygous for 21-hydroxylase deficiency (v), and classical 21-hydroxylase deficient patients (c). The data include males and females regardless of phase of the menstrual cycle or age. ACTH was administered intravenously as a 250-μg bolus. (From New MI, Lorenzen F, Lerner AJ, et al. Genotyping steroid 21-hydroxylase deficiency: Hormonal reference data. J Clin Endocrinol Metab 1983; 57:320. © 1983, by The Endocrine Society.)

tantly, the response to an ACTH bolus also usually distinguishes carriers from noncarriers of the gene abnormality.

Other Adrenal Disorders

A number of other causes of adrenal hyperandrogenism may occur but are relatively rare. Adrenal tumors can produce androgens and lead to virilization.[79] They are more common in the first decade of life and, in approximately one half of cases, are benign. Malignant ad-

renal tumors occur more commonly in toddlers and younger children, and both carcinomas and adenomas may be bilateral in their presentation. They may be associated with hemihypertrophy, Beckwith-Wiedemann syndrome, or other syndromes that predispose to neoplasia or malformations of the genitourinary system.[80] Furthermore, the location of virilizing adrenal tumors can be unusual; a case with associated glucocorticoid excess has even been reported to arise within an adrenal rest tumor of the ovary.[81]

The presence of an adrenal tumor must be suspected in a child with rapid progression of virilization. There is often pubic hair development, clitoral enlargement, acne, and an increase in the rate of growth and of skeletal maturation. When associated with Cushing's syndrome, the excess glucocorticoid production blunts the growth spurt typical of prepubertal virilization.[82] Occasionally, these tumors can develop in utero and produce clitoral hypertrophy and labial fusion in the newborn.

The diagnosis of adrenal tumor is usually easily made on the basis of the clinical presentation and elevated urinary 17-ketosteroid, plasma testosterone, and/or plasma DHEAS levels. DHEAS values greater than 600 μg/dl should dictate consideration of an adrenal tumor as the cause.[79] Occasionally, dexamethasone suppression is required to differentiate a congenital tumor from CAH. Some degree of ACTH dependency[70] or gonadotropin dependency[83] may be found in adrenal virilizing tumors.

Cortisol resistance may cause premature pubarche or late-onset hirsutism.[67, 84] In these patients, a functional abnormality of the glucocorticoid receptor leads to compensatory hypersecretion of ACTH and hypercortisolemia without other clinical or biochemical findings of Cushing's syndrome. The clinical findings are due to the overproduction of nonglucocorticoid adrenal steroids, and hypertension with hypokalemia may accompany the syndrome. Congenitally rapid cortisol metabolism resulting from 11β-hydroxysteroid dehydrogenase deficiency may resemble mild cortisol resistance.[85]

Several other clinical disorders may present with adrenal hyperandrogenism and resemble PCO syndrome. Hyperprolactinemia may present with hirsutism, acne, amenorrhea, and, in approximately one half of cases, galactorrhea.[8, 86] DHEA and DHEAS levels are elevated, as is plasma free testosterone, in part because of a direct effect of hyperprolactinemia on adrenocortical function.[86] Acromegaly may also be associated with PCO syndrome, either because of a direct effect of the elevated IGF I levels on ovarian androgen production or because of adrenal androgenic hyperfunction.[87]

Ovarian Disorders

Ovarian hyperandrogenism is most often the result of functional disorders that equate with PCO syndrome (see Table 16–3).[9, 33] According to this theory, polycystic ovaries represent a severe form of the syndrome, while less severe cases have no ovarian anatomic abnormality. Experience in adults and adolescents indicates that approximately two thirds of hyperandrogenic women have functional ovarian hyperandrogenism indicative of dysregulation of androgen secretion, and a similar number have adrenal hyperandrogenism of a similar type (exaggerated adrenarche). Half the time, the ovarian and adrenal sources coexist.[9] Less than 10% have late-onset CAH or other causes of hyperandrogenemia. Ovarian hyperandrogenism, however, can occasionally result from benign or malignant ovarian tumors. Even more rare is true hermaphroditism.[88]

PCO Syndrome

In 1935 Stein and Leventhal described a syndrome, now known as PCO syndrome, characterized by bilateral polycystic ovaries associated with amenorrhea, hirsutism, and obesity.[89] Subsequent clinical, biochemical, and morphologic studies have underscored the heterogeneity of this functional disorder, raising considerable controversy regarding its definition, pathophysiology, clinical presentation, and treatment.[33, 90–92] A conference held in 1990 by the National Institute of Child Health and Human Development indicated that otherwise unexplained chronic hyperandrogenism, in association with anovulation, is the common denominator in what most investigators consider to be PCO syndrome.

PCO syndrome is the most common cause of hyperandrogenism of peripubertal onset in females, with symptoms typically beginning at about the time of menarche.[33, 92, 93] In 43 volunteers 10 to 16 years of age, PCO syndrome was documented by dexamethasone suppression testing criteria in 2.3% and was possibly present in another 4.6%. The frequency of PCO syndrome in adults has been estimated at between 0.6% and 4.3%, with a 1.4% incidence of polycystic ovaries found on laparoscopy and a 3.5% incidence on autopsy.[91] These data suggest that PCO syndrome has the same overall incidence (about 3%) in both adolescents and adults. However, the incidence is even higher in patients with certain clinical disorders, such as insulin resistance syndromes, where PCO syndrome seems to be a uniform finding.[33, 92] Taken together, this evidence is compatible with PCO syndrome's being caused by congenital disorders of ovarian function first appearing at adolescence.

In its full-blown state, PCO syndrome presents with symptoms of oligo-ovulation, hyperandrogenemia, and obesity.[33, 93] Classically, the anovulation is expressed as oligoamenorrhea and the hyperandrogenism as hirsutism, and the ovaries can be seen by ultrasound to be bilaterally enlarged, with thecal-stromal hyperplasia and 10 or more subcapsular cystic follicles (characteristically less than 10 mm in diameter).[90] More often, however, the clinical findings are more variable and subtle, depending not only on the severity of hyperandrogenism (which is typically modest), but also on the sensitivity of peripheral target organs to androgenic stimulation. Thus, patients may present with acne without hirsutism, with dysfunctional uterine bleeding or normal menstrual cycles, and with no sonographic abnormalities. A high index of suspicion is therefore warranted if any of these milder symptoms are present.

The etiology of PCO syndrome has been a matter of considerable debate.[33, 66, 90–92, 94] Part of the controversy surrounds the issue of whether hyperandrogenism in PCO syndrome arises from adrenal or ovarian sources. In any model, a vicious cycle of hyperandrogenism

seems to be established; as a result, the primary abnormality initiating the development of PCO syndrome may be difficult to delineate. Because of the frequent adrenal 17-ketosteroid hyperresponsiveness to ACTH, some investigators believe that PCO syndrome originates as an adrenal disorder during puberty. According to this theory, adrenal hyperandrogenism is central to the pathogenesis via a complex cycle of events in which secretion of androstenedione and its peripheral conversion to estrone initiate the syndrome (Fig. 16–9).[66] Yen has suggested that exaggerated adrenarche initiates this process.[92] More specifically, increased secretion of androstenedione by the adrenal gland leads to increased concentrations of estrogen, primarily estrone, through its peripheral conversion in adipose and other tissues. The elevated androgen levels also decrease SHBG concentrations, further increasing the concentration of estrone that is free and biologically active. The increase in the plasma concentration of estrone sensitizes the pituitary to secrete excessive LH, resulting in a high LH-to-FSH ratio, which leads to excessive stimulation of ovarian thecal androstenedione production and deficient granulosa cell aromatase activity. The resulting increase in ovarian androgens leads to polycystic ovaries

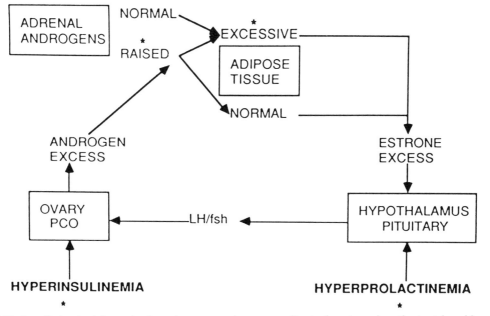

FIGURE 16–9 ••• Pathophysiology of polycystic ovary syndrome according to the estrone hypothesis. Adrenal hyperandrogenemia leads to excess estrone, which preferentially stimulates pituitary luteinizing hormone (LH) secretion and results in secondary ovarian hyperandrogenism. The asterisk indicates that more than one potential initiating event may occur in a given patient. (From McKenna TJ. Pathogenesis and treatment of polycystic ovary syndrome. N Engl J Med 1988; 318:558. Reprinted with permission of The New England Journal of Medicine.)

and at the same time contributes further to the circulating pool of androgens, thereby perpetuating the vicious cycle of hyperandrogenism.

This theory, while plausible, is not universally accepted for several reasons. Estrone is a weak estrogen, and attempts to reproduce gonadotropin secretory abnormalities through exogenous estrone administration have not led to increased LH concentrations.[95] In addition, not all cases of PCO syndrome have gonadotropin secretory abnormalities characterized by either an elevated LH level or an abnormal LH-to-FSH ratio.[33] Furthermore, suppression of ovarian steroid production through the use of GnRH agonist therapy leads to a reduction in the plasma concentration of androstenedione and testosterone but not of DHEA or DHEAS, suggesting that the ovary itself is at least partly responsible for the elevated androgen levels in PCO syndrome, independent of adrenal androgen production.[96]

A new model has been proposed in which functional ovarian hyperandrogenism is the common denominator of PCO syndrome (Fig. 16–10).[6, 33] The disorder is functional, as there is no necessary anatomic basis for it, and it is gonadotropin dependent. It is postulated that PCO syndrome arises from those heterogeneous disorders that increase either the intraovarian concentration of androgen or the process of follicular atresia. An increase in one of these can then induce abnormalities in the other, establishing a vicious cycle of increased androgen production. In about half the cases of PCO syndrome, an elevated serum LH level is probably the factor initiating ovarian hyperandrogenism. In other cases of PCO syndrome, gonadotropin abnormalities are absent,[97] and the pathogenetic mechanisms appear related to intraovarian factors, some of which seem to act by amplifying the action of LH on the ovary.[98] Furthermore, exogenous androgen administration has been shown to produce the anatomic changes of Stein-Leventhal syndrome—namely, cortical sclerosis, cysts, and hyperthecosis—probably because of the great increase in the intraovarian concentration of androgen.[99] A similar mechanism would seem to account for polycystic ovaries in poorly controlled virilizing CAH.

The increased serum LH in PCO syndrome results from a combination of abnormalities. Determinations of gonadotropin levels at frequent intervals for extended periods of time indicate that the gonadotropin secretory pattern of adolescent PCO syndrome is characterized by an abnormal diurnal rhythm, with peak LH secretion at midday.[98, 100] The pulse frequency in PCO syndrome is increased to some extent by the lack of nocturnal slowing of gonadotropin secretion, as should occur during the normal early follicular phase, and there may be increases in LH pulse amplitude as well. Because gonadotropin secretion is ultimately controlled by the secretion of GnRH produced in the hypothalamus, these changes in gonadotropin secretion are very likely the result of alterations at the level of the hypothalamic GnRH pulse generator.[101] The basis for the abnormalities of GnRH secretion is not known but may involve alterations in dopamine or endogenous opioid production. The elevated ratio of LH to FSH may well be accounted for by a combination of increased GnRH pulse frequency and inhibition of FSH secretion by the hyperestrogenic state.[24, 33] In patients with CAH and PCO syndrome, it is possible that abnormalities in the GnRH pulse generator are programmed by perinatal androgen exposure.[102]

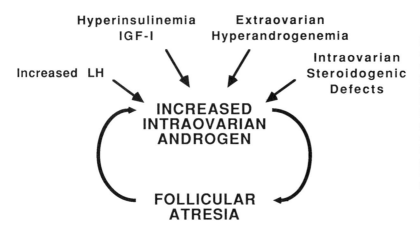

FIGURE 16–10 ••• Pathophysiology of polycystic ovary (PCO) syndrome as functional ovarian hyperandrogenism. PCO syndrome is postulated to result from those factors that either increase intraovarian androgen concentrations or cause premature follicular atresia. An increase in either of these can then induce abnormalities in the other in a to-and-fro manner. The known causes of these processes are indicated.

Women with ovarian hyperandrogenism typically have a characteristic pituitary-gonadal response to testing with the GnRH agonist nafarelin (Fig. 16–11).[7, 94] Their gonadotropin responses often resemble those of males in that they have significantly greater early LH and lesser FSH responses. Regardless of whether LH and FSH responses are elevated, however, they have greater 17-hydroxyproges-

terone and, to a lesser extent, androgenic responses than those of normal women.[7, 9] 17-Hydroxypregnenolone and DHEA responses are less consistently elevated, and pregnenolone is not elevated at all in PCO syndrome patients. There is rarely evidence of a discrete block in the steroidogenic pathway, as the responses of all steroids on the pathway from 17-hydroxyprogesterone to estrone and estra-

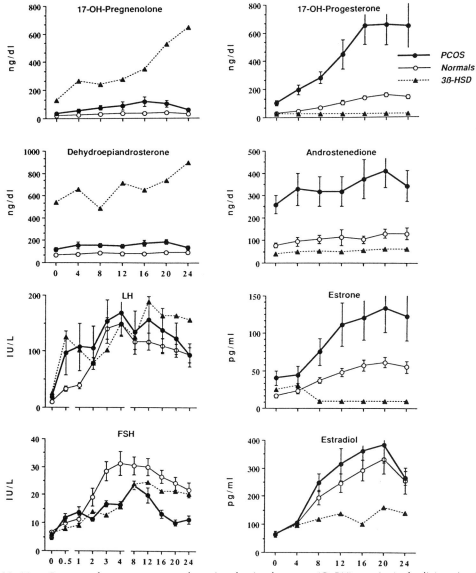

FIGURE 16–11 ••• Patterns of response to gonadotropin-releasing hormone (GnRH) agonist (nafarelin) testing in patients with the functional ovarian hyperandrogenism (PCO syndrome [PCOS]) and a patient with late-onset 3β-hydroxysteroid dehydrogenase deficiency (3β-HSD) in comparison with normal early follicular phase females (Normals). PCO syndrome patients have significantly greater early (30 to 60 minutes) LH responses and lesser mean FSH responses than normal women. Their 17-hydroxyprogesterone responses ($P < .001$) and androstenedione responses ($P < .05$) are significantly increased. Estrogen responses tend to be greater. This steroidogenic pattern is different from that found with an intraovarian steroidogenic block, as exemplified by the patient with 3β-HSD deficiency (3β-ol). (From Rosenfield RL. Hyperandrogenism in peripubertal girls. Pediatr Clin North Am 1990; 37:1333.)

diol are normal or elevated. Dexamethasone suppression of adrenal function does not alter the results.[6, 24] The elevated responses of 17-hydroxyprogesterone and androstenedione, without evidence of a block in the subsequent steroidogenic steps or consistent abnormalities in the earlier steps in the steroidogenic pathway, suggest increased ovarian 17α-hydroxylase and 17,20-lyase (desmolase) activities.

Abnormal regulation of these activities can result from overstimulation by LH, as discussed earlier. In addition, we postulate that in cases of PCO syndrome in which LH abnormalities are not found, there is dysregulation of androgen secretion, either as the result of intrinsic defects in the enzyme or as the result of endocrine, paracrine, or autocrine factors that modulate the ovarian androgen response to LH (see Fig. 16–5). Thus, we suspect that the abnormal regulation (dysregulation) of apparent $P-450_{c17}$ activities within the ovary underlies most cases of PCO syndrome, preventing the normal coordination of intraovarian androgen with estrogen production that is so important for the proper function of the ovaries.[6, 7]

We have postulated that similar intrinsic abnormalities in the regulation of $P-450_{c17}$ within the adrenal cortex could explain the coexistence of adrenal 17-ketosteroid hyperresponsiveness to ACTH in half the cases of PCO syndrome[6, 9] (see "Exaggerated Adrenarche"). Others might consider women with oligomenorrhea and isolated exaggerated adrenarche to have an "adrenal" form of PCO syndrome.[66, 67]

PCO syndrome secondary to the buildup of androgenic precursors caused by inefficient estradiol biosynthesis within the ovary is rare but can result from congenital defects in the activity of ovarian 3β-HSD (see Fig. 16–11)[24] or 17-ketosteroid oxidoreductase (see Fig. 16–1).[94] These enzyme deficiencies can be diagnosed on the basis of the abnormal ovarian steroid response to GnRH agonist stimulation and the associated adrenal enzyme abnormalities as elucidated by ACTH testing. There has been considerable interest in the possibility that aromatase deficiency may cause PCO syndrome, but whatever aromatase deficiency is present typically appears to be reversible and secondary to the FSH deficit.[103]

A premature commitment of follicles to atresia seems characteristic of PCO syndrome and is usually secondary to the etiologic factors mentioned earlier that in one way or another increase the concentration of androgens within the ovary. However, in some cases, follicular atresia may be the primary event leading to PCO syndrome, as in the case of insulin resistance syndromes (see later discussion). Importantly, atretic follicles are relatively androgenic and hypoestrogenic; this imbalance between the production of androgen and estrogen perpetuates the cycle of hyperandrogenism and follicular maturational arrest.[33]

One of the most common conditions associated with PCO syndrome is insulin resistance. Virtually every form of severe insulin resistance—whether caused by antiinsulin receptor antibodies, insulin receptor defects, or postreceptor defects—has been reported to be associated with PCO syndrome.[104, 105] It is not clear whether insulin resistance is directly responsible for the development of PCO syndrome or is secondary to the hyperandrogenism or the obesity associated with this condition. The modest hyperandrogenism of PCO syndrome does not seem likely to be causative, since a reduction in the concentration of androgens does not always lead to an increase in insulin sensitivity, and not all subjects with PCO syndrome and insulin resistance are obese.[106, 107] Rather, it is likely that insulin resistance itself contributes to the development of PCO syndrome.[105] It is known that insulin (and IGF I) synergize with FSH in stimulating granulosa cell growth and function, increasing FSH-mediated induction of aromatase activity.[108, 109] Thus, deficiency of insulin action may initiate PCO syndrome by arresting granulosa cell maturation or decreasing aromatase activity, thus increasing the intraovarian androgen concentration that brings about premature follicular atresia. Alternatively, the hyperinsulinemia of insulin resistance syndromes may cause ovarian hyperandrogenism by acting through the IGF I receptor or a spared insulin receptor to synergize with LH in stimulating excessive androgen production by ovarian thecal cells[34, 35, 104] or by altering the intraovarian synthesis or secretion of IGF I or IGF-binding proteins.[92]

The diagnosis of PCO syndrome often presents difficulties because of heterogeneity in clinical presentation and the variability in severity of presenting signs and symptoms. The difficulty is compounded by the fact that the criteria for diagnosis are not specific among disorders causing hyperandrogenic amenorrhea. Whereas elevated baseline or GnRH-stimulated LH levels have been mainstays of diagnosis, a prolactinoma may be associated with polycystic ovaries and LH hyperresponsiveness.[110, 111] Similarly, women with virilizing CAH may have polycystic ovaries and high serum LH levels.[112] Paradoxically, multicystic or polycystic ovaries may be visualized by ultrasound examination in apparently normal adolescents or adult women, respectively,[90] yet polycystic ovaries are not necessary for the diagnosis of PCO syndrome.[97]

Ovarian Tumors

Virilizing ovarian tumors may be malignant or benign and are frequently suspected on the basis of rapidly progressive virilization, testosterone concentrations greater than 200 ng/dl, and characteristic ultrasound or computed tomographic (CT) findings. The most common virilizing ovarian tumor is the Sertoli-Leydig cell tumor (arrhenoblastoma), which is occasionally gonadotropin responsive.[8, 113] Ovarian lipid cell tumors are also typically gonadotropin responsive and dependent in part on ACTH as well.[114] Ovarian virilizing tumors typically secrete predominantly androstenedione and are thus characterized by a disproportionate elevation of plasma androstenedione relative to testosterone. Mild elevation of urinary 17-ketosteroid excretion is characteristic.

Peripheral Overproduction of Androgen

Obesity can cause hyperandrogenemia and amenorrhea, thus mimicking PCO syndrome.[4, 33, 115, 116] Because testosterone formation from androstenedione is increased and SHBG is suppressed, testosterone production is increased, and plasma free testosterone levels are high. Estrone formation from androstenedione is also increased,[4] and estradiol metabolism is diverted to active rather than inactive metabolites.[117] Insulin resistance also commonly occurs.[4]

Approximately 10% of a series of hyperandrogenemic women had idiopathic hyperandrogenemia—that is, hyperandrogenemia for which an intensive search revealed no clear adrenal or ovarian source for the androgen excess.[9] This probably arose from increased peripheral metabolism of inactive steroid precursors to active androgens. Such an abnormality has been postulated in subjects who present with postmenarchal acne or hirsutism and who demonstrate a persistent elevation of plasma free testosterone with a normal 24-hour gonadotropin profile and normal steroid responses to ACTH and GnRH agonist testing. Either dexamethasone or estrogen-progestin combinations usually suppress the plasma free testosterone to normal levels.

DIAGNOSIS OF HYPERANDROGENIC STATES

The diagnosis of hyperandrogenism requires a high index of suspicion, as well as a thorough and systematic approach by the physician. A careful history should be taken including the timing and progression of puberty, the timing and progression of the signs and symptoms of hyperandrogenism, the use of medications, and the presence of similar complaints in other family members. Particular attention should be paid to the menstrual history. The physical examination should concentrate on the scoring of hirsutism and acne and assessing the extent of virilization and estrogenization. When appropriate, a complete gynecologic examination should be performed and adnexal and/or adrenal masses carefully searched for. Judgment must be exercised in the decision to perform a full pelvic examination in a teenager; assessment of the anatomy of internal organs may be complemented by abdominal ultrasound. Ancillary diagnostic procedures, such as an adrenal CT scan, should be obtained as indicated by the history and physical examination.

Key elements in the history and physical examination may provide important clues to the diagnosis. Onset of virilization in the neonatal period with labial fusion and clitoromegaly suggests in utero onset, as often seen in CAH or, more rarely, in congenitally virilizing tumors. Isolated pubic hair development in a young girl suggests precocious adrenarche, whereas more extensive pubic or axillary hair development, acne, growth spurt, and advancement in bone age suggest a frankly virilizing disorder such as late-onset CAH. Rapidly progressive virilization, especially if associated with markedly elevated androgen levels or signs of Cushing's syndrome, should alert the physician to the possibility of an adrenal or ovarian tumor. PCO syndrome is suggested by the peripubertal onset of hirsutism, acne, obesity, or menstrual abnormalities associated with normal estrogenization.

The laboratory evaluation of hyperandrogenism should include determinations of plasma total testosterone, free testosterone, androstenedione, and DHEAS.[22] Determinations of urinary 17-hydroxycorticoids and 17-ketosteroids are seldom helpful. Random 17-hydroxyprogesterone levels are usually normal in girls with late-onset CAH and thus are usually of limited diagnostic utility. Baseline plasma testosterone values in the frankly male range (i.e., more than 350 ng/dl) are pathognomonic for ovarian or adrenal virilizing tumors, whereas levels of around 200 ng/dl strongly suggest the presence of such lesions. A basal DHEAS level that is very high (more than 600 μg/dl) suggests an adrenal neoplasm. In such cases, ultrasound, a CT scan, or a magnetic resonance imaging (MRI) scan will usually demonstrate the mass and establish the diagnosis.

Much more commonly, especially in cases of functional adrenal or ovarian hyperandrogenism, the baseline plasma testosterone may be normal or only minimally elevated. In most cases, however, the free testosterone is usually elevated or the SHBG level is low, reflecting the hyperandrogenic state of the individual. It is thus important to measure both the total and free testosterone, since a normal plasma total testosterone level does not rule out an important hyperandrogenic disorder. Because the assay of plasma free testosterone is not well standardized among laboratories, some investigators prefer ancillary measurement of plasma androstenedione.

Hyperandrogenemia is present in most severe cases of hirsutism or acne and about half of the mild cases.[54, 56] Because of episodic and cyclic secretions of androgens, however, a random value may be misleadingly normal. Clearly it is both costly and impractical to measure many steroids on multiple occasions; a strategy must be used to derive maximal diagnostic information from limited sampling. If key historical, physical, and/or laboratory features do not point to a specific diagnosis (such as an ovarian or adrenal tumor) and serum LH, FSH, prolactin, and thyroxine do not yield diagnostic information, diagnostic screening usually is reasonably accomplished using dexamethasone suppression testing.[22]

Dexamethasone suppression testing is performed by administering a "low" dose of 1 mg/m² daily in divided doses orally for 5 days (or longer in patients who are very obese or have relatively high DHEAS levels). The pattern of response of plasma free testosterone, DHEAS, and cortisol usually segregates patients diagnostically, as shown in Figure 16–

12. Normal suppression of androgens is most specifically indicated by a reduction of the plasma free testosterone into the normal range for dexamethasone-suppressed, nonhirsute women. Dexamethasone suppressibility is considered normal in a peri- or postmenarchal female if the plasma free testosterone level is less than 8 pg/ml. Normal adrenal suppression is indicated by a reduction of both DHEAS and cortisol to levels below the normal range for adult controls (<70 and <3 μg/dl, respectively). Lack of suppression of cortisol usually indicates the presence of adrenal virilizing tumors, Cushing's syndrome, or noncompliance with dexamethasone therapy.

The vast majority of patients with normal adrenal suppression but subnormal suppression of free testosterone after dexamethasone administration have PCO syndrome.[22, 33] It must be borne in mind, however, that a specific diagnostic study for establishing this diagnosis is not presently available. An elevated serum LH level may be a useful corroborative test (type I PCO syndrome), but elevation of serum LH is not specific for PCO syndrome, and many patients have LH levels that are normal (type II PCO syndrome).[97] The presence of bilateral polycystic ovaries on pelvic ultrasound examination may be supportive of the diagnosis, but the sensitivity and specificity are relatively low; both false-negative and false-positive results are relatively common. Suppression of plasma free testosterone after a therapeutic trial of combination estrogen-progestin is highly suggestive of PCO syndrome, but it must be kept in mind that gonadotropin dependence has been occasionally reported with virilizing ovarian[113] and adrenal[83] tumors. Preliminary studies suggest that GnRH agonist testing may be useful in confirming the diagnosis of PCO syndrome; a serum 17-hydroxyprogesterone level of more than 224 ng/dl in response to a 100-μg subcutaneous test dose of the GnRH agonist nafarelin seems promising as a specific test for PCO syndrome.[7]

Normal suppression of androgens after dexamethasone administration requires ruling out the presence of CAH. The diagnosis can be confirmed in most cases by measuring steroid intermediates after an intravenous bolus of ACTH, as acute stimulation of adrenocortical steroid production will yield a steroid pattern indicative of the nature and severity of the enzyme defect. New and colleagues have developed a nomogram based on ACTH testing that delineates the type of steroid response for

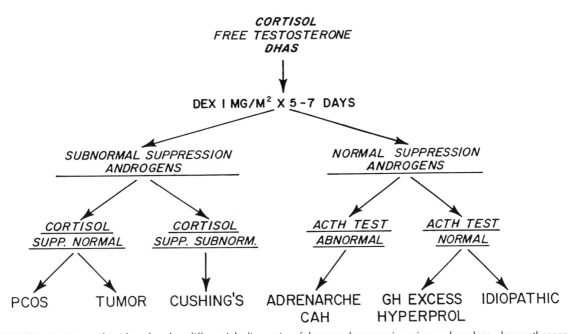

FIGURE 16–12 ••• Algorithm for the differential diagnosis of hyperandrogenemia using a low-dose dexamethasone suppression test. After 5 to 7 days of dexamethasone (1 mg/m²/day), subnormal suppression of plasma free testosterone points toward PCO syndrome (PCOS) (if both dehydroepiandrosterone sulfate [DHEAS] and cortisol suppress normally), tumor (if only cortisol suppresses normally), or Cushing's syndrome (if cortisol does not suppress normally). Normal suppression of hyperandrogenemia is an indication for ACTH testing. GH, growth hormone; HYPERPROL, hyperprolactinemia. (From Rosenfield RL. The ovary and female sexual maturation. In: Kaplan SA (ed). Clinical Pediatric Endocrinology. 2nd ed. Philadelphia: WB Saunders, 1989:259.)

the classic and nonclassic forms of CAH caused by 21-hydroxylase deficiency (see Fig. 16–8).[76] An increase in 17-hydroxyprogesterone of more than 1200 ng/dl 60 minutes after intravenous injection of 250 μg of cosyntropin is diagnostic of virilizing CAH; the late-onset types of CAH typically are indicated by levels greater than 1200 ng/dl, while the classic types are indicated by levels greater than 12,000 ng/dl.

As previously noted, the criteria for distinguishing mild 3β-HSD deficiency from exaggerated adrenarche on the basis of the ACTH stimulation test are in dispute. Some investigators believe that Δ^5-steroid responses greater than those of Tanner stage II–III controls indicate the presence of 3β-HSD deficiency. We accept the diagnosis of 3β-HSD deficiency only if Δ^5-steroids (such as 17-hydroxypregnenolone and DHEA) increase to more than twice normal in response to ACTH, while Δ^4-steroids (such as 17-hydroxyprogesterone and androstenedione) increase subnormally (see Table 16–4). Otherwise, the steroid response is typical of what we refer to as exaggerated adrenarche. It is anticipated that molecular biologic identification of genetic 3β-HSD de-

ficiency will lead to improved diagnostic criteria for this disorder.

At the end of this sequence of testing, very few cases of hyperandrogenemia remain unexplained. Idiopathic hyperandrogenemia may be accounted for in some patients by abnormal peripheral androgen metabolism, in which case it is suppressible by either dexamethasone and/or estrogen-progestin. Experience with GnRH agonist testing suggests that many cases of hyperandrogenemia currently considered idiopathic are actually mild cases of functional ovarian hyperandrogenism. If androgens are persistently normal in a patient with hirsutism, the diagnosis is truly idiopathic hirsutism, a cosmetic problem caused by an apparently increased sensitivity of pilosebaceous units to androgen.

TREATMENT OF HYPERANDROGENISM

Treatment of hyperandrogenism in adolescence must be directed at the underlying cause and be undertaken with an understanding of its pathophysiology. Surgical extirpation is the treatment of choice for adrenal and ovarian tumors. In the case of adrenal tumor, care must be taken to examine both adrenal glands at the time of surgery to evaluate the possibility of bilateral lesions and to search for the presence of remaining functional adrenal tissue.[79] Coverage with glucocorticoids is important both at the time of surgery and postsurgically if there is glucocorticoid secretion by the tumor. Surgical correction results in normalization of plasma and urinary steroid abnormalities within days. When surgery is not successful or not possible because of metastases, chemotherapy may be attempted but has generally had limited success.

In classic virilizing CAH, as in all types of CAH, provision of the missing end product— namely, glucocorticoid, mineralocorticoid, or both—results in amelioration of adrenal insufficiency, inhibition of trophic hormone stimulation, and suppression of elevated steroid levels. Glucocorticoid replacement is usually accomplished by the administration of hydrocortisone (15–25 mg/m^2/day divided in three doses). Mineralocorticoid replacement, necessary in all salt-losing and in those non–salt-losing patients with elevated plasma renin activity, is usually achieved with fludrocortisone acetate (Florinef) (0.05 to 0.2 mg/day). In adolescents and older individuals, normalization of ACTH and plasma androgen levels can usually be achieved by the use of prednisone (5 to 7.5 mg/day given in two divided doses, with the larger fraction at bedtime). Adequate control is typically associated with 17-hydroxyprogesterone levels approximating high normal values (200 ng/dl). Failure to normalize menses in an adolescent suggests incomplete control of progesterone levels or coincident PCO syndrome.[65, 118]

Clinical remission of hyperandrogenic signs and symptoms typically occurs with adequate replacement therapy. However, treatment must be individualized and closely monitored and adjusted, as both excessive and insufficient therapy are associated with adverse effects. In this regard, and especially in younger individuals, particular attention must be given to the growth and developmental pattern as well as bone age progression.

Glucocorticoids are also indicated for some patients with other forms of functional adrenal hyperandrogenemia, but are generally less effective.[47] The sequelae of glucucorticoid therapy can be minimized by using a modest bedtime dose (5 mg prednisone or 0.25 mg dexamethasone) to selectively reduce adrenal

androgen secretion without causing adrenal insufficiency.[119] More than 0.25 mg dexamethasone are likely to cause cushingoid side effects. Neither glucocorticoids nor mineralocorticoids are indicated for premature adrenarche, which should be considered simply a normal phenomenon occurring prematurely.

The treatment of functional ovarian hyperandrogenism, including PCO syndrome, is directed at correcting menstrual irregularities, alleviating symptoms of androgen excess, and, when appropriate, inducing ovulation. There is no treatment that is ideal or universally successful, and therapy must be individualized according to the needs and desires of the individual.

In general, cyclic progestin administration is the method of choice for the treatment of adolescent menstrual irregularities when hirsutism is absent and fertility is not an issue. Medroxyprogesterone acetate (Provera) is used in dosages of 10 mg daily at bedtime for 5 days, commencing at intervals of 3 weeks to 2 months. More frequent administration is chosen for patients with intractable dysfunctional uterine bleeding and less frequent administration for patients with amenorrhea, with the increased time between dosing permitting the clinician to ascertain the possibility of spontaneous menses. Adolescents who are sexually active need to be warned about the need for barrier contraception while on cyclic medroxyprogesterone therapy.

In patients with dysfunctional uterine bleeding in whom menstrual regularity cannot be achieved with progestin alone, oral contraceptives are usually of benefit. An estrogen-progestin combination contraceptive pill that contains low androgenic activity is generally recommended (see later discussion). Modest breakthrough bleeding can be managed by adding conjugated estrogens (Premarin), 2.5 mg daily for 10 days.

If progestin or oral contraceptive therapy fails to control dysfunctional uterine bleeding or bleeding is severe and rapid, causing significant anemia, conjugated estrogens (Premarin) can be administered in a dose of 10 to 25 mg intravenously every 4 hours until bleeding ceases. The patient may then be maintained for 3 weeks on Premarin, 10 mg orally daily; if breakthrough bleeding occurs during this time, the dose is increased in 5-mg increments to a maximum of 20 mg/day. On the last 5 days of this 3-week regimen, medroxyprogesterone should be added to prevent endometrial hyperplasia and further breakthrough bleeding. If these regimens fail, dilatation and curettage or suction curettage should be performed. If medical management fails, a genital tract tumor must be considered.

When functional hyperandrogenism is associated with hirsutism and/or acne, treatment should be directed at interrupting one or more of the steps leading to the expression of symptoms: (1) inhibition of adrenal or ovarian androgen synthesis and secretion; (2) alteration of binding of androgens to SHBG; (3) impairment of the peripheral conversion of androgen precursors to active androgen; and (4) inhibition of androgen action at the target level.[22] Because the maximal effect of pharmacologic agents on hair growth takes 9 to 12 months and is sometimes not totally effective, concomitant treatment with local cosmetic measures (including bleaching, plucking, waxing, and electrolysis) is usually necessary.

When there are no specific contraindications or associated cardiovascular risk factors, the treatment of choice for hyperandrogenism producing mild hirsutism in a teenager with PCO syndrome is combination estrogen-progestin therapy. This therapy will lower free testosterone levels by reducing serum gonadotropins, increasing SHBG levels, and modestly decreasing DHEAS levels. Estrogen-progestin therapy can be expected to arrest hirsutism but may not lead to substantial improvement. Furthermore, the choice of progestin is important; ethynodiol diacetate has the least and norgestrel the greatest androgenic potential.[120] (See Chapter 18.)

Moderate or severe hirsutism and/or acne can be improved by treatment with antiandrogens, a class of hormone antagonists that inhibits the binding of androgens to the androgen receptor. Agents in this category include spironolactone, cyproterone acetate, and flutamide. Spironolactone (Aldactone) is most widely used in the United States and is clinically antiandrogenic and progestational in doses of 50 to 100 mg bid. Simultaneous administration of cyclic estrogen-progestin is indicated to ensure a regular menstrual cycle and prevent potential problems with the fetus should the teenager become pregnant. Side effects of spironolactone include initial diuresis, irregular uterine bleeding, hyperkalemia, and postural hypotension, which may limit the long-term use necessary to sustain improvement. Serum chemistry panels should be monitored at regular intervals.

Cyproterone acetate is a potent progestational and antiandrogenic agent that has proven to be very successful in the treatment of hirsutism and menstrual irregularity.[121] It is administered in a cyclic manner, generally in a dose of 50 mg per day during the first 10 days of a 21-day course of estrogen. It has limited adverse effects but is not presently available in the United States because of its association with breast cancer when administered to dogs. Flutamide is a potent nonsteroidal agent with selective antiandrogenic properties that is currently under investigation. Preliminary data indicate that it is efficacious in the therapy of hirsutism. Cusan et al. successfully treated hirsute women with flutamide (250 mg bid) in combination with an estrogen-progestin without complications.[122] After 7 months, the mean Ferriman-Gallwey score decreased by half, and marked improvement in acne and seborrhea was also noted. Whereas cimetidine has reportedly been successful in the treatment of hirsutism, its use is limited because of its frequent side effects.

Other measures used in the treatment of functional ovarian hyperandrogenism include weight reduction in obese hyperandrogenemic patients. This is sometimes successful in reversing hyperandrogenemia and menstrual disorders.[115, 116] There is virtually no place for wedge resection in the management of adolescent PCO syndrome except as an incidental procedure when ovarian tumor is suspected.

PROGNOSIS OF HYPERANDROGENIC DISORDERS

The long-term prognosis of hyperandrogenism depends on its underlying cause. A report by Ibañez et al.[123] provided the first available data on long-term prognosis of patients with precocious adrenarche. These authors performed a retrospective study of 127 females with typical precocious adrenarche. They observed a transient acceleration of growth and bone maturation in their patients but found no negative effects on the timing of gonadarche or final adult height. However, information regarding future reproductive function in patients with precocious adrenarche is still lacking.

Considerable information is available regarding the prognosis of those with congenital adrenal hyperplasia. The outcome depends greatly on the adequacy of hormonal replacement therapy and surgical correction of the underlying sexual ambiguity. Lack of prompt institution of glucocorticoid or mineralocorticoid therapy in the newborn with salt-losing congenital adrenal hyperplasia is associated with substantial morbidity and mortality, primarily because of the severe underlying adrenal insufficiency. Later in childhood and adolescence, inappropriate glucocorticoid or mineralocorticoid replacement therapy may be associated with growth attenuation and Cushing's syndrome (in cases of overtreatment) or with adrenal crises, excessive virilization, exaggerated bone maturation, and short adult stature (in cases of undertreatment). Adult height has been reported to be below average in both males and females with congenital adrenal hyperplasia,[124] and the fertility rate is low.[125] To a great extent, fertility is dependent on proper surgical correction of the external genitalia, hormone therapy, and psychological support.[126] However, preliminary data suggest that perinatal masculinization of the neuroendocrine system results in a high incidence of PCO syndrome in spite of the best medical management.[102]

The long-term prognosis for patients with adrenal neoplasms, like those with ovarian neoplasms, depends on the tumor's histologic characteristics. Those with benign lesions have an excellent prognosis, whereas those with malignant lesions typically have a poor long-term outcome, primarily because of the aggressive nature of such tumors and lack of response to radiation and chemotherapy.[79]

The irregular menstrual cycles in and virilization of the majority of patients with functional ovarian hyperandrogenism can be controlled with the previously outlined regimens, but reliable data on long-term prognosis as it relates to the reinitiation of ovulatory cycles and fertility is lacking. One theory considers PCO syndrome to be the result of chronic anovulation. Although ovulation induction improves ovarian hyperandrogenism,[127] it does not seem to be effective as a long-term form of therapy. The diagnosis of PCO syndrome has been made as early as 11 years of age (in premenarchal girls). They have ongoing menstrual abnormalities and hirsutism. Our experience is consistent with that of Southam and Richart,[128] who reported that an irregular menstrual cycle persisting for 2 years after menarche was predictive of a 50% incidence of ongoing menstrual abnormality. Clomiphene citrate has been successful in reinstating ovulatory cycles in approximately 75% of subjects.[129] Other therapies—including the combination of clomiphene citrate and human menopausal gonadotropin–human chorionic gonadotropin (hMG-hCG) or glucocorticoids, or GnRH agonist pulsatile therapy—have been successful in establishing ovulatory cycles in patients resistant to clomiphene citrate alone.[92] Weight control is an important adjuvant to medical therapy; weight reduction and increased exercise, by themselves, improve hyperandrogenism and lead to ovulatory cycles in approximately one third of patients.[130]

References

1. Miller WL. Molecular biology of steroid hormone synthesis. Endocr Rev 1988; 9:295.
2. Schweikert HU, Milewich L, Wilson JD. Aromatization of androstenedione by isolated human hairs. J Clin Endocrinol Metab 1975; 40:413.
3. Rivarola MA, Singleton RT, Migeon CJ. Splanchnic extraction and interconversion of testosterone and androstenedione in man. J Clin Invest 1967; 46:2095.
4. Glass AR. Endocrine function in human obesity. Metabolism 1981; 30:1.
5. Zuber MX, John ME, Okamura T, et al. Bovine adrenocortical cytochrome $P450_{17\alpha}$–regulation of gene expression by ACTH and elucidation of primary sequence. J Biol Chem 1986; 261:2475.
6. Rosenfield RL, Barnes RB, Cara JF, Lucky AW. Dysregulation of cytochrome P450c17α as the cause of polycystic ovary syndrome. Fertil Steril 1990; 53:785.
7. Rosenfield RL, Ehrmann DA, Brigell DF, et al. Gonadotropin releasing hormone agonist as a probe for the pathogenesis and diagnosis of ovarian hyperandrogenism. Ann NY Acad Sci, in press, 1993.
8. Rosenfield RL. The ovary and female sexual maturation. In: Kaplan SA (ed). Clinical Pediatric Endocrinology. 2nd ed. Philadelphia: WB Saunders, 1989, p 259.
9. Ehrmann D, Rosenfield RL, Barnes RB, et al. Detection of functional ovarian hyperandrogenism in women with androgen excess. N Engl J Med 1992; 327:157.
10. Payne AH, Quinn PG, Rani CSS. Regulation of microsomal cytochrome P450 enzymes and testosterone production in Leydig cells. Recent Prog Horm Res 1985; 41:153.
11. Abraham GE. Ovarian and adrenal contributions to peripheral androgens during the menstrual cycle. J Clin Endocrinol Metab 1974; 39:340.
12. Parker LN. Adrenarche. Endocrinol Metab Clin North Am 1991; 20:71.
13. Rich BH, Rosenfield RL, Lucky AW, et al. Adrenarche: Changing adrenal response to ACTH. J Clin Endocrinol Metab 1981; 52:1129.
14. Rosenfield RL, Rich BH, Lucky AW. Adrenarche as a cause of benign pseudopuberty in boys. J Pediatr 1982; 101:1005.
15. Dickerman Z, Grant DR, Faiman C, Winter JSD. Intraadrenal steroid concentrations in man: Zonal differences and developmental changes. J Clin Endocrinol Metab 1984; 59:1031.
16. Schiebinger RJ, Albertson BD, Cassorla FG, et al. The developmental changes in plasma adrenal andro-

gens during infancy and adrenarche are associated with changing activities of adrenal microsomal 17-hydroxylase and 17,20-desmolase. J Clin Invest 1981; 67:1177.

17. Byrne GC, Perry YS, Winter JSD. Kinetic analysis of adrenal 3β-hydroxysteroid dehydrogenase activity during human development. J Clin Endocrinol Metab 1985; 60:934.

18. Kennerson AR, McDonald DA, Adams JB. Dehydroepiandrosterone sulfotransferase localization in human adrenal glands: A light and electron microscopic study. J Clin Endocrinol Metab 1983; 56:786.

19. Dhom G. The prepubertal and pubertal growth of the adrenal (adrenarche). Beitr Pathol 1973; 150:357.

20. Grumbach MM, Richards GE, Conte FA, et al. Clinical disorders of adrenal function and puberty. An assessment of the role of the adrenal cortex in normal and abnormal puberty in man and evidence for an ACTH-like pituitary adrenal androgen stimulating hormone. In: James VHT, Serio M, Giusti G, Martini L (eds). The Endocrine Function of the Human Adrenal Cortex. London: Academic Press, 1978, p 583.

21. Parker L, Odell WD. Control of adrenal androgen secretion. Endocr Rev 1980; 1:392.

22. Ehrmann DA, Rosenfield RL. An endocrinologic approach to the patient with hirsutism. J Clin Endocrinol Metab 1990; 71:1.

23. Sklar CA, Kaplan SL, Grumbach MM. Evidence for dissociation between adrenarche and gonadarche: Studies in patients with idiopathic precocious puberty, gonadal dysgenesis, isolated gonadotropin deficiency, and adolescence. J Clin Endocrinol Metab 1980; 51:548.

24. Barnes RB, Rosenfield RL, Burstein S, Ehrmann DA. Pituitary-ovarian responses to nafarelin testing in the polycystic ovary syndrome. N Engl J Med 1989; 320:559–565.

25. Cumming DC, Rebar RW, Hopper BR, Yen SSC. Evidence for an influence of the ovary on circulating dehydroepiandrosterone sulfate levels. J Clin Endocrinol Metab 1982; 54:1069.

26. Ryan KJ. Granulosa-thecal cell interaction in ovarian steroidogenesis. J Steroid Biochem 1979; 11:799.

27. Hsueh AJW, Adashi EY, Jones PBC, Welsh TH. Hormonal regulation of the differentiation of cultured ovarian granulosa cells. Endocr Rev 1984; 5:76.

28. Erickson GF, Magoffin DA, Dyer CA, Hofeditz C. The ovarian androgen producing cells: A review of structure/function relationships. Endocr Rev 1985; 6:371.

29. Conway BA, Mahesh VB, Mills TM. Effect of dihydrotestosterone on the growth and function of ovarian follicles in intact immature female rats primed with PMSG. J Reprod Fertil 1990; 90:267.

30. McFarland KC, Sprengel R, Phillips HS, et al. Lutropin-choriogonadotropin receptor: An unusual member of the G protein-coupled receptor family. Science 1989; 245:494.

31. Hillier S, Ross GT. Effects of exogenous testosterone on ovarian weight, follicular morphology and intra-ovarian progesterone concentration in estrogen-primed hypophysectomized immature female rats. Biol Reprod 1979; 20:261.

32. Hoffman F, Meger C. On the action of intraovarian injection of androgen on follicle and corpus luteum maturation in women. Geburtshilfe Frauenheilkd 1965; 25:1132.

33. Barnes RB, Rosenfield RL. Polycystic ovary syndrome: Pathogenesis and treatment. Ann Intern Med 1989; 110:386.

34. Cara JF, Rosenfield RL. Insulin-like growth factor I and insulin potentiate luteinizing hormone-induced androgen synthesis by rat ovarian thecal-interstitial cells. Endocrinology 1988; 123:733.

35. Hernandez ER, Resnick CE, Holtzclaw WD, et al. Insulin as a regulator of androgen biosynthesis by cultured rat ovarian cells: Cellular mechanism(s) underlying physiological and pharmacological hormonal actions. Endocrinology 1988; 122:2034.

36. Hillier SG, Yong EL, Illingworth PJ, et al. Effect of recombinant inhibin on androgen synthesis in cultured human thecal cells. Mol Cell Endocrinol 1991; 75:R1–R6.

37. Rosenfield RL, Moll GW Jr. The role of proteins in the distribution of plasma androgens and estradiol. In: Molinatti G, Martini L, James VHT (eds). Androgenization in Women. New York: Raven Press, 1989, p 25.

38. Hammond GL. Molecular properties of corticosteroid binding globulin and sex-steroid binding proteins. Endocr Rev 1990; 11:65.

39. Moll GW Jr, Rosenfield RL. Estradiol inhibition of pituitary luteinizing hormone release is antagonized by serum proteins. J Steroid Biochem 1986; 25:309.

40. Ekins R. Measurement of free hormones in blood. Endocrinol Rev 1990; 11:5.

41. Gershagen S, Lundwall A, Fernlund P. Characterization of the human sex hormone binding globulin (SHBG) gene and demonstration of two transcripts in both liver and testis. Nucleic Acids Res 1989; 17:9245.

42. Nestler JE, Powers LP, Matt DW, et al. A direct effect of hyperinsulinemia on serum sex hormone binding globulin levels in obese women with the polycystic ovary syndrome. J Clin Endocrinol Metab 1991; 72:53.

43. Moll GW Jr, Rosenfield RL. Plasma free testosterone in the diagnosis of adolescent polycystic ovary syndrome. J Pediatr 1983; 102:461.

44. Lubhan DB, Joseph DR, Sullivan PM, et al. Cloning of human androgen receptor complementary DNA and localization to the X chromosome. Science 1988; 240:327.

45. Rosenfield RL. Pilosebaceous physiology in relation to hirsutism and acne. Clin Endocrinol Metab 1986; 15:341.

46. Lobo RA, Paul WL, Gentzschein E, et al. Production of 3α-androstanediol glucuronide in human genital skin. J Clin Endocrinol Metab 1987; 65:711.

47. Rittmaster RS, Thompson DL. Effect of leuprolide and dexamethasone on hair growth and hormone levels in hirsute women: The relative importance of the ovary and the adrenal in the pathogenesis of hirsutism. J Clin Endocrinol Metab 1988; 70:1096.

48. Kuttenn F, Mowszowicz G, Shaison G, Mauvais-Jarvis P. Androgen production and skin metabolism in hirsutism. J Clin Endocrinol Metab 1977; 75:83.

49. Kaufman FR, Gentzschein E, Stanczyk FZ, et al. Dehydroepiandrosterone and dehydroepiandrosterone sulfate metabolism in human genital skin. Fertil Steril 1990; 54:251.

50. Forman GM, Samuels HH. Interactions among a subfamily of nuclear hormone receptors: The regulatory zipper model. Mol Endocrinol 1990; 4:1290.

51. Carson-Jurica MA, Schrader WT, O'Malley BW. Steroid receptor family: Structure and function. Endocr Rev 1990; 11:201.

52. Bläuer M, Vaalasti A, Pauli S-L, et al. Location of androgen receptor in human skin. J Invest Dermatol 1991; 97:264.

53. McPhaul MJ, Marcelli M, Zoppi S, et al. The spec-

trum of mutations in the androgen receptor gene that causes androgen resistance. J Clin Endocrinol Metab 1993; 76:17.

54. Reingold SB, Rosenfield RL. The relationship of mild hirsutism or acne in women to androgens. Arch Dermatol 1987; 123:209.

55. Biffignandi P, Molinatti GM. Antiandrogens and hirsutism. Horm Res 1987; 28:242.

56. Marynick SP, Chakmakjian ZH, McCaffree DL, et al. Androgen excess in cystic acne. N Engl J Med 1983; 308:981.

57. Temeck JW, Pang S, Nelson C, New MI. Genetic defects of steroidogenesis in premature pubarche. J Clin Endocrinol Metab 1987; 64:609.

58. Oberfield SE, Mayes DM, Levine L. Adrenal steroidogenic function in a black and Hispanic population with precocious pubarche. J Clin Endocrinol Metab 1990; 70:76.

59. Morris AH, Reiter EO, Geffner ME, et al. Absence of nonclassical congenital adrenal hyperplasia in patients with precocious adrenarche. J Clin Endocrinol Metab 1989; 60:709.

60. Ghizzoni L, Virdis R, Ziveri M, et al. Adrenal steroid, cortisol, adrenocorticotropin, and β-endorphin responses to human corticotropin-releasing hormone stimulation test in normal children and children with premature pubarche. J Clin Endocrinol Metab 1989; 69:875.

61. Siegel SF, Finegold DN, Urban MD, et al. Premature pubarche: Etiological heterogeneity. J Clin Endocrinol Metab 1992; 74:239.

62. Saenger P, Reiter EO. Premature adrenarche: A normal variant of puberty? Editorial. J Clin Endocrinol Metab 1992; 74:236.

63. Rosenfield RL, Rich BH, Wolsdorf JI, et al. Pubertal presentation of congenital Δ5-3β-hydroxysteroid dehydrogenase deficiency. J Clin Endocrinol Metab 1980; 51:345.

64. Lucky AW, Rosenfield RL, McGuire J, et al. Adrenal androgen hyperresponsiveness to ACTH in women with acne and/or hirsutism: Adrenal enzyme defects and exaggerated adrenarche. J Clin Endocrinol Metab 1986; 62:840.

65. Barnes RB, Ehrmann DA, Brigell DF, Rosenfield RL. Ovarian steroidogenic responses to gonadotropin-releasing hormone testing with nafarelin in hirsute women with adrenal responses to ACTH suggestive of 3β-hydroxysteroid dehydrogenase (3β-HSD) deficiency. J Clin Endocrinol Metab 1993, in press.

66. McKenna TJ. Pathogenesis and treatment of polycystic ovary syndrome. N Engl J Med 1988; 318:558.

67. Lobo RA. The role of the adrenal in polycystic ovary syndrome. Reprod Endocrinol 1984; 2:251.

68. Miller WL, Levine LS. Molecular and clinical advances in congenital adrenal hyperplasia. J Pediatr 1987; 111:1.

69. White PC, New MI, Dupont B. Congenital adrenal hyperplasia. N Engl J Med 1987; 316:1519.

70. Rosenfield RL. Congenital adrenal hyperplasia and reproductive function in females. In: Flamigni C, Venturoli S, Givens J (eds). Adolescence in Females. Chicago: Year Book Medical, 1985, p 373.

71. Rosenfield RL. Hyperandrogenism in peripubertal girls. Pediatr Clin North Am 1990; 37:1333.

72. Müller J. Aldosterone biosynthesis in bovine, rat, and human adrenal: Commonalities and challenges. Mol Cell Endocrinol 1991; 78:C119.

73. Cara JF, Moshang T Jr, Bongiovanni AM, Marx BS. Elevated 17-hydroxyprogesterone and testosterone in a newborn with 3β-hydroxysteroid dehydrogenase deficiency. N Engl J Med 1985; 313:618.

74. Pang S, Levine LS, Stoner E, et al. Non salt-losing congenital adrenal hyperplasia due to 3β-hydroxysteroid dehydrogenase deficiency with normal glomerulosa function. J Clin Endocrinol Metab 1983; 56:808.

75. Zachman M, Völlman A, New MI, et al. Congenital adrenal hyperplasia due to deficiency of 11β-hydroxylation of 17α-hydroxylated steroids. J Clin Endocrinol Metab 1971; 33:501.

76. New MI, Lorenzen F, Lerner AJ, et al. Genotyping steroid 21-hydroxylase deficiency: Hormonal reference data. J Clin Endocrinol Metab 1983; 57:320.

77. Pollack MS, Levine LS, Pang S, et al. Prenatal diagnosis of congenital adrenal hyperplasia (21-hydroxylase deficiency) by HLA typing. Lancet 1979; 1:1107.

78. Forest MG, Betuel H, David M. Traitement antenatal de l'hyperplasie congenitale des surrenales pare deficit en 21-hydroxylase: Etude multicentrique. Ann Endocrinol (Paris) 1987; 48:31.

79. Lee PDK, Winter RJ, Green OC. Virilizing adrenocortical tumors in childhood: Eight cases and a review of the literature. Pediatrics 1985; 76:437.

80. Fraumeni JM, Miller RW. Adrenocortical neoplasms with hemihypertrophy, brain tumors and other disorders. J Pediatr 1967; 70:129.

81. Adeyemi SD, Grange AO, Giwa-Osagie OF, Elesha SO. Adrenal rest tumour of the ovary associated with isosexual precocious pseudopuberty and cushingoid features. Eur J Pediatr 1986; 145:236.

82. Vouilainen R, Leisti S, Perheentupa J. Growth in Cushing syndrome. Eur J Pediatr 1985; 144:141.

83. Werk EE, Sholiton LJ, Kalejs L. Testosterone-secreting adenoma under gonadotropin control. N Engl J Med 1973; 289:767.

84. Malchoff CD, Javier EC, Malchoff DM, et al. Primary cortisol resistance presenting as isosexual precocity. J Clin Endocrinol Metab 1990; 70:503.

85. Phillipou G, Higgins BA. A new defect in the peripheral metabolism of cortisone to cortisol. J Steroid Biochem 1985; 22:435.

86. Glickman SP, Rosenfield RL, Bergenstal RM, Helke JC. Multiple androgenic abnormalities, including elevated free testosterone, in hyperprolactinemic women. J Clin Endocrinol Metab 1982; 55:251.

87. Lim NY, Dingman JF. Androgenic adrenal hyperfunction in acromegaly. N Engl J Med 1964; 271:1189.

88. Talerman A, Jarabak J, Amarose AP. Gonadoblastoma and dysgerminoma in a true hermaphrodite with 46,XX karyotype. Am J Obstet Gynecol 1981; 140:475.

89. Stein IF, Leventhal ML. Amenorrhea associated with polycystic ovaries. Am J Obstet Gynecol 1935; 29:181.

90. Franks S. Polycystic ovary syndrome: A changing perspective. Clin Endocrinol 1989; 31:87.

91. Goldzieher JW. Polycystic ovarian disease. Clin Obstet Gynecol 1973; 16:82.

92. Yen SSC. Chronic anovulation caused by peripheral endocrine disorders. In: Yen SSC, Jaffe RB (eds). Reproductive Endocrinology. 3rd ed. Philadelphia: WB Saunders, 1991, p 576.

93. Goldzieher JW, Axelrod LR. Clinical and biochemical features of polycystic ovarian disease. Fertil Steril 1963; 14:631.

94. Pang SY, Softness B, Sweeney WJ III, New MI. Hirsutism, polycystic ovarian disease, and ovarian 17-ketosteroid reductase deficiency. N Engl J Med 1987; 316:1295.

95. Chang RJ, Manfdel FP, Lu JK, Judd HL. Enhanced

disparity of gonadotropin secretion by estrone in women with polycystic ovarian disease. J Clin Endocrinol Metab 1982; 54:490.

96. Chang RJ, Laufer LR, Meldrum DR, et al. Steroid secretion in polycystic ovarian disease after ovarian suppression by a long-acting gonadotropin-releasing hormone agonist. J Clin Endocrinol Metab 1983; 56:897.

97. Berger MJ, Taymor ML, Patton WC. Gonadotropin levels and secretory patterns in patients with typical and atypical polycystic ovarian disease. Fertil Steril 1975; 26:619.

98. Zumnoff B, Freeman R, Coupey S, et al. A chronobiologic abnormality in luteinizing hormone secretion in teenage girls with the polycystic-ovary syndrome. N Engl J Med 1983; 309:1206.

99. Futterweit W, Deligdisch L. Histopathological effects of exogenously administered testosterone in 19 female to male transsexuals. J Clin Endocrinol Metab 1986; 62:16.

100. Porcu E, Venturoli S, Magrini O, et al. Circadian variations of luteinizing hormone can have two different profiles in adolescent anovulation. J Clin Endocrinol Metab 1987; 65:488.

101. Marshall JC. Regulation of gonadotropin secretion. In: DeGroot L (ed). Endocrinology. 2nd ed. Philadelphia: WB Saunders, 1989, p 1903.

102. Barnes RB, Rosenfield RL. Masculinization of the human pituitary-ovarian axis by perinatal androgen exposure: Polycystic ovary syndrome (PCOS) in congenital adrenal virilizing disease (CAVD). Endocrinology 1991; 128(suppl):335.

103. Erickson GF, Hsueh AJ, Quigley ME, et al. Functional studies of aromatase activity in human granulosa cells from normal and polycystic ovaries. J Clin Endocrinol Metab 1979; 49:851.

104. Moller DE, Flier JS. Insulin resistance—mechanisms, syndromes, and implications. N Engl J Med 1991; 325:938.

105. Barbieri RL, Smith S, Ryan KJ. The role of hyperinsulinemia in the pathogenesis of ovarian hyperandrogenism. Fertil Steril 1988; 50:197.

106. Dunaif A, Green G, Futterweit W, Dobrjansky A. Suppression of hyperandrogenism does not improve peripheral or hepatic insulin resistance in the polycystic ovary syndrome. J Clin Endocrinol Metab 1990; 70:699.

107. Dunaif A, Segal KR, Futterweit W, Dobrjansky A. Profound peripheral insulin resistance, independent of obesity, in polycystic ovary syndrome. Diabetes 1989; 38:1165.

108. Adashi EY, Resnick CE, D'Ercole AJ, et al. Insulin-like growth factors as intraovarian regulators of granulosa cell function. Endocr Rev 1985; 6:400.

109. Poretsky L, Kalin MF. The gonadotropic function of insulin. Endocr Rev 1987; 8:132.

110. Futterweit W, Krieger DT. Pituitary tumors associated with hyperprolactinemia and polycystic ovary disease. Fertil Steril 1979; 31:608.

111. Monroe SE, Levine L, Chang J, et al. Prolactin-secreting pituitary adenomas. V. J Clin Endocrinol Metab 1981; 52:1171.

112. Dewailly D, Vantyghem-Haudiquet MC, Sainsard C, et al. Clinical and biological phenotype in late-onset 21-hydroxylase deficiency. J Clin Endocrinol Metab 1986; 63:418.

113. Hatch R, Rosenfield RL, Kim MH, Tredway D. Hirsutism: Implications, etiology, and management. Am J Obstet Gynecol 1981; 140:815.

114. Rosenfield RL, Cohen RM, Talerman A. Lipid cell tumor of the ovary in reference to adult-onset congenital adrenal hyperplasia and polycystic ovary syndrome. J Reprod Med 1987; 32:363.

115. Kopelman PG, White N, Pilkington FRE, Jeffcoate SL. The effect of weight loss on sex steroid secretion and binding in massively obese women. Clin Endocrinol 1981; 14:113.

116. Bates GW, Whitworth NS. Effect of body weight reduction on plasma androgens in obese, infertile women. Fertil Steril 1982; 38:406.

117. Lustig RH, Bradlow HL, Fishman J. Estrogen metabolism in disorders of nutrition and dietary composition. In: Pirke KM, Wuttke WW, Schweiger U (eds). The Menstrual Cycle and Its Disorders. Berlin: Springer-Verlag, 1989, p 119.

118. Rosenfield RL, Bickel S, Razdan AK. Amenorrhea related to progestin excess in congenital adrenal hyperplasia. Obstet Gynecol 1980; 56:208.

119. Rittmaster RS, Givner ML. Effect of daily and alternate day low dose prednisone on serum cortisol and adrenal androgens in hirsute women. J Clin Endocrinol Metab 1988; 67:400.

120. Dickey RP. Managing Contraception Pill Patients. 5th ed. Durant, OK: Creative Infomatics, 1986, p 206.

121. Kuttenn F, Rigaud C, Wright F, Mauvais-Jarvis P. Treatment of hirsutism by oral cyproterone acetate and percutaneous estradiol. J Clin Endocrinol Metab 1980; 51:1107.

122. Cusan L, Dupont A, Tremblay R, Labrie F. Treatment of hirsutism with the pure antiandrogen flutamide. Rec Res Gynecol Endocrinol 1988; 1:577.

123. Ibañez L, Virdis R, Potau N, et al. Natural history of premature pubarche: An auxological study. J Clin Endocrinol Metab 1992; 74:254.

124. Styne DM, Richards GE, Bell JJ, et al. Growth patterns in congenital adrenal hyperplasia. Correlation of glucocorticoid therapy with stature. In: Lee PA, Plotnick LP, Kowarski AA, Migeon CJ (eds). Congenital Adrenal Hyperplasia. Baltimore: University Park Press, 1977, p 247.

125. Mulaikal RM, Migeon CJ, Rock JA. Fertility rates in female patients with congenital adrenal hyperplasia due to 21-hydroxylase deficiency. N Engl J Med 1987; 316:178.

126. Money J, Schwartz M. Dating, romantic and nonromantic friendships, and sexuality in 17 early-treated adrenogenital females aged 16–25. In: Lee PA, Plotnick LP, Kowarski AA, Migeon CJ (eds). Congenital Adrenal Hyperplasia. Baltimore: University Park Press, 1977, p 419.

127. Blankstein J, Rabinovici J, Goldenberg M, et al. Changing pituitary reactivity to follicle-stimulating hormone and luteinizing hormone after induced ovulatory cycles and after anovulation in patients with polycystic ovarian disease. J Clin Endocrinol Metab 1987; 65:1164.

128. Southam AL, Richart RM. The prognosis for adolescents with menstrual abnormalities. Am J Obstet Gynecol 1966; 94:637.

129. Futterweit W. Polycystic Ovarian Disease. New York: Springer-Verlag, 1984.

130. Pasquali R, An·enucci D, Casimirri F, et al. Clinical and hormonal characteristics of obese amenorrheic hyperandrogenic women before and after weight loss. J Clin Endocrinol Metab 1989; 68:173.

CHAPTER 17

Adolescent Sexuality

ROBERT T. BROWN

BARBARA A. CROMER

Little is more basic to the nature of human beings than sexuality. The melding of parental gametes assigns us our genotypic sex, and then other physiologic, cultural, and societal factors help us shape our phenotypic expression of that chromosomal "throw of the dice." From the earliest moments out of the uterus, the shaping begins. With that first question, "Is it a girl or a boy?," a host of forces begins to direct the kind of woman or man an infant will become. This chapter will examine the contributions of the various factors that shape humans as men and women and will explore the results of that shaping in terms of how adolescents express their sexuality. In addition, the chapter will look at how Americans formally transmit knowledge of sexuality to their children and adolescents by means of sex/sexuality education.

Human sexuality includes the physical characteristics of and capacities for specific sex behaviors, together with psychosocial values, norms, attitudes, and learning processes that influence these behaviors. It also includes a sense of gender identity and related concepts, behaviors, and attitudes about the self and others as men or women in the context of one's society.[1] Whereas biologic factors such as genotype and hormonal influences on the developing brain affect sexuality from the moment of conception, other extrinsic factors begin to exert their influences from birth. The family's perception of maleness and femaleness, rooted as it is in the norms and expectations of their culture and of society in general, is expressed to the infant from the start. Because we are a species in which assignment of gender is basic, it may be difficult to discern the various factors that make humans women and men. Therefore, it is instructive to look at an analogous species in which gender is not existent. This can be done only through literature, and the novel in which it is best expressed is *The Left Hand of Darkness* by Ursula LeGuin.[2] In this novel, LeGuin introduces a species that is similar to humans but has no sex differentiation until individuals go "into heat" to procreate. Therefore, all children and adolescents are treated equally, and the concept of gender difference is unnecessary and unknown. All relationships in this society exist without the constant influence of gender as we know it.

In addition to elucidating the factors that affect adolescent sexuality, this chapter will discuss the consequences of the expression of sexuality, the epidemiology of and risk factors for early adolescent sexual activity, and sexual dysfunction and homosexuality (Table 17–1).

TABLE 17–1 ••• MAJOR FACTORS INFLUENCING DEVELOPMENT OF SEXUALITY

Biology
Family
Culture
Society

BIOLOGY

Biology determines a person's genotype and the major factors in that genotype's phenotypic expression. If a girl has two X chromosomes but an enzymatic defect is present in her adrenal glands, she may be born with masculinized genitalia. The reaction of her family to this defect will influence greatly this girl's self-concept as a woman. Even if the girl is not fully masculinized, she may have severe acne and/or hirsutism, which undoubtedly will influence her self-image. Similarly, if a girl born with a missing X chromosome (i.e., with Turner syndrome) is perceived at birth as undeniably female, she may be treated for the rest of her life as a girl rather than as a woman, because, without pharmacologic assistance, she will not mature.

Because of as-yet-undetermined influences of androgens on the fetal brain, a particular girl may be more "boyish" than her peers, or a combination of genetic factors may make her more adept at sports. This physical capability may make her seem more "masculine" and will influence how she is perceived by others and, ultimately, by herself.

FAMILY

A child's first sense that he or she is a boy or girl and exactly what that means is conveyed by the parents early in childhood.[3] As the child develops, she witnesses how the mother behaves as a woman, how the father behaves as a man, and how they behave toward each other. These impressions go a long way in helping the child define what a man or woman should be.[4] Modifications of these images come from other members of the family such as grandparents and siblings. Absence of one of the parents or of someone who assumes that parental role can make it difficult for a child to understand how women and men behave with each other. Girls "test" how to behave as a woman with their fathers or another close adult male. Without that input, many girls may go "looking for Daddy" and may engage in considerable risk-taking behavior toward that end.[5] Such behavior may lead to adolescent parenthood or abusive situations. Inappropriate behavior on the part of a girl's male authority figure may also color her view of sexuality. A girl who has been sexually abused is likely to have a significantly impaired self-image. Many of these victims may attempt suicide or become prostitutes.[6] On the other hand, a girl who is reared in a home in which her parents are caring, loving, supportive, and affectionate toward each other and in which the bounds of propriety are observed will be able, in all likelihood, to enter into a mature relationship when she reaches adulthood.

CULTURE

Cultural attitudes toward sexuality greatly influence the manner in which an adolescent can express her sexuality. This is exemplified in several ways. First, the culture assigns men and women specific roles. When these roles are sharply delimited, the choices open to the adolescent to express manhood or womanhood are few. Cultural ambiguity regarding sexual behavior leaves the adolescent with many options but little guidance. Similarly, the culture dictates how sexual feelings may be expressed; there are four basic types in this regard: sexually repressive, sexually restrictive, sexually permissive, or sexually supportive.[7] Each type of culture has a distinctive approach to the emergent sexuality of its youth.

A sexually repressive culture attempts to limit sexuality. The Puritans of New England are an example of such a culture. Sexual play among the young is not allowed, and premarital chastity is required. Sexuality is associated with guilt, fear, and anger. Sexual pleasure has little value.

A sexually restrictive culture also attempts to limit sexuality. These cultures are common; the United States during the first 60 years of this century is a fairly typical example. In such a culture there is little sexual play in childhood, and premarital chastity is required of at least one of the sexes. These cultures are typically ambivalent about sex, and sex tends to be feared primarily for the problems that it can cause.

Tolerance of sexuality is characteristic of a sexually permissive culture. This culture exhibits loose enforcement of formal prohibitions. Children may participate in sexual play as long as adults do not see it overtly. Sexual activity among adolescents and before marriage is the norm, and sex is considered a normal and valued part of human life. Although somewhat common in non-European cultures, this approach to sexuality appeared in the United States in the early 1960s and lasted to the mid

1980s. Because of the problems associated with this approach (acquired immunodeficiency syndrome [AIDS], other sexually transmitted diseases, and adolescent pregnancy), American culture is attempting to revert to a restrictive approach to sexuality.

Sexually supportive cultures have been especially common among the peoples of Oceania. These cultures cultivate sexuality. Sex is seen as indispensable for human happiness, and sexual experimentation is encouraged in the young. Customs and institutions supply sexual information and experience to young people of all ages, and there is no sexually latent period in a child's life.

The United States consists of a mix of cultures and therefore has a great variety of approaches toward and opinions about child and adolescent sexuality. One of the problems American youth may encounter is conflict between the culture within which they were raised and that of others with whom they interact. One of the effects of the "global village" produced by the media is the blurring of the differences between many of the cultures in our country. Youth who spend a great deal of time in front of the television may question much more readily the values imparted to them by their natal culture.

SOCIETY

In some instances, culture is uniform throughout society, but this is not the case in the United States, in which various cultures blend into a (hopefully) harmonious whole, but each component stays distinct. With children growing up in many, at times disparate, cultures, conflict between the sexuality values with which adolescents are raised and those that they confront in society at large are inevitable. Comfort and security with their own sexuality as learned in the home might enable adolescents to negotiate the conflicting messages that are confronted as they mature.

One of the predominant ways in which current societal norms of sexual roles and behaviors are conveyed to adolescents is via the media, particularly television. The media exert a powerful influence on adolescents by exposing them to an adult world of which they were formerly unaware.[8] Many parents abdicate their responsibility to teach their children about sex and sexuality, and television, movies, and magazines are increasingly important

sources of information about "normal" behavior.[9]

No other leisure activity is more widely pursued than television watching, especially among children. Adolescents watch less television than children,[10] but what they do watch is heavily laden with messages about sexual roles and sexual behaviors. Further discussion about the possible influence of media on adolescent sexual behavior is presented later.

DEVELOPMENT OF ADOLESCENT SEXUALITY

It is the mix of the described influences that determines how an adolescent will develop as a sexual being, in terms of both self-image and behavior. To understand the sequence, it is necessary to understand basic adolescent development.

Adolescents develop in three primary arenas: organic, cognitive, and psychosocial. Organic development is puberty, which is discussed in Chapter 4. Cognitive development, as delineated by Piaget, occurs in age-specific stages.[11] Children begin to think in an adult fashion at about the age of 12 years. Piaget calls this type of thinking formal operational thought. Full capacity to think in this manner is not reached, however, until at least 15 or 16 years of age. Early (10- to 13-year-old) and middle (14- to 16-year-old) adolescents cannot be expected to function in an adult fashion most of the time. They need explicit examples to understand ideas. In the medical setting, for example, history taking must be specific and directive. In the same vein, instructions to the teenager should also be very concrete.

Psychosocial development encompasses an adolescent's ability to view him- or herself realistically and relate to others. A convenient way of understanding this facet of development is to divide it into four tasks that the adolescent must achieve before he or she can be said to have entered adulthood effectively:

1. The achievement of effective separation, or *independence*, from the family of origin;
2. The achievement of a realistic *vocational* goal;
3. The achievement of a mature level of *sexuality*;
4. The achievement of a realistic and positive *self-image*.[12]

Sexuality refers to more than just the capacity to participate in physical sexual behavior. It includes the way a person views her- or himself as a woman or a man in our society and how that person relates to other women and men in general and to one particular person specifically. Sexuality includes the ability of a person to enter and maintain an intimate relationship on a giving and trusting basis.

Early adolescents express sexuality in ways that are humorous to adults but painful to the adolescent. Adolescents think about the opposite sex a great deal but rarely do much with their thoughts, given appropriate adult supervision. Although they have many fantasies about the opposite sex and contact in school, social contact occurs primarily in situations created by and supervised by adults (e.g., school dances). School dances are classic situations for the study of early adolescent sexuality behavior. At junior high dances the girls form a mass in the middle of the dance floor that bounces in time to the music, while the boys, averaging a head shorter than the girls, circle around the outside and now and then dart toward the middle to "count coup." The girls try to ignore these forays while occasionally sending off "scouting" parties of at least three girls to the bathroom.

As boys or girls grow into middle adolescence, their efforts at relating to those to whom they are romantically inclined center more on group dating and social activities. Teenagers at this stage of development are more secure in their physical self-image and are more prone to spend time with others in their peer group. Any romantic involvement they may have is normally with a partner who is of similar age and is characterized not by the giving nature of a mature relationship, but by more selfish motivations. A girl is preoccupied with how her partner matches up to her image of the ideal "catch," and a boy is preoccupied with how far he can go sexually with this girl. Feelings are intense and all encompassing to the teenager involved. The partner, however, can never really match up to the image that the teenager has created, so the relationship has a very short life span by adult standards. By late adolescence, the young person usually has grown to the point where he or she can enter into a relationship in a more adult fashion. These relationships usually are characterized by greater concern of the participants for the feelings and welfare of their partners. The capacity for true intimacy has begun to develop, and the adolescents are capable of adult

type relationships. While this internal process is proceeding, it is subject to all the forces that were outlined previously and to the conditioning the adolescent received as a child.

SEXUAL ACTIVITY

Epidemiology

There is surprisingly little accurate information on the profile of teenage sex behavior in this country. Most of the data discussed to this point were obtained before 1983 (Table 17–2). Results from these surveys should be interpreted with a certain amount of caution because of various biasing influences. For example, fewer than 50% of contacted households participated in a number of the surveys.[13–15] Second, some of the data were obtained from a single geographic area, such as North Carolina[16] or Michigan.[17] Given these limitations, one can say that the information derived is applicable to those particular samples but is not necessarily representative of other adolescent populations. Third, the reliability of responses about sexuality is an unavoidable potential bias. In an attempt to minimize this effect, all the surveys used questionnaires completed in private by the adolescent.

Information about sexual activity is most limited for adolescents younger than 15 years of age. Vener et al. reported in 1972 that 20% and 7% of 13-year-old boys and girls, respec-

TABLE 17–2 ••• PREVALENCE OF SEXUAL ACTIVITY*

Type	Age	Gender	Rate
Masturbation	13	Both	54%
Masturbation	18	Both	82%
Kissing	13	Both	67%
Kissing	15	Both	97%
Breast fondling	13	Boys	20% to 40%
Breast fondling	13	Girls	25% to 31%
Breast fondling	18	Boys	75%
Breast fondling	18	Girls	67%
Penile/vaginal play	13	Both	20%
Penile/vaginal play	17	Male	60%
Sexual intercourse	13	Male	13%
Sexual intercourse	13	Female	7%
Sexual intercourse	18	Male	13%
Sexual intercourse	18	Female	60%

*Prevalence data for all nonintercourse behaviors are derived from Sorenson,[14] and prevalence data for intercourse are drawn from Vener et al.[17]

tively, admitted to having had sexual intercourse.[17] However, this sample was drawn from a solely white population in the midwest. By age 15, the percentage of sexually active adolescents ranges from 14% to 44% in males and from 7% to 30% in females in national samples.[13, 14, 18] At the same age and for both sexes, blacks are more than twice as likely as whites to have experienced sexual intercourse.[14, 18] By 18 years of age, the racial and gender gaps begin to close. About 80% of males and 60% of females are sexually active by this age; rates for blacks are 2% to 5% higher than these figures.[18] The sparse data available for Hispanic teenagers suggest that rates for sexual activity lie somewhere between those of whites and blacks.[18]

Since the 1960s, a climate of increasing sexual liberalism has been reflected in increasing prevalences of sexual activity in adolescents. Chilman noted that in one group of white high school seniors, the prevalence of coital activity in the late 1960s had increased 300% in girls and 50% in boys compared with figures obtained during the 40 previous years.[19] Moreover, during the relatively short period between 1969 and 1973, Vener and Stewart reported a 6% increase (to 33% in males and 22% in females) in the prevalence of coital activity among white high school students.[20] Using three repeated samplings during the 1970s, Zelnik and Kantner demonstrated an increase from 52% to 64% in black females and from 23% to 42% in white females age 15 to 19 years living in urban areas. These numbers had dropped to 53% and 40%, respectively, by 1982.[21]

There are even fewer data regarding the prevalence of sexual behaviors other than sexual intercourse. The first sexual behavior to consider is masturbation. Although it is almost 20 years old, the national survey by Sorenson provides the best information about the incidence of this activity in young people.[14] Only 11% of the sample population stated that they had begun to masturbate at younger than 12 years of age, but this number rose to 54% by age 13 and 82% by age 15. Across all age groups, males were more likely to have masturbated, and with greater frequency. About half of those practicing masturbation, regardless of sex, reported at least some guilt or anxiety associated with the activity. Nonvirgins were twice as likely to engage in masturbation as virgins, and among virgins, those who had experienced some heterosexual foreplay were twice as likely to masturbate than those who

had not. One interesting finding was that girls who had had intercourse were more likely to have masturbated than boys with a similar behavioral profile (39% vs. 36%, respectively). This may be related to the frequent lack of orgasm during intercourse in female adolescents and the subsequent need to release physical tension.

The following data were pooled from three surveys that included information about sexual activity with a partner other than sexual intercourse.[12, 14, 20] About two thirds of 13-year-old teenagers reported that they had been kissed, whereas up to 97% reported being kissed by 15 years of age. Some 20% to 40% of 13-year-old boys had engaged in breast fondling, and 25% to 31% of 13-year-old girls had had their breasts fondled. By 15 and 18 years of age, up to two thirds and three fourths of adolescent girls and boys, respectively, had practiced this behavior. The prevalence of vaginal and penile play was fairly similar between the sexes, with about 20% at age 13 years and 60% at age 17 years performing these behaviors. About 20% of adolescents reported the practice of cunnilingus and/or fellatio.

It has traditionally been assumed that sexual intercourse represents the end result of a progression of intimate behaviors over time. Although this appears to be true for white females, one author suggests that black girls may skip the early stages;[14] this may be one reason for the earlier initiation of sexual intercourse in the black population.[19] Interestingly, Vener and Stewart found that, over 3 years, although the degree of "light petting" (kissing and fondling above the waist) did not change, there was an increase in the prevalence of "heavy petting" (fondling below the waist) and sexual intercourse.[20] Thus, the changing mores in sexual behavior may serve to attenuate the early stages of sexual activity and hasten the onset of sexual activity.

Risk Factors

Early Puberty. There is some evidence that early sexual maturation is associated with early sexual activity. First, a positive correlation has been demonstrated between gynecologic age and sexual debut.[22, 23] Second, girls with precocious puberty tend to initiate sexual activity at a younger age than their normally maturing peers.[24] Although a direct hormonal effect is implicated in the development of libido, the onset of sexual behavior in early maturers is also probably determined by a complex array of psychosocial influences. For example, a girl who has advanced secondary sex characteristics may attract older boys who are more sexually experienced or, because she is assumed to be socially mature by parents, is given less restrictive curfews. Udry found that serum testosterone along with a variety of behavioral variables (e.g., attitudes toward sexual permissiveness) were the major components affecting the level of sexuality in teenage girls, thereby supporting a biosocial model for sexual initiation.[16] In contrast, Udry found a more strictly hormonal explanation for the same behavior in teenage boys (Table 17–3).

Demographic Background. Low socioeconomic status is associated with higher prevalences of sexual activity. Hayes reported higher rates in adolescents whose mothers had not finished high school than in those whose mothers had received some postgraduate education.[18] Vener et al. found lower rates in a community of mostly professional wage earners than in a nearby area populated by mostly blue-collar workers.[17] Poverty, with its attendant lack of opportunities for educational and professional advancement, is a clear risk factor for early sexual activity and explains at least some increased levels of sexual activity in the black population. However, even after controlling for the statistical effects of socioeconomic status, black adolescents still have higher prevalences (>10% difference) than white adolescents.[18, 25] These differences may be due to additional influences from the sociocultural environment, such as community attitudes toward teenage childbearing and forbearance toward life-styles outside the traditional norm.[19, 25] Further research is needed to disentangle the complex web of environmental and personal variables determining sexual behavior in each ethnic group.

Personality Characteristics. Adolescents who admit to sexual activity are more likely than their virginal peers to have low future

TABLE 17–3 ••• RISK FACTORS FOR SEXUAL ACTIVITY

Developmental
Socioeconomic factors
Personality characteristics
Family characteristics
Peer influences
Media

and educational achievement orientation; they also are more likely to display attitudes of alienation, nontraditional attitudes toward sex, and other socially experimental behaviors.[19] Although virginal adolescents are more likely to report high religiosity, this source of influence is related more to the perceived importance of religion in their lives than to the precepts taught in any individual denomination.[26] There is also a positive relationship between substance abuse and sexual activity. Using data from a national survey, Mott and Haurin reported that adolescents who used marijuana or alcohol, when compared with those who did not, were more likely to initiate sexual intercourse within the following year; the converse was also true. In addition, marijuana use was more strongly associated with subsequent sexual debut than regular alcohol use.[27] Interestingly, despite the increased prevalence of sexual activity in the 1970s, the personality characteristics of virgins and nonvirgins did not appear to change. Jessor and Jessor found that the personality features that distinguished virgins from nonvirgins in 1979 were the same as those that had been found in the two groups 4 years earlier.[28]

Family Characteristics. In the United States, it is generally observed that even in families with effective lines of communication, parents and teenagers feel uncomfortable discussing sexuality.[29] As a result, there is often little direct parental input in the initial development of an adolescent's attitudes toward sexuality. However, that is not to say that family characteristics do not exert significant influence on an adolescent's sexual attitudes and behavior. First, there is some evidence to suggest that the earlier the mother and older sister's sexual debut, the earlier that of a younger adolescent will be.[18] In addition, a higher degree of parental supervision and consistent limit setting have been associated with delay in the sexual initiation of the adolescent,[15] whereas permissive parental attitudes toward sexuality and other nonnormative behaviors have been associated with an early sexual initiation.[15, 19] Although teenagers whose parents are separated or divorced are more likely to be sexually active than their peers with intact families,[13] the specific source of this influence is unclear. The association could be related to the adolescent's feeling a sense of physical or emotional isolation from a parent struggling with marital issues.[21] Brooks-Gunn and Furstenberg emphasize the importance of further elucidation of family impact on sexual behavior in the adolescent, including study of social and cognitive development related to family styles of decision making and moral judgments.[29]

Peer Influences. Considering the frequent lack of home education and the developmentally appropriate progressive separation from the family, it is not surprising that adolescents obtain most of their information about sex from peers. In addition, the literature implies that a positive relationship exists between being sexually active and having sexually active friends. However, most of the studies have been marred by having adolescents estimate the level of peer sexual activity, which frequently is unreliable. Billy et al., who obtained direct information from both adolescent subjects and their friends, found that males did not choose and did not appear to be influenced by friends based on their level of sexual activity.[30] Girls, on the other hand, tended to name friends with the same profile of sexual behaviors. Unfortunately, whether sexual activity represented a criterion for friendship or a behavioral response to peer group norms could not be determined. Hayes adds that male partners also may exert a significant amount of influence on the sexual attitudes and behaviors of adolescent girls.[18]

Media. Visual media (i.e., television and film) represent an important resource of information about some sexual behaviors. It is a potentially powerful influence, as the average teenager spends a minimum of 12 hours a week watching television, and young people are the primary target of many movies. Certainly, these media also provide models of sexual attractiveness; for example, up to one third of commercials have sex appeal as their major selling point.[31] Display of different types of sexual activity is common in all the visual media but is almost always lacking in any allusion to pregnancy or other adverse consequences, such as sexually transmitted diseases. However, a causal relationship between media exposure and subsequent sexual behavior should not be assumed. Some data suggest a media influence on adolescents' perceptions of sexual activity in the real world, reinforcement of sex-role stereotyping, and effects on attitudes toward sexual beauty. However, there is no convincing evidence for a causal effect on actual teenage sexual behavior in any form. It has been reported that adolescents who watch a great deal of television are more likely to be sexually active, but this relationship may simply reflect a third linking variable, such as socioeconomic status or lack of parental supervision.

SEXUAL DYSFUNCTION

Sexual dysfunction has been defined as any "condition considered by the affected individual or those around him/her to inhibit sexual functioning physically or psychologically."[32] Certainly, any type of dysfunction that occurs in adults can occur in adolescents, but there is little objective information regarding the prevalences and prognostic implications of these types of disorders in this age group. The traditional observation is that the majority of adolescents experience some form of sexual dysfunction and that the prognosis is usually good for ultimate normal function. In most cases, the problems arise from a naiveté about sexual technique.[32]

Although premature ejaculation is the most common type of sexual dysfunction in males, affecting up to 15% to 20%, only a small minority seek professional help.[33] Premature ejaculation has been defined as ejaculation either within 2 minutes of penetration or before adequate sexual satisfaction of the partner. Given the usual low level of knowledge regarding sexual matters in teenagers, the prevalence of this disorder would be expected to be high. In one survey, 22% of college students reported a history of premature ejaculation.[34] The overwhelming majority of such episodes are caused by psychological factors.

The other common type of sexual dysfunction in males is lack of adequate erection, or impotence. Of a large group of adolescents seen for clinical evaluation of sexual dysfunction, the majority had impotence as the presenting complaint.[35] Reassurance that physiologic function remains intact is found by a positive history of nocturnal tumescence and periodic nocturnal emissions; in these cases, the cause is psychological. Other diagnostic considerations in this age group include prostatic enlargement from sexually transmitted disease or substance abuse, particularly alcohol, amphetamines, and heroin.[32] Farrow offers a list of etiologic factors (Table 17–4).[36]

Types of sexual dysfunction in females may be divided into two similar categories: disorders of arousal and disorders of orgasm (Table 17–5). Study of problems related to arousal has been sparse, partly because the process does not interfere with the ability to engage in

TABLE 17-4 ••• COMMON ETIOLOGIC FACTORS IN ADOLESCENT MALE SEXUAL DYSFUNCTION

Nonorganic Conditions (more common)
  Sexual partner dysfunction
  Performance anxiety/guilt
  Environmental factors—lack of privacy
  History of sexual abuse
  Sexual identity disorders and sexual role confusion
  Affective disorder
  Anxiety
  Alcohol-/drug-induced
Primary Medical Conditions (less common)
  Cardiovascular: Aortic coarctation, internal iliac/
    pudendal artery stenosis, priapism
  Metabolic: Diabetes mellitus, sickle cell disease,
    chronic renal and hepatic disorders
  Endocrine: Addison's disease, hyperprolactinemia,
    hypothyroidism, hypogonadism
  Systemic infections: Infectious mononucleosis,
    hepatitis, genitourinary infection, prostatitis,
    urethritis
  Neurologic: Spinal cord injury, CNS lesions,
    peripheral neuropathy (metabolic drug-induced),
    head injury, epilepsy
  Drug-related: Antihypertensive medications, CNS
    depressants, phenothiazines, imipramine, cimetidine,
    amphetamines, propranolol, spironolactone
  Secondary medical conditions: Abdominal surgery,
    trauma, radiation, cancer chemotherapy, chronic
    illnesses, genital surgery
  Local conditions: Congenital hypospadias, epispadias

Adapted by permission of Elsevier Science Publishing Co., Inc. from An approach to the management of sexual dysfunction in the adolescent male, by Farrow JA, Journal of Adolescent Health Care, Vol. No. 6, p 397. Copyright 1985 by The Society for Adolescent Medicine.

coitus or reproduction.[33] More attention has been paid to orgasmic insufficiency, defined as persistent orgasmic delay or absence after a normal excitement stage. This disorder is the most common sexually related problem in women of all ages. In a group of female college students, 44% complained of anorgasmia. Orgasmic dysfunction is usually a function of insufficient knowledge about arousal patterns. Greydanus et al. note that adolescents of both

TABLE 17-5 ••• TYPES OF ADOLESCENT FEMALE SEXUAL DYSFUNCTION

Disorders of arousal
Disorders related to orgasm
  Orgasmic insufficiency: Persistent delay or absence
    after a normal excitement stage. This is the most
    common sexually related problem in women of all
    ages and is usually a function of insufficient
    knowledge about arousal patterns.
Dyspareunia
  Inadequate vaginal lubrication
  Associated with pelvic pathology

sexes display considerable ignorance regarding orgasm in the female.[32]

Dyspareunia, or pain on vaginal intercourse, is another type of sexual dysfunction that occurs in both sexes but is much more common in females. In the adolescent girl, this is usually caused by a lack of sex education about the need for, and techniques to elicit, vaginal lubrication. Therefore, the most common cause of dyspareunia in the female is inadequate lubrication, which leads to vaginismus on insertion of the penis. Vulvovaginitis is the other major cause.

HOMOSEXUALITY

Homosexuality has been defined as a persistent pattern of sexual arousal in response to persons of the same sex along with a persistent pattern of absent or weak heterosexual arousal.[37] As an alternative choice of sexual expression, it has not been considered a psychopathologic condition by the American Psychiatric Association since 1973. Progress in the understanding of adolescent homosexuality, especially lesbianism, has lagged behind that of the adult population. Most of our information is derived from clinical anecdotes from homosexual adults recalling their adolescence.[38]

In the Kinsey survey of adult women, 10% admitted to homosexual arousal by age 15; 4% to 5% had had a homosexual experience by that age, and 2% to 3% had reached orgasm by homosexual stimulation.[39] These figures doubled by age 20. The estimated prevalence of exclusive lesbianism in adults is 5%. Unlike in girls, the rate of homosexual activity in boys decreases from a peak of 29% at age 12 to 12% by age 15.[40] However, by age 15, 27% of the same sample of men recalled having had such activity to orgasm at least once. The estimated prevalence of exclusive homosexuality in adult men is 10%.

There is a low correlation between homosexual behavior during adolescence and that during adulthood. However, from a developmental perspective, what distinguishes homosexuality from heterosexuality is unclear. The differences are probably present early in life, as the majority of homosexual adults report having homosexual attachments before the onset of adolescence.[37] The evolution of theory regarding the causes and development of homosexuality has been reviewed by Roessler and Deisher.[41] Although the physical and cognitive development of homosexual adolescents is the same as that of their heterosexual peers, their psychosocial development can be more turbulent.[42] This is probably because of the additional developmental task of adapting to a socially stigmatized identity.[43] The process may be somewhat less turbulent for the teenage lesbian, as close relationships and some demonstrative affection are more socially acceptable for girls. Fewer behavioral restrictions also allow for more experience in developing a stable intimate relationship among lesbian teenagers, when compared with their gay male peers. After interviewing a small sample of gay teenage boys, Remafedi reported high rates of substance use, school dropout, conflicts with the law, and psychiatric hospitalizations.[43] However, these figures may be inflated, as adjustment problems are more prevalent among teenagers who "come out" because of the risk of ostracization by family and peers. It may actually be more functional for the homosexual to delay the natural developmental progression toward a full homosexual identity (which includes coming out) until he or she is financially self-sufficient and has an alternative supportive network. The usual developmental stages toward full homosexual identity in teenagers are further discussed by Hetrick and Martin.[42]

SEX EDUCATION

The negative consequences of adolescents' expression of their sexuality (e.g., adolescent pregnancy and sexually transmitted diseases [STDs], particularly AIDS) has emphasized as never before the need for sex education. This fact is understood by the American public, which overwhelmingly supports sex education for children and youth.[44] However, although the need for young people to be better educated in this area is not disputed, there is still considerable discussion as to the content of such education and where it is best to provide it.

As can be seen from the previous section, sexuality is an essential component of all human beings. Our self-perceptions color all of our relationships and influence many of our behaviors. With this in mind, education about sexuality should take a broad focus. It should include not only the mechanics of sexual behavior, but also material designed to help children and adolescents understand themselves as men and women and to help them learn how to express their sexuality in positive ways. Unfortunately, however, this is not the case in most instances. Traditionally, sex education provided by parents has been limited to "the birds and the bees," sex education in religious institutions has been limited to "don't do it until you're married," and sex education in schools has concentrated on the biology of reproduction. Another sex educator in this country, the media (especially television), has dealt with what men and women are and how they behave toward each other, but mostly in a negative fashion.[45]

If parents do educate their children and adolescents about sexuality, it is usually done in a cursory manner, with little information given about relationships and behavior as men and as women. Instead, mechanical facts are conveyed, along with a sense of guilt.[46] However, even if they never mention the word "sex," parents, by example, are the primary sexuality educators of their children. For the most part, parents want to be the sexuality educators of their children, but they feel they are not able to be for several reasons: their own lack of information; their discomfort in discussing sexual issues; confusion about their own beliefs, feelings, and attitudes; and potential conflict with their children over those same attitudes, feelings, values, and beliefs.[47] Parents can be their children's best source of sexuality education if they are trained properly in that role.

Because of parental default in this arena, the schools have become the primary conveyors of formal sex education in this country. Most states require or heavily encourage sex and/or AIDS education,[48] and at least 60% of American teenagers receive some sex education during their school years.[49] Sex education in the schools definitely increases adolescents' knowledge about sex,[48] and it does not encourage adolescents to initiate sexual activity.[50] Whether it influences behavior is unclear.[51–54]

Although most sex education courses include the essential facts about human reproduction and discuss AIDS and the major STDs, until recently, few dealt with contraception, and many do not include content about interpersonal relationships and acceptance of one's own sexuality.[48] One of the problems with sex education in the schools is that certain topics, such as contraception, are taught in high school, but students are initiating sexual activity during the elementary and middle school years.[55-57] Therefore, they start out with no information or with erroneous information passed on by their peers. Adolescents with unreliable knowledge or no knowledge develop inappropriate attitudes about sex, and these attitudes correlate with high-risk sexual behavior.[56] Sexuality education provided earlier in the school years might help to alleviate this problem.

Although schools are increasingly providing sex education, the medium through which children and adolescents get most of their information, whether good or bad, is the media, specifically television.[58] Television contains at least 14,000 sexual references, innuendoes, and behaviors each year, few of which involve the use of birth control, self-control, abstinence, or responsibility.[59] "Soap operas," a favorite of female teenagers, contain at least eight episodes of extramarital sex for every episode of sex between married spouses. Public service announcements about AIDS are relatively common, but there are few announcements about how sex can be performed while preventing AIDS (i.e., by using condoms). There are still no advertisements for contraceptives on network television.

Whatever the biases of educators (i.e., whether educators feel that sex education should be abstinence based or comprehensive), all agree that education is needed, and the best place to provide it is in the home. Other industrialized countries have as much teenage sexual activity as the United States, but much lower rates of adolescent pregnancy and sexually transmitted disease. Americans must develop a uniform approach to teenage sexuality while recognizing the many cultural differences in our society.

References

1. Chilman CS. Adolescent Sexuality in a Changing American Society—Social and Psychological Perspectives. Bethesda, MD: US Department of Health, Education, and Welfare, Center for Population Research, 1980, p 3.
2. LeGuin UK. The Left Hand of Darkness. New York: Ace Books, 1969.
3. Moore RE. Normal childhood and early adolescent sexuality: A psychologist's perspective. Semin Adolesc Med 1985; 1:97.
4. Strasburger VC. Normal adolescent sexuality: A physician's perspective. Semin Adolesc Med 1985; 1:101.
5. Gordon S, Scales P, Everly K. The Sexual Adolescent. 2nd ed. North Scituate, MA: Duxbury Press, 1979.
6. Hibbard RA, Orr DP. Incest and sexual abuse. Semin Adolesc Med 1985; 1:153.
7. Currier RL. Juvenile sexuality in global perspective. In: Constantine LL, Martinson FM (eds). Children and Sex, New Findings, New Perspectives. Boston: Little, Brown, 1981, pp 9–19.
8. Meyrowitz J. Where have the children gone? Newsweek, August 30, 1982. p 13.
9. Strasburger VC. Normal adolescent sexuality: A physician's perspective. Semin Adolesc Med 1985; 1:101.
10. AC Nielsen Co. Report on television. 1984.
11. Piaget J: The intellectual development of the adolescent. In: Caplan G, Lebovici E (eds). Adolescence—Psychosocial Perspectives. New York: Basic Books, 1969.
12. Brown RT: Assessing adolescent development. Pediatr Ann 1978; 7:16.
13. Coles R, Stokes G. Sex and the American Teenager. New York: Harper & Row, 1985.
14. Sorenson RC. Adolescent Sexuality in Contemporary America. New York: World Publishing, 1973.
15. Jessor SL, Jessor R. Transition from virginity to nonvirginity among youth: A social-psychological study over time. Dev Psychol 1975; 11:473.
16. Udry JR. Biological predispositions and social control in adolescent sexual behavior. Am Sociol Rev 1988; 53:709.
17. Vener AM, Stewart CS, Hager DL. The sexual behavior of adolescents in middle-America: Generational and American-British comparisons. J Marriage Fam 1972; 34:696.
18. Hayes CD (ed). Risking the Future. Washington, DC: National Academy Press, 1987.
19. Chilman CS. Adolescent Sexuality in a Changing American Society. 2nd ed. New York: John Wiley & Sons, 1983.
20. Vener AM, Stewart CS. America revisited: 1970–1973. J Marriage Fam 1974; 36:728.
21. Zelnik M, Kantner JF. Sexual activity, contraceptive use and pregnancy among metropolitan-area teenagers: 1971–1979. Fam Plann Perspect 1980; 12:230–231, 233–237.
22. Brooks-Gunn J, Furstenberg FF Jr. Coming of age in the era of AIDS: Puberty, sexuality, and contraception. Milbank Q 1990; 68:59.
23. Doyle LL, Hogue CJR. The relation between age at menarche and age at first intercourse in users of public health facilities. Adolesc Pediatr Gynecol 1988; 1:252.
24. Sonis WA, Comite F, Blue J, et al. Behavior problems and social competence in girls with true precocious puberty. J Pediatr 1985; 106:156.
25. Furstenberg FF. Race differences in teenage sexuality, pregnancy, and adolescent childbearing. Milbank Q 1987; 65:381.
26. Grant LM, Demetriou E. Adolescent sexuality. Pediatr Clin North Am 1988; 35:1271.
27. Mott FL, Haurin RJ. Linkages between sexual activity and alcohol and drug use among American adolescents. Fam Plann Perspect 1988; 20:128.
28. Jessor SL, Jessor R. The time of first intercourse: A prospective study. J Pers Soc Psychol 1983; 44:608.
29. Brooks-Gunn J, Furstenberg FF Jr. Adolescent sexual behavior. Am Psychol 1989; 44:249.
30. Billy JOG, Rodgers JL, Udry JR. Adolescent sexual behavior and friendship choice. Soc Forces 1984; 62:652.
31. Brown JD, Childers KW, Waszak CS. Television and adolescent sexuality. J Adolesc Health Care 1990; 11:62.
32. Greydanus DE, Demarest DS, Sears JM. Sexual dysfunction in adolescents. Semin Adolesc Med 1985; 1:177.

33. Katchadourian H. Sexual dysfunction and therapy. In: Katchadourian H (ed). Fundamentals of Human Sexuality. 5th ed. Fort Worth, TX: Holt, Rinehart & Winston, 1989, p 411.

34. Miller GD, Cirone J. Sexual dysfunction in college sexuality course attenders and course treatment benefits: A preliminary report. J Am Coll Health Assoc 1978; 27:107.

35. Johnson R, Stanford P. Sexual dysfunction in adolescent males with prostatic enlargement. J Curr Adolesc Med 1980; 2:31.

36. Farrow JA. An approach to the management of sexual dysfunction in the adolescent male. J Adolesc Health Care 1985; 6:397.

37. Remafedi G, Blum R. Working with gay and lesbian adolescents. Pediatr Ann 1986; 15:773.

38. Remafedi G. Male homosexuality: The adolescent's perspective. Pediatrics 1987; 79:326.

39. Kinsey AC, Pomeroy WB, Martin CE, et al. Sexual Behavior in the Human Female. Philadelphia: WB Saunders, 1953.

40. Kinsey AC, Pomeroy WB, Martin CE. Sexual Behavior in the Human Male. Philadelphia: WB Saunders, 1948.

41. Roessler T, Deisher RW. Youthful male homosexuality. Homosexual experience and the process of developing identity in males aged 16 to 22 years. JAMA 1972; 219:1018.

42. Hetrick ES, Martin AD. Developmental issues and their resolution for gay and lesbian adolescents. J Homosex 1987; 14:25.

43. Remafedi G. Adolescent homosexuality: Psychosocial and medical implications. Pediatrics 1987; 79:331.

44. Louis Harris and Associates. Public Attitudes Toward Teenage Pregnancy, Sex Education, and Birth Control. New York, 1988, p 24.

45. Strasburger VC. Adolescent sexuality and the media. Pediatr Clin North Am 1989; 36:747.

46. Kelly GF. Parents as sex educators. In: Brown L (ed). Sex Education in the Eighties. New York: Plenum Press, 1981, p 101.

47. Vincent ML, Clearie AF, Schluchter MD. Reducing adolescent pregnancy through school and community-based education. JAMA 1987; 257:3382–3386.

48. The Alan Guttmacher Institute. Risk and Responsibility: Teaching Sex Education in America's Schools Today. New York, 1989.

49. Kenney AM, Guardado S, Brown L. What states and school districts want students to be taught about pregnancy prevention and AIDS. Fam Plann Perspect 1989; 21(2):56. Published erratum, 1989; 21(3):133.

50. Marsiglio W, Mott FL. The impact of sex education on sexual activity and contraceptive use, and premarital pregnancy among American teenagers. Fam Plann Perspect 1986; 18:151.

51. Anderson JD, Kann L, Holtzman D, et al. HIV/AIDS knowledge and sexual behavior among high school students. Fam Plann Perspect 1990; 22:252.

52. Scott-Jones D, Turner SL. Sex education, contraceptive and reproductive knowledge, and contraceptive use among black adolescent females. J Adolesc Research 1988; 3:171.

53. Laszlo AT, Johnson J (eds). AIDS Education for High-Risk Youth: Assessing the Present, Planning for the Future. Rockville, MD: Community Research Branch, National Institute on Drug Abuse, 1990, pp 41–42.

54. Furstenberg FF Jr, Moore KA, Peterson JL. Sex education and sexual experience among adolescents. Am J Publ Health 1985; 75:1331.

55. Banks IW, Wilson PI. Appropriate sex education for black teens. Adolescence 1989; 93:233.

56. Brooks-Gunn J, Furstenberg FF Jr. Adolescent sexual behavior. Am Psychol 1989; 44:249.

57. Melchert T, Burnett KF. Attitudes, knowledge, and sexual behavior of high-risk adolescents: Implications for counseling and sexuality education. J Counsel Develop 1990; 68:293.

58. Sprafkin J, Silverman LT. Sex on prime-time. In: Schwartz M (ed). TV and Teens. Reading, MA: Addison-Wesley, 1982, p 130.

59. Lou Harris and Associates. Sexual Material on American Network Television During the 1987–1988 Season. New York: Planned Parenthood Federation of America, 1988.

○○○

CHAPTER 18

Contraception

RAMONA I. SLUPIK

Of the 25 million teenagers in the United States, 4 million are sexually active. Fifty percent have had intercourse before the age of 17, and the average age at time of first coitus for both sexes is 16.[1] Fifty percent of all initial adolescent pregnancies occur within 6 months of initiating intercourse—20% conceive in the first month alone.[2] The resultant teenage birth rate is 1.2 million pregnancies per year, 82% of which are unintentional.[2] Furthermore, the U.S. adolescent pregnancy rate is twice that of Britain and France, three times that of Sweden, and seven times that of the Netherlands (Fig. 18–1). The extent of the problem has continued to increase, even in the past decade; the birth rate in 15- to 17-year-olds rose by 10% to 33.8 per 1000.[3, 4]

To understand the predicament of contraception for the teenager, the entire scope of psychosocial dilemmas facing teenagers in today's society must be appreciated, including the initial motivation behind engaging in sexual intercourse, as well as reasons for not desiring, not using, or discontinuing contraceptive methods. In addition, the physician has a responsibility to educate these young patients in regard to the risk of sexually transmitted diseases and the failure rates associated with each contraceptive method. The gynecologist's relative inaccessibility to the male patient, with the resultant lack of proper education for this population, is a constant source of frustration.[5]

The fast-paced world of the late twentieth century has led teenagers into a physically adult life-style before any emotional maturity has been attained. The media have propagated an attitude of sexual promiscuity such that impulsive responses are popularized without an attendant sense of social responsibility or self-control. Teenagers are led to believe that they are free to live "for the moment" and so are deceived into thinking there are no long-term consequences to their immediate actions. This sense of invincibility pervades their attitudes toward both pregnancy and sexually transmitted diseases (STDs) (i.e., "It won't happen to me," at least "not this time"). Widespread use of alcohol and drugs in recreational settings has likewise enhanced extempore behavior.[6]

Unfortunately, ignorance and denial have been dominant traits for much of the century. Despite advances in scientific technology and research, the topic of sexual intercourse is taboo in most American households, and few schools have an adequate sex education program.[7, 8] As a result, most American youth first learn about sex outside the home, and thus attitudes toward birth control are less influenced by parental standards than by a misinformed, misguided peer group.[9–12] This unwillingness to confront the issue of sex education persists, despite the fact that numerous studies have demonstrated that teenagers armed with basic knowledge of reproductive biology and contraceptive methods are less likely to become sexually promiscuous, to conceive, or to contract venereal disease.[2, 13, 14] In a home in which sexual behavior is discussed openly and honestly and where parents are receptive to the special needs of their adolescents, a teenager is much less likely to have

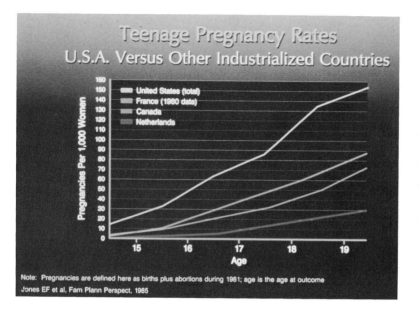

FIGURE 18–1 ••• Pregnancy and abortion rates for teenagers aged 15 to 19 years by country (1980–1981). (Adapted with the permission of The Alan Guttmacher Institute from EF Jones, JD Forrest, N Goldman, SK Henshaw, R Lincoln, JI Rosoff, CF Westoff, and D Wulf, "Teen pregnancy in developed countries: Determinants and policy implications." Family Planning Perspectives, Vol. 17, No. 2, March/April 1985.)

an undesired, out-of-wedlock pregnancy, to drop out of school, or to become a runaway. Other studies have demonstrated the usefulness of adolescent participation in small socioeducational groups as a forum for discussion of sexuality and dispelling of major myths regarding pregnancy and parenting. Long-term results indicate that emphasizing the right to self-determination and contraception can have a significant impact on promoting responsible sexual behavior.[15]

The health care professional's realistic, pragmatic approach to the individual female adolescent and her life-style will result in a contraceptive choice that optimizes that method's effectiveness (Table 18–1). It is essential to foster a supportive attitude of trust and confidentiality; encouraging follow-up ensures patient satisfaction with her chosen method, early detection of side effects or complications, and the opportunity to select another type of contraception when appropriate.

COUNSELING THE ADOLESCENT

The clinician must be able to properly communicate with the teenager, especially in discussions relating to sexuality. General principles include focusing on "responsible sexuality," establishing a "safe and comfortable"

environment for teenagers to discuss sexuality, and learning the fallacies and myths concerning ways to prevent pregnancy and the problems related to communication with parents and other adults.[14] One 3-year study indicated that participation in small socioeducational groups provided an excellent forum for opening the lines of communication between a health care provider and a teenager either contemplating becoming sexually active or already sexually active.[14] The program focused on problems between the adolescent and parents, the right to self-determination, and contraception.

TABLE 18–1 ••• FACTORS TO REMEMBER WHEN CHOOSING A CONTRACEPTIVE METHOD FOR THE ADOLESCENT

1. Acceptability: Is it a method the patient will continue to use consistently?
2. Effectiveness of method and frequency of intercourse: Does the method lend itself to the "unplanned" coital episode often seen in this age group?
3. Number of partners/concerns of sexually transmitted disease: Is the patient adequately protected?
4. Cost/access to medical care: Can the patient afford the method on a long-term basis?
5. Motivation/self-discipline of patient and male partner: Will reluctance to interrupt foreplay result in nonuse of the method?
6. Safety/risk: Will short-term convenience result in long-term drawbacks?
7. Personal and family religious and ethical philosophy: Will it influence usage?

Strong emphasis was placed on postponement of sexual intercourse until after high school or marriage. Each adolescent was an integral part of the decision-making skills program; the result of the 3-year study indicated that participation in such groups has had a significant impact on promoting responsible sexual behavior.

ORAL CONTRACEPTIVES

Oral contraceptives (OCs) may well be the method of choice for most adolescents. Advantages include a high efficacy (98% to 99%), even with an occasional "missed" or "late" pill, and a relative degree of safety in this age group. Multiple noncontraceptive health benefits increase their attractiveness (Table 18–2). They afford a measure of protection, although admittedly not the best, against pelvic inflammatory disease (PID) and STDs because of their effect on cervical mucus. Drawbacks to be considered include the motivation required to take a pill daily, cost of the initial visit to the prescribing physician, and monthly expenditure per pill pack (although the latter can be overcome in certain situations through public aid, Planned Parenthood, or university health care clinics). However, in view of the fact that this is probably the only method available for this age group that does not require interruption of foreplay or cooperation of the male partner, the positive aspects far outweigh the negative. Absolute medical contraindications are listed in Table 18–3. With the advent of low-dose and multiphasic OCs, however, patients with controlled diabetes mellitus, mi-

TABLE 18–2 ••• NONCONTRACEPTIVE HEALTH BENEFITS OF ORAL CONTRACEPTIVES

Increased menstrual cycle regularity
Decreased incidence of:
 • Menorrhagia
 • Iron-deficiency anemia
 • Dysmenorrhea
 • Dysfunctional uterine bleeding
 • Premenstrual syndrome
Decreased incidence of:
 • Fibrocystic breast disease
 • Fibroadenomas
Decreased incidence of pelvic inflammatory disease and sequelae, including ectopic pregnancy
Decreased incidence of functional ovarian cysts
Decreased risk of ovarian cancer
Decreased risk of endometrial cancer
Decreased incidence of rheumatoid arthritis

TABLE 18–3 ••• ABSOLUTE CONTRAINDICATIONS TO ORAL CONTRACEPTIVES

Present or past history of deep vein thrombophlebitis or thromboembolic disease
Cerebral vascular disease
Coronary artery or cardiac valvular disease
Breast carcinoma
Endometrial carcinoma
Undiagnosed abnormal uterine bleeding
Cholestatic jaundice of pregnancy
Hepatic tumor
Known or suspected pregnancy

graines, and mild smoking habits (<10 cigarettes/day) are now potential users of OCs, provided they continue to be medically supervised.

Oral Contraceptive Formulations

All OCs currently available in the United States are referred to as "combined"—i.e., all contain both estrogen or progestin in each tablet, with the exception of the "minipill," which contains progestin only. (The latter is not to be confused with the "morning-after" pill or with triphasics—see later discussion.) The estrogenic component is in the form of ethinyl estradiol (EE) or mestranol (ME), and the two are roughly equivalent in terms of potency (Table 18–4). The progestin component varies from pill to pill, containing norgestimate, desogestrel or gestodene, ethynodiol diacetate (EDDA), norethindrone (NET), norethindrone acetate (NETA), norgestrel (NG), or levonorgestrel (LNG), in order of increasing androgenicity (Table 18–5). Androgenicity is measured in the laboratory by parameters such as prostatic growth, steroid displacement, and sex hormone–binding globulin levels[16] and is clinically observable via side effects such as acne and hirsutism.

A number of new progestins are rapidly becoming available, including norgestimate, desogestrel, and gestodene, as noted above. The newer progestins appear to have less adverse effect on the lipid profile compared with the more traditional progestins.[17] The mechanism of action of these new pills is similar, for the most part, to that of the combination pill in that there is inhibition of ovulation. The progestational agent suppresses luteinizing hormone (LH) secretion, while the estrogenic agent suppresses follicle-stimulating hormone (FSH) secretion. The former component also

TABLE 18–4 ••• ORAL CONTRACEPTIVE FORMULATIONS

Brand Name	Manufacturer	Estrogen	Dose (μg)	Cycle Days	Progestin	Dose (μg)	Cycle Days
Monophasic*: Estrogen, 20–35 μg ("low-dose")							
Brevicon	Syntex	EE	35	1–21	NET	0.5	1–21
Demulen	Searle	EE	35	1–21	EDDA	1.0	1–21
Levlen	Berlex	EE	30	1–21	LNG	0.15	1–21
Loestrin 1/20	Parke-Davis	EE	20	1–21	NETA	1.0	1–21
Loestrin Fe 1/20†	Parke-Davis	EE	20	1–21	NETA	1.0	1–21
Loestrin 1.5/30	Parke-Davis	EE	30	1–21	NETA	1.5	1–21
Loestrin Fe 1.5/30†	Parke-Davis	EE	30	1–21	NETA	1.5	1–21
Lo/Ovral	Wyeth-Ayerst	EE	30	1–21	NG	0.3	1–21
Modicon	Ortho	EE	35	1–21	NET	0.5	1–21
Nordette	Wyeth-Ayerst	EE	30	1–21	LNG	0.15	1–21
Norinyl 1 + 35	Syntex	EE	35	1–21	NET	1.0	1–21
Ortho-Novum 1/35	Ortho	EE	35	1–21	NET	1.0	1–21
Ovcon 35	Mead-Johnson	EE	35	1–21	NET	0.4	1–21
Marvelon		EE	35	1–21	DES	0.15	1–21
Mercilon		EE	20	1–21	DES	0.15	1–21
Minulet‡		EE	30	1–21	GES	0.075	1–21
Ortho-Cyclen	Ortho	EE	35	1–21	NGM	0.25	1–21
Monophasic*: Estrogen, 50 μg							
Demulen 1/50	Searle	EE	50	1–21	EDDA	1.0	1–21
Norinyl 1/50	Syntex	ME	50	1–21	NET	1.0	1–21
Norlestrin 1/50	Parke-Davis	EE	50	1–21	NETA	1.0	1–21
Norlestrin Fe 1/50†	Parke-Davis	EE	50	1–21	NETA	1.0	1–21
Ortho-Novum 1/50	Ortho	ME	50	1–21	NET	1.0	1–21
Ovcon 50	Mead Johnson	EE	50	1–21	NET	1.0	1–21
Ovral	Wyeth-Ayerst	EE	50	1–21	NG	0.5	1–21
Biphasic*							
Ortho-Novum 10/11	Ortho	EE	35	1–21	NET	0.5	1–10
						1.0	11–21
Triphasic*							
Ortho-Novum 7/7/7	Ortho	EE	35	1–21	NET	0.5	1–7
						0.75	8–14
						1.0	15–21
Tri-Levlen	Berlex	EE	30	1–6	LNG	0.05	1–6
			40	7–11		0.075	7–11
			30	12–21		0.125	12–21
Tri-Norinyl	Syntex	EE	35	1–7	NET	0.5	1–7
			35	8–16		1.0	8–16
			35	17–21		0.5	17–21
Triphasil	Wyeth-Ayerst	EE	30	1–6	LNG	0.05	1–6
			40	7–11		0.075	7–11
			30	12–21		0.125	12–21
TriMinulet		EE*	30	1–6	LNG	0.05	1–6
			40	7–11		0.075	7–11
			30	12–21		0.125	12–21
Tri-Nova		EE*	30	1–6	LNG	0.05	1–6
			40	7–11		0.075	7–11
			30	12–21		0.125	12–21
Tri-Cyclen	Ortho	EE	35	1–7	NGM	0.180	1–7
				8–15		0.215	8–15
				16–21		0.280	16–21
Progestin Only							
Micronor§	Ortho				NET	0.35	
Nor-Q.D. ‖	Syntex				NET	0.35	
Ovrette ‖	Wyeth-Ayerst				NG	0.075	

*All are available in 21- or 28-day pill packages.
†Last seven pills in 28-day pack contain 75 mg ferrous fumarate.
‡Other trade names are Femodene, Femovan, Ginoden, Gynera.
§Available in 28-day pill package.
‖Available in 42-day pill package.
DES, Desogestrel; EDDA, ethynodiol diacetate; EE, ethinyl estradiol; GES, gestodene; LNG, levonorgestrel; ME, mestranol; NET, norethindrone; NETA, norethindrone acetate; NG, norgestrel; NGM, norgestimate.
See Appendix F for additional oral contraceptive formulations.

TABLE 18–5 ••• ANDROGENIC PROGESTIN
POTENCY*

Gestodene	<1
Desogestrel	<1
Norgestimate	<1
Norethindrone	1
Norethindrone acetate	1
Norgestrel	5–10
Levonorgestrel	10–20

Adapted from Dorflinger LJ. Relative potency of progestins used in oral contraceptives. Contraception 1985;31:557.
*The potency of each substance is compared to that of norethindrone (1).

produces an endometrium that is not conducive to implantation and thickens the cervical mucus, thus inhibiting sperm transport.

Most healthy young patients do well on almost any low-dose pill, whether monophasic or multiphasic. After the first two to three cycles, however, persistent side effects may require a change in OC formulation (Table 18–6). For example, young women who continue to complain about nausea or breast tenderness may benefit from a change to a lower potency estrogen or higher potency progestin formula. (Ingestion with meals or at bedtime will also minimize nausea.) Subjects with acne, in contrast, will improve on a pill with a higher estrogen-to-progestin ratio (e.g., Demulen 1/35 or Ovcon 35). Initial breakthrough bleeding may signify a compliance problem or simply forgetting to take the pill at the same time daily. However, patients who experience breakthrough bleeding while on multiphasic OCs, especially if it continues past the first few cycles, despite proper intake, will benefit from a change to a monophasic formulation. At times, side effects may be idiosyncratic, and the best pill formulation will be found only by trial and error.

Generic OCs may contain an unpredictable amount of hormone, as the FDA considers a 25% deviation as still acceptable (i.e., an individual pill may contain 75% to 125% of the labeled dose).[18] In view of the sometimes erratic pill-taking habits of adolescents (frequent missed or late pills), this may result in breakthrough ovulation and accidental pregnancy; thus, generic OCs are not recommended, particularly in this age group.

Patients can be reassured that there is no long-term fertility impairment after discontinuing oral contraceptives.[17] New-start patients in this age group require particularly detailed instructions on beginning their therapy and on possible nuisance side effects (e.g., break-

through bleeding, nausea, breast tenderness) to lessen the risk of confusion, frustration, pill failure, or discontinuance in the future. The combined use of OCs with condoms to prevent venereal disease transmission would be ideal in this age group,[19, 20] but hope for long-term compliance is admittedly unrealistic.

Before initiating OC therapy in the adolescent, one would prefer that there be evidence of appropriate maturation of the hypothalamic-pituitary-ovarian (HPO) axis, as manifested by a minimum of three (ideally regular) menstrual periods.[21] (Some researchers believe that maturation of the HPO axis is manifested by 12 to 18 months of regular menstrual periods.[22, 23]) By setting such limits, however, we run the risk of the adolescent's becoming pregnant while waiting to reach "pill eligibility." Many experts take the opinion that only medical contraindications to OCs need to be considered; teenagers and their parents can be reassured that the low-dose OC formulations are the most extensively studied, safest medications in history.[24] Young girls with evidence of an endocrinopathy, reproductive or otherwise, need to be appropriately evaluated and treated before institution of OC therapy.

It is imperative that the patient be informed of the side effects and appropriate management. With regard to breakthrough bleeding, the patient should be reassured that bleeding will cease as the patient continues to take the OCs, usually after the first two to three cycles. Better compliance will be the end result of a properly informed patient. Persistent breakthrough bleeding in a patient who desires to continue the same OC can be addressed with supplementation of additional estrogens (conjugated estrogens, 2.5 mg/day × 7 to 10 days, or a second OC pill daily for 7 to 10 days). It may be helpful to recommend to the adoles-

TABLE 18–6 ••• SIDE EFFECTS OF ORAL
CONTRACEPTIVES

Estrogenic side effects
    Breast tenderness/swelling
    Nausea
    Fluid retention
    Hypertension
    Mood changes/depression
Progestational side effects
    Acne
    Weight gain/increased appetite
    Nervousness
    Amenorrhea
    Glucose intolerance

TABLE 18–7 ••• ORAL CONTRACEPTIVE–DRUG INTERACTIONS

Reduced OC Efficacy	
Effect Well-Established	*Data Conflicting*
Rifampin	Tetracycline, doxycycline
Griseofulvin	Ampicillin, penicillin
Phenytoin	Carbamazepine
Phenobarbital	Primidone
	Ethosuximide
Drugs Potentiated by OCs	
Effect Established/Suspected	*Data Conflicting*
Imipramine	Other tricyclics
Diazepam	Other benzodiazepines
Aminophylline, theophylline	
Corticosteroids	

cent starting on OCs that she wear a panty liner for the first several weeks of her OC course.

The issue of weight gain and bloating should be discussed openly. The adolescent should be advised that the incidence of weight gain is significantly less with the lower dose pills than was seen with higher dose pills in the past.[23, 24] She should be informed that her weight gain will be monitored at each visit, and if it should become a problem, a change in pill formula, an exercise program, and/or a low-salt diet will usually resolve the problem.[25]

Many drugs have been reported to interact with OCs, either by decreasing the contraceptive effect or by potentiating the concomitant drug.[26] Not all reports contain firm pharmacokinetic evidence (Table 18–7). In general, certain antibiotics and anticonvulsants may speed OC metabolism; patients taking such medications should use a 50-µg estrogen OC, especially if spotting occurs on a lower dose. Conversely, OCs may increase the effect of some antidepressants, tranquilizers, and bronchodilators, and the dosages of these drugs usually need to be decreased.

After the Initial Follow-Up

Follow-up for adolescents receiving the pill should be scheduled in 6 weeks and again in 3 months. Younger patients and high-risk patients should be seen more often. At each visit, weight and blood pressure are measured. The patient is interviewed regarding compliance, side effects of the medication, and satisfaction with the method. Questions are answered and "missed pill" episodes reviewed. At the initial follow-up, visits can be scheduled as needed but probably should take place every 6 to 12 months, depending on the individual patient.[27]

Progestin-only "Minipill"

The progestin-only pill, also termed the "minipill" (Micronor, Nor-Q, Ovrette), contains a reduced amount of progestin (see Table 18–4) and no estrogen. It is taken continuously (daily) instead of cyclically, as with other OCs. The mechanism of preventing pregnancy is similar to that of other oral contraceptives—altered cervical mucus, antiimplantation progestational effect on endometrium—but ovulation is less completely suppressed, resulting in a lower effectiveness rate (92% to 95%) and a higher incidence of side effects such as breakthrough bleeding (20% to 30% of users) and irregular cycle length. It has no advantage over combined oral contraceptives except that it may be used in situations where estrogen is contraindicated.

"Morning-after" Pill

The "morning-after" pill is not intended for routine use, but rather is reserved for emergency situations such as rape. The risk of pregnancy from a single act of coitus at midcycle has been estimated at 14%.[28] In the past, diethylstilbestrol (DES) or conjugated estrogens were prescribed in high doses. Currently, the simplest regimen consists of two 1-mg progestin–50-µg estrogen pills (e.g., Ovral) taken within 72 hours of unprotected coitus and repeated in 12 hours. Effectiveness averages 98%, and side effects are minimal.[29] An antiemetic may also be prescribed.

CONDOMS

At first glance, condoms would seem to be the perfect contraceptive method for adolescents. They would appear to be ideal for occasional sexual activity and for teens who might begin sexual activity before a physician visit or before OCs become effective. Because this age group tends to engage in sporadic interludes with a series of single partners, prophylactics provide protection against STD transmission. Over-the-counter availability and low cost are added benefits. In actuality, it is the male partner's unwillingness to utilize this method that makes it a less desirable choice (Table 18–8). Even an increase in acquired immunodeficiency syndrome (AIDS)

TABLE 18–8 ••• REASONS GIVEN BY ADOLESCENTS FOR NOT USING CONDOMS

1. Need to interrupt foreplay to apply
2. Decreased penile sensation during coitus
3. Lack of availability if coitus is unplanned or takes place in unusual location
4. Ignorance regarding potential for pregnancy
5. Female partner's misplaced trust in promise of coitus interruptus
6. Female partner's fear that requesting a condom may result in loss of male's affection/interest
7. Reluctance of male to accept responsibility for contraception
8. Implication that one or both partners may be an STD carrier

awareness has not substantially changed condom usage, possibly because the emphasis of human immunodeficiency virus (HIV) transmission via homosexual behavior has created a false sense of security in heterosexual teenagers.[8] When properly used, condoms' effectiveness rates approach 90% to 98%, especially when combined with a spermicide.[19, 20] Thus, it is still an appropriate primary choice for the properly motivated couple; it also can be recommended as a backup method for patients who take OCs haphazardly or as additional STD prevention in patients on another form of birth control.[19, 20]

DIAPHRAGM

The diaphragm is a relatively inexpensive form of birth control that still affords some STD protection. It can be a suitable option for a well-motivated teenager in a stable relationship. It requires fitting by a physician and may disrupt foreplay to a lesser extent than condoms, for instance, although patients should be reminded that insertion of additional spermicide before each coital episode is required for optimal effectiveness (81% to 98%), and it must remain in place for 6 hours after sexual contact. Still, the requirement for an initial fitting by a health care professional and the attendant cost may be a hindrance, and the bulky packaging makes it difficult to camouflage discreetly. In addition, some teens may choose to ignore the recommendation for yearly replacement, another potential failure factor (Table 18–9). The rare reports of toxic shock syndrome associated with diaphragm use should not discourage the physician from recommending it in this age group.[30]

CERVICAL CAP

The cervical cap is similar to the diaphragm except that it covers only the cervix. For this reason, it is slightly more difficult to insert. Many young patients will not be comfortable enough with their own anatomy to check high in the vagina for proper cervical coverage or dislodgement. Forgetting to fill the cap (one third full) with spermicide or removing the cap less than 8 hours after coitus are other possible causes of user failure. As a result, effectiveness varies from 88% to 94%.[25] A backup method of contraception is recommended for the first one to two cycles. There is also a theoretical risk of accelerated cervical dysplasia, and the cap is contraindicated in the presence of an abnormal Pap smear or lower genital tract infection. Although no cases have been reported, the cap carries the same potential risk of toxic shock syndrome as the diaphragm[30] and should not be used during menstruation. All these variables make the cervical cap a less than perfect choice for most teenagers.

SPONGE

The sponge is one of only a few effective over-the-counter female contraceptive devices.

TABLE 18–9 ••• PATIENT INSTRUCTIONS FOR USE OF DIAPHRAGM

1. Contraceptive jelly is first applied to the rim of the diaphragm and centrally, where it will be in contact with the cervix.
2. The diaphragm (with contraceptive jelly) can be inserted up to 6 hours before intercourse. If more than 6 hours have elapsed or if intercourse is repeated, an extra applicator full of jelly is inserted into the vagina, without removing the diaphragm.
3. After insertion of the diaphragm, the patient must check to be sure the cervix is fully covered by the diaphragm.
4. The diaphragm must be left in place for at least 6 hours after intercourse, but it should not be left in place for more than 12 hours after intercourse. Douching should be avoided for at least 6 hours after intercourse.
5. After the diaphragm is removed, it should be washed with mild soap and dried completely.
6. Before each use, the diaphragm must be checked for holes by being held up to a light; the rim also should be checked for any cracks or puckers.
7. The diaphragm should be replaced every year or any time a tear or crack is discovered.
8. Because of the risk of toxic shock syndrome, the diaphragm should not be used during the menstrual period.
9. If the patient has a weight change of 15 pounds or more, or if she becomes pregnant, the diaphragm should be refitted.

The unique advantage of not requiring a health care professional prescription makes it an excellent backup method for the teenager who cannot afford a visit to a contraceptive clinic, is concerned about possible lack of confidentiality, or thinks it unwise to rely on her male partner's promises to use another method. Effectiveness is relatively good (80% to 91%), and it does provide some protection against STDs. The fact that the device provides contraception for 24 hours and can remain in place for a total of 30 hours enhances its desirability, in that only the initial coital episode during this time frame need be interrupted. However, there is a learning curve; patients must familiarize themselves with proper insertion technique (i.e., with the loop oriented to the distal vagina). Failure to do so may result in difficult removal, with fragmentation of the device and the attendant theoretical risk of toxic shock syndrome.[31] In addition, because water is required to activate the spermicide before insertion, its effectiveness can be decreased by the less than optimal physical locations some adolescents choose for coitus.

VAGINAL SPERMICIDAL INSERTS

Vaginal spermicidal inserts include several barrier methods of contraception such as foam, jellies, creams, suppositories, and films. The most widely used of these spermicidal agents are nonoxynol-9 and octoxynol-9. They are available over the counter at a reasonable cost, which is the main advantage for their use in adolescent patients. Notably, the suppositories are small enough to fit discreetly into a purse, and the film can be carried easily in a wallet or in a pocket. Elimination of clumsy applicators should make films and suppositories even more attractive to adolescents.

The principal foam products on the market are Emko, Ortho-Gynol, and Delfen. The commonly available suppositories include Encare Oval, Semicid, Intercept, and vaginal contraceptive film (VCF) (Table 18–10). It is wise to have samples of these products, especially those that require an applicator, so that proper placement can be demonstrated. The patient should be encouraged to read the package insert and to discuss any questions she might have about the product. Ideally, a condom should be used in conjunction with vaginal spermicidals.

TABLE 18–10 ••• PATIENT INSTRUCTIONS FOR USE OF SPERMICIDES

1. Insert the contraceptive foam, suppository, or film high into the vagina so that it will cover the cervix. Use the foam 30 minutes or less before (*not* after) intercourse.
2. Do not douche for at least 6 hours after intercourse.
3. Keep an extra condom with the contraceptive foam, as use of the combination lessens the risk of failure.

THE FEMALE CONDOM

The female condom is a soft, loose polyurethane sheath with two flexible rings, one of which functions as an insertion device covering the cervix internally like a diaphragm. The second ring remains outside the vagina to protect the labia. Insertion is said to be similar to that of a tampon, as the precise positioning required with the diaphragm and cervical cap is unnecessary.[32] The female condom can be inserted any time before intercourse, is disposable, and is intended for one-time use only. It is intended to be sold over the counter. The female condom has been approved by the FDA only for the prevention of STDs, not for contraception. Research trials of the female condom are being conducted in the United States by Wisconsin Pharmaceuticals (WPC-333) and in England (Femshield), Denmark, and Sweden, as well as in 15 other countries under the direction of the World Health Organization.

INTRAUTERINE DEVICE

During the 1970s, many young women selected the intrauterine device (IUD) over other contraceptive methods, with the major advantages being the lack of a need to interrupt foreplay, lack of maintenance expenditures (beyond what was required for initial insertion), and high effectiveness rate (95% to 98%). However, adolescents' tendency toward either multiple partners or a series of single partners and the inherent risk of PID, ectopic pregnancy, and subsequent infertility contraindicate use of the IUD. At one time the IUD was espoused as the method of choice for the severely mentally disabled patient, but the inability of these patients to cope with the pain of insertion and the increased difficulty that caretakers may have dealing with the associated menorrhagia make it a less practical option. Preferred alternatives for the mentally disabled are medroxyprogesterone acetate or the levonorgestrel implant.

MEDROXYPROGESTERONE ACETATE (DEPO-PROVERA)

A standard 150-mg dose of medroxyprogesterone acetate (Depo-Provera), administered intramuscularly every 3 months, exerts contraceptive action by suppression of the HPO axis and prevention of the midcycle LH surge, with an additional atrophic effect on the endometrium and increased cervical mucus viscosity. Pregnancy rates are less than 0.5 per 100 women annually.[8, 19] Contraindications include a present or past history of thrombophlebitis or thromboembolic disease, carcinoma of the breast, undiagnosed vaginal bleeding, or suspected pregnancy.[33]

Although medroxyprogesterone's high effectiveness rate and relatively long duration of action would seem to make it a feasible contraceptive choice for adolescents, its usefulness is limited by a 20% to 30% incidence of breakthrough bleeding in the first year of use. Although many patients achieve an amenorrheic state after this period, additional drawbacks are the need for physician visits every 3 months and the associated cost. The American Academy of Pediatrics has endorsed the use of this drug in certain situations, such as in the mentally disabled; however, its implementation gradually may be superseded by other agents such as the levonorgestrel implant.

LEVONORGESTREL IMPLANTS (NORPLANT)

The levonorgestrel implant (Norplant) is a sustained-release, subdermally placed progestin contraceptive consisting of six thin, flexible, Silastic membrane capsules (34 mm long and 2.4 mm wide), each filled with 36 mg of levonorgestrel and designed to remain in place for up to 5 years. The progestin exerts its contraceptive effect by decreasing gonadotropin output (FSH and LH) and thus suppressing ovulation. Additional actions include a progestin-induced thickening of the cervical mucus to retard sperm migration and an adverse effect on the endometrium to prevent implantation.

The levonorgestrel implant is highly effective; reported failure rates are 4.5/1000 users

TABLE 18–11 ••• CONTRAINDICATIONS FOR THE LEVONORGESTREL IMPLANT (NORPLANT)

Pregnancy
Undiagnosed genital bleeding
Active thrombophlebitis or thromboembolic disease
Acute liver disease
Benign or malignant liver tumors
Known or suspected breast cancer

annually,[34] and its contraceptive effect is reversible. Of those desiring to conceive after implant removal, 50% become pregnant within 3 months, and 86% within 1 year.[35] Absolute contraindications are few (Table 18–11).

The most prevalent side effect is irregular menstrual bleeding; at least one episode of menorrhagia occurs in 44% of patients in the first year of use, but there is a decrease in the mean number of bleeding days per year as the duration of use is extended.[36]

A Norplant-2 rod system has been investigated in Singapore. This method, involving only two rods placed subdermally, has proved to be quite efficacious, safe, and acceptable. The 2.4- and 4.4-mm rods result in release of levonorgestrel in such a way as to maintain adequate levels of the progestin in the circulation. One hundred patients were evaluated by Seng and coworkers[37]; no accidental pregnancies occurred in the series reported. Apparently, the only significant side effect was menstrual irregularity, although one patient noted slight weight loss. There were also a number of nonspecific complaints such as abdominal pain, weakness, fatigue, and hematoma at the site of placement of the Norplant-2 system. Return of fertility compared quite favorably with that of the six-rod Norplant preparation.[37]

Although levonorgestrel implants are by no means the method of choice for many adolescents, an irrefutable advantage is the enhanced long-term compliance, with need for replacement only once every 5 years. In the future this may become the best contraceptive option for a severely mentally disabled and/or institutionalized teenager.

STERILIZATION

The tragic consequences of an undesired pregnancy in a severely mentally disabled adolescent—namely, inadequate antenatal care, potential inheritance of genetic and/or physical defects or mental retardation, risks of maternal morbidity and mortality, and lack of childrearing capabilities—cannot be understated.

If it can be unequivocally decided that the patient suffers from a devastating mental and/or physical disability that is irremediable and renders her forever incapable of suitably raising a child, sterilization is appropriate.[38] The medical record must document the irreversibility of the condition and reasons that other forms of contraception (e.g., Depo-Provera, Norplant) cannot be used. In addition, the legal guardian must understand that sterilization is intended to be permanent and must be told the measurable failure rate.[39]

By performing these procedures in carefully considered circumstances, the rights of the individual are not being ignored, but rather protected.

References

1. Special Task Force of Committee on Adolescent Health Care, American College of Obstetricians and Gynecologists. Adolescent Sexuality: Guides for Professional Involvement. Washington, DC: ACOG, 1990.
2. Zabin L, Kantner J, Zelnick M. The risk of adolescent pregnancy in the first months of intercourse. Fam Plann Perspect 1979; 11(14):215.
3. National Center for Health Statistics. Advance report of final natality statistics 1988. Monthly Vital Statistics Report 1990; 39(4)(suppl).
4. American College of Obstetricians and Gynecologists. The adolescent obstetric-gynecologic patient. ACOG technical bulletin no. 45. September, 1990.
5. Strasburger V. Adolescent sexuality and the media. Pediatr Clin North Am 1989; 36(3):747.
6. Repke JT. Adolescent pregnancy: Can we solve the problem? Editorial. Mayo Clin Proc 1990; 65:1152.
7. Benson MD, Perlman C, Sciarra JJ. Sex education in the inner city. JAMA 1986; 255(1):43.
8. Grace E, Emans SJ, Woods ER. The impact of AIDS awareness on the adolescent female. Adolesc Pediatr Gynecol 1989; 2(1):40.
9. Jay MS, Bridges CE, Gottlieb AA, et al. Adolescent contraception: An overview. Adolesc Pediatr Gynecol 1988; 1(2):83.
10. Jay MS, DuRant RH, Litt TF. Female adolescents' compliance with contraceptive regimens. Pediatr Clin North Am 1989; 36(3):731.
11. Stewart DC. Sexuality and the adolescent: Issues for the clinician. Primary Care 1987; 14(1):83.
12. Dawson DA. The effects of sex education on adolescent behavior. Fam Plann Perspec 1986; 18(4):162.
13. Marsiglio W, Mott FL. The impact of sex education on sexual activity, contraceptive use, and premarital pregnancy among American teenagers. Fam Plann Perspec 1986; 18(4):151.
14. Moyse-Steinberg D. A model for adolescent pregnancy prevention through the use of small groups. 9th Annual Symposium of the Committee for the Advancement of Social Work with Groups, 1987. Soc Work Groups 1990; 13(2):57, 68.
15. Dorflinger LJ. Relative potency of progestins used in oral contraceptives. Contraception 1985; 31:557.
16. Lobo RA. The androgenicity of progestational agents. Int J Fertil 1987; 33(suppl):6.
17. Godsland IF, Crook D, Wynn V. Clinical and metabolic considerations of long-term oral contraceptive use. Am J Obstet Gynecol 1992; 166(suppl)(6 pt2):1955–1963.
18. Ansbacher R. Interchangeability of low-dose oral contraceptives. Are current bioequivalent testing measures adequate to ensure therapeutic equivalency? Contraception 1991; 43(2):139–147.
19. Werner MJ, Biro FM. Contraception and sexually transmitted diseases in adolescent females. Adolesc Pediatr Gynecol 1990; 3(3):127.
20. Davis AJ. Teenagers, sexuality & contraception. Dialog Contraception 1990; 3(2):1.
21. Brenner P, Misherz P. Contraception. In: Glass RH (ed). Office Gynecology. 3rd ed. Baltimore: Williams & Wilkins, 1988, pp 53–85.
22. Shearin R, Boehkle J. Hormonal contraception. Pediatr Clin North Am 1989; 36(3):697–715.
23. Speroff L, Glass RH, Kase NG. Clinical Gynecologic Endocrinology and Infertility. 4th ed. Baltimore: Williams & Wilkins, 1989, pp 461–498.
24. Sanfilippo J. Adolescents and oral contraceptives. Int J Fertil 1991; 36(suppl)(2):65–79.
25. Emans SJ, Goldstein D. Pediatric and Adolescent Gynecology. Boston: Little, Brown, 1990, pp 451–503.
26. Drug interactions with oral contraceptives: A review of known and suspected interacting agents. The Contraception Report 1992; 111(5):9–12.
27. Strasburger V. Prescribing oral contraceptives. In: Strasburger VC (ed). Basic adolescent gynecology: An office guide. Baltimore: Urban & Schwarzenberg, 1990, pp 23–44.
28. Hatcher RA, Guest F, Stewart F, et al. Contraceptive Technology 1988–1989. 14th ed. New York: Livingston Publishers, 1988.
29. Korba VD, Heil CG. Eight years of fertility control with norgestrel-ethinyl estradiol (Ovral): An updated clinical review. Fertil Steril 1975; 26(10):973–981.
30. Slupik RI. Toxic shock syndrome and contraceptive methods. In: Sciarra JJ (ed). Gynecology and Obstetrics. Vol 6. Philadelphia: JB Lippincott, 1990.
31. Faich G, Pearson K, Fleming D, et al. Toxic shock syndrome and the vaginal contraceptive sponge. JAMA 1986; 255:216–218.
32. Kulig JW. Adolescent contraception: Non-hormonal methods. Pediatr Clin North Am 1989; 36(3):717–730.
33. Zatuchni GI, Slupik RI. Drug Handbook for the Obstetrician and Gynecologist. St. Louis: Mosby–Year Book, 1990.
34. Bardin C. Long acting steroidal contraception: An update. Int J Fertil 1989; 34(suppl):88.
35. Shoupe D, Mishell D. Norplant: Subdermal implant system for long-term contraception. Am J Obstet Gynecol 1989; 160:1286.
36. Darney PD, Klaisle CM, Tanner S, et al. Sustained-released contraceptives. Curr Prob Obstet Gynecol Fertil 1990; XIII(3):90.
37. Seng K, Viegas O, Ratnah S. Norplant contraceptive implants—a comparison of capsules vs. rods in Singapore. Singapore Med J 1990; 316:368–372.
38. Schor DP. Sex and sexual abuse in developmentally disabled adolescents. Semin Adolesc Med 1987; 3(1):1.
39. ACOG Committee on Ethics. Ethical considerations in sterilization. ACOG committee opinion no. 73. September, 1979.

CHAPTER 19

Adolescent Pregnancy

PATRICK J. SWEENEY

The United States has one of the highest adolescent pregnancy rates in the world. This has been true for more than two decades, and it would appear unlikely that any significant improvement will occur in the foreseeable future. Adolescent pregnancy in the United States has been variously referred to as a problem, an epidemic, and even an embarrassment. While there is general agreement concerning the magnitude of the problem, there is considerable disagreement with respect to possible solutions. Most authorities concur that there is no single solution, or "quick fix." Adolescent pregnancy is a multifaceted problem with long-term medical, social, educational, economic, and political implications.

During the latter part of the 1960s, young maternal age increasingly came under suspicion as a risk factor for poor pregnancy outcome. Numerous literature reviews and statistical reports claimed that adolescent mothers were at increased risk for any of several prenatal or obstetric complications, including anemia, hypertension, preterm labor, prolonged labor, cephalopelvic disproportion, low-birth-weight infants, and sexually transmitted diseases.[1-4] Subsequently, researchers began to question the implied, and often stated, assumption that teenage mothers suffered from some biologic disadvantage, possibly because their own bodies were still maturing. The fact that teenagers often received inadequate or no prenatal care also began to receive increasing attention. Consequently, in the early 1970s numerous special teenage pregnancy projects were initiated at medical centers throughout the country. These special projects were designed to provide pregnancy testing, counseling, and comprehensive prenatal services to pregnant teens in a nonthreatening, nonjudgmental, supportive environment. The health care providers, nutritionists, and social workers recruited for these projects were selected on the basis of their desire to work with adolescents and their knowledge of an adolescent's special needs. Intensive outreach programs encouraged pregnant teens to seek early care.

Many of these teen pregnancy programs reported marked improvements in several pregnancy outcome parameters.[5, 6] Initially these improved outcomes were credited to the multidisciplinary approach and the special services that were the hallmark of these programs. Later studies, however, suggested that adequate prenatal care was the crucial variable in these adolescent pregnancy programs and attributed much of the success of these programs to their ability to recruit pregnant adolescents early and to achieve compliance with subsequent prenatal visits.[7-11] Although early and continuous prenatal care is associated with improved perinatal outcomes, it does not fully explain the markedly higher low-birth-weight rates experienced by adolescents.[12]

In the late 1970s the social and economic consequences of adolescent childbearing received as much, if not more, attention than the medical complications. Politicians and educators realized that 80% of teenagers who became pregnant while in high school never completed their secondary education.[13] Without a high school diploma or marketable skill, these young, single mothers and their children entered a vicious cycle of welfare dependency and repeat pregnancy. The incidence of repeat pregnancy within 1 year of an adolescent's first delivery has been reported to range from 17% to 40% and increases to 28% to 50% for repeat pregnancy within 2 years.[14]

As we entered the 1980s, many of the adolescent pregnancy programs enlarged their scope of services to include the provision of parenting education. Some researchers had reported that even normal, healthy infants born to teenage mothers were more likely to die in their first year of life than were infants of older mothers.[15, 16] These higher postneonatal mortality rates were predominantly a result of infections, violence, accidents, and sudden infant death syndrome and may have been secondarily related to the young mother's social, economic, or educational limitations. Child abuse and neglect have also been reported to be more prevalent in teen parent families.[17-20] Thus, the goal of parenting education classes was to help these teen parents to maintain their child's immunization status, to recognize the signs and symptoms of early infections, to prevent household accidents and poisonings, and to know when and where to seek medical assistance. In addition, information on basic developmental milestones was often provided.

More recently, the emphasis has switched once again to primary prevention. The past decade has witnessed countless debates over the advisability, legality, and morality of providing sex education in the public schools. The American government not only ignores the documented success of public education programs in other countries, but continues to consider legislation that would severely restrict the access of minors to contraceptive and abortion services. School-based clinics are even more controversial. The inability of our nation—with its outstanding educational and health care resources—to effectively respond to such an obvious need is indeed tragic.

INCIDENCE

In 1976 the Alan Guttmacher Institute published a statistical compilation of what was then known about adolescent sexuality, contraceptive use, pregnancy, childbirth, and abortion.[21] At that time, more than 1 million teenagers in the United States became pregnant each year. Unfortunately, that number has remained stable for more than a decade (Table 19–1).[22] Until 1986, many people had been encouraged by the fact that the teenage birth rate had steadily decreased since 1970—a fact often quoted by those opposed to sex education and contraceptive services for teens, claiming that the problem was well on its way to resolution. However, although it was true that the birth rate was decreasing, the pregnancy rate continued to increase, with the difference being the increased number of teen pregnancies that terminated in an elective or spontaneous abortion. In addition, examination of the birth rates by age group revealed that most of the decrease occurred in the 18- to 19-year-old age group (Table 19–2)[23]—individuals who are "teenagers" by definition, but for whom the medical and social disadvantages of childbearing appear to be much less significant than for school-age teens. The decrease in the 15- to 17-year-old age group was much less dramatic, and there was essentially no change at all for the youngest teens (ages 10 to 14). These facts convincingly demonstrate that the adolescent pregnancy problem is definitely not headed toward resolution. In fact, there is evidence to the contrary; the birth rate for young teenagers (ages 15 to 17) increased 6% in 1988 to 33.8%—the highest rate since 1977.

Historically, the problem of adolescent pregnancy seemed to become a "problem" in the 1960s and 1970s, largely because of the changing mores of the nation, the increased sexual freedom of adolescents, the availability of contraceptives, and the legalization of abortion. It is interesting to note that in 1960, births to teenagers accounted for only 13.9% of all U.S. births, and many of these were to young, married women. Very little research had been done on adolescent pregnancy before this time,

TABLE 19–1 ••• NUMBERS OF BIRTHS, ABORTIONS, AND PREGNANCIES TO TEENAGERS, UNITED STATES, 1985

Age Group	Births	Abortions	Pregnancies
<15	10,220	16,970	30,930
15–17	167,789	165,630	383,540
18–19	299,696	233,570	616,570
Total	477,705	416,170	1,031,040

Adapted with permission of The Alan Guttmacher Institute from Stanley K. Henshaw, Asta M. Kenney, Debra Somberg and Jennifer Van Vort, *Teenage Pregnancy in the United States: The Scope of the Problem and State Responses*, New York 1989.

TABLE 19–2 ••• BIRTH RATES ACCORDING TO AGE OF MOTHER, UNITED STATES, 1970–1990

Year	Age of Mother (yr)		
	10–14	*15–17*	*18–19*
1970	1.2	38.8	114.7
1971	1.1	38.2	105.3
1972	1.2	39.0	96.9
1973	1.2	38.5	91.2
1974	1.2	37.3	88.7
1975	1.3	36.1	85.0
1976	1.2	34.1	80.5
1977	1.2	33.9	80.9
1978	1.2	32.2	79.8
1979	1.2	32.3	81.3
1980	1.1	32.5	82.1
1981	1.1	32.1	81.7
1982	1.1	32.4	80.7
1983	1.1	32.0	78.1
1984	1.2	31.1	78.3
1985	1.2	31.1	80.8
1986	1.3	30.6	81.0
1987	1.3	31.8	80.2
1988	1.3	33.8	81.7
1989	1.4	36.4	84.2
1990	1.4	37.5	88.6

National Center for Health Statistics. Advance report of final natality statistics, 1990. Monthly Vital Statistics Report, 1993; 41(9):21, 31.

and rarely was an article in the medical literature devoted to this topic. The *Index Medicus* did not even list "adolescent pregnancy" as a separate classification. By 1975, the percentage of teenage births had increased to 18.9%, with a much larger proportion to unmarried mothers and very young teenagers.[24] From 1975 to 1985, the *Index Medicus* catalogued 878 articles under "pregnancy in adolescence."

OBSTETRIC RISKS OF ADOLESCENTS: THE IMPACT OF AGE AND SOCIOECONOMIC FACTORS

When large population groups are studied, teenage mothers consistently have poorer pregnancy outcomes than mothers who are in their twenties. Whether this increased risk is due to psychosocial or biologic factors remains controversial, and there is a considerable amount of information in the literature to support both hypotheses.

As early as 1962, a standard textbook on obstetrics and gynecology stated:

In terms of large population groups, there is a definitively higher incidence of maternal and fetal neonatal mortality among girls who deliver before seventeen years of age. The higher mortality rate undoubtedly is due to social and psychologic factors. . . . It has been shown repeatedly that from the standpoint of parturition alone the young gravida does as well as, or better than, her older sister when she has adequate prenatal care and competent obstetrical attention.[25]

Pregnant teenagers, particularly those younger than 15, have higher rates of certain complications (e.g., anemia and pregnancy-induced hypertension), maternal mortality, and premature and/or low-birth-weight infants than women in their twenties.[26–28] Although the overall maternal mortality rate in the United States has plummeted from 660 per 100,000 live births in 1930[29] to 7.9 per 100,000 live births in 1982,[30] the rate for young adolescents has remained significantly higher. One report stated that the risk of maternal death is 60% higher for pregnant girls younger than 15 compared with women in their early twenties;[26] another claimed that mothers younger than 15 experience a rate of maternal death that is 2.5 times that for mothers aged 20 to 24.[21] In a review of teenage pregnancy and maternal mortality in New York state, McLean et al.[31] reported that 87.5% of the adolescent maternal deaths were classified as preventable.

When one examines the overall birth statistics for individual states or the entire nation, it is clear that teenagers continue to have a higher incidence of low-birth-weight infants. Eisner et al.,[32] using data from more than 500,000 single live births in the United States in 1974, performed multivariate analyses to determine the correlates of low birth weight. They reported that when other factors were held constant, nonwhite race, previous reproductive loss, short interpregnancy interval, out-of-wedlock birth, lack of prenatal care, and maternal age under 18 or over 35 *each* increased the risk of having a low-birth-weight infant.

For decades, race has been one of the most significant correlates of low birth weight in the United States, with the incidence of low birth weight being more than twice as high for black infants as for white infants. Nevertheless, even within racial groups, there is a direct correlation between young maternal age and percentage of low birth weight (Table 19–3).[23]

Several reports based on U.S. vital statistics data have examined the association between maternal age and low birth weight, attempting to control for other variables. These reports

TABLE 19–3 ••• PERCENTAGE OF LOW-BIRTH-WEIGHT INFANTS ACCORDING TO AGE OF THE MOTHER AND RACE OF THE CHILD, UNITED STATES, 1990

Age of Mother (yr)	Race of Child	
	White	Black
<15	10.2	15.7
15	9.1	14.8
16	8.6	13.4
17	7.8	13.5
18	7.5	13.2
19	6.9	12.6
20–24	5.7	12.0
25–29	5.0	12.7
30–34	5.3	13.9
35–39	6.2	15.0
40–44	7.0	14.6
45–49	9.8	15.8
All ages	5.7	12.9

National Center for Health Statistics. Advance report of final natality statistics, 1990. Monthly Vital Statistics Report, 1993; 41(9):21, 31.

consistently demonstrated a direct relationship between low birth weight and young maternal age, even when controlled for marital status,[33] prenatal care,[34] and short interpregnancy interval.[35]

A series of studies spanning 20 years all reported the incidence of low birth weight to be higher in the adolescent population. Klein's[36] population included 1824 births to young women 16 years of age or less during 1971–1972. The premature birth rate was significantly higher for girls delivering at age 16 or less (17.7%) than for older teenagers (14.5%) or women older than 20 (13.7%).

A summary of the findings of the Louisiana Infant Mortality Study[37] compared mortality and low-birth-weight rates for the very young teenager (414 births to girls ages 10 to 14) to women ages 20 to 24 and found that the perinatal mortality rate was much higher in the young girls (56.5 per 1000 vs. 23.4 per 1000), as was the incidence of prematurity (15% vs. 8%).

In a retrospective study, Spellacy et al.[38] compared the pregnancy outcomes of 144 adolescent (ages 10 to 15) and 877 mature (ages 20 to 24) women. The racial distribution was significantly different between the groups; 81.3% of the adolescents were black, compared with only 36.9% of the mature women. Holding race constant, the adolescents had a significant increase in the incidence of low-birth-weight infants (20.2% vs. 8.7%).

Mangold[39] reviewed matched birth and death certificates for all 36,341 births to Arkansas residents in 1978. He found that younger teenagers (≤17 years of age) had a higher incidence of low-birth-weight infants and perinatal mortality; he suggested, however, that the increased obstetric risk was an artifact of the teenagers' generally lower socioeconomic status and inferior access to health care. He also restricted his analysis to first births to eliminate the potentially confounding effects of parity on pregnancy outcome. Several other researchers reported an increased incidence of low-birth-weight infants among the adolescent mothers—differences that they felt were primarily, if not entirely, explainable by social and behavioral variables.[9, 40–43]

Although it is true that teenage births in the United States occur disproportionately to young women who are socially and/or economically disadvantaged, it is difficult to attribute poor pregnancy outcomes entirely to socioeconomic status. Studies from large urban hospitals, whose patients are often predominantly from low-income populations, continue to demonstrate an increased incidence of low birth weight and preterm labor in adolescent mothers when compared with older women, even when prenatal care, ethnicity, and other factors have been controlled.[44]

Even in countries where teenage childbearing is not concentrated in the lower socioeconomic classes, adolescents have disproportionately high rates of low-birth-weight infants. In Saudi Arabia, for example, where the teaching of Islam advises an early marriage, teenage pregnancies are common in all socioeconomic groups; nevertheless, Al-Sibai et al.[45] reported that the incidence of low-birth-weight infants born to mothers ≤17 was 23%. A study from Ireland that compared the birth outcomes of more than 800 teenage mothers with those of mothers aged 20 to 29 years found that prematurity, stillbirth, and first-week neonatal mortality rates all were higher for the teenage group.[46]

Some of the obstetric complications previously reported to be increased in adolescents have subsequently been found to be no more prevalent in adolescents than in older women; these include prolonged labor, cephalopelvic disproportion, and cesarean section rates. Other medical complications have maintained their strong association with adolescent pregnancy, even though the adolescent's biologic age is not the sole risk factor responsible for the association. Included in this latter group are low birth weight, preterm birth, poor maternal weight gain, pregnancy-induced hypertension, anemia, and sexually transmitted diseases.[47–49] Brown et al.[50] reported that the incidence of preterm labor and delivery of a low-birth-weight infant was significantly higher in 286 teenaged primigravidas (≤16 years old) when compared with an equivalent number of adult primigravidas ages 21 to 25. Interestingly, the teenagers in their study were more likely to have a low-birth-weight infant (11.5% vs. 5.3%), despite the fact that they were also significantly more likely to have received adequate prenatal care.

Based on information available in 1989, the American Academy of Pediatrics (AAP) stated that the greater frequency of low-birth-weight infants is the only major pregnancy complication unquestionably related to maternal age. It admitted that preeclampsia could "possibly" be age dependent, but all other complications were most likely explainable on the basis of socioeconomic status.[51]

Much of the confusion and controversy surrounding the potential increased medical risk to teenage mothers may be due, in part, to faulty study designs (e.g., lack of control groups, inappropriate control groups, and inability to control for several other variables known to be associated with poor pregnancy outcome). One of the major inconsistencies is the varying age limits used by researchers to define a "teenager." Many of the early reports included all teenagers, ages 13 through 19; in such cases, the older teens far outnumbered the younger ones, severely skewing the results. The AAP has recognized that adolescent pregnancy has different implications for the 18- or 19-year-old high school graduate than for the 13- or 14-year-old student. Its Committee on Adolescence has stated that their "primary concern is the individual in early to middle adolescence (younger than the age of 18 years) who is biologically and/or psychosocially immature."[51] Authors and statisticians have begun to separate the 18- to 19-year-olds from teens who are 17 and under; when numbers have been large enough for statistical significance, results have been reported for each year of age. As a result of this more precise reporting, the very young teenagers (≤15) consistently appear to be at increased risk for suboptimal perinatal outcomes, regardless of racial and socioeconomic factors.[52]

EFFECTS OF PARITY ON PREGNANCY OUTCOME IN ADOLESCENTS

A 1980 government report stated, "Both mother's age and the birth order of the child are independently related to birth weight, but the interaction of these two factors may strengthen or moderate their individual effects."[53] Several studies have indicated that multiparous adolescents are at even greater risk of bearing low-birth-weight infants than their age-matched, primiparous controls.[54–57] However, studies investigating the effect of parity on pregnancy outcome should be interpreted with caution; many such studies compare all first births to all second births, ignoring the fact that these births are to different groups of women, and that teenagers who have repeat pregnancies may have multiple other factors that place their pregnancies at increased risk. Aside from possible differences in social and economic factors, repeat pregnancy in adolescence is likely to be associated with a short interpregnancy interval—itself a risk factor for low birth weight.[35]

Some studies have attempted to isolate the effects of parity on pregnant adolescents by comparing the outcome of first and subsequent births to the same teenage mothers. Jekel et al.[58] reported that in their group of multiparous adolescents, the incidence of low birth weight was 2 1/2 times greater and perinatal mortality was nine times greater for the subsequent-birth group than for the first-birth group. Although their sample size was small (N = 103) and tended to be older teens (≤18 at time of first birth), their results raised serious concerns about the potential additional risks a second pregnancy might pose to a group of young women whose pregnancy outcomes already appeared to be compromised by age and/or socioeconomic disadvantages. Sukanich et al.,[59] in a retrospective review of 139 teenagers who had had two deliveries, reported that the mean maternal ages at the time of the first and second deliveries were 15.2 and 18.3 years, respectively. Although there was a greater incidence of pregnancy-induced hypertension in the first pregnancies, there were no statistically significant differences between first and second births with respect to low birth weight or gestational age as determined by newborn examination.

Sweeney[60] compared the first and second

birth outcomes of 407 teenage mothers, all of whom were 17 years of age or less at the time of the second birth. He found that the mean birth weight was significantly lower for the first birth group ($P = <.0001$), even though the mothers were more likely to have initiated prenatal care earlier with their first pregnancy than they did with their second ($P = .001$). Ninety-five percent of these young mothers were black, single, and unemployed. With a mean interpregnancy interval of less than 1 year, it is unlikely that the mothers' socioeconomic status or general health habits changed significantly between births. The one factor that consistently varied from first birth to second was maternal age; obviously all mothers were younger at the time of their first birth. This study strongly suggests that a second pregnancy during young adolescence—while clearly undesirable for many social, psychological, and educational reasons—does not have a greater risk of a poor medical outcome than the first pregnancy. However, given the higher incidence of low birth weight and perinatal mortality associated with teenage pregnancy in general, the knowledge that a second pregnancy should fare no worse than the first is of little consolation.

NUTRITION AND WEIGHT GAIN

Maternal nutritional status is an important determinant of birth weight. The Institute of Medicine's report, *Preventing Low Birthweight*, clearly implicated both low maternal prepregnancy weight and poor weight gain during pregnancy as risk factors for low birth weight.[61] A later study confirmed and quantified this relationship in adolescents.[62] This association of maternal weight gain and infant birth weight appears to be even stronger for adolescents than it is for women ages 20 to 24.[63] In fact, adolescent mothers apparently must gain more weight than adult mothers to accomplish similar increases in infant birth weight.[64–67] Scholl et al.[68] suggest that comprehensive prenatal care programs for adolescents exert their beneficial effects on infant birth weight indirectly by improving maternal weight gain and prolonging gestation.

Although the direct relationship between maternal weight gain and infant birth weight has been known for years, bigger is not always better, as evidenced by the morbidity and mortality associated with macrosomia. Interestingly, one study of pregnancy weight gain in adolescents reported that the risk of a macrosomic infant was 13.1 times higher in adolescents gaining 20 kg or more, yet there was no increased risk of cesarean section or perinatal mortality.[69] Some researchers have recommended caution in attempting to decrease the incidence of low-birth-weight infants by increasing maternal weight gain.[70] Such a solution is probably oversimplistic, and the benefit of increased infant birth weight may well be overshadowed by known and unknown risks associated with excessive maternal weight gain. In addition, the potential long-term effects on general health status (e.g., adult obesity) should be considered.

Research on adolescents has suggested that although inadequate weight gain during pregnancy is associated with low birth weight, its underlying cause may differ depending on whether the poor weight gain occurred early or late in gestation. Early inadequate weight gain was associated with a significantly increased risk of a small-for-gestational age (SGA) infant, whereas late inadequate gains were associated with preterm delivery. In both instances, the risk of low birth weight persisted, even when the total weight gain was adequate for gestation.[71] Another study by the same authors reported on the possible predictive ability of early weight gain in adolescents. At 16 weeks' gestation, gains below the 25th percentile were associated with an increased risk of low birth weight, while weight gains above the 75th percentile doubled the risk of macrosomia.[72] The low-birth-weight phenomenon in young teenagers may be secondary to inadequate maternal fat stores and/or excessive mobilization of fat during pregnancy as measured by anthropometrics (midarm circumference and triceps skinfold).[73]

CONGENITAL MALFORMATIONS

Congenital malformations have also been reported to occur with greater frequency in infants born to young teenagers. The combination of small numbers of births to very young mothers ($\leq$16 years old) and a low incidence of major malformations in the general population makes it difficult to perform significant statistical analyses on this group. Pooling data on all teenage births to obtain sufficient case numbers, however, may mask higher rates of abnormalities in the very young. Those who have been able to report their data for each year of maternal age have demonstrated some definite trends. Erickson[74] has suggested that girls younger than 16 may have a risk of having a child with Down syndrome that is comparable to that of women older than 35. Grazi et al.[75] reviewed the records of 925 infants born to teenage mothers in Buffalo, New York, during 1976–1978. They not only found significantly higher incidences of perinatal mortality and low birth weight in the offspring of teenagers, but also found that major and multiple malformations occurred with significantly greater frequency in the teenage group.

OTHER FACTORS COMPLICATING ADOLESCENT PREGNANCY

There are many other aspects of adolescent pregnancy that deserve attention. Some of these, known to be associated with poor pregnancy outcomes regardless of maternal age, may be particularly problematic for teenage mothers, whose pregnancies may already be compromised by biologic and/or emotional immaturity. These include the following:

- Smoking
- Abuse of alcohol and other drugs
- Sexually transmitted diseases
- Small physical stature
- Inadequate prenatal care
- Stress, emotional instability, isolation from family

In addition, those who care for pregnant adolescents need to be aware of, and sensitive to, the multiple other, "less medical" problems faced by their patients, including:

- Family relationships
- Completion of high school
- Job training, vocational skills, and employment
- Child care
- Family planning and prevention of early subsequent pregnancy

DEVELOPMENT OF INFANTS OF ADOLESCENT MOTHERS

Given that neonatal, postneonatal, and infant mortality rates are higher for infants born to young teenage mothers, what is known about the health and development of the survivors? This chapter cannot sufficiently address this question, and studies are inconsistent. There is evidence to suggest that children born to teenage mothers are more likely to be behaviorally, socially, intellectually, and even physically disadvantaged compared with children born to older mothers.[76] Others believe that maternal age per se is not the critical variable in determining child health and development, and when relevant background characteristics are controlled, offspring of teenage mothers are as healthy and develop as well as controls born to older mothers.[77, 78] This apparent disagreement is reminiscent of arguments elucidated earlier describing the association between adolescent pregnancy and poor pregnancy outcome. Once again, the question is not so much whether these children suffer behaviorally and intellectually, but rather how much, if any, of these developmental problems are due to maternal age or socioeconomic status. As already stated, teenage mothers are more likely to be from low-income and/or minority families, have lower educational attainment, and be single parents, each of which creates a suboptimal environment for child development, regardless of the mother's age.

NONMEDICAL CONSEQUENCES OF ADOLESCENT PREGNANCY

Although teenage childbearing often results in incomplete secondary education, decreased employment opportunities, repeat pregnancies, and economic dependence, it is possible for teenage mothers to escape this unfortunate legacy. Furstenberg et al.[79] reported on a longitudinal study of more than 300 primarily urban black women who gave birth as adolescents in the 1960s. Despite the disadvantages of the early pregnancy, a substantial majority completed high school and found regular employment. Economic independence was associated with having had economically secure, better educated parents and greater personal educational motivation.

SPECIAL CLINICS FOR TEENS

There has been a resurgence of interest in the multiple benefits provided by specialized programs for pregnant and parenting adolescents. It appears that attempts to improve adolescent birth outcomes simply by promoting early entry into prenatal care may fail to capitalize on the additional benefits to be derived from educational, social, and other support services, particularly if coordinated through individual case management.[80] In evaluating the effects of a specialized prenatal educational program for adolescents, Slager-Earnest et al.[81] investigated the incidence of perinatal and newborn complications in two groups of adolescents who delivered at term. Both groups attended the same prenatal clinic, presented for care at similar stages of gestation, and were delivered at the same hospital; in addition, they were homogeneous for age, race, income, education, and marital status. The experimental group attended a specialized educational program for pregnant adolescents; the control group did not. The attenders had significantly lower incidences of several prenatal, intrapartum, and newborn complications compared with the controls. Other researchers, reporting on their 6-year experience with nearly 4500 pregnant adolescents, found that the obstetric outcome for those attending the special program was superior to that of the control group.[56] The special program patients gained more weight; had lower incidences of anemia, preeclampsia, and low birth weight; and demonstrated a threefold improvement in neonatal mortality compared with controls. Additional evidence to suggest the importance of special services to pregnant teens comes from a study comparing the pregnancy outcomes of adolescents living in a maternity shelter to those of a group of adolescents living in their own homes but receiving identical medical care. Despite the fact that the shelter adolescents were a particularly high-risk group (i.e., predominantly black, single, receiving public assistance, and registering late for prenatal care), they delivered significantly fewer low-birth-weight and preterm infants than did the control group.[82]

Elster et al.[83] reported that a comprehensive prenatal care program for teens probably has little effect on pregnancy outcome when compared with standard prenatal care and nutrition services; however, teens who attended the special prenatal program scored significantly better on several measures designed to evaluate parenting abilities. Data collected at 12 and 26 months postpartum revealed that those in the intervention group had a greater knowledge of infant development and were more likely to have completed infants' immunizations, more likely to have remained in school, and less likely to have had a repeat pregnancy.

SCHOOL-BASED CLINICS

The number of school-based clinics in the United States has grown exponentially from 10 in 1980 to 138 in 1988, with an additional 65 in the planning stages.[84] Despite the fact that only 10% to 25% of all school-based clinic visits are for family planning services, the controversy surrounding such clinics centers on the issue of reproductive health care, specifically contraception. According to a 1987 report, although 48% of these clinics offer gynecologic examinations and prescribe contraceptives, only 21% are actually permitted to dispense contraceptives on site.[85] The success of school-based clinics in decreasing pregnancy rates and encouraging school completion may well be directly linked to the comprehensiveness of the services provided, including the provision of child care. Consequently, any plan of evaluation must control for the degree to which reproductive health services are offered. Administrators responsible for these school-based programs must set realistic goals. It would be unfair, for example, to consider a school-based initiative a failure in reducing teen pregnancy rates if the funding agency or board of education had imposed service and/or counseling restrictions with respect to the provision of contraceptive services.

ECONOMICS OF TEEN PREGNANCY

In 1985, the United States spent $16.65 billion on families that were begun when the mother was in her teens.[86] This figure includes direct payments for services and the administrative costs associated with Aid to Families with Dependent Children (AFDC), Medicaid, and food stamps but does not include services such as housing, special education, child protection services, foster care, day care, and other social services. The estimated public cost of a single birth to a teenager who is receiving welfare is $36,508 by the time the child reaches age 20. Although comprehensive adolescent pregnancy prevention programs require significant funding,[87] they appear to be very cost effective. It is estimated that for every dollar spent on a teenager by the federal family planning program (Title X), three dollars can be saved in the next year alone. Unfortunately, not only has funding for the Title X program decreased, but various legislative efforts have been made to further restrict access of adolescents to family planning services by attempting to require parental consent or notification.

CONCLUSION

The United States has one of the highest adolescent pregnancy rates in the developed world, a situation that has remained unchanged for at least two decades. Teenage pregnancy is a multifaceted problem for which there is no simple solution. It will require the continued perseverance of dedicated and knowledgeable individuals from all areas of society. Members of the political arena must understand the long-term detrimental effects of adolescent pregnancy and be willing to commit the necessary resources to support programs designed to prevent or delay early childbearing. Educators must recognize the need for sensitive yet informative sex education programs and be willing to fight for their implementation. Health care institutions must provide a full range of reproductive health services for adolescents, and public health officials must continue to oppose regulations that would restrict services to this very needy group. Parents must realize that, like it or not, their children are growing up in a society that encourages and promotes sexual freedom, and the peer pressure to participate can be overwhelming. Finally, individuals in positions of authority must be willing and able to face reality. Although delaying age at first intercourse is an admirable goal—one to which we should all aspire—we must deal with the facts. Fifty percent of U.S. teenagers become sexually active by the age of 17, and their use of effective contraception is sporadic at best, particularly in the first few months after the initiation of sexual intercourse. While new ways to change this behavior are being explored, its existence and its consequences cannot be ignored. We must provide these young people with comprehensive reproductive health services, including prenatal care, parenting education, and family planning.

References

1. Battaglia FC, Frazier TM, Hellegers AE. Obstetrics and pediatric complications of juvenile pregnancy. Pediatrics 1963; 32:902.
2. Osofsky HJ. The Pregnant Teenager. Springfield, IL: Charles C Thomas, 1968.
3. Duenhoelter JH, Jimenez JM, Baumann G. Pregnancy performance of patients under fifteen years of age. Obstet Gynecol 1975; 46:49.
4. Stepto RC, Keith L, Keith D. Obstetrical and medical problems of teenage pregnancy. In: Zackler J, Brandstadt W (eds). The Teenage Pregnant Girl. Springfield, IL: Charles C Thomas, 1975, p 83.
5. Smith PB, Wait RB, Mumford DM, et al. The medical impact of an antepartum program for pregnant adolescents: A statistical analysis. Am J Public Health 1978; 68:169.
6. Youngs DD, Niebyl JR, Blake DA, et al. Experience with an adolescent pregnancy program. Obstet Gynecol 1977; 50:212.
7. Dwyer JF. Teenage Pregnancy. Springfield, IL: Charles C Thomas, 1974.
8. Ryan GM, Schneider JM. Teenage obstetric complications. Clin Obstet Gynecol 1978; 27:1191.
9. Davidson EC, Fukushima T. The age extremes for reproduction: Current implications for policy change. Am J Obstet Gynecol 1985; 152:467.
10. Sherline DM, A-Davidson R. Adolescent pregnancy: The Jackson, Mississippi experience. Am J Obstet Gynecol 1978; 132:245.
11. Slap GB, Schwartz JS. Risk factors for low birthweight to adolescent mothers. J Adolesc Health Care 1989; 10:267.
12. Stickle G. Overview of incidence, risks, and consequences of adolescent pregnancy and childbearing. Birth Defects 1981; 17:5.
13. Fielding JE. Adolescent pregnancy revisited. N Engl J Med 1978; 299:893.
14. Stevens-Simon C, Parsons J, Montgomery C. What is the relationship between postpartum withdrawal from school and repeat pregnancy among adolescent mothers? J Adolesc Health Care 1986; 7:191.
15. Babson SG, Clarke NG. Relationship between infant death and maternal age. J Pediatr 1983; 103:391.
16. Shapiro S, McCormick MC, Starfield BH, et al. Relevance of correlates of infant deaths for significant morbidity at 1 year of age. Am J Obstet Gynecol 1980; 136:363.
17. Zuravin SJ. Child maltreatment and teenage first births: A relationship mediated by chronic sociodemographic stress? Am J Orthopsychiatry 1988; 58:91.
18. Kinard EM, Klerman LV. Teenage parenting and child abuse: Are they related? Am J Orthopsychiatry 1980; 50:481.
19. Johnson CF. Sudden infant death syndrome vs. child abuse: The teenage connection. J Pedod 1983; 7:196.
20. Sahler OJ. Adolescent parenting: Potential for child abuse and neglect? Pediatr Ann 1980; 9:67.
21. Alan Guttmacher Institute. Eleven Million Teenagers. 1976.
22. Henshaw SK, Kenney AM, Somberg D, Van Vort J. Teenage Pregnancy in the United States. New York: The Alan Guttmacher Institute, 1989.
23. National Center for Health Statistics. Advance report of final natality statistics, 1990. Monthly Vital Statistics Report 1993; 41(9):21, 31.
24. Lee K, Paneth N, Gartner LM, et al. Neonatal mortality: An analysis of the recent improvement in the United States. Am J Public Health 1980; 70:15.
25. Huffman JW. Gynecology and Obstetrics. Philadelphia: WB Saunders, 1962, p 112.
26. Carey WB, McCann-Sanford T, Davidson EC. Adolescent and obstetric risk. Semin Perinatol 1981; 5:9.

27. National Research Council. Risking the Future: Adolescent Sexuality, Pregnancy, and Childbearing. Washington, DC: National Academy Press, 1987.

28. Davis S. Pregnancy in adolescents. Pediatr Clin North Am 1989; 36:665.

29. Wallace HM. Maternal and child health in the United Kingdom. In: Wallace HM (ed). Health Care of Mothers and Children in National Health Services: Implications for the United States. Cambridge, MA: Ballinger, 1975, p 13.

30. National Center for Health Statistics. Vital Statistics of the United States, 1982. Volume II: Mortality. Part A. DHHS publication no. PHS 86–1122. Washington, DC: US Government Printing Office, 1986.

31. McLean RA, Mattison ET, Cochrane NE, Fall KL. Maternal mortality study: Teenage pregnancy and maternal mortality in New York State. NY State J Med 1979; 79:226.

32. Eisner V, Brazie JV, Pratt MW, Hexter AC. The risk of low birthweight. Am J Public Health 1979; 69:887.

33. National Center for Health Statistics. Trends in Teenage Childbearing, United States, 1970–81. Vital and Health Statistics. Series 21, no. 41. DHHS publication no. (PHS) 84–1919. Public Health Service. Washington, DC: US Government Printing Office, 1984.

34. Taffel S. Prenatal Care: United States, 1969–1975. DHEW publication no. 78–1911. Hyattsville, MD: Public Health Service, 1978.

35. Spratley E. Interval Between Births: United States, 1970–77. DHHS publication no. PHS 81–1917. Washington, DC: US Government Printing Office, 1981.

36. Klein L. Early teenage pregnancy, contraception, and repeat pregnancy. Am J Obstet Gynecol 1974; 120:249.

37. Dott AB, Fort AT. Medical and social factors affecting early teenage pregnancy. Am J Obstet Gynecol 1976; 125:532.

38. Spellacy WN, Mahan CS, Cruz AC. The adolescent's first pregnancy: A controlled study. South Med J 1978; 71:768.

39. Mangold WD. Age of mother and pregnancy outcome in the 1981 Arkansas birth cohort. Soc Biol 1983; 30:205.

40. Merritt TA, Lawrence RA, Naeye RL. The infants of adolescent mothers. Pediatr Ann 1980; 9:100.

41. Geronimus AT. The effects of race, residence, and prenatal care on the relationship of maternal age to neonatal mortality. Am J Public Health 1986; 76:1416.

42. Poma PA. Effect of maternal age on pregnancy outcome. J Natl Med Assoc 1981; 73:1031.

43. Zuckerman B, Alpert JJ, Dooling E, et al. Neonatal outcome: Is adolescent pregnancy a risk factor? Pediatrics 1983; 71:489.

44. Leppert PC, Namerow PB, Barker D. Pregnancy outcome among adolescent and older women receiving comprehensive prenatal care. J Adolesc Health Care 1986; 7:112.

45. Al-Sibai MH, Khwaja SS, Al-Suleiman SA, Magbool G. The low birthweight infants of Saudi adolescents: Maternal implications. Aust NZ J Obstet Gynaecol 1987; 27:320.

46. Kelly AW, Al-Bassam S, Kevany J. Teenage mothers: Pregnancy performance and newborn status. Ir J Med Sci 1985; 154:390.

47. Saller DN, Crenshaw MC. Medical complications in adolescent pregnancy. Md Med J 1987; 36:935.

48. McAnarney ER, Hendee WR. Adolescent pregnancy and its consequences. JAMA 1989; 262:74.

49. Lavery JP. Obstetric problems. In: Sanfilippo JS, Lavery JP (eds). Pediatric and Adolescent Obstetrics and Gynecology, New York: Springer-Verlag, 1985, p 285.

50. Brown HL, Fan Y, Gonsoulin WJ. Obstetric complications in young teenagers. South Med J 1991; 84:46.

51. American Academy of Pediatrics, Committee on Adolescence. Adolescent pregnancy. Pediatrics 1989; 83:132.

52. McAnarney ER. Young maternal age and adverse neonatal outcome. Am J Dis Child 1987; 141:1053.

53. National Center for Health Statistics. Factors associated with low birthweight: United States, 1976. DHEW publication no. PHS 80–1915. Hyattsville, MD: Public Health Service, 1980.

54. McCormick MC, Shapiro S, Starfield B. High-risk young mothers and infant mortality and morbidity in four areas in the United States: 1973–1978. Am J Public Health 1984; 74:18.

55. Massad LS, Hage ML. The impact of prior pregnancy on adolescent pregnancy. Adolesc Pediatr Gynecol 1990; 3:71.

56. Hardy JB, King TM, Repke JT. The Johns Hopkins adolescent pregnancy program: An evaluation. Obstet Gynecol 1987; 69:300.

57. Elster AB. The effect of maternal age, parity, and prenatal care on perinatal outcome in adolescent mothers. Am J Obstet Gynecol 1984; 149:845.

58. Jekel JF, Harrison JT, Bancroft DRE, et al. A comparison of the health of index and subsequent babies born to school-age mothers. Am J Public Health 1975; 65:370.

59. Sukanich AC, Rogers KD, McDonald HM. Physical maturity and outcome of pregnancy in primiparas younger than 16 years of age. Pediatrics 1986; 78:31.

60. Sweeney PJ. A comparison of low birth weight, perinatal mortality, and infant mortality between first and second births to women 17 years old and younger. Am J Obstet Gynecol 1989; 160:1361.

61. Institute of Medicine, Committee to Study the Prevention of Low Birthweight. Preventing Low Birthweight. Washington DC: National Academy Press, 1985, p 242.

62. McAnarney ER, Bayer CA, Kogut CF, et al. Adolescent coitus and infant birthweight. J Adolesc Health Care 1986; 7:96.

63. Horon IL, Strobino DM, MacDonald HM. Birthweights among infants born to adolescent and young adult women. Am J Obstet Gynecol 1983; 146:444.

64. Naeye RL. Teenaged and pre-teenaged pregnancies: Consequences of the fetal-maternal competition for nutrients. Pediatrics 1981; 67:146.

65. Frisancho AR, Matos J, Flegel P. Maternal nutritional status and adolescent pregnancy outcome. Am J Clin Nutr 1983; 38:739.

66. Frisancho AR, Matos J, Leonard WR, Yaroch LA. Developmental and nutritional determinants of pregnancy outcome among teenagers. Am J Phys Anthropol 1985; 66:247.

67. Haiek L, Lederman SA. The relationship between maternal weight for height and term birth weights in teens and adult women. J Adolesc Health Care 1988; 10:16.

68. Scholl TO, Miller LK, Salmon RW, et al. Prenatal care adequacy and the outcome of adolescent pregnancy: Effects on weight gain, preterm delivery, and birthweight. Obstet Gynecol 1987; 69:312.

69. Scholl TO, Salmon RW, Miller LK, et al. Weight gain during adolescent pregnancy. J Adolesc Health Care 1988; 9:286.

70. Stevens-Simon C, McAnarney ER. Adolescent maternal weight gain and low birth weight: A multifactorial model. Am J Clin Nutr 1988; 47:948.

71. Hediger ML, Scholl TO, Belsky DH, et al. Patterns of weight gain in adolescent pregnancy: Effects on birth weight and preterm delivery. Obstet Gynecol 1989; 74:6.

72. Scholl TO, Hediger ML, Ances IG, et al. Weight gain during pregnancy in adolescence: Predictive ability of early weight gain. Obstet Gynecol 1990; 75:948.

73. Maso MJ, Gong EJ, Jacobson MS, et al. Anthropometric predictors of low birthweight outcome in teenage pregnancy. J Adolesc Health Care 1988; 9:188.

74. Erickson JD. Down syndrome, paternal age, maternal age, and birth order. Ann Hum Genet 1978; 41:289.

75. Grazi RV, Redheendran R, Mudaliar N, Bannerman RM. Offspring of teenage mothers: Congenital malformations, birth weight, and other findings. J Reprod Med 1982; 27:89.

76. Roosa MW, Fitzgerald HE, Carson NA. Teenage and older mothers and their infants. Adolescence 1982; 17:1.

77. McAnarney ER, Lawrence RA, Alten MJ, Iker HP. Adolescent mothers and their infants. Pediatrics 1984; 73:358.

78. Rothenberg PB, Varga PE. The relationship between age of mother and child health and development. Am J Public Health 1981; 71:810.

79. Furstenberg F, Brooks-Gunn J, Morgan SP. Adolescent mothers and their children in later life. Fam Plann Perspect 1987; 19:142.

80. Korenbrot CC, Showstack J, Loomis A, Brindis C. Birth weight outcomes in a teenage pregnancy case management project. J Adolesc Health Care 1989; 10:97.

81. Slager-Earnest SE, Hoffman SJ, Beckmann CJA. Effects of a specialized prenatal adolescent program on maternal and infant outcomes. J Obstet Gynecol Neonatal Nurs 1987; 16:422.

82. LaGuardia KD, Druzin ML, Eades C. Maternity shelter care for adolescents: Its effect on incidence of low birthweight. Am J Obstet Gynecol 1989; 161:303.

83. Elster AB, Lamb ME, Tavare J, Ralston CW. The medical and psychosocial impact of comprehensive care on adolescent pregnancy and parenthood. JAMA 1987; 258:1187.

84. Dryfoos JG. School-based health clinics: Three years of experience. Fam Plann Perspect 1988; 20:193.

85. Lovick S. The School-Based Clinic Update, 1987. Houston: Support Center for School-Based Clinics, 1987.

86. Burt MR. Estimates of Public Costs for Teenage Childbearing: A Review of Recent Studies and Estimates of 1985 Public Costs. Washington, DC: Center for Population Options, 1986.

87. Zabin LS. The Baltimore pregnancy prevention program for urban teenagers: II. What did it cost? Fam Plann Perspect 1988; 20:188.

CHAPTER 20

Sexually Transmitted Diseases in Childhood

KRISTI MORGAN MULCHAHEY

The diagnosis of a sexually transmitted disease (STD) is fortunately rare in childhood. However, STDs may be diagnosed in both symptomatic children with genitourinary complaints [1-3] and asymptomatic children who have been sexually abused.[4-6] In sexually abused children, survey studies have estimated the incidence of STDs to range from 1% to 26%, with most studies indicating an incidence of 1% to 5%. All STDs that have been reported in adults have also been reported in the pediatric population.[7]

When a clinician is faced with the task of screening a symptomatic child or a child with a history of sexual abuse, many factors need to be considered. The bulk of published data dealing with STDs is from adult populations; however, there are a number of factors unique to childhood that are diagnostically and therapeutically important. The histology and physiology of the genital tract in children is markedly different from that in adults, affecting the presentation of STDs in childhood. The choice of an appropriate diagnostic test should take into account the unique characteristics of the pediatric age group. Mode of transmission is also an extemely important issue. Both perinatal (i.e., vertical) transmission and sexual transmission have been reported in pediatric

STDs. The possibility of fomite and casual transmission must also be considered, although these appear to be quite uncommon.

PEDIATRIC GENITAL TRACT PHYSIOLOGY AND HISTOLOGY

The genital tract of the prepubertal girl is dramatically influenced by the presence or absence of estrogen. In the neonatal period, transplacental passage of maternal hormones results in a thickened vaginal epithelium that accumulates intracellular glycogen. An acidic pH results from the metabolism of this glycogen by the abundant *Lactobacillus* organisms that are present. Normal pediatric vaginal flora is often similar to maternal vaginal flora. As estrogens are metabolized, however, the vaginal epithelium takes on the characteristic thin appearance found during childhood. On cytologic examination, the epithelial cells are smaller than the estrogenized epithelial cells of adults, with a higher nucleus-to-cytoplasm ratio. Histologic sections show a thinner epithelium with an alkaline pH and the typical basal and parabasal cells seen in the unestrogenized vaginal epithelium of the postmenopausal women (Figs. 20–1, 20–2). This changes with the onset of puberty and the production of estrogen, when the vaginal epithelium again thickens and accumulates *Lactobacillus* and glycogen, and the pH falls.[2]

There are also anatomic differences in the genital tract of prepubertal and postpubertal females. In childhood, the cervix comprises a relatively larger portion of the uterus; with puberty, differential growth results in a relatively larger uterine fundus. In the estrogenized genital tract, the portio of the cervix contains endocervical glands that are susceptible to infection by organisms such as *Neisseria gonorrhoeae* and *Chlamydia trachomatis*. In contrast, the prepubertal child usually has no endocervical glands on the ectocervix, thereby protecting the upper genital tract from infection with these organisms (Fig. 20–3).[8] The thin, unestrogenized vaginal epithelium is much more susceptible to infection resulting in a true vaginitis with these organisms.[2]

TESTING FOR STDs IN CHILDREN

Diagnostic testing for STDs in the pediatric age group is another situation in which clinical data known for the adult population must be interpreted with caution. Children are anatomically and physiologically different from adults. Cultures in children need to be obtained from the anatomic sites where infection with these sexually transmitted organisms is most likely. In the prepubertal girl, cultures for gonococcal and chlamydial infection may be obtained from the vagina rather than the cervix. In prepubertal boys, as in adult males, the rectum is more likely than the urethra to be the site of infection.

The use of antigen detection testing methods has been increasingly popular in adult populations. These diagnostic tools are widely available, simple to perform, and cost effective. They also offer a more rapid diagnosis than the direct culture testing methods. However, it is important to critically compare these indirect testing methods with the culture techniques that have long been the "gold standard." Most of the sensitivity and specificity data that have been generated with the nonculture methods are from high-prevalence populations. Adults attending an STD clinic, for example, will obviously have much higher rates

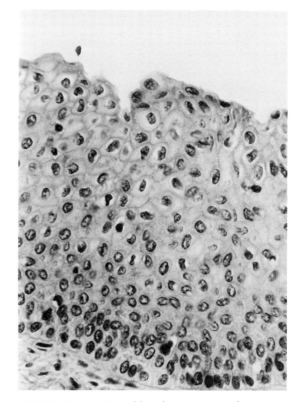

FIGURE 20–1 ••• Vaginal histologic specimen from a prepubertal child (hematoxylin and eosin stain).

of infection than children being screened for STDs because of genitourinary complaints or sexual abuse.[9] In addition, nonculture methods in adults have been used to test samples from anatomic sites such as cervix or urethra. These are different from the sites where infection is found in the pediatric age group. For these reasons, nonculture testing methods are not recommended for use in children.[10]

SOURCES OF TRANSMISSION OF PEDIATRIC STDs

In recent years, the role of nonsexual transmission of STDs in children has gained more attention. In 1982, the Centers for Disease Control Sexually Transmitted Disease Guidelines stated, "Diagnosis of any sexually transmitted infection in a child who is prepubertal but not neonatal raises the strong possibility of sexual abuse unless proven otherwise. The presence of an STD may be the major or only physical evidence of sexual abuse and may be asymptomatic."[11] Contrast this with the 1989

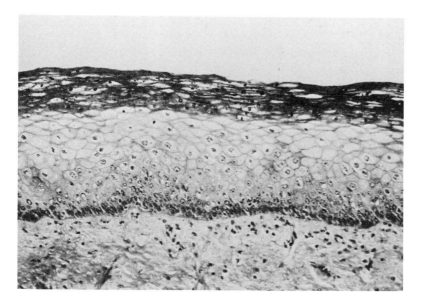

FIGURE 20–2 ••• Vaginal histologic specimen from an adult.

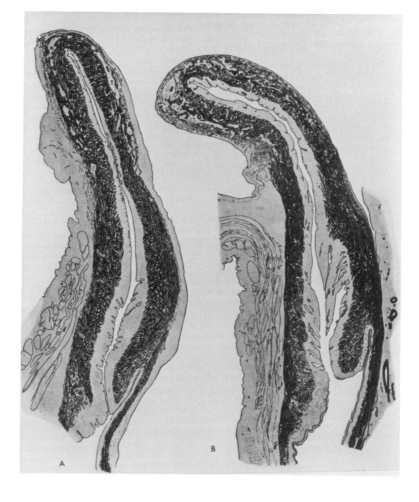

FIGURE 20–3 ••• Structure of the uterus of a 7-year-old child (A) and a 9-year-old child (B). (From Huffman JW. Anatomy and physiology. In: Huffman JW, Dewhurst J, Capraro JV [eds]. Physiology. The Gynecology of Childhood and Adolescence. 2nd ed. Philadelphia: WB Saunders, 1981.)

Sexually Transmitted Disease Guidelines, which state "The identification of a sexually transmissible agent from a child beyond the neonatal period suggests sexual abuse. However, exceptions do exist. . . . When the only evidence of sexual abuse is the isolation of an organism or the detection of antibodies, findings should be carefully confirmed."[12]

When the possibility or actual diagnosis of an STD is considered for any child, it is essential to take into account all possible sources of infection. Acquisition through sexual contact, vertical transmission at birth, nonsexual casual contact, and fomite transmission should all be considered. It may be more realistic, especially in the pediatric age group, to use the term *sexually transmissible disease* rather than *sexually transmitted disease*.

SEXUALLY TRANSMISSIBLE DISEASES

Gonorrhea

Biology

N. gonorrhoeae is a gram-negative diplococcus responsible for some of the most commonly reported STDs in adults.[13] It is also one of the most extensively studied sexually transmissible agents responsible for infection in childhood. This organism enters the body through mucous membrane surfaces such as those in the mouth, urethra, vagina, endocervix, and anorectal canal.[14] In children, the most commonly infected sites are the vagina, rectum, pharynx, and conjunctiva. The vaginal epithelium of the prepubertal girl is composed of relatively few layers of unestrogenized cells. Unlike the adult vaginal epithelium, which is resistant to infection with *N. gonorrhoeae*, the vaginal epithelium of the prepubertal child may be infected if exposed to this organism. However, the absence of endocervical glands on the ectocervix of the prepubertal child makes the cervix more resistant to infection. For this reason, ascending genital tract infection with *N. gonorrhoeae* is rare in children. Most of the reports of gonococcal peritonitis in children precede the widespread availability of antibiotics.[15] Infection of Bartholin's duct gland is also quite rare in prepubertal girls.

Demographics

The overall incidence of gonorrheal infection in children is relatively low, although it depends on the population of children being evaluated. The overall incidence of gonococcal infection (Fig. 20–4) in the 0- to 9-year-old age group was reported at 6.5 per 100,000 in both 1980 and 1985.[16] Included in this group are neonates with gonococcal infection, most commonly ophthalmia neonatorum. From 1 % to 7.5% of pregnant women attending public health obstetric clinics have been found to have positive cervical cultures for *N. gonorrhoeae*, with a 30% risk of neonatal transmission.[17, 18]

Gonococcal infections may occasionally be detected in both asymptomatic children and in those with genitourinary complaints. In prepubertal girls with symptomatic vaginitis, cultures positive for *N. gonorrhoeae* have been reported in 5% to 7%.[1, 19] In healthy children being screened during routine pediatric visits, the incidental finding of *N. gonorrhoeae* was very low, 1% or less.[3, 20]

The greatest concern about the possibility of gonococcal infection exists among children who are possible victims of sexual abuse. In children being screened for STDs because of a report of suspected sexual abuse, the incidence of positive gonococcal cultures has ranged from 4.7% to 11%. DeJong found an overall incidence of 4.7% in children who had been sexually abused. This incidence rose to 7.4% in children when there had been a delay in reporting and to 8.1% in children who had experienced multiple episodes of abuse.[5] White et al. have reported an 11% incidence of gonococcal infection in a population of 409 sexually abused children.[4] A 5.57% incidence of gonococcal infection was noted by Cupoli and Sewell in a series of 1059 children in Tampa, Florida.[6] Siblings of children with gon-

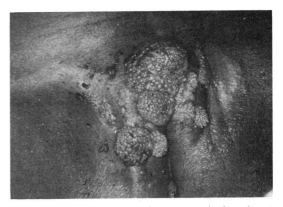

FIGURE 20–4 ••• Extensive vulvar, periurethral, and perianal condyloma in a prepubertal girl. (Courtesy of Dr. David Muram, Memphis, TN)

ococcal infections may be at increased risk for infection. Farrell found that 17% of children with positive gonococcal cultures also had one or more siblings with positive cultures. After the neonatal period, the vagina is the most commonly reported site for gonococcal cultures, followed by the rectum, pharynx, and conjunctiva. Although Groothius et al.[21] reported a 54% incidence of pharyngeal gonorrhea in a series of 16 sexually abused children, the 0.4% incidence reported by Weiss and DeJong[22] in a series of 461 sexually abused children is more in keeping with other reports in the literature.

It has been suggested that the incidence of gonorrheal infections in children may be increasing; however, the increase in reported cases most likely represents increased detection efforts and improved reporting of confirmed cases.[23]

Presentation

The incubation period for *N. gonorrhoeae* is roughly 1 week, with symptoms generally appearing in 2 to 7 days. Neonates most commonly present within 3 to 4 days of birth with ophthalmia neonatorum, although gonococcal arthritis, meningitis, and sepsis have also been reported.[17]

Children with symptomatic gonococcal infection usually present with a vulvovaginitis accompanied by erythema, purulent vaginal discharge, and pruritus. Dysuria may result from the vulvitis or from urethritis. An 18-institution cooperative study of children with symptomatic gonococcal infection found erythema in 40%, pruritus in 22%, and dysuria in 8%.[24] If untreated, this purulent vaginal discharge may be replaced by a serous discharge that may persist for several months. Older studies of the natural history of untreated gonococcal vaginitis in girls have reported cases in which the discharge resolved without treatment, leaving the children colonized (and, therefore, infectious) for up to 6 to 7 months. After this time, some children became culture negative without treatment. Populations of children studied in the preantibiotic era also indicated a 9% incidence of peritonitis.[15]

Children may also have asymptomatic colonization with *N. gonorrhoeae*. Several studies have reported a relatively high incidence of gonococcal infection in asymptomatic sexually abused children. In DeJong's 1986 review, 44% of the positive gonococcal cultures were from asymptomatic children.[5] Along with other studies,[4] this points out the importance of culturing even asymptomatic children when there is a possibility of sexual abuse.

In prepubertal boys, urethritis may be the only presenting symptom.[25] Pharyngitis and proctitis have been reported in children of both sexes. However, colonization of the pharynx and anorectum is more common than symptomatic infection.[26, 27] Gonococcal conjunctivitis after the neonatal period has also been reported and generally presents with a febrile illness accompanied by hyperpurulent conjunctivitis and periorbital cellulitis. This potentially severe infection may result in visual impairment if not diagnosed promptly and treated appropriately.[28]

Infection at more than one anatomic site is also quite common. In a series of 108 children, Nelson et al. found that 50% of girls with positive vaginal cultures also had positive rectal cultures, and 15% had simultaneous positive vaginal and pharyngeal cultures. Only 3% had positive rectal cultures as the sole finding.[24] Ingram et al. found that 41% of girls with positive vaginal cultures were also colonized with *N. gonorrhoeae* in the anorectal canal, and 19% had pharyngeal colonization.[27] In Silber and Controni's report of six children with asymptomatic pharyngeal gonorrhea, four of the children also had vaginal colonization with *N. gonorrhoeae*.[26] DeJong also reported in his study of 532 sexually victimized children that 32% of the positive cultures for *N. gonorrhoeae* were from anatomic sites not disclosed in interviews.[5] This clearly demonstrates the importance of culturing all three sites (pharynx, vagina, and rectum) when screening for *N. gonorrhoeae* and of culturing other sites if an unanticipated positive culture is obtained.

Source of Transmission

Beyond the neonatal period, sexual contact is nearly the exclusive cause of gonococcal infections in children. Because of the incubation period of *N. gonorrhoeae*, perinatally acquired infection usually presents in the first week(s) of life. In several carefully evaluated series, the strong likelihood of sexual transmission of pediatric gonococcal disease has been demonstrated. Branch and Paxton found a history of sexual abuse in 160 of 161 cases reported in 1- to 14-year-old children.[29] In a later study, Ingram et al.[27] found a history of sexual contact in all children between the ages of 5 and 12 years with gonococcal infection. In children younger than 4 years, he could document sexual abuse in only 35%. However, he stressed the difficulty of detecting sexual abuse in young children, especially during the preverbal years. For well-documented reasons, older children also may have difficulty disclosing sexual abuse. Only 17% of the older children in this study disclosed a history of sexual abuse during the first interview after the gonococcal infection was diagnosed.[27] In fact, two of the children did not disclose a history of sexual abuse until 8 years after completion of the study.[30] Farrell et al. also stress the need for a multidisciplinary approach in the evaluation of a child with gonococcal infection, as the majority of the sexually abused children in his study did not disclose such abuse during the initial interview.[31]

When a child who is beyond the neonatal period is younger than 4 years presents with a gonococcal infection, sexual contact remains the most likely origin, although it is difficult to prove. In this age group especially, questions about transmission by fomites and close, nonsexual contact are often raised. The gonococcal organisms may remain viable in water for 2 hours and on towels for 24 hours.[30] There is only one documented case of an identified fomite transmitting *N. gonorrhoeae* to a child: the child of a laboratory worker developed pharyngeal gonococcal infection after eating a Thayer-Martin plate containing *N. gonorrhoeae* colonies.[32] The question of fomite transmission was raised but never answered in an outbreak of gonococcal infection in infants kept on the same hospital ward in 1927.[33] Rice et al. failed to demonstrate either positive cultures from toilet seats or transmission to non-infected children in a hospital ward where children with untreated gonococcal vaginal discharge shared bathroom facilities with healthy children.[34]

The transmission of gonococcal infection from one child to another through genital exploratory behavior has been reported. Potterat et al. described one case of a 5-year-old girl who infected her 4- and 7-year-old playmates.[35] This is probably an uncommon occurrence; an earlier study of 160 cases of pediatric gonococcal infection by Branch and Paxton could identify no children under the age of 10 who were infected by their peers.[29]

Although gonococcal conjunctivitis is the least common gonorrheal infection in children, it may be one exception to the strong relationship between infection with *N. gonorrhoeae* and sexual contact. Accidental gonococcal conjunctivitis has been reported in adult laboratory workers.[36, 37] However, most cases of gonococcal conjunctivitis in adolescents and adults are thought to be due to direct contact with infected urine or genital secretions.[38, 39] Studies of childhood gonococcal conjunctivitis have been hampered by the unsuspected nature of the infection. Children were usually treated empirically with antibiotics before identification of the responsible organism, making culturing of other sites impossible. However, in a study of four children with gonococcal conjunctivitis, two parents were found to carry identical isolates. In each case, the child slept with the parent, and no sexual contact could be documented.[28] Again, the inherent difficulties of obtaining an adequate history from small children warrant caution.

Diagnosis

The correct choice of diagnostic test(s) is crucial in avoiding the possibility of either a false-negative or false-positive result, with either type of error having serious consequences. The use of indirect testing methods for *N. gonorrhoeae* is not recommended in children; both false-positive and false-negative tests have been reported with monoclonal antibody and direct fluorescent antibody testing methods used in preadolescent children.[10, 40] Although the presence of gram-negative intracellular diplococci on Gram stain has been used by some as a diagnostic tool for *N. gonorrhoeae*, false-positive results have also been reported with this method. Farrell et al. found that 14% of prepubertal patients with a positive Gram stain actually had a negative culture.[31] For that reason, it is suggested that the use of Gram-stained secretions be confined to situations where therapy must be initiated in a symptomatic child before receiving culture results.[10]

Even with the use of culture techniques to isolate *N. gonorrhoeae*, possible sources of error still exist. In a low-prevalence population, presumptive criteria for identification of organisms from positive cultures will have a low predictive value. Nongonococcal *Neisseria* organisms may be part of the normal flora in children, especially in the pharynx. The use of nonselective media is quite common, especially if gonococcal infection is unsuspected. For this reason, confirmation of organisms presumptively identified as *N. gonorrhoeae* is necessary, using methods such as carbohydrate degradation, enzyme substrate, or immunologic testing. Of 40 pediatric gonococcal isolates submitted to the Centers for Disease Control for confirmatory testing, 14 were found to be nongonococcal *Neisseria*. It is also recommended that isolates obtained from children be stored at −70°C for additional confirmatory testing, should this be needed at a subsequent date.[10]

Treatment

The Centers for Disease Control currently recommends the use of ceftriaxone in children with gonococcal infections. Children weighing more than 45 kg are treated as adults, and children weighing less than 45 kg with uncomplicated infection (vulvovaginitis, urethritis, pharyngitis, or proctitis) may be treated with a single 125-mg intramuscular dose of ceftriaxone. Spectinomycin (40 mg/kg) may be used intramuscularly in children who cannot tolerate ceftriaxone. It is recommended that children older than 8 years also receive a 7-day course of doxycycline. Children with complicated gonococcal infections (conjunctivitis, peritonitis, arthritis, or meningitis) should undergo a more prolonged course of parenteral ceftriaxone.[12]

Successful single-dose oral antibiotic therapy with amoxicillin and probenecid for culture-confirmed, uncomplicated childhood gonococcal infection has also been reported. In a multicenter study, this regimen was as efficacious as intramuscular penicillin G procaine and probenecid.[24] Although the endemic rise of penicillinase-producing *N. gonorrhoeae* may limit the usefulness of this therapy, the low cost and high patient acceptance of an oral regimen is attractive in situations when culture and sensitivity results are available. Although some data in adults suggest that the oral regimen is less effective in pharyngeal and rectal gonococcal infections,[41] Nelson et al. did not have any treatment failures using an oral amoxicillin-probenecid regimen in children with positive pharyngeal or rectal cultures.[24]

Prophylactic treatment for gonococcal infection in asymptomatic children being evaluated for possible sexual abuse is not recommended.[5] Kramer and Jason have calculated that 96% of children receiving prophylactic treatment receive such unnecessarily.[42] The rare nature of upper tract genital disease in children supports this stance.

One final aspect of treatment of gonococcal infection in children that should be stressed is follow-up. Follow-up cultures after treatment are important to document complete eradication of the organism. Some researchers have suggested a second set of follow-up cultures 6 to 8 weeks after documented cure to determine any reinfection. This is especially important when the source of infection was not identified or casual contact or fomite transmission was believed to be the source. In some cases, the assistance of Child Protective Services may be necessary. Farrell et al. noted that 92% of children treated as outpatients were lost to follow-up.[31] Clearly, a multidisciplinary approach is helpful in ensuring proper compliance and follow-up.

Chlamydia Trachomatis Infection

Biology

C. trachomatis is an obligate intracellular parasite with 15 serotypes currently identified. The less common serotypes, L1, L2, and L3, are responsible for lymphogranuloma venereum; the serotypes D through K are responsible for inclusion conjunctivitis, pneumonia, vaginitis, nongonococcal urethritis, cervicitis, and salpingitis. This obligate intracellular organism can be cultured only in a living cell host, not in artificial culture media.

Inclusion conjunctivitis is primarily a disease of the neonatal period, with chlamydial pneumonitis occuring during infancy. In adulthood, genital tract infection is the usual clinical presentation. Beyond infancy, chlamydial infection in children is uncommon and generally presents as genital tract infection. *C. trachomatis* directly infects the squamocolumnar junction epithelial cells, causing extensive cellular damage in its life cycle. In adults, the urethra of the man and the endocervix of the woman are the most common primary sites of infection. As with gonococcal infection of the prepubertal genital tract, the "atrophic," unestrogenized vaginal epithelium may be directly infected with this organism, causing a true vaginitis. This organism is never considered part of the normal flora but may often produce colonization without symptoms.[43]

Demographics

Infection with *C. trachomatis* is one of the most common sexually transmitted diseases in the adult population, with an estimated 4 million new cases occurring annually.[44] The significant cost and lack of availability of chlamydial cell cultures have resulted in underdiagnosis of this infection in the adult population. The more recent development of antigen detection testing methods has improved the ease of diagnosis in adults, although these testing methods are not recommended for use in pediatric populations. It should also be remembered that infections with *C. trachomatis* are not "reportable" infections in most areas, making underreporting more likely.

No overall figures are available regarding the incidence of chlamydial infection in children. However, a number of studies have suggested that vertical transmission during the perinatal period is quite common. Many studies have found that 6% to 10% of pregnant women are infected with *C. trachomatis*, with high-risk populations having infection rates of 22% to 26%. Pregnant adolescents have shown infection rates as high as 37%. Vertical transmission is very common in infants delivered through an infected genital tract. The risk of inclusion conjunctivitis ranges from 18% to 50%; chlamydial pneumonitis occurs in 10% to 22% of exposed infants; and 60% to 70% of exposed infants will demonstrate serologic evidence of infection by 12 months of age.[17, 18, 45–47]

Infection of the genital tract is the most common presentation in children after infancy. As with gonococcal infection, the incidence will vary greatly according to the population being studied. Hammerschlag et al. found a 1% incidence of positive vaginal chlamydial cultures in a population of nonselected girls being screened in an ambulatory pediatric clinic as part of a study examining normal vaginal flora.[3] Paradise et al. found no positive chlamydial cultures in their population of girls with vaginitis, although 2.8% of the control population of asymptomatic girls had positive cultures.[1] In a study by Bump, 20% of girls with symptoms of vaginitis were found to have chlamydial infection; there was a 44% positive culture rate in children whose presenting complaint was vaginal bleeding.[48]

When a population of suspected sexually abused children is examined, the overall incidence of chlamydial infection is generally reported to be between 2% and 6%.[5, 6, 49, 50] This relatively low incidence has led to a description of genital chlamydial infection in childhood as "statistically nonsignificant but clinically important."[51] However, the incidence varies greatly in different areas, which many authors have attributed to high rates of chlamydial infection in the adult population. The highest reported incidence was found by Keskey et al., who reported 43% positive cultures in preadolescent sexually abused children.[52] Case-control studies have often been confounded by the appearance of chlamydial infection in the control population, with unsuspected abuse often detected after investigation.[49, 50]

As with gonococcal infection, multisite infection with *C. trachomatis* has been reported. In Ingram et al.'s population of suspected sexual abuse victims, 8% of children had positive vaginal cultures. They also found 2.4% positive rectal and 0.8% positive pharyngeal cultures in this group; in addition, 1.4% of pharyngeal cultures were positive in children who were at risk for abuse.[53] An earlier study by Ingram et al. noted a 3% incidence of positive pharyngeal and concomitant vaginal and rectal cultures in a population of abused children.[49] In children with a very high incidence of chlamydial genital infection, 53% had multiple positive culture sites.[52] As with gonococcal infection, many of these positive cultures were obtained from anatomic sites not mentioned by children in their disclosures of abuse.

Presentation

In the neonatal period, infection with *C. trachomatis* most commonly presents with the development of inclusion conjunctivitis at 5 to 7 days of age. A mucoid discharge is initially present and may become purulent within a few days. Without treatment, colonization of the conjunctiva may persist for up to 2 years. Contrary to what was once thought, untreated conjunctival infection may produce chronic sequelae. Perinatal exposure to *C. trachomatis* may also result in pneumonitis presenting at 3 to 11 weeks of age with a history of prolonged cough and congestion. Some, but not all, infants may have a history of conjunctivitis.[45]

Perinatal exposure may also result in colonization of the vagina and rectum.[54] Longitudinal studies of infants exposed to *C. trachomatis* at birth have shown carriage of the organism up to 55 weeks in the rectum and 53 weeks in the vagina.[55] One study has demonstrated rectal colonization for up to 2 years after perinatal exposure.[56] In these studies, the majority of the infants were asymptomatic.

C. trachomatis is also known to cause symptomatic vaginitis in infected children. Even before the organism was identified, there were case reports of vaginitis in prepubertal girls caused by the same organism responsible for inclusion conjunctivitis.[57] Unlike in adult women, where this organism infects the squamocolumnar epithelium of the cervix, prepubertal children are infected in the atrophic, unestrogenized squamous epithelium of the vagina. When symptomatic, children usually present with vaginitis, urethritis, and/or pyuria.[48] *C. trachomatis* has also been reported as a cause of symptomatic urethritis in prepubertal boys.[58] In their series of children with genital chlamydial infection, Fuster and Neinstein found that 44% of children presented with vulvar erythema, 24% with vaginal discharge, 25% with rectal pain, and 12% with vaginal bleeding.[59] Bump found a 44% incidence of positive chlamydial cultures in children presenting with vaginal bleeding.[48] Many studies have confirmed the common occurrence of asymptomatic colonization in children. In Ingram et al.'s study, 60% of children with positive vaginal cultures were asymptomatic. All of the children in this study who had a positive oral or rectal culture were asymptomatic.[53]

Although nongonococcal urethritis in men usually develops within 2 weeks of exposure,[43] many reports of chlamydial infection in children have suggested the possibility of a long latent period. In Hammerschlag et al.'s case-control study of prepubertal girls with chlamydial infection, positive cultures in the control group were attributed to sexual abuse 3 years before the study.[50]

In children infected with chlamydia by sexual contact, evidence of vaginal penetration is not always present on physical examination. As with gonococcal infection in children, this suggests that the organism may be spread by vulvar contact with infected secretions or an infected body part. Ingram et al. found that 60% of sexually abused children who had positive vaginal chlamydial cultures had no evidence of vaginal penetration.[53] Fuster and Neinstein also found evidence of hymenal tears in only 26% of prepubertal girls with positive vaginal chlamydial cultures.[59] Chronic *C. trachomatis* infection has been reported in infants.[60] In a series of 22 infants studied at the University of Washington, it was noted that many infants infected with *C. trachomatis* remained infected for months or even years in the absence of specific antimicrobial therapy.

Furthermore, such infections may be confused with those acquired by sexual abuse.

Concomitant infection with *C. trachomatis* and *N. gonorrhoeae* has also been a fairly common finding. Many of the early reports of pediatric chlamydial vaginitis were in children whose symptoms persisted after treatment for documented gonococcal vaginitis and who were subsequently found to have positive chlamydial cultures. In a study of prepubertal children with gonococcal infection, Rettig and Nelson found that 27% were also positive for *C. trachomatis*.[58]

Mode of Transmission

The primary modes of transmission of *C. trachomatis* all involve direct contact rather than fomite transmission. Given the obligate intracellular nature of this parasite, transmission via fomites is extremely unlikely in theory and has never been documented.

At birth, the neonate is innoculated by contact with infected secretions. Perinatal exposure has been well documented to result in spread of the organism to the eyes, nasopharynx, vagina, and rectum. Vertical transmission at the time of cesarean section performed after the rupture of membranes has also been reported.[17, 18, 45–47] It appears that each site may be separately innoculated at birth, in addition to autoinnoculation from one site to the other. Bell et al. found that the majority of infants infected with *Chlamydia* organisms at birth demonstrated positive nasopharyngeal cultures several months before positive vaginal and/or rectal cultures were documented.[56]

The potential for prolonged colonization with perinatally acquired *C. trachomatis* may complicate determination of the source of infection in the toddler, where obtaining a history from the child is limited. Perinatal colonization to the age of 2 years has been reported, as in the case of a 16-month-old girl with symptomatic chlamydial vaginitis following untreated perinatally acquired inclusion conjunctivitis.[51]

In children older than 24 to 36 months, genital infection with *C. trachomatis* has been highly associated with sexual abuse.[49] In Hammerschlag et al.'s case-control study, a diagnosis of chlamydial vaginitis strongly correlated with a history of sexual abuse.[50] Even in unsuspected cases of chlamydial vaginitis in the control group, careful investigation revealed histories of sexual abuse. As with gonococcal infection, it is important to remember that a history of abuse may not be obtained on the first (or even second) interview with a child. Bump found an initial history of sexual abuse in only 25% of girls with chlamydial vaginitis; subsequent interviewing discovered a history of abuse in all but one child.[48] Again, a multidisciplinary approach and a high index of suspicion are appropriate.

Diagnosis

Choosing the correct diagnostic test is essential. Cell culture is regarded as the "gold standard" and the most optimal method of diagnosing the presence of this obligate intracellular organism. The most commonly employed technique involves a monolayer of susceptible cells (e.g., McCoy cells). Because this organism is intracellular, it is important to obtain epithelial cells for the culture, rather than simply culturing any discharge that is present.[44] In adults this would involve a careful endocervical or urethral culture. In prepubertal children, a careful vaginal or urethral culture is necessary. As discussed earlier, prepubertal girls may be infected with *C. trachomatis* without evidence of vaginal penetration or symptoms of vaginitis. Therefore, cultures should not be omitted simply because the child is asymptomatic or has normal hymenal anatomy. Although culturing the rectum and pharynx will not often yield positive results, infection and colonization at both sites have been documented, and culturing these areas is currently recommended by the Centers for Disease Control.[12]

The use of correct growth and/or transport media is necessary to obtain accurate results. The correct choice of swab type is also important to avoid toxic effects of the cell culture.[61] Urethral swabs with calcium alginate (Calgi swabs) are often useful in obtaining cultures from children because of their small diameter; these swabs may be batch tested to ensure there is no toxicity to the growth of *C. trachomatis* in cell culture. When positive culture results are obtained, freezing of the specimen at $-70°C$ may be indicated. This is especially important if later forensic confirmation may be indicated.[61]

Antigen detection testing has become increasingly popular in response to the expense and limited availability of cell cultures for *C. trachomatis*. These testing methods employ either a direct fluorescent monoclonal antibody (e.g., Microtrak) or an enzyme-linked immunosorbent assay (ELISA) (e.g., Chlamydiazyme). The antigen detection methods were developed and sensitivity and specificity data generated in high-prevalence populations, such as adult STD clinics, and used in the cervix and urethra.[44] The Centers for Disease Control recommend against the use of these testing methods in prepubertal children.[12] The low prevalence of *C. trachomatis* infection in sexually abused children and the need to test anatomic sites other than the cervix and urethra contribute to unacceptable sensitivity and specificity rates. False-positive and false-negative rates of up to 50% have been reported with the use of antigen detection methods in children. The specificity and sensitivity rates reported for adults are not applicable in children, where the prevalence rate for *C. trachomatis* infection is much lower and cross-reacting organisms (e.g., *Escherichia coli*, group B streptococci, and *Actinobacter*) are present in oral and fecal flora.[59, 62, 63]

Serologic testing for the presence of antibodies to *C. trachomatis* has not been clinically useful in children, as seroconversion is common during the childhood years. In a study of well children, 15% of those between 9 months and 15 years of age demonstrated antibodies against *C. trachomatis*. Seropositivity increased with age: 2.7% of those younger than 6 years were positive, compared with 23% of those between 6 and 15 years. This seroconversion is greater than would be expected from perinatal exposure.[64]

Treatment

Treatment of choice for pediatric genital chlamydial infection is erythromycin in children 8 years and younger, with tetracycline recommended in children older than 8 years. *C. trachomatis* is also susceptible to sulfonamides and trimethoprim; however, trimethoprim has not been widely used for *C. trachomatis* because of its lack of activity against other organisms known to cause genital disease, particularly other sexually transmitted diseases.

Prophylactic treatment for *C. trachomatis* in children is not indicated. As with gonococcal infection, the low prevalence and minimal risk for the development of upper genital tract disease allows the practitioner to wait for culture results before instituting treatment. Given the high false-positive rates of antigen detection methods, it would also seem reasonable to wait for culture results before treating a child with a positive antigen detection test. Because of the relatively high association of infection with *N. gonorrhoeae* and *C. trachomatis* in children, coverage for *C. trachomatis* should be included in treatment for children with gonococcal infection if chlamydial cultures are not available.[48]

After treatment, reevaluation should include a test of cure. Again, this should be performed using a cell culture method. Dead antigen may be responsible for a false-positive test by the antigen detection method. As with gonococcal infection, testing for reinfection in 2 to 3 months may be reasonable with *C. trachomatis* in prepubertal children. This is especially helpful in situations where abuse is suspected but not proven or when a prepetrator cannot be identified.

Trichomoniasis

Infection with the single cell protozoa, *Trichomonas vaginalis*, is an uncommon finding in prepubertal children beyond the neonatal period. It appears that the unestrogenized vagina with its alkaline pH is relatively resistant to infection and colonization with this organism.[65, 66] A review of the literature since 1956 reveals only scattered case reports of trichomoniasis in groups of symptomatic and asymptomatic girls.[7] Studies of pediatric vulvovaginitis by Paradise et al. and Gerstner et al. did not identify *T. vaginalis* in the symptomatic girls studied.[1, 20] The protozoa was found in only 1% of sexually abused girls studied by White et al.[4]

In contrast, the organism is a relatively common cause of vaginitis during the neonatal period, being isolated in from 4% to 17% of infants examined because of vaginal discharge during the first few days of life.[67] This is probably attributable to the effect of maternal estrogen on the vagina of the neonate and the resulting acidic pH.

In Jones et al.'s review of 18 girls with *T. vaginalis* isolated from the vagina, 65% were symptomatic. In two girls evaluated after being sexually abused, symptoms developed within 7 to 10 days of the abuse.[68] When symptomatic, girls usually present with a copious frothy discharge often described as yellow-gray in color. There are often accompanying complaints of vulvar pruritus and dysuria.[2] Because the prepubertal vagina is less likely to support

growth of this organism, the urinary tract may be the primary source of infection.[69] In these situations, the protozoa may not be identified in vaginal specimens but may be noted on urinalysis.[66] In the neonate, isolation of *T. vaginalis* in specimens obtained from both the vagina and the nasopharynx has been reported.[70]

Earlier reports of trichomoniasis in children did not address the issue of source of transmission. However, sexual transmission is the most common source of infection in both adults and children.[7, 66, 68, 71] Furthermore, perinatal acquisition is the most common form of nonvenereal transmission.[69] Approximately 5% of neonates born to mothers with vaginal trichomoniasis become infected.[72–74] Many of these infections will spontaneously resolve as maternal estrogen effect diminishes and vaginal pH rises. It is unknown whether *T. vaginalis* infection in childhood could be related to neonatal exposure.[66]

The possibilities of fomite transmission and acquisition by nonsexual contact are unclear but appear unlikely. The organism is very sensitive to dessication but may survive for several hours on moist surfaces and in body fluids.[75] Although spread by way of wet, contaminated clothes in crowded, unhygienic conditions[71]; infected water from toilets[76]; and sleeping with an infected mother[77] has been suggested, well-documented cases of trichomoniasis in childhood as a result of fomite transmission have not been reported.[7, 69]

Diagnosis of trichomoniasis is usually made by the appearance of the motile organism on a wet preparation of secretions. At higher levels of magnification, the flagellum of the organism may be visualized. Significant numbers of leukocytes often accompany the organism, making careful inspection of the wet preparation important.[65] Culture of the organism is both more sensitive and more specific in making the diagnosis but is not widely available or used.[78]

Metronidazole has been well described as an effective method of treatment in adults, and initial concerns of carcinogenicity of this antibiotic do not appear clinically warranted.[79] Neonatal infection may often be managed expectantly, with the infection usually spontaneously subsiding with loss of maternal estrogen. However, newborns may require treatment of more severe infections, such as those worsened by the presence of severe candidiasis.[80] In these infants, as well as older children who require treatment, metronidazole may be given in three divided doses of 15 mg/kg/day (maximum dose, 250 mg) for 7 days. The safety of metronidazole treatment in children has been evaluated in the treatment of amebiasis. Single-dose treatment, as frequently used in adulthood, has not been evaluated in children.[2, 81]

Condyloma Acuminatum

Biology

In both adults and children, condylomata acuminata are caused by infection with the human papillomavirus (HPV). More than 50 subtypes of this double-stranded DNA virus have been identified. As shown in Table 20–1, each viral subtype is somewhat site specific, infecting either skin or mucosal surfaces. The virus infects the germinal layer of the epithelium, and it has been suggested that it enters through a traumatic break in the epithelium. Viral subtypes also differ in their association with the development of neoplasia.[82, 83]

Demographics

The prevalence of infection with HPV is difficult to determine. One conservative estimate suggests that 2% of reproductive-age women are infected with this virus.[82] A dramatic increase in the number of clinical cases of HPV has been reported in adults. The number of office visits for condylomata in adults increased 459% between the years of 1966 and 1981. In adult females, this increase was 684%.[84] Although exact statistics are not

known for the pediatric population, the proliferation of case reports of pediatric HPV infection suggests an increase paralleling that seen in adults.[85–91]

Presentation

Anogenital condyloma in children generally presents as flesh-colored verrucous growths. Lesions have also been reported in the moist mucosal membranes of the urethra, bladder, mouth, and eye.[92] The condyloma may be friable and easily traumatized, especially in moist areas. The typical keratinized or "warty" appearance of the condyloma may not be present in diaper-age children because of exposure of the condyloma to continuous moisture. Children with condyloma generally present with asymptomatic lesions noted by their caretaker during diapering and bathing. However, the friable and vascular nature of pediatric condylomata may result in vaginal or rectal bleeding, dysuria, vaginal discharge, or painful defecation.[93]

The anatomic distribution of genital condylomata may vary between adults and children. In adults, labial lesions are most common in women, while penile lesions are the predominant site of infection in men. In contrast, prepubertal children are much more likely than adults to present with periurethral and perianal condylomata. In one study of prepubertal boys, 77% were found to have perianal condyloma; 16% had involvement of the urethral meatus, and only 3% had involvement of the penile shaft.[94] Similar findings have been noted in prepubertal girls, with several authors reporting a 30% to 70% incidence of perianal warts and a 19% to 33% incidence of periurethral warts.[95, 96]

The majority of women with external condylomata have upper genital tract disease; one study noted a 68% incidence of vaginal and cervical lesions in women with external condylomata.[94] This is of particular concern, given the association of certain HPV subtypes (16, 18, 31, and 33) with high-grade neoplasia of the vagina and cervix.[97–100] However, studies examining the upper genital tract of prepubertal girls for the presence of HPV lesions have shown this to be unusual.[96, 101] In contrast, the clinical finding of perianal condylomata has been strongly associated with the presence of additional HPV lesions in the anal canal.[96] This may represent a focus of untreated disease and a source for recurrence. Parallels drawn

TABLE 20–1 ••• HPV TYPES AND ASSOCIATED LESIONS

Type	Lesion
1a–c	Plantar warts
2a–e	Common warts
3a,b	Flat warts
4	Plantar warts
10a,b	Flat warts
11a,b	Condylomata acuminata
	Cervical dysplasia
	Laryngeal papillomatosis
16, 18, 31, 33, 35	Condylomata acuminata
	Cervical dysplasia
	Squamous cell carcinomas

From Shah KV. Biology of human genital tract papillomaviruses. In: Holmes KK (ed). Sexually Transmitted Diseases. 2nd ed. New York: McGraw-Hill, 1990, pp 425–431.

between cervical intraepithelial neoplasia and anal intraepithelial neoplasia in the adult population are an additional cause for concern in infected children.[102] From these data, clinicians should consider the urethra and the anal canal as potential sites of infection.[103]

Sexually abused children presenting with genital condylomata are also at significant risk for other STDs. Herman-Giddens et al. found a 50% incidence of other STDs in sexually abused girls.[104] The risk was greatest in the subset of girls who had had multiple abusers. Genital condylomata that are refractory to standard treatment have also been reported in children with human immunodeficiency virus (HIV) infection.[105, 106]

Perioral condylomata have also been reported in children with documented sexual abuse. This is an unusual finding, representing only 3% of cases in a review of several series of case reports.[94] More commonly reported is juvenile laryngeal papillomatosis. This generally presents in children younger than 5 years with hoarseness and, rarely, respiratory obstruction. These HPV lesions are often asymptomatic, making a true estimate of their prevalence difficult. However, it has been suggested that this well-studied form of pediatric HPV infection may serve as a model for the study of genital HPV in children.[107]

Mode of Transmission

Vertical transmission at birth, casual transmission, and sexual transmission have all been implicated as possible modes of infection in children with HPV. Vertical transmission of juvenile respiratory papillomatosis has been the most thoroughly studied. Nearly all pediatric laryngeal HPV lesions that have been typed have shown types 6 and 11, which are commonly responsible for genital disease. Epidemiologic studies of these children have shown that fewer than 1% were delivered abdominally, and up to 60% of these mothers were known to have HPV lesions at the time of delivery.[108]

Genital HPV is a very common finding in women of childbearing age, with cervical specimens testing positive for HPV DNA in more than 10% of some obstetric populations. In a study of healthy mothers and infants without known HPV infections, HPV DNA was found in 4.3% of foreskin specimens obtained at circumcision of these healthy newborns.[109] In these cases, exposure to the virus is speculated

to occur directly during passage through an infected genital tract. The possibility of hematogenous spread has been suggested by a case report of a premature newborn who was delivered by cesarean section, before known rupture of membranes, with genital condylomata noted at birth.[110] The risk of hematogenous spread must be exceedingly low, given the rarity of congenital condylomata acuminata and the widespread presence of genital HPV in obstetric populations. In this case report, the possibility of occult rupture of fetal membranes as the cause of premature labor was not excluded, making ascending infection a possibility.

Vertical transmission of HPV resulting in laryngeal lesions has been well documented and probably occurs through aspiration of infected secretions into the upper airway of the newborn at birth. Presumed vertical transmission of genital HPV in infants and toddlers has also been reported. Although it is unclear why these anatomic sites are the most commonly reported sites of perinatally acquired HPV, it is possible that these mucosal surfaces are subjected to trauma at birth, resulting in epithelial cell damage that allows entry of the virus. Boyd found that 19% of cases of pediatric genital HPV infection had been attributed to perinatally acquired disease.[94] The majority of presumed perinatally transmitted HPV cases have been reported in children younger than 2 years,[89, 90] which is in keeping with data suggesting an incubation period of up to 20 months in children.[95] It is important to remember the inherent difficulties in evaluating children of this age group for possible sexual abuse (i.e., the absence of a history from a preverbal child and the infrequent finding of genital trauma and other STDs in this age group).

Sexual transmission of HPV has been well documented in adults, with the usual incubation periods ranging from 4 weeks to 3 months.[111–113] In several reviews, transmission by sexual abuse was documented in 50% to 80% of children evaluated.[90, 94, 114] In a series excluding children less than 2 years of age, abuse was documented in as many as 90% of the children evaluated.[104] Demographic studies comparing route of delivery, maternal history of HPV, history of sexual abuse, evidence of genital trauma, and the presence of other STDs have shown significant differences between children younger than 3 years and those older than 3 years with condyloma.[115] Studies that "rule out" sexual abuse in older children with condyloma based on the presence of genital HPV lesions in parents should be interpreted with caution; it is well known that the maternal sexual partner is frequently the perpetrator of sexual abuse, and partners of women with HPV are very frequently infected with the virus. It is essential to stress that each child, regardless of age, who presents with condyloma acuminatum deserves a thorough and careful evaluation to assess the possibility of sexual abuse.[116, 117]

Reviews of cases of pediatric genital HPV have also included a significant number of children in whom the source of infection was unknown (i.e., 10% to 37% of reported cases)[90, 94, 104] and have raised questions about the possibility of casual spread of HPV or spread of warts by autoinoculation. In the adult population, the spread of genital condyloma via casual contact or autoinoculation is considered highly unlikely. Studies have failed to show an increased incidence of genital condyloma in adults with other cutaneous HPV lesions.[118] Whether these data are applicable to the pediatric population has recently been questioned. Some authors have suggested that casual contact may be responsible for some genital HPV lesions in children, citing that normal contact involved in the care of small children is much less "casual" than contact between adults. Fleming has reported one case of genital HPV in a 5-year-old boy that was thought to be due to autoinoculation from cutaneous warts.[119] Hansen et al. have also noted the presence of HPV-2 in genital warts of two children, with sexual transmission later documented in one case. Another child in the series was also found to have HPV-2 and HPV-18 coexisting in a single specimen.[90] Obalek and colleagues have reported HPV-2 in 21% of children evaluated for genital condyloma.[89] Because HPV-2 is generally associated with cutaneous warts, they concluded that casual contact or autoinoculation was responsible for disease in these children. Again, caution is warranted in excluding the possibility of abuse based on HPV DNA type alone; factors such as cross-reactivity of HPV types on DNA probes, the knowledge that condyloma may express different viral types at different times, and the finding of HPV-1 and HPV-2 in genital specimens of adult condylomata are extremely important to consider.[120] Each child with genital condyloma deserves careful evaluation for the possibility of sexual abuse.

Diagnosis

The diagnosis of genital condylomata acuminata in children can generally be established by careful clinical inspection. The application of 3% to 5% acetic acid on a compress for 10 to 15 minutes may elicit the classic acetowhite appearance of condyloma familiar to clinicians experienced in the care of adult HPV. In general, 3% acetic acid is sufficient for mucosal lesions and will cause less discomfort than the 5% solution frequently required to obtain an acetowhite appearance in keratinized lesions.[94] On mucosal surfaces, the typical "warty" appearance is less common than a pink or red fleshy growth, often with marked vascularity. Careful inspection of the perianal and periurethral area is important and often reveals lesions initially missed.

The differential diagnosis of genital lesions in children should include condylomata lata of secondary syphilis, generally having a less raised and "velvety" appearance; perineal tumors; urethral prolapse, easily confused with infected and traumatized periurethral condyloma; rhabdomyosarcoma (sarcoma botryoides); and molluscum contagiosum. Biopsy may be indicated in cases in which the diagnosis is in question.[93] A thorough evaluation of the vagina, cervix, periurethral area, and anal canal should also be performed with the patient anesthetized.

Microscopic examination of condyloma will generally reveal the classic findings of a hyperplastic squamous epithelium with acanthosis, hyperkeratosis, and parakeratosis. Koilocytosis is often present. Specimens should also be evaluated for findings of atypia. Immunoperoxidase staining has been used in an attempt to improve the specificity of the diagnosis by biopsy. However, when compared with testing for HPV DNA, immunoperoxidase is relatively nonspecific. In pediatric populations, a positive immunoperoxidase stain has been reported in only 30% to 40% of lesions known to contain HPV DNA.[87, 96]

Several series have examined the role of DNA typing in the assessment of pediatric genital condyloma. In these cases, HPV-6/11 is most commonly reported, with occasional reports of HPV-2 and an infrequent report of HPV-16/18. The presence of an "as-yet-uncharacterized" HPV type has also been mentioned in several reports.[87–91, 94, 96] The clinical usefulness of HPV typing of pediatric lesions is not clearly defined. In adults, HPV typing is more specific than histology alone in determining diagnosis, although lesions with the classic appearance of condyloma occasionally may not type with any available DNA probes. This may be due to the as-yet-uncharacterized HPV types. Several articles have reported the use of typing in an attempt to determine the source of transmission of the virus. Until more data are available, this should be done with great caution.[121] In adults, it is well known that some cross-reactivity exists between different types and that a single wart may express more than one type of HPV DNA at different times. Although the viral subtypes are considered relatively site specific, HPV-1 and HPV-2 have been reported in anogenital condyloma in adults.[120] HPV-16 has also been reported in periungual squamous cell carcinoma in adults.[122] Clearly, a great disservice may be done to the pediatric patient by relying on only one piece of information when drawing conclusions in this complex problem.

Although most of the HPV typing data collected in children have been positive for the "low risk" viral types of HPV-6 and HPV-11, HPV-16 and HPV-18 have also been reported in prepubertal children.[87, 88, 90] In adults, these viral types have been associated with an increased risk of high-grade intraepithelial lesions and squamous cell carcinomas.[98, 99, 118, 123] There has been some concern that children infected with these viral types may have a similar increased risk of neoplasia. There are two reports in the literature of squamous cell carcinoma of the vulva in young, nonsexually active females. One report by Lister and Akinla describes the development of vulvar carcinoma in a 14-year-old girl with a history of genital condyloma since infancy.[124] The previously discussed high incidence of anal canal disease in children with perianal condyloma[96] and the similarities between cervical intraepithelial neoplasia and anal intraepithelial neoplasia in adults[102] are of great concern. There are presently no standard recommendations for follow-up of children exposed to HPV, although most concern centers around those children exposed to the subtypes with oncogenic potential.[94] It is clear that these children deserve careful follow-up so that the long-term risks of neoplasia can be more clearly defined.[85]

Treatment

Any clinician who is experienced in the long-term care of adults infected with HPV is familiar with the frustrations associated with treatment. The special needs of children often compound these treatment difficulties. An ideal treatment for children would be inexpensive, effective, atraumatic, and widely available, but unfortunately, all treatment regimens available to children are associated with relatively high recurrence risks, the need for close supervision by the clinician, and the possibility of physical discomfort or emotional trauma as a result of frequent genital examinations. Although spontaneous regression of condyloma has been well described in adults, this is not recommended as a treatment of choice in children.[94]

Podophyllin resin is widely available as a 20% to 25% solution combined with tincture of benzoin, and its use has been described in the pediatric age group. When podophyllin resin is used in children, it is essential that the clinician be assured of careful compliance. The caretaker of the child must remove the solution by washing with soap and water approximately 4 hours after application. Systemic absorption of podophyllin resin and resultant neurotoxicity have been described in adults and adolescents.[125–127] In pregnant adult women, deaths have been reported when large areas of abraded condylomata were painted with podophyllin resin and covered with an occlusive dressing.[128] These data should encourage clinicians to use this substance cautiously in children. Clinicians accustomed to treating adults should remember that painting a given surface area in a child with podophyllin resin will expose a much higher percentage of the total body surface area than in an adult. A 1 cm^2 area on the skin of an average sized 3-year-old represents the same percentage of body surface area as a 3 cm^2 area in an adult. Systemic absorption may also be increased by the use of an occlusive dressing or disposable diapers. For this reason, it has been suggested that more dilute solutions (e.g., 5% to 15%) may be more appropriate for use in children.[95] As in adults, a relatively high recurrence rate has been reported, with treatment failures and/or recurrences noted in 43% of the pediatric population treated by Stringel et al.[103, 129]

Cryotherapy using a probe or direct application of liquid nitrogen has also been described in the treatment of condyloma in adults and children. There is some theoretical concern about the effectiveness of cryotherapy in the treatment of condyloma, as data suggest that viable virus will persist in tissue after treatment.[100] As in the topical application of caustic solutions such as trichloroacetic or bichloroacetic acid, the therapeutic value of these agents is limited by the discomfort or actual pain involved in their use. An older child with a few condylomata may tolerate these treatment modalities well. However, in children with more extensive disease, their usefulness will be limited by the need for frequent treatments.

The topical use of 5-fluorouracil cream has been reported in adults as a cost-effective treatment of condyloma.[130] This relatively low-cost drug may be applied externally by a parent or caregiver. Although careful follow-up by a clinician is necessary, less frequent follow-up may be required once treatment is under way and the caregiver has been educated in proper use. The most common side effect noted is inflammation of the skin surrounding the condyloma. However, this may be controlled by titrating the amount of cream and frequency of use as appropriate for each child.

In the past, electrosurgical fulguration was commonly employed in the treatment of more severe condyloma. The use of anesthesia is required, thereby increasing both the medical risk and the financial cost of the procedure. Unfortunately, fulguration does not have a significantly lower recurrence rate than less invasive treatment methods, with up to a 50% recurrence rate noted.[90] The use of electrosurgical fulguration has also been associated with significant tissue damage and may cause scarring and stricture formation.[103, 129] The potential damage from electrosurgical fulguration, particularly in children with perianal and periurethral condyloma, should be carefully considered in planning their treatment.

The carbon dioxide (CO_2) laser has become increasingly popular in the treatment of genital condyloma. Like electrosurgical fulguration, it requires general anesthesia. However, careful use of the laser allows control over the depth of tissue destruction and avoids much of the scarring associated with electrosurgery.[94] The CO_2 laser may also be used to treat lesions in the periurethral and perianal area, as well as in the anal canal, where other modalities are more difficult to use. Gale and Muram also noted fewer subjective complaints of postoperative discomfort in their series of children treated with the CO_2 laser. They also noted a 29% recurrence rate, again supporting the advantages of laser over electrosurgical fulguration.[131]

Success with the use of interferon in adults with genital condyloma has led several investigators to use interferon in children. The most extensive use of interferon in children has been reported in the treatment of laryngeal papillomatosis.[132] The safety of interferon was demonstrated in these children, although its use was associated with reversible elevation of liver enzyme levels and neutropenia. Clinical side effects of fever, anorexia, and nausea and vomiting were noted. Linear growth was carefully followed and remained unaffected. However, 6-month follow-up of the groups comparing surgical and interferon treatment did not demonstrate any improvement in recurrence rate.[132] Persistent viral infection during clinical remission after interferon treatment has been demonstrated in biopsy studies of laryngeal papillomatosis.[133]

The use of interferon in the treatment of genital condyloma in children has not yet been extensively studied, although case reports of its use are appearing in the literature. These case reports suggest that much of the data collected on interferon use in laryngeal papillomatosis is applicable to children with condyloma. Similar laboratory and clinical side effects have been reported.[101, 105] There are no long-term studies of the effectiveness of interferon in children with genital condyloma. However, studies of adults suggest that significant numbers of patients will experience recurrence after termination of treatment. Intralesional interferon has also been reported to be more effective than systemic administration,[134] and the majority of studies demonstrating efficacy in adults have used intralesional interferon. The difficulties associated with multiple intralesional injections in the pediatric age group and the lower effectiveness of systemic interferon may ultimately limit the usefulness of this modality in children.

Clinical experience and literature review clearly indicate that there is no single "correct" treatment for children with condyloma. Instead, clinicians should be familiar with a number of treatment modalities so that therapy for each child may be individualized. Education of parents regarding the biology of the virus and the chronic nature of the infection may be helpful in dealing with the natural frustrations associated with the high recurrence rate of lesions.

The oncogenic potential of the HPV is also a cause for concern in long-term management of these children. Although there are no long-term studies in children, studies in adults have raised concerns about the risk of later development of neoplastic lesions in children exposed to HPV.[98, 99, 118] Many authors have emphasized the importance of long-term follow-up in these children, especially those exposed to the "high-risk" viral subtypes. However, until long-term studies can be performed, the exact nature of this follow-up remains undefined.[94]

Genital Herpes

Biology

Genital herpes is caused by infection with the double-stranded DNA herpes simplex virus (HSV), which occurs in two subtypes, HSV-1 and HSV-2.[135] Although it was once thought that HSV-1 occurred only in oral lesions and HSV-2 in genital lesions, it has been well documented that infection with a particular HSV type is not site specific. Each HSV type will generate its own specific antibody response, with antibody against one HSV type not providing immunity to the other type.[10]

Presentation

During childhood, herpes simplex virus infection most commonly presents as gingivostomatitis. Taieb et al.'s series of 50 children with primary HSV infection found oral lesions in 96%.[136] This may appear as a mild gingivitis or as a more severe infection with painful vesicular lesions of the lips and oral cavity that later ulcerate. Pharyngitis may also develop, again ranging from a mild to a more severe ulcerative form. HSV types 1 and 2 have both been isolated as the cause of childhood gingivostomatitis. Pharyngitis has also been noted in 10% of adults with primary genital herpes.[137]

Multifocal disease appears surprisingly common in children with primary HSV infection. Taieb et al. found multifocal disease in 36% of the children in their series. Herpetic whitlow was present as a painful vesicular lesion, usually along the edge of the nail. Lesions were also reported at other cutaneous sites.[136]

Genital herpes lesions caused by both HSV-1 and HSV-2, have been reported in children,[138–141] although genital lesions accounted for only 6% of lesions in Taieb's series.[136] The clinical presentation of primary genital herpes is very similar to that described in adults. After an incubation period of between 2 and 20 days,[139] painful vesicular lesions develop. These later ulcerate and are often accompanied by systemic symptoms. Inguinal adenopathy, fever, malaise, nausea, and headache may occur, and urinary retention may develop. Lesions caused by HSV-1 and HSV-2 may be clinically indistinguishable, but HSV-2 is four times more likely to cause recurrent genital herpes. Secondary lesions are generally less severe, with less viral shedding and no systemic symptoms.[135]

Transmission

Herpes simplex virus is transmitted by close contact with an individual who is shedding the virus, with the virus entering mucosal surfaces through an epithelial break.[137] The virus has been shown to survive in water and on plastic surfaces for several hours,[142] but fomite transmission has never been documented. The possibility of nonsexual transmission through close contact has been implicated by the high incidence of antibodies to HSV-2 in children in certain geographic areas.[143] However, the casual transmission of genital herpes to a child through nonsexual contact has not been proven.

Perinatal transmission of HSV has been well studied. Congenital HSV infection may occur from transplacental passage, although this is uncommon. Vertical transmission of the virus at the time of vaginal delivery has been described as the cause of the potentially devastating neonatal herpes infection.[135] Perinatal transmission is an uncommon cause of childhood genital herpes, but if the genitals are the site of neonatal cutaneous infection, the possibility of recurrent genital lesions exists.[66]

Autoinoculation from nongenital lesions has been documented as a source of genital herpes during childhood. However, transmission by sexual contact is the most common source of childhood genital herpes.[141, 144] Only small series of children with genital herpes have been reported in the literature. However, in Kaplan et al.'s study of six children, sexual contact was responsible for transmission in four.[140] In Nahmias et al.'s series of five children, three had a history of sexual abuse or physical findings consistent with sexual abuse.[138]

When a child presents with genital herpes, other sites should be carefully inspected for lesions, which sometimes may be asymptomatic. In particular, the oropharynx and hands should be carefully inspected. When both oral and genital lesions are present, the likelihood of autotransmission increases. However, cases of sexual transmission have been documented in children with simultaneous oral and genital herpes lesions.[138, 145]

Diagnosis

The diagnosis of genital herpes in a child is best made by viral culture of suspicious lesions.

Differential diagnosis of ulcerative and vesicular lesions includes varicella and recurrent herpes zoster, ammonia dermatitis, trauma, syphilis, Stevens-Johnson syndrome, condyloma, impetigo, erythema multiforme, and candidiasis, among others.[138]

Cell culture is the most accurate method of diagnosing genital herpes. However, false-positive culture results may occur in children with herpes zoster as a result of the similar cytopathic effects of herpes simplex and herpes zoster in cell culture. For this reason, it is recommended that positive herpes culture results in children be subjected to confirmatory testing.[10] False-negative culture results may occur if specimens are obtained from lesions with decreased viral shedding (e.g., recurrent lesions or those that are ulcerated or crusted).[135]

Antigen detection testing has not been evaluated in children and is not recommended. The concerns for specificity and sensitivity in testing are the same as for *C. trachomatis*.[10]

Treatment

There are no available specific treatment guidelines for children with genital herpes infection. It is unknown whether the data regarding the use of antiviral agents, such as acyclovir, in adults are pertinent in children. Acyclovir is a competitive inhibitor of viral DNA polymerase, inhibiting viral DNA synthesis. The use of acyclovir in adults has been demonstrated to be effective in the symptomatic treatment of primary outbreaks and suppressive treatment of secondary lesions.[135] Because the therapeutic safety of acyclovir in children has been demonstrated with neonatal herpes simplex and childhood herpes zoster, some clinicians use acyclovir to treat children with genital herpes. Others prefer to use symptomatic treatment of the genital lesions with local care, sitz baths, and drying agents. Bacterial superinfection may require antibiotics, although this is uncommon except in the immunocompromised[137] and those with epithelial skin breaks caused by other dermatologic conditions such as atopic dermatitis or diaper dermatitis.[136]

Bacterial Vaginosis

Bacterial vaginosis generally presents as a thin, white vaginal discharge with a "fishy" odor. On culture of the vaginal discharge, a mixed collection of organisms is seen; these include *Gardnerella vaginalis*, anaerobes such as *Bacteroides* species and *Mobiluncus*, and sometimes genital mycoplasmas.[146] In the mid 1980s, case reports began to appear describing a similar clinical presentation in children, especially among sexually abused children.[147] In 1984, Muram and Buxton reported three cases of vaginitis caused by *G. vaginalis* in prepubertal girls who had been sexually abused and suggested that "the isolation of *Gardnerella vaginalis* should alert the physician to the probability of sexual abuse."[148]

In both adults and children, bacterial vaginosis is best diagnosed by the finding of clue cells on wet preparation, accompanied by the release of an amine odor with application of an alkaline solution (potassium hydroxide). In adults, microscopic examination of a wet preparation was found to be the most specific (94%) and sensitive (98%) single method for diagnosis of bacterial vaginosis. The specificity increased to 99% when the alkalinization of vaginal secretions was used. Gram stain was found to be less specific and less sensitive.[149] Diagnosis based solely on the isolation of *G. vaginalis* from culture of vaginal secretions has not been found to be accurate, with *G. vaginalis* isolated in 50% of adult women who did not otherwise meet diagnostic criteria for bacterial vaginosis.[150] This appears to also be true in children, with Hammerschlag et al.'s findings of a 13.5% incidence of vaginal colonization with *G. vaginalis* (then called *Corynebacterium vaginale*) in healthy asymptomatic children. The frequency of colonization was age dependent; 18% of children younger than 2 years were colonized, with a 2.5% incidence in those 3 to 10 years old, and 63% in those 11 to 15 years old.[151] Bartley et al. also found clinical evidence of bacterial vaginosis in only 3 of 25 prepubertal girls with positive culture results for *G. vaginalis*. They also found that the presence of *G. vaginalis* did not correlate with clinical symptoms such as pain or pruritus or clinical findings such as bleeding, discharge, or vulvar erythema.[152]

It is unclear exactly how often bacterial vaginosis is responsible for vaginitis in the pediatric age group. In Paradise et al.'s study of symptomatic girls with vaginitis, no cases of bacterial vaginosis or positive cultures for *G. vaginalis* were identified, although selective media for *G. vaginalis* were not used.[1] However, other studies have identified cases of bacterial vaginosis, meeting the described clinical criteria, in prepubertal children.[152, 153]

Controversy exists regarding the mode of transmission of bacterial vaginosis in the postpubertal female. While the incidence of bacterial vaginosis is higher in sexually experienced women, it may also be present in virginal women.[146] Bump and Bueschling found a 12% incidence of bacterial vaginosis in virginal adolescents.[154] However, when bacterial vaginosis is studied in prepubertal populations, data suggest that it is usually sexually transmitted. Hammerschlag et al.'s case-control study examined sexually abused girls and a matched control population; they considered a diagnosis of bacterial vaginosis "definite" when both clue cells and an amine odor were present, and "possible" when either clue cells or an amine odor were present. A statistically significant difference in the incidence of bacterial vaginosis was found in the two groups of girls, with a 4% incidence of possible bacterial vaginosis in the nonabused controls and no definite cases. In the abused girls, they found a 25% incidence of possible or definite bacterial vaginosis, with 12.9% meeting definite criteria. They concluded that bacterial vaginosis, especially in those cases meeting definite criteria, is usually sexually transmitted in the prepubertal child.[153] It is unknown whether bacterial vaginosis can be perinatally transmitted.[66]

The study by Hammerschlag et al. also suggests another interesting finding in the natural history of bacterial vaginosis after sexual assault. In the children meeting clinical criteria for bacterial vaginosis, none met these criteria on initial evaluation shortly after the abuse episode. However, on later evaluation, vaginal wash specimens demonstrated clue cells and an amine odor along with clinical symptoms in 60% of those meeting criteria.[153] This is very similar to findings by Jenny et al. in adult women after sexual assault; they found a statistically significant increase in bacterial vaginosis when initial and follow-up examinations were compared.[155]

There are no formal published guidelines for the treatment of bacterial vaginosis in the pediatric age group. Hammerschlag et al. refer to the use of metronidazole in symptomatic children.[153] The use of ampicillin and amoxicillin has also been described in adults and may be of some benefit in the pediatric age group.[146]

Syphilis

Infection with *Treponema pallidum* has increased dramatically in the pediatric population, reflecting the increase in syphilis seen in women of childbearing age. Perinatal transmission of syphilis occurs most often by hematogenous transplacental passage of the organism, rather than by direct exposure at the time of birth.[156] Congenital and acquired syphilis may usually be distinguished by examining results of maternal serologic tests and cord blood/neonatal serologic tests obtained at the time of birth. However, there is a latent period between infection and conversion to positive serology. If the infant is delivered during this "window" of time, congenital syphilis may result despite a negative perinatal serologic result. This possibility should be considered when a child less than 1 year old presents with possible acquired syphilis.[157, 158]

Primary syphilis has very similar presentations in the pediatric and adult populations, generally appearing as a painless genital chancre at an average of 21 days after exposure. Primary lesions may also present in the oral cavity and perianal area. Perianal chancres have been confused with simple perianal fissures.[159] Differential diagnosis of these lesions can include condylomata acuminata, trauma, and ulcerative lesions such as those caused by herpes simplex.[160] At this stage, serologic tests are frequently negative. Nontreponemal testing, such as rapid plasma reagin (RPR) and VDRL, generally takes 4 to 8 weeks to convert after initial exposure; these tests may be positive during the first week after the chancre is present. Results of microhemagglutination–*Treponema pallidum* (MHA-TP) and flourescent treponemal antibody absorption tests may also be negative during the incubation period in early primary syphilis. For this reason, the clinician faced with a possible syphilitic chancre in a child should perform a darkfield examination.[158]

Secondary syphilis has also been reported in children. It often presents as a skin rash within 1 to several months after exposure. Differential diagnosis of such a rash includes pityriasis rosea, psoriasis, and tinea versicolor, as well as viral illnesses and drug reactions. Again, a relatively high index of suspicion is necessary to accurately diagnose the very infrequent condition of secondary syphilis in the pediatric population.[159]

In the absence of perinatal transmission,

syphilis is nearly always sexually transmitted. Accidental transmission in laboratory accidents and during surgery on infected individuals has been described.[71] Transmission during transfusion of blood, by contact with syphilitic lesions on the breast of a nursing mother, and by "nonsexual" kissing have all been described; however, these forms of transmission are very rare.[66]

Except in rare situations, syphilis in a child after the neonatal period is acquired through sexual abuse. Fortunately, this is one of the least common STDs noted among sexually abused children. White et al.'s series reported six cases of positive serologic tests in the 108 children screened; this is one of the highest syphilis rates noted in the literature.[4] Much lower prevalence rates of positive syphilis serologic tests in sexually abused children have been reported; one positive test was reported in 532 children evaluated by DeJong.[5] Cupoli and Sewell found only 1 in 1059 serologic tests to be positive[6]; and the Center for Child Protection in San Diego found only two positive serologic tests in more than 6000 children screened.[161] This clearly indicates that syphilis is one of the most uncommon STDs transmitted to children during sexual abuse.

The Centers for Disease Control currently recommend that cerebrospinal fluid samples be obtained in children to rule out congenital syphilis. They recommend that any child with congenital syphilis or evidence of neurologic involvement be treated with aqueous crystalline penicillin G (200,000 to 300,000 U/kg/day) for 10 to 14 days. If congenital and neurosyphilis can be ruled out, children may be treated with 50,000 U/kg of intramuscular benzathine penicillin, not to exceed 2.4 million U.

Human Immunodeficiency Virus

Acquired immunodeficiency syndrome (AIDS), caused by infection with the RNA retrovirus, human immunodeficiency virus (HIV), has been well described in the pediatric population.[162–165] Among the 1995 cases reported to the Centers of Disease Control as of February 1990 that met the diagnostic criteria for AIDS, vertical transmission was responsible for infection in 81%. Transmission via transfusion of blood or its components was responsible for 11% of cases, while 5% of children had coagulation disorders and 3% had an undetermined source of infection. In 1985,

Osterholm and MacDonald raised the "unanswered question" of the possibility of HIV transmission in the pediatric population from childhood sexual abuse.[166] Since that time, scattered case reports have described HIV-infected children in whom the method of transmission was thought to be sexual abuse.[161, 167–169]

It is difficult to determine the prevalence of HIV infection in childhood victims of sexual abuse. Dattel et al. reported only one HIV-positive child in 161 children screened in San Francisco County; this was an adolescent male who had been sexually abused and subsequently worked as a prostitute, engaging in high-risk sexual behavior.[170] Gutman et al. reported a history of sexual abuse in 14.6% of 96 HIV-positive prepubertal children evaluated at Duke University. Of these 15 children, four were determined to have acquired their HIV infection from sexual abuse; in another six, abuse was a "possible" source; two had received infected blood components; and in the remaining three, vertical transmission was documented.[171] In a phone survey of child abuse programs, Gellert et al. noted six HIV-positive children in 300 screenings performed from a total of 26,000 children evaluated by these centers.[172]

In the limited number of children described who have acquired HIV infection from sexual abuse, many of the same risk factors described in the adult population are noted among these young patients. Fischl et al. noted that 10% of the children in her series lived with caregivers who engaged in high-risk behaviors.[173] Gutman also frequently identified the risk factors of substance abuse, alcoholism, prostitution, and poverty among the caregivers of the HIV-positive children in her series. She noted an

TABLE 20–2 ▪▪▪ HIV ANTIBODY INDICANTS IN SEXUALLY ABUSED CHILDREN

Victim
Clinical profile consistent with AIDS/AIDS-related complex
Behavioral profile of high-risk adolescent (e.g., prostitute, gay, drugs)
Parent/adolescent insistent on test
Assailant
HIV seropositive
Clinical profile consistent with AIDS/AIDS-related complex
High-risk behavioral profile (e.g., gay, drugs)

Adapted with permission from Child Abuse and Neglect, Vol. 14, Gellert GA, Durfee MJ, Berkowitz CD. Developing guidelines for HIV testing among victims of pediatric sexual abuse., © 1990, Pergamon Press.

TABLE 20–3 ••• TRANSMISSION OF STDs TO CHILDREN

	Sexual	Perinatal	Casual/Fomite
N. gonorrhoeae	High	Possible	Rare
C. trachomatis	High	Common	Very rare
T. pallidum	High	Possible	Rare
Herpes simplex	Possible	Possible	?
Bacterial vaginosis	High	?	Rare
HPV	High	Possible	Uncommon
T. vaginalis	High	Possible	?

HPV, human papillomavirus.

Adapted from Ingram DL. Controversies about the sexual and nonsexual transmission of adult STDs to children. In: Krugman RD, Leventhal JM (eds). Child Sexual Abuse. Report of the 22nd Ross Roundtable on Critical Approaches to Common Pediatric Problems. Columbus, OH: Ross Laboratories, 1991, p 21.

increased incidence of HIV infection in children who were victims of anal-receptive or oral-receptive sexual activity, known to be a risk factor among adults.[171, 174, 175] HIV-positive patients also had a higher incidence of genital injury, as manifested by bleeding, discharge, and genital lesions.[171]

Observations such as these, along with recommendations from the Centers of Disease Control for the consideration of HIV screening in child abuse victims, have led to discussions about the development of protocols for HIV screening. Gellert et al. conducted an extensive survey of child protection programs in 1990, finding that none had defined protocols in place at that time.[172] It appeared that screening was performed in selected cases at the discretion of the clinican; testing appeared to occur most frequently in situations where the alleged perpetrator was known to be HIV

TABLE 20–4 ••• CDC RECOMMENDED LABORATORY PROCEDURES AT INITIAL AND FOLLOW-UP EVALUATION OF SEXUALLY ABUSED PREPUBERTAL CHILDREN

Gram stain of any genital or anal discharge
Culture for Neisseria gonorrhoeae†
Culture for Chlamydia trachomatis†
Wet preparation of vaginal secretion for trichomonads
Culture of lesions for herpes simplex virus
Serologic test for syphilis
Serologic test for HIV‡
Frozen serum sample

*Care should be taken in the interpretation of results of any Gram stain of any anal discharge.

†Culture of pharynx, rectum, and vagina/urethra should be done.

‡Testing for HIV should be based on the prevalence of infection and on suspected risk.

Note. Syphilis and HIV serologic tests should be repeated in 12 weeks. All other tests should be repeated 10 to 14 days after the initial examination.

From Centers for Disease Control. 1989 sexually transmitted diseases treatment guidelines. MMWR 1989; 38(S8):11–38.

positive or in high-risk sexual assault, such as anal intercourse. Based on their survey, they recommended a protocol to be used in assessing the need for HIV screening among victims of child abuse (Table 20–2).[172]

Many authors have stressed the importance of a thoroughly evaluated testing program, informed consent of the parent or guardian, and the need for follow-up testing in acutely abused children with initially negative serologic test results. As is often seen with testing for STDs in children, compliance with follow-up is poor. Dattel reported that only 5% of the children in need of follow-up HIV testing actually returned for care.[176] Another author has suggested that testing of alleged perpetrators may be more appropriate, especially HIV-positive individuals who admit to abusing multiple victims.[175] Because many programs selectively screen children based, at least in part, on the history disclosed, Hammerschlag has suggested obtaining a frozen serum sample from all children.[40] This sample could be screened at a later date if additional "at risk" history was disclosed by the child.[40] However, not all investigators agree that screening sexually abused children for HIV infection is advisable or cost effective. Fost estimates that $25,000 would be spent in screening costs for each HIV-positive child identified.[177] He also points out that HIV screening in sexually abused children does not fulfill the standard criteria usually applied to screening programs.

CONCLUSION

The correct diagnosis of a pediatric STD involves a thorough understanding of the complexities of possible sources of transmission, unique aspects of clinical presentation, correct diagnostic procedures, and specialized treatment issues (Tables 20–3, 20–4). A multidisplinary approach is also essential in the often difficult process of evaluating the possibility of sexual abuse. These children deserve a humane approach to their care and treatment, as many of them have already faced sexual abuse. It is important to avoid retraumatizing them by the medical process.

References

1. Paradise JE, Campos JM, Friedman HM, Frishmuth G. Vulvovaginitis in premenarcheal girls: Clinical features and diagnostic evaluation. Pediatrics 1982; 70:193–198.
2. Arsenault PS, Gerbie AB. Vulvovaginitis in the preadolescent girl. Pediatr Ann 1986; 15:577–585.
3. Hammerschlag MR, Alpert S, Rosner I, et al. Microbiology of the vagina in children: Normal and potentially pathogenic organisms. Pediatrics 1978; 62:57–62.
4. White ST, Loda FA, Ingram DL, Pearson A. Sexually transmitted diseases in sexually abused children. Pediatrics 1983; 72:16–21.
5. DeJong AR. Sexually transmitted diseases in sexually abused children. Sex Transm Dis 1986; 13:123–126.
6. Cupoli JM, Sewell PM. One thousand fifty-nine children with a chief complaint of sexual abuse. Child Abuse Neglect 1988; 12:151–162.
7. Jenny C. Child sexual abuse and STD. In: Holmes KK (ed). Sexually Transmitted Diseases. 2nd ed. New York: McGraw-Hill, 1990, pp 895–900.
8. Huffman JW. Anatomy and physiology. In: Huffman JW, Dewhurst J, Capraro VJ (eds). The Gynecology of Childhood and Adolescence. 2nd ed. Philadelphia: WB Saunders, 1981, pp 24–69.
9. Schachter J. Rapid diagnosis of sexually transmitted diseases—speed has a price. Diagn Microbiol Infect Dis 1986; 4:195–189.
10. Whittington WL, Rice RJ, Biddle JW, Knapp JS. Incorrect identification of *Neisseria gonorrhoeae* from infants and children. Pediatr Infect Dis J 1988; 7:3–10.
11. Centers for Disease Control. Sexually transmitted diseases treatment guidelines. MMWR 1982; 31:595–605.
12. Centers for Disease Control. 1989 sexually transmitted diseases treatment guidelines. MMWR 1989; 38(S8):11–38.
13. Sweet RL, Gibbs RS. Sexually transmitted diseases. In: Sweet RL, Gibbs RS (eds). Infectious Diseases of the Female Genital Tract. 2nd ed. Baltimore: Williams & Wilkins, 1990, pp 109–143.
14. Singleton AF. An approach to the management of gonorrhea in the pediatric age group. J Natl Med Assoc 1981; 73:207–218.
15. Benson RA, Steer A. Vaginitis of children. Am J Dis Child 1937; 53:806.
16. Gutman LT, Wilfert CM. Gonococcal diseases in infants and children. In: Holmes KK (ed). Sexually Transmitted Diseases. 2nd ed. New York: McGraw-Hill, 1990, pp 803–810.
17. Frau LM, Alexander ER. Public health implications of sexually transmitted diseases in pediatric practice. Pediatr Infect Dis 1985; 4:453–467.
18. Alexander ER. Maternal and infant sexually transmitted diseases. Urol Clin North Am 1984; 11:131–139.
19. Lang WR. Pediatric vaginitis. N Engl J Med 1955; 253:1153.
20. Gerstner GJ, Grunberger W, Boschitsch E, Rotter M. Vaginal organisms in prepubertal children with and without vaginitis. Arch Gynecol 1982; 231:247–252.
21. Groothuis JR, Bischoff MC, Jauregui LE. Pharyngeal gonorrhea in young children. Pediatr Infect Dis 1983; 2:99–101.
22. Weiss JC, DeJong AR. Gonococcal infection and sexual abuse. Pediatr Infect Dis 1983; 2:415.
23. McClure EM, Stack MR, Tanner T, et al. Pharyngeal culturing and reporting of pediatric gonorrhea in Connecticut. Pediatrics 1986; 78:509–510.
24. Nelson JD, Mohs E, Dajani AS, Plotkin SA. Gonorrhea in preschool and school-aged children: Report of the prepubertal gonorrhea cooperative study group. JAMA 1976; 236:1359–1364.
25. Ingram DL, White ST, Durfee MF, Pearson AW. Sexual contact in children with gonorrhea. Am J Dis Child 1982; 136: 994–996.
26. Silber TJ, Controni G. Clinical spectrum of pharyngeal gonorrhea in children and adolescents. J Adolesc Health Care 1983; 4:51–54.
27. Ingram D, White S, Durfee M. The association of gonorrhea (GC) in children and sexual contact. Ambulatory Pediatr Assoc Program Abstr 1982 number 33.
28. Lewis LS, Glauser TA, Joffe MD. Gonococcal conjunctivitis in prepubertal children. Am J Dis Child 1990; 144:546–548.
29. Branch G, Paxton R. A study of gonococcal infections among infants and children. Publ Health Rep 1965; 80:347–352.
30. Ingram DL. The gonococcus and the toilet seat revisited. Pediatr Infect Dis 1989;8:191.
31. Farrell MK, Billmire E, Shamroy JA, Hammond JG. Prepubertal gonorrhea: A multidisciplinary approach. Pediatrics 1981; 67:151–153.
32. Lipsitt HJ, Parmet AJ. Nonsexual transmission of gonorrhea to a child. N Engl J Med 1984; 311:470.
33. Cooperman MB. Gonococcal arthritis in infancy. Am J Dis Child 1927; 33:932–948.
34. Rice JL, Cohn A, Steer A, Adler EL. Recent investigation of gonococcic vaginitis. JAMA 1941; 117:1766–1769.
35. Potterat JJ, Markewich GS, King RD. Child-to-child transmission of gonorrhea: Report of asymptomatic genital infection in a boy. Pediatrics 1986; 78:712.
36. Diena BB, Wallace R, Ashton FE, et al. Gonococcal conjunctivitis: Accidental infection. CMA 1976; 115:609–610.
37. Bruins SC, Tight RR. Laboratory-acquired gonococcal conjunctivitis. JAMA 1979; 241:274.
38. Wan WL, Farkas GC, May WN, Robin JB. The clinical characteristic and course of adult gonococcal conjunctivitis. Am J Opthalmol 1986; 102:575–583.
39. Legido A, Joffe M. Gonococcal conjunctivitis mimicking orbital cellulitis in a young adolescent. Am J Dis Child 1989; 143:443–444.
40. Hammerschlag M. Pitfalls in the diagnosis of sexually transmitted diseases in children. ASPAC News 1989; 4–5.

41. Hammerschlag MR, Rawstron SA, Bromberg K. A commentary on the 1989 sexually transmitted diseases treatment guidelines. Pediatr Infect Dis 1990; 9:382–384.

42. Kramer DG, Jason J. Sexually abused children and sexually transmitted diseases. Rev Infect Dis 1982; 4(suppl):S883–S890.

43. Schachter J. Biology of chlamydia trachomatis. In: Holmes KK (ed). Sexually Transmitted Diseases. 2nd ed. New York: McGraw-Hill, 1990, pp 167–180.

44. Sweet RL, Gibbs RS. Chlamydial infections. In: Sweet RL, Gibbs RS (eds). Infectious Diseases of the Female Genital Tract. 2nd ed. Baltimore: Williams & Wilkins, 1990, pp 45–74.

45. Harrison HR, Alexander ER. Chlamydial infections in infants and children. In: Holmes KK (ed). Sexually Transmitted Diseases. 2nd ed. New York: McGraw-Hill, 1990, pp 811–820.

46. Hammerschlag MR, Chandler JW, Alexander ER, et al. Longitudinal studies on chlamydial infections in the first year of life. Pediatr Infect Dis 1982; 1:395–401.

47. Schachter J, Grossman M, Sweet RL. Prospective study of perinatal transmission of C. trachomatis. JAMA 1986; 255:3374–3377.

48. Bump RC. *Chlamydia trachomatis* as a cause of prepubertal vaginitis. Obstet Gynecol 1985; 6:384–388.

49. Ingram DL, Runyan DK, Collins AD, et al. Vaginal *Chlamydia trachomatis* infection in children with sexual contact. Pediatr Infect Dis 1984; 3:97–99.

50. Hammerschlag MR, Doraiswamy B, Alexander ER, et al. Are rectogenital chlamydial infections a marker of sexual abuse in children? Pediatr Infect Dis 1984; 3:100–104.

51. Rettig PJ. Pediatric genital infection with *Chlamydia trachomatis*: Statistically nonsignificant, but clinically important. Pediatr Infect Dis 1984; 3:95–96.

52. Keskey TS, Suarez M, Gleicher N, et al. *Chlamydia trachomatis* infection in sexually abused children. Mt Sinai J Med 1987; 54:129–134.

53. Ingram DL, White ST, Occhiuti AR, Lyna PR. Childhood vaginal infections: Association of *Chlamydia trachomatis* with sexual contact. Pediatr Infect Dis 1986; 5:226–229.

54. Schachter J, Grossman M, Holt J. Infection with *Chlamydia trachomatis*: Involvement of multiple anatomic sites in neonates. J Infect Dis 1979; 139:232.

55. Bell TA, Stamm WE, Kuo CC. Chlamydial Infections. Cambridge, England: Cambridge University Press, 1986; pp 305–308.

56. Bell TA, Stamm WE, Kuo C-C, et al. Delayed appearance of *Chlamydia trachomatis* infections acquired at birth. Pediatr Infect Dis 1987; 6:928–931.

57. Thygeson P, Stone W. Epidemiology of inclusion conjunctivitis. Arch Ophthalmol 1942; 27:91.

58. Rettig PJ, Nelson JD. Genital tract infection with *Chlamydia trachomatis* in prepubertal children. J Pediatr 1981; 99:206–210.

59. Fuster CD, Neinstein LS. Vaginal *Chlamydia trachomatis* prevalence in sexually abused prepubertal girls. Pediatrics 1987; 79:235–238.

60. Bell T, Stamm W, Wang S, et al. Chronic *Chlamydia trachomatis* infections in infants. JAMA 1992; 267:400.

61. Mahony JB, Chernesky MA. Effect of swab type and storage temperature on the isolation of *Chlamydia trachomatis* from clinical specimens. J Clin Microbiol 1985; 22:865–867.

62. Alexander ER. Misidentification of sexually transmitted organisms in children: Medicolegal implications. Pediatr Infect Dis 1988; 7:1–2.

63. Hammerschlag MR, Rettig PJ, Shields ME. False positive results with the use of chlamydial antigen detection tests in the evaluation of suspected sexual abuse in children. Pediatr Infect Dis 1988; 7:11–14.

64. Black SB, Grossman M, Cles L, Schachter J. Serological evidence of chlamydial infection in children. J Pediatr 1981; 98:65–67.

65. Sweet RL, Gibbs RS. Infectious vulvovaginitis. In: Sweet RL, Gibbs RS (eds). Infectious Diseases of the Female Genital Tract. 2nd ed. Baltimore: Williams & Wilkins, 1990, pp 216–228.

66. Ingram DL. Controversies about the sexual and nonsexual transmission of adult STDs to children. In: Krugman RD, Leventhal JM. Child Sexual Abuse. 22nd Ross Roundtable on Critical Approaches to Common Pediatric Problems. Columbus, OH: Ross Laboratories, 1991, pp 14–27.

67. Lang WR. Premenarchal vaginitis. Obstet Gynecol 1959; 13:723.

68. Jones JG, Yamauchi T, Lambert B. *Trichomonas vaginalis* infection in sexually abused girls. Am J Dis Child 1985; 139:846.

69. Rein MF, Muller M. *Trichomonas vaginalis* and trichomoniasis. In: Holmes KK (ed). Sexually Transmitted Diseases. 2nd ed. New York: McGraw-Hill, 1990, pp 481–492.

70. Blattner RJ. *Trichomonas vaginalis* infection in a newborn infant. J Pediatr 1967; 71:608.

71. Neinstein LS, Goldenring J, Carpenter S. Nonsexual transmission of sexually transmitted diseases: An infrequent occurrence. Pediatrics 1984; 74:67–76.

72. Al-Salihi FL. Neonatal *Trichomonas vaginalis*: Report of three cases and review of the literature. Pediatrics 1974; 53:196.

73. Bramley M. Study of female babies of women entering confinement with vaginal trichomoniasis. Br J Vener Dis 1976; 52:58.

74. Robinson SC, Halifax NS. Observations on vaginal trichomoniasis. I. In pregnancy. Can Med Assoc J 1961; 84:948.

75. Lossick JS. Trichomonads Parasitic in Humans. New York: Springer, 1989, p 237.

76. Burgess JA. *Trichomonas vaginalis* infection from splashing in water closets. Br J Vener Dis 1963; 39:248.

77. Orley J, Florian E, Juranji R. Vaginal discharge in puberty. Gynaecologia 1969; 168:191–202.

78. Fouts AC, Kraus SJ. Trichomonas vaginitis: Reevaluation of its clinical presentation and laboratory diagnosis. J Infect Dis 1980; 141:137–143.

79. Beard CM, Noller KL, O'Fallon WM. Lack of evidence for cancer due to use of metronidazole. N Engl J Med 1979; 301:519.

80. Williams TS, Callen JP, Owen LG. Vulvar disorders in the prepubertal female. Pediatr Ann 1986; 15:588–605.

81. Alchek A. Pediatric vulvovaginitis. J Reprod Med 1984; 29:359–375.

82. Sweet RL, Gibbs RS. Perinatal infections. In: Sweet RL, Gibbs RS (eds). Infectious Diseases of the Female Genital Tract. 2nd ed. Baltimore: Williams & Wilkins, 1990, pp 290–319.

83. Shah KV. Biology of human genital tract papillomaviruses. In: Holmes KK (ed). Sexually Transmitted Diseases. 2nd ed. New York: McGraw-Hill, 1990, pp 425–431.

84. Centers for Disease Control. Condyloma acuminatum—United States, 1966–1981. MMWR 1983; 32:306–308.

85. Bender ME. New concepts of condyloma acuminata in children. Arch Dermatol 1986; 122:1121–1123.

86. Seidel J, Zonana J, Totten E. Condylomata acuminata as a sign of sexual abuse in children. J Pediatr 1979; 22:553–554.

87. Vallejos H, Mistro AD, Kleinhaus S, et al. Characterization of human papilloma virus types in condylomata acuminata in children by in situ hybridization. Lab Invest 1987; 56:611–615.

88. Rock B, Naghashfar Z, Barnett N, et al. Genital tract papillomavirus infection in children. Arch Dermatol 1986; 122:1129–1132.

89. Obalek S, Jablonska S, Favre M, et al. Condylomata acuminata in children: Frequent association with human papillomaviruses responsible for cutaneous warts. J Am Acad Dermatol 1990; 23:205–213.

90. Hanson RM, Glasson M, McCrossin I, et al. Anogenital warts in childhood. Child Abuse Neglect 1989; 13:225–233.

91. Goerzen JL, Robertson DI, Inoue M, Trevenen CL. Detection of HPV DNA in genital condylomata acuminata in female prepubertal children. Adolesc Pediatr Gynecol 1989; 2:224–229.

92. Clark DP. Condyloma acuminata in children. Curr Concepts Skin Disord 1985; 6:10–17.

93. Cohen PR, Young AW. Genital warts in children: Diagnosis, treatment, and legal implications. Med Aspects Hum Sex 1989; Oct: 22–28.

94. Boyd AS. Condylomata acuminata in the pediatric population. Am J Dis Child 1990; 144:817–824.

95. DeJong AR, Weiss JC, Brent RL. Condyloma acuminata in children. Am J Dis Child 1982; 136:704–706.

96. Mulchahey KM. Genital findings in prepubertal girls with human papilloma virus infection. Abstract. Presented at the Fourth Annual Meeting of North American Society for Pediatric Adolescent Gynecology, 1990, Costa Mesa, CA.

97. McCance DJ. Human papillomaviruses and cancer. Biochem Biophys Acta 1986; 823:195.

98. Macnab B. Human papillomavirus in clinically and histologically normal tissue of patients with genital cancer. N Engl J Med 1986; 315:1052.

99. McCance DJ. Human papillomavirus types 16 and 18 in carcinomas of the penis in Brazil. Int J Cancer 1986; 37:55.

100. Nuovo GJ, Pedemonte BM. Human papillomavirus types and recurrent cervical warts. JAMA 1990; 263:1223–1226.

101. Trofatter KF, English PC, Hughes CE, Gall SA. Human lymphoblastoid interferon (Wellferon) in primary therapy of two children with condylomata acuminata. Obstet Gynecol 1986; 67:137–140.

102. Scholefield JH, Sonnex C, Talbot IC, et al. Anal and cervical intraepithelial neoplasia: Possible parallel. Lancet 1989; ii:765–769.

103. Stringel G, Mercer S, Corsini L. Condyloma acuminata in children. J Pediatr Surg 1985; 20:499–501.

104. Herman-Giddens ME, Gutman LT, Berson NL. Association of coexisting vaginal infections and multiple abusers in female children with genital warts. Sex Transm Dis 1988; 6:63–67.

105. Laraque D. Severe anogenital warts in a child with HIV infection. Letter. N Engl J Med 1989; 320:1220–1221.

106. Forman AB, Prendiville JS. Association of human immunodeficiency virus seropositivity and extensive perineal condylomata acuminata in a child. Arch Dermatol 1988; 124:1010–1011.

107. Kashima HK, Shah K, Goodstein M. Recurrent respiratory papillomatosis. In: Holmes KK (ed). Sexually Transmitted Diseases. 2nd ed. New York: McGraw-Hill, 1990, pp 889–893.

108. Shah K, Kashima H, Polk BF. Rarity of cesarean delivery in cases of juvenile-onset respiratory papillomatosis. Obstet Gynecol 1986; 68:795.

109. Fife KH, Rogers RE, Zwickl BW. Symptomatic and asymptomatic cervical infections with human papillomavirus during pregnancy. J Infect Dis 1987; 156:904.

110. Tang C-K, Shermeta DW, Wood C. Congenital condylomata acuminata. Am J Obstet Gynecol 1978; 131:912–913.

111. Oriel JD, Almeida JD. Demonstration of virus particles in human genital warts. Br J Vener Dis 1970; 46:37.

112. Oriel JD. Natural history of genital warts. Br J Vener Dis 1971; 47:1–13.

113. Teokharov BA. Non-gonococcal infections of the female genitalia. Br J Vener Dis 1969; 45:334–340.

114. Goldenring JM. Condylomata acuminata: Still usually a sexually transmitted disease in children. Letter. Am J Dis Child 1991; 145:600–601.

115. Mulchahey KM. Characteristics of children with genital human papilloma virus infection. North American Society for Pediatric Adolescent Gynecology, 1990, Costa Mesa, CA.

116. Gutman L, Herman-Giddens M, Prose NS. Diagnosis of child sexual abuse in children with genital warts. Letter. Am J Dis Child 1991; 145:126.

117. Schachner L, Hankin D. Assessing child abuse in childhood condyloma acuminatum. J Am Acad Dermatol 1985; 12:157–160.

118. Gissman L, Schwartz E. Papillomaviruses. New York: John Wiley, 1986, p 190.

119. Fleming KA. DNA typing of genital warts and a diagnosis of sexual abuse in children. Lancet 1987; ii:454.

120. Krzyzek RA, Watts SL, Anderson DL, et al. Anogenital warts contain several distinct species of human papillomavirus. J Virol 1980; 36:236–244.

121. Norins AL, Caputo RV, Lucky AW, Krafchik BR. Genital warts and sexual abuse in children: American Academy of Dermatology Task Force on Pediatric Dermatology. J Am Acad Dermatol 1984; 11:529–530.

122. Moy RL, Eliezri YD, Nuovo GJ, et al. Human papillomavirus type 16 DNA in periungual squamous cell carcinomas. JAMA 1989; 261:2669–2673.

123. Marx JL. How DNA viruses may cause cancer. Science 1989; 243:1012–1013.

124. Lister UM, Akinla O. Carcinoma of the vulva in childhood. J Obstet Gynecol Br Comm 1972; 79:470–473.

125. Stoehr GP. Systemic complications of local podophyllin therapy. Ann Intern Med 1978; 89:362.

126. Slater GE. Podophyllin poisoning: Systemic toxicity

following cutaneous application. Obstet Gynecol 1978; 52:94.

127. Moher LM, Maurer SA. Podophyllin toxicity: Case report and literature review. J Fam Pract 1979; 9:237.

128. Ward JW, Clifford WS, Monaco AR, Bickerstaff HJ. Fatal systemic poisoning following podophyllin treatment of condyloma acuminatum. S Med J 1954; 47:1204–1206.

129. Stringel G, Spence J, Corsini L. Genital warts in children. Can Med Assoc J 1985; 132:1397–1398.

130. Pride GL. Treatment of large lower genital tract condylomata acuminata with topical 5-fluorouracil. J Reprod Med 1990; 35:384–387.

131. Gale C, Muram D. The surgical treatment of condyloma acuminata in children. Adolesc Pediatr Gynecol 1990; 3:189–192.

132. Healy GB, Gelber RD, Trowbridge AL, et al. Treatment of recurrent respiratory papillomatosis with human leukocyte interferon. N Engl J Med 1988; 319:401–407.

133. Steinberg BM, Topp WC, Schneider PS, Abramson AL. Laryngeal papillomavirus infection during clinical remission. N Engl J Med 1983; 308:1261–1264.

134. Friedman-Kien AE, Eron LJ, Conant M, et al. Natural inferferon alfa for treatment of condylomata acuminata. JAMA 1988; 259:533–538.

135. Sweet RL, Gibbs RS. Herpes virus infection. In: Sweet RL, Gibbs RS (eds). Infectious Diseases of the Female Genital Tract. 2nd ed. Baltimore: Williams & Wilkins, 1990, pp 144–157.

136. Taieb A, Body S, Astar I, et al. Clinical epidemiology of symptomatic primary herpetic infection in children. Acta Paediatr Scand 1987; 76:128–132.

137. Corey L. Genital herpes. In: Holmes KK (ed). Sexually Transmitted Diseases. 2nd ed. New York: McGraw-Hill, 1990, pp 391–413.

138. Nahmias AJ, Dowdle WR, Naib ZM, et al. Genital infection with herpesvirus hominis types 1 and 2 in children. Pediatrics 1968; 42:659–666.

139. Gardner M, Jones J. Genital herpes acquired by sexual abuse of children. J Pediatr 1984; 104:243–244.

140. Kaplan KM, Fleisher GR, Paradise JE, Freidman HN. Social relevance of genital herpes simplex in children. Am J Dis Child 1984; 138:872–874.

141. Gushurst CA. The problem of genital herpes in prepubertal children. Am J Dis Child 1985; 139:542–545.

142. Nerurkar LS, West F, May M, et al. Survival of herpes simplex virus in water specimens collected from hot tubs in spa facilities and on plastic surfaces. JAMA 1983; 250:3081–3083.

143. Douglas JM, Corey L. Fomites and herpes simplex viruses: A case of nonvenereal transmission? JAMA 1983; 250:3093.

144. Hibbard RA. Herpetic vulvovaginitis and child abuse. Am J Dis Child 1985; 139:542.

145. Miller RG, Whittington WL, Coleman RM, Nigida SM. Acquisition of concomitant oral and genital infection with herpes simplex virus type 2. Sex Transm Dis 1987; 14:41–43.

146. Hillier S, Holmes KK. Bacterial vaginosis. In: Holmes KK (ed). Sexually Transmitted Diseases. 2nd ed. New York: McGraw-Hill, 1990, pp 547–559.

147. DeJong AR. Vaginitis due to *Gardnerella vaginalis* and to *Candida albicans* in sexual abuse. Child Abuse Neglect 1985; 9:27–29.

148. Muram D, Buxton BH. *Gardnerella vaginalis* in children: An indicator of sexual abuse. Pediatr Adolesc Gynecol 1984; 2:197–200.

149. Thomason JL, Gelbert SM, Anderson RJ, et al. Statistical evaluation of diagnostic criteria for bacterial vaginosis. Am J Obstet Gynecol 1990; 162:155–160.

150. Eschenbach D. Diagnosis and clinical manifestation of bacterial vaginosis. Am J Obstet Gynecol 1988; 158:819.

151. Hammerschlag MR, Alpert S, Rosner I, et al. Microbiology of the vagina in children: Normal and potentially pathogenic organisms. Pediatrics 1978; 62:57–62.

152. Bartley DL, Morgan L, Rimsza ME. *Gardnerella vaginalis* in prepubertal girls. Am J Dis Child 1987; 141:1014–1017.

153. Hammerschlag MR, Cummings M, Doraiswamy B, et al. Nonspecific vaginitis following sexual abuse in children. Pediatrics 1985; 75:1028–1031.

154. Bump RC, Bueschling WJ. Bacterial vaginosis in virginal and sexually active adolescent females: Evidence against exclusive sexual transmission. Am J Obstet Gynecol 1988; 159:935.

155. Jenny C, Hooton TM, Bowers A, et al. Sexually transmitted diseases in victims of rape. N Engl J Med 1990; 322:713–716.

156. Zenker PN, Berman SM. Congenital syphilis: Trends and recommendations for evaluation and management. Pediatr Infect Dis 1991; 10:516–522.

157. Dorfman DH, Glaser JH. Congenital syphilis presenting in infants after the newborn period. N Engl J Med 1990; 323:1299–1302.

158. Sanchez P, Wendal G, Norgard MV. Congenital syphilis associated with negative results of maternal serologic tests at delivery. Am J Dis Child 1991; 145:967–969.

159. Ginsburg CM. Acquired syphilis in prepubertal children. Pediatr Infect Dis 1983; 2:232–234.

160. Horowitz S, Chadwick DL. Syphilis as a sole indicator of sexual abuse: Two cases with no intervention. Child Abuse Neglect 1990; 14:129–132.

161. Gellert GA, Durfee MJ. HIV infection and child abuse. N Engl J Med 1989; 321:685.

162. Ammann AJ. The acquired immunodeficiency syndrome in infants and children. Ann Intern Med 1985; 103:734–737.

163. Shannon KM, Ammann AJ. Acquired immune deficiency syndrome in childhood. J Pediatr 1985; 106:332–342.

164. Rogers MF. AIDS in children: A review of the clinical, epidemiologic and public health aspects. Pediatr Infect Dis 1985; 4:230–236.

165. Okeske J, Minnefor A, Cooper R, Thomas K. Immune deficiency syndrome in children. JAMA 1983; 249:2345–2349.

166. Osterholm MT, MacDonald KL. Facing the complex issues of pediatric AIDS: A public health perspective. JAMA 1987; 258:2736–2737.

167. Leiderman IZ, Grimm KT. A child with HIV infection. JAMA 1986; 256:3094.

168. Rubinstein A. Pediatric AIDS. Curr Probl Pediatr 1986; 16:362–409.

169. Thomas PA, Lubin K, Miblerg J, et al. Cohort comparison study of children whose mothers have acquired immunodeficiency syndrome and children of well inner city mothers. Pediatr Infect Dis 1987; 6:247–251.

170. Dattel BJ, Coulter K, Grossman M, Hauer LB. Presence of HIV antibody (Ab) in sexually abused children (SAC). IV International Conference on Aids, 1988.

171. Gutman LT, St Claire KK, Weedy C, et al. Human immunodeficiency virus transmission by child sexual abuse. Am J Dis Child 1991; 145:137–141.

172. Gellert GA, Durfee MJ, Berkowitz CD. Developing guidelines for HIV testing among victims of pediatric sexual abuse. Child Abuse Neglect 1990; 14:9–17.

173. Fischl MA, Dickinson GM, Scott GB, et al. Evaluation of heterosexual partners, children, and household contacts of adults with AIDS. JAMA 1987; 257:640–644.

174. Padian N, Marquis L, Francis DP. Male-to-female transmission of human immunodeficiency virus. JAMA 1987; 258:788–790.

175. Fuller AK, Bartucci RJ. HIV transmission and childhood sexual abuse. JAMA 1988; 259:2235–2236.

176. B. J. Dattel, MD, personal communication.

177. Fost, N. Ethical considerations in testing victims of sexual abuse for HIV infection. Child Abuse Neglect 1990; 14:5–7.

CHAPTER 21

○○○ # Sexually Transmitted Diseases in Adolescence

EDWIN M. THORPE, Jr.
DAVID MURAM

The increasing incidence of sexually transmitted diseases (STDs) among persons 13 to 19 years of age raises significant concerns about the overall reproductive health status of adolescents in the United States. Epidemiologic surveys of teenagers indicate that the initiation of sexual activity is occurring at an earlier age and often is not accompanied by methods for pregnancy or STD prevention (Fig. 21–1).[1] Adolescents who initiate sexual intercourse at younger ages are more likely to have multiple partners, thus increasing their chance of becoming infected with a sexually transmitted disease. Every year 2.5 million teenagers are infected with an STD; this number represents approximately one of every six sexually active teens and one fifth of the national STD cases.[2] In 1990, the highest age-specific rates for gonorrhea were found in sexually experienced female adolescents (1172 per 100,000); the second highest rates were in sexually experienced male adolescents (954 per 100,000).[3] Behaviors that are typical of adolescents, such as denying the possibility of harm, lead to increased sexual risk taking. Furthermore, many teenagers are often uninformed of symptoms or signs of acute infections and are less likely to seek treatment for an STD. The sequelae of undiagnosed and untreated STD

(i.e., pelvic inflammatory disease, infertility, ectopic pregnancy, cervical cancer, and facilitation of HIV transmission) exact a considerable cost. Risk behavior and threats to health are amplified by the use of alcohol, drugs, and tobacco, which may impair adolescents' ability to make judgments about sex and contraception, thereby placing them at increased risk of pregnancy or infection. This chapter will explore current trends regarding the major STDs found in adolescents.

EPIDEMIOLOGY OF STDs IN ADOLESCENTS

Because of reporting ability and numerical significance, the best estimates of STD morbidity patterns among adolescents are obtained by examining trends for gonorrhea. In 1991, approximately 609,459 cases of gonorrhea (233 per 100,000 population) were reported to the Centers for Disease Control (CDC), reflecting a continuing decline since 1980.[3] However, rates in adolescents have declined more slowly than those in any other age group and have actually increased from 881 per 100,000 to 954 per 100,000 in black adolescent males.[3] A

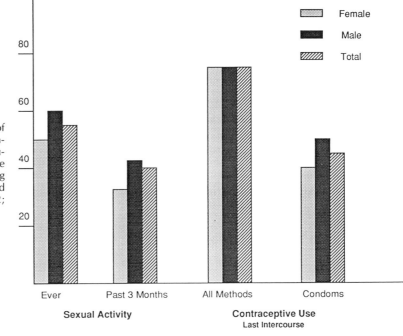

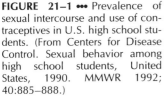

FIGURE 21–1 ••• Prevalence of sexual intercourse and use of contraceptives in U.S. high school students. (From Centers for Disease Control. Sexual behavior among high school students, United States, 1990. MMWR 1992; 40:885–888.)

racial trend is apparent, with an incidence in black male and female teenagers nearly 44-fold greater and 16-fold greater, respectively, than that in white teenagers. It has been speculated that prevention messages have been less successful and that diverted partner notification efforts and overburdened public clinics have disproportionately affected minority populations.[4] Furthermore, the use of illicit drugs, particularly crack cocaine, is associated with high levels of sexual activity and risk taking. In one study, one third of black adolescent male crack users reported 10 or more sexual partners in the preceding year.[5–8]

Chlamydia is one of the most prevalent STDs in the United States, affecting an estimated 4 million people each year.[3] Among adolescents, chlamydial infections are diagnosed more commonly than gonorrhea.[9] In one study, chlamydia was detected in 8% to 40% of teenage females during the routine gynecologic examination, a rate twice that for gonorrhea.[10] Because infections caused by chlamydia are not reportable diseases throughout the United States, the true incidence is unknown. This further complicates efforts for control and increases the risk for associated complications such as pelvic inflammatory disease, ectopic pregnancy, and infertility.

Infections caused by viral STDs, human pap-

illomavirus (HPV), and herpes simplex virus (HSV) are probably the most common in the United States. Using sensitive detection techniques, studies of the prevalence of HPV report infection rates as high as 38% to 46% in adolescents and sexually active young adult females.[11, 12] Additionally, asymptomatic cervical infection is nearly three times more common than reported external genital warts.[13] Serologic studies of HSV antibody have revealed widespread asymptomatic infection among a representative cohort of patients in the United States.[14] Approximately 4% of white teenagers and 17% of black teens have been infected, as determined by HSV-2 antibody, by the age of 19.

Clearly, adolescents participate in significant risk-taking behavior. To reduce the incidence of human immunodeficiency virus (HIV) infection and STDs, programs and policies must address adolescent decision making regarding sexual activity and the psychosocial dynamics influencing these decisions. Chapter 22 provides a discussion of risk determinants of STDs and HIV infections in adolescents.

GONORRHEA

Gonorrhea is an infection of the mucous membrane of the urethra and genital tract caused by *Neisseria gonorrhoeae*, a gram-negative diplococcus. Clinical illness caused by *N. gonorrhoeae* was described in ancient literature as early as 2637 BC. The organism itself was described by Albert Neisser from stained smears of exudates from urethras, cervices, and neonatal ophthalmic tissue and first cultured by Leistkow in 1882.[15] Because the gonococcal organisms infect columnar and transitional epithelia, the vaginal mucosa in an adult is resistant to infection with *N. gonorrhoeae*.

The incubation period for *N. gonorrhoeae* is roughly 1 week, with symptoms generally appearing in 2 to 7 days after exposure. Asymptomatic infections are not uncommon, particularly in females, only 10% to 20% of whom will have a mucopurulent cervical discharge.[16] Other related symptoms in women include urethritis, increased vaginal discharge, dysuria, intermenstrual bleeding, and menorrhagia.[17, 18] Urogenital involvement in females may extend to the vestibular glands, Skene's glands, and Bartholin's ducts and glands, in which case purulent secretions may be expressed from the infected site (Fig. 21–2). In males, local complications include epididymitis, posterior urethritis, lymphangitis, and prostatitis. The majority of infections of the anal canal present with nonspecific symptoms such as irritation and tenesmus or are asymptomatic. The natural history of these infections is not well understood, but isolated rectal infections in women are uncommon, occurring in less than 5% of patients with gonorrhea.[19] However, rectal infection is relatively common in patients with urogenital infections, occurring in 35% to 50% of female patients with cervicitis[20, 21] and in 40% of sexually active homosexual men.[22, 23] Most rectal infections in females are assumed to occur by local spread of infected cervical secretions, in contrast to male homosexuals, in whom rectal gonorrhea is due to direct inoculation through receptive anal intercourse.

Despite the development of a wide variety of new methods to detect *N. gonorrhoeae* (e.g., DNA probes and antigen detection methods), a Gram-stained smear or culture obtained by direct inoculation onto selective media remains the method of greatest utility. The presence of morphologically typical, gram-negative intracellular diplococci is sufficiently sensitive (90% to 95%) and specific (95% to 100%) to establish the diagnosis of gonorrhea in symptomatic males.[24] Gram-stained smears are relatively insensitive in women (30% to 60%), and interpretation may be hampered by vaginal bacterial contamination.[19, 21] For this reason, the use of Gram-stained smears for treatment determination should be confined to situations in which therapy must be initiated in a high-risk patient before culture results are received.[16] These include suspected pelvic inflammatory disease, history of exposure to gonorrhea, and the presence of mucopurulent cervical discharge. Likewise, stained smears of urethral and anal specimens, with the exception of mucopurulent anal discharge, are too nonspecific for routine use. Because of the expense of confirmation, the lack of symptoms, spread to exposed persons, and the often self-limited nature of the infection, an argument has been made to forego routine culture from the pharynx.[16] Currently, none of the newer diagnostic technologies has demonstrated cost or performance advantages over Gram-stained smears and culture.

Disseminated Gonococcal Infection

Disseminated gonococcal infections (DGIs) occur in 0.5% to 3% of patients with untreated urogenital gonorrhea.[25, 26] It is the most common systemic complication of acute gonorrhea. Typical clinical manifestations, in addition to malaise and fever, include skin lesions, arthralgia, and tenosynovitis. Classically, the arthritis is a migrating polyarthritis involving the wrists, metacarpals, ankles, and knees. The typical skin lesion of DGI consists of a necrotic pus-

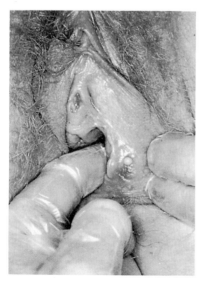

FIGURE 21–2 ••• Gonococcal bartholinitis.

tule on an erythematous base (Fig. 21–3). The number of lesions may vary, but most patients have fewer than 30, and these may evolve from or present as macules, pustules, ecchymoses, petechiae, or bullae.[27, 28] DGI occurs more commonly in females, and the onset of symptoms follows the menstrual period in approximately 50% of patients.[25–29] Pregnancy and pharyngeal gonorrhea have also been cited as risk factors. Gonococcal strains that bejcome blood borne tend to be nutritionally deficient auxotypes, AHU/1A-1 and AHU/1A-2.[18] These strains are more likely to cause asymptomatic infections and to be susceptible to penicillin, more difficult to culture, and more resistant to the complement-mediated bactericidal activity of human sera.[25, 27, 30]

The definitive diagnosis of DGI is based on isolation of the gonococcus from the blood, skin lesions, synovial fluid, or the cerebrospinal fluid; this can be done in 10% to 30% of patients early in the course of the disease.[25–28] In some patients, the diagnosis is established based on the typical clinical manifestations and concurrent isolation of *N. gonorrhoeae* from the lower genital tract, the rectum, or, at times, from a sexual partner.

Treatment

Although the incidence of gonorrhea has been declining since 1975, the emergence of antimicrobial-resistant gonorrhea has created a complex problem for clinicians and monitors of resistant patterns. By 1990, antimicrobial-resistant strains accounted for 8.4% of all reported cases of gonorrhea.[3] Gonococcal re-

sistance to antimicrobial agents has been evolving since the availability of sulfonamides and penicillin in the 1940s. In 1976, penicillinase-producing *Neisseria gonorrhoeae* (PPNG) was discovered, marking an accelerated trend toward antibiotic resistance because of the mechanism by which resistance is acquired: a new plasmid that carried genes for production of a β-lactamase capable of disrupting the β-lactam ring of the penicillin molecule. Plasmid-mediated resistance is responsible for the increasing numbers of tetracycline-resistant gonorrhea (TRNG) strains and combined PPNG-TRNG resistance. Resistant gonorrhea resulting from random selection of mutants from the huge gonoccocal population has been termed *chromosome-mediated–resistant gonorrhea* (CRNG). Recognizing the importance of these changing microbial trends, the CDC created a sentinel surveillance system to monitor antimicrobial-resistant *N. gonorrhoeae.* The Gonococcal Isolate Surveillance Project (GISP) consists of 24 sentinel STD clinics that submit isolates to five regional laboratories on a monthly basis for susceptibility testing.

Because of widespread and steadily increasing resistance to penicillin, the CDC's *1989 STD Treatment Guidelines* recommended the use of penicillinase-resistant regimens (e.g., ceftriaxone combined with doxycycline).[30] As a result, treatment regimens consisting of second- and third-generation cephalosporins (cefuroxime axetil, ceftizoxime, cefotaxime), and fluorinated quinolones (ciprofloxacin, norfloxacin) have become standard throughout the United States. For patients who cannot take ceftriaxone, the preferred alternative is spectinomycin, 2 gm intramuscularly in a single dose.[30] Amoxicillin combined with probenecid is still useful if the source of the infection is proven not to be penicillin resistant. The recommended treatment of patients with systemic infections (DGI, meningitis, endocarditis) is high-dose, intravenous ceftriaxone or an equivalent β-lactam–resistant antibiotic.

Additional Considerations

Patients infected with gonorrhea are at risk for infection with other STDs. Thus, the diagnosis of one infection should initiate a search for concurrent infections. Patients should undergo serologic testing for syphilis and should be offered counseling and testing for HIV infection. Patients with incubating syphi-

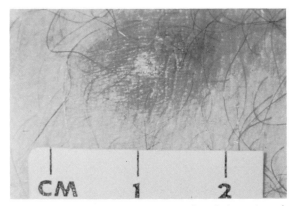

FIGURE 21–3 ••• Hemorrhagic pustule of disseminated gonococcal infection.

lis may be cured by β-lactam antibiotics combined with tetracycline. However, patients treated with regimens utilizing spectinomycin or fluoroquinolones require further testing and appropriate therapy for syphilis.

Prevention

Treatment of asymptomatic carriers and of sexual partners may reduce the pool of infected individuals who may in turn infect others. Routine screening for cervical gonococcal infection was found to be cost effective in communities with a high prevalence of asymptomatic infections.[30a] The study supported the use of widespread gonococcal screening as an essential part of a gonorrhea prevention program. In addition, patients who received therapies that are not effective against PPNG must be tested for cure. Concurrent treatment with doxycycline or tetracycline for coexistent chlamydia is recommended.[25] Because STDs are indicators of unsafe sex practices and risk-taking behavior, educational programs must be developed to alter such behavior.

CHLAMYDIAL INFECTIONS

In the United States, infection caused by *Chlamydia trachomatis* is the most common of the bacterial STDs. Conservative estimates indicate that at least 4 million cases occur annually.[2] As many as 75% of women and 25% of men with uncomplicated chlamydial infection have no symptoms or signs of infection. Recognition of the association between infection with *C. trachomatis* and tubal infertility and subfertility in the form of ectopic pregnancy has been one of the most important advances in the field of reproductive health. In addition, perinatal chlamydial infections are a common cause of infant pneumonia and the most common cause of neonatal conjunctivitis. Because of these issues, widely available screening programs are crucial for chlamydia prevention. Control measures, however, are severely hampered by the expense of laboratory tests for chlamydia, a factor that restricts the ability to screen effectively in facilities where funding is limited. Also, *C. trachomatis* infections are not reportable in all states, which significantly limits the impact of traditional disease intervention efforts and partner notification for treatment. Thus, spread of asymp-

tomatic infections with profound long-term consequences, particularly in females and infants, is common.

C. trachomatis is an obligate intracellular parasite with 17 different immunotypes currently identified.[31, 32] Types A, B, Ba, and C are most commonly associated with ocular trachoma and types L1, L2, and L3 are the cause of lymphogranuloma venereum. Immunotypes D through K are responsible for the majority of sexually transmitted infections; types D, E, and F are the most common.[33] An in-depth discussion of the biology, host response, and pathogenesis of chlamydial infections is beyond the scope of this chapter, and interested readers are encouraged to consult Schacter's work.[34]

Clinical Manifestations

In females, the endocervix is the organ most commonly infected with *C. trachomatis*. Most of these infections are asymptomatic and can only be detected by screening pelvic examinations, as the majority of chlamydial infections of the endocervix fail to demonstrate sufficient inflammation to result in clinical signs.[35] The most common clinical signs, when present, are a yellow or green mucopurulent endocervical discharge[36] and hypertrophic ectropion (Fig. 21–4).[37] (*Hypertrophic ectopy* refers to an area of cervical ectopy that is edematous, congested, and bleeds easily on manipulation.) These clinical signs have been correlated with the number of polymorphonuclear (PMN) leukocytes (10 to 30 per 1000 fields) obtained from a carefully collected endocervical Gram-stained smear.[35–38]

Results of screening studies in STD clinics have shown that the urethra is a common site for *C. trachomatis* infection.[39, 40] Among women with symptoms of dysuria and frequency of urination, urine cultures for other common urinary tract pathogens are often negative, whereas chlamydial organisms can be isolated in as many as 65% of patients.[41] Studies have shown that simultaneously culturing both the urethra and the cervix increases the yield of culture-positive females by as much as 20%.[42]

Upper Genital Tract Infection

C. trachomatis may ascend from the endocervix into the upper genital tract, leading to

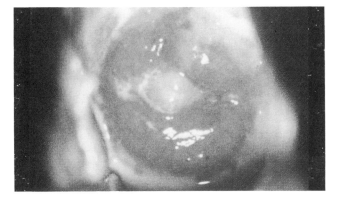

FIGURE 21–4 ••• Mucopurulent cervicitis due to C. *trachomatis*.

asymptomatic or symptomatic pelvic inflammatory disease (PID). Early studies of symptomatic patients with PID showed that cervical cultures of many were positive for *C. trachomatis*.[43] In later studies utilizing laparoscopy to directly obtain specimens from the fallopian tubes, *C. trachomatis* was recovered in about 30% of patients.[44] Clinically, the presentation of PID caused by *C. trachomatis* is similar to that caused by *N. gonorrhoeae*, although the symptoms may be less severe,[45] consisting only of menorrhagia and metrorrhagia.[46] Serologic studies have suggested that *C. trachomatis* is also a common cause of perihepatitis.[47]

Diagnosis

Although chlamydial culture is expensive and technically difficult, it remains the "gold standard" for clinical purposes and the procedure against which new diagnostic methods are measured. In untreated patients, 70% to 80% have positive results when cultured repetitively, and culture-negative patients usually remain so on repeated culture.[48–50] The low sensitivity of chlamydial cultures is affected by several factors, including specimen collection techniques, sites of sampling, the number of sites sampled, and specimen transport and storage conditions.[51] Newer techniques using vortexing and sonication of specimens resulted in recovery of organisms in up to 96% of specimens.[52] Serologic testing has little or no role in the diagnosis of acute chlamydial infections.

The financial and technical constraints on routine testing for *C. trachomatis* have fueled attempts to generate a sensitive set of predictors of chlamydial infection based on nonlaboratory data (i.e., data from patient histories or physical examinations). Antigen detection

methods, such as direct fluorescent antibody staining and enzyme-linked immunosorbent assays, have offered appealing alternatives to the use of bacteriologic cultures. These tests are less expensive, more rapid, and can be used in any physician's office. However, the sensitivity of direct fluorescent antibody screening tests ranges from 60% to 100% and that of enzyme-linked immunosorbent assay from 48% to 98%.[53] The highest sensitivity and specificity rates are found in patients from high prevalence settings (e.g., STD clinics). The use of nonculture tests in low-risk populations may not be appropriate when the prevalence of *C. trachomatis* is less than 10%.[53]

In most circumstances, the diagnosis is made in some patients based solely on clinical grounds and the presence of reported risk factors. Risk factors include young age, nonwhite race, single marital status, and use of oral contraceptives.[39, 54–56] The incidence of chlamydia infection is also high in pregnant women, women with acute PID, and sex partners of men with urethritis or of women with mucopurulent cervicitis. Screening should be expanded to include sexually active young women who have had a new sex partner or more than two partners in the previous 2 months.[57]

Treatment

Drugs with the greatest activity against *C. trachomatis* in tissue culture are rifampin and the tetracyclines, followed by macrolides and azalides, sulfonamides, some fluoroquinolones, and clindamycin.[58] On the basis of efficacy and cost, the tetracyclines continue to be the drugs of choice for the treatment of chlamydial infections.[51] In particular, doxycycline (100 mg orally twice daily for 7 days) is currently recommended because of improved patient compliance and an excellent pharmacokinetic profile.[59] Unlike *N. gonorrhoeae*, no clinically significant evidence of *C. trachomatis* resistance has been noted. Alternatively, an erythromycin base or an equivalent (sulfisoxazole or amoxicillin) are recommended. Considerable interest has been generated by published studies evaluating single-dose oral azithromycin for uncomplicated genital chlamydial infections.[60, 61]

The recommended therapy for chlamydial infection during pregnancy consists of an erythromycin base or equivalent, 500 mg orally four times daily for 7 days. However, in one study, cure rates among pregnant patients treated with amoxicillin were similar to those of erythromycin-treated pregnant women.[62] In addition, gastrointestinal side effects requiring cessation of therapy were significantly more common with erythromycin. Oral clindamycin has also demonstrated effectiveness in eradicating cervical chlamydial infection in pregnant patients.[63]

Lymphogranuloma Venereum

Lymphogranuloma venereum (LGV) is an uncommon infection caused by *C. trachomatis* immunotypes L1 through L3. Fewer than 100 cases are reported annually.[64] Although included in the differential diagnosis for genital ulcer disease, ulcers are a minor feature of LGV. The incidence of acute LGV in males outnumbers that in females by as much as 5:1,[65] principally because symptomatic infection is much less common in females. The ulcer presents in several different forms but typically is small, shallow, and painless; in females, the endocervix appears to be the most common initial site of infection.[66] Lymphadenopathy is the principal feature of LGV and appears 7 to 30 days after the ulcer. Inguinal adenopathy occurs as a result of multiple enlarged, matted, and tender nodes, which may coalesce with suppuration and bubo formation (Fig. 21–5). When left untreated, these swollen glands can rupture and form draining sinuses. Systemic signs—fever, malaise, and myalgia—are commonly seen in this stage. In addition, women infected with LGV often develop acute proctocolitis, with fever, tenesmus, and rectal pain. Even without treatment, most LGV infections resolve spontaneously after this stage. In some patients, however, healing is associ-

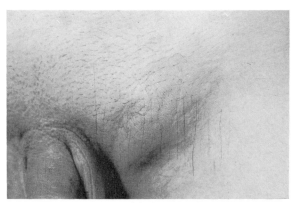

FIGURE 21–5 ••• Inguinal bubo caused by lymphogranuloma venereum.

ated with scarring and fibrosis that may lead to rectal strictures and to chronic genital edema (elephantiasis). Genital ulcers and sinuses may persist. Such deformities may require extensive reconstructive surgery.

The diagnosis can often be established by the typical clinical features, when present, but usually a complement fixation serologic titer ≥1:64 is diagnostic.[64] The specific diagnosis requires isolation of *C. trachomatis* from infected tissue and subsequent immunotyping or microimmunofluorescence to distinguish type-specific immune responses. Despite their limitations, other techniques (e.g., monoclonal antibodies or histologic identification of *C. trachomatis* in infected material) may also be used.

Effective treatment of lymphogranuloma venereum consists of oral tetracycline and erythromycin therapy. It is recommended that the treatment period be extended to 3 weeks regardless of the regimen used.[67] Alternative medications include sulfisoxazole, chloramphenicol, and rifampin. As mentioned previously, reconstructive surgery may be required to correct anogenital deformities.

PELVIC INFLAMMATORY DISEASE

Acute PID is a major public health problem, affecting 1 of 10 American women during their reproductive years.[68] It has been estimated that 1 million females are treated annually for PID at a cost of $4.2 billion dollars when the costs of the sequelae are included.[69] A 1% increase in the incidence of PID will increase this cost two-fold by the year 2000. As a complication of sexually transmitted organisms, PID exacts a more significant toll on adolescent females because of the sequelae of tubal infertility, ectopic pregnancy, and chronic pelvic pain at an earlier stage of reproductive life.[70]

PID is an acute syndrome attributed to the ascending spread of microorganisms from the vagina and endocervix to the endometrium, fallopian tubes, and contiguous structures. The etiology of the offending organisms reflects geographic variations and is also dependent on the sites that are cultured. Various studies have shown that *N. gonorrhoeae* may be recovered from 5% to 81% of patients with acute PID and that *C. trachomatis* has been recovered from 6% to 68% of such patients.[71] However, studies utilizing laparoscopy for recovery of organisms from the fallopian tube have demonstrated that mixed bacteria are often present.[72–75] The most common aerobic organisms include *Escherichia coli, Haemophilus influenzae*, group B streptoccoci, and *Gardnerella vaginalis*. Anaerobic bacteria recovered most frequently include the *Bacteroides* sp., *Peptostreptococcus*, and *Peptococcus*. Genital mycoplasms have been recovered infrequently from patients with acute PID, and their exact role in the etiology of PID has not been determined.

Several other factors may influence the ability of microorganisms to ascend from the endocervix into the uterus and fallopian tubes. Cervicovaginal bacteria are introduced into the uterus and tubes during menses. Specific mucosal immune mechanisms (e.g., secretory immunoglobulin A [IgA]) may be inactivated by *N. gonorrhoeae* proteases, thereby immobilizing an important host defense.[76] The relationship between use of the intrauterine contraceptive device (IUD) and the development of PID remains controversial, despite more than 25 studies addressing this subject.[77] The presence of an IUD tail and its ability to "wick" bacteria into the uterine cavity, the formation of microulcers, conversion of the vaginal (bacterial) environment to a predominantly anaerobic flora, and the foreign body inflammatory reaction produced by the device have all been postulated as mechanisms for an increased risk of upper genital tract infection.[71] Recognized risk factors for the development of PID are summarized in Table 21–1.

Clinical Manifestations

Patients presenting with PID may be asymptomatic patients or have severe peritonitis.

TABLE 21–1 ••• RISK INDICATORS ASSOCIATED WITH THE DEVELOPMENT OF PID

Demographic and social indicators
  Age
  Socioeconomic status
  Single marital status
Contraceptive practice
  Intrauterine contraceptive device
Health care behavior
  Evaluation of symptoms
  Compliance with treatment instructions
  Partner notification
Others
  Douching
  Smoking
  Temporal relationship to menstrual cycle

From Centers for Disease Control. Pelvic inflammatory disease: Guidelines for prevention and management. MMWR 1991; 40(RR-5):1–25.

Abdominal pain, usually of less than 10 days duration, is the most common symptom encountered. Other symptoms of varying significance include recent onset of menses, increased dysmenorrhea with previous period, irregular menses (menorrhagia), recent pelvic dyspareunia, and proctitis symptoms. Gastrointestinal symptoms such as nausea and vomiting, diarrhea, and anorexia are related to bowel inflammation caused by free pus in the abdomen.

Clinical signs that have the strongest degree of correlation with laparoscopically proven PID include abnormal vaginal discharge, elevated temperature above 38°C, and a palpable adnexal mass.[78, 79] Additionally, up to 15% of patients with PID present with perihepatitis (Fitz-Hugh-Curtis syndrome) as part of the clinical picture.

Clinical Diagnosis

The clinical diagnosis of acute PID is based primarily on a history of abdominal pain and the presence of tenderness to motion of the cervix and adnexae on bimanual examination. If signs of a lower genital tract infection (more leukocytes on a wet-mount specimen than any other cellular component) are present, along with abdominal pain and motion tenderness, the diagnosis of PID is correct in only 60% of patients.[80] All patients should undergo cervical cultures for *N. gonorrhoeae* and cultures or nonculture tests for *C. trachomatis*. Additional criteria useful for the diagnosis of PID are listed in Table 21–2. The lack of substantial

TABLE 21–2 ••• CRITERIA FOR DIAGNOSING PID

Routine
    Oral temperature >38.3°C
    Abnormal cervical or vaginal discharge
    Elevated erythrocyte sedimentation rate and/or
        C-reactive protein
    Culture or nonculture* evidence of cervical infection
        with *N. gonorrhoeae* or *C. trachomatis*
Elaborate
    Histopathologic evidence on endometrial biopsy
    Tubo-ovarian abscess on sonography
    Laparoscopy

*Gram stain antigen detection assay.
From Centers for Disease Control. Pelvic inflammatory disease: Guidelines for prevention and management. MMWR 1991; 40(RR-5):1–25.

clinical signs dictates that clinicians have a high index of suspicion when evaluating young women at risk for PID. Atypical features such as menorrhagia, mucopurulent cervicitis, or both in women not using oral contraceptives should be considered as signs indicating upper genital tract infection,[46] and a more thorough workup and therapy are required.

Management

An appropriate plan of management requires a thorough assessment of the severity of infection. Hospitalization should be utilized liberally, although there is no objective evidence that parenteral antimicrobial therapy results in better long-term outcomes. Indications for hospitalization are listed in Table 21–3. Because bacteriologic data suggest a mixed infection in many patients, administration of broad-spectrum antibiotics is required, along with adequate support with intravenous fluids and analgesia. Patients managed on an outpatient basis require close follow-up (within 72 hours) for response to therapy and compliance with medication instructions.[81] This opportunity should be used to emphasize the need to avoid sexual intercourse and to refer sexual partners for evaluation and treatment.

Treatment and Prevention

Many different treatment regimens have been evaluated and proved to be highly effective in achieving clinical cure. No single regimen has been shown to be clearly superior, but two basic regimens have been recommended by the Centers for Disease Control to provide broad-spectrum coverage for the pathogens most likely to be encountered (Table 21–4). A discussion of treatment considerations is provided in Peterson et al.[82]

Effective stategies are crucial for preventing PID and thereby protecting women from the adverse reproductive consequences and avoiding substantial economic losses. The best strategies for preventing PID are prevention of lower genital tract infection with *C. trachomatis* and *N. gonorrhoeae* in both men and women.[81] Early detection, followed by prompt and effective treatment of lower genital tract infections, must be employed if prevention fails.

TABLE 21–3 ••• INDICATIONS FOR HOSPITALIZATION OF PATIENTS WITH PID

Uncertain diagnosis
Suspected pelvic abscess
Pregnancy
Adolescent patient
Severe illness precluding outpatient treatment
Inability to tolerate or comply with outpatient regimen
Failure to respond to outpatient treatment
Clinical follow-up within 72 hours if starting antibiotics
    cannot be arranged

From Centers for Disease Control. 1989 sexually transmitted diseases treatment guidelines. MMWR 1989; 38:27–39.

TABLE 21–4 ••• RECOMMENDED TREATMENT OF HOSPITALIZED PATIENTS WITH PID

Recommended Regimen A:

    Cefoxitin (2 gm IV every 6 hours) or cefotetan (2 gm
    IV every 12 hours)

plus

    Doxycycline (100 mg PO or IV every 12 hours)

Recommended Regimen B:

    Clindamycin (900 mg IV every 8 hours)

plus

    Gentamicin (2.0 mg/kg loading dose followed by a
    1.5-mg/kg maintenance dose every 8 hours)

Intravenous regimens are given for at least 48 hours after
    the clinical signs and symptoms have improved.
    Following discharge, patients should be given:

    Doxycycline (100 mg PO every 12 hours)

or

    Clindamycin (450 mg PO every 6 hours)

Oral medications should be continued for a total of 10 to
    14 days of therapy

From Centers for Disease Control. 1989 sexually transmitted diseases treatment guidelines. MMWR 1989; 38:27–39.

SYPHILIS

Historically, syphilis has been a major cause of morbidity and mortality worldwide. The implementation of public health initiatives and the availability of penicillin initially led to a significant decline in syphilis-related consequences. However, since 1986, the incidence of primary and secondary syphilis has increased yearly to a rate of 20 per 100,000, the highest level since 1949.[83, 83a] These most recent increases have been most prevalent in non-white heterosexuals and have been closely linked to illicit drug use, particularly the use of crack cocaine.[83a] Although the highest rates for early syphilis occur in adults age 20 to 24, in women the rate of increase has been greater for adolescent females during the 1990s.[3] Of grave concern is the risk of congenital syphilis in a population in which pregnancy rates continue largely unabated. The association between increased HIV transmission and genital ulcer disease in heterosexuals[9] amplifies the current risk environment for both teenagers and adults.

Syphilis is caused by *Treponema pallidum*, a spirochete that measures 6 to 20 μm by 0.1 to 0.18 μm, making it too narrow to be seen by light microscopy.[83b] It has a characteristic corkscrew motility that allows identification by darkfield examination. Because the spirochete cannot survive outside the body, contracting the disease by modes other than intimate contact is rare. The organism usually enters the body through invisible breaks in the skin or through intact mucous membranes lining the mouth, rectum, or genital tract. Approximately one third of individuals exposed to a sexual partner with syphilis will acquire the disease.[84] Other potential routes of transmission include perinatal transmission and transmission through transfusion of infected blood. Serologic tests for syphilis are performed routinely in blood banks, and thus transfusion of blood or blood products is a remote mode of transmission. Hematogenous spread through infected needles shared by intravenous drug users represents a theoretical concern. Syphilis infection in children is discussed in detail in Chapter 20.

Clinical Manifestations

The clinical features of untreated syphilis are divided into a series of clinical stages that are used as indicators of the length of infection and as a guide for therapy. However, overlap among the various stages occurs frequently, and at times, the features of a specific stage are mild or even absent.

Primary Syphilis

Approximately 3 weeks after inoculation, the patient develops a macule or papule at the site of entry.[85] The lesion is usually found around the genitalia but is sometimes seen on the lips or mouth, on the breasts, or around the rectum. The ulcer is a painless, usually solitary lesion, with raised, well-defined borders and a clean, indurated base. The chancre contains large numbers of spirochetes and is highly contagious. It is usually associated with nontender regional adenopathy, which may be unilateral or bilateral. Although the external genitalia is the most common site for ulcers in females, the cervix and vagina are frequently involved (Fig. 21–6).[86] Even without treatment, the chancre slowly heals in several weeks; the spirochetes, however, spread throughout the body.

Secondary Syphilis

Between 4 and 10 weeks after the appearance of the chancre, secondary syphilis occurs. This stage is characterized by an array of clinical manifestations. Systemic complaints such as low-grade fever, myalgia, and arthralgia are common, as is generalized adenopathy. The most prominent feature is a painless, nonpruritic maculopapular rash that typically affects the limbs, including the palms and soles, and the trunk (Fig. 21–7). Alternatively,

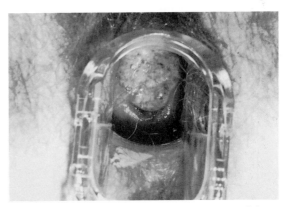

FIGURE 21–6 ••• Cervical chancre of primary syphilis.

lesions described as pustular, eczematous, nodular, and plaquelike may present in secondary syphilis. Lesions presenting as mucous patches form in the mouth and around the vagina and anus. Other anogenital lesions, called *condylomata lata*, are broad-based, flat, beefy lesions that are pearly gray in color and highly contagious (Fig. 21–8). The reader is urged to consult a dermatologic reference or a comprehensive review of syphilis for additional descriptions, including ocular and neurologic manifestations. These symptoms and the lesions eventually resolve, and the disease enters its latent phase.

Latent Syphilis

During latency, serologic tests for syphilis are reactive, but there are no clinical signs of the disease. Latent syphilis of less than 1 year duration is considered early latent, while late-latent syphilis is syphilis with a latent phase longer than 1 year. The World Health Organization (WHO) designates a 2-year period for differentiation of early and late syphilis. Differentiation of these two phases is designed to reflect differences in infectivity and to serve as a guide for therapy. Recurrent early manifestations are seen primarily in the first year after secondary syphilis, and the infectious potential for sexual partners during that year is assumed to be greater; infectious potential is less for

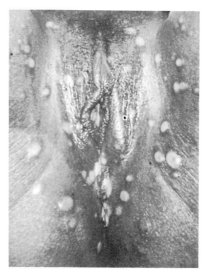

FIGURE 21–8 ••• Condylomata lata of secondary syphilis involving the perineum.

partners of patients with disease of long-standing duration.[80] The rationale for a longer duration of therapy in patients with late-latent syphilis is that treponemes are assumed to be dividing at a slower rate and thus require higher teponemocidal levels of antibiotic.

Tertiary Syphilis

Approximately two thirds of syphilitic patients who enter late latency have no further clinical illness and are no longer infectious. However, the disease may cause serious complications several months to years later. The more common cardiovascular manifestations of tertiary syphilis include aortic aneurysm, aortic insufficiency, and coronary ostial occlusion. Gummata, the chronic inflammatory lesions of tertiary syphilis, affect primarily the skin, subcutaneous tissues, and bone. Initially, the lesions appear as nodules and slowly progress to form granulomatous lesions that may ulcerate. These lesions destroy normal surrounding tissues, and the clinical features vary with the organs affected. CNS involvement occurs at all stages of syphilis. Asymptomatic CNS disease, confirmed by cerbrospinal fluid cell and serologic abnormalities, may also be present in some individuals. Involvement of the brain and spinal cord (neurosyphilis) occurs in some persons, causing mentation impairment and difficulties with sensation and movement. The reader is encouraged to seek a more comprehensive review of cardiovascu-

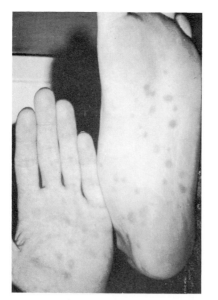

FIGURE 21–7 ••• Palmar-plantar rash of secondary syphilis.

lar and CNS manifestations of late syphilis for a more detailed discussion of these subjects.

Diagnosis

The diagnosis of syphilis is based on characteristic clinical features in conjunction with positive results on appropriate serologic tests. During the primary and secondary stages, *T. pallidum* can be observed on darkfield examination of chancres, condylomata lata, and mucous patches. Reactive nonspecific serologic tests (the rapid plasma reagin [RPR] or the Venereal Disease Research Laboratory [VDRL] test) must be confirmed with specific antibody tests for *T. pallidum*. Commonly employed specific tests include the flourescent treponemal antibody absorption test (FTA-ABS), the microhemagglutination–*T. pallidum* test (MHA-TP), or the hemagglutination treponemal test for syphilis (HATTS). Patients with suspected CNS involvement may require an evaluation of the cerebrospinal fluid.

Treatment

Penicillin remains the cornerstone of therapy for syphilis. It has remained effective because of the persistent sensitivity of *T. pallidum* to penicillin. The benzathine formulation readily achieves the sustained, moderately low serum levels required to eradicate the spirochete, which has a long division time. Treatment regimens are based on the stage of the disease at diagnosis. Benzathine penicillin (2.4 million U intramuscularly in two separate injections) is the recommended treatment for patients with primary, secondary, and early-latent disease.[67] For patients who are allergic to penicillin, doxycycline (100 mg orally twice daily for 14 days) or tetracycline (500 mg orally four times daily for 14 days) may be used. Patients with late-latent syphilis, syphilis of unknown duration, or tertiary syphilis other than neurosyphilis should receive a longer course of therapy for reasons mentioned earlier. Benzathine penicillin (7.2 million U administered in 2.4 million–U doses at weekly intervals for 3 weeks) is currently recommended.[67] Treatment of patients who are allergic to penicillin is with doxycycline or tetracycline, although 4 weeks of such therapy is recommended.[67] Patients with neurosyphilis should be given aqueous crystalline penicillin G, (12 to 24 million U intravenously daily [2 to 4 million U intravenously every 4 hours] for 10 to 14 days) or procaine penicillin G (2.4 million U intramuscularly daily), given together with probenecid (500 mg orally four times daily) for the same length of time.

Additional Considerations

Pregnant adolescents with syphilis should be given penicillin at the dosage appropriate for the stage of disease.[67] Because tetracyclines are contraindicated in pregnancy and because of unacceptably high failure rates to prevent congenital syphilis when using alternative drugs (erythromycin), pregnant women who are allergic to penicillin should undergo skin testing and desensitization to receive penicillin.[80]

Patients should be cautioned regarding Jarisch-Herxheimer reactions after treatment for early syphilis. These self-limited manifestations include myalgias, chills, headache, and postural hypotension. Management consists of hydration and aspirin. Pregnant patients may experience preterm labor or fetal distress and should be observed for such.

To assess response to treatment, follow-up serologic testing should be performed at 3-, 6-, and 12-month intervals after treatment. At least a fourfold (two-dilution) decline in titer is generally regarded as an appropriate response.[87, 88] Sexual partners of individuals with early syphilis should be assumed to have incubating syphilis and therefore should be treated as patients with early disease. All infected persons and their sexual contacts should be encouraged to undergo HIV counseling and testing.

GENITAL HERPES SIMPLEX INFECTION

Genital HSV infection is a common sexually transmitted viral disease in all populations of sexually active persons.[14, 89] Although symptomatic disease in adults is self-limiting, the first episode of genital HSV may be associated with considerable medical morbidity, including hospitalization for aseptic meningitis and urinary retention. Recurrent episodes exact a significant toll psychologically and economically.[90] A high proportion of seropositive persons in both

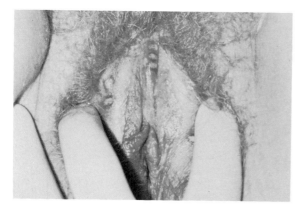

FIGURE 21–9 ••• First episode of genital herpes of the vulva.

high- and low-prevalence populations have unrecognized HSV-2 infection.[91] In addition, current strategies for diagnosing genital HSV infections, including colposcopy, Pap smears, and viral cultures of lesions, fail to identify many cases.[92] Without greater emphasis on prevention and risk reduction, the spread of this incurable disease may remain unchecked, which may have significant implications regarding the transmission of HIV.

HSV is a member of the herpesvirus family, which includes the Epstein-Barr, cytomegalovirus, and varicella zoster viruses. Two major serotypes of HSV cause genital infection in humans: HSV-1, responsible primarily for oral and some genital infections, and HSV-2. The subtypes are similar in their DNA content but exhibit differences in their infective properties and clinical manifestations.[93] Although the majority of genital infections are caused by HSV-2, HSV-1 can be isolated from 10% to 25% of genital lesions in with primary, first-episode HSV and in 1% of patients with nonprimary, first-episode HSV.[90] HSV has a predilection for cutaneous and mucous membrane sensory ganglia and persists in this neural tissue in a dormant state. The risk of recurrence after primary, first-episode genital herpes is more than 80% with HSV-2 infection and approximately 50% with HSV-1.[90, 94]

Primary infection occurs in patients with no previous exposure to HSV and thus no circulating HSV antibodies. The initial episode is associated with significant vulvar pain, dysuria, and, at times, urinary retention. Tender inguinal lymphadenopathy is typically present. Systemic symptoms are common, with patients complaining of fever, headaches, malaise, and myalgia. Severe complications such as menin-gitis are rarely encountered. Early in the course of the disease, the infected area shows vesicular lesions with associated inflammation and edema. With time, these vesicles break, forming ulcerative lesions with an erythematous base, often covered with a purulent exudate (Fig. 21–9). The ulcers may coalesce and form a larger ulcer with a covering crust. Complete healing of the lesions usually occurs within 2 weeks, although it may take as long as 4 to 6 weeks. Recurrent episodes of the disease are typically less painful and have minimal systemic signs, a smaller mean number of lesions, and a shorter mean duration of viral shedding.

Diagnosis

Viral culture of the lesions is the most sensitive and specific method of diagnosis of mucocutaneous HSV.[93] Vesicles and pustular lesions have the highest viral isolation rates; up to 90% will produce positive cultures.[95] Ulcers demonstrate positive cultures in 70% of cases, whereas crusted lesions yield positive cultures in only 30% of cases.[95] Cytologic examination of lesional exudate using Tzanck preparations or Papanicolaou smears is much less sensitive and provides less definitive information regarding viral type. Serologic testing is not useful for the diagnosis of HSV in adults, because commercially available tests do not reliably differentiate between type-specific and type-common antigens.[95] Except to document seroconversion in primary genital herpes infection or screen for evidence of past HSV infection, serologic testing should not be performed.

Treatment

Antiviral therapy with oral or parenteral acyclovir is currently recommended for primary genital herpes infections. Acyclovir has been shown to accelerate healing of genital lesions and decrease the duration of viral shedding, and parenteral therapy has been shown to limit local and systemic symptoms.[96] Treatment should be initiated as soon as the diagnosis is suspected, as the benefits usually outweigh the risks incurred while waiting for culture results and the toxicity of acyclovir is quite low, especially with oral therapy. The recommended therapy for the first episode of genital herpes is oral acyclovir (200 mg five times daily for 10 days).[67]

Local adjunctive treatment of the vulvovaginal lesions is important. Sitz baths using tepid water and Burow's solution are soothing to the inflamed perineum. Wet areas are then patted dry or dried with a hair dryer on a low setting, followed by application of topical lidocaine gel or ointment. Patients can be encouraged to void in the bath or tub to limit urine contamination of the lesions. Occasionally catheterization is needed if urinary retention is present or appears likely.

With recurrent genital HSV, initiation of oral therapy at the first sign of prodrome or lesions is only moderately effective in reducing the number of symptomatic days.[97] Episodic therapy should be reserved for patients with infrequent but moderately or prolonged recurrences. Patients with frequent recurrences generally benefit from prolonged suppressive therapy, regardless of the severity of recurrences.[98, 99]

HUMAN PAPILLOMAVIRUS INFECTION

The incidence of HPV infections has increased dramatically since the 1970s. Using more sensitive detection techniques (e.g., polymerase chain reaction), it has been estimated that at least 24 million persons are currently infected.[3] First visits to private physicians for a genital wart, a likely indicator of new cases, nearly tripled between 1966–1970 and 1986–1990.[3] It has been estimated that genital warts account for approximately 5% of all STD clinic visits, and in some clinics, cases of genital warts outnumber cases of gonorrhea.[3] More than 60 subtypes of HPV have been identified to date, and approximately 20 of these have been associated with genital infection.[100] Research into the biology of HPV has revealed that certain serotypes of the virus are likely to induce premalignant and malignant lesions in previously infected areas. The long-term potential for genital and/or anal neoplasia is of particular concern in affected individuals.

Papillomaviruses are members of the papovavirus family, which also includes simian virus 40 and the polyomaviruses. Structurally, they are unencapsulated, have an icosahedral virion capsid, and contain a double-stranded DNA genome. The early transcription regions, E6 and E7, are important for transformation, and the late (L) region is responsible for viral capsid formation.[101] Although it is known that the virus is transmitted sexually, the exact mechanism of infection at the molecular level is unknown. It is assumed that the virus gains entry to the basal cell layer of the surface epithelium through microscopic abrasions, leading to transformation of one or more basal cells.[102] Genital lesions usually appear after an incubation period of approximately 3 months (range, 3 weeks to 8 months). The natural history of HPV infection is remarkably variable, ranging from spontaneous regression to persistent infection and, in cases, neoplastic progression.[102] Evidence of a role of host cell–mediated immunity in controlling HPV infections has been gained from examining immunodeficient patients. Several studies have documented an increased incidence of genital neoplasia in renal transplant patients and in patients with lymphoma, Hodgkin's disease, chronic lymphocytic leukemia, and HIV infection.[103] It is well appreciated that HPV infections worsen during pregnancy, but it is not clear whether this is due to alterations in cell-mediated immunity, hormonal changes, or other factors.[104]

Clinical Manifestations

Genital warts can be symptomatic or asymptomatic. They are usually multifocal and frequently involve large areas of the genital tract. The most common sites in females are the posterior fourchette, adjacent labia and perineum, vaginal introitus, vagina, and cervix. Approximately 5% of men and women with genital warts also have perianal and anal warts that may or may not be associated with anal intercourse.[105] Three types of lesions are commonly seen: exophytic warts, papules, and macules (flat condylomas). Condyloma acuminatum is the most widely recognized manifestation of anogenital HPV infection. A disorder characterized by a subset of pigmented condylomatous papules is referred to as *bowenoid papulosis*; these lesions are associated with low-grade intraepithelial neoplasia.[106] The giant condyloma (Buschke-Löwenstein tumor) is an uncommon, locally invasive, nonmetastasizing tumor originating from genital warts.

Diagnosis

A variety of clinical and laboratory methods are currently available to diagnose genital warts. Inspection with the unaided eye will readily discern the typical cauliflower-like projections and, occasionally, flat, papular lesions. Application with 5% acetic acid for 5 minutes may augment the identification of flat lesions that are not readily apparent.[107, 108] Tissue infected with HPV often undergoes epithelial hyperplasia and has a shiny white appearance (acetowhitening) after soaking with acetic acid (Fig. 21–10). Distal urethroscopy is important for the diagnosis of meatal and distal urethral warts in men. Anoscopy and proctoscopy are often necessary for the diagnosis of anal warts, which can extend beyond the dentate line.

Aside from clinical observation, cytology and histology are the only laboratory methods available to nearly all clinicians. Koilocytosis, which is highly characteristic of HPV-induced lesions, is described cytologically as a large epithelial cell with a hyperchromatic nucleus and perinuclear ring in the cytoplasm.[109] Immunohistochemistry may become a more useful method when type-specific HPV antisera becomes available. DNA hybridization currently is the most sensitive and specific, widely available method for detecting HPV.[103] Commercially available kits for dot-blot hybridization have not been subjected to large-scale trials to determine their utility in clinical practice. Polymerase chain reaction has great potential, as it amplifies a small segment of HPV DNA if present in the specimen.[110] However, this technique is currently limited to research settings.

Treatment

Genital warts are difficult to treat and commonly recur. A variety of treatment modalities

TABLE 21–5 ••• TREATMENT MODALITIES FOR GENITAL WARTS

Topical cytotoxic agents
  Podophyllin, 10% to 25% solution
  Podophyllotoxin, 0.5% solution
  Trichloroacetic acid, 75% and 85% solution
  5-Fluorouracil, 5% cream
Surgical therapy
  Cryotherapy
  Electrocautery
  Laser
Immunomodulators
  Interferon

are available, but no single treatment or combination is completely satisfactory (Table 21–5). The ideal therapy for HPV should be rapid, easy to administer, and relatively inexpensive and have minimal, if any, side effects. Unfortunately, none of the available therapies fulfills these criteria. While the overall goal is to eradicate warts and dysplastic tissue, reduce symptoms, and reduce transmission of HPV to noninfected individuals, elimination of HPV is virtually impossible because of the inability to completely detect latent virus at all infected sites. In addition, each treatment modality is associated with certain adverse effects. Nonetheless, given the risk of anogenital neoplasia associated with HPV, treatment should be offered to all patients.[103]

MEDICAL IMPLICATIONS OF STDs IN ADOLESCENTS

STDs in adolescents have significant importance because of the high rates of infections in this group and because many of these infections will have the greatest health impact in the future. Many teenagers infected with STDs are asymptomatic, do not recognize symptoms when they are present, or fail to associate symptoms with a disease that has potentially severe complications. The significance of lower genital tract infections and their sequelae disproportionately affects females and future reproduction. In females, several biologic characteristics function to increase susceptibility to STDs and their sequelae.

Female teenagers comprise approximately 20% of the 1 million women diagnosed annually with PID in the United States.[111] Sexually active adolescents have a particularly high rate of PID when rates are statistically adjusted for sexual activity. Conversely,

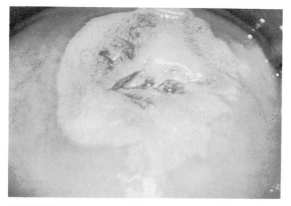

FIGURE 21–10 ••• Aceto-white appearance of the transformation zone with application of acetic acid caused by HPV infection.

women age 15 to 24 with PID appear to have less PID-associated tubal damage and incidence of infertility than do older women with PID.[80, 112] However, the infertility rate increases approximately threefold with each recurrent infection. Along with age-related sexual behaviors, physiological characteristics that increase the risk for PID in adolescents are a lower prevalence of antichlamydial antibodies and greater penetrability of cervical mucus.[70]

During adolescence, the squamocolumnar junction is extruded onto the portio of the cervix. This zone of ectopy (or ectropion) consists primarily of columnar epithelial cells, which are particularly susceptible to both chlamydial and gonococcal infections. Cervical mucus acts as a mechanical barrier to the ascent of pathogens into the upper genital tract. This function is enhanced by the progestin component of oral contraceptives, which promote formation of a thick, tenacious mucus. Impedance to the attachment of bacteria to epithelial cells and neutralization of bacterial activity is provided by secretory immunoglobulin A (SigA) in cervical mucus. Conversely, oral contraceptive use promotes ectopy, thereby increasing the risk of cervical infection with *C. trachomatis*.[35] Because cervicitis is often asymptomatic or unrecognized by patients and practitioners, these infections act as reservoirs for pathogens that may ascend to cause upper genital tract infection (e.g., PID, chorioamnionitis, and postpartum endometritis).[113] The alteration of humoral defenses by STD pathogens may be the first phase of the development of lower genital tract infection and subsequent upper tract involvement.

The relationship between oral contraceptive use and risk of genital tract infection is complex. A two- to threefold increase in the recovery of *C. trachomatis* from the cervix of oral contraceptive users has been repeatedly documented.[35, 112, 113] However, rates of PID have been shown to be reduced by up to 50% in oral contraceptive users compared with non–oral contraceptive users.[115] This apparent paradox is explained by the effect of oral contraceptives on the development of cervical ectopy, which increases the attachment and subsequent recovery of chlamydia. Conversely, the thick cervical mucus and relative atrophy of the endometrial cavity produced by oral contraceptives act to reduce upper genital tract invasion and proliferation of pathogens. Local immune responses and mucosal cell susceptibility may be altered by oral contraceptive use.[116]

The prevalence of cervical ectopy in adolescent females and the association between cervical infections and ectopy have important implications for the transmission of HIV. Prospective studies of sexually active women in Africa have shown that HIV seroconversion is nearly six times more likely in women with cervical infections caused by STD pathogens (including *C. trachomatis* and *N. gonorrhoeae*) than in women without these infections.[117, 118] The use of oral contraceptives and adolescent age have been independently associated with HIV infection.[118, 119] In addition, a cross-sectional study of couples in Kenya demonstrated that after controlling for confounding variables, cervical ectopy remained the only independent predictor of HIV seropositivity.[120] The authors hypothesized that vascularity of ectopy and the ease of bleeding with trauma may facilitate entry of the virus into the blood stream or the target cells of the mucosa or surrounding tissue. The prevalence of cervical ectopy in pregnancy and the increased possibility of transmission of HIV during pregnancy and of subsequent perinatal transmission thus are significant issues.

Evidence linking the presence of genital ulcer disease (GUD) with HIV infection is more compelling than that for nonulcerative STD. Although a detailed discussion of this subject has been published,[121] it is important to emphasize that both prospective and cross-sectional studies of GUD (syphilis, chancroid, HSV, etc.) have shown a strong association between HIV seroconversion and GUD.[117, 122, 123] In addition, evidence of an increased number of clinical recurrences or persistent lesions, atypical lesions, and treatment failures with recommended antimicrobial therapy has emerged from studies of heterosexual and homosexual cohorts.[121] The relatively recent resurgence of genital ulcer–producing diseases in heterosexuals in the United States and the increases in new cases of genital HSV raise the specter of HIV-related illnesses that may overwhelm all efforts for control.[124]

The relationship between HPV infection and the development of genital neoplasia raises particular concerns for adolescents. The alarming prevalence (nearly 50%) in a cohort of sexually active teenagers indicates that subclinical infections comprise the major portion of HPV infections.[125] Current theory identifies HPV as an essential prerequisite for neoplasia.[125] Other factors, including cigarette smoking, HPV DNA type (16, 18, 31, 33, 35, etc.), oral contraceptive use, and host immune alterations are associated with genital neoplasia.[125, 126] Prospective studies of the risk of cervical cancer after cytologic detection of HPV demonstrate an increased risk of progression to cervical cancer in women younger than age 25.[127, 128]

The limitation of Papanicolaou smears in detecting HPV disease was demonstrated in a study of 9000 women with normal Pap smears, 10% of whom tested positive for HPV-16.[129] In 70% of patients, in situ hybridization failed to detect persistent HPV-16 in follow-up Pap smears, and some patients with negative smears subsequently tested positive for HPV.[130] These findings amplify concerns regarding latent viral infections acquired relatively early in life and the potential for neoplastic transformation at an earlier age.

Infection with HIV may affect the natural history of HPV infection in two principal ways. First, infection with multiple HPV types and the development of multicentric lesions have been described in women.[131–133] Second, HIV-related immunosuppression may augment development of anogenital neoplasia. Despite the confounding influence that stage of infection may have on HPV detection, several studies have shown a significant association between abnormal results on cervical cytologic tests and infection with HIV.[134–136] Although well-designed prospective studies are needed to establish the nature of these interactions, implications for the health of sexually active individuals are of grave concern.

References

1. Centers for Disease Control. Premarital experience among adolescent women—United States, 1970–1988. MMWR 1991; 39:929–932.
2. Centers for Disease Control. Division of STD/HIV Prevention Annual Report, 1990. Atlanta: US Department of Health and Human Services, Public Health Service, 1991.
3. Centers for Disease Control. Division of STD/HIV Prevention Annual Report, 1991. Atlanta: US Department of Health and Human Services, Public Health Service, 1992.
4. Cates W. Teenagers and sexual risk taking: The best of times and the worst of times. J Adolesc Health 1991; 12:84–94.
5. Fullilove RE, Fullilove MT, Bowser BP, et al. Risk of sexually transmitted disease among black adolescent crack users in Oakland and San Francisco, California. JAMA 1990; 263:851–855.
6. Reference deleted.
7. Reference deleted.
8. Reference deleted.
9. Batteiger BE, Jones RB. Chlamydia infections. Infect Dis Clin North Am 1987; 1:55–81.
10. Shafer M-A, Moscicki AB. Sexually transmitted diseases. In: Hendee WR, Wilford B (eds). Health of Adolescents: Adolescent Health Issues. San Francisco: Jossey-Bass, 1991.
11. Rosenfeld WD, Vermund SH, Wentz SJ, et al. High prevalence rate of human papillomavirus infection and associated abnormal Papanicolau smears among sexually active adolescents. Am J Dis Child 1989; 143:1443–1447.
12. Bauer HM, Ting Y, Greer CE, et al. Genital human papillomavirus infection in female university students as determined by a PCR-based method. JAMA 1989; 265:472–477.
13. Stone KM. Epidemiologic aspects of genital HPV infection. Clin Obstet Gynecol 1989; 32:112–116.
14. Johnson RE, Nahmias A, Madger LS, et al. A seroepidemiologic survey of the prevalence of herpes simplex virus type 2 infection in the United States. N Engl J Med 1989; 321:7–12.
15. Kampareier RH. Identification of the gonococcus by Albert Neisser. Sex Transm Dis 1978; 5:71–73.
16. Judson FN. Gonorrhea. Med Clin North Am 1990; 74:1353–1366.
17. McCormack M, et al. Clinical spectrum of gonococcal infection in women. Lancet 1977; 2:1182–1185.
18. Hook EW, Hansfield HH. Gonococcal infections in the adult. In: Holmes KK, et al (eds). Sexually Transmitted Diseases. 2nd ed. New York: McGraw-Hill, 1990, pp 149–165.
19. Barlow D, Phillips I. Gonorrhea in women: Diagnostic, clinical, and laboratory aspects. Lancet 1978; 1:761–764.
20. Schmake JD, et al. Observation on the culture diagnosis of gonorrhea in women. JAMA 1969; 210:312–315.
21. Thin RN, Shaw EJ. Diagnosis of gonorrhea in women. Br J Vener Dis 1979; 55:434–438.
22. Lebedoff DA, Hochman EB. Rectal gonorrhea in men: Diagnosis and treatment. Ann Intern Med 1980; 92:463–467.
23. Quinn TC, et al. The polymicrobial origin of intestinal infections in homosexual men. N Engl J Med 1983; 309:576–580.
24. Jacobs NF, Krans SJ. Gonoccocal and nongonococcal urethritis in men. Clinical and laboratory differentiation. Ann Intern Med 1975; 82:7–11.
25. O'Brien JA, et al. Disseminated gonococcal infection. A prospective analysis of 49 patients and a review of the pathophysiology and immune mechanisms. Medicine 1983; 2:395–397.
26. Holmes KK, et al. Disseminated gonococcal infection. Ann Intern Med 1979; 74:979–982.
27. Mase AT, Einstein BI. Disseminated gonococcal infection (DGI) and gonococcal arthritis (GCA): II. Clinical manifestations, diagnosis, complications, treatment and prevention. Semin Arthritis Rheum 1981; 10:173–180.
28. Hansfield HH, et al. Treatment of the gonococcal arthritis–dermatitis syndrome. Ann Intern Med 1976; 95:175–179.
29. Weisner PJ, et al. The clinical spectrum of pharyngeal gonococcal infections. N Engl J Med 1973; 288:181–185.
30. Dice PA, Goldenberg DL. Clinical manifestations of disseminated gonococcal infection caused by *Neisseria gonorrhoeae* are linked to differences in bacterial reactivity of infecting strains. Ann Intern Med 1985; 95:175–180.

30a. Pederson AHB, Bonin P. Screening females for asymptomatic gonorrhea infection. Northwest Med 1971; 70:255–259.

31. Wang SP, Grayston JT. Immunological relationship between genital TRIC, lymphogranuloma venereum, and related organisms in the new microtiter indirect immunofluorescence test. Am J Ophthalmol 1970; 70:367–371.

32. Wang SP, Kno CC, Barnes RC, et al. Immunotyping of *Chlamydia trachomatis* with monoclonal antibodies. J Infect Dis 1985; 152:791–794.

33. Kuo CC, Wang SP, Holmes KK, et al. Immunotypes of *Chlamydia trachomatis* isolates in Seattle, Washington. Infect Immun 1983; 41:865–868.

34. Schacter J. Biology of *Chlamydia trachomatis*. In: Holmes KK (ed). Sexually Transmitted Diseases. 2nd ed. New York: McGraw-Hill, 1990, pp 167–180.

35. Harrison JR, Costia M, Meder JB, et al. Cervical *Chlamydia trachomatis* infection in university women: Relationship to history, contraception, ectopy and cervicitis. Am J Obstet Gynecol 1985; 153:244–249.

36. Brunham RC, Paavonen J, Stevens CE, et al. Mucopurulent cervicitis: The ignored counterpart in women of urethritis in men. N Engl J Med 1984; 311:1–8.

37. Rees E, Tait IA, Hobson D, et al. Chlamydia in relation to cervical infection and pelvic inflammatory disease. In: Hobson D, Holmes KK (eds). Nongonococcal Urethritis and Related Infections. Washington, DC: American Society for Microbiology, 1977, p 67.

38. Katz BP, Caine VA, Jones RB. Diagnosis of mucopurulent cervicitis among women at risk for *Chlamydia trachomatis* infection. Sex Transm Dis 1988; 16:103–106.

39. Brunham RC, et al. Epidemiologic and clinical correlates of *C. trachomatis* and *N. gonorrhoeae* infection among women attending an STD clinic. Clin Res 1981; 29:474–494.

40. Paavonen J. *Chlamydia trachomatis*–induced urethritis in female partners of men with nongonococcal urethritis. Sex Transm Dis 1979; 6:69–72.

41. Stamm WE, Wagner KF, Amsel R, et al. Causes of the acute urethral syndrome in women. N Engl J Med 1980; 303:409–414.

42. Jones RB, Katz BP, Vanderpol B, et al. Effect of blind passage and multiple sampling in recovery of *Chlamydia trachomatis* from urogenital specimens. J Clin Microbiol 1986; 24:1029.

43. Eschenbach DA, Buchanan TM, Pollock HM, et al. Polymicrobial etiology of acute pelvic inflammatory disease. N Engl J Med 1975; 293:166–171.

44. Mardh PA, Ripa KT, Svensson L, et al. *Chlamydia trachomatis* infection in patients with acute salpingitis. N Engl J Med 1977; 296:1377.

45. Svensson L, Westrom L, Ripa KT, et al. Differences in some clinical and laboratory parameters in acute salpingitis related to culture and serologic findings. Am J Obstet Gynecol 1980; 138:1017–1021.

46. Wolner-Hansen P, Kiviat N, Holmes KK. Atypical pelvic inflammatory disease: Subacute, chronic or subclinical upper genital tract infection in women. In: Holmes KK (ed). Sexually Transmitted Diseases. 2nd ed. New York: McGraw-Hill, 1990, pp 615–620.

47. Wang SP, Eschenback DA, Holmes KK, et al. *Chlamydia trachomatis* infection in Fitz-Hugh-Curtis syndrome. Am J Obstet Gynecol 1980; 138:1034–1038.

48. Schacter J. Chlamydial infections. N Engl J Med 1978; 298:428–434.

49. Paavonen J, et al. Treatment of NGU with trimethoprim-sulfadiazine and with placebo: A double blind placebo controlled study. Br J Vener Dis 1980; 56:101–105.

50. Stamm WE, et al. Treatment of the acute urethral syndrome. N Engl J Med 1981; 304:956–961.

51. Martin DH. Chlamydial infections. Med Clin North Am 1990; 74:1367–1387.

52. Barnes RC. Laboratory diagnosis of human chlamydial infections. Clin Microbiol Rev 1989; 2:119–131.

53. Stamm WE. Diagnosis of chlamydia trachomatis genitourinary infection. Ann Intern Med 1988; 108:710–720.

54. Richmond J, et al. Value and feasibility of screening women attending STD clinics for cervical chlamydia infections. Br J Vener Dis 1980; 56:92–96.

55. Sultz GR, et al. *Chlamydia trachomatis* infections in female adolescents. J Pediatr 1981; 98:981–989.

56. Bowie WR, et al. Prevalence of *C. trachomatis* and *N. gonorrhoeae* in two populations of women. Can Med Assoc J 1981; 124:1477–1481.

57. Handsfield HH, Jasman LL, Roberts PL, et al. Criteria for selective screening for *Chlamydia trachomatis* infection in women attending family planning clinics. JAMA 1986; 255:1730–1738.

58. Stamm WE, Holmes KK. *Chlamydia trachomatis* infections of the adult. In: Holmes KK (ed). Sexually Transmitted Diseases. 2nd ed. New York: McGraw-Hill, 1990, pp 181–193.

59. Toomey KE, Barnes RC. Treatment of chlamydia trachomatis genital infection. Rev Infect Dis 1990; 12(suppl 6):5645–5653.

60. Stamm WE. Azithromycin in the treatment of uncomplicated genital chlamydial infection. Am J Med 1991; 91(suppl A):195–205.

61. Martin DH, Mroczkowski TF, Dalu ZA, et al. A controlled trial of a single dose of azithromycin for the treatment of chlamydial urethritis and cervicitis. N Engl J Med 1992; 327:921–925.

62. Cromblehome WR, Schacter J, Grossman M, et al. Amoxicillin therapy for *Chlamydia trachomatis* infection in pregnancy. Am J Obstet Gynecol 1990; 75:752–756.

63. Alger LS, Lovchik JC. Comparison of efficacy of clindamycin versus erythromycin in eradication of antenatal *Chlamydia trachomatis*. Am J Obstet Gynecol 1991; 165:23–27.

64. Schmid G. Approach to the patient with genital ulcer disease. Med Clin North Am 1990; 74:1556–1572.

65. Schacter J. Lymphogranuloma venereum and other nonocular *Chlamydia trachomatis* infections. In: Hobson D, Holmes KK (eds). Nongonococcal Urethritis and Related Infections. Washington, DC: American Society for Microbiology, 1977, pp 91–97.

66. Perina P, Osoba AD. Lymphogranuloma venereum. In: Holmes KK (ed). Sexually Transmitted Diseases. 2nd ed. New York: McGraw-Hill, 1990, pp 195–204.

67. Centers for Disease Control. 1989 sexually transmitted diseases treatment guidelines. MMWR 1989; 38:27–39.

68. Aral SO, Mosher WD, Cates W Jr. Self-reported pelvic inflammatory diseases in the United States. JAMA 1991; 266:2570–2573.

69. Washington AE, Katz D. Cost and payment services for pelvic inflammatory disease: Trends and projections, 1983 through 2000. JAMA 1981; 266:2581–2586.

70. Cates W, Rolfs RT, Aral SO. Sexually transmitted diseases, pelvic inflammatory disease and infertility: An epidemiologic update. Epidemiol Rev 1990; 12:199–220.

71. Eschenbach DA. Acute pelvic inflammatory disease. In: Sciarra J (ed). Gynecology and Obstetrics. Vol I. Hagerstown, MD: Harper & Row, 1988.

72. Eschenbach DA, Buchanon TM, Pollock HM, et al. Polymicrobial etiology of acute pelvic inflammatory disease. N Engl J Med 1975; 293:166.

73. Paavonen J, Teisala K, Heinoven PK, et al. Microbiological and histopathological findings in acute pelvic inflammatory disease. Br J Obstet Gynaecol 1987; 94:454–460.

74. Wasserheit JN, Bele TA, Kivrat NB, et al. Microbiological causes of proven pelvic inflammatory disease and efficacy of clindamycin and tobramycin. Ann Intern Med 1986; 104:187–193.

75. Sweet RL, Mille J, Hadley K, et al. Use of laparoscopy to determine the microbiologic etiology of acute salpingitis. Am J Obstet Gynecol 1979; 134:781.

76. Rice DA, Schacter J. Pathogenesis of pelvic inflammatory disease: What are the questions? JAMA 1991; 266:2587–2593.

77. Washington AE, Aral SO, Wolner-Hanssen P, et al. Assessing risk for pelvic inflammatory disease and its sequelae. JAMA 1991; 266:2581–2586.

78. Jacobson L, Wertrom L. Objectivized diagnosis of acute pelvic inflammatory disease: Diagnostic and prognostic value of laparoscopy. Am J Obstet Gynecol 1969; 105:1088–1098.

79. Kahn JG, Walker CK, Washington AE, et al. Diagnosing pelvic inflammatory diseases: A comprehensive analysis and considerations for developing a new model. JAMA 1991; 266:2594–2604.

80. Westrom L, Mardh PA. Acute pelvic inflammatory disease (PID). In: Holmes KK (ed). Sexually Transmitted Diseases. 2nd ed. New York: McGraw-Hill, 1990, pp 593–613.

81. Centers for Disease Control. Pelvic inflammatory disease: Guidelines for prevention and management. MMWR 1991; 40(RR-5):1–25.

82. Peterson HB, Walker CK, Kahn JG, et al. Pelvic inflammatory disease: Key treatment options. JAMA 266:2605–2611.

83. Centers for Disease Control: Primary and secondary syphilis—United States, 1981–1990. MMWR 1991; 40:314–315, 322–323.

83a. Rolff RT, Nakashima AK. Epidemiology of primary and secondary syphilis in the United States, 1981–1989. JAMA 1990; 264:1432–1437.

83b. Hutchins CM, Hook EW. Syphilis in adults. Med Clin North Am 1990; 74:1389–1416.

84. Schroeter AL, Turner RH, Lucas JB, et al. Therapy for incubating syphilis effectiveness of gonorrhea treatment. JAMA 1971; 218:711–713.

85. Chapel TA. The variability of syphilitic chancres. Sex Transm Dis 1978; 5:68–70.

86. Mindel A, Tovey SJ, Timmins DJ, et al. Primary and secondary syphilis, 20 years' experience. 2. Clinical features. Genitourin Med 1989; 65:1–3.

87. Fiumara NJ. Treatment of secondary syphilis: An evaluation of 204 patients. Sex Transm Dis 1977; 4:92–95.

88. Fiumara NJ. Treatment of seropositive primary syphilis: An evaluation of 196 patients. Sex Transm Dis 1977; 4:96–99.

89. Siegal D, Golden E, Washington AE, et al. Prevalence and correlates of herpes simplex infections: The Population-based AIDS in Multiethnic Neighborhoods Study. JAMA 1992; 268:1702–1708.

90. Corey L, Adams HG, Brown ZA, et al. Genital herpes simplex virus infections: Clinical manifestations, course, and complications. Ann Intern Med 1983; 98:958–972.

91. Koutsky LA, Ashley RL, Holmes KK, et al. The frequency of unrecognized type 2 herpes simplex infection among women. Sex Transm Dis 1990; 17:90–94.

92. Koutsky LA, Stevens CE, Holmes KK, et al. Underdiagnosis of genital herpes by current clinical and viral-isolation procedures. N Engl J Med 1992; 326:1533–1539.

93. Mertz GJ. Genital herpes simplex virus infections. Med Clin North Am 1990; 74:1433–1454.

94. Reeves WC, Corey L, Adams HG, et al. Risk of recurrence after first episodes of genital herpes: Relationship to HSV type and antibody response. N Engl J Med 1981; 305:315–319.

95. Fife KH, Corey L. Herpes simplex virus. In: Holmes KK (ed). Sexually Transmitted Diseases. 2nd ed. New York: McGraw-Hill, 1990, pp 941–952.

96. Corey L, Benedetti JK, Critchlow C, et al. Treatment of primary first-episode genital herpes simplex virus with acyclovir: Results of topical, intravenous and oral therapy. J Antimicrob Chemother 1983; 12(suppl B):79.

97. Reichman RC, Badger GJ, Mertz GJ, et al. Treatment of recurrent genital herpes simplex infections with oral acyclovir: A controlled trial. JAMA 1984; 251:2103–2108.

98. Mertz GJ, Eron L, Kaufman R, et al. Prolonged continuous versus intermittent acyclovir treatment in normal adults with frequently recurring genital herpes simplex virus infection. Am J Med 1988; 85(suppl 2A):14–19.

99. Mertz GJ, Jones CC, Mills J, et al. Long-term acyclovir suppression of frequently recurring genital herpes simplex virus infection. A multicenter double-blind trial. JAMA 1988; 260:201–206.

100. de Villers E-M. Heterogeneity of the human papillomavirus group. J Virol 1989; 63:4898–4903.

101. Neary K, Horwitz BH, DiMaio D. Mutational analysis of open reading frame E4 of bovine papillomavirus type 1. J Virol 1987; 61:1248–1252.

102. Oriel JD. Natural history of genital warts. Br J Vener Dis 1971; 47:1–13.

103. Brown DR, Fife KH. Human papillomavirus infections of the genital tract. Med Clin North Am 1990; 74:1455–1485.

104. Schwartz DB, Greenberg MD, Daoud Y, et al. The management of genital condylomas in pregnancy. Obstet Gynecol Clin North Am 1987; 14:589–599.

105. Oriel D. Genital human papillomavirus infection. In: Holmes KK (ed). Sexually Transmitted Diseases. 2nd ed. New York: McGraw-Hill, 1990, pp 433–441.

106. Stoltz E, Memke HE, Vuzeviski VD. Other genital dermatoses. In: Holmes KK (ed). Sexually Transmitted Diseases. 2nd ed. New York: McGraw-Hill, 1990, pp 717–735.

107. Aho M, Vesterinen E, Myer B, et al. Natural history of vaginal intraepithelial neoplasia. Cancer 1991; 68:195–202.

108. Cone R, Beckmann A, Aho M, et al. Subclinical manifestations of vulvar human papillomavirus infections. Int J Gynecol Pathol 1991; 10:26–31.

109. Koss LG, Durfee GR. Unusual patterns in squamous epithelium of the uterine cervix and pathologic study

of koilocytotic atypia. Ann NY Acad Sci 1956; 63:1245–1251.

110. Shibata DK, Arnheim N, Martin WJ. Detection of human papillomavirus in paraffin-embedded tissue using the polymerase chain reaction. J Exp Med 1988; 167:225–230.

111. Washington AE, Sweet RL, Shafer M-A. Pelvic inflammatory disease and its sequelae in adolescents. J Adolesc Health Care 1985; 6:298–310.

112. Westrom L. Influence of sexually transmitted diseases on sterility and ectopic pregnancy. Acta Eur Fertil 1985; 16:21–32.

113. Holmes KK. Lower genital tract infections in women: Cystitis, urethritis, vulvovaginitis, and cervicitis. In: Holmes KK, et al (eds). Sexually Transmitted Diseases. 2nd ed. New York: McGraw-Hill, 1990, pp 527–545.

114. Cromer BA, Heald FP. Pelvic inflammatory disease associated with *Neisseria gonorrhoeae* and *Chlamydia trachomatis:* Clinical correlates. Sex Transm Dis 1987; 14:125–129.

115. Washington AE, Gove S, Schacter J, Sweet RL. Oral contraceptives, *Chlamydia trachomatis* infection, and pelvic inflammatory disease: A word of caution about protection. JAMA 1985; 253:2246–2250.

116. Wolner-Hanssen P, Eschenbach DA, Paavonen J, et al. Decreased risk of symptomatic pelvic inflammatory disease associated with oral contraceptive use. JAMA 1990; 263:54–59.

117. Laga M, Nzila N, Manoka AT, et al. Nonulcerative sexually transmitted diseases (STD) as risk factors for HIV infection. Abstract Th.C.97. In: Program and Abstracts: Sixth International Conference on AIDS, San Francisco, June, 1990.

118. Plummer FA, Simonsen NJ, Cameron DW, et al. Co-factors in male-to-female transmission of human immunodeficiency virus type I. J Infect Dis 1991; 163:233–239.

119. N'Galy B, Ryder RW. Epidemiology of HIV infection in Africa. J Acquir Immune Defic Syn 1988; 1:551–558.

120. Moss GB, Clemetson D, D'Costa L, et al. Association of cervical ectopy with heterosexual transmission of human immunodeficiency virus: Results of a study of couples in Nairobi, Kenya. J Infect Dis 1991; 164:588–591.

121. Wasserheit JN. Epidemiological synergy: Interrelationships between human immunodeficiency virus infection and other sexually transmitted diseases. Sex Transm Dis 1992; 19:61–77.

122. Cameron DW, Lourdes JD, Gregory MM, et al. Female-to-male transmission of human immunodeficiency virus type 1: Risk factors for seroconversion in men. Lancet 1989; 2:403–407.

123. Holmberg SD, Stewart JA, Gerber AR, et al. Prior

herpes simplex virus type 2 infection as a risk factor for HIV infection. JAMA 1988; 59:1048–1050.

124. Aral SO, Holmes KK. Sexually transmitted diseases in the AIDS era. Sci Am 1991; 264:62–69.

125. Wright TC, Richart RM. Review: Role of human papillomavirus in the pathogenesis of genital tract warts and cancer. Gynecol Oncol 1990; 37:151–164.

126. Ritter DB, Kadish AS, Vermund SH, et al. Detection of human papillomavirus deoxyribonucleic acid in exfoliated cervicovaginal cells as a predictor of cervical neoplasia in a high-risk population. Am J Obstet Gynecol 1988; 159:1517–1525.

127. Mitchell H, Drake M, Medley G. Prospective evaluation of the risk of cervical cancer after cytological evidence of human papillomavirus infection. Lancet 1986; 1:573–575.

128. Kurman RJ, Schiffman MH, Lancaster WD, et al. Analysis of individual papillomavirus types in cervical neoplasia: A possible role for type 18 in rapid progression. Am J Obstet Gynecol 1987; 156:212–216.

129. De Villers EM, Wagner D, Schneider A, et al. Human papillomavirus infections in women with and without abnormal cervical cytology. Lancet 1987; 1:703–705.

130. Moscicki A-B, Winkler B, Irwin CE Jr, Schacter J. Differences in biological maturation, sexual behavior, and sexually transmitted disease between adolescents with and without cervical neoplasia. J Pediatr 1989; 115:487–493.

131. Byrne MA, Taylor-Robinson D, Munday PE, et al. The common occurrence of human papillomavirus infection and intraepithelial neoplasia in women infected with HIV. AIDS 1989; 3:379–382.

132. Caube P, Poulques H, Katlama C. Multifocal human papillomavirus infection of the genital tract in HIV seropositive women. NY State J Med 1990; 90:162–163.

133. Feingold AR, Vermund SH, Burk RD, et al. Cervical cytologic abnormalities and papillomavirus infection in women infected with human immunodeficiency virus. J Acquir Immune Defic Syn 1990; 3:2911–2916.

134. Schrager LK, Friedland GH, Maude D, et al. Cervical and vaginal squamous abnormalities in women infected with human immunodeficiency virus. J Acquir Immune Defic Syn 1989; 2:570–575.

135. Vermund SH, Kelley DF, Burk RD, et al. Risk of human papillomavirus (HPV) and cervical intraepithelial lesions (SIL) highest among women with advanced HIV disease. Abstract no. S.B. 517. In: Program and Abstracts: Sixth International Conference on AIDS. San Francisco, June, 1990.

136. Crocchiolo P, Lizioli A, Goisis F, et al. Cervical dysplasia and HIV infection. Lancet 1988; 2:238–239.

CHAPTER 22

HIV Infection in Adolescents

EDWIN M. THORPE, Jr.

DAVID MURAM

Human immunodeficency virus (HIV) infection and acquired immunodeficiency syndrome (AIDS) are not widespread within the adolescent population but are increasing. Adolescents 13 to 19 years of age comprise less than 1% of AIDS victims (Table 22–1).[1] The incidence of AIDS in this age group has increased 19% between 1989 and 1990; the incidence in 10- to 19-year-olds has increased 40% during the same period. Because of the length of time between infection with HIV and the diagnosis of AIDS, many of the 38,226 patients diagnosed in the 20- to 29-year-old age group were infected during their adolescence.[2] Clearly, the formative period of adolescence often involves participation in significant sexual risk-taking behavior. During the 1980s, teens reported higher levels of sexual activity at earlier ages, experienced more than 1 million pregnancies annually, and suffered from persistently high rates of sexually transmitted diseases (STDs).[2] These factors have prompted the U.S. Public Health Service to make teenagers a central target of HIV prevention strategies.[3] To reduce the incidence of AIDS in this risk group, policies and programs must address adolescent decision making regarding sexual activity and substance abuse. This effort will also afford an opportunity to confront the more visible crises of unwanted teen pregnancy and STD infection.

HIV INFECTION AND AIDS

AIDS follows infection with HIV, a RNA retrovirus. Aside from a mononucleosis-like illness that accompanies the initial infection with HIV, it is virtually asymptomatic. The significant morbidity and mortality related to HIV infection are produced by progressive deterioration of the cellular immune system and resulting opportunistic infections and cancers. HIV infection and AIDS have been well described among the world population, where it has reached epidemic proportions in sub-Saharan Africa, Thailand, and India.

HIV was first isolated in 1983 from patients with AIDS and the AIDS-related complex (ARC). Initially, various names were ascribed to the virus (e.g., type III [HTLV III] and AIDS-associated retrovirus [ARV]).[4–6] The virus became known as HIV in 1986 when an international committee on taxonomy recommended distinguishing this virus as a newly recognized human pathogen.[7] The virus was thought to infect peripheral mononuclear cells, primarily the T-helper lymphocytes.[4–6] Subsequently, HIV was recovered from macrophages and was noted to be capable of infecting a variety of other human cells, including B lymphocytes, promyelocytes, and epidermal Langerhans' cells.[8, 9] The virus has also been isolated from brain tissue[10] and the epithelium of the bowel.[11] HIV has been recovered from numerous body fluids, such as plasma, serum, cerebrospinal fluid, vaginal and cervical secretions, urine, breast milk, tears, saliva, semen, and bronchial fluids.[8, 12]

In the United States, HIV type 1 (HIV-1) is the most prevalent serotype and can be transmitted by sexual activity. A closely related

TABLE 22–1 ••• CHARACTERISTICS OF U.S. AIDS CASES REPORTED IN 1990 AND PERCENTAGE CHANGE 1989–1990

	Number	%	Rate*	% Change
Sex				
Male	38,082	87.9	30.9	21.7
Female	5,257	12.1	4.1	33.2
Age (years)				
0–4	622	1.4	3.3	16.7
5–9	120	0.3	0.6	34.8
10–19	208	0.5	0.6	39.6
20–29	8,338	19.2	19.7	19.3
30–39	19,722	45.5	46.8	21.3
40–49	10,026	23.1	33.5	31.2
50–59	3,013	7.0	13.4	19.7
60+	1,290	3.0	3.1	23.0
Race/ethnicity†				
White	22,342	51.6	11.8	19.7
Black	13,186	30.4	42.5	27.6
Hispanic	7,322	6.9	31.9	25.6
Asian/Pacific Islander	260	0.6	3.8	8.8
American Indian/Alaskan native	71	0.2	4.0	12.7
Region				
Northeast	13,572	31.3	26.7	26.7
Midwest	4,068	9.4	6.8	16.5
South	14,331	33.1	16.8	30.2
West	9,624	22.2	18.2	13.1
U.S. territories	1,744	4.0	46.2	15.6
HIV exposure category				
Men who had sex with men	23,738	54.8	—	19.3
History of IV drug use				
Women and heterosexual men	10,018	23.1	—	23.8
Homosexual and bisexual men	2,295	5.3	—	3.7
Persons with hemophilia				
Adult/adolescent	340	0.8	—	17.6
Child	31	0.1	—	24.0
Transfusion recipients				
Adult/adolescent	866	2.0	—	11.5
Child	39	0.1	—	−2.5
Heterosexual contacts	2,289	5.3	—	40.3
Born in a pattern II country‡	422	1.0	—	11.3
Perinatal transmission	681	1.6	—	20.5
No identified risk	2,620	6.0	—	—
Total	43,339	100.00	17.2	23.0

*Per 100,000 population.
†Excludes persons with unspecified race/ethnicity.
‡Persons born in countries where heterosexual transmission predominates.
From Centers for Disease Control Update: Acquired immunodeficiency syndrome—United States, 1981–1990. MMWR 1991; 40:362.

virus that also causes AIDS, HIV-2, has been identified in western Africa, Europe, and parts of South America.[13] This serotype has also been detected in the United States but is not as prevalent as HIV-1. HIV has an affinity for receptors that are present on helper (CD4) lymphocytes as well as on circulating cells that migrate to the brain. When helper cells are infected with HIV-1, either they are destroyed or their function is significantly impaired, rendering the infected person susceptible to unusual infections and malignancies. Affected cells that migrate into the brain may cause CNS infections with subsequent neurologic or psychiatric disorders (e.g., dementia and encephalitis).[14]

Clinically, infection with HIV is variably manifested in individuals, and rapidity of disease progression is not uncommon.[15] At any given point, an individual may be infected by a population of viruses, rather than by a single virus.[16] In addition, the biologic properties of HIV can change, as evidenced in viral isolates recovered over time from the same individual.[16, 17] This may be explained in part by the high spontaneous mutation rate of the virus.

Because infection with HIV requires exposure to infected blood or body fluids, the major modes of transmission are exposure to contaminated blood and blood products (transfusion, needle sharing), intimate sexual contact, and perinatal transmission. STDs such as genital ulcers (syphilitic, chancroid, herpetic) and gonococcal or chlamydial cervicitis may also facilitate transmission of the virus.[18, 19] However, it is possible that these diseases simply identify those persons who engage in risk-taking behavior.

Initially, HIV affected primarily homosexual males and intravenous drug users. However, worldwide, heterosexual transmission is currently the most frequent route for the transmission of HIV. In HIV-infected persons who report only heterosexual contact as a risk factor, women have outnumbered men since 1981.[1] This can be explained by the greater ease of male-to-female transmission[20] and the greater number of men who are infected.[21] The increased numbers of infected women increase the likelihood of perinatal transmission of HIV. Maternal-fetal transmission rates of 25% to 35% have been consistently reported by prospective studies,[22–26] although one investigation reported a rate of 13%,[27] citing maternal P24 antigenemia and CD4 counts of less than 700/μl as major factors associated with transmission. Most HIV-infected infants are asymptomatic at birth and are diagnosed within the first 2 years of life. They usually die within the subsequent 2 years.[26, 28–30]

SIGNS AND SYMPTOMS

In adults and adolescents, the course of HIV infection can be divided into three distinct stages. The first is characterized by an acute, mononucleosis-like illness that usually begins 2 to 4 weeks after infection.[31] However, incubation periods as short as 5 days and as long as 3 months have been noted.[32, 33] The more prominent manifestations are sore throat, fever, fatigue, headache, and swollen lymph nodes. Antibodies can usually be detected in most infected persons 6 to 12 weeks after initial exposure.[34] This initial illness is not severe and generally lasts from 3 to 14 days. After seroconversion, an asymptomatic period of variable length begins. The mean time to development of AIDS is 7 to 9 years but may be delayed as much as 15 years or longer.[35–37]

In the next stage, AIDS-related complex,

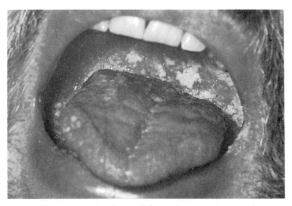

FIGURE 22–1 ••• Oral candidiasis in a patient with HIV infection.

the patient presents with complaints of fatigue, weight loss, chronic headache, fever, and generalized lymphadenopathy. In rare instances, the patient suffers from AIDS-related dementia, characterized by personality changes, mood swings, memory loss, or other cognitive disorders. The neurologic defects may be related to meningitis or to encephalitis, the latter representing a more diffuse brain disease.[14]

The third stage of the disease process is characterized by the onset of opportunistic infections or malignancies. AIDS itself is a clinical diagnosis based on the presence of one or more of a defined group of opportunistic infections and neoplasms.[38] The diseases most often associated with AIDS include *Pneumocystis carinii* infection, some uncommon fungal infections, and, recently, tuberculosis (Figs. 22–1 and 22–2). Neoplasms that are often associated with AIDS include Kaposi's sarcoma and lymphoma (Fig. 22–3). The course of disease is highly variable and is determined by the occurrence of infections, cancers, and

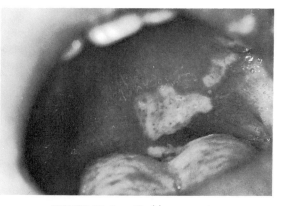

FIGURE 22–2 ••• Oral herpes zoster.

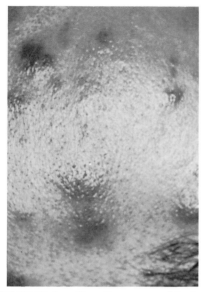

**FIGURE 22–3 ••• ** Kaposi's sarcoma of the face.

those symptoms directly attributable to HIV per se, such as generalized wasting and dementia.

DIAGNOSIS AND TREATMENT

Diagnosis of HIV infection depends on demonstration of the virus or antibodies against it in blood or other tissues. Measurable antibodies against the virus usually appear within 2 months after infection.[34, 39] Within 6 months, 95% of infected individuals have antibodies against the virus.

Unfortunately, there is no curative therapy for the disease. In 1987, the first report appeared demonstrating the efficacy of zidovudine (AZT or ZDV) in prolonging the survival of patients with AIDS or ARC.[40] Subsequent clinical trials revealed that zidovudine slows the progression of AIDS and provides a reasonable degree of prophylaxis against *P. carinii* pneumonia (PCP).[41–43] Additional observational evidence[44, 45] clearly demonstrates that zidovudine prolongs survival in patients with AIDS and that early treatment associated with prophylaxis against PCP slows progression of AIDS.[46] Other nucleoside analogues, dideoxycytidine (DDC) and dideoxyinosine (DDI), have recently been approved by the U.S. Food and Drug Administration for use in persons who do not respond to zidovudine therapy. Other antiviral agents, including vaccines, are currently under investigation.

HIV INFECTION IN TEENAGERS

It is difficult to determine the prevalence of HIV-infection in teenagers, because of the prolonged latent period between seroconversion and the onset of symptoms. As stated earlier, AIDS is not widespread in the adolescent population, representing less than 1% of reported AIDS cases in the United States. Unlike in adults, a larger proportion of adolescents with AIDS are female (27% vs. 10% in adults), black or Hispanic (56% vs. 44%), and were infected with HIV through heterosexual contact (14% vs. 5%).[1] Among teenagers who applied for military service between 1985 and 1989, 3 of every 10,000 tested positive for HIV.[47] The infection rate for black teens was 1 in 1000. An HIV seroprevalence survey conducted at 19 universities throughout the United States revealed that 30 (0.2%) of the 16,861 students, or 1 in 500, tested positive for HIV.[48] The seroprevalence of HIV among a particularly high-risk group of runaway and homeless youth at a shelter facility revealed that 142 (5.3%) of 2667 teens were infected.[49] A large, blinded serosurvey was conducted by the Centers for Disease Control (CDC) between 1988 and 1989 at STD clinics, women's health clinics, and drug treatment centers in 38 metropolitan areas.[50] Among 15- to 19-year-olds, the rate of seropositivity was 0.4%, compared with 1.4% for the 20- to 24-year-old age group. Although the highest rates were found in male patients who reported having sex with males (9.7% to 55.6%), affected female heterosexuals significantly outnumbered heterosexual males.[51]

Similarly, 488 of 137,209 (3.6 per 1000) Job Corps students between ages 16 and 21 tested positive for HIV-1.[52] The results were part of a routine screening of applicants conducted between March 1987 and February 1990. Seroprevalence increased with year of age and was highest among black and Hispanic teenagers from large Northeastern cities. The authors also noted the disproportionately high seroprevalence among students from rural areas and small towns in the Southeast. In addition, among 16- to 17-year-olds, the seropositivity rate was higher in females (2.3 per 1000) than in males (1.5 per 1000) (Fig. 22–4), although the overall rate was slightly higher for males.

Cumulatively, these data indicate that the HIV infection rate is particularly high in teenagers engaging in high-risk behavior. To re-

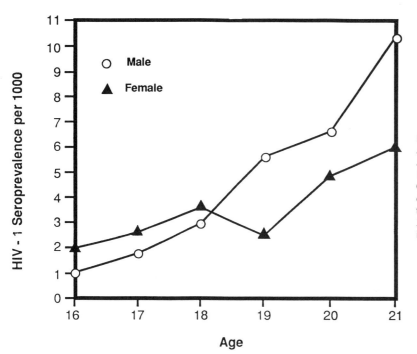

FIGURE 22–4 ••• HIV-1 seroprevalence in Job Corps students by sex and age, 1987–1990. (From St. Louis ME, Conway GA, Haymon CR, et al. Human immunodeficiency virus infection in disadvantaged adolescents. JAMA 1991; 266:2390. Copyright 1991, American Medical Association.)

duce the incidence of HIV in adolescents, a more complete understanding of factors related to decisions regarding risk taking is required.

RISK DETERMINANTS OF STD AND HIV IN ADOLESCENTS

Adolescence represents an important period of transition for developing humans, and it is during this time that behavior that may lead to disease promulgation is established. Rates of STDs in adolescents are influenced by a wide variety of factors, including frequency of sexual activity and number of partners, physical and psychological development, education, peers, parents, religion, and culture. Thus, a critical prelude to the development of successful disease prevention programs is a more complete appreciation of determinants of risk-related behavior in adolescents. Information on the premarital sexual experience of teenagers, as evidenced by the age at initiation of intercourse and reported sexual activity, indicates that most adolescents are sexually active by age 19.[52, 53] At all ages, greater proportion of males than females engage in sexual intercourse, and black teenagers report an earlier onset of sexual activity. These factors pose

great concern because of the cumulative impact that early initiation of intercourse has on the number of sexual partners and the degree of exposure to different sexual partners. Recent CDC findings suggest a decline in the proportion of high school students who report engaging in behaviors that put them at risk for HIV infection (Fig. 22–5).[54]

Compounding the reality of sexual activity in adolescents is the fact that the use of contraceptives is infrequent and often inconsistent. Although periodic condom use offers more protection than none, intermittent use in settings of significant risk often leads to STD acquisition.[55, 56] It has been reported that despite high levels of knowledge about modes of HIV transmission exhibited by adolescents, few sexually active teens change their behavior based on factual information alone.[57] Sexually active teens appear more likely to use condoms consistently (when available) if they feel personally at risk, if they believe condoms are effective in preventing HIV infection, and if they have consulted a physician about condom use. In addition, having communication skills with which to negotiate condom use with a partner increases the likelihood of compliance. One study reported success in reducing high-risk behavior and increasing condom use in 157 inner-city minority males, thereby demonstrating the value of prevention efforts.[58]

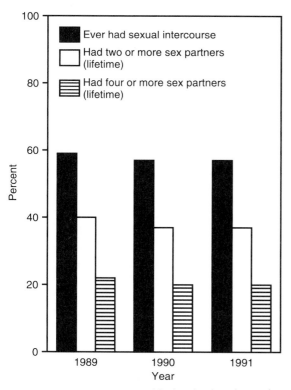

FIGURE 22–5 ••• Percentage of high school students who reported ever having had sexual intercourse and having had sexual intercourse with multiple sex partners in the United States, 1989 through 1991. (Adapted from Centers for Disease Control: MMWR 41:866–868, 1992.)

Paralleling the increase in sexual activity, experimentation with tobacco, alcohol, and illicit drugs has increased in adolescents over the last 2 decades (Fig. 22–6).[59, 60] More than 4.5 million adolescents between 12 and 17 years of age report having tried an illicit drug.[61] The increased rates of adolescent substance use and sexual activity may be linked, either because similar factors influence both, or because engaging in one behavior increases the likelihood of participating in the other. Studies of sexually active teens have shown that condoms are significantly less likely to be used after drinking alcohol or using drugs.[57, 61] Among inner-city youth who were highly informed about HIV transmission, occasional alcohol and marijuana use were found to be strong predictors of high-risk sexual activity. Although intravenous drug use provides a direct route for HIV transmission, nonintravenous drugs and alcohol can impair judgment, thereby reducing the likelihood that a young person will make appropriate decisions about

avoiding activity in which HIV transmission is likely.

The number of homeless and runaway youth in the United States has reached crisis proportions. Approximately 3 million young people run away from home each year because of family conflicts, violence, and abuse.[61] Nearly one in four girls and one in six boys are sexually assaulted before the age of 18, and a history of sexual abuse is associated with behavioral outcomes that place these individuals at risk for STDs.[62] Having severed their principal means of support, these youth turn to prostitution for survival. A shelter serving runaway and homeless youngsters in New York City reported that 91% of the responders acknowledged being sexually active, with an average of nearly three sexual partners a week.[63] Thirty-eight per cent reported having used crack cocaine, and nearly one third admitted to having exchanged sex for food, money, shelter, or drugs. Although a significant proportion of males engage in homosexual or bisexual activity, exchange of sex for survival in homeless youth more commonly involves females.[64] These relationships are often an exploitation of psychological trauma from previous abuse at home and are perpetuated by intimidation and drug dependency. Although these youth represent a small proportion of sexually active adolescents, they have the greatest risk for disease acquisition.

Adolescents are often reluctant to seek regular reproductive health care or treatment for an STD. Most adolescents learn that they have an STD only after they have sought health care for some other reason, most often contraception or prenatal care. Furthermore, only half of all teenagers diagnosed with an STD complete the full treatment prescribed.[65] Low compliance with treatment regimens has been partly attributed to adolescent concern about confidentiality.[66]

IMPLICATIONS FOR INTERVENTION AND PREVENTION

Strategies for intervention require a comprehensive and coordinated effort to involve all facets of adolescent life. A more complete understanding of the complexities of teenage sexual behavior and the dynamics surrounding initiation of sexual activity serves as a basis for targeting prevention efforts. The role of peer

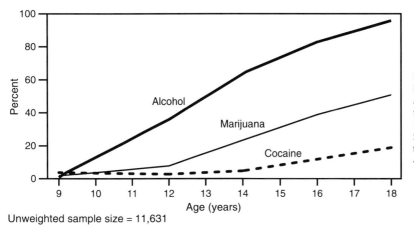

FIGURE 22–6 ••• Percentage of high school students who first used alcohol, marijuana, or cocaine before reaching selected ages in the United States, Youth Risk Behavior Study, 1990. (Adapted from Centers for Disease Control: MMWR 40:776–784, 1991.)

influences and identification of modifiable determinants in the lives of teens may allow development of specific strategies tailored to diverse groups.

Prevention of STDs and HIV infection in sexually active adolescents is dependent on identifying teenagers at risk and eliciting their trust and cooperation in disease management.[67] A willingness to cooperate is critical for identification of potentially infected partners, compliance with treatment regimens, and reduction in risk behavior.

Because many of the consequences of teenage sexual activity are the result of uninformed decisions, early unbiased sex education can provide a foundation for analyzing and coping with situations in which the pressure to become sexually involved is significant. In addition to teaching recognition of signs and symptoms of acute infection, education should also stress appropriate health care behavior, emphasizing the need for periodic examinations for early disease detection.

For the psychologically and emotionally vulnerable adolescent, messages that reinforce self-esteem and empowerment of partner selection and sex negotiation may help overcome barriers among patients, their peers, and health care providers. Discussing options, including sexual abstinence and contraceptives, and general health maintenance may assist teenagers in responsible decision making.

References

1. Centers for Disease Control. HIV/AIDS surveillance report. July, 1992.
2. Centers for Disease Control. Division of STD/HIV prevention annual report, 1991. Atlanta: US Department of Health and Human Services, Public Health Service, 1992.
3. Centers for Disease Control. Strategic plan for preventing human immunodeficiency virus (HIV) infection. Atlanta: US Department of Health and Human Services, Public Health Service, July, 1992.
4. Barre-Simonssi F, Nugeyre M, Dauget C, et al. Isolation of a T-lymphocytopic retrovirus from a patient at risk for acquired immunodeficiency syndrome. Science 1983; 220:868.
5. Gallo R, Salahuddin S, Popovic M, et al. Frequent detection and isolation of cytopathic retrovirus (HTLV-III) from patients with AIDS and at risk for AIDS. Science 1984; 224:500.
6. Levy JA, Hoffman AD, Kranier SM, et al. Isolation of lymphocytopathic retroviruses from San Francisco patients with AIDS. Science 1984; 225:840.
7. Coffin J, Haase A, Levy JA, et al: Human immunodeficiency viruses. Science 1986; 232:697.
8. Levy JA, Kaminsky LS, Morror WJW, et al. Infection by the retrovirus associated with the acquired immunodeficiency syndrome. Ann Intern Med 1985; 103:694.
9. Tschachler E, Groh V, Popovic M, et al. Epidermal Langerhans cells: A target for HTLV-III/LAV infection. J Invest Dermatol 1987; 88:233.
10. Shaw G, Harper M, Hahn B, et al. HTLV-III infection in brains of children and adults with AIDS encephalopathy. Science 1985; 227:177.
11. Nelson JA, Wiley CA, Reynolds-Kohler C, et al. Detection of the human immunodeficiency virus in bowel epithelium. Lancet 1988; 1:259.
12. Levy JA, Shimabukuro J. Recovery of AIDS-associated retroviruses from patients with AIDS, related conditions, and clinically healthy individuals. J Infect Dis 1985; 152:734.
13. Clavel F, Guetard D, Brun-Vezinet F, et al. Isolation of a new human retrovirus from West African patients with AIDS. Science 1986; 233:343.
14. Navia BA, Cho ES, Petito CK, et al. The AIDS dementia complex: II. Clinical features. Ann Neurol 1986; 19:517.
15. Clameck N, Taelman P, Hermans P, et al. A cluster of HIV infection among heterosexual people without apparent risk factors. N Engl J Med 1989; 321:1460–1478.
16. Hahn BH, Shaw GM, Tayler ME, et al. Genetic

variation in HTLV-III/LAV overtime in patients with AIDS or at risk for AIDS. Science 1986; 232:1548–1553.

17. Cheng-Mayer C, Seto D, Levy JA. Biological features of HIV that correlate with virulence. Science 1988; 240:1522–1525.

18. Laga M, Nzila N, Manoka AT, et al. Nonulcerative sexually transmitted diseases (STD) as risk factors for HIV infection. Abstract Th.C.97. In: Program and Abstracts: Sixth International Conference on AIDS, San Francisco, June 1990.

19. Plummer FA, Simonsen NJ, Cameron DW, et al. Cofactors in male-to-female transmission of human immunodeficiency virus type I. J Infect Dis 1991; 163:233–239.

20. Padian NS, Shiboski SC, Jewell NP. Male-to-female transmission of human immunodeficiency virus. JAMA 1991; 266:1664–1667.

21. Gainan ME. HIV, heterosexual transmission and women. JAMA 1992; 268:520–521.

22. European Collaborative Study. Mother-to-child transmission of HIV infection. Lancet 1988; 2:1030–1042.

23. Italian Multicentre Study. Epidemiology, clinical features, and prognostic factors of paediatric HIV infection. Lancet 1988; 2:1043–1046.

24. Cowan MJ, Walker C, Culver K, et al. Maternally transmitted HIV infection in children. AIDS 1988; 2:437–441.

25. Ryder R, Nsa W, Hassig SE, et al. Perinatal HIV transmission in two African hospital: One-year follow-up. Abstract 4128. In: Final Program and Abstracts of the IV International Conference on AIDS. Book I. Stockholm, Sweden: Swedish Ministry of Health and Social Affairs, National Bacteriologic Laboratory, Karolinska Institute, World Health Organization, 1988, p 291.

26. Blanche S, Rouzioux C, Moscato MLC, et al. A prospective study of infants born to women seropositive for human immunodeficiency virus type 1. HIV infection in newborns, French Collaborative Study Group. N Engl J Med 1989; 320:1643–1648.

27. European Collaborative Study. Children born to women with HIV-1 infection: Natural history and risk of transmission. Lancet 1991; 2337:253–260.

28. Reference deleted.

29. Halsey NA, Boulous R, Holt E, et al. Transmission of HIV-1 infections from mothers to infants in Haiti: Impact on childhood mortality and nutrition. JAMA 1990; 264:2088–2092.

30. Scott GB, Hulto C, Mukuch RW, et al. Survival in children with perinatally acquired human immunodeficiency virus type I infection. N Engl J Med 1989; 321:1791–1796.

31. Cooper DA, Gold J, McLeana P, et al. Acute AIDS retrovirus infection. Definition of a clinical illness associated with seroconversion. Lancet 1985; 1:537–540.

32. Centers for Disease Control. Public Health Service guidelines for counseling and antibody testing to prevent HIV infection and AIDS. MMWR 1987; 36:509–515.

33. Ranki A, Valle SL, Krohn M, et al. Long latency precedes overt seroconversion in sexually transmitted human-immunodeficiency virus infection. Lancet 1987; 2:589–593.

34. Hessol NA, Lifson AR, O'Malley PM, et al. Prevalence, incidence, and progression of human immunodeficiency virus infection in homosexual and bisexual men in hepatitis B vaccine trials, 1978–1988. Am J Epidemiol 1989; 130:1167–1175.

35. Goedert JJ, Biggar RJ, Weiss SH, et al. Three-year incidence of AIDS in five cohorts of HTLV-III-infected risk group members. Science 1986; 231:992–995.

36. Lifson AR, Rutherford GW, Jaffe HW. The natural history of human immunodeficiency virus infection. J Infect Dis 1988; 158:1360–1367.

37. Goedert JJ, Kessler CM, Aledort LM, et al. A prospective study of human immunodeficiency virus type I infection and the development of AIDS in subjects with hemophilia. N Engl J Med 1989; 321:1141–1148.

38. Centers for Disease Control. Revision of the CDC surveillance case definition for acquired immunodeficiency syndrome. MMWR 1987; 36(1S):1s–15s.

39. Horsburgh CR, Jason J, Longini IM, et al. Duration of human immunodeficiency virus infection before detection of antibody. Lancet 1989; 1:637–639.

40. Fischl MA, Richman DD, Grieco MH, et al. The efficacy of azithothymidine (AZT) in the treatment of patients with AIDS and AIDS-related complex: A double-blind, placebo-controlled trial. N Engl J Med 1987; 317:185–191.

41. Fischl MA, Richman DD, Hansen N, et al. The safety and efficacy of zidovudine (AZT) in the treatment of subjects with mildly symptomatic human immunodeficiency type 1 (HIV) infection: A double-blind, placebo-controlled trial. Ann Intern Med 1990; 112:737.

42. Volverding PA, Lagokos SW, Koch MA, et al. Zidovudine in asymptomatic human immunodeficiency virus infection: A controlled trial in persons with fewer than 500C D4-positive cells per cubic millimeter. N Engl J Med 1990; 322:941–949.

43. Graham NMH, Zeger SL, Park LP, et al. Effect of zidovudine and *Pneumocystis carinii* pneumonia prophylaxis on progression of HIV-1 infection to AIDS. Lancet 1991; 338:265–269.

44. Moore RD, Hidalgo J, Sugland BW, Chaisson RE. Zidovudine and the natural history of the acquired immunodeficiency syndrome. N Engl J Med 1991; 324:437–443.

45. Swanson CE, Cooper DA. Factors influencing the outcome of treatment with zidovudine of patients with AIDS in Australia. AIDS 1990; 4:749–757.

46. Graham NMH, Zeger SL, Parker LP, et al. The effects on survival of early treatment of human immunodeficiency virus infection. N Engl J Med 1992; 326:1037–1042.

47. Burke DS, Brundage JF, Herbold JR, et al. Human immunodeficiency virus infections in teenagers. JAMA 1990; 263:2074.

48. Gayle HD, Kelling RP, Garcia-Tunon M, et al. Prevalence of the human immunodeficiency virus among university students. N Engl J Med 1990; 323:1538–1541.

49. Stricof RL, Kennedy JT, Nattell TC, et al. HIV seroprevalence in a facility for runaway and homeless adolescents. Am J Public Health 1991; 81(suppl):50–53.

50. Centers for Disease Control. Premarital experience among adolescent women—United States, 1970–1988. MMWR 1991; 39:929–932.

51. Wendell DA, Oranto IM, McCray E, et al. Youth at risk: Sex, drugs, and human immunodeficiency virus. Am J Dis Child 1992; 146:76–81.

52. St. Louis ME, Conway GA, Haymon CR, et al. Human immunodeficiency virus infection in disadvantaged adolescents. JAMA 1991; 266:2387–2391.

53. Centers for Disease Control. Sexual behavior among high school students. MMWR 1992; 40:885–888.

54. Centers for Disease Control. HIV instruction and selected HIV-risk behaviors among high school students—United States. MMWR 1992; 41:866–868.

55. Fineberg HV. Education to prevent AIDS: Prospects and obstacles. Science 1988; 239:592–596.

56. Centers for Disease Control. Selected behaviors that increase risk for HIV infection among high school students—U.S., 1990. MMWR 1992; 41:231, 237–240.

57. Hingson RW, Strunin L, Berlin BM, Herren T. Beliefs about AIDS, use of alcohol and drugs, and unprotected sex among Massachusetts adolescents. Am J Public Health 1990; 80:295–299.

58. Jemmott JB, Jemmott LS, Fong GT. Reductions in HIV-associated sexual behaviors among black male adolescents: Effects of an AIDS prevention intervention. Am J Public Health 1992; 82:372–377.

59. Centers for Disease Control. Tobacco use among high school students—United States, 1990. MMWR 1991; 40:617–619.

60. Centers for Disease Control. Alcohol and other drug use among high school students—United States, 1990. MMWR 1991; 40:776–777, 783–784.

61. Network of Runaway and Youth Services. Cited in AIDS Education: Programs for Out-of School Youth Slowly Evolving. US General Accounting Office publication HRD-90-III. Washington, DC: US Government Printing Office, 1990.

62. Keller SE, Bartlett JA, Schleifer SJ, et al. HIV-related sexual behavior among a healthy inner-city heterosexual adolescent population in an endemic area of HIV. J Adolesc Health 1991; 12:44–48.

63. Zierler S, Fiengold L, Laufer D, et al. Adult survivors of childhood sexual abuse and subsequent risk of HIV infection. Am J Public Health 1991; 81:572–575.

64. Margetson N, Lipman C. Children at risk: The impact of poverty, the family and the street on homeless and runaway youth in New York City. Presented at the National Symposium on Youth Victimization, Atlanta, April 27, 1990.

65. Bidwell RJ, Deisher RW. Adolescent sexuality: Current issues. Pediatr Ann 1991; 20:298–302.

66. Jay S, Litt IF, Durant RH. Compliance with therapeutic regimens. J Adolesc Health Care 1984; 5:124–126.

67. Beck-Sprague C, Alexander ER. Sexually transmitted diseases in children and adolescents. Infect Dis Clin North Am 1987; 1:277–304.

CHAPTER 23

Child Sexual Abuse

DAVID MURAM

Child sexual abuse is recognized as a common and serious problem that affects children regardless of their age, sex, socioeconomic class, or geographic location.[1] Children from infancy to young adulthood have been victims of abuse, with the average reported age at first incident ranging between 8 and 11 years.[1, 2] Other investigators have suggested that younger children (4 to 9 years) may be at a higher risk because of a naive and trusting approach to adults and a vulnerability to being misled regarding the meaning of various sexual activities.[3] Although the actual number of child victims is unknown, percentage estimates range from 1% to 38% of all females younger than 18.[2, 4–6] It is well accepted that the number of reported incidents of child sexual abuse represents only a portion of the actual number of victims. The National Center on Child Abuse and Neglect (NCCAN) estimates the number of child victims to be more than 200,000 per year.[7]

Some states have introduced child protection laws. One example is Tennessee, which introduced such a law in 1985. Among its provisions, the law requires that "Any person, physicians included, who knows or has reasonable cause to suspect, that a child has been sexually abused shall report such knowledge or suspicion to the department." During the first 2 years of the registry, the number of validated incidents of abuse involving minors rose from an average of 15 reports per month in 1984 to 60 validated incidents per month in 1986.[8] However, during the following 3-year period from October 1986 through September 1989,

the number of validated incidents of abuse remained relatively stable at about 30 to 35 per month.[9] Reported abuse rates were higher for girls than for boys; of 1985 separate incidents involving minors, 1600 involved females and 385 involved males. The validation rate in Shelby County, Tennessee, remained stable, at about 57%. In this particular study, the ratio of female to male victims was 4:1. Previous retrospective studies have shown the ratio to be about 2:1. It is possible that this higher ratio represents misdiagnosis and underreporting of male victims. Furthermore, the increased female-to-male ratio over a 5-year period reflects better recognition by professionals of signs and symptoms of abuse in female victims.[9]

In a number of areas throughout the country, special multidisciplinary facilities have been developed to provide care for these young victims of abuse.[10, 11] Still, many of these children are brought to emergency department facilities or to their private physician's office for evaluation. Many physicians have difficulty correctly identifying and managing victims of child sexual abuse.[12–15]

DEFINITIONS

The literature contains considerable variation and inconsistency in the descriptions and definitions of child sexual abuse and incest. Terms such as *molestation, sexual abuse, child rape, sexual victimization,* and *incest* often have been used interchangeably and without adequate specification. Furthermore, sexual interaction between two minors is considered by many to represent sexual experimentation and not abuse. Some authors have suggested that a 5-year age difference between the two minors is sufficient for the activity to be considered abusive,[16] but an exact age discrepancy for determination of abuse has not been established.

In an effort to reduce the inconsistency and confusion, the NCCAN adopted the following definition of child sexual abuse[7]:

Contact or interaction between a child and an adult, when the child is being used for the sexual stimulation of that adult or another person. Sexual abuse may also be committed by another minor, when that person is either significantly older than the victim, or when the abuser is in a position of power or control over that child.

This definition was purposely written to encompass all forms of sexual abuse and exploitation perpetrated on children by adults.

Incest, a major subcategory of sexual abuse, consists of inappropriate sexual behavior within the context of a preexisting family relationship. It includes relatives of various types and degrees of relatedness and individuals of the same or opposite sex. Because the stepparent and stepchild relationships are frequently indistinguishable from those maintained by natural parents, sexual activity between established steprelatives often is placed in the incest category. Sexual companions of a parent, such as a common-law spouse or a paramour living in the home, are placed in the incest category only if there is a longstanding relationship and that person is functioning as a surrogate parent. Such inclusion has practical implications, because in incestuous relationships, the home becomes an unsafe environment for the victim.

The legal definitions for crimes of sexual assault vary from state to state. Despite these differences, most authorities agree that for rape to have taken place, the following four components must be present:

1. A victim
2. Lack of consent or inability to consent (e.g., child, mental disability)
3. Threats or the actual use of force
4. Penetration

Not all sexual assaults are defined as rapes.[1] The physician treating victims of sexual assault should be familiar with the various definitions determined by his or her state. A list of definitions is included in Appendix 1.

THE ABUSIVE RELATIONSHIP

Child sexual abuse is a sexual relationship imposed on a child by an all-powerful and dominant perpetrator. Authority and power enable the perpetrator to coerce the child into compliance. Although in some instances the perpetrator selects the victim by chance (e.g., abduction), in most cases the perpetrator has known the child for a period of time, has easy access to him or her, and has opportunities to be alone with the victim. By using inducement (e.g., small gifts or special attention) the perpetrator engages the child in a relationship that gradually evolves into sexual behavior. Physical force is rarely used by a family member but may be used by a perpetrator who is not known to the child.

Initially the sexual acts are limited to exposure, light touch, etc. These rapidly progress to overt sexual acts, the most common of which is oral penetration. If another area of the child's body is to be penetrated, the next most likely opening is the anus. Vaginal penetration in very young children is limited, but the perpetrator will often rub his penis against the genital area of the child, an act known as *dry intercourse*. The hymen and the fossa navicularis may be injured during dry intercourse, but the extent of these injuries is rather limited. However, direct penetration of the vagina of a young child by an erect penis will cause significant injury.

As the sexual relationship develops, the perpetrator persuades or pressures the child to keep the activity secret. The child is made to feel guilty, ashamed, and responsible for this undesirable relationship. At times, threats, demonstration of force, or even the use of force are used to secure the child's silence. Usually, the child does not reveal details of the abusive relationship.

Disclosure of the abuse is often accidental, and the secret is usually revealed as a result of external circumstances. Someone may observe an abnormal pattern of behavior, or physical injury may bring the child to a physician's attention. Less frequently, the participant conscientiously tells an outsider about the abuse, either to share the experience or because the youngster wishes to discontinue the abusive relationship. After disclosure, the child may be under pressure to suppress publicity, information, and intervention, particularly if he or she has been a victim of an incestuous relationship. The perpetrator and other family members induce feelings of guilt and isolation in the child with the intention of forcing him or her to withdraw the complaint and stop cooperating with outsiders.

MEDICAL EVALUATION

History

When the victim is a young child, additional information is required. Victims of physical or sexual abuse must be removed from an unsafe environment, and thus it is extremely important to know who the perpetrator is, and how the child sustained the injury. The questions must be open ended and not leading. For example, it is preferable to ask, "Why are you here?" instead of "Who hurt you?" The information should be recorded carefully, using the victim's own words and not adult terms (Appendix 2). Although a detailed history is desirable, the patient should not be made to repeat the story of the incident over and over again. To overcome deficiencies that arise from the limited verbal skills of the young victims, other interviewing techniques, such as play-interviews, and the use of anatomically detailed dolls have been developed (Fig. 23–1).[17–19] The use of drawings often facilitates communication with these young patients and is discussed in greater detail in Chapter 24. When these techniques are used, the interviewer must be experienced, ask open-ended questions, and not lead the child to predetermined answers

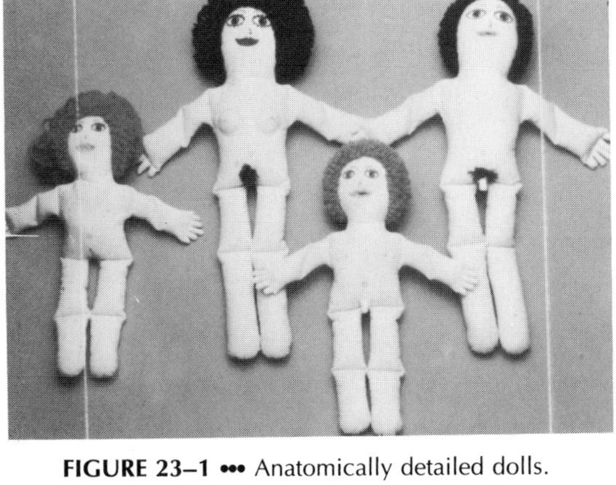

FIGURE 23–1 ••• Anatomically detailed dolls.

TABLE 23–1 ••• OBTAINING A HISTORY FROM CHILD VICTIMS OF SEXUAL ABUSE

General measures
  Provide a comfortable environment.
  Language and technique should be developmentally appropriate.
  Allow sufficient time to avoid any coercive quality to the interview.
  Establish a rapport with the child.
Questioning
  The initial questions should be nondirective to elicit spontaneous responses.
  Leading questions should be avoided. If such questions are used, responses should be carefully evaluated.
  Nonverbal tools (e.g., anatomically detailed dolls or drawings) may be used to assist the child in communication.
  Anatomically detailed dolls should be used primarily for the identification of body parts and clarification of previous statements.
  Psychological testing is not required for the purpose of proving sexual assault.
  At some point, the child should be questioned directly about the abusive relationship.

(Table 23–1). Even with these techniques, it is sometimes impossible to obtain a detailed history from a very young victim. The physician is then compelled to accept an account of the incident from relatives, police officers, neighbors, and other children. Throughout the encounter with the child, the physician should be aware of signs and symptoms commonly associated with child abuse (e.g., night terrors, change in sleeping habits, clinging behavior). The examiner should note the child's composure, behavior, and mental state, as well as the child's interaction with parents and other persons (Table 23–2).

Physical Examination

Most children can be fully evaluated in an office that is properly equipped to examine young children. The evaluation is well tolerated by most children. In rare instances, often after penile penetration of the vagina, a significant degree of trauma is present (Fig. 23–2), and a properly equipped operating room and general anesthesia are required for a thorough evaluation and repair.[20, 21] However, in most children the physical findings are less dramatic or absent altogether. Some forms of abuse do not cause injury, and in these circumstances an examination is not expected to detect any physical evidence of abuse.

Even when injured, many of these children

TABLE 23–2 ••• NONSPECIFIC SYMPTOMS SEEN IN CHILD VICTIMS OF SEXUAL ABUSE

Behavioral
   Anxiety, fearfulness
   Sleep disturbances
   Withdrawal
   Somatic complaints
   Increased sexual play
   Inappropriate sexual behavior
   School problems
   Acting-out behaviors
   Self-destructive behaviors
   Depression, low self-esteem
Physical
   Unexplained vaginal injuries
   Unexplained vaginal bleeding
   Bruising, bites, scratches
   Pregnancy
   Sexually transmitted diseases
   Recurrent vaginal infections
   Pain in the anal or genital area
   Recurrent atypical abdominal pain

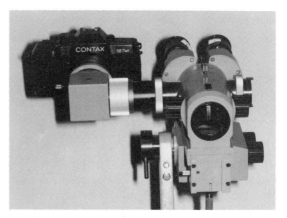

FIGURE 23–3 ••• A colposcope equipped with photographic equipment. The attachment allows the physician to use any type of camera, including a video camera.

may not be seen for weeks, months, or even years after the incident occurs. This delay allows semen and debris to wash away and most, if not all, injuries to heal. Physical findings, when present, vary with the degree of trauma sustained by the victim. Minimal trauma results in minor injuries that heal in a short time and leave no permanent scars. Deep lacerations take longer to heal and often leave scars that can be seen even after a relatively long period.

The use of magnifying devices to enhance anogenital findings is well accepted. Investigators have reported using a simple magnifying glass, otoscope, and/or colposcope (Fig. 23–3). The colposcope currently appears to be the instrument of choice for the examination of child victims of sexual abuse.[22–26] Colposcopy allows a detailed magnified inspection of the vulva to search for physical signs of abuse that may have escaped detection by unaided examination (Fig. 23–4). In this technique, the external genitalia are inspected through a colposcope under magnification. The labia are gently retracted downward and laterally to expose the hymenal ring and the posterior vaginal wall.[27] The Valsalva maneuver and the knee-chest position can be used in some patients to better visualize the lower vaginal walls. The genitalia are inspected both under regular illumination and through a green filter that better demonstrates vascular patterns. No solutions or dyes need to be applied to the genitalia during the examination.

Although the use of colposcopy may enhance the physical findings, most physicians'

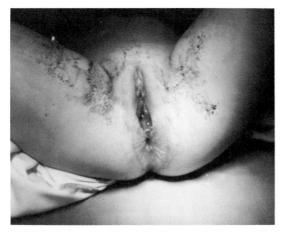

FIGURE 23–2 ••• A 20-month-old girl who sustained a significant vaginal injury from sexual assault.

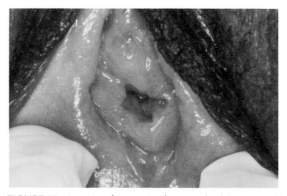

FIGURE 23–4 ••• A colposcopic photograph of the external genitalia. An intact hymen is noted.

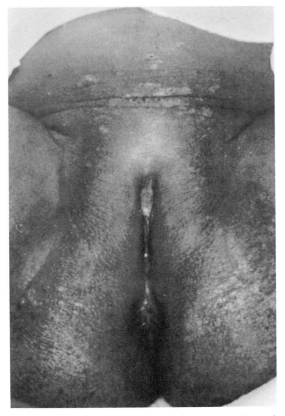

FIGURE 23–5 ••• A 14-month-old infant referred for evaluation of possible sexual abuse. Severe diaper rash was mistaken as representing genital injuries.

experience in the use of the colposcope for this purpose is limited, and thus the colposcopic findings should be interpreted with caution. Small areas of skin irritation and superficial abrasions that cannot be detected with the naked eye may be identified under magnification. Some of these lesions may not be the result of sexual abuse. Vulvar irritation is fairly common in small children as a result of poor local hygiene, maceration of the skin due to wetness from diapers, or self-scratching due to local infection (Fig. 23–5). Such nonspecific findings, enhanced by the colposcope, should not be regarded as definitively diagnostic of sexual abuse. Despite its limitations, colposcopy improves the examiner's diagnostic skills by providing an opportunity to review the physical findings under magnification. In addition, when equipped with a camera attachment, the colposcope allows the physician to obtain adequate photographs that can then be added to the medical record or used for education or peer review. Finally, when legal action is taken, these pictures can be reviewed

to refresh the examiner's memory and may be introduced as evidence. However, the evaluation of child sexual abuse victims and the use of a colposcope requires experience and training; otherwise, misdiagnosis is likely to occur.[15]

Some investigators have found the colposcope extremely useful.[25, 26] In one series, only colposcopic examination was able to identify signs of genital trauma in 59 of 500 (11.8%) patients. However, that particular series was comprised primarily of adult patients, and it is difficult to extrapolate from this series the usefulness of colposcopy in children.[25] In a prospective study limited to prepubertal children, other investigators have concluded that colposcopy does not substantially enhance the accuracy of detecting signs of sexual abuse in prepubertal children when compared with a careful unaided physical examination.[22] Most importantly, regardless of whether a colposcope is used, the physician must conduct a thorough examination and objectively record the findings. Unfortunately, consensus has not been reached regarding the meaning of the various specific findings observed in child victims of abuse.[28]

Abnormal Physical Findings

There are no well-defined criteria or accepted terminology by which to classify physical findings of sexual abuse; different terms are used to describe the same findings. A simplified classification of the physical findings observed in prepubertal girls has been developed (Table 23–3). This classification distinguishes nonspecific findings from those that

TABLE 23–3 ••• MEDICAL EVALUATION: CLASSIFICATION OF ABNORMAL FINDINGS

Category	Abnormalities
1: Normal examination	No abnormalities detected Variations of normal
2: Nonspecific abnormalities	Redness, irritation, abrasions Friability of the posterior fourchette Labial adhesions, hymenal tags, hymenal bumps and clefts Nonspecific infections Bruising of the external genitalia
3: Specific findings	Hymenal-vaginal tear Hymenal-perineal tear Sexually transmitted disease Bite marks on the genitalia
4: Definitive abnormalities	Presence of sperm Pregnancy in an adolescent

are highly suggestive or definitively related to abuse and has proved useful in subsequent legal proceedings. All physical findings are classified into one of the following four categories[29, 30]:

1. Normal-appearing genitalia
2. Nonspecific findings. These are abnormalities of the genitalia that could have been caused by sexual abuse, but are also often seen in girls who are not victims of sexual abuse (e.g., inflammation and scratching). These findings may be the sequelae of poor perineal hygiene or nonspecific infection. Included in this category are redness of the external genitalia (Fig. 23–6), increased vascular pattern of the vestibular and labial mucosa, presence of purulent discharge from the vagina, small skin fissures or lacerations in the area of the posterior fourchette (Fig. 23–7), and agglutination of the labia minora (Fig. 23–8).
3. Specific findings. This is the presence of one or more abnormalities strongly suggesting sexual abuse. Such findings include recent or healed lacerations of the hymen and vaginal

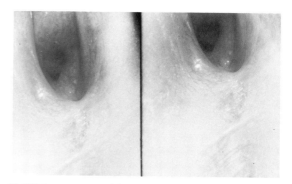

FIGURE 23–7 ••• Friability of the posterior fourchette. Notice the fissures caused by separation of the labia.

mucosa (Figs. 23–9, 23–10), enlarged hymenal opening of 1 cm or more, proctoepisiotomy (a laceration of the vaginal mucosa extending to the rectal mucosa) (see Fig. 23–2), and indentations in the skin indicating teeth marks (bite marks). This category also includes patients with laboratory confirmation of a sexually transmitted disease.

4. Definitive findings. Definitive findings consist of the presence of sperm.

Many injuries are superficial and are often limited to the vulvar skin. Within a few days the healing process is complete, and when the child is examined at a later date, the anatomic features of the anogenital area appear normal.[31] It has been shown that even in girls in whom sexual abuse has been documented, the medical evaluation fails to reveal specific findings in 50% of victims.[30, 31]

In a large prospective study, 205 prepubertal girls who were determined by child protective services to be victims of sexual abuse were evaluated.[30] Sixty-five (32%) had normal-appearing genitalia and failed to show any sign

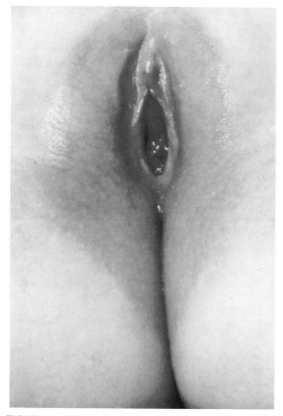

FIGURE 23–6 ••• Vulvar redness and irritation caused by nonspecific vulvovaginitis.

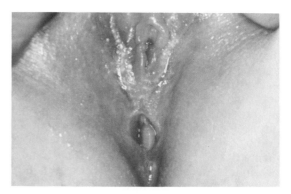

FIGURE 23–8 ••• Agglutination of the labia minora.

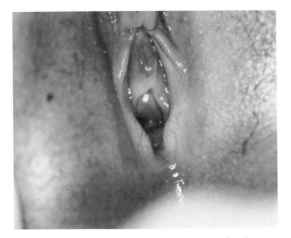

FIGURE 23–9 ••• Vagina of a 9-year-old girl who was assaulted 2 weeks before the examination. Notice a healing tear of the hymen and vaginal wall.

of previous injury. Nonspecific abnormalities were present in 45 (22%), and 95 (46%) had abnormalities considered specific for sexual abuse. Hymenal-vaginal lacerations were detected in 68 of these young girls (Table 23–4). In three, the examination revealed extensive lacerations through the posterior vaginal wall, with extension into the rectum. Two patients were found to have motile sperm in the vaginal fluid or on the vulvar skin. Venereal disease was noted in 31 girls; in the majority of these (25), there were no other signs of genital injury (see Table 23–4).

In general, the external genitalia and the anal area can be manipulated by oral, digital,

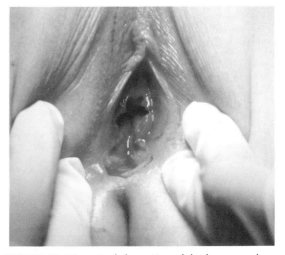

FIGURE 23–10 ••• Fresh laceration of the hymen and vagina after an assault.

and genital contact. Unless vaginal penetration occurs, injury is limited to the vulvar region. When the perpetrator rubs his penis on the child's vulva (dry intercourse), erythema, swelling, skin bruising, and excoriations are found on the labia and vestibule. Similar findings can be expected when the perpetrator digitally manipulates the vulva or introitus without vaginal penetration. These injuries are superficial and often limited to the vulvar skin. Within a few days the healing process is complete, and when the child is examined at a later date, the anatomic features of the anogenital area appear normal.[31]

The relationship between the size of the hymenal aperture and sexual abuse allegations remains controversial, and normative data concerning nonabused children are few or deficient. Observations by Cantwell documented that 74% of female pediatric victims with hymenal orifice diameters >4 mm had a history of sexual abuse.[32] The same author later described a decrease in hymenal orifice diameter, attributed to healing, after reexamination of 20 sexually abused girls.[33] In another study, Adams and colleagues reported average hymenal orifice diameters exceeding 6 mm in 23 abused girls who denied penetrating sexual contact (Table 23–5).[34] The investigators observed that hymenal orifice diameters increased as a function of both advancing age and degree of sexual contact. Emans et al. noted that a group of sexually abused girls had larger hymenal orifice diameters than a group that had not been abused. The average difference in diameter between the two groups was 1.6 mm, which is perhaps within the range of measurement error. Furthermore, only 7% of the abused girls had measurements exceeding the range observed in the nonabused girls.[35] In another study the investigators noted that 53% of sexually abused girls, including 26% of those who specifically described digital or penile penetration, had hymenal orifice diameters <4 mm. The study concluded that introital diameter is a specific (>90%) but not highly sensitive test (6% to 48%).[36]

The absence of physical findings should not be construed to suggest that the history obtained from the child is incorrect. One study correlated the physical findings and histories obtained from the victims with confessions obtained from the perpetrators.[31] The study documented the reliability of the histories obtained from the children. In only six instances did the assailant not confirm the child's story, but even in these instances, the assailant ad-

TABLE 23–4 ••• GENITAL FINDINGS IN PREPUBERTAL GIRLS (N = 205) WHO WERE VICTIMS OF SEXUAL ABUSE

Category	Findings	No. of Patients
1	No abnormalities	65
2	Redness and irritation	16
	Redness, irritation, and skin lacerations	12
	Skin lacerations only	8
	Labial adhesions	8
	Redness, irritation, and labial adhesions	1
3	Laceration of hymen	28
	Venereal disease	24
	Lacerations of hymen and enlarged hymenal opening (≥ 1 cm)	12
	Laceration of hymen, redness, and irritation	6
	Laceration of hymen, venereal disease	5
	Laceration of hymen, redness, irritation, and skin lacerations	5
	Proctoepisiotomy	3
	Laceration of hymen and skin lacerations	3
	Laceration of hymen, venereal disease, and labial adhesions	2
	Laceration of hymen, redness, irritation, and labial adhesions	2
	Laceration of hymen, enlarged hymenal opening, and irritation	2
	Bite marks	1
4	Motile sperm in vaginal fluid and laceration of hymen	1
	Semen on vulva, redness, and irritation	1

From Muram D. Child sexual abuse—genital tract findings in prepubertal girls. I. The unaided medical examination. Am J Obstet Gynecol 1989; 160(2):328–333.

mitted to sexually assaulting the child and confirmed penile contact, although penetration was denied. All the patients in that study were confirmed victims of sexual abuse by the perpetrators' admission, but the medical examination failed to detect abnormalities in 29% of the patients. Of all abnormal findings, hymenal-vaginal tear (HVT) was the most common finding observed in girls who described penile or digital penetration. Of the 18 girls in whom vaginal penetration was described, only 11 were found to have HVT (Table 23–6).[31]

Anal abuse is a common form of sexual assault against children, especially in male victims.[37, 38] Although genital injuries are often recognized as possible signs of abuse, anal and perianal injuries are sometimes dismissed by physicians as being associated with common bowel disorders (e.g., constipation or diarrhea).[39, 40] A number of studies have examined the issue of perianal abnormalities caused by sexual assault. In one study,[41] the authors attempted to collect normative data regarding anogenital anatomy from a sample of 267 nonabused prepubertal children ranging in age from 2 months to 11 years. In a significant number of these children, the investigators observed perianal erythema, increased pigmentation, smooth areas on or near the anal verge in the midline, and skin tags or folds. They failed to notice fissures, abrasions, lacerations, or hematomas in any of the subjects.

TABLE 23–5 ••• MEAN HYMENAL DIAMETER RELATED TO AGE AND TYPE OF ABUSE ALLEGED

| Type of Abuse | Age (yr) | | |
	1–5	*6–9*	*10–12*
Total group	n = 42	n = 29	n = 15
	0.54 ± 0.35 cm	0.97 ± 0.41 cm	1.17 ± 0.39 cm
Fondling only	n = 10	n = 12	n = 3
	0.62 cm	0.85 cm*	0.90 cm
Digital penetration	n = 3	n = 5	n = 3
	0.75 cm	0.91 cm	1.17 cm
Penile penetration	n = 2	n = 12	n = 5
	1.10 cm	1.29 cm*	1.45 cm

*Significant difference, $P < 0.0002$

From Adams J, Ahmad M, Phillips P. Anogenital findings and hymenal diameter in children referred for sexual abuse examination. Adolesc Pediatr Gynecol 1988; 1:123–127.

TABLE 23–6 ••• RELATIONSHIP BETWEEN GENITAL FINDINGS AND CONFESSION OF VAGINAL PENETRATION BY THE PERPETRATOR

Findings (Category)	Vaginal Penetration		
	Yes	No	Total
Normal-appearing genitalia	2	7	9
Nonspecific abnormalities (e.g., inflammation, labial adhesions)	5	3	8
Abnormalities suggestive of abuse (e.g., vaginal tears, venereal disease)	11	3	14
Total	18	13	31

Reprinted from Muram D. Child sexual abuse: Relationship between sexual acts and genital findings. Child Abuse Negl 1989; 13(2):211–216. Copyright 1989, with kind permission from Pergamon Press Ltd, Headington Hill Hall, Oxford OX3 OBW, UK.

Interestingly, the investigators observed anal dilatation, which was more prevalent the longer the child remained in a knee-chest position. With this dilatation, the investigators observed the loss of the slightly puckered anal verge and the flattening or smoothing out of the folds, which was attributed to the relaxation of anal sphincter muscles (Table 23–7).

Other studies have considered anal dilatation and soft tissue changes to be associated with sexual abuse. In one study, 143 children were evaluated and the following abnormalities observed: fissures or tears (n = 53), red-

ness and other minor skin changes (n = 53), reflex anal dilatation (n = 42), laxity of the sphincter (n = 38), venous congestion (n = 24), scars or skin tags (n = 8), and human papilloma virus (HPV) lesions (n = 4)[38] (Table 23–8). Further observations allowed the authors to conclude that virtually complete healing, even in very young children, is to be expected. This may take from weeks to years, with some anal appearances remaining permanently abnormal with scarring. Swelling of the anal margin largely disappears within 7 to 10 days. Anal dilatation commonly disappears in 1 to 6 weeks, deep fissures may take months to heal, and distended veins are one of the last signs to disappear. Anal dilatation in some children remains many months after abuse has ceased.[38]

Similar abnormalities were observed in another group of 310 sexually abused children.[42] Abnormal findings were present in 104 children (34%); anal dilatation in 61 (19.7%); skin tags in 44 (14.2%); rectal tears in 33 (10.6%); sphincter tears in 15 (4.8%); HPV lesions in 4 (1.3%); perineal scarring in two (0.6%); and bite marks in one (0.3%). Anal and perianal abnormalities were observed in 59 of 70 children (84%) with obvious indications for anal assault, but in only 25 of 175 (14%) who denied such abuse. Failure to document perianal abnormalities in almost two thirds of the patients may be the result of the healing process.

TABLE 23–7 ••• FREQUENCY OF PERIANAL FINDINGS

Findings	Number of Subjects Observed*	Subjects With Positive Findings	Percentage With Positive Findings
Erythema	168	68	41%
Pigmentation	251	74	30%
Venous congestion			
Beginning	113	8	7%
Midpoint	113	59	52%
End	113	83	73%
Anal dilatation	267	130	49%
Intermittent anal dilatation	130†	81	62%
Configuration during dilatation			
Oval	94	84	89%
Round	94	8	9%
Irregular	94	2	2%
Smooth area	81	21	26%
Dimple/depression	81	15	18%
Skin tags	164	18	11%
Scars	240	4‡	2%

*The number of observed subjects varied because of missing data as a result of changes over time in the number of variables assessed.
†Includes only those subjects whose anus dilated.
‡May include "smooth area" on anal verge, no photographs available to recheck findings.
Note: No abrasions, hematomas, fissures, or hemorrhoids were discovered in the 267 subjects.
Reprinted from McCann J, Simon M, Voris J, Wells R. Perianal findings in prepubertal children selected for nonabuse: A descriptive study. Child Abuse Negl 1989; 13:179–193. Copyright 1989, with kind permission from Pergamon Press Ltd, Headington Hill Hall, Oxford OX3 OBW, OK.

TABLE 23–8 ••• PERCENTAGE FREQUENCY OF ANAL SIGNS IN CHILDREN

Physical Sign	All Ages (N = 143)	0–5 (N = 69)
Fissures or tears	53	59
Reflex and dilatation	42	53
Reddening/skin changes	53	43
Laxity	38	37
Venous congestion	24	21
Tear	8	19
Scars/tags	8	3
Warts	4	6

Reprinted from Hobbs CJ, Wynne JM. Sexual abuse of English boys and girls: The importance of anal examination. Child Abuse Negl 1989; 13:195–210. Copyright 1991, with kind permission from Pergamon Press Ltd, Headington Hill Hall, Oxford OX3 OBW, UK.

Other disorders may cause perianal abnormalities. Such abnormalities are often seen in children suffering from Crohn's disease or Hirschsprung's disease. In children with significant constipation, the anal canal gapes when the buttocks are gently drawn apart. This is a normal anorectal reflex initiated by the distended rectum. Usually, stool may be seen in the anal canal. After defecation, minor small fissures may be seen for 2 to 3 weeks (Fig. 23–11). Reddening of the perianal area may be noted in children with fecal soiling.[41] Unfortunately, children who have been abused often suffer from functional constipation, and a damaged anal sphincter often causes fecal soiling.

The absence of abnormal perianal findings is easily explained. Many victims of anal assault do not sustain significant physical injuries, because the anal sphincter and anal canal are capable of dilatation. Penetration, even by an adult male penis, may occur without significant injury. The pain that follows anal assault may cause spasm of the anal sphincter and result in functional constipation, thus providing an explanation for the child's complaints of pain and rectal bleeding. Most children do not immediately disclose incidents of sexual abuse, and many victims are not brought for an examination for weeks, months, or even years after the abuse occurs. By that time, the injuries often have healed completely, and the physical examination reveals few, if any, abnormalities.

Although the literature describes large series of children who were evaluated after anal assault, it is difficult to conclude which findings are caused by abuse. More controlled studies are required to identify the specific findings indicative of anal assault.

It is estimated that there is a 20% likelihood that a sibling of an abused child has also been abused at some time.[43] In intrafamilial abuse, incestuous fathers may abuse more than one child, and some cases have been cited in which the father begins with the oldest child and abuses other children as they reach a certain age.

Since the 1980s, groups of children who have become victims of sexual molestation in ritualistic settings, with more than one perpetrator involved, have been described.[44, 45] Not surprisingly, these investigators have recommended that siblings of such sexual assault victims be evaluated as well.[43–45] In one study, investigators evaluated 247 young females, age 12 and under, who were referred for medical evaluation.[46] One hundred and eighty-eight girls were suspected victims of sexual assault (primary victims); 59 were closely associated with known victims of abuse and were referred only because of a request by child protective agencies (secondary victims). The two patient groups were similar in age and race distribution. Of the 247 girls, 174 were found to have abnormal genital findings. Nonspecific findings were present in 55 of 247, and findings considered specific for sexual abuse were observed in 119 of 247. The remaining 73 patients had normal-appearing genitalia and failed to show any sign of previous injury. Of the 59 girls in the associate group, 45 (76%) were found to have abnormal genital findings. Nonspecific findings consisting of inflammation were present in 5 (8%), and findings considered specific for sexual abuse were observed in 40 (68%). All 40 girls with abnormalities suggestive of abuse had HVTs. In 28, only remnants of the hymenal ring were observed. When compared with the primary victims, girls in the secondary

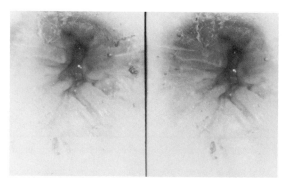

FIGURE 23–11 ••• Fine perianal fissures indicative of mucocutaneous injury. In this particular instance, the origin of the injury was unknown.

TABLE 23–9 ••• GENITAL FINDINGS IN SIBLINGS AND FRIENDS OF CHILD VICTIMS OF SEXUAL ASSAULT

Findings	Entire Group (N = 247)	Primary Victims (N = 188)	Associates (N = 59)
Specific	119 (48%)	79 (42%)	40 (68%)
Nonspecific	55 (22%)	50 (27%)	5 (8%)
Normal	73 (30%)	59 (31%)	14 (24%)

Reprinted from Muram D, Speck P, Gold S. Genital abnormalities in female siblings and friends of child victims of sexual abuse. Child Abuse Negl 1991; 15:105–110. Copyright 1989, with kind permission from Pergamon Press Ltd, Headington Hill Hall, Oxford OX3 OBW, UK.

group were more likely to demonstrate genital abnormalities suggestive of sexual abuse (x^2 = 13.7; P = .0011) (Table 23–9). There was no correlation between the age of the child and the presence or absence of genital abnormalities. Of the 59 secondary victims, 50 girls were interviewed by child protective agencies, and 24 of these (48%) disclosed that they were also victims of assault. However, the presence or absence of genital abnormalities on examination did not predict which girls were more likely to disclose abuse.[46]

Collection of Evidence

Although the primary objective of the physical examination is to attend to the medical needs of the victim, the examination has a secondary purpose as well: to collect samples that can later be used as evidence. Specimens should be collected from all victims for proper medical management of the patient. Furthermore, if the assault occurred within 72 hours of the examination, samples should be collected for the forensic laboratory and handled separately. The specimens collected for forensic purposes must be noted in the record, with a description of the location from which they were obtained and any associated findings (e.g., saliva collected from the patient's neck near a bite mark). All items collected must be individually packaged and clearly labeled and the containers and envelopes sealed and signed by the examiner. The evaluator may wish to use a commercially available collection kit (Fig. 23–12). Each label must include the following:

- Patient identification
- Specimen
- Site from which the specimen was collected
- Date and time collected
- Examiner's initials

All specimens must be placed in a container and sealed with special evidence tape, properly labeled, and with a routing slip attached. The physician may wish to use commercially available kits specially designed for this purpose.

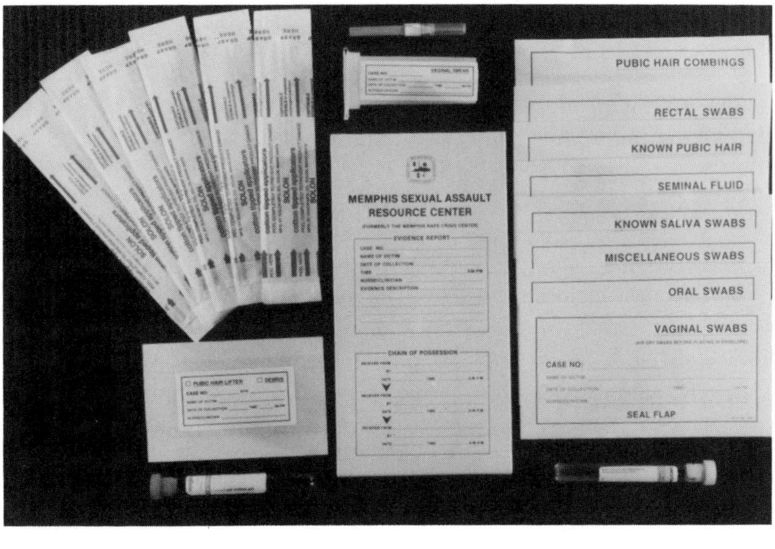

FIGURE 23–12 ••• Commercially available kit for the collection of evidence in sexual assault cases. The kit includes swabs, glass slides, envelopes, containers, labels, and sealing tape.

The kit is then given to the police investigator, who signs for it in the record and on the routing slip. All persons handling the materials must sign the routing slip. Such a system is necessary to maintain the chain of evidence; otherwise, results obtained from these specimens may not be admissible in court. If the kit must be stored in the physician's office, it should be placed in an inaccessible area, preferably locked, until it can be given to the police investigator or the forensic laboratory.

The clothing worn by the patient during the assault is collected and placed in a properly labeled bag. A description and condition of the clothes should be attached. During the general inspection, all foreign material (e.g., sand, grass, etc.) should be removed and placed in clearly labeled envelopes. Scrapings from underneath the fingernails and loose hairs on the skin are collected. A Wood lamp can be used to detect the presence of seminal fluid on the patient's body, as the ultraviolet light causes semen to fluoresce. The stain may be lifted off the skin with moistened cotton swabs for further analysis.

If vaginal penetration is suspected, vaginal fluid is collected and sent for culture, wet preparation, cytologic examination, and acid phosphatase determination. An immediate wet mount preparation performed by the examining physician can detect the presence of sperm. Culture swabs are obtained from the rectum, vagina, urethra, and the pharynx, even if the patient denies orogenital contact. When the cost is prohibitive, selective cultures may be obtained in asymptomatic children with a remote history of abuse. The specimens required are listed in Table 23–10.

TREATMENT

The following objectives must be addressed when treating a child who is a victim of sexual abuse:

1. Repair of injuries and treatment of sexually transmitted disease
2. Protection against further abuse
3. Psychological support for the victim and family

Repair of Injuries

Many sexual assault victims do not sustain serious physical injury, particularly if they

TABLE 23–10 ••• THE FORENSIC EVALUATION SPECIMENS TO BE COLLECTED

General
  Outer and underclothing if worn during or immediately after the assault
  Fingernail scrapings
  Dried and moist secretions and foreign material observed on the patient's body. Use Wood lamp to detect semen
Oral cavity
  Swabs for semen (two) if within 6 hours of the assault
  Culture for gonorrhea and other sexually transmitted diseases
  Saliva (for reference)
Genital area
  Dried and moist secretions and foreign material
  Comb pubic hair; collect all loose hair and foreign material
  Vaginal swabs (three)
  Wet mount
  Dry mount slides (two)
  Culture for gonorrhea and other sexually transmitted diseases
Anus
  Dried and moist secretions and foreign material
  Rectal swabs (two)
  Dry mount slides (two)
  Culture for gonorrhea and other sexually transmitted diseases
Blood
  Blood type
  RPR
  Pregnancy test (blood or urine)
  Alcohol/toxicology evaluation (blood or urine)
Urine
  Urinalysis
Blood or urine
  Pregnancy test
  Alcohol/toxicology evaluation
Other
  Saliva: use clean gauze or filter paper
  Head hair: cut and remove sample
  Pubic hair: cut and remove sample

were sexually active before the assault. Superficial injuries (bruises, edema, local irritation) resolve within a few days and require no special treatment. Meticulous perineal hygiene is important to prevent secondary infections. Sitz baths should be utilized to remove secretions and contaminants. In some patients with extensive skin abrasions, broad-spectrum antibiotics should be given as prophylaxis. In most patients, vulvar hematomas do not require special treatment. Small hematomas can usually be controlled by pressure with an ice pack, and even massive swelling of the vulva usually subsides promptly when cold packs and external pressure are applied (Fig. 23–13). Occasionally, large hematomas continue to increase

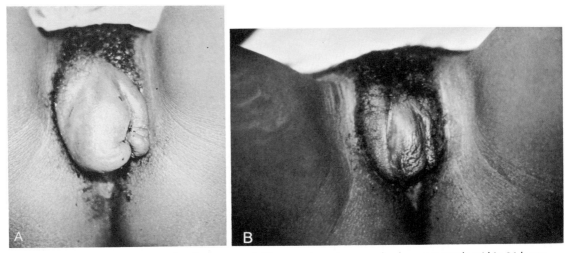

FIGURE 23–13 ••• *A,* A large vulvar hematoma. *B,* The same hematoma resolved spontaneously within 36 hours.

in size and should be incised, with the clots removed and bleeding points identified and ligated. Large vulvar tears require suturing, which is best accomplished under general anesthesia, using fine, absorbable suture material.

Bite wounds should be irrigated copiously and necrotic tissue cautiously debrided. A non-infected fresh wound can often be closed primarily, but most bite wounds should be left open. Closure is completed when granulation tissue is formed. After 3 to 5 days, secondary debridement may be required to remove necrotic tissue. Antitetanus immunization should be provided if the child is not already immunized. Broad-spectrum antibiotics should be prescribed for therapy rather than prophylaxis.

Although vulvar injuries are easily accessible for repair, injuries of the vagina or rectum may present surgical difficulties because of the small caliber of the organs involved. Special instruments, as well as proper exposure and assistance, are required. Many vaginal lacerations are superficial and limited to the mucosal and submucosal tissues. Such tears are repaired with fine suture material after complete hemostasis is secured. Vaginal wall hematomas form when bleeding persists underneath the repaired vaginal mucosa. The internal pressure created by the blood clot often controls the bleeding. If the bleeding continues, the overlying mucosa is incised, the blood clot evacuated, and the bleeding points identified and ligated.

Treatment of Sexually Transmitted Disease

If the child is asymptomatic, prophylactic antibiotic therapy is not necessary.[11] Instead, treatment should be deferred until the results of cultures and serologic tests for syphilis become available so that optimal therapy can be instituted. If vulvovaginitis is clinically suspected on the initial visit, appropriate antibiotic therapy is administered. When the infection is severe, a short course of topical estrogen cream promotes healing of vulvar and vaginal tissues. When irritation is intense, hydrocortisone cream (1%) may be necessary to alleviate the pruritis. A repeat Venereal Disease Research Laboratory (VDRL) test is required 6 weeks later to detect seroconversion.

Protection Against Further Abuse

It is imperative that the child's safety be assured. Is the perpetrator known? Can the child be safely discharged home? Sometimes it is advisable to admit the child to the hospital or provide temporary placement until these questions can be confidently answered. All patients who are suspected to be victims of child sexual abuse should be referred to child protective services for further evaluation.

Psychological Support for the Victim and Family

In the period immediately following sexual assault or disclosure, the victim and family often require intensive day-to-day support, counseling, and guidance. The therapist must be prepared to assist them to cope with the examination, the medical treatment, the investigative interviews, child protective services, and law enforcement agencies.

After sexual abuse, child victims often complain of depression, feelings of guilt, fear, and low self-esteem. The major thrust of emotional therapy involves strengthening the child's ego, improving self-image, and enabling him or her to learn to trust others and feel secure again. Appropriate referral for counseling is imperative. To begin the strengthening process, children need to realize that they are victims. They must ventilate their feelings of anger and hurt so that these feelings may be later expressed without experiencing additional guilt. Children often have both positive and negative feelings toward the perpetrator and often require help in sorting out these feelings. Sometimes children blame their parents for not protecting them. The parent-child relationship and intrafamilial structure are critical areas that require restructuring. After this crisis intervention phase, a treatment program using individual and peer group therapy is initiated. The patient and family should be offered treatment as required.[3, 47]

References

1. Kemp C. Sexual abuse, another hidden pediatric problem. Pediatrics 1978; 62:382.
2. Kemp C. Incest and other forms of sexual abuse. In: Kemp CE, Helfer RE (eds). The Battered Child. Chicago: University of Chicago Press, 1980.
3. Gelinas D. The persisting negative effects of incest. Psychiatry 1983; 46:312.
4. Russell D. The incidence and prevalence of intrafamilial and extrafamilial sexual abuse of female children. Child Abuse Negl 1983; 7:133.
5. Sarafino E. An estimate of nationwide incidence of sexual offenses against children. Child Welfare 1979; 58:127.
6. Weinberg S. Incest Behavior. New York: Citadel, 1955.
7. National Center on Child Abuse and Neglect (NCCAN). Child sexual abuse: Incest, assault and exploitation. Special report. Washington, DC: HEW, Children's Bureau, August 1978.
8. Muram D, Weatherford T. Child sexual abuse in Shelby county. Two years of experience. Adolesc Pediatr Gyncol 1988; 1:114–118.
9. Muram D, Dorko B, Brown J, Tolley E. Child sexual abuse in Shelby county, Tennessee: A new epidemic? Child Abuse Negl 1991; 15:523–529.
10. Muram D, Rivara F, Buxton B. Comment on current practice: Management of sexual abuse in prepubertal children. Pediatr Adolesc Gynecol 1984; 2:191.
11. Stovall T, Muram D, Wilder M. Sexual abuse and assault: A comprehensive program utilizing a centralized system. Adolesc Pediatr Gynecol 1988; 1:248–251.
12. James J, Womack W, Strauss F. Physician reporting of sexual abuse of children. JAMA 1978; 240:1145.
13. Ladson S, Johnson C, Doty R. Do physicians recognize sexual abuse? Am J Dis Child 1987; 141:411–415.
14. Orr D. Limitations of emergency room evaluations of sexually abused children. Am J Dis Child 1978; 132:873.
15. Brayden R, Altemeier W, Yeager T, Muram D. Interpretation of colposcopic photographs: Evidence for competence in assessing sexual abuse? Child Abuse Negl 1991; 15:69–76.
16. Finkelhor D. Sexually Victimized Children. New York: Free Press 1979.
17. Eaddy VB GC. Play with purpose. Public Welfare 1981; 39:43.
18. Goodwin J. The use of drawings in incest cases. In: Goodwin J (ed). Sexual Abuse Incest Victims and Their Families. Boston: John Wright PSG, 1982.
19. Cohn DS. Anatomical doll play of preschoolers referred for sexual abuse and those not referred. Child Abuse Negl 1991; 15:455–466.
20. Muram D. Pediatric and adolescent gynecology. In: Pernoll ML (ed). Current Gynecologic and Obstetric Diagnosis and Treatment. 7th ed. Norwalk, CT: Appleton & Lange, 1991, pp 629–656.
21. Muram D. Genital tract injuries in the prepubertal child. Pediatr Ann 1986; 15(8):616–620.
22. Muram D, Elias S. Child sexual abuse—genital tract findings in prepubertal girls. II. Comparison of colposcopic and unaided examinations. Am J Obstet Gynecol 1989; 160(2):333–335.
23. McCann J. Use of the colposcope in childhood sexual abuse examinations. Pediatr Clin North Am 1990; 37(4):863–880.
24. Slaughter L, Brown C. Colposcopy to establish physical findings in rape victims. Am J Obstet Gynecol 1992; 166:83–86.
25. Teixeira W. Hymenal colposcopic examination in sexual offenses. Am J Forens Med Pathol 1981; 2:209–215.
26. Heger A. Child Sexual Abuse: A Medical View. Los Angeles: United Way Children's Institute International, 1985.
27. McCann J, Voris J, Simon M, Wells R. Comparison of genital examination techniques in prepubertal girls. Pediatrics 1990; 85(2):182–187.
28. Adams J, Phillips P, Ahmad M. The usefulness of colposcopic photographs in the evaluation of suspected child sexual abuse. Adolesc Pediatr Gynecol 1990; 3:75–82.
29. Muram D. Classification of genital findings in prepubertal girls who are victims of sexual abuse. Adolesc Pediatr Gynecol 1988; 2:149.
30. Muram D. Child sexual abuse—genital tract findings in prepubertal girls. I. The unaided medical examination. Am J Obstet Gynecol 1989; 160(2):328–333.
31. Muram D. Child sexual abuse: Relationship between sexual acts and genital findings. Child Abuse Negl 1989; 13(2):211–216.
32. Cantwell H. Vaginal inspection as it relates to child sexual abuse in girls under thirteen. Child Abuse Negl 1983; 7:171–176.
33. Cantwell H. Update on vaginal inspection as it relates to child sexual abuse in girls under thirteen. Child Abuse Negl 1987; 11:545–546.

34. Adams J, Ahmad M, Phillips P. Anogenital findings and hymenal diameter in children referred for sexual abuse examination. Adolesc Pediatr Gynecol 1988; 1:123–127.
35. Emans SJ, Woods E, Flagg N. Genital findings in sexually abused, symptomatic, and asymptomatic girls. Pediatrics 1987; 79:778–786.
36. White S, Ingram D, Lyna PR. Vaginal introital diameter in the evaluation of sexual abuse. Child Abuse Negl 1989; 13:217–224.
37. Hobbs CJ, Wynne JM. Buggery in childhood—a common syndrome of child abuse. Lancet 1986; II:792–796.
38. Hobbs CJ, Wynne JM. Sexual abuse of English boys and girls: The importance of anal examination. Child Abuse Negl 1989; 13:195–210.
39. Clayden G. Anal appearances and child sexual abuse. Lancet 1987; I:620–621.
40. Roberts R. Examination of the anus in suspected child sexual abuse. Lancet 1986; II:1100.
41. McCann J, Simon M, Voris J, Wells R. Perianal findings in prepubertal children selected for nonabuse: A descriptive study. Child Abuse Negl 1989; 13:179–193.
42. Muram D. Anal and perianal abnormalities seen in prepubertal victims of abuse. Am J Obstet Gynecol 1989; 161:278–281.
43. Schmitt B, Grosz C, Carroll C. The child protection team: A problem oriented approach. In: Helfer R, Kemp C (ed). Child Abuse and Neglect: The Family and the Community. Cambridge, MA: Ballinger Publishing, 1976, p 95.
44. Haugaard J, Reppucci N. The Sexual Abuse of Children. San Francisco: Jossey-Bass, 1988, pp 155–156.
45. Green A. Special issues in child abuse. In: Schetcky D, Green A (ed). Child Sexual Abuse: A Handbook for Health Care and Legal Professionals. New York: Brunner/Mazel Publishers, 1988, pp 133–134.
46. Muram D, Speck P, Gold S. Genital abnormalities in female siblings and friends of child victims of sexual abuse. Child Abuse Negl 1991; 15:105–110.
47. Sgroi S. Handbook of Clinical Intervention in Child Sexual Abuse. Lexington, MA: Lexington Books, 1982.

Definitions

Intimate parts include the primary genital area, groin, inner thigh, buttock, or breast of a human being.

Sexual contact includes the intentional touching of the victim's, the defendant's or any other person's intimate parts or the intentional touching of the clothing covering the immediate area of the victim's, the defendant's, or any other person's intimate parts, if that intentional touching can be reasonably construed as being for the purpose of sexual arousal or gratification.

Sexual penetration means sexual intercourse, cunnilingus, fellatio, anal intercourse, or any intrusion, however slight, of any part of a person's body or of any object into the genital or anal openings of the victim's, the defendant's, or any other person's body; emission of semen is not required. In some states, **sodomy** is no longer separated from the above definition. It remains a legal term pertaining to a variety of sexual acts involving orifices other than the vagina.

Rape is the unlawful sexual penetration of the victim by the defendant, or of the defendant by the victim.

Sexual battery is unlawful sexual contact of the victim by the defendant, or vice versa.

Statutory rape is the sexual penetration of the victim by the defendant, or of the defendant by the victim, when the victim is at least 13 but less than 18 years of age and the defendant is at least 4 years older than the victim.

Medical Interview of Sexually Abused Children

1. Obtain information from the parent, social worker, or significant other, without the child present. Ask the child's terminology for genitalia.

2. Interview the child alone in a nonthreatening room, preferably not an examination room.

- Establish a rapport (let the child color, play with toys, etc.)
- Be unhurried, calm, nonjudgmental

3. Begin the actual interview:

- "Do you know why you are here?"
  OR
- "Some children who come to see me tell me that someone has touched them in a way that made them uncomfortable. Has anything like that happened to you?"
  OR
- "I am a doctor who looks at little girl/boy parts. We're concerned that someone has touched (hurt) your girl/boy parts that you didn't want to. Would anything like that have happened to you?"

4. What happened?

- Use dolls
- "Can you show me what happened?"
- "Did he/she touch you here or here?"
- "And then what happened?"
- "What were you wearing?"
- "What was she (he) wearing?"
- "Did he (she) take your clothes off?"
- "Were you on your side? your back? your tummy?"

5. Who did this?

- Even 2-year-olds can identify people.

- Repeat the question later in the interview for clarification.

6. Where did this happen?

- Four- to 5-year-olds are the youngest children who are able to answer "where?"
- "Where was your mother when this happened?"
- "Where were your family members when this happened?"

7. When did this happen?

- Seven- to 8-year-olds are the youngest children who are able to answer "when"?
- Ask younger patients: "Was it light or dark outside?"
- Use holidays—Christmas or summer, for instance—for a reference point.

8. Reassure the patient after the interview:

- "Thank you for telling me."
- "I believe what you said."
- Acknowledge that the patient is not at fault but will need to tell more people so that it doesn't happen again.

9. Explain the examination:

- "We need to check your girl/boy parts to make sure they are okay. Can you help with that?"

Note:

1. Do *not* ask leading questions. (*Hint:* These start with "Is," "Are," "Were," "Do," "Did.")

2. Dictate the history verbatim. Quote the child's answers in his or her own words.

CHAPTER 24

Expressive Therapy

LISA A. TURNER-SCHIKLER
KENNETH SCHIKLER

Physicians who provide gynecologic care to children and adolescents are likely to be familiar with an array of behaviors in their patients. This may potentially limit the scope of the examination and affect the condition of the patient. Whether the patient is an infant exhibiting normal stranger anxiety or a toddler recalling a recent visit to the pediatrician for immunizations that were painful, many normal younger children may be either mildly uncooperative because of apprehension or wildly resistant with terror. Also, when the indication for a gynecologic evaluation has provoked uncomfortable feelings in the parents, as may happen with ambiguous genitalia or sexual abuse, these feelings may be transmitted to the child, making initiation of a routine and painless evaluation difficult.

The toddler and preschool child frequently have "physician's office–phobia" and, in addition, are typically learning about privacy and body parts. The idea of a stranger examining their "private parts" can be overwhelming for some young patients.

The school-age child being evaluated for precocious puberty may be embarrassed about the examination. The sexually abused youngster may exhibit a wide range of behaviors at the time of examination; these are associated with feelings of apprehension regarding loss of control, embarrassment, anger, sadness, fear of pain, and fear of the potential implications of more questions, more examinations, and more strangers.

The adolescent female patient may have to deal with the frustration and anger associated with chronic medical conditions that might affect her ideal plans for future fertility (ovarian dysgenesis). The physician may also see patients whose behaviors become an issue after the examination. The adolescent with a diagnosis of pregnancy or a sexually transmitted disease may be shocked, distraught, angry, or seemingly blasé. In any case, in addition to requiring objective informational counseling, the patient's psychosocial needs must be addressed.

The adolescent with chronic pelvic pain may not obtain complete relief of symptoms from medical or surgical intervention. These patients can be expected to be frustrated and angry and to feel helpless.

These situations are daily occurrences for the health care provider evaluating children and adolescents, yet quite often the treatment of these behavioral needs is not addressed in traditional residency training. Even when the physician has an interest in providing for these needs, time constraints make such treatment less feasible. In addition, many of the fears, apprehensions, recollections, and emotions may be too sensitive for the youngster to comfortably verbalize. In light of this denial or repression, traditional interviewing/verbal counseling may seem too threatening for the initiation of a therapeutic relationship.

An expressive therapist may well assist in patient preparation for the gynecologic examination by gathering accurate information for diagnosis, by aiding patients dealing with issues regarding their long-term or short-term diagnosis and pain, and also by attempting to learn more about the patients. A number of expressive therapy programs exist in the United States.

HISTORY

Art therapy evolved from the discipline of psychiatry and was particularly influenced by both Sigmund Freud and Carl Jung, who placed immense significance on symbolism. Freud developed the concept of consciousness, expressed particularly vividly in the symbolic imagery of dreams. Jung postulated a "universal unconscious," with common symbols appearing among different cultures through various epochs.[1] As a result, Jungian psychiatrists have been especially interested in the art of many cultures.

The roots of art date back to prehistoric eras, when our predecessors expressed their relationship to their world in cave drawings and explored the meaning of existence in imagery. The use of art expression as a therapeutic modality did not come into its own until the 1940s through the pioneering efforts of Margaret Naumburg.[2] Relying heavily on psychoanalytic theory and practice, she encouraged clients to draw spontaneously and to free associate their pictures. She entered the world of therapy through her contacts with psychoanalysts whose children were students of the progressive school she directed. She was followed in the 1950s by Edith Kramer,[3] who worked extensively with children. Kramer's approach was different from Naumburg's in that she emphasized the integrative and healing properties of the creative process itself, which does not require verbal reflection. This differentiation of emphasis continued to polarize the profession, with one extreme placing emphasis on art, and the other on therapy. In the former, the creative process of the client is stressed; in the latter, the art forms the basis for insight.[4]

In the 1960s art therapy became a recognized branch of the health sciences. At that time, two events were significant in its development: the creation of the *American Journal of Art Therapy* and the establishment of the American Art Therapy Association. The first 2-year master's program in expressive therapies in the United States was established in 1969 at the University of Louisville.

Expressive therapy, which is used both diagnostically and therapeutically, recognizes and utilizes the value of artistic creative expression as a means of communication in the following ways: drawing, painting, sculpting, and creative writing. Each modality allows a nonthreatening outlet for emotional and psychological concerns. Thus, coping strategies are developed and/or strengthened.

COMMON TOOLS

Human Figure Drawing. The art therapist has multiple tools from which to choose. The human figure drawing (HFD) is one helpful diagnostic tool.[5] The total drawing and the combination of various signs and indicators should always be considered and should then be analyzed on the basis of the child's age, maturation, emotional status, and cultural background. It is not possible to make a meaningful diagnosis or evaluation of a child's behavior on the basis of any single sign on an HFD. To complete an HFD, the patient is given an 8½″ × 11″ sheet of paper and a no. 2 pencil and is asked to "draw a person."

Emotional indicators are reflective of a child's anxieties, concerns, and attitudes.[5] Examples include slanting figures, absent facial features, omission of body parts, and excessive shading. The three criteria for emotional indicators are as follows:

1. The indicator must be clinically valid (i.e., it must differentiate between HFDs of children with and without emotional problems).
2. The indicator must be unusual and occur infrequently in the HFDs of normal children who are not psychiatric patients (i.e., the sign must be present in less than 16% of the HFDs of children at a given age level).
3. It must not be related to age and maturation (i.e., its frequency of occurrence in HFDs must not increase solely on the basis of children's increase in age).

The materials for a house-tree-person (HTP) drawing are 8½″ × 11″ sheets of paper and a no. 2 pencil (Figs. 24–1 through 24–4).[6] The instructions are to "draw a house," "draw a tree," "draw a person," and "draw a person who is of the opposite sex from the first person you drew."

Text continued on page 389

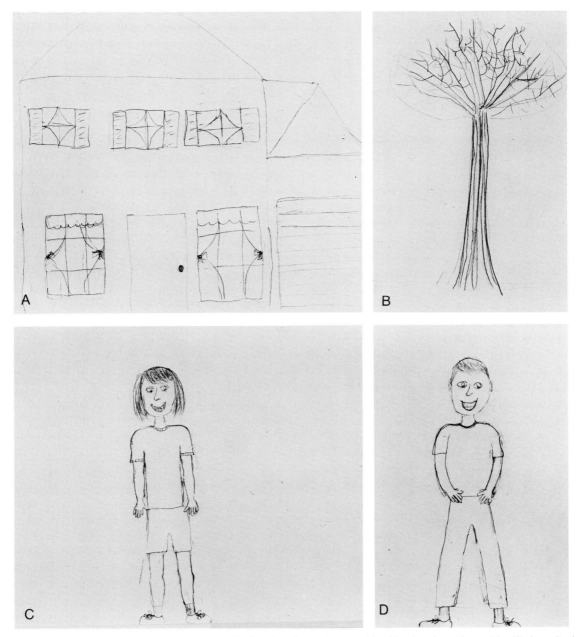

FIGURE 24–1 ••• *A–D,* House-tree-person (HTP) drawings by a 12-year-old white female with no identified medical problems suggest overcompensation (large house), anxiety (excessive erasures), aggression (teeth in drawings of people), strong need for privacy, and emotional trauma (scarring on bark of tree).

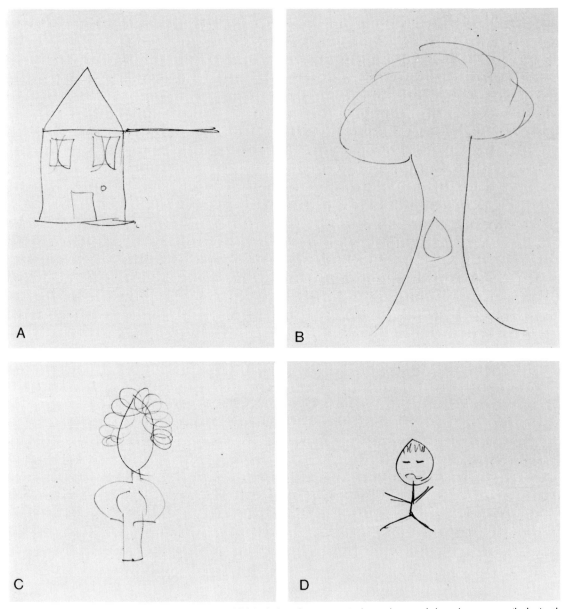

FIGURE 24–2 ••• *A–D,* Drawings by a 13-year-old black female suggest independence of thought, trauma (hole in the tree trunk), regression of figures (particularly the male figure), and helplessness (omission of feet and hands). Omission of female facial features is an indicator of an emotional problem.

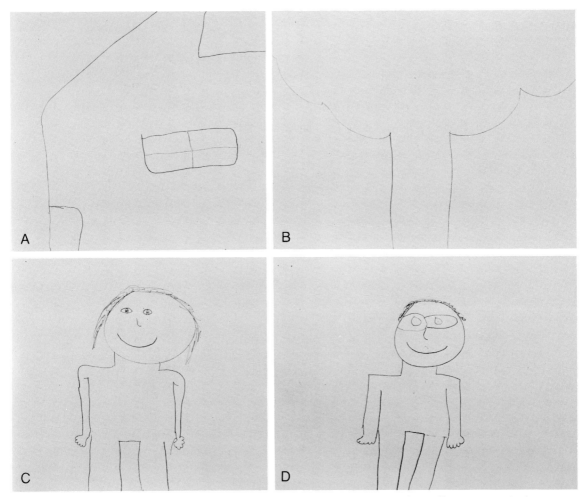

FIGURE 24–3 ●●● *A–D,* HTP drawings by a 12-year-old female suggest depression, low self-esteem, poor body concept, an aggressive tendency or attempts to overcompensate (large house and tree), and helplessness (omission of feet).

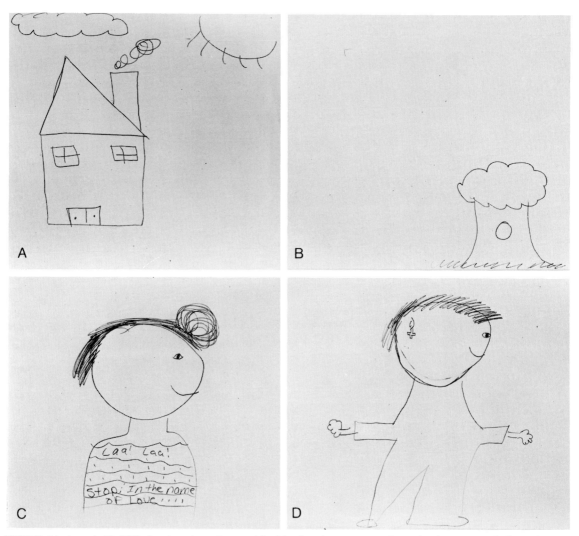

FIGURE 24–4 ••• *A–D,* HTP drawings by a 9-year-old white female suggest anxiety (clouds), trauma (hole in the tree trunk), denial (profile view of people), helplessness (omission of hands, legs, and feet of female person), and regression between people drawings.

Houses by normal patients (6 years and older) include one door, one window, one wall, and one roof. The tree drawing should be considered the productive gestalt. Some of the most penetrating psychological analyses of intrapersonal, interpersonal, and environmental adjustment can be made from drawn trees. Tree drawings by normal patients are expected to contain a trunk and at least one branch.

Person or human figure drawings are widely held to represent the drawer's self-perception and/or perception of his or her body image. Figures considered normal will be 6 or 7 inches tall on 8½" × 11" paper and will take about 10 to 12 minutes to complete. The head and face will be attended to first; figures will be near normal in proportion and will manifest some spontaneity. Erasing will be minimal; and line quality will be consistent with steady pressure. Self-sex is most commonly drawn first. Clothing will be present. Feet and ears will not be emphasized. Placement on the page illustrates feelings regarding self-esteem, with the bottom of the page suggesting low self-esteem (Figs. 24–5 through 24–8).

Kinetic Family Drawing. A third tool is the kinetic family drawing (KFD).[7] Instructions are to "draw your family doing something together." Analysis examines placement, barriers, omissions, elevations, action, light source, and rotated figures. This tool gives us an indication of how the family members relate to one another. Family-centered circle drawings[8] are also helpful in gaining insight into family dynamics.

Although HFDs, HTP drawings, and KFDs are helpful tools for assessment, many professionals outside the field of art therapy have questioned their reliability. Authors such as Palmer,[9] Cummings,[10] Golumb,[11] and Martin[12] have written articles addressing the strengths and shortcomings of projective drawing tests.

GRAPHIC DEVELOPMENT

Graphic development is a series of stages of graphic growth through which a child evolves as he or she matures.[13] During the disordered scribbling stage, the child experiments with holding the crayon and is excited by the random erratic movements. Pleasure comes purely from the motion. Children of all ethnicities and nationalities begin with scribbling. It is apparent that scribbling is a natural part of the total development of children, reflecting their physiologic and psychological growth.[13]

Controlled scribbling brings smaller movement in which children watch what they are doing. Visual control begins at this stage.

At about 3 years of age, naming of scribbles occurs with language development. Images can symbolize something else. Encephalopods, or head-foot-people, symbolize the human form. This, too, occurs across cultures.

Preschematic graphic development involves

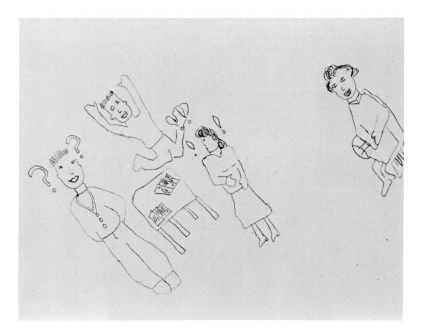

FIGURE 24–5 ••• Kinetic family drawing (KFD) by a 15-year-old black female suggests a barrier between patient, who is sitting contemplating a basketball, and family members. The mother figure suggests denial (profile of face). Questions and exclamation marks suggest chaos and ambivalence. The family's being drawn diagonally also suggests chaos and instability.

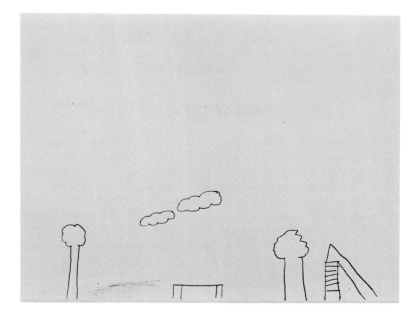

FIGURE 24–6 ••• KFD by a 16-year-old black female depicting a "picnic in the park" suggests anxiety (clouds, erasure) and low self-esteem. The family is absent from the drawing (isolation).

FIGURE 24–7 ••• KFD by 16-year-old white female depicting "family cookout." The slanting figures are an indicator of an emotional problem. The drawer is absent from picture. Anxiety is suggested. Regression of younger sibling is shown (omission of feet). The barrier is between the sibling and a man.

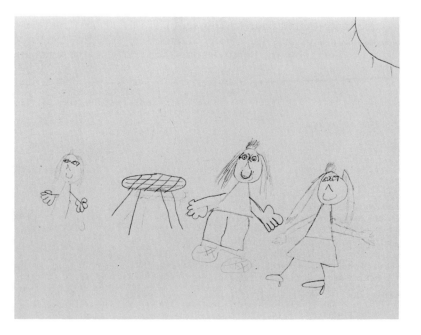

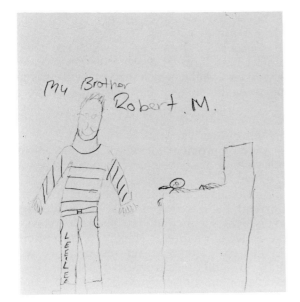

FIGURE 24–8 ••• KFD by 13-year-old black female of "cooking eggs" suggests low self-esteem and lack of family unity. The patient is absent from drawing, and only the brother is depicted as "family doing something together."

form and closure (line as pathway vs. line as boundary). The child at this level is beginning to understand symbolic play.

The schematic child has definite concepts of self. These symbols are used repeatedly. The more detailed the drawing, the more environmentally aware the child is. Piaget believed that environmental awareness was equivalent to intelligence. All forms, everything from people to houses to trees, have a particular schema. Things are put in order with a baseline and skyline and have a left-to-right orientation. This orientation occurs in Western culture because children learn to read in a left-to-right direction. Schema deviations occur because of a strong emotional reaction or experience that caused the child to deviate from his or her normal schema. If a child is scared, he or she may omit eyes from the figure; this is usually done unconsciously.

Dawning realism, or gang age, is the stage at which the child begins to separate from parents. Peers are important to the child, and he or she begins to draw differences between boys and girls, men and women. Children begin to understand the emotional use of color, and drawings contain overlapping of forms to show depth of field. Most adults draw at this level.

The pseudonaturalistic stage is characterized by children wanting things to look real. They blend colors and express sexuality in drawings, although on an unconscious level.

Adolescent graphic development becomes more symbolic. The adolescent's art work becomes a personal statement. It may stress resentment against society or sexuality and typically is very emotional. With an understanding of graphic development, the therapist can recognize regression.

APPLICATIONS

Expressive therapy, or art therapy, refers to the use of artistic expression for many purposes in a great variety of settings. There are art therapists in private practice whose work with clients is insight oriented on a long-term basis. Art therapy may be used for clarification purposes in a short-term crisis intervention center. Drug and alcohol addiction centers use art therapy to help addicts examine their lives. Art therapy is also being used increasingly with physically and mentally disabled people.[4]

Art therapy is probably used most extensively in hospital psychiatric wards and psychiatric outpatient settings where patients may be seen individually or in groups. In group settings, the shared art expression becomes an important vehicle of communication.[14] Patients may also participate in family art therapy, where family members draw their perceptions of the family and make joint pictures to explore family dynamics. This can be especially helpful for families facing issues regarding sexual abuse. Individual and family art therapy procedures are used for diagnostic and evaluative purposes as well as for treatment.

Hospitals and outpatient facilities employ art therapists to work with patients who have chronic illnesses or life-threatening illnesses such as cancer. The traditional application of art therapy for chronic pain extends to the patient with chronic pelvic pain, including the patient with dysmenorrhea. One useful tool in dealing with patients with chronic pain is a pain scale. The patient is encouraged to graphically represent her pain, thus gaining a sense of control or mastery over it by being able to establish boundaries for the pain's magnitude. Relaxation techniques and self-guided imagery are also useful for these patients.

The art therapist is called on to alleviate preexamination anxiety. Relaxation and guided imagery are employed. In guided imagery, patients are asked to visualize a calm, secure, safe environment; this is reinforced by having them graphically represent this haven. Patients are encouraged to allow their minds to wander back to that secure environment during the examination. The therapist also encourages fearful patients to draw their perceptions of the examination. These techniques were employed with "Janice," an early adolescent who came to our center for dysfunctional uterine bleeding. She had a great deal of anxiety regarding her first gynecologic examination and refused the examination. The expressive therapist worked with Janice, utilizing relaxation techniques and guided imagery, after which she completed the examination.

Hibbard and Hart[15] published their results of a replication study confirming previous reports of an association between children's HFDs and alleged sexual abuse. In cases in which children and adolescents are suspected of having been sexually abused, graphic representations, including the presence of genitalia on HFDs, are sought for diagnostic purposes because of their association with sexual abuse. The therapist also examines phallic symbolism in HTP drawings. The majority of the patients older than 3 years of age are seen by the art therapist. Typically these drawings indicate helplessness, with hands and feet—features expected to be included in drawings of normal children—omitted from the human figure drawing (see Figs. 24–2*C*, 24–3*C*). Further investigation often reveals a history of nightmares.

One early adolescent drew her recurring nightmare: a man telling her, "You die." The therapist enhanced the patient's coping skills in the following manner. The patient was asked to consider and draw ways in which she could protect herself in her dream. She devised and portrayed a plan in which she recruited a friend and brought along a baseball bat to restore her own sense of safety. In essence, by recognizing a coping fantasy, she attained a sense of control over her fears.

Another problem for which the therapist's skills are used is unplanned pregnancies, which continue to be a major concern of health professionals dealing with adolescent females. Currently, KFDs are being used in an attempt to discover factors that may be associated with the choice of whether to employ contraception. At this early stage in our research, we can draw no significance from our numbers. However, an interesting and unexpected association may be occurring. Of the contraceptors, almost half depict themselves as independent from the family—that is, either absent from the drawing or separated by distance or a physical barrier from the rest of the family members (see Figs. 24–5 through 24–8). In the drawings collected from those adolescents choosing not to contracept, the patients have consistently placed themselves within the family structure.

DRAWINGS DURING OFFICE EVALUATION

Obtaining drawings from the patient assists in the assessment of her concerns, thus allowing the opportunity to better address psycho-

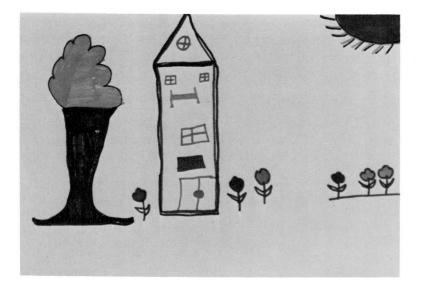

FIGURE 24–9 ••• Free drawing by 10-year-old white female. Note the differences between trees in Figures 24–9 and 24–10*B*.

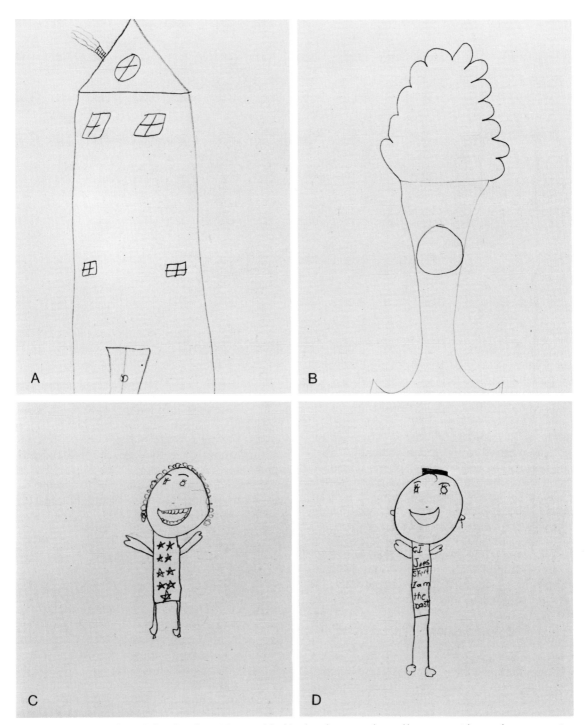

FIGURE 24–10 ••• *A–D,* HTP drawings by a 10-year-old white female suggest low self-esteem, evidence of trauma, anxiety (excessive erasure), poor body concept, and aggression. Note also the ''empty eyes'' in the people.

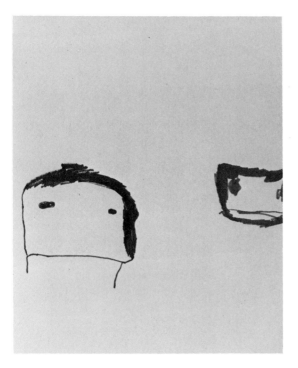

FIGURE 24–11 ••• Free drawing by 3-year-old white female.

logical manifestations. A helpful vehicle for communication is the "free drawing," in which the patient is instructed to draw anything she wants to draw. The free drawing in Figure 24–9 was completed by a 10-year-old white female using markers on paper. When she finished, the therapist asked her to talk about her drawing. She pointed to the green structure "floating" around the second story of the house she had drawn and said, "This is a bed with a magic little girl in the bed, and she disappears." She appeared proud of her drawing, which is schematically normal for her age. Further exploration by the physician revealed the following: "Two years ago, Daddy tied my hands to the bed and pulled down my swimsuit and put his thing inside me." Apparently, the patient's father had moved several states away and she finally felt safe enough to tell her mother what had happened. This patient also completed an HTP drawing during this session (Fig. 24–10).

In another instance, a free drawing was obtained from a 3-year-old patient who was not being very verbal with any of the staff. After she completed her drawing (Fig. 24–11), she pointed to the figure in black and said, "This is my Dad. He hurt me. He stuck a pencil somewhere." The patient then pointed to the purple drawing and said, "This is my Mom." Note the differences in size and dis-

tance between the two figures. After this drawing, the patient scribbled lines on paper, and although she appeared content, she did not verbalize anything further.

The drawings in Figure 24–12 were completed by a 15-year-old black female. Figure 24–12E depicts what the patient feared her mother would do to the boy who had allegedly raped her. At this point, we were able to problem solve and discuss how to handle the situation. This patient also completed an HTP drawing (see Fig. 24–12A–D).

CONCLUSION

Having the services of an expressive therapist available for patients has been a productive and enlightening experience. The application of therapeutic techniques from the field of art therapy has yielded the immediate benefit of reducing anxiety in patients and the long-term benefit of assisting patients to develop coping mechanisms to deal with a myriad of psychobiologic issues. Art therapy is a potential research tool that will allow us to learn more about the neurodevelopmental and psychosocial aspects of female health issues in children and adolescents.

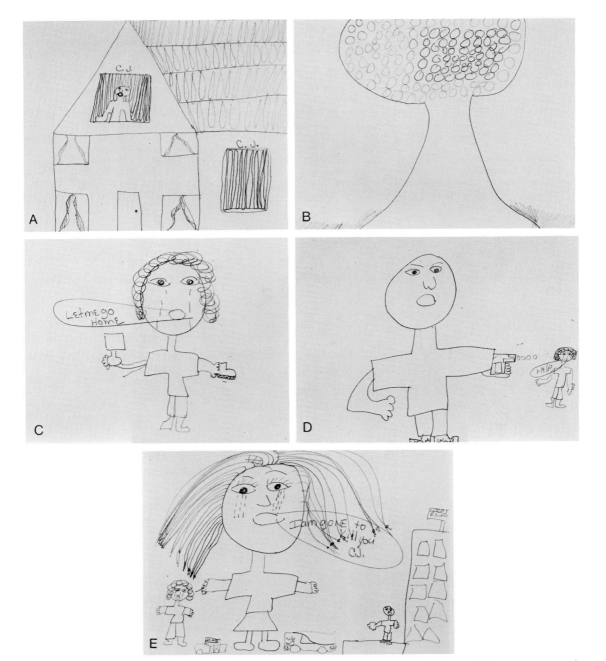

FIGURE 24–12 ••• *A–D*, HTP drawings by a 15-year-old black female suggest low self-esteem, high nurturance needs, feelings of fear, and anxiety. *E*, Free drawing by 15-year-old black female who chose pencil over markers to illustrate this emotional scene.

References

1. Jung C. Man and His Symbols. New York: Doubleday, 1964.
2. Naumburg M. Dynamically Oriented Art Therapy: Its Principles and Practice. New York: Grune & Stratton, 1966.
3. Kramer E. Art as Therapy With Children. New York: Schocken Books, 1971.
4. Wadeson H. Arts Psychotherapy. New York: John Wiley & Sons, 1980, pp 13–14.
5. Koppitz E. Psychological Evaluation of Children's Human Figure Drawings. New York: Grune & Stratton, 1968, p 36.
6. Odgon D. Psychodiagnostics and Personality Assessment: A Handbook. 2nd ed. Los Angeles: Western Psychological Services, 1986, p 66.
7. Burns R, Kaufman S. Actions, Styles and Symbols in Kinetic Family Drawings (K-F-D): An Interpretive Manual. New York: Brunner/Mazel, 1972.
8. Burns R. A Guide to Family Centered Circle Drawings. New York: Brunner/Mazel, 1990.
9. Palmer JO. The Psychological Assessment of Children. New York: John Wiley & Sons, 1983.
10. Cummings JA. (1986). Projective drawings. In: Knoff H (ed). The Assessment of Child and Adolescent Personality. New York: Guilford Press, 1986, pp 199–244.
11. Golumb C. The Child's Creation of a Pictorial World. Berkeley, CA: University of California Press, 1992.
12. Martin RP. The ethical issues in the use and interpretation of the Draw-a-Person test and other similar projective procedures. School Psychologist 1983; 38(6):8.
13. Lowenfeld V, Brittain W. Creative and Mental Growth. New York: MacMillan, 1987, pp 191, 474–479.
14. Sinrod H. Communication through painting in a therapy group. Bull Art 1964; 3:133–147.
15. Hibbard R, Hart G. Genitalia in human figure drawings: Childrearing practices and child sexual abuse. J Pediatr 1990; 116:5.

CHAPTER 25

Eating Disorders

PAULINE S. POWERS

The primary care physician is often the first physician consulted by a patient with an eating disorder. Approximately 95% of anorexia nervosa patients and 80% of bulimia nervosa patients are female. The disease process typically begins in adolescence with a bimodal risk at ages 14 and 18.[1] Secondary amenorrhea is a classic finding among anorexics. Primary amenorrhea and short stature may occur among anorexics whose weight loss or failure to gain in height or weight begins before or during the adolescent growth spurt. Menstrual irregularities also occur among bulimia nervosa patients but are an inconsistent finding. Patients with chronic eating disorders may consult a gynecologist for infertility and conditions related directly or indirectly to low estrogen levels (e.g., osteoporosis). The role of the physician dealing with the pediatric and adolescent gynecologic patient with an eating disorder and facilitating entry into appropriate psychiatric treatment cannot be overemphasized. The clinician must be able to recognize the common history of sexual abuse and the impact this may have on the physician-patient relationship.

DIAGNOSTIC AND CLINICAL FEATURES

Anorexia Nervosa

Anorexia nervosa is the most common cause of significant weight loss in adolescent girls in the United States. Among the general population, the incidence ranges from 0.45 to 1.6 per 100,000.[2, 3] However, among a high-risk population of adolescent girls in private schools in Britain, a prevalence of 1 in 100 was found.[4] The current diagnostic criteria (*DSM III-R*[5]) include weight loss of 15% or more below ideal body weight (IBW), a morbid unreasonable fear of obesity, body image disturbance (e.g., misperception of size as larger than in reality and negative attitudes toward one's appearance), and, in females, amenorrhea of at least 3 months duration. In patients whose weight loss (or failure to gain weight) starts before or during the adolescent growth spurt, linear growth may be impaired. The current criteria account for this possibility by specifying that there may also be a failure to achieve weight gain during a period of growth, leading to a body weight 15% below predicted levels.

Although the usual age of onset is between 10 and 25, patients as young as 4[6] and as old as 94[7] years have been described. In female prepubertal anorexics, primary amenorrhea occurs. In a series of 600 patients, 3% were prepubertal,[8] and 73% were female, compared with approximately 95% of adolescent and adult-onset anorexia nervosa patients. Eating disturbances in children aged 5 to 10 at the Piagetian stage of concrete thinking have been described[9]; these children may conceptualize food and water as one entity and restrict both, quickly becoming dehydrated and critically ill. The outcome in prepubertal anorexics is similar to that in adolescent and adult-onset anorexics: 62% show improvement, 10% are slightly improved, 24% are not improved, and 4% die.[6] However, even patients who improve often have a late onset of menarche and permanent interference with growth in stature and breast development.[10]

Bulimia Nervosa

Bulimia nervosa is characterized by recurrent episodes of binge eating of varying duration (from minutes to hours) and frequency (often up to many times a day); this binge eating is accompanied by feelings of loss of control. There are regular efforts to counter the effects of the binge eating by dieting or fasting, self-induced vomiting, laxatives, diuretics, diet pills, overexercise, and, rarely, abuse of enemas or thyroid medications or phlebotomy. Bulimia nervosa occurs across the weight spectrum. Approximately 50% of patients with anorexia nervosa also have bulimia nervosa,[11] and 30% of obese patients who present for treatment also meet the criteria for bulimia nervosa.[12] Binge-eating obese patients are more likely to try to counter its effects with dieting or fasting than with other purge methods. In addition, among patients of normal weight who have bulimia nervosa, up to 50% have a past history of anorexia nervosa.[13]

The current diagnostic criteria for bulimia are imprecise, and the level of severity ranges from clinically insignificant (e.g., infrequent binge eating followed by brief self-limited episodes of restrictive dieting) to life threatening (e.g., a patient who binge eats multiple times daily, purges by multiple methods, and has physiologic complications, including hypokalemia, hyperamylasemia, gastric erosions, and hematemesis).

Prevalence rates as high as 19% have been reported among female college students using self-report forms.[14] However, studies that have included patient interviews as well as certain frequency criteria (for example, binge eating at least three times per week) and purging criteria (e.g., by self-induced vomiting or laxative or diuretic abuse) have found the prevalence rate to vary between 1% and 2% of females age 18 to 30.[15] Although the usual age of onset is several years later than among anorexia nervosa patients, prepubescent patients with typical symptoms of bulimia nervosa have been described.

PHYSIOLOGIC ABNORMALITIES

Multiple physiologic abnormalities have been identified in both anorexia and bulimia nervosa patients. Problems commonly seen by obstetricians and gynecologists (e.g., infertility and amenorrhea), as well as other primary care physicians, are described in detail in later sections. Because at least 50% of the patients have both anorexia and bulimia, signs and symptoms of semistarvation, binge eating, and purging often occur in the same individual. The severity of the physiologic complications appears to depend on the innate vulnerability of the patient, as well as the duration and intensity of the abnormal behavior. For example, a 16-year-old girl who was 5'3" (1.6 m) tall lost weight from 115 to 88 lb (52.3 to 40 kg) in 6 months by severely restricting her food intake and severely overexercising; she presented with amenorrhea, cachexia, dehydration, low serum potassium, supraventricular tachycardia, "euthyroid sick syndrome," low serum protein, mitral valve prolapse, and both pneumothorax and pneumomediastinum. Another patient, age 32 and with a 16-year history of bulimia nervosa and subsyndromal anorexia nervosa, presented at 5'2" (1.57 m) tall and weighing 98 lbs (44.5 kg), with infertility, menstrual irregularities, enlarged parotid glands, mild cachexia but no dehydration, nomal serum electrolytes and proteins, elevated parotid amylase isoenzyme, and osteopenia. The difference in presentation of these two patients is partly related to the different methods used to achieve or maintain low body weight and the duration of the disorder. Rapid weight loss or very severe binge eating or purging are more likely to result in acute problems such as cardiac arrhythmias and electrolyte disturbances, whereas slow weight loss or prolonged but less intense binge eating or purging is more likely to result in chronic problems such as parotid gland enlargement, hyperamylasemia, or osteoporosis. The nature of the purge behavior is also very significant. For example, severe abuse of laxatives or diuretics is likely to be associated with acute electrolyte or cardiac problems.

In the following discussion, the physiologic complications of these disorders will be reviewed in terms of semistarvation, abnormal food or fluid intake, purge behavior, and overexercise. For each of these abnormal behaviors aimed at weight loss, the common complications and the relationship to presenting signs, symptoms, or laboratory data will be discussed. Certain clinical findings may relate to different weight loss methods. For example, low serum potassium may occur as a consequence of semistarvation or purging by any method. Another example is pneumothorax or pneumomediastinum; although this is more commonly found in patients who have purged (and thus cause elevated intrathoracic pressure), in the patient described earlier, it was related to a combination of factors, including overexercise and semistarvation. As a final example, hyperamylasemia and enlarged parotid glands are more commonly found in patients who chronically induce vomiting, but they can also occur during severe semistarvation, in patients who binge eat and do not purge, or during the weight gain phase in recovery from anorexia nervosa.

Semistarvation

Cardiac abnormalities are common in patients with low weight.[16, 17] Prolonged QT intervals and ventricular arrhythmias are the most dangerous of these and are usually associated with electrolyte disturbances, especially low potassium levels. Purging by vomiting and particularly by laxative or diuretic abuse can also result in electrolyte disturbances, which are usually, but not always, reflected in low serum levels. Total body potassium stores may fall significantly before serum levels fall.[18] Electrocardiographic changes include ST-T wave abnormalities and U waves when serum potassium is low. Decreased cardiac performance and decreased exercise tolerance also occur.

Classic endocrine abnormalities include the "euthyroid sick syndrome"; amenorrhea associated with decreased serum levels of luteinizing hormone (LH), follicle-stimulating hormone (FSH), and estradiol; and elevated cortisol levels; these abnormalities are described in detail later in this chapter. Skeletal complications, including early osteopenia and osteoporosis with atraumatic fractures, are also common. The most frequent gastrointestinal consequence of semistarvation is delayed gastric emptying[19]; the associated postprandial discomfort often facilitates continued weight loss.

Imaging studies of the brain have documented mild to moderate cerebral atrophy and enlarged ventricles in up to a third of patients[20]; these abnormalities normalize in some, but not all, patients after weight restoration.[21] One positron emission tomography study of five anorexic patients who did not binge or purge found glucose hypermetabolism in the head of the caudate that normalized with weight gain.[22] Although neuropsychological abnormalities (including abnormalities on sections of the Wechsler Adult Intelligence Scale[23]) have been found in anorexics, it is unknown whether these abnormalities correlate with the changes noted in various radiographic studies of the brain.

Hematologic abnormalities[24] include leukopenia, anemia, mild thrombocytopenia, and bone marrow hypoplasia. Immunologic studies have found a wide variety of abnormalities, most notably decreased complement components (especially, complement factor 3 [C–3]), often not associated with decreased albumin.[25] One interesting finding is that some semistarved anorexia nervosa patients seem to be relatively resistant to viral infections until weight falls below 60% of IBW.[26] Decreased fat and muscle content are hallmarks of the disorder and are etiologically related to a number of the physiologic and cognitive complications, including skeletal, cardiac, and (probably) central nervous system changes.

Abnormal Food and Fluid Intake

Binge eating is a subjective term that includes a range of behaviors from consumption of a trivial number of calories (for example, consumption of a carrot stick labeled a "binge" by the patient), to normal food consumption, to consumption of enormous quantities of food (up to 20,000 calories at a time). Binge eating of large quantities can result in gastric dilatation or perforation.[27] More commonly, binge eating carbohydrates contributes to the dental caries that occur in bulimia.[28] Benign parotid hypertrophy[29, 30] may also develop, resulting in swollen cheeks; this condition is usually, but not always, painless. Binge eating usually results in an increase in fat content, even when associated with purge behavior, since it is primarily the components of lean body stores that are depleted with purging.

Unusual eating habits aimed at attenuating hunger may also result in significant complications. For example, patients may drink large quantities of water and develop decreased concentrating capacity of the kidneys.[31] Large quantities of low-calorie, carotene-containing foods (e.g., green vegetables) may be consumed and result in a yellowish skin tone, particularly of the soles and palms, as well as elevated serum carotene levels.[32]

Purge Behavior

The wide range of purge behaviors used results in a variety of clinical presentations. Electrolyte abnormalities may include hypokalemia, hyponatremia, and hypomagnesemia. Dental complications include loss of enamel and dentin on teeth contacting the lingual surfaces of the tongue.[28] Buccal erosions may develop from regurgitated hydrochloric acid. Dry mouth, associated with a decrease in pH, decreased buffering capacity, and decreased quantity and quality of the saliva, may also occur,[33] and benign parotid hypertrophy may develop secondary to purging by vomiting.[29] Pneumothorax, pneumomediastinum, or subcutaneous emphysema may result from increased intrathoracic pressure caused by induced vomiting.[34]

Overexercise

As discussed in detail later, overexercise, particularly when associated with less than optimal fat content, may be related to an increased risk of osteopenia or osteoporosis. Exercise is used by many eating disorder patients as a way to facilitate weight loss and counter anticipated weight gain after binge eating.

MENSTRUAL FUNCTION: ENDOCRINE AND NEUROCHEMICAL PARAMETERS

Of female anorexia nervosa patients who develop anorexia nervosa after menarche, at least 25% develop amenorrhea before significant weight loss.[35, 36] This finding has prompted numerous endocrine studies of patients with anorexia nervosa. Since the late 1980s, research has also focused on the endocrine abnormalities of patients with bulimia nervosa, both those at normal weight and those with coexisting anorexia nervosa.

Part of the fascination with the endocrine changes that occur in anorexia nervosa is the fact that patients who are semistarved and regain weight often progress from prepubertal through pubertal to adult stages of hormonal development and thus provide a clinical model for understanding puberty. Boyer and colleagues[37] demonstrated a regression in the circadian secretory pattern of LH to prepubertal levels at the nadir of weight loss; with weight gain, the change in the LH secretory pattern progressed from the prepubertal pattern (low levels of LH throughout the 24-hour period) to early premenarchal patterns (increased levels of LH secretion during sleep) and then to late pubertal patterns (a marked increase of LH secretion during sleep and episodic secretion of LH during waking) and to the normal adult pattern (episodic secretion of LH of equal magnitude during sleep and waking). Although only a few patients were studied, this report set the stage for using the weight recovery phase of anorexia nervosa as a model for the changes that occur during puberty in the normal female. Clinically, this is a useful model, because patients with anorexia nervosa who gain weight have signs and symptoms that parallel (but do not duplicate) normal puberty; for example, acne begins, and breast enlargement and tenderness develop during weight restoration.

Hypothalamic-Pituitary-Ovarian Axis in Anorexia Nervosa

Abnormalities of the hypothalamic-pituitary-ovarian (HPO) axis include low estradiol levels, often below 10 pg/ml,[38] although levels as high as 32 pg/ml have been reported.[39] The lowest levels are noted in patients who restrict their caloric intake, higher levels are noted in patients who purge, and intermediate levels occur in patients who alternate between the two methods. Gonadotropin levels (LH and FSH) are routinely low.[39] The response of LH and FSH to gonadotropin-releasing hormone (GnRH) may be normal, absent, or blunted; qualitatively normal but delayed; or present only after repeated injections of GnRH.[40]

Although weight loss may partly explain the endocrine changes, there is evidence that other factors are involved. Weiner[40] has estimated that only 50% of the variance in response to GnRH is accounted for by weight loss alone. Vigersky and colleagues[41] found that dieting women who lost an average of 19.5% of IBW and developed amenorrhea had normal LH levels. In another study of five healthy women who fasted for 21 days (average weight loss, 8 kg), two continued to have adult LH patterns.[42] Other factors[43] that may contribute to the endocrine abnormalities include changes in fat content, restriction of carbohydrates, vitamin deficiency, binge eating, altered timing of eating, electrolyte imbalance, volume depletion, hyperactivity, sleep disturbance, substance abuse (including diet pills, thyroid medications, diuretics, and laxatives), alcohol, caffeinism (i.e., consumption of large quantities of beverages containing caffeine to assuage hunger), and psychological stress. The rapidity and severity of weight loss, purging by vomiting, and the duration of any of these factors may also affect hormonal levels.

Not all weight-restored anorexics resume menses.[44] During weight recovery, estradiol increases in some, but not all, patients, even though gonadotropin levels rise.[45] Adult circadian patterns of gonadotropins also resume in some, but not all, patients.

Several problems have beset studies of the resumption of menses. First, some patients have been declared weight restored even when they were 15% below IBW. Second, it is unclear whether some patients may require higher weights for normal endocrine function (i.e., they may have a physiologic "set point" that is above normal on the usual height-weight tables); therefore, they may not actually be weight restored when in the IBW range. Meyer and colleagues[46] have found that weight-restored anorexics who regain menses have fewer preoccupations with food and weight than weight-restored patients who do not regain menses. Perhaps these patients are not at their own IBW.

HPO Axis in Bulimia Nervosa

Menstrual irregularities occur in 20% to 64% of bulimics. In one study,[43] 18 of 28 female patients had a history of an episode of amenorrhea lasting 3 months or longer. Pirke and colleagues[47] found inadequate follicular development as evidenced by low estradiol levels in mildly underweight bulimic patients; in normal and slightly overweight bulimic patients, they found luteal phase dysfunction as evidenced by low serum progesterone levels.

Reports on LH and FSH in bulimia nervosa patients are conflicting. For example, normal plasma LH and FSH levels have been reported in women who purge by vomiting, but elevated levels have been reported in women who purge by laxative abuse.[48] In another study,[49] no significant differences were found between bulimics and normal controls in the nocturnal secretion of LH, but there were highly significant differences in the secretion of FSH; in addition, plasma LH and FSH levels were significantly reduced in bulimics with evidence of decreased caloric intake. Kiriike et al.[50] found low basal LH levels in four of nine bulimics with oligomenorrhea or amenorrhea, but normal responses of LH to GnRH; there was a significant correlation between basal LH levels and body weight (which ranged from 86% to 108% of IBW).

Part of the difficulty in assessing these studies is that bulimia nervosa occurs in patients across the weight spectrum, with varying degrees of semistarvation determined only in part by weight. For example, in the study by Fichter and colleagues,[49] the weight range was 84% to 113% of IBW, which may well include patients who would also meet the criteria for anorexia nervosa. They found lower levels of LH and FSH in bulimics who had low triiodothyronine (T_3) levels and low caloric intake during the week preceding the testing. Another complicating factor is a previous history of anorexia nervosa. For example, Russell[13] reported that when weight-recovered anorexia nervosa patients develop bulimic symptoms, age-inappropriate LH patterns persist. Gonadotropin secretion has also been studied in bulimia nervosa by Schweiger and coworkers.[51] In a series of 22 normal-weight bulimic patients, an increased rate of ovarian dysfunction and decreased pulsatile LH secretion appeared to be important mechanisms associated with the disease process. Furthermore, it was hypothesized that the observed increased serum cortisol levels indicated activation of the hypothalamic-pituitary-adrenal axis and were believed to be associated with the pathogenesis of gonadal dysfunction in bulimics (Fig. 25–1).

Thus, there is some evidence that HPO axis abnormalities occur in bulimia nervosa patients, although generally the abnormalities are less pronounced and less consistent than those in anorexia nervosa patients. Detailed studies involving dynamic testing of the HPO axis of normal-weight bulimia patients have yet to be done. In addition, complications induced by a previous history of anorexia nervosa or a cur-

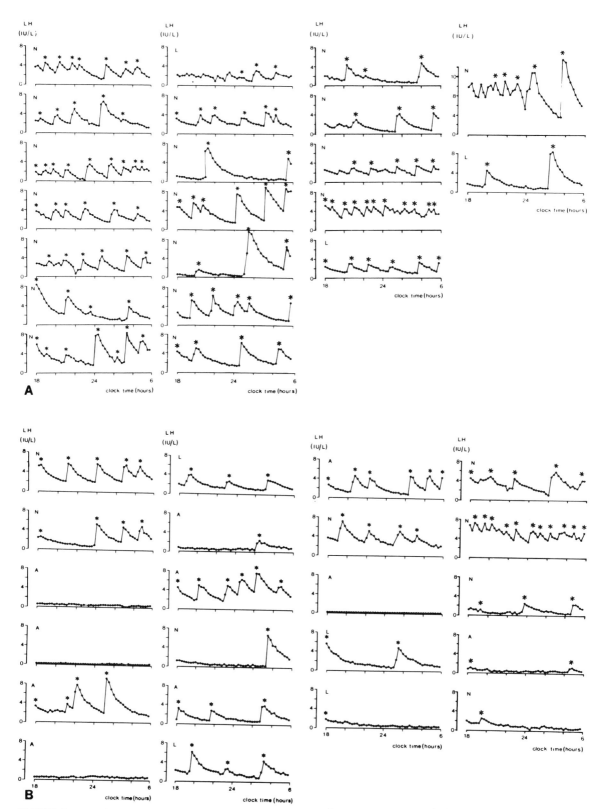

FIGURE 25–1 ••• Mean serum LH concentrations (IU/L) measured at 15-minute intervals for 12 hours during the early follicular phase for each subject. *A*, Normal controls. *B*, Bulimic women. The asterisks indicate significant pulses, detected by the Pulsar program. (From Schweiger U, Pirke KM, Laessle RG, Fichter MM. Gonadotropin secretion in bulimia nervosa. J Clin Endocrinol Metab 1992; 74(5):1124. © The Endocrine Society.)

rent state of semistarvation (not necessarily related to whether the patient is at or near IBW) makes studies of bulimia nervosa difficult.

Future studies will need to control for the presence of semistarvation.[52] During the first hours of starvation, glycogen body reserves are depleted. Next, muscle tissue is consumed, and amino acids form the substrate for gluconeogenesis. Finally, free fatty acids serve as the energy supply in many tissues, including muscle. However, free fatty acids cannot cross the blood-brain barrier, and the energy supply of the brain, usually supplied by glucose, is instead supplied by ketones, the metabolites of free fatty acids. After several days of starvation, plasma levels of the ketone bodies β-hydroxybutyric acid (β-HBA) and acetoacetate rise. Thus, measurement of β-HBA has been used as one index of starvation. In anorexia nervosa patients, β-HBA levels are very significantly elevated at low weights but quickly fall during the first few weeks of nutritional rehabilitation.[53] T_3 levels have also been used as an index of semistarvation (see "Hypothalamic-Pituitary-Thyroid Axis Abnormalities").

Premenstrual Exacerbation of Binge Eating

Some bulimic patients may have an increase in binge eating before menses. Animal studies have documented a relationship between food intake and the menstrual cycle.[54] In a pilot study of eight normal women, there was an average daily caloric increase of 500 calories during the 10 days after ovulation compared with the 10 days before.[55]

Although Leon and colleagues[56] did not find an association between menstrual phase and frequency of binge eating, a study by Gladis and Walsh[57] found a modest but statistically significant premenstrual exacerbation of binge eating. The subjects in the two studies were drawn from different clinical situations, and the former study compared group differences, whereas the latter study compared menstrual phase differences within the same subject, which is probably a more relevant comparison.

OTHER ENDOCRINE ABNORMALITIES

Hypothalamic-Pituitary-Thyroid Axis Abnormalities

The hypothalamic-pituitary-thyroid (HPT) axis has been particularly well studied in an-orexia nervosa patients.[43] The majority of patients with anorexia nervosa have the "euthyroid sick syndrome," characterized by T_3 in the hypothyroid range, elevated reverse T_3 (rT3, the metabolic inactive isomer of T_3), normal or slightly decreased serum thyroxine (T_4) levels but normal free T_4 levels, and a normal baseline thyroid-stimulating hormone (TSH) level. Low concentrations of T_3 are the most frequently encountered abnormality found in nonthyroidal disease and have been correlated with degree of weight loss. About 80% to 90% of T_3, which is the more active thyroid hormone, is derived from the peripheral conversion of T_4. The low serum T_3 level represents a protective metabolic adaptation of the body to starvation or carbohydrate restriction. Most of these changes return to normal with nutritional rehabilitation.

The thyrotropin-releasing hormone (TRH) stimulation test is abnormal in some anorexia nervosa patients. The normal response to TRH is a surge of TSH, released from the pituitary, that peaks in 15 to 20 minutes. In anorexics there is a delayed response in about 50% of patients and a blunted response in about 15%.[43] This abnormality is not typical of primary hypothyroidism (which produces an exaggerated response) and is probably a reflection of hypothalamic dysfunction.

Findings have been variable in bulimia nervosa patients, with some studies showing normal baseline T_3, T_4, rT_3, and TSH levels and other studies finding significantly lower levels. One important difference between anorexia nervosa and bulimia nervosa is that rT_3 levels are not elevated in bulimia nervosa.[58] Another difference is that the TSH response to TRH is not usually delayed but is blunted more often than in anorexia nervosa patients.[59, 60] Blunting of the TSH response to TRH has been associated with other psychiatric disorders, particularly depression.[61]

Abnormalities of the Hypothalamic-Pituitary-Adrenal Axis

Elevated free urinary cortisol levels[62] and elevated mean 24-hour total cortisol levels[63] have been documented in anorexia nervosa patients. The 24-hour secretory pattern of cortisol is also disturbed, with elevated levels occurring during the evening and first half of the night, when values normally are low or undetectable.[63] The plasma half-life of cortisol is also prolonged[64] as a result of decreased hepatic metabolism of cortisol. It may be that the cortisol production rate does not increase absolutely, but rather in relationship to body weight and body surface area, although this would not account for the changes in secretory pattern.[65] The precise location of the abnormality in the HPA axis is unknown, but the normal adrenal response to adrenocorticotropic hormone (ACTH) administration, coupled with normal pituitary responses to glucocorticoids (inferred from the study by Gold et al.,[66] who found a blunted ACTH response to corticotropin-releasing hormone in the presence of increased glucocorticoids), suggests that the abnormality is at the level of the hypothalamus or above.

The overnight dexamethasone suppression test (DST) is easily performed to test for HPA overactivity. More than 90% of patients with anorexia nervosa demonstrate nonsuppression of the DST on the DST,[67] which generally reverts to normal with only a 10% weight gain.[64] These studies, taken together, provide convincing evidence for HPA hyperactivity in anorexia nervosa patients.

In bulimia nervosa patients, nonsuppression of the DST is demonstrated in 20% to 50%.[43, 68] This rate of nonsuppression is very similar to that found in patients with major depression.[69] In a study comparing 24 women with bulimia to normal controls, Fichter and colleagues[49] did not find elevated nocturnal cortisol plasma levels.

FAT CONTENT

Critical Fat Content Theory

Frisch[70] has argued that adequate fat content, rather than adequate body weight per se, is the crucial factor regulating menstrual function. In an early study, Frisch and Revelle[71] found that onset of menses occurred at the same average weight (47 kg, or 103 lb) for both early and late maturers. They then studied body fat content among these girls, using calculations dependent on height and weight measures, and found that at menses the average body fat content was 24%.

Frisch and McArthur[72] found that in order to have menarche, young girls whose height growth was nearly complete (which is usually the case before menarche) had to gain enough weight in relationship to their height to de-

crease their percentage of water content to 59.8%, which would mean that at least 17% of their weight was fat. These investigators also found that after simple weight loss, women with secondary amenorrhea needed to obtain a weight that was about 10% heavier than the menarchal threshold to restore and maintain normal ovulation; body fat in these patients accounted for about 22% of total body weight. Frisch and McArthur concluded that a minimum of 17% body fat is required for menarche, and 22% body fat is required for normal ovulation at the end of growth in height (at about age 18). Normal adolescents gain fat between menarche and age 18, when they have typically completed the phase of adolescent subfertility during which the ovary, uterus, and fallopian tubes are still growing and there are many anovulatory cycles. Frisch[70] has proposed a nomogram that can be used to predict the minimum weight needed for a female of a given height to have menarche and the probability of regaining menses after secondary amenorrhea at certain weights (Fig. 25–2). Frisch has also hypothesized[73] that both the relative and absolute fat contents are important, because the woman must be large enough to reproduce.

The main drawback to Frisch's theory[74] is that it uses formulas that depend solely on measures of height and weight, and these measures do not necessarily reflect fat content. For example, Welham and Behnke[75] studied football players who were clearly overweight using standard height and weight tables and found that these athletes had a lower than average fat content. Similarly, Abraham and colleagues[76] studied a group of ballet dancers with high muscle content who were normal in weight but had low fat content. Meyer and colleagues[46] reported that in anorexia nervosa patients studied an average of 8 years after treatment, Frisch's critical weight threshold divided most, but not all, patients into groups according to whether menses had restarted; unfortunately, fat content was not reported in their study.

Fat Content in Eating Disorder Patients

Several observations regarding fat content in anorexics and bulimics are relevant to integrating the concept of critical fat content into a useful clinical guideline for setting target

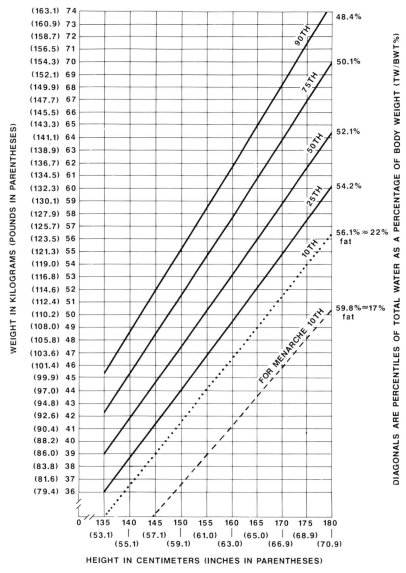

FIGURE 25–2 ••• Nomogram proposed by Frisch and McArthur indicating the threshold, or minimum weight, a female of a given completed height must attain to have normal menstrual cycles. The dashed line shows the minimum weight necessary for menarche. The dotted line shows minimum weight for correcting secondary amenorrhea. The top five diagonal lines indicate percentiles of total water as a percentage of weight—which is an index of fatness—for fully grown, mature women in a normal sample; the dotted line is the 10th percentile. The dashed line represents the 10th percentile for the same sample at menarche. The 50th-percentile line indicates the normal weight for height of mature women 18 to 25 years old. (Adapted from Frisch RE. Fatness and fertility. Sci Am 1988; 258:88.)

weights for these patients. Normal-weight bulimics often weigh more than before the onset of their disorder, have a higher fat content than age- and weight-matched peers, and require significantly fewer calories (about 200 fewer per day)[77] to maintain their weight than controls. These data have been interpreted in a variety of ways, but one likely contributing factor is that repeated weight gain–weight loss cycles (associated with binge-purge-binge episodes) may result in a continuously increasing fat content. On the other hand, anorexia nervosa patients without bulimia nervosa who are weight restored require approximately 200 calories more per day to maintain a restored

weight than would be predicted, at least in the first few months after weight restoration.[77]

Many methods are available to assess fat content, including underwater weighing, electrical impedance, and skinfold measures. Of these techniques, skinfold measures are both the easiest and least expensive to use, at least in normal and underweight subjects. Skinfolds are measured at four sites—triceps, biceps, subscapular, and suprailiac—and total fat content can be determined using the nomogram devised by Durnin and Womersely[78] for females age 16 to 50 (Table 25–1). Proposed reference values using the four-site caliper method in younger girls have recently been

TABLE 25–1 ••• PERCENTAGE OF BODY WEIGHT AS FAT IN FEMALES AGE 13 AND OLDER*

Skinfolds (mm)	Age in Years			
	16–29	*30–39*	*40–49*	*50+*
15	10.5			
20	14.1	17.0	19.8	21.4
25	16.8	19.4	22.2	24.0
30	19.5	21.8	24.5	26.6
35	21.5	23.7	26.4	28.5
40	23.4	25.5	28.2	30.3
45	25.0	26.9	29.6	31.9
50	26.5	28.2	31.0	33.4
55	27.8	29.4	32.1	34.6
60	29.1	30.6	33.2	35.7
65	30.2	31.6	34.1	36.7
70	31.2	32.5	35.0	37.7
75	32.2	33.4	35.9	38.7
80	33.1	34.3	36.7	39.6
85	34.0	35.1	37.5	40.4
90	34.8	35.8	38.3	41.2
95	35.6	36.5	39.0	41.9
100	36.4	37.2	39.7	42.6
105	37.1	37.9	40.4	43.3
110	37.8	38.6	41.0	43.9
115	38.4	39.1	41.5	44.5
120	39.0	39.6	42.0	45.1
125	39.6	40.1	42.5	45.7
130	40.2	40.6	43.0	46.2
135	40.8	41.1	43.5	46.7
140	41.3	41.6	44.0	47.2
145	41.8	42.1	44.5	47.7
150	42.3	42.6	45.0	48.2
155	42.8	43.1	45.4	48.7
160	43.3	43.6	45.8	49.2
165	43.7	44.0	46.2	49.6
170	44.1	44.4	46.6	50.0
175	—	44.8	47.0	50.4
180	—	45.2	47.4	50.8
185	—	45.6	47.8	51.2
190	—	45.9	48.2	51.6
195	—	46.2	48.5	52.0
200	—	46.5	48.8	52.4
205	—	—	49.1	52.7
210	—	—	49.4	53.0

*The equivalent fat content, as a percentage of body weight, for a range of values for the sum of four skinfolds (biceps, triceps, subscapular, and suprailiac) of females of different ages.
Modified from Durnin J, Womersely J. Body fat assessed from total body density, and its estimation from skinfold thickness: Measurements on 481 men and women aged from 16 to 72 years. Br J Nutr 1974; 32:77.

TABLE 25–2 ••• PERCENTAGE OF BODY FAT IN FEMALES*

Age (yr)	Skinfolds (mm)				
	15%	*20%*	*25%*	*30%*	*35%*
0	17	22	30	40	52
1	18	24	32	43	58
2	18	25	34	45	60
4	18	25	34	46	62
6	19	25	35	47	63
8	19	26	35	48	65
10	19	27	37	51	69
12	21	30	42	58	80
14	23	33	47	66	92
16	25	37	53	75	106
18	27	40	58	85	122

Data from 2285 Dutch children aged 0–18 years. Skinfolds (in millimeters) are the sum of biceps, triceps, suprailiac, and subscapular skinfold thicknesses.
From Westrate JA, Deurenberg P. Body composition in children: Proposal for a method for calculating body fat percentage from total body density or skinfold-thickness measurements. Am J Clin Nutr 1989; 50:1104.

scribed by Fomon and colleagues[80] for females age 10 and younger (Table 25–3) are also useful.

Although a number of technical errors can occur with the caliper method, including misplacement of the calipers, the measures are replicable in experienced hands. A more serious problem is that the nomograms make certain assumptions about the relationship between peripheral fat content (as estimated by

TABLE 25–3 ••• PERCENTAGE OF BODY WEIGHT AS FAT IN FEMALES FROM BIRTH TO AGE 10

Age	Length/Height		Weight		Fat
	cm	*in*	*kg*	*lbs*	*%*
Birth	50.5	19.98	3.325	7.315	14.9
1 mo	53.4	21.02	4.131	9.098	16.2
3 mo	59.6	23.46	5.743	12.63	23.8
6 mo	65.8	25.91	7.250	15.95	26.4
9 mo	70.4	27.72	8.270	18.19	25.0
12 mo	74.3	29.25	9.180	20.20	23.7
18 mo	80.2	31.57	10.78	23.72	21.8
24 mo	85.5	33.66	11.91	26.20	20.4
3 yr	94.1	37.05	14.10	31.02	18.5
4 yr	101.6	40.00	15.96	35.11	17.3
5 yr	108.4	42.68	17.66	38.85	16.7
6 yr	114.6	45.12	19.52	42.94	16.4
7 yr	120.6	47.48	21.84	48.05	16.8
8 yr	126.4	49.76	24.84	54.65	17.4
9 yr	132.2	52.05	28.46	62.61	18.3
10 yr	138.3	54.45	32.55	71.61	19.4

From Fomon SJ, Ziegler EE, Nelson SE. Body composition of reference children from birth to age 10 years. © Am J Clin Nutr 1982; 35:1169. American Society for Clinical Nutrition.

published by Westrate and Deurenberg[79] (Table 25–2). The estimation of fat content in this study utilized formulas dependent on certain unproven assumptions about the relationship between body density and skinfold measures; however, as a first estimate, Table 25–2 is a useful guide for determining the fat content of younger girls using skinfold measures. The issue of "normal" fat content in younger girls is even less well understood. The data de-

fatfold measures) and visceral fat content, assumptions that may not be correct in eating disorder patients, particularly during quick weight changes.

In summary, fat content is probably an important factor in the regulation of menses and ovulation. Frisch's theory that 17% total body fat is necessary for menarche and 22% total body fat is needed for normal ovulation is an elegant hypothesis that deserves further study.[70] Use of height and weight measures (including the currently popular body mass index) will not be adequate to prove or disprove the theory. Use of more sophisticated measures of fat content (including skinfold and possibly noninvasive radiologic measures) will contribute significantly to an understanding of disturbances in body composition that occur in both anorexia nervosa and bulimia and the relationship between changes in body composition and hormonal regulation.

OVARIAN AND UTERINE CHANGES

Treasure and colleagues[81] studied 11 patients with anorexia nervosa using sequential pelvic ultrasounds during the course of weight restoration. Initially, ovarian volume was small, and the internal ovarian structure was amorphous. With weight gain, multiple small cysts (i.e., polycystic ovaries) developed in 10 of 11 patients. Five of the patients continued to gain weight, and there was an increase in the size of the cysts; in three patients a dominant cyst subsequently developed after further weight gain. It was proposed that a critical nutritional threshold must be achieved before a dominant cyst can develop. These authors found no significant change in uterine size with weight gain, although there was a trend for an increase in uterine size.

Increase in ovarian size and development paralleled the changes documented to occur in LH and FSH with weight gain. Specifically, the changes in ovarian structure and size with weight gain replicate normal pubertal development, albeit at a more rapid pace. In a later study,[82] three stages of ovarian development were confirmed during weight restoration: amorphous, multifollicular (previously termed multicystic or polycystic), and a final stage of a single dominant follicle. Characteristic endocrine findings were noted in each stage. In the amorphous stage, LH, FSH, and estradiol levels were low; in the multifollicular stage, FSH rose significantly, but LH levels increased only moderately, and estradiol levels remained low. In the single dominant follicle stage, LH increased, FSH increases were small or absent, and estradiol levels rose until follicular size was >22 mm and then fell. Uterine size is thought to be mediated by estradiol, and in this study, uterine growth was associated with an increase in plasma estradiol.

Treasure[82] also studied 20 normal-weight bulimics (i.e., weight ranging from 85% to 105% IBW) with amenorrhea and found decreased ovarian volume, multifollicular ovaries, and a marked decrease in uterine area. He also studied five normal-weight bulimics with oligomenorrhea and found normal ovarian size with the development of one dominant follicle but failure to ovulate and inadequate corpus luteum function. In this study, 41% of the patients who were discharged with multifollicular ovaries (and at lower weights) were readmitted with a severe relapse, whereas only 16% who were discharged with a dominant follicle (and at higher weights) were readmitted.

INFERTILITY AND EATING DISORDERS

Bates and colleagues[83] studied 47 females aged 16 to 36 who presented to a reproductive endocrinologic clinic for assessment of infertility (29 patients) or menstrual dysfunction (18 patients). Those in the infertile group were an average of 9% below IBW, and those with menstrual irregularities were an average of 11% below IBW. Four patients were diagnosed as having anorexia nervosa. Among the women who agreed to increase their weight to predicted IBW, 19 of 26 infertile women conceived spontaneously, and 9 of 10 with secondary amenorrhea resumed menstruation. Eleven of the women refused to accept low weight as a cause of reproductive failure and refused to participate in the study.

In a study by Stewart and colleagues,[84] 11 (16.7%) of 66 women aged 21 to 39 evaluated in a university hospital fertility clinic had *DSM III-R* eating disorders (one had anorexia nervosa, four had bulimia nervosa, and six had atypical eating disorders). Furthermore, the 12 amenorrheic women in the sample had a higher prevalence of eating disorders (58%) than did women with normal cycles (7%). These eating disorder prevalences are significantly higher than the 4% reported in a careful survey of women aged 16 to 35 attending a family practice clinic.[85] Thus, infertile women with menstrual abnormalities may be particularly likely to have an eating disorder.

PREGNANCY AND EATING DISORDERS

Kohmura and colleagues[86] reported that 81% of 21 patients with anorexia nervosa studied 10 years after treatment had regained menses and developed normal eating behavior; 14 patients became pregnant (11 spontaneously and three as a result of induction), and 12 had a term delivery. Body weight was not statistically significantly different between patients in whom menses was restored and those in whom menses was not restored, suggesting that other factors (e.g., fat content or psychological status) may influence resumption of menses. Treasure and Russell[87] studied six anorexic women (mean duration, 15 years) who had seven pregnancies while at low weights. A subnormal intrauterine growth rate was observed during the third trimester, but "catch-up" growth was noted during the first 2½ months after birth.

In a more detailed report,[88] 74 women previously treated for anorexia nervosa or bulimia were studied; 15 had conceived 23 pregnancies. Women who were in remission at the time of follow-up had greater maternal weight gain, infants with higher birth weights, and higher 5-minute Apgar scores than women who conceived while still symptomatic. Furthermore, women who had symptoms of either anorexia nervosa or bulimia continued to have symptoms during pregnancy and the first year postpartum. The authors recommend delaying pregnancy until there is a full recovery from the eating disorder. Smith and Hanson[89] reported that some women with anorexia nervosa may underfeed their children. In a report[90] of 12 patients who had anorexia or bulimia nervosa, significant disturbances in parenting skills were noted, with two of those patients abandoning their children.

OSTEOPOROSIS

Several studies have documented that patients with anorexia nervosa often have osteopenia (significantly reduced bone mass) and, occasionally, osteoporosis (osteopenia associated with atraumatic fractures).

In an early report,[91] significantly reduced radial bone density was found in 18 anorectic women (two of whom developed vertebral compression fractures) compared with 28 normal controls; in this study, bone density was not related to estradiol levels, a finding that has been confirmed by others.[92] Treasure and colleagues[93] studied 31 adult anorexia nervosa women (three of whom had vertebral crush fractures) and 31 age-matched controls and found that anorexia nervosa patients had significantly reduced bone mineral density of the lumbar spine and femoral neck compared with normal controls. Biller and colleagues[94] found that spinal osteopenia was severe in more than 50% of the women studied and that spinal bone density was lowest in those women whose amenorrhea began in adolescence.

A study by Bachrach and colleagues[95] addressed the issue of osteopenia in adolescent anorexia nervosa patients. They studied 18 anorexia nervosa girls aged 12 to 20 and found significantly lower whole-body bone mass and lumbar vertebral bone density than in 25 normal controls. The decrement in bone density was more than two standard deviations below normal values for age. Body mass index was significantly correlated with bone density in both anorexics and normal controls. Bone density measures were also correlated with age of onset and duration of anorexia nervosa but were not correlated with duration of amenorrhea or activity levels. Half of the adolescent girls who developed osteopenia in this study had been diagnosed as anorexic for 1 year or less, and the authors suggest that osteopenia may occur early in the disorder.

Mazess and colleagues[96] studied total skeletal mineral in 11 anorexia nervosa patients and found it was approximately 25% less than in normal controls; this study also noted a 10% reduction in overall bone density, with an even greater diminution of bone density in the thoracolumbar region (27% less than normal controls). These investigators used the dual photon absorptiometry (DPA) method to assess total-body soft tissue composition, as well as bone mineral content and bone mineral density, and detected a fivefold decrease in subcutaneous fat and a twofold decrease in intraabdominal fat compared with normal controls.

Davies and colleagues[97] compared 11 normal-weight bulimic patients, 26 anorexia nervosa patients, 26 patients with both anorexia nervosa and bulimia, and 211 normal controls. They found that patients in both anorexia nervosa groups had spinal and proximal forearm densities that were significantly below those of normal controls, but the normal-weight bulimics did not. In this study, estrogen status was not significantly associated with the measures of bone mineral content. (Estrogen deficient was defined as no menses for 3 or more months, and estrogen replete was defined as either normal menses or receiving oral contraceptives.)

In one study (Anderson AE, LaFrance ND, unpublished data, 1991), 96 female eating disorder patients were divided into four groups: restricting anorexia nervosa (n = 27); anorexia nervosa with bulimic features (n = 27); normal-weight bulimia nervosa with a past history of anorexia nervosa (n = 15); and normal-weight bulimia nervosa without a past history of anorexia nervosa (n = 13). Bone mineral density was lowest in the anorectic group with bulimic complications and significantly low in the restricting anorectic group. Normal-weight bulimic patients with a previous anorectic episode had significantly lower bone densities than those without a past anorectic episode. Thus, a past episode of anorexia nervosa may result in lowered bone density.

Physiology of Bone

Bone mass increases throughout childhood with nearly half of the adult skeletal mass laid down during adolescence. The age at which bone accretion is completed is uncertain, but it may continue in females until age 35.[98] The balance between bone formation and bone resorption is a dynamic one that is influenced by both nutritional and endocrine factors. Hormones that increase bone resorption, and thus bone loss, include low estrogen and elevated glucocorticoids (both of which are prominent features of anorexia nervosa). Estrogen prevents bone resorption and decreases remodeling; progesterone has been reported to promote bone formation and accelerate remodeling.

Effect of Exercise

The effect of exercise on bone density is unclear. An early study[91] hypothesized that exercise protected against bone loss, but several other studies[94, 95, 99] found no correlation between levels of exercise and bone loss. The issue of exercise is probably quite complex. Joyce and colleagues[100] reported that moderate exercise is beneficial in preventing bone loss, but strenuous exercise is detrimental to bone mineral density among eating disorder patients. However, Prior and colleagues[99] compared three groups of normal-weight patients without eating disorders who were sedentary, normally active, or preparing for a marathon. They assessed hormonal levels (LH, FSH, estrogen, and progesterone) in the midfollicular and midluteal phases and compared bone density changes over the course of a year. They found statistically significant correlations between changes in bone density during the year and the annual luteal phase index (mean ratio of the length of the luteal phase to the length of the menstrual cycle), as well as the estimated serum luteal phase of progesterone. They concluded that short luteal phases, especially anovulatory cycles, may increase bone loss in women. Interestingly, women in training for a marathon did not have greater bone loss than those in the other two groups.

In a review of various theories accounting for the discrepant findings regarding exercise and bone density in anorexics, Dalsky[101] posited that in the presence of estrogen deficiency, moderate physical activity decreases the rate of bone turnover and then increases bone formation, but endurance exercise training does not have these effects.

Glucocorticoids

Excess glucocorticoid levels decrease bone formation; osteoporosis occurs with long-term corticosteroid therapy, and elevated cortisol levels are one of the hallmarks of anorexia nervosa. The osteoporosis associated with hypercortisolism affects primarily trabecular bone (such as the spine), which has a more rapid turnover rate. One proposed mechanism for this decreased bone formation is inhibition of collagen production and osteoblast precursor replication and differentiation. Savvas and colleagues[102] studied the relationship between skin thickness, bone density, and collagen content in anorexics and found an association between bone loss, thin skin, and skin collagen content. They postulated that estrogen has a direct effect on collagen metabolism and contended that estrogen deficiency reduces bone collagen and thus results in osteoporosis. In a study of anorexics, Biller and colleagues[94] found a significant negative correlation between the urinary cortisol-to-creatine ratio and bone mass measures.

Effect of Treatment

The question of whether restoration of menses, ovulation, IBW, adequate calcium intake, or various activity levels improve bone density in anorexia nervosa patients has yet to be resolved. In a longitudinal study,[103] 27 female anorexics were followed for a mean of 27 months (range, 9 to 53 months) with initial and repeat single photon absorptiometry (SPA) of the forearm. Initially, bone density measures of the forearm were low and did not improve or significantly decrease at follow-up. Two patients had clinically apparent fractures at the time of the initial assessment; at follow-up, three new fractures had occurred. One problem with this study is that only 7 of the 27 patients weighed more than 85% of IBW (hence the 20 other patients may have met formal *DMS III-R* criteria for anorexia nervosa). Second, the issue of restoration of ovulation among those patients who were weight restored was not addressed.

Assessment of Bone Density

The studies noted have used a variety of different methods to assess bone density, including SPA using a ^{125}I source,[95, 97] single energy quantitative computed tomography,[99] and DPA using a gadolinium ^{53}Gd source.[95, 102] Although SPA of the radius has been found to differentiate normal controls from postmenopausal osteoporotic women,[104] studies of anorectic women[96] found significantly lower bone density in the lumbar spine (and normal bone density in the forearm) using DPA. Thus the forearm SPA probably has less clinical relevance, at least for anorexia nervosa patients. The disadvantage of the spinal DPA is that it is relatively imprecise. Precision is defined as the coefficient of variation (standard deviation over a short period of time divided by the mean) for repeated measures. Factors that contribute to the imprecision of the spinal DPA include distortion of the measurement by fat content (including fat in the bone mar-

row) and absence of bone density standards. Problems that arise in selecting the bone site include (1) selecting spinal bone sites that are as large as possible, but with reference material near the selected site unattenuated by bone mineral; and (2) selecting bone that is free from other disturbing bones in the projection of the beam. Of the two sites that meet these criteria, the best are the lumbar spine and femoral neck. The crucial advantage of these sites is that they are often affected by osteopenia in patients with anorexia nervosa. The main drawback to the quantitative computed tomography (QCT) technique is that marrow fat influences the measurements obtained; the resultant inaccuracy is at least five times greater with this method than with DPA.[105]

Thus, of the two commonly used methods that have been used to assess eating disorder patients, one (SPA) is not as clinically relevant, and the other (DPA of the spine) is relatively imprecise, theoretically requiring large subject groups in follow-up studies to detect small changes in the bone mineral density. To assess the longitudinal effect of treatment, reproducible and precise techniques are needed.

A new method, dual energy x-ray absorptiometry (DEXA), has been developed that may offer more precision in assessing bone density of the lumbar spine. Multiple studies of older women with osteoporosis have been performed using this method, and DEXA has been found to be more precise.[106] However, this method has not yet been used in studies of osteopenia among eating disorder patients.

CONCLUSION

Osteopenia is a common complication of anorexia nervosa in females, occurs early in the course of the disorder (within the first year), may be particularly likely to develop in adolescents (the age at greatest risk for the onset of anorexia nervosa), and has not been shown to improve with weight restoration or return of menses. The factors that probably contribute to the development of osteopenia in anorexia nervosa include decreased body mass, low fat content, decreased estrogen and progesterone levels, elevated cortisol levels, abnormal activity levels (either over- or underexertion), and inadequate calcium intake. Assessment of the effects of treatment on the osteopenia that occurs so regularly in anorexia is hampered by the currently available techniques, which are either inaccurate (e.g., the QCT) or sufficiently imprecise (e.g., DPA) as to require large sample sizes to detect what may be clinically relevant changes in bone density. Osteoporosis currently occurs in more than 20 million postmenopausal women in the United States at an annual cost of $7 to $10 million.[107] Because anorexia nervosa is a risk factor for osteoporosis and is increasing in prevalence, the long-term impact may be particularly important.

SEXUAL ABUSE AND EATING DISORDERS

The prevalence of sexual abuse before age 18 in the general female population has been estimated to range between 19% and 30%.[108, 109] The prevalence of father-daughter incest (including stepfathers) ranges from 1% to 5%.[108] Although it is possible that these community-based samples overestimate prevalence (e.g., patients stating that they have been abused when they have not been), it is more likely that these percentages are underestimates, since the most common mechanisms for coping with sexual abuse include the intrapsychic defense mechanisms of denial, dissociation, and minimization (all of which might result in "forgetting" the experiences). Prevalence of a history of sexual abuse among female psychiatric inpatients ranges from 22% to 46%,[110, 111] which is higher than the base rate among the general population. Psychiatric patients have been studied by diagnostic groups. Several studies have documented a very high prevalence of sexual abuse history (75% to 90%) in female patients with multiple personality disorders.[112, 113] On the other hand, a history of sexual abuse is found in only about 20% of female patients with schizophrenia.[112] The prevalence of a history of sexual abuse in patients with eating disorders has been studied extensively and seems to be higher than the reported base rate in the population, but not as high as among patients with multiple personality disorder.[114–117] Female inpatients with anorexia nervosa, bulimia, or both have prevalence rates ranging from 30% to 55%, whereas among female eating disorder outpatients, the reported prevalence rates are somewhat lower (30% to 40%).

Abuse History and Eating Pathology

The correlation between abuse history and eating pathology has also been addressed. In a study of 706 junior high school students,[118] 18.3% had a history of physical or sexual abuse or both; 76% of the students who had been both sexually and physically abused had considered harming themselves, and those who had been sexually abused were nearly five times as likely to use laxatives or induce vomiting. In a study of 635 high school students,[119] those with a physical abuse history were six times more likely to induce vomiting than nonabused high school students. Finally, of 348 female college students,[120] 23% had been victims of child sexual abuse experiences; those who had histories of abuse had statistically significantly higher scores on a self-report form assessing eating disorder symptoms than those with no such history.

Despite multiple methodologic problems (including assessment of those who have not yet passed through the age at risk for child or adolescent sexual abuse and the use of different methods of assessment), several conclusions seem warranted. First, there is a high base rate of a history of sexual abuse in the general female population; second, the prevalence rate is probably higher in female psychiatric patients, especially inpatients, and in certain psychiatric diagnostic groups, notably those with multiple personality disorder, anorexia nervosa, or bulimia. Finally, abnormal eating behavior and various purging behaviors are correlated with a history of sexual abuse (and physical abuse) in general studies of those in early, middle, and late adolescence.

Effects on Patient Care

Because more than one third of the patients who have eating disorders also have a history of sexual abuse, the health care professional who assesses a patient with anorexia nervosa or bulimia should suspect this possibility. Some patients may volunteer the information, but it is much more likely that sexual abuse will not be mentioned. Asking the patient if she has been sexually or physically abused will often result in the patient acknowledging this history. The initial response should be to validate the reality of the abuse and to indicate that these experiences have probably had a profound influence on the patient's life, including her sexual functioning. The physician can then inquire about any anxiety regarding the pelvic examination that may be related to this history and suggest various strategies to relieve this anxiety, including the presence of a relative, a detailed description of the examination, or any other necessary procedures. Some patients may be so anxious that a consultation with a psychiatrist may be needed before the examination.

Some patients who have been abused may not acknowledge it, even when questioned in an empathic and understanding manner. Usually this means that the patient is not emotionally prepared to cope with her feelings about the experience, and the physician should not query the patient further. Patients with anorexia nervosa or bulimia should be evaluated and treated by mental health professionals, and the history of sexual abuse may emerge after several years of treatment.

TREATMENT

Both anorexia nervosa and bulimia nervosa require prompt psychiatric intervention. It is well established that in patients with anorexia nervosa, prognosis worsens with duration of the illness and severity of weight loss.[121, 122] The added development of bulimia nervosa in a patient with anorexia nervosa worsens the prognosis.[121] In some semistarved patients, bulimia starts when the drive to eat overwhelms the patient. In other anorexic patients, the onset of bulimia is related to iatrogenic factors. Patients who are urged to gain weight without attending to the psychological issues may comply and then begin purging when no longer under medical observation.

Most patients with anorexia nervosa require inpatient treatment at some point during recovery. Weight restoration is a crucial aspect of treatment. Several methods have been used, but the effectiveness of behavior modification programs based on operant conditioning is well established.[123] Long-term individual psychotherapy, starting in the hospital and usually continuing for at least 2 years after hospitalization, is an essential part of treatment. Family therapy is an important aspect of a comprehensive treatment plan.[124, 125] Patients who are 25% or more below IBW, who also have bulimia nervosa (or purging without binge eat-

ing), who have been ill more than 6 months, or who have any of the well-known physiological complications of semistarvation need hospitalization to achieve and maintain IBW, as well as to establish a positive relationship with an individual therapist.

Normal-weight patients with bulimia nervosa can usually be treated as outpatients using a combination of individual or group psychotherapy and antidepressant medication. Although a relationship between the affective disorders (particularly depression) and anorexia nervosa has been suspected, in bulimia nervosa patients this idea has been repeatedly investigated.[126] Patients with bulimia nervosa often (but not always) present with symptoms of major depression, have family histories replete with affective disorders and alcoholism, and often improve significantly with antidepressant medication. Fluoxetine has been the best studied antidepressant; in a multicenter trial of more than 200 patients,[127] there was a significant reduction in the frequency of binge eating on 60 mg of fluoxetine daily regardless of whether the patient met criteria for major depression.

Role of the Physician

The physician rendering care to young, underweight, amenorrheic females should have a high index of suspicion for anorexia nervosa and in such cases should facilitate prompt assessment and treatment by mental health professionals. One of the most effective strategies available is to stress to the patient (and her family) the long-term physiologic complications of eating disorders. Although the long-term psychological consequences are equally devastating, early in the course of these conditions (at the very time when early intervention is likely to be most effective), the patient may feel better, because the underlying psychodynamic conflicts have been temporarily alleviated by the symptoms. Thus, early in the disorder, the patient is less likely to appreciate the deleterious effects of these behaviors on her own emotional growth and development.

It is often useful to provide the patient and her family with information on the long-term outcome. Early mortality occurs in 15% to 20% of anorexia nervosa patients followed over 20 years.[121, 122] The mortality rate seems to be lower (approximately 5%) with current treatment methods, although in these studies, follow-up has been only 4 to 5 years.[128] Although the initial reduction in symptoms in bulimia nervosa is often quite positive, with many patients improving with short-term intervention, the long-term outcome of bulimia nervosa is not known.

References

1. Halmi K, Casper R, Eckert E, et al. Unique features associated with age of onset of anorexia nervosa. Psychiatry Res 1979; 1:209.
2. Willi J, Grossman S. Epidemiology of anorexia nervosa in a defined region of Switzerland. Am J Psychiatry 1983; 140:564.
3. Kendell RE, Hall DJ, Hailey A, Babigian HM. The epidemiology of anorexia nervosa. Psychol Med 1973; 3:200.
4. Crisp AH, Palmer RL, Kalucy RS. How common is anorexia nervosa? A prevalence study. Br J Psychiatry 1976; 128:549.
5. Diagnostic and Statistical Manual. 3rd ed. Revised (DSM-III-R). Washington, DC: American Psychiatric Association Press, 1987, p 65.
6. Gislason IL. Eating disorders in childhood. In: Blinder BJ, Chaitin BF, Goldstein RS (eds). The Eating Disorders: Medical and Psychological Bases of Diagnosis and Treatment. New York: PMA Publishing, 1988, p 285.
7. Bernstein IC. Anorexia nervosa: 94-year-old woman treated with electroshock. Minn Med 1972; 55:552.
8. Goodman S, Blinder BJ, Chaitin BF, Hagman J. Atypical eating disorders. In: Blinder BJ, Chaitin BF, Goldstein RS (eds). The Eating Disorders: Medical and Psychological Bases of Diagnosis and Treatment. New York: PMA Publishing, 1988, p 393.
9. Chatoor I, Egan J. Nonorganic failure to thrive and dwarfism due to food refusal: A separation disorder. J Am Acad Child Adolesc Psychiatry 1983; 22:294.
10. Russell GFM. Premenarchal anorexia nervosa and its sequelae. J Psychiatr Res 1985; 19:363.
11. Casper RC, Eckert ED, Halmi KA. Bulimia: Its incidence and clinical importance in patients with anorexia nervosa. Arch Gen Psychiatry 1980; 37:1030.
12. Gormally J, Black S, Dastun S, Rardin D. The assessment of binge-eating severity among obese persons. Addict Behav 1982; 7:47.
13. Russell G. Bulimia nervosa: An ominous variant of anorexia nervosa. Psychol Med 1979; 9:429.
14. Halmi KA, Falk JR, Schwartz E. Binge-eating and vomiting: A survey of a college population. Psychol Med 1981; 11:706.
15. Pyle RL, Mitchel JE. The epidemiology of bulimia. In: Blinder BF, Chaitin BF, Goldstein RS (eds). The Eating Disorders: Medical and Psychological Bases of Diagnosis and Treatment. New York: PMA Publishing, 1988, p 259.
16. Schocken DD, Holloway JD, Powers PS. Weight loss and the heart. Arch Intern Med 1989; 149:877.
17. Powers PS, Schocken DD, Feld J, et al. Cardiac function during weight restoration in anorexia nervosa. Int J Eat Disord 1991; 10:521.
18. Forbes GB. Lean body mass-body fat interrelationships in humans. Nutr Rev 1987; 45:225.
19. Dubois A, Gross HA, Ebert MH, Castell DO. Altered gastric emptying and secretion in primary anorexia nervosa. Gastroenterology 1979; 77:319.
20. Kohlmeyer K, Lehmkuhl F, Poustka F. Computed tomography in patients with anorexia nervosa. AJNR 1983; 4:437.
21. Heinz ER, Martinez J, Haenggeli A. Reversibility of cerebral atrophy in anorexia nervosa and Cushing's syndrome. J Comput Assist Tomogr 1977; 1:415.
22. Hernholz K, Krieg JC, Emrick HM, et al. Regional cerebral glucose metabolism in anorexia nervosa measured by positron emission tomography. Biol Psychiatry 1987; 22:43.
23. Fox C. Neuropsychological correlates of anorexia nervosa. Int J Psychiatry Med 1981; 11:285.
24. Kay J, Stricker R. Hematologic and immunologic abnormalities in anorexia nervosa. South Med J 1983; 76:1008.
25. Palmblad JA, Fohlin L, Nurberg R. Plasma levels of complement factors 3 and 4. Acta Paediatr Scand 1979; 6G8:617.
26. Pertschuk M, Crosby L, Barot L, Mullen J. Immunocompetency in anorexia nervosa. Am J Clin Nutr 1982; 35:968.
27. Mitchell JE, Pyle RL, Miner RA. Gastric dilatation as a complication of bulimia. Psychosomatics 1982; 23:96.
28. Wolcott RB, Yager J, Gordon G. Dental sequelae to the binge-purge syndrome (bulimia); report of cases. J Am Dent Assoc 1984; 109:723.
29. Levin P, Falko J, Dixon K, et al. Benign parotid enlargement in bulimia. Ann Intern Med 1980; 93:827.
30. Blinder BJ, Hagman J. Serum salivary isoamylase levels in patients with anorexia nervosa, bulimia or bulimia nervosa. Hillside J Clin Psychiatry 1986; 8:152.
31. Mecklenburg R, Loriaux D, Thompson R, et al. Hypothalamic dysfunction in patients with anorexia nervosa. Medicine 1974; 523:147.
32. Casper R, Kirschner B, Sanstead H, et al. An evaluation of trace metals, vitamins and taste function in anorexia nervosa. Am J Clin Nutr 1980; 33:1801.
33. Levinson NA. Oral manifestations of eating disorders: Indications for a collaborative treatment approach. In: Blinder BJ, Chaitin BF, Goldstein RS (eds). The Eating Disorders: Medical and Psychological Bases of Diagnosis and Treatment. New York: PMA Publishing, 1988, p 405.
34. Al-Muffy N, Bevan D. A case of subcutaneous emphysema, pneumomediastinum and pneumothorax associated with functional anorexia. Br J Clin Pract 1977; 31:160.
35. Halmi KA. Anorexia nervosa: Demographic and clinical features in 94 cases. Psychosom Med 1974; 38:18.
36. Warren MP, Vande Wiele RL. Clinical and metabolic features of anorexia nervosa. Am J Obstet Gynecol 1973; 117:435.
37. Boyar RM, Katz JL, Finkelstein JW, et al. Anorexia nervosa: Immaturity of the 24-hour luteinizing hormone secretory pattern. N Engl J Med 1974; 291:861.
38. Eisenberg E. Toward an understanding of reproductive function in anorexia nervosa. Fertil Steril 1981; 36:543.
39. Wakeling A, DeSouza VFA. Differential endocrine and menstrual responses to weight changes in an-

orexia nervosa. In: Darby PL, Garfinkel PE, Garner DM, Coscina DV (eds). Anorexia Nervosa: Recent Developments in Research. New York: Alan R. Liss, 1983, p 271.

40. Weiner H. Psychoendocrinology of anorexia nervosa. Psychiatr Clin North Am 1989; 12:187.
41. Vigersky RA, Anderson AE, Thompson RH, Loriaux DL. Hypothalamic dysfunction in secondary amenorrhea associated with simple weight loss. N Engl J Med 1977; 297:1141.
42. Pirke KM, Fichter MM, Warnhoff M, et al. Hypothalamic regulation of gonadotropin secretion in anorexia nervosa and starvation. Int J Eating Dis 1983; 2:151.
43. Hudson JI, Hudson MS. Endocrine dysfunction in anorexia nervosa and bulimia: Comparison with abnormalities in other psychiatric disorders and disturbances due to metabolic factors. Psychiatr Dev 1984; 4:237.
44. Falk JR, Halmi KA. Amenorrhea in anorexia nervosa: Examination of the critical weight hypothesis. Biol Psychiatry 1982; 17:799.
45. Sherman BM, Halmi KA, Zamudio R. LH and FSH response to gonadotropin releasing hormone in anorexia nervosa: Effect of nutritional rehabilitation. J Clin Endocrinol Metab 1975; 41:135.
46. Meyer A, von Holtzapfel B, Deffner G, et al. Psychoendocrinology of amenorrhea in the late outcome of anorexia nervosa. Psychother Psychosom 1986; 45:174.
47. Pirke KM, Fichter MM, Chlond C, et al. Disturbances of the menstrual cycle in bulimia nervosa. Clin Endocrinol 1987; 27:245.
48. Friedman EJ, Stolar M, Kramer M, Gerner RH. Psychological and endocrine evaluation of bulimia. Presented at the Annual Meeting of the American Psychiatric Association, Los Angeles 1984.
49. Fichter MM, Pirke KM, Pöllinger J, et al. Disturbances in the hypothalamo-pituitary-adrenal and other neuroendocrine axes in bulimia. Biol Psychiatry 1990; 27:1021.
50. Kiriike N, Nishiwaki S, Nagata T, et al. Gonadotropin response to LH-RH in anorexia nervosa and bulimia. Acta Psychiatr Scand 1988; 77:420.
51. Schweiger U, Pirke KM, Laessle RC, Fichter MM. Gonadotropin secretion in bulimia nervosa. J Clin Endocrinol Metab 1992; 74:1122.
52. Pirke KM, Pahl J, Schweiger U, Warnhoff M. Metabolic and endocrine indices of starvation in bulimia: A comparison with anorexia nervosa. Psychiatry Res 1985; 15:33.
53. Ploog DW, Pirke KM. Psychobiology of anorexia nervosa. Psychol Med 1987; 17:843.
54. Czaja JA. Food rejection by female rhesus monkeys during the menstrual cycle and early pregnancy. Physiol Behav 1975; 14:579.
55. Dalvit SP. The effect of the menstrual cycle on patterns of food intake. Am J Clin Nutr 1981; 34:1811.
56. Leon GR, Phelen PW, Kelly JT, Patten SR. The symptoms of bulimia and the menstrual cycle. Psychosom Med 1986; 48:415.
57. Gladis MM, Walsh BT. Premenstrual exacerbation of binge-eating in bulimia. Am J Psychiatry 1987; 144:1592.
58. Kiyohara K, Tamai H, Kobayaski N, Nakagawa T. Hypothalamic-pituitary axis alterations in bulimic patients. Am J Clin Nutr 1988; 47:805.
59. Vigersky RA, Loriaux DL, Anderson AE, Lipsett MB. Anorexia nervosa: Behavioral and hypothalamic aspects. Clin Endocrinol Metab 1976; 5:517.
60. Mitchell JE, Bantle JP. Metabolic and endocrine investigations in women at normal weight with the bulimic syndrome. Biol Psychiatry 1983; 18:355.
61. Targum SD, Sullivan AC, Byrnes SM. Neuroendocrine interrelationships in major depressive disorder. Am J Psychiatry 1982; 139:282.
62. Walsh BT, Katz JK, Levin J, et al. Adrenal activity in anorexia nervosa. Psychosom Med 1978; 40:499.
63. Boyar RM, Hellman LD, Roffwarg H. Cortisol secretion and metabolism in anorexia nervosa. N Engl J Med 1977; 296:190.
64. Doerr P, Fichter M, Pirke KM, Lund R. Relationship between weight gain and hypothalamic pituitary adrenal function in patients with anorexia nervosa. J Steroid Biochem 1980; 13:529.
65. Weiner H, Katz JL. The hypothalamic-pituitary-adrenal axis in anorexia nervosa: A reassessment. In: Darby PL, Garfinkel PE, Garner DM, Coscina DV (eds). Anorexia Nervosa: Recent Developments in Research. New York: Alan R Liss, 1983, p 249.
66. Gold PW, Gwirtsman H, Augerinos PC. Abnormal hypothalamic-pituitary-adrenal function in anorexia nervosa. N Engl J Med 1986; 314:1335.
67. Gerner RH, Gwirtsman HE. Abnormalities of dexamethasone suppression test and urinary MHPG in anorexia nervosa. Am J Psychiatry 1981; 138:650.
68. Gwirtsman HE, Roy-Byrne P, Yager S, Gerner RH. Neuroendocrine abnormalities in bulimia. Am J Psychiatry 1983; 140:559.
69. Gwirtsman HE, Gerner RH, Sternbach H. The overnight dexamethasone suppression test: Clinical and theoretical review. J Clin Psychiatry 1982; 43:321.
70. Frisch RE. Fatness and fertility. Sci Am 1988; 258:88.
71. Frisch RE, Revelle R. The height and weight of adolescent boys and girls at the time of peak velocity of growth in height and weight: longitudinal data. Hum Biol 1969; 41:536.
72. Frisch RE, McArthur JW. Menstrual cycles: Fatness as a determinant of minimum weight for height necessary for their maintenance or onset. Science 1974; 185:949.
73. Frisch RE. The right weight: Body fat, menarche and ovulation. Clin Obstet Gynecol 1990; 4:419.
74. Mellits ED, Cheek DB. The assessment of body water and fatness from infancy to childhood. Monogr Soc Res Child Dev 1970; 35:12.
75. Welham WC, Behnke AR. The specific gravity of healthy men; body weight divided by volume and other physical characteristics of exceptional athletes and of naval personnel. JAMA 1942; 118:498.
76. Abraham SF, Beaumont PJV, Fraser TS, Llewellyn-Jones D. Body weight, exercise and menstrual status among ballet dancers in training. Br J Obstet Gynaecol 1982; 89:507.
77. Kaye W, Hansen D. Introduction to the psychobiology of eating disorders: Part II. Presented at the annual meeting of the ANAS, Columbus, OH, 1989.
78. Drunin J, Womersely J. Body fat assessed from total body density and its estimation from skinfold thickness: Measurements on 481 men and women aged from 16 to 72 years. Br J Nutr 1974; 32:77.
79. Westrate JA, Deurenberg P. Body composition in children: Proposal for a method for calculating body fat percentage from total body density or skinfold-thickness measurements. Am J Clin Nutr 1989; 50:1104.
80. Fomon SJ, Haschke F, Ziegler EE, Nelson SE. Body

composition of reference children from birth to age 10 years. Am J Clin Nutr 1982; 35:1169.

81. Treasure JL, Gordon PAL, King EA, et al. Cystic ovaries: A phase of anorexia nervosa. Lancet 1985; 2:1379.

82. Treasure JL. The ultrasonographic features in anorexia nervosa and bulimia nervosa: A simplified method of monitoring hormonal states during weight gain. J Psychosom Res 1988; 32:623.

83. Bates GW, Bates SR, Whiteworth NS. Reproductive failure in women who practice weight control. Fertil Steril 1982; 37:373.

84. Stewart DE, Robinson GE, Goldbloom DS, Wright C. Infertility and eating disorders. Am J Obstet Gynecol 1990; 163:1196.

85. King MB. Eating disorders in general practice. Br Med J 1986; 293:1412.

86. Kohmura H, Miyake A, Aono T, Tanizawa O. Recovery of reproductive function in patients with anorexia nervosa: A 10 year follow-up study. Eur J Obstet Gynecol Reprod Biol 1986; 22:293.

87. Treasure JL, Russell GFM. Intrauterine growth and neonatal weight gain in babies of women with anorexia nervosa. Br Med J 1988; 296:1038.

88. Stewart DE, Raskin J, Garfinkel PE, et al. Anorexia nervosa, bulimia and pregnancy. Am J Obstet Gynecol 1987; 157:1194.

89. Smith SM, Hanson R. Failure to thrive and anorexia nervosa. Postgrad Med J 1972; 48:382.

90. Woodside DB, Skekter-Wolfson LF. Parenting by patients with anorexia nervosa and bulimia nervosa. Int J Eating Disord 1990; 9:303.

91. Rigotti NA, Nussbaum SR, Herzog DB, Neer RM. Osteoporosis in women with anorexia nervosa. N Engl J Med 1984; 311:1601.

92. Treasure JL, Russell GFM, Fogelman I, Murby B. Reversible bone loss in anorexia nervosa. Br Med J 1987; 295:474.

93. Treasure J, Fogelman I, Russell GFM. Osteopenia of the lumbar spine and femoral neck in anorexia nervosa. Scott Med J 1986; 31:206.

94. Biller BMK, Saxe V, Herzog DB, et al. Mechanism of osteoporosis in adult and adolescent women with anorexia nervosa. J Clin Endocrinol Metab 1989; 68:548.

95. Bachrach LK, Guido D, Katzman D, et al. Decreased bone density in adolescent girls with anorexia nervosa. Pediatrics 1990; 86:447.

96. Mazess RB, Barden HS, Ohlrich ES. Skeletal and body-composition effects of anorexia nervosa. Am J Clin Nutr 1990; 52:438.

97. Davies KM, Pearson PH, Huseman CA, et al. Reduced bone mineral in patients with eating disorders. Bone 1990; 11:143.

98. Kreipe RE, Forbes GB. Osteoporosis: A "new morbidity" for dieting female adolescents. Pediatrics 1990; 86:478.

99. Prior JC, Vigna YM, Schechter MT, Burgess AE. Spinal bone loss and ovulatory disturbances. N Engl J Med 1990; 323:1221.

100. Joyce JM, Warren DL, Humphries LL, et al. Osteoporosis in women with eating disorders: Comparison of physical parameters, exercise and menstrual status with SPA and DPA evaluation. J Nucl Med 1990; 31:325.

101. Dalsky GP. Effect of exercise on bone: Permissive influence of estrogen and calcium. Med Sci Sports Exerc 1990; 22:281.

102. Savvas M, Treasure J, Studd J, et al. The effect of

anorexia nervosa on skin thickness, skin collagen and bone density. Br J Obstet Gynaecol 1989; 96:1392.

103. Rigotti NA, Neer RM, Skates SJ, et al. The clinical course of osteoporosis in anorexia nervosa: A longitudinal study of cortical bone mass. JAMA 1991; 265:1133.

104. Johnston CC, Slemenda CW, Melton LJ. Clinical use of bone densitometry. New Engl J Med 1991; 324:1105.

105. Genant HK, Block JE, Steiger P, Glüer CC. Quantitative computed tomography in the assessment of osteoporosis. In: Genant HK (ed). Osteoporosis Update 1987. Perspectives for Internists, Gynecologists, Orthopaedists, Radiologists and Nuclear Physicians. San Francisco: Radiology Research and Education Foundation, 1987, p 49.

106. Kellie SE. Diagnostic and Therapeutic Technology Assessment (DATTA): Measurement of bone density with dual-energy x-ray absorptiometry (DEXA). JAMA 1992; 267:287.

107. Culliton BJ. Osteoporosis reexamined: Complexity of bone biology is a challenge. Science 1987; 235:833.

108. Russell DEH. The Secret Trauma: Incest in the Lives of Girls and Women. New York: Basic Books, 1987.

109. Finkelhor D. Child Sexual Abuse. New York: Free Press, 1984.

110. Sansonnet-Heyden H, Haley G, Marriage K, Fine S. Sexual abuse and psychopathology in hospitalized adolescents. J Am Acad Child Adolesc Psychiatry 1987; 26:753.

111. Beck JC, van der Kolk B. Reports of childhood incest and current behavior of chronically hospitalized women. Am J Psychiatry 1987; 144:1472.

112. Coons PM, Bowman ES, Pellow TA, Schneider P. Post-traumatic aspects of the treatment of victims of sexual abuse and incest. Psychiatr Clin North Am 1989; 12:325.

113. Putnam FW, Guroff JJ, Silberman EK, et al. The clinical phenomenology of multiple personality disorder: A review of 100 recent cases. J Clin Psychiatry 1986; 47:285.

114. Hall RC, Tice L, Beresford TP, et al. Sexual abuse in patients with anorexia nervosa and bulimia. Psychosomatics 1989; 30:73.

115. Powers PS, Coovert DL, Brightwell DR. Sexual abuse history in three eating disorders. Presented at the annual meeting of the American Psychiatric Association, Montreal, May, 1988.

116. Sloan G, Leichner P. Is there a relationship between sexual abuse or incest and eating disorders. Can J Psychiatry 1986; 31:656.

117. Oppenheimer R, Howells K, Palmer RL, Challener DA. Adverse sexual experience in childhood and clinical eating disorders: A preliminary description. J Psychiatr Res 1985; 9:357.

118. Hibbard RA, Brack GJ, Rauch S, Orr DP. Abuse, feelings and health behaviors in a student population. Am J Dis Child 1988; 142:326.

119. Riggs S, Alario AJ, McHorney C. Health risk behaviors and attempted suicide in adolescents who report prior mistreatment. J Pediatr 1990; 116:815.

120. Smolak L, Levine MP, Sullins E. Are child sexual experiences related to eating disordered attitudes and behaviors in a college sample? Int J Eating Disord 1990; 9:167.

121. Hsu LKG, Crisp AH, Harding B. Outcome of anorexia nervosa. Lancet 1979; I:61.

122. Morgan HG, Purgold J, Welbourne J. Management and outcome in anorexia nervosa: A standardized prognostic study. Br J Psychiatry 1983; 143:282.

123. Powers PS. Anorexia nervosa: Evaluation and treatment. Compr Ther 1990; 16:24.

124. Minuchin S, Rosman BL, Baker L. Psychosomatic Families: Anorexia Nervosa in Context. Cambridge, MA: Harvard University Press, 1978.

125. Selvini-Palazzoli M, Viaro M. The anorectic process in the family: A six-stage model as a guide for individual therapy. Fam Process 1988; 17:129.

126. Strober M, Katz JL. Do eating disorders and affective disorders share a common etiology? Int J Eating Disord 1987; 6:171.

127. The Fluoxetine Bulimia Nervosa Collaborative Study Group. Fluoxetine in the treatment of bulimia nervosa: A multicenter placebo-controlled, double-blind trial. Arch Gen Psychiatry. 1992; 49:139.

128. Hsu LKG. The outcome of anorexia nervosa: A reappraisal. Psychol Med 1988; 18:807.

CHAPTER 26

○○○ # Depression and Suicide

DENISE FORD-NEPA

CHILDHOOD DEPRESSION

The concept of childhood depression is a relatively new one in the psychiatric literature. Toolan[1] states that as recently as 1962, the existence of depression in children was not widely accepted by the medical and psychiatric community. The prevailing idea at the time was that to experience depression, a well-developed superego was required; children were thought not to have such a well-developed superego. According to Toolan, depression exists in children but is manifested differently depending on the age of the child. Hughes et al.[2] reported that major depressive disorder occurs in children from 6 to 12 years old and is similar to the syndrome seen in adults in terms of family history, dexamethasone suppression, response to antidepressant therapy, and phenomenology. Simeon[3] described the prevalence of depressive disorders as ranging from 0.14% to 1.9% in the general population. Petti[4] indicated that depression occurs in 60% of hospitalized child psychiatric patients. Carlson and Cantwell[5] reported that 27% of those in an outpatient child psychiatric population were clinically depressed.

Diagnostic Indicators of Depression in Children

The ability of the primary care physician to diagnose depression in the children that he or she sees in clinical practice is an extremely important quality and skill, because most depressed children are seen by primary care physicians before they are referred for psychiatric evaluation. The physician can be an effective tool in ensuring that the child and family receive needed treatment for depression.

Several researchers have noted the specific diagnostic indicators of depression in children and infants. Spitz[6] described the syndrome of "anaclitic depression" occurring in infants and toddlers when these young children were separated from their mothers after 6 months of age. The young child responded to the separation from the primary caretaker with sadness and tearfulness. The child withdrew from the social environment, lost weight, and developed slowness of movement, loss of appetite, and difficulty in sleeping. According to Spitz,[6] this syndrome is reversible if the mother-child bond can be reinstated within 3 months. Another pioneer in the area of human attachment and loss and its relationship to the etiology of childhood depression is John Bowlby.[7] Bowlby believes that the separation of a child from its mother is of paramount importance in the development of depressive symptomatology in children. He has identified three phases in the response of a young child to separation from its primary caretaker. The first phase is protest, in which the child responds by emotional affective "storms" in an effort to restore the mother. The next stage is despair, in which the child affectively withdraws in sadness because of the separation from the parent. The third stage is detachment, in which the child

TABLE 26–1 ••• ATTACHMENT-RELATED RESPONSE TO SEPARATION OF A YOUNG CHILD FROM ITS PRIMARY CARETAKER

Phase	Emotional Response
Protest	Emotional affective storms in an effort to restore the parent
Despair	Withdrawal in sadness because of separation from the parent
Detachment	Emotional detachment indicating resignation to loss of the parent

eventually becomes resigned to the loss of the maternal object. Even when the child is reunited with the mother figure, the process of detachment continues for a period of time until the child is psychologically able to emotionally reattach to the maternal figure (Table 26–1).

The American Psychiatric Association has classified mental disorders in the *Diagnostic and Statistical Manual-III-R* (*DSM-III-R*). The most common forms of childhood depression are major depressive disorder, dysthymia, and adjustment disorder with depressed mood. The *DSM-III-R*[8] is very specific in terms of the symptoms related to each diagnostic category.

Major Depressive Disorder

Major depressive disorder is a very serious disorder that occurs in children, adolescents, and adults. A predominantly dysphoric mood is evident for at least 2 weeks. The child may be irritable, hopeless, despairing, and sad. For the diagnosis to be definitive, five of the symptoms listed in Table 26–2 must be seen every day for at least 2 weeks.

TABLE 26–2 ••• *DSM-III-R* SYMPTOMS OF A MAJOR DEPRESSIVE DISORDER

Change in appetite as reflected by weight gain or weight loss
Insomnia or hypersomnia
Psychomotor agitation or hyperactivity in children
Fatigue or lack of energy—apathy can be noted in children
Feelings of worthlessness, reproach, and guilt
Difficulty concentrating or thinking
Depressed or irritable mood
Recurrent thoughts of death, suicidal ideation, or suicidal attempts
Loss of interest in pleasure or loss of pleasure in usual activities

Data from Diagnostics and Statistical Manual of Mental Disorders. 3rd ed, Revised. Washington: American Psychiatric Association, 1987, pp 222–224.

TABLE 26–3 ••• *DSM-III-R* SYMPTOMS OF DYSTHYMIC MOOD DISORDER

Depressed or irritable mood
Two of the following symptoms: appetite disturbance, sleep disturbance, fatigue, hopelessness, poor concentration, or low self-esteem
Symptoms have been experienced for at least a year with no relief for more than 2 months

Data from Diagnostics and Statistical Manual of Mental Disorders. 3rd ed, Revised. Washington: American Psychiatric Association, 1987, pp 216–224.

Dysthymia

Dysthymia is a depressive syndrome in children characterized by a depressed and irritable mood and at least two of the symptoms that characterize the depressive syndrome (Table 26–3). However, the magnitude of symptoms is not great enough for the condition to qualify as major depressive disorder. The child must also have experienced these symptoms for at least a year, with no relief from these symptoms for longer than 2 months.

Adjustment Disorder With Depressed Mood

In adjustment disorder with depressed mood, the symptoms are depression, despair, and hopelessness, but in these cases, there is an identifiable psychosocial stressor, and the depressive symptomatology has its onset within 3 months of the psychological stressor.

A study by Mitchell et al.[9] demonstrated several findings that are relevant to the relationship between depression and childhood. These researchers found that the criteria used to diagnose depression in adults can be used also to diagnose depression in children and adolescents. Depressed children and depressed adolescents did not differ significantly from each other in terms of depressive symptomatology, but there were some differences between depressed children and depressed adults. The adults reported more insomnia, depressive feelings in the early morning, and eating disturbances (weight loss and lack of appetite). Mitchell et al. also found that depressed children think about and attempt suicide as often as depressed adolescents. There is a relationship between major depressive disorder in children and separation anxiety, as well as between depressed preadolescent boys and conduct disorders. Thus young boys who are quite depressed will often present with conduct disorders.

Hughes et al.[2] discussed the descriptive profile of the depressed child from ages 6 to 12. They believe that the descriptive profile of the depressed child is very similar to that of the adult. The most prominent symptoms include sadness, hopelessness, and dysthymia, along with vegetative symptoms of fatigue, loss of appetite, and difficulty sleeping. Suicidal ideation and attempts are also prevalent. Depressed children had difficulties in school and family histories that included psychiatric disorder adjustment problems.

In summary, there are several specific diagnostic indicators for depression in children. Several research studies were reviewed in an effort to discuss the most recent research findings regarding childhood depression.

Several clinical vignettes that typify clinical examples of childhood depression follow. The pediatric adolescent gynecologist will very likely have an opportunity to intervene in such cases in a timely and important way.

Clinical Vignette ••• A Case of Anaclitic Depression

Laura was a very frail, thin 9-month-old infant who presented to the pediatrician via a social worker from the Department of Human Services. Laura had been placed in an orphanage 2 months previously and was awaiting placement in a therapeutic foster home. The social worker described the infant as being inconsolably sad, with a large number of unremitting crying episodes. She also described the infant as withdrawn from her social environment, and she did not appear to want to interact with any of her caretakers at the orphanage. The social worker was further alarmed by the infant's lack of appetite, refusal to eat, and loss of weight, and for these reasons sought a consultation with the pediatrician. After a thorough medical evaluation, the pediatrician could not find any physical or medical explanations for the child's symptoms. The pediatrician told the social worker that the infant appeared anaclitically depressed and suggested that the social worker get in contact with appropriate mental health/psychiatric services so that the infant could be reunited with an appropriate maternal figure, if not with her own mother.

History. Laura had been a full-term infant who was cheerful, healthy, and very well bonded with her mother from the time of her birth until the age of 7 months, when her mother had to be hospitalized for a serious physical illness. Ordinarily the infant would have been placed with a very supportive maternal grandmother, but Laura had to be placed in an orphanage because of her maternal grandmother's health. The child's symptoms after separation from her mother were indicative of severe anaclitic depression. The social worker, who was very concerned about the emotional and physical welfare of this infant, kept in contact with the child's mother and maternal grandmother.

Outcome. The social worker was exceptionally responsive to the pediatrician's recommendation. The infant was able to be returned to the mother within 3 months of being separated from her. With the help of continued follow-up by the pediatrician and by mental health services, the child returned to her former state of good emotional and physical health within 6 months.

Clinical Vignette ••• A Case of Major Depression in an 11-Year-Old Girl

Mariana was an 11-year-old girl who was brought to the family practice physician's office by her mother. The mother indicated that during the preceding month, the child had demonstrated a severely depressed mood and was frequently both tearful and irritable. The mother described the child's mood as hopeless, despairing, and sad and indicated the presence of vegetative signs of major depression such as a 20-pound weight gain in the previous month and a great deal of difficulty sleeping. In interviewing the child, the family practice physician was able to determine that the child had felt very tired and fatigued for the previous month and had withdrawn from social activities that she had previously enjoyed. She had also been experiencing suicidal ideation for the past month. Mariana stated that she had difficulty concentrating in school. Her mother indicated that she was very concerned about her child and sought recommendations from the physician. Her sincere concern for her child was heightened by the fact that the patient's maternal grandmother and maternal aunt had both been diagnosed as being biologically depressed. The family practice physician decided to refer the patient for psychiatric evaluation, because the child appeared to be experiencing a major depression and required psychiatric evaluation and intervention.

Clinical Vignette ••• A Case of Adjustment Disorder With Depressed Mood in a 7-Year-Old Girl

Charlene was an attractive 7-year-old girl with bright red hair and freckles who was brought to the pediatrician by her recently divorced mother. The mother stated that before her divorce, the child had had a sunny disposition and abundant energy; since the divorce, she had been a very irritable, disagreeable child who cried a great deal and was having difficulty in her second-grade class. The mother stated that Charlene had been very close to her father and was having a great deal of difficulty adjusting to seeing her father only on weekends. Charlene told the pediatrician that she missed her father very much and related that her depressed mood and social difficulties began shortly after her father left. The mother confirmed the child's self-report. The pediatrician evaluated the child both physically and emotionally and decided to refer both Charlene and her mother for mental health services in an effort to assist them in dealing with the adjustment disorder with depressed mood related to the recent divorce.

Importance of the Primary Care Physician in Providing Intervention

The primary care physician is very important in terms of assessing and diagnosing childhood depression in the family practice patient population. Blumenthal[10] indicated in her research that primary care physicians see more psychiatric patients in day-to-day practice than do psychiatrists. Many psychiatric patients are either unwilling to receive or unaware that they require psychiatric care and instead are assessed by the primary care physician. Thus,

the physician has a very important role in intervening with these patients and making the appropriate referral to mental health services. Blumenthal[10] also indicated that more than 80% of psychiatric patients who are in their first major psychiatric crisis seek out their primary care physician rather than a psychiatrist. If patients have legitimate psychiatric problems, the physician should refer them for psychiatric evaluation and follow-up mental health care. Many depressed children and adults would not receive appropriate mental health care in a timely way if it were not for perceptive primary care physicians who made the appropriate referral.

Etiology of Childhood Depression

Several variables are related to childhood depression. Goodyer et al.[11] indicated that the presence of stressful events in the mother's life, a parent's poor marital relationship with his or her partner, and the presence of parental emotional distresses are all significantly related to emotional disorders in the school-age child. Puig-Antich et al.[12] found that prepubertal onset of major depression is significantly more prevalent when alcoholism, major depression, or other psychiatric disorders are present in first- and second-degree relatives.

Clinical Vignette ••• Relationship Between a Family History of Major Depressive Disorder and the Presence of Such a Disorder in an 11-Year-Old Girl

Cassandra, an 11-year-old girl, was brought to the pediatrician by her mother. The patient was extremely pale and frail, and she had deep black circles under her eyes. The mother reported that during the preceding 2 months, the child had begun to manifest mood swings and irritability. The mother had also noticed insomnia and nightmares, as well as a severe decrease in weight and appetite. The child complained of fatigue and a lack of interest in activities that she had previously enjoyed. She had been involved in cheerleading activities in school and had participated in several extracurricular clubs at school, but for the previous 2 months, she had refused to participate in any of these activities. Both Cassandra and her teachers reported that she had significant difficulty concentrating in class. The mother reported to the pediatrician that there was a strong family history of major depression. Cassandra's maternal grandmother had been diagnosed as having major depressive disorder in her early twenties. She had been hospitalized twice for treatment of depression and was receiving outpatient psychotherapy and antidepressant medication to maintain the stabilization of her depression. The mother also indicated that two of the child's maternal uncles had been diagnosed with major depressive disorder, and the mother had also received treatment for depression as a young adult. The pediatrician believed Cassandra was also expressing signs and symptoms of a major depressive disorder and referred her for psychiatric evaluation. The diagnosis of major depressive disorder was confirmed by the psychiatrist. The child responded very well to a combination of individual, family, and antidepressant therapy.

Clinical Vignette ••• Relationship Between Traumatic Victimization and Depression in a 9-Year-Old Girl

Many clinically depressed children have family histories that include traumatic victimization—specifically, alcoholism, sexual abuse, physical abuse, and emotional abuse that occur with regularity. In fact, many of these depressed children come from families where these problems have occurred in many members over several generations.

Mary was a 9-year-old girl who was brought to the family practice physician by her social worker. The child had recently been removed from her family because of allegations of sexual and physical abuse. There was also a strong history of alcoholism in several members of the child's family, including her father, who was accused of sexually abusing her. The social worker was very concerned about the child's depression, irritability, poor peer relations, and difficulty adjusting to her placement at the children's shelter. The child reported experiencing these symptoms for more than a year.

The family practice physician believed the most appropriate diagnosis was dysthymia and referred Mary for mental health evaluation and care. The child responded to intervention and was ultimately placed in a very therapeutic foster home, where her depression stabilized.

In summary, there are several issues that are directly related to the etiology of depression in childhood. Primary ones include a family history of biologic depression, a history of traumatic victimization, and a history of distress in the mother of the depressed child.

Treatment Modalities for the Depressed Child

It is very important that the physician understand the treatment modalities for the depressed child. The primary intervention strategies include play therapy, individual therapy, group therapy, expressive art therapy, and family therapy. If the child is experiencing biologic depression, an antidepressant may be utilized as part of the therapeutic regime.

Play Therapy

Play therapy is generally utilized with very young children (ages 4 to 8) whose verbal skills are not fully developed. Children in this age range express their intrapsychic conflicts through the medium of play. The therapist (usually a child psychologist or a child psychiatrist) engages the child in therapeutic play, and through this modality, the depressed child can express and deal with the issues related to the depression.

Individual Therapy

Individual therapy is a modality that can be used with the older child who possesses verbal skills and also with the latency-aged child (ages 5 through 11). Individual therapy involves having the depressed child develop a trusting relationship with the therapist so that he or she feels able to discuss the issues related to the depressive condition. The child's expression of feelings and conflicts in a warm, supportive context is thought to be an important part of the therapeutic process. The ability of the child to receive support and feedback from the therapist is also important.

Group Therapy

Group therapy is often used in the treatment of depressed children. The group provides an interpersonal context for these children that is very helpful, because most children with depressive symptomatology have either withdrawn from peers or have very poor peer relationships. A play group is utilized for very young children (ages 4 to 7). In this play group, the children work on depressive issues and social relationships through the medium of play. The group therapist encourages expression of feelings and conflicts through the modality of play. Children are also encouraged to relate constructively to each other; social interaction and a sense of being a part of the group are extremely helpful in the treatment of childhood depression. For older children (ages 8 to 12), group therapy is used to assist the children to talk about feelings and problems related to their depression. Constructive feedback and problem solving are provided by peers and the group therapist. Such supportive interactions are invaluable for the depressed child and assist in ameliorating feelings of despair and social isolation.

Family Therapy

Family therapy is an extremely important part of working with depressed children. Family therapy allows the child and the parents to constructively discuss the problems in the family that are related to the child's depression. This approach allows parents and children to constructively work through conflicts and issues, which leads to healthier functioning within the whole family.

Antidepressant Therapy

If the psychiatrist considers the child to be biologically depressed, a trial of antidepressant medication may be prescribed as an adjunct to other therapy modalities. A therapeutic response to the medication often reduces the vegetative symptoms of the depression (i.e., sleep disturbance, eating disturbance, lethargy, and inability to concentrate) so that the child is more psychologically capable of working on the issues involved. Thus, this therapy is an extremely helpful part of the total treatment regime of the biologically depressed child.

ADOLESCENT DEPRESSION

Adolescent depression remains a major problem in American society. Violence, suicide, and substance abuse are prevalent among teenagers. Many of these sociologic problems with teenagers have their origin in depressive symptomatology. Kanashani et al.,[13] in a study of the prevalence of depression in adolescents, found that 4.7% had a major depressive disorder and 3.3% had a dysthymic disorder. Depression is thus considered a significant problem for adolescents. Simeon[3] indicated that the morbidity and mortality rates of adolescent depression have increased 11% since the 1970s. Depression is a key factor in the problems of victimization, teenage pregnancy, drug and alcohol abuse, runaways, delinquency, and other forms of aberrant behavior. Diagnosis and treatment of teenage depression are important ways to intervene in a variety of sociologic problems.

Diagnostic Indicators of Depression in Adolescents

According to Mitchell et al.,[9] the criteria used to diagnose depression in adults can also be used to diagnose depression in adolescents. A major depressive episode is a common diagnostic category of depression in this age group. The primary symptoms include severe depressive feelings, an eating disturbance involving either an increase or a decrease in appetite, and difficulty sleeping. Other symptoms include psychomotor activity, difficulty concentrating, fatigue, loss of interest in usual activities, and suicidal ideation. Definitive diagnosis requires the major depressive episode to be evident for at least 2 weeks.

Another major category of depression in adolescents is dysthymia. Like in children, symptoms include most or all of the symptoms that characterize the major depressive syndrome, but the magnitude of these symptoms is not severe enough for the condition to qualify as a major depressive episode. In adolescents, a dysthymic disorder is considered to be a long-term depression, and the symptoms must have been experienced for at least a year.

Inamdar et al.[14] found that adolescents reported more suicidal acts than did adults. Conversely, adults reported more symptoms related to insomnia, appetite reduction, and weight loss than did adolescents.

Two commonly seen symptom complexes in adolescents are dysthymic disorder with acting-out equivalents and dysthymic disorder with acting-in equivalents. Both symptom complexes include a chronic long-standing depression. The dysthymic disorder with acting-out equivalents involves angry acting-out symptoms. The dysthymic disorder with acting-in equivalents is characterized by withdrawal and isolation.

Clinical Vignette ••• Dysthymic Disorder With Acting-Out Equivalents in a 15-Year-Old Adolescent Female

Joan was a 15-year-old adolescent female. Her mother contacted the pediatrician because Joan was experiencing rapidly declining grades and numerous instances of truancy. The mother stated that these problems had been occurring during the preceding year but had reached a crisis state when the adolescent was expelled from school. Other symptoms included depression, constant irritability, and very poor peer relations. When Joan was questioned about her depression, truancy, poor peer relations, and declining grades during the preceding year, she responded by saying that she "just did not care." Joan further shared her feelings of depression and hopelessness with the pediatrician. The physician recommended that Joan be evaluated by a psychiatrist. Ultimately Joan was diagnosed as manifesting a dysthymic disorder with acting-out equivalents and underwent outpatient individual and family therapy.

Clinical Vignette ••• Dysthymic Disorder With Acting-In Equivalents in a 14-Year-Old Adolescent Female

Mara was a 14-year-old adolescent female. She had been a vivacious teenager who was full of life and interested in everything around her, but approximately a year before seeing the physician, she began to withdraw gradually from the many activities that she was involved in at school. She told her mother she was not interested in these activities, and they bored her. Soon her grades began to drop, and she complained that she had difficulty concentrating. Then she began to isolate herself from her family by spending long periods of time in her room with the curtains drawn. She then began to eat dinner in her room and refused to come to the dinner table with the family. Mara's mother noticed that she lost about 35 pounds during the year before pediatric consultation. Other symptoms included severe emotional lability and crying spells. Mara complained of extreme fatigue and was absent from school a great deal because of this complaint. Mara's friends said she had changed, and they felt they didn't even know her because she was so frail and depressed. Mara told her mother often that she wished to be dead. Mara's mother found letters discussing suicide in her room. Mara's mother sought consultation with the pediatrician because of the depressive symptomatology and the severely withdrawn and isolating behavior. The pediatrician evaluated Mara completely and ruled out any physical illness. He felt that she was severely depressed and referred her for a psychiatric evaluation. The psychiatrist diagnosed Mara as having dysthymic disorder with acting-in equivalents. Mara underwent individual, group, and family therapy and responded well, making good progress within 2 months of treatment.

Intervention Strategies for the Primary Care Physician

Many adolescents come to the attention of primary care physicians because of somatic complaints related to depressive symptomatology. It is very important, therefore, that primary care physicians be extremely aware of the signs and symptoms of depression in adolescents so that appropriate referrals for psychiatric evaluation and mental health services can be made. Many pediatricians and family practice physicians, as well as obstetricians-gynecologists, have depressed teenagers brought to them because parents feel that some of the depressive symptoms are related to a physical condition. Weight gain and weight loss are symptoms that often are brought to the attention of the primary care physician. Also, other depressive symptoms such as insomnia, difficulty concentrating, psychomotor agitation, and fatigue are often first brought to the attention of the primary care physician rather than the psychiatrist. Many times, despite severe depressive symptoms, neither the adolescent nor the family is aware that the teenager is depressed. The primary care physician must be educated in terms of assessing diagnostic indicators for adolescent depression so that the correct referral for psychiatric evaluation and mental health services can be made. Because depression in adolescents tends to be more destructive and lethal than that in younger patients (e.g., violence, substance abuse, and suicide), it is especially important for the primary care physician to be aware of diagnostic cues of depression in teenagers so that proper intervention can be made.

Etiology of Depression in Adolescents

Several variables have been found to be related to depression in adolescents. Bowlby[7] indicated that loss of important attachment figures is often related to the onset of depressive symptomatology. Many such losses are found in the history obtained in severely depressed adolescents. Marton et al.[15] found that many depressed adolescents manifested a borderline personality disorder. The diagnosis of antisocial personality was also found to be related to depression in adolescents. Puig-Antich and coworkers[12] discovered that a history of depression and alcoholism in biologic relatives was also related to the onset of depressive symptomatology in young people. A history of family dysfunction and traumatic victimization (physical or emotional abuse) is also related to depression in adolescents.

Clinical Vignette ••• Relationship Between a Clinical History of Significant Loss of a Parental Figure and Major Depressive Disorder in a 15-Year-Old Girl

Melissa was an extremely obese 15-year-old female who was brought to the primary care physician because of rapidly deteriorating behavior during the preceding 2 months. When obtaining the family history, the family practice physician was told by Melissa's social worker that the adolescent's mother had died when Melissa was 5 years old. At that time, Melissa and her two younger brothers were left in the care of their biologic father. Initially the father was able to adequately care for the children, but after about 6 months, the father began to abuse drugs and neglect the children both physically and emotionally. At age 8, Melissa and her brothers were abandoned by their father. The Department of Human Services was called in to take custody of the children. Thus, by the age of 8, Melissa had lost her mother through death and her father through substance abuse. Melissa was finally placed with an extremely supportive foster mother who took a real interest in her and wanted to adopt her. The patient adjusted well and lived with her foster mother until she was 14 years old. The mother was in the process of adopting Melissa and her brothers when she had a severe heart attack and died. Thus, Melissa lost another maternal figure in her young life. Melissa was placed in a residential treatment center, where she appeared to become severely depressed. Severe mood lability, irritability, tearfulness, and suicidal ideation were noted in this patient, as were a 50-pound weight gain and severe insomnia during the previous 6 months. The family practice physician ruled out any physical problems and felt that referral to a child psychiatrist for evaluation of Melissa's depression was appropriate. Melissa was evaluated, and it was felt that she was severely depressed and was diagnosed as manifesting a major depressive episode. The child psychiatrist also recommended inpatient hospitalization because of the severity of her depression and the suicidal ideation. The patient responded well to inpatient hospitalization and antidepressant medication. After 60 days in the adolescent psychiatric program, Melissa was discharged and placed in a group home setting, where she did well with outpatient psychotherapy and continuation of antidepressant medication.

This clinical vignette indicates the importance of the relationship between significant parental losses and the onset of major depressive episode in a teenager. It also highlights the importance of asking questions pertaining to the loss of parental figure(s) when obtaining a patient history.

Clinical Vignette ••• Relationship Between a Family History of Alcoholism and the Development of Dysthymia in a 15-Year-Old Girl

Clarissa was an extremely thin 15-year-old girl with blonde hair, dark circles under her eyes, and complaints of fatigue, sleeplessness, and loss of appetite. Her mother indicated to the pediatrician that Clarissa had been experiencing these symptoms for the previous year, but the mother had become alarmed at Clarissa's 25-pound weight loss during this period, as well as her insomnia and level of fatigue. She was concerned that something was physically wrong with Clarissa. Clarissa had been extremely perfectionistic in terms of her grades and grooming, but during the preceding year, Clarissa complained of not being able to concentrate on her studies, and her previous intense interest in her appearance had given way to a nearly total lack of interest in dress and hygiene. It did not occur to her mother that Clarissa might be depressed, and she sought a pediatric consultation to determine a physical cause for the patient's symptoms. In taking a careful family history, the pediatrician found that both of Clarissa's parents were alcoholics, and Clarissa had to take on many of the parental responsibilities within the home. The mother described the father as "violent and unreasonable" when he drank and herself as "very withdrawn and quiet." Clarissa's mother stated that during the previous year both her and her husband's drinking had become more severe, and there was much more stress within the family and increased pressure on Clarissa. In fact, Clarissa was called on to take on the responsibilities of both her parents, as well as to deal with the "life tasks" of a 15-year-old girl. There was a strong family history of alcoholism on both the maternal and paternal sides of the family; two maternal uncles and her paternal grandmother were alcoholics. The pediatrician ruled out any physical problems and referred Clarissa to a psychiatrist, who began treating her on an outpatient basis for dysthymia. As part of family therapy, outpatient alcoholism treatment was recommended for both parents. The parents were willing to participate in outpatient treatment for alcoholism and responded well to therapy for their addiction. Clarissa was asked to attend Alateen, a treatment modality for children of alcoholic parents. Both Clarissa and her parents responded well to mental health intervention. Because of the timely intervention of the physician, Clarissa and her family were able to obtain help.

Personality Disorders

Marton et al.[15] reported that personality disorders are often found in adolescents with depressive disorders. Large numbers of dysphoric adolescents are considered "delinquent," "bad," "sociopathic," and "irresponsible" by parents, social workers, or other persons who have custody of these teenagers.

Conduct Disorder

One personality disorder commonly found in depressed teenagers is conduct disorder. Many teenagers who appear to be delinquent and have behavior disorders are also experiencing a depressive condition for which they also need treatment.

DSM III-R describes conduct disorder in the following manner. Three of the following symptoms must be noted for at least 6 months:

- Two instances of runaway behavior
- Stealing behavior
- Stealing involving confrontation of a victim
- Physical aggression and cruelty
- Fighting
- Lying
- Fire-setting behavior
- Truancy
- Breaking and entering
- Destruction of the property of others
- Forced sexual behavior with others
- Animal cruelty
- Use of a weapon in more than one fight

These symptoms are indicative of a behavioral pattern that violates the basic rights of others and of society. Conduct disorders are more prevalent in males than in females.

Clinical Vignette ••• Dysthymic Disorder With Concomitant Conduct Disorder in a 14-Year-Old Male

Mario, a 14-year-old Mexican American male, was referred for pediatric evaluation by his juvenile probation officer. He was brought in by his anxious and intimidated mother, who described Mario as unruly and defiant for the previous 2 years. The mother described his behavior as antisocial and said that Mario had been noted to steal, be extremely physically aggressive with his peers, and engage in truancy, and destroy the property of others. The mother further described Mario as "having no respect for the rights of others or their property." She indicated that Mario had been quite depressed for more than a year since his father had abandoned the family. Mario had previously been very close to his father, and the father's absence had had an extremely negative effect on him. Mario said he didn't care about anything after his father left. The pediatrician ruled out any physical problems and referred Mario to a child psychiatrist; he felt Mario was very depressed, in addition to having significant behavioral problems. Mario was diagnosed as having a dysthymic disorder along with an additional conduct disorder. Because of Mario's severe acting-out behavior, he was placed in a residential treatment setting where he could receive individual, group, and family therapy while in a structured group setting where he could also learn some internal controls and receive help in terms of his conduct disordered behavior.

Borderline Personality Disorder

Another extremely important personality disorder that is found with great frequency in depressed adolescents is borderline personality disorder. It is very important that the primary care physician be aware of the frequency of borderline personality disorder in depressed adolescents; these teenagers are likely to be brought to the attention of the primary care physician because of the intense and unstable character of such adolescents' interpersonal relationships and the emotional difficulty they cause parents and other authority figures. Many depressed adolescents also manifest a concomitant borderline personality disorder. The *DSM III-R* defines borderline personality disorder as being characterized by severe instability of interpersonal relationships, mood, and self-image. Five of the following symptoms must be present for the diagnosis of the borderline personality disorder:

- Extreme anxiety related to abandonment issues
- Extreme feelings of boredom and emptiness

- Recurrent suicidal threats, self-mutilation, or other suicidal behavior
- Severe affective lability
- Extreme difficulty controlling anger
- Poor impulse control in two of the following areas: sexuality, drug and alcohol abuse, eating, stealing, or driving
- Identity disturbance
- Severe abandonment anxiety

Because borderline adolescents are difficult for parents and authority figures to manage, it is very likely that such adolescents will be brought to the primary care physician with a request for evaluation and referral. In addition to borderline personality disorder, many of these teenagers also manifest a depressive disorder.

Clinical Vignette ••• Major Depression and Borderline Personality Disorder in a 17-Year-Old Female

Brandy, a rather angry-appearing 17-year-old teenager, was brought to the pediatrician by her adoptive mother. The mother stated that Brandy had always been a rather difficult child to manage because of her temper and poor impulse control. However, during the preceding 6 months, her mood swings had become extremely severe. Within a span of hours, she would go from acting like a relatively normal teenager to fits of screaming and throwing things, with no apparent external provocation for these affective changes. Brandy would also mutilate her arms when she was extremely upset, and her pale arms were covered with red marks from this self-mutilative behavior.

The adoptive mother was especially upset by Brandy's self-mutilation and suicidal threats when she became angry and frustrated. Brandy also appeared to be exceedingly frightened by issues that related to separation and abandonment. Therefore, friendships were hard for her to deal with, because she could not tolerate abandonment or even brief separations. Brandy also had difficulty in terms of impulse control (sexual promiscuity and substance abuse). The adoptive mother was extremely frustrated with Brandy's promiscuity and her drinking, which had escalated during the previous 6 months. It was very hard to interest Brandy in constructive activities, because she complained of pervasive feelings of boredom and emptiness. The pediatrician ruled out any physical problem, and referral for a mental health evaluation was made. The psychiatrist diagnosed Brandy as manifesting major depressive disorder and borderline personality disorder. A recommendation was made to place Brandy in a structured residential treatment setting for adolescents where both disorders could be treated.

Treatment Modalities for the Depressed Adolescent

It is very important that primary care physicians be aware of the different treatment modalities used with the depressed adolescent. The most frequently utilized modalities are individual therapy, group therapy, residential treatment, and acute inpatient hospitalization.

Individual Therapy

Individual therapy, usually on an outpatient basis, is a therapeutic modality in which the adolescent develops a trusting relationship with the therapist. Through this relationship, the adolescent is able to explore and express conflicts related to depressive issues. Development of a trusting relationship with a depressed teenager has its unique challenges. It is necessary for the therapist to be viewed as an ally and not just "another dominating parental figure." However, if the therapist is to help the adolescent, there also must be a good therapist-parent alliance. Essentially the therapist's job is to help parents understand and manage the adolescent more effectively.

Family Therapy

Family therapy is a very important therapeutic modality used with adolescents. Many adolescents' problems are directly related to difficulties within the family system. Family therapy enables all family members, including the adolescent, to express and work on problems related to the family.

Group Therapy

Group therapy is an extremely powerful modality to use with adolescents. Because of their stage of development, adolescents often discount and rebel against feedback given by parents and adults. However, feedback that is given by peers is given great respect and attention. Many adolescents are also more open with their peers because of their difficulty trusting adults. Group therapy consists of a group of adolescent peers (6 to 10 members) and a group therapist. The group therapist's role is to facilitate group discussion and work on individual issues within a group setting.

Residential Treatment

Residential treatment consists of a structured residential living arrangement in which the adolescent is placed for a period ranging from 2 months to 1 year. Residential treatment is recommended for adolescents who would not be able to function on an outpatient basis because of severe impulse control or judgment problems. Often, teenagers whose problems include runaway behavior, drug and alcohol abuse, stealing, and severe aggression are placed in a residential treatment setting. While in such a setting, the adolescent also receives individual, family, and group therapy.

Acute Inpatient Hospitalization

When the adolescent's depression is severe and dangerous, acute inpatient hospitalization is likely to be recommended. If an adolescent's depression renders him or her a danger to self or others, then admission to an inpatient facility is often sought for safe treatment of the adolescent. Inpatient hospitalization involves 24-hour supervision in a protected environment. While hospitalized, adolescents usually receive educational and recreational therapy, as well as individual, family, and group treatment. Antidepressant therapy is also often utilized to stabilize depressed adolescents while they are hospitalized.

CHILD AND ADOLESCENT SUICIDE

Blumenthal[10] reported that suicide is the second most frequent killer of young people, and the rate of suicide for America's adolescent population has tripled since the 1970s. Suicidal ideation is common in depressed children, but children rarely commit suicide. Suicide is more common in adolescents, and teenagers—especially depressed and psychologically stressed individuals—are considered to be at risk for suicidal ideation and behavior. Blumenthal[10] further indicates that most (75%) completed suicides (i.e., those resulting in death) are carried out by males; 50% of these involve firearms. Boyd[16] reported an alarming increase in the use of firearms in suicide among younger people. Frederick[17] indicated that male adolescents are three times more likely to complete suicide than females, but females are three times more likely to attempt suicide than males. For several decades, suicide has ranked second or third as the leading cause of death in teenagers.

It is very important for the physician to understand that suicide is a significant cause of death in adolescents. Adolescent males are at greater risk for completing suicide than adolescent females and more often commit suicide with firearms.

Diagnostic Indicators of Suicide in Adolescents and Children

The ability of the primary care physician to identify and diagnose a suicidal child or adolescent is extremely important, as these patients often come to the attention of the physician before they are directed to mental health services. Blumenthal[10] reported that most physicians see at least six "extremely suicidal" patients with suicidal ideation. Many suicidal patients use medication prescribed by their primary care physician to commit suicide and often have seen their physician within weeks of the suicide. Eighty percent of patients experiencing their first psychiatric crisis go to a physician rather than a psychiatrist, and therefore, it is extremely important that physicians be aware of the signs of suicide in adolescents so that appropriate intervention can be achieved.

A history of a previous suicide attempt is one of the most important indicators of suicide.[10] It is important to inquire about previous suicide attempts in patients assessed as being very depressed. Patients with certain psychiatric disorders have been found to have a higher incidence of suicide. Major depressive disorders, psychoses, and drug and alcohol abuse are also found to be related to suicidal behavior. In teenagers, manifestation of a depressive disorder combined with either a con-duct disorder or a borderline personality disorder has been found to be related to suicidal behavior. A family history of affective illness or of relatives who have committed suicide is also related to the incidence of suicide in children and adolescents. Bowlby[7] reported that the loss of an important attachment figure is also a factor in suicidal ideation and behavior in children and adolescents. Kosky et al.[18] identified family dysfunction, alcoholism, and the disruption of attachments as factors related to suicidal behavior in adolescents. These authors found that the disruption of attachments was a particularly important issue in adolescent males who attempted suicide. Like Frederick,[17] Kotila and Lonnqvist[19] indicated that adolescent boys committed suicide three times more often than adolescent girls, although girls were noted to attempt suicide 10 times more often than boys. These authors noted that adolescent boys who attempted suicide were frequently under the influence of alcohol when the suicide attempt was made. In fact, in adolescent males, drug or alcohol abuse often precipitated the suicide attempt. The suicide attempts of adolescent females were often found to be an immediate response to crisis or frustration.

Frederick[17] identified several indicators of youth suicide. Suicide is likely to occur when an adolescent feels that a series of negative life events have happened. Another indicator is a feeling of helplessness or inability to deal with stressful life events. The inability of adolescents to feel that they have some control over events in their lives is related to these feelings of helplessness. A final indicator of suicide in adolescents is a feeling of hopelessness, often diagnosed by the physician as clinical depression.

Clinical Vignette ••• A 17-Year-Old Suicidally Depressed Adolescent

Amy was an extremely pale and thin adolescent who appeared to be approximately 4 years younger than her stated age. She was brought to her family practice physician because her mother was very concerned about several suicide notes that had been found in Amy's bedroom and purse. The mother was especially concerned because Amy had attempted suicide 1 year previously and had been hospitalized for 2 months in an adolescent inpatient facility. There was a family history of depression on the maternal side, and Amy's maternal grandfather had committed suicide. The patient had recently had several interpersonal losses; her boyfriend had stopped seeing her, and her best friend had moved away. Amy had recently told her mother that she felt very depressed, and her life was no longer worth living. The primary care physician ruled out any physical causes and proceeded to interview the patient. Amy was asked if she was considering suicide at the present time. She answered affirmatively. After completing the interview, the physician met with Amy's mother and recommended that Amy's mother take her to a psychiatrist immediately after leaving the physician's office to evaluate Amy's suicide potential and determine whether inpatient hospitalization was indicated. The mother complied. The child psychiatrist who evaluated Amy indicated that she was very depressed and suicidal. The psychiatrist felt that Amy presented a danger to herself. She was admitted to an adolescent facility for inpatient treatment for 30 days and responded well to a combination of individual, family, group, and antidepressant therapy. She was discharged in stable condition and placed on weekly outpatient psychotherapy with medication and follow-up.

This is an example of how a primary care physician can intervene to save the life of a seriously depressed and suicidal adolescent. Without the timely intervention of the primary care physician, this patient may have attempted suicide.

Role of the Primary Care Physician in Intervention

The primary care physician is in a unique position to assess depression and suicidal ideation in the child and adolescent patient. The physician must be aware of the diagnostic indicators of suicide in children and adolescents. The physician also needs to ask the patient direct questions concerning issues related to previous suicide attempts and current suicidal ideation.

After the physician has determined that the child or adolescent is suicidal, he or she should meet with the parents or legal guardian of the child. The physician must then inform the family of the patient's depression and suicidal ideation, explaining them to the family in understandable terms. The physician should recommend to the family that the young person be taken for an emergency evaluation by a mental health specialist, specifically a psychiatrist who can assess the suicide potential of the child or adolescent. The psychiatrist will then make appropriate recommendations for the treatment of the patient.

Crisis Intervention in the Suicidal Child or Adolescent

The most important ability the primary care physician must have is the ability to assess the indicators of lethality in a child or adolescent. Specifically, the physician should be aware of major diagnostic indicators of suicide in children and adolescents so that he or she can make appropriate psychiatric referral for emergency evaluation and intervention. Once the child or adolescent has been assessed as being a danger to him- or herself by a psychiatrist, usual treatment involves placing the youth in an inpatient facility so that individual, family, group, and possibly antidepressant therapy can take place in a safe environment. For an extremely suicidal youth, placing the patient in a safe environment where he or she can have 24-hour supervision until suicidal behavior is stabilized is very important. The psychotherapeutic modalities of individual, family, and group therapy take a slightly different focus when dealing with a suicidal youth; these will be described in the following section.

Treatment Modalities For the Suicidal Adolescent

Individual Therapy

Individual therapy for a suicidally depressed adolescent involves having the therapist develop a trusting relationship with the adolescent so that he or she will feel able to explore the issues and feelings related to his or her suicidal impulses. Because many suicidal adolescents have experienced numerous losses of significant interpersonal relationships, much of the therapeutic work often involves assisting adolescents through the grieving process and thus helping them to emotionally resolve these losses. Assisting the adolescent to deal with overwhelming feelings of hopelessness and helplessness is also often involved in the individual therapy.

Family Therapy

Family therapy is a very important part of treatment for the suicidal adolescent, because many times much of the patient's depression and desire to commit suicide has to do with severe family dysfunction. In family therapy, the adolescent's problems with his or her family are brought out and worked on. Family problems that are often related to adolescent suicidal ideation include alcoholism in or substance abuse by one or both of the parents, parental depression, physical abuse, and sexual abuse. It is very important that the family issues related to the patient's suicidal ideation and behavior be worked on in the family context.

Group Therapy

Group therapy is also an important therapeutic modality for the suicidal adolescent. Many of these patients feel extremely hopeless and helpless in relation to the parental figure. Their only hope may be related to constructive feedback offered by peers. The group often offers the suicidally depressed adolescent an optimistic viewpoint. Group therapy enables the patient to understand how problems that he or she felt were hopeless or insolvable can actually be solved in a hopeful and constructive manner. In addition, suicidal teenagers are often very withdrawn and constricted, and the group format encourages them to open up to an audience of their peers, something that is often less threatening to the adolescent than talking to an adult.

Clinical Vignette ••• Crisis Intervention in a Suicidal Adolescent by a Primary Care Physician

Dr. B. was contacted at his private practice office by Mrs. S., who was hysterical and sobbing. She stated that her 15-year-old daughter Sally had just locked herself in the bathroom and was threatening to slash her wrists with a knife. Mrs. S. stated that Sally had been depressed for the past several months. The precipitating event for this suicide threat was the breakup between Sally and her boyfriend. Sally had come home from school despondent after the breakup and run into the bathroom with a knife several minutes before the mother contacted Sally's pediatrician. Dr. B. told Sally's mother to get Sally out of the bathroom immediately, either by talking her out or by calling the police so that they could get her out. Afterward, Dr. B. directed Sally's mother to take her to the emergency department so that she could be evaluated by a psychiatrist and a recommendation made for treatment. The mother was told to allow the police to escort her and Sally to the hospital if she couldn't do it alone. The mother was asked to call Dr. B. from the emergency department to let him know of the outcome of the evaluation. At the emergency department, the attending psychiatrist diagnosed Sally as having major depressive disorder and felt that she was a danger to herself because of suicidal intent. The psychiatrist admitted her to an adolescent facility on an emergency basis. The attending psychiatrist was extremely complimentary of Dr. B.'s clear and appropriate intervention in the situation. Dr. B. was relieved to hear from the mother that Sally had been admitted to an adolescent inpatient unit and was adjusting well.

References

1. Toolan J. Depression and suicide in children. In: Lesse S (ed). What We Know About Suicide and How to Treat It. Northvale, NJ: Jason Aronson, 1988.
2. Hughes CW, Preskorn SH, Weller E, Hassanein R. A descriptive profile of the depressed child. Psychopharmacol Bull 1989; 25(2):232–237.
3. Simeon JG. Depressive disorder in children and adolescents. Psychiatr J Univ Ottawa 1989; 14:356–361.
4. Petti TA. Depression in hospitalized child psychiatry patients. J Am Acad Child Adolesc Psychiatry 1978; 17:49–58.
5. Carlson G, Cantwell D. A survey of depressive symptoms in a child and adolescent psychiatric population. J Am Acad Child Psychiatry 1979; 18:587–599.
6. Spitz RA. Anaclitic depression. Psychoanal Study Child 1946; 2:313–342.
7. Bowlby J. Attachment and Loss. Vol. 2. Separation, Anxiety, and Anger. London: Hogarth Press, 1973.
8. Diagnostic and Statistical Manual of Mental Disorders (DSM-III-R). 3rd ed. Washington, DC: American Psychiatric Association, 1987.
9. Mitchell J, McCauley E, Burke PM, Moss S. Phenomenology of depression in children and adolescents. J Am Acad Child Psychiatry 1988; 27(1):12–20.
10. Blumenthal SJ. Suicide: A guide to risk factors, assessment, and treatment of suicidal patients. Med Clin North Am 1988; 72(4):937–964.

11. Goodyer IM, Wright C, Altham PM. Maternal adversity and recent stressful life events in anxious and depressed children. J Child Psychol 1988; 29(5):651–667.

12. Puig-Antich J, Goetz D, Davies M, et al. A controlled family history study of prepubertal major depressive disorder. Arch Gen Psychiatry 1989; 46:406–418.

13. Kashani JH, Gabrielle A, Beck NC, et al. Depression, depressive symptoms, and depressed mood among a community sample of adolescents. Am J Psychiatry 1987; 144:931–934.

14. Inamdar S, Siomopoulous G, Osborn M, Bianchi E. Phenomenology associated with depressed mood in adolescents. Am J Psychiatry 1979; 136:156–159.

15. Marton P, Korenblum M, Dutcher S, et al. Personality dysfunction in depressed adolescents. Can J Psychiatry 1989; 34:810–813.

16. Boyd J. The increasing rate of suicide by firearms. N Engl J Med 1983; 308:872–874.

17. Frederick CJ. An introduction and overview of youth suicide. In: Peck ML, Farberow NL, Litman RE (eds). Youth Suicide. New York: Springer, 1985.

18. Kosky R, Silbern S, Zubrick SR. Are children and adolescents who have suicidal thoughts different from those who attempt suicide? J Nervous Mental Dis 1990; 178:38–43.

19. Kotila L, Lonnqvist J. Adolescent suicide attempts: Sex differences predicting suicide. Acta Psychiatr Scand 1988; 77:264–270.

CHAPTER 27

Adolescent Drug Abuse

PAUL KING

Although there is evidence of a general decline in illegal drug abuse since its peak in the early 1970s, chemical abuse still remains a major problem in adults and adolescents. According to the National Household Survey, illegal drug abuse declined from 12% of the population in 1985 to 7% in 1988. Alcohol abuse declined from 59% to 53% and cigarette smoking from 32% to 25% during the same period.[1]

The high school senior survey conducted by the National Institute on Drug Abuse (NIDA) likewise showed an adolescent decline.[2] Abuse of illegal drugs declined from 21.3% of seniors in 1988 to 19.3% in 1989. Marijuana abuse was down to 17% in 1989, a marked change from the peak of 37% in 1978. Declines in abuse were specifically noted for "crack" cocaine, tranquilizers, and barbiturates. Increased efforts by the government, prevention programs, and treatment professionals have helped to improve attitudes about drugs, with the goal being the repudiation of drug abuse among the vast majority of young people. In 1979, only 34.2% of seniors felt negatively about experimentation with marijuana; 10 years later, 64.6% of seniors disapproved of marijuana abuse. Fifty-four percent of seniors indicated that cocaine abuse is risky and an even greater percentage have similar feelings about crack cocaine. The decline in abuse among teens is clearly a result of reduced demand, as the easy availability of drugs continues to be a widespread problem.

Several trends, however, continue to be alarming. Inhalant abuse remains a steady problem, and phencyclidine (PCP) abuse is increasing. Old drugs are finding new and dangerous uses, such as abuse of steroids by young athletes. Alcohol abuse remains a significant problem, and cigarette smoking rates remain high. There are several new drugs produced in homemade laboratories and known as "designer drugs"; an example is "ecstasy" (methylenedioxy methamphetamine). Lysergic acid diethylamide (LSD) is making a comeback (Table 27–1). Another problem is the high high school dropout rate, currently approaching 30%.[3] Dropouts, of course, are not included in the senior drug and alcohol surveys.

SIGNS AND SYMPTOMS OF ADOLESCENT SUBSTANCE ABUSE

The following signs of substance abuse must be viewed as a constellation leading to a strong

---

TABLE 27–1 ••• SIGNS OF DRUG ABUSE

Hallucinogens: Hallucinations ("tripping"); dilated pupils, memory loss, time distortion.
Marijuana: Rapid heart beat, euphoria, relaxation, increased appetite, disorientation.
Stimulants: Increased alertness, excitation, euphoria, increased pulse rate and blood pressure, insomnia, loss of appetite.
Inhalants: Excitement, euphoria, drunken behavior, confusion, hallucinations.

Adapted from Kaufman E. Help at Last. A Complete Guide to Chemically Dependent Men. New York: Gardner Press, 1991.

suspicion that chemicals are the cause; a single sign is not sufficient for diagnosis.

1. Changes in patterns of behavior. The young person develops an ongoing, persistent negative attitude. There are fewer and fewer periods of positive thinking. There is increased defiance at home.

2. Decreased interest in school and school work. The usual complaint is boredom. Grades that once were adequate deteriorate to Ds and Fs in less than a year.

3. Increased irritability. Violence toward family members is an especially ominous sign.

4. Lack of motivation. This sign is most specific in marijuana smokers who lose ambition in school, motivation in sports, and involvement in positive activities.

5. Stolen money. Adolescent females may support a boyfriend's drinking or drug habit with money stolen from home. Of course, forged checks, unaccountable items purchased on credit cards, and missing valuables may be used to buy drugs.

6. Involvement in the occult. Satanic rites and rituals often involve group sex, drinking, and drug abuse.

7. Physical signs such as slurred speech, pallor, red eyes, and dilated pupils. Many over-the-counter pills—diet aids, sleeping aids, motion sickness pills, and cough medicines—when taken in large enough quantities, can cause a wide variety of symptoms.

8. A new set of friends who appear to have a negative attitude and/or unkempt appearance.

9. A substance-abusing boyfriend. Boyfriends have a major influence on the attitudes of teenage girls. If the boyfriend has a drinking or drug problem, the girl will either be pulled into the same pattern or will lose positive interests as she tries to help him. Both patterns are destructive to the development of a young girl.

10. Date rape or party rape. These often occur in a context of heavy drinking or drug abuse.

ALCOHOL ABUSE

Alcohol remains by far the most popular drug among teenagers, as it is legal for those who are of age. Pressure to drink begins as early as the fourth grade.[3] Alcohol is a central nervous system depressant and, in low doses,

produces excitement by depressing the reticular activating system of the brain stem. The resulting cortical disinhibition and excitement are similar to the effects produced by general anesthetics; judgment is also impaired. Because of this disinhibition and impairment of judgment, alcohol is often used before sexual activity. The term currently used by teenagers to refer to abusive drinking is *partying*. In previous years, a party was a social gathering in which alcohol might or might not be present. This has changed. In "partying," the primary goal is to drink until drunk, and the beverage consumed may be beer, pure grain alcohol (PGA) mixed in a punch, or mixed drinks. Alcohol may also be used along with other central nervous system depressants, such as benzodiazepine, tranquilizers, or marijuana. The end result in "partying" is to be completely out of control and therefore not assume any responsibility for one's behavior.

Another effect of alcohol is an increase in aggressive behavior as a result of impairment of the neurotransmitter serotonin. Blackouts, which consist of memory loss and uncontrollable behavior, may occur with heavy drinking. In fact, many teenagers who drink heavily talk about the number of blackouts that they have experienced. It is almost as if they are proud that they have drunk enough to have had blackouts. Unfortunately, however, blackouts are a sign of a serious drinking problem. "Partying" teenagers tend to drink like alcoholic individuals until they are intoxicated, sick, or the alcohol is gone. This is the reason that teenagers can develop a dependence on alcohol within months, whereas in adults the same process often takes years. Most professionals in the drug abuse field have abandoned the concept of teaching adolescents how to drink responsibly. The immaturity of teenagers, the striving to look and act as adults, and the inability to handle mood-altering substances create a situation in which adolescents are extremely vulnerable to becoming dependent on alcohol. If a parent is an alcoholic, this increases both genetic risk and vulnerability to many social and psychological problems from growing up in a home with an alcoholic.[4] Adolescents see their parents and other adults drinking, and they know about college students and drinking parties, whether from seeing it in movies or hearing about it from older brothers and sisters. Commercials show young adults having fun and associate fun with beer consumption. Drinking alcohol is associated with acting silly and having a good time. Teens see alcohol as a socially acceptable thing to do. Some popular songs may glorify and glamorize drinking. Beer is considered an integral part of America. It is sold in grocery stores and at football, baseball, and basketball games. Rarely is a sporting event televised without numerous beer commercials. Drinking by teens is a problem, not a phase of growing up, especially when a teenager is drinking abusively and getting into trouble.[5, 6]

Alcohol is a powerful substance that gives a sense of power and esteem. Young people drink alcohol to feel powerful and in control. It removes feelings of inadequacy and insecurity. Boys feel strong or macho; girls feel adult and feminine. Everyone wants to be powerful, secure, and glamorous, and very few adolescents have those feelings.

MARIJUANA ABUSE

Marijuana—also known as grass, tetrahydrocannabinol (THC), Acapulco gold, pot, and hash—was the drug of the 1960s. At that time, marijuana was considered a relatively safe drug that enhanced music and the expansion of the mind. Timothy Leary talked about the mind expansion of hallucinogens, and the use of psychedelics gained society's approval; marijuana was not thought to be harmful. However, times have changed, and so has the concept of marijuana. When marijuana is inhaled, it produces about 2000 chemicals. It acts on the limbic system to produce a dreamy, relaxed state, although depending on the concentration of the active chemical, THC, it may instead produce feelings of panic and dread. THC decreases the release of acetylcholine at the neuromuscular junction.[7] The dreamy state is so pleasant to chronic smokers that, when deprived of marijuana, they become angry and irritable. The problem attitude of teens who are marijuana smokers may be caused by the discomfort of not being "stoned," not by the state of intoxication.

Marijuana also affects the central nervous system and slows things down. The young person feels tired, moody, and passive, feelings known collectively as an *amotivational state*. He or she does not feel motivated to perform in school, sports, or activities. There is an "I don't care" attitude.[8] There is also an emotional movement away from the family in a drive to stay mellow, which means keeping the brain level of marijuana up high. Senses are enhanced, but the ability to act on these sensations is gone, and short-term memory is impaired.[8] There is a sense of enhancement and enjoyment of food and music, all of which are part of the fantasy state created by the drug.

Research on the effects of marijuana on the reproductive system shows an increased number of spontaneous abortions, toxic effects on the fetus, and a reduction in testosterone in male fetuses.[9] Although this research was done with laboratory mice, it is worthy of recognition. In a large sample of junior and senior high school students, a relationship was noted between marijuana abuse, heavy drinking, and a lack of church involvement. Friends had the greatest influence on attitudes; these young people perceived a great social pressure to use alcohol and other drugs and had great tolerance for deviant ideas and unconventional attitudes. Behaviors associated with marijuana abuse include abusive problem drinking, delinquent behavior, and precocious sexual behavior.[10] Other research on attitudes among adolescent drug abusers has found precocious sexuality, aggressive behavior, and a preference for heavy metal music.[11] Disaffection from prosocial institutions begins in adolescence and continues into young adulthood. This leads to greater participation in deviant activities, involvement in a subculture, and increased abuse of other drugs.[12] The result is a significant percentage of adolescents who are unlikely to become productive adults.

ALCOHOL, DRUGS, AND SUICIDE

There is a statement in Alcoholics Anonymous that with alcohol consumption one either becomes sobered up or you get locked up or covered up. In a study of juvenile delinquents, alcohol and drug abuse was found to be the most common psychiatric diagnosis in 63% of the sample. Several studies have shown an association between interpersonal disruption, alcoholism, and suicide.[13] The abuse of alcohol or drugs was a significant factor in 67% of 133 suicides in young people (<30 years old) studied at the University of San Diego.[14] This study also included 150 suicides in subjects older than 30. Alcoholism and substance abuse were so closely intertwined, especially in the young population, that pure alcoholics or pure substance abusers accounted for only a small minority of the patients. Eighty-four percent used both alcoholic and nonalcoholic substances. Substance abuse was a factor in 67% of the suicides in those younger than 30, compared with 46% of suicides in those older than 30. Recent interpersonal loss was a greater factor in suicide in substance abusers than in those with pure affective disorders.[15] Results clearly show that a history of alcoholism, substance abuse, and interpersonal loss puts an adolescent at high risk for suicide. Brent studied 156 suicide victims, age 10 to 19, who killed themselves between 1960 and 1983.[16] The percentage of those who were "high" or intoxicated rose from 3.4% in 1960 to 31% in 1983. Suicide carried out by firearms was five times more likely in those who had been drinking, showing the correlation with violent behavior and intoxication.

STIMULANTS, COCAINE, AND CRACK

Stimulants, or "speed," comprise a large class of drugs that vary from over-the-counter stimulants (also known as look-alikes), considered low in potency and available without prescription, to "ice," the newest and extremely powerful, smokable form of methamphetamine. Over-the-counter stimulants are legal, self-administered, and available in pharmacies and supermarkets. Many of these substances contain phenylpropanolamine, caffeine, and ephedrine. These drugs initially appear harmless, but a young person can seriously overdose on these products and become quite agitated, experiencing hypertension, palpitations, and psychotic episodes.[17] Many such preparations are sold in magazine advertisements as look-alike drugs. They are cheap and carry such names as 20/20s, 30/30s, 357s, pink footballs, or white crosses. These drugs are used by younger adolescents and sometimes in combination with other drugs by older adolescents. Advertisements are careful not to mislead the reader into thinking that the drugs are amphetamines, which fall under the Controlled Substance Drug Act of 1970. Young teenage girls may use these substances for appetite suppression.

In 1980, over-the-counter weight control preparations containing phenylpropanolamine, ephedrine, or pseudoephedrine, entered the market. A Food and Drug Administration (FDA) advisory panel concluded that they were safe and effective, although the FDA itself does not approve or endorse that conclusion. Several subsequent reports have warned about side effects such as palpitations, tachycardia, and hypertension. Phenylpropanolamine directly stimulates adrenergic receptors and indirectly stimulates alpha- and beta-adrenergic receptors, releasing norepinephrine; long-term use may deplete norepinephrine stores and adversely affect central nervous system activity. The perception by teens that these drugs are safe leads to self-administration to achieve weight loss, and taking these drugs in large quantities may result in toxicity.[18]

Amphetamines include amphetamine, methamphetamine, dextroamphetamine, and benzamphetamine (street names: black beauties, dexies, speed, crystal meth, ice, and crank). Depending on the chemistry, these drugs may be taken orally, inhaled (snorted), or injected. They were originally approved for the medical treatment of obesity on a short-term basis, for narcolepsy, and for attention deficit disorder. This last disorder is a common childhood problem marked by inattention and impulsive behavior, with the child easily distracted. Amphetamines and related drugs such as methylphenidate improve attention and increase impulse control. There are other sympathomimetic drugs related to amphetamines and with a similar mechanism of action that are used for short-term weight reduction; these include phenmetrazine. The amphetamines exert their central nervous system effects primarily by enhancing the release of neurotransmitters from presynaptic neurons. Neurotransmitters affected by amphetamines include norepinephrine, dopamine, and 5-hydroxytryptamine (5-HT, or serotonin). This accounts for the increased alertness, locomotor stimulating action, and anorexia. Other central nervous system effects include paranoia and psychotic behavior. Peripherally, there are both alpha and beta effects causing elevated blood pressure, tachycardia, slowing of gastrointestinal motility, and smooth muscle contractions, often leading to difficulty in voiding.

Other forms of stimulants include the previously mentioned "designer drugs." One injectable form is called crank, which is a form of methamphetamine. Poisoning with amphetamines may result in coma, convulsions, or death.

The drug abuse warning network is a system consisting of emergency department recordings of drug reactions. All forms of "speed" (amphetamines, methylphenidate) account for nearly 3% of the emergency department drug reactions. Look-alike drugs account for 1.6%.[19]

Treatment of amphetamine toxicity involves acidification of the urine with ammonium chloride, which accelerates the excretion of the drug. Antipsychotic drugs are helpful in alleviating central nervous system effects such as autonomic hyperarousal and paranoid delusions; either haloperidol or chlorpromazine may be used. However, the latter drug, when given in too large a dose, can result in severe orthostatic hypertension. Beta blockers may be helpful for managing hypertension.

Amphetamine, cocaine, and crack abusers are irritable, with feelings of omnipotence and paranoia when using these drugs in high dosage. A "crash" ensues when drug use ceases, leading to apathy, depression, and a suicide risk. The greatest "crash" occurs with drugs that are injected or smoked.

Cocaine is a naturally occurring substance that comes from the coca plant grown in Peru and the Andes mountains. Cocaine hydrochloride has relatively little toxicity because it is snorted. The resulting vasoconstriction prevents the accumulation of high concentrations of the drug within the blood stream and brain. Users become psychologically rather than physically addicted to a euphoria causing a direct effect on the dopamine system. However, this changed with the introduction of free-basing and crack. In free-basing, the alkaloid is changed into a form that is smoked using an organic solvent such as ether. When nonflammable solvents were found to accomplish the same result at less risk, a new form was created: crack. The use of crack brought with it serious and lethal effects. Crack enters the blood stream in extremely high concentrations through the lung's capillary surfaces. This tremendous increase in concentration in a short period of time is the "rush" that gives an intense euphoria. This creates possible lethal conduction problems.

A number of NIDA-sponsored studies have given insight into the mechanisms of cardiovascular abnormalities and sudden death associated with cocaine use. Cocaine causes vasoconstriction and increased sympathetic tone and has anesthetic effects. Susceptible persons may suffer from dysrhythmia, decreased cardiac output, and myocardial infarction.[20]

A new smokable form of methamphetamine known as "ice" has become popular primarily in Hawaii and California. Ice, a designer drug, is a different problem in that it is produced and consumed here in America. Other designer amphetamines include "ecstasy" and "Eve" (3,4-methenediopyethamphetamine); young people believe these are safe until proven dangerous.[21] The danger of violence is very real with the use of stimulant drugs such as amphetamines and cocaine.[22]

The widespread use of cocaine and crack has led to new problems involving pregnancy and fetal, neonatal, and neurologic development. Postmortem cesarean sections necessitated by cocaine-related cardiac arrhythmias and deaths in pregnant women have been reported.[23] Other significant problems include intrauterine growth retardation and/or prematurity. There have also been reports of increases in congenital anomalies involving the genitourinary tract, the gastrointestinal tract, and the cardiovascular system.[24, 25]

Drug abuse in pregnant women crosses economic and racial lines. In a study of 715 pregnant women in Pinellas County, Florida, more than 13% of private obstetric patients tested positive for drugs, compared with 16% receiving prenatal care at public clinics. Tests were done for cocaine, marijuana, and alcohol. The same study found that the rate of drug use in pregnant white women was 15%, compared with 14% in pregnant black women.

Other effects of cocaine include vasoconstriction leading to a decreased blood supply, especially to the distal phalanges, causing limb reduction deformities. Other problems include periventricular-intraventricular hemorrhage. There is an increased rate of spontaneous abortion as a result of uterine muscle contraction, placental abruption, and intrauterine growth retardation. Infants suffer from prematurity and low birth weight, decreased head circumference, and decreased length. Children show a variety of neurobehavior problems in orientation, state regulation, and motor development. In addition, when the infant doesn't respond normally, the mother withdraws her attention, leading to further withdrawal and neglect, possibly abuse by the mother.[26] Others disagree, stating that there is insufficient evidence because of methodologic problems. Social issues such as poverty, violence, and parental neglect or violence should also be considered.[27]

INHALANTS

There have been scattered reports of adolescents dying of cardiac arrhythmia or other sudden causes after inhalation of a volatile substance. Adhesive tape remover[29] and typewriter correction fluid containing 1,1,1,-trichloroethane and trichloroethylene have been linked to a number of deaths.[29, 30] Cardiac deterioration has been reported in patients given halothane anesthetic who had a history of exposure to trichloroethane.[30] Chemical abusing youngsters deliberately soak a rag with a chemical and place it over the face or inhale the fumes from a paper or plastic bag, a process called "huffing." Inhalants are very popular drugs, especially among younger adolescents. Their greatest appeal is among poverty stricken children. According to one rural drug counselor, "The kids are simple, the drug is cheap and easily available, and the high is powerful." One rural adolescent who used Freon stated, "It is the cheapest and easiest way to get drunk." Other young people point out how easy it is to "get off," with an almost immediate high. The changes in consciousness are analogous to those produced by anesthesia, with excitation, euphoria, and exhilaration. There is a rapid onset of action within a few minutes. Inhalants traverse the blood-brain barrier very quickly, because they are lipid soluble and accumulate in brain tissue, producing loss of inhibitions, confusion, and disorientation. Young people describe the sensation as similar to being drunk, but different. Excessive inhalation results in progressive depression of the central nervous system, with ataxia, hyporeflexia, stupor, seizures, or cardiorespiratory arrest. One rural youngster with little to no supervision described taking a drum of Freon into a car, closing the windows, and just laying back as he got progressively more stuporous.

The most commonly inhaled substances are glues, paints, and aerosols that contain toluene, or "tolley." Many clinical syndromes (e.g., encephalopathies, hallucination, coma, and cerebellar damage) have been directly related to both acute and chronic toluene abuse. Gasoline inhalation causes nausea and loss of consciousness. Neurologic symptoms occur with both chronic and acute gasoline sniffing; these include encephalopathy and ataxia. Freon, which is a halogenated hydrocarbon, is commonly used as a propellant in air conditioners. It produces significant depression of the cardiovascular system, cardiotoxicity, ventricular tachycardia, and fibrillation.[31] Nitrous oxide is another inhalant that is commonly used as a propellant for whipping cream. Finally, there are a number of substances found in "head shops" where drug abuse paraphernalia is sold. Aliphatic nitrites, called "rush," "poppers," and "snappers," are smooth muscle relaxants that cause vasodilatation. Medical complications result from vasodilatation and the formation of methemoglobin.

Inhalants are not a fad, although the particular types of inhalants used may change depending on availability; abuse of these substances will continue. Adults who work with young people need to be aware of this. If substances such as acrylic markers or typewriter correction fluid are missing from school supplies, youngsters may be using them. Hardware store managers need to be wary of youngsters buying Freon, solvents, or Scotchgard (isoparaffinic hydrocarbon).

DRUG SCREENING TESTS

The urine drug screen is a valuable diagnostic tool for both assessment and planning ongoing management. As a general rule, adolescents who present in an office or clinic setting will not have obvious physical symptoms. Toxicology screening tests may then be of tremendous importance in identifying abusers of marijuana, alcohol, sedatives, or stimulants. Comprehensive screening procedures consist of two parts: a primary screen and gas chromatography/mass spectrometry. The primary screen is usually an enzyme immunoassay or thin-layer chromatography (TLC). Such screens are quick and economical, and a positive result is then confirmed by a more specific and sensitive test. Gas chromatography/mass spectrometry is the most specific test but is too time consuming and expensive to be used as a primary screen.

It is not feasible for every adolescent to undergo drug screening. Indications for a urine screen include the following:

1. Adolescents with conduct problems (i.e., runaways)
2. Adolescents with psychiatric symptoms
3. Acute-onset behaviors or mood swings
4. Recurrent respiratory ailments
5. Recurrent accidents or unexplained somatic symptoms[32]

In most situations, urine tests are preferred over serum tests because of higher concentrations in the urine. An exception is phencyclidine piperidine (PCP), in which the drug remains in the blood stream for several days before being excreted. If the patient presents in a toxic state, both the blood and the urine may need to be tested. THC metabolites may be detected for up to several weeks after marijuana is smoked. Sensitivity may vary, but a given screen should detect at least 50 ng/ml, with an even greater sensitivity preferred. Cocaine is metabolized to benzoylecgonine and is easily detected. Heroin is difficult to detect but is most often "cut" with quinine, which is easily detected. In addition, although heroin breaks down to morphine, so does codeine, and therefore the presence of morphine may be misleading.

The most common presumptive tests are the enzyme-multiplied immunoassay technique (EMIT), thin-layer chromatography (TLC), and gas-liquid chromatography (GLC). EMIT utilizes an enzyme-substrate reaction, but because of the significant number of false-positive results, a confirmatory test is necessary. TLC identifies drugs by comparing the drug's distance from the point of origin with that of a solvent. The gas chromatography mass spectrometry, as stated earlier, is the most sensitive and specific confirmatory test. This technique uses ionized substances separated electromagnetically and identified by a specific mass spectrum. This high sensitivity is combined with the separation technique of capillary gas chromatography. A positive result using this technique is admissible as legal evidence in court.

The drugs most commonly found in drug poisoning cases are different from those used recreationally. The drugs seen most often in poisonings are aspirin, tranquilizers, sedatives, and antidepressants/stimulants.[33] Another study of a pediatric hospital population identified over-the-counter preparations and prescription drugs as the most common poisoning agents.[34]

TREATMENT

Recovery for an adolescent who is chemically dependent requires a long-term commitment on the part of the teenager and the family. The form of treatment (inpatient, outpatient, day care) often is less important than involvement for an extended period of time. One study of a day-care program proved that success depended on involvement for at least 1 year.[35] Another important factor is the acceptance by the adolescent that his or her life was unmanageable because of chemical abuse and that he or she is powerless over alcohol and/or drugs. This admission is the first step of the 12 Steps of Alcoholics Anonymous (Table 27–2). Working the steps in a self-help 12-step program requires that the drug abuser admit that he or she is compelled to use drugs, and that such use is different from social use. Giving up egocentrism is vital for recovery. Elkind has examined two aspects of this self-centeredness.[36] First, adolescents have a tendency to exaggerate how much attention they are receiving for behavior. Second, they feel they are unique ("Others may get hooked on drugs, but not me."). The adolescent feels that he or she will not experience negative consequences. This reasoning is also a factor in the failure of many adolescent girls to use contraception when they are sexually involved.[37]

TABLE 27–2 ••• TWELVE STEPS OF ALCOHOLICS ANONYMOUS

1. We admitted we were powerless over alcohol—that our lives had become unmanageable.
2. Came to believe that a Power greater than ourselves could restore us to sanity.
3. Made a decision to turn our will and our lives over to the care of God *as we understood Him.*
4. Made a searching and fearless moral inventory of ourselves.
5. Admitted to God, to ourselves, and to another human being the exact nature of our wrongs.
6. Were entirely ready to have God remove all these defects of character.
7. Humbly asked Him to remove our shortcomings.
8. Made a list of all persons we had harmed and became willing to make amends to them all.
9. Made direct amends to such people wherever possible, except when to do so would injure them or others.
10. Continued to take personal inventory, and when we were wrong, promptly admitted it.
11. Sought through prayer and meditation to improve our conscious contact with God *as we understood Him,* praying only for knowledge of His will for us and the power to carry that out.
12. Having had a spiritual awakening as the result of these steps, we tried to carry this message to alcoholics and to practice these principles in all our affairs.

Step 1 of Alcoholics Anonymous (AA) places the responsibility squarely on the adolescent. Denial by the patient and enabling by the parents are destroyed. When in front of other alcoholics, the adolescent states: "My name is _____, and I am an alcoholic." This establishes an identity of being chemically dependent. Taking a white poker chip at an AA meeting demonstrates the willingness, at least for that day, to begin the journey toward recovery. Any program with a 12-step orientation must be sure to help adolescents adjust and involve themselves in the self-help offered by Alcoholics Anonymous or Narcotics Anonymous. "Defeat of a narcissistic or self-centered orientation is the goal of primary treatment for adolescents and a necessary prerequisite for taking Step One."[38]

Outpatient treatment can be effective if two prerequisites are met. First, the parents must have control over the child and must not be afraid that the child will run away, become violent, or attempt suicide. Otherwise, inpatient treatment may be necessary. Outpatient treatment should avoid any therapy that indulges the adolescent and makes the parent feel responsible for the adolescent's chemical abuse. Avoid a therapist who feels that a confidential relationship is more important than sharing vital information with parents. Stripping away an antisocial belief system is necessary for successful treatment. The therapist and family must be allies in this endeavor, or treatment will fail. If group or multifamily treatment is a part of the outpatient program, this is much better for the patient and more effective. Group therapy encourages honesty among peers. Multifamily therapy breaks down the feelings of isolation parents have and provides a new bonding, with a feeling of not being alone.

Other prerequisites for success in outpatient treatment are encouragement in AA meetings, obtaining a sponsor in a 12-step program, and setting up a schedule of meetings with parental support. A 12-step self-help group called Al-Anon helps parents understand their child's disease and what they need to do to aid recovery. In addition, it is important for parents to understand that this is a relapsing illness, and they need to continue to encourage their child in some form of treatment, intervention, or 12-step involvement.

Inpatient treatment programs may be multidisciplinary or follow the Minnesota model. Multidisciplinary programs are led by a child psychiatrist and combined with a 12-step program. In this approach, a child psychiatrist, psychologist, counselors, and educators draw up an individualized treatment plan. This is known as problem-oriented treatment planning and addresses developmental problems, family issues, and coexisting psychopathology in addition to drug and alcohol problems. In the Minnesota model programs, the program milieu is coordinated around working the first several steps of the 12-step program. Many of the counselors are recovering alcoholics or addicts who have received degrees or counselor certification in substance abuse. The most effective programs combine the multidisciplinary approach with the Minnesota model. Quality programs have a qualified staff and a child psychiatrist who are trained and experienced in the treatment of chemically dependent adolescents.

Other important aspects of treatment programs include family treatment and physical rehabilitation. The family program should include some combination of parental education, family therapy, and multifamily therapy and should encourage involvement in those self-help groups that are free and community based. These include Al-Anon, Toughlove, and Parents Anonymous. Vigorous cardiovascular fitness programs improve health and muscle tone and increase self-esteem. At the same time, stimulation of the brain's natural endorphins gives a feeling of well-being and, later, a sense of calm and relaxation. The program must be strict, with no tolerance for aggression or sexual acting out.

Many excellent adolescent programs are not located within medical complexes, but at free-standing psychiatric hospitals. Therefore, it may be helpful to visit such a program so that referrals may be made with confidence, as parents are often in an emotional crisis at the time of referral. Parents should be advised to meet the treatment team and discuss all family concerns before admission. Inpatient treatment is an important decision, but if all goes well, it can make a profound difference in the lives of both the adolescent and other family members. A new spiritual identity develops with a relationship to God unfettered by theology or dogmatic practices. Acceptance of a higher power by a teenager or young adult sets the stage for improvement in all relationships and enables them to have the proper attitude to be successful in society. The dismal alternative is disconnection from society as a result of drugs, pregnancy, and dropping out of school.[39]

Treatment programs are quite varied but may be summarized as follows:

1. Outpatient treatment: School-based counseling, community hotlines, self-help groups (AA), social service agencies, structured outpatient programs.

2. Day treatment: Therapy for the adolescent and the family.

3. Halfway house treatment: Often staffed with recovering addicts who serve as role models for the 12-step program.

4. Inpatient treatment: Minnesota model with multidisciplinary treatment led by a physician who has training and expertise in treatment of substance abuse disorders.[40]

5. Residential treatment: 24-Hour program with nearly all staff members consisting of recovering addicts who serve as role models for the adolescent.

References

1. National Household Survey on Drug Abuse, 1988. In: Drug Abuse Update, no. 31. Decatur, GA: Families in Action, December, 1989.
2. NIDA Update: News from the National Institute on Drug Abuse. In: Drug Abuse Update, no. 32. Decatur, GA: Families in Action, March, 1990.
3. The Commercial Appeal, Memphis, Tennessee. July 31, 1989.
4. Gordis E. "Children of alcoholics: Are they different?" Alcohol Alert. Washington, DC: NIAA, 9, 7/90, p 3.
5. MacDonald DI. Patterns of alcohol and drug abuse among adolescents. Pediatr Clin North Am 1987; 34(2):275–288.
6. MacDonald DI. Drugs, drinking and adolescents. Am J Dis Child 1984; 138:117–125.
7. Dilsaver, SC. The pathophysiologies of substance abuse and affective disorders—an integrative mode? J Clin Psychopharmacol 1987; 7(1):1–10.
8. Schwartz RH. Marijuana: An overview. Pediatr Clin North Am 1987; 34(2):305–317.
9. Dalterio SL. Marijuana and the unborn. In: Drug Awareness Information Newsletter. Danvers, MA: Connie & Otto Molton, 1989.
10. Jessor R, Chase JA, Donovan JE. Psychosocial correlates of marijuana use and problem drinking in a national sample of adolescents. Am J Public Health 1980; 70(6):604–613.
11. King P. Correlation of heavy metal music and substance abuse among adolescents. Postgrad Med 1988; 83:295–304.
12. Kandel DB. Marijuana users in young adulthood. Arch Gen Psychiatry 1984; 41:200–209.
13. Murphy GE. Suicide and substance abuse. Arch Gen Psychiatry 1988; 45(6):593–594.
14. Rich CL, Young D, Fowler RC., San Diego suicide study in young vs. old subjects. Arch Gen Psychiatry 1986; 43:577–582.
15. Rich CL, Fowler RC, Fogarty LA, Young D. San Diego suicide study III: Relationships between diagnoses and stressors. Arch Gen Psychiatry 1988; 45:589–594.
16. Brent DA, Perper JA, Allman CJ. Alcohol, firearms and suicide among youth. Temporal trends in Allegheny County, Pennsylvania, 1960–1983. JAMA 1987; 257(24):3369–3372.
17. Dietz AJ. Amphetamine—the reactions to phenylpropanolamine. JAMA 1981; 245(6):601–602.
18. King P, Coleman JH. Stimulants and narcotic drugs. Pediatr Clin North Am 1987; 34(2):349–362.
19. National Institute on Drug Abuse. Drug Abuse Warning Network, series G, no. 14, U.S. Department of Health and Human Services, January to June, 1984.
20. Goodwin FK. From the Alcohol Drug Abuse and Mental Health Administration. JAMA 1990; 264(15):1928.
21. Gold M. 1985, Ecstasy, etc. Alcoholism Addiction Mag 1985; Sept/Oct. 1:11.
22. Lerner MA. The fire of ice. Newsweek, Nov. 27, 1989.
23. Banstra ES. Cocaine use in pregnancy: Neonatal manifestations. Symposium at LeBonheur Children's Hospital, Memphis, TN, October 11, 1990.
24. Chasnoff IJ, Griffith DR, MacGregor S, et al. 1989, Temporal patterns of cocaine use in pregnancy: Perinatal outcome. JAMA 1989; 261:1741–1744.
25. Chavez GF, Mulinare J, Cordeo JF, et al. Maternal cocaine use during early pregnancy as a risk factor: Congenital anomalies. JAMA 1989; 262:795.
26. Chasnoff IJ. 1990, Cocaine, pregnancy and the child. Symposium at LeBonheur Children's Hospital, Memphis, TN, October 11, 1990.
27. Mayes LC, Granger RH, Borenstein MH, et al. 1992. The problem of prenatal cocaine exposure. A rush to judgment. JAMA 1992; 267(3):406.
28. Zipp TM. Sniffing up trouble: Adhesive tape remover pads. JAMA 1986; 256:39–40.
29. Smialek JE, Troutman WG. 1985, Sniffing up trouble: Inhalation of volatile substances. JAMA 1985; 254:1721–1722.
30. McLeod AA, Marjot R, Monaghan MJ, et al. Chronic cardiac toxicity after inhalation of 1,1,1-trichlorethane. Br Med J 1987; 294:727–729.
31. McHugh MJ. The abuse of volatile substances. Pediatr Clin North Am 1987; 34(2):333–340.
32. Gold MS, Dackis CA. Role of the laboratory in the evaluation of suspected drug abuse. J Clin Psychiatry 1986; 47(suppl):17–23.
33. MacKenzie RG, Cheng M, Hafte AJ, et al. The clinical utility and evaluation of drug screening techniques. Pediatr Clin North Am 1987; 34(2):423–436.
34. Trinkoff AM, Baker SP. Poisonings and hospitalization and death from solids and liquids among children and adolescents. Am J Public Health 1986; 76:657–660.
35. Feigelman W. Treating Teenage Drug Abuse in a Day Care Setting. New York: Praeger, 1990.
36. Elkind D. Egocentrism in adolescence. Child Dev 1967; 38:1025–1034.
37. Arnett J. Contraceptive use, sensation seeking and adolescent egocentrism. J Youth Adolesc 1990; 19(2).
38. King P. Sex, Drugs and Rock-n-Roll: Healing Today's Troubled Youth. Redmond, WA: Professional Counselor Books, 1988.
39. Vobejda B. Millions of teens disconnected from society. Washington Post, November 2, 1985.
40. Bailey GW. Current perspectives on substance abuse in youth. J Am Acad Child Adolesc Psychiatry 1989; 28(2):151–162.

CHAPTER 28

Diagnostic Imaging

LUIGI FEDELE
MILENA DORTA

The use of invasive instrumental diagnostic investigations such as hysterosalpingography, hysteroscopy, and pelvic pneumography in children and adolescents is limited, but occasionally a serious organic disease may be present that requires a precise diagnosis to avoid inappropriate interventions and plan definitive therapy. In such situations, ultrasonography (USG) should be an integral component of pelvic exploration. However, USG has proved to have limitations, especially in the precise characterization of tissues. The vaginal probe is of limited benefit in pediatric patients because of its invasive nature. This explains the use of abdominal USG, as well as of more sophisticated noninvasive investigation methods such as magnetic resonance imaging (MRI) in pediatric gynecology, and also the frequent recourse to diagnostic endoscopy despite its invasiveness and cost.

IMAGING OF THE NORMAL FEMALE PELVIS IN CHILDREN AND ADOLESCENTS

USG provides immediate real-time images of the pelvic structures in multiple planes. Real-time, preferably linear, probes of 3.5, 7.5, or 10 MHz are used, according to the patient's habitus. Generally, sagittal or transverse images are obtained, but additional images may be generated by angling the transducer on the sagittal, coronal, and transverse planes. Children usually have minimal periviseral fat and thus are excellent subjects for USG. The absence of ionizing radiation means that the examination can be repeated without biologic effects.

An inconvenience of abdominal USG is the need for a full bladder to act as an ultrasonic window. It elevates the small bowel, which, when filled with air, reflects the echoes and obscures the structures posterior. If necessary, sterile water can be instilled as contrast medium to outline the bladder, vagina (water vaginography), or rectum (water enema technique). It can also be used to fill other structures such as a cloaca or utricle. Patients should be well hydrated before the examination to facilitate the procedure, and bladder filling should be avoided by catheterization. Neonates should be placed comfortably on an examination table and the room well heated to prevent rapid loss of body heat.

Another difficulty in pediatric USG is patient movement, and thus the parents should be allowed to remain close to the child during the examination. Sedation is occasionally required; chloral hydrate (50 mg/kg), given orally 30 minutes before the study begins, may be used. However, the best sedation for a neonate or small child is often a full stomach.

Transvaginal USG does not require a full bladder. It uses a 5- or 6-MHz transducer placed in the vagina, and therefore the technique cannot be applied in children or in adolescents with an intact hymen. These high-frequency probes provide excellent resolution 2 to 7 cm from the transducer. This pelvic USG modality, which represents an important advance, is often fundamental in the evaluation of cul-de-sac masses and the adnexa, as it is not affected by the patient's habitus or abdominal surgical scars, and the probe can be placed very close to the structures to be investigated. With a transvaginal probe, it is easy to differentiate solid masses from cystic ones and to recognize septa, vegetations, and calcifications in cystic masses.

Computed tomography (CT) generally provides poor density resolution of the gynecologic structures. Nevertheless, it does offer some advantages: great spatial resolution, short imaging time, and low cost. It uses ionizing radiation and requires preimaging patient preparation such as opacification of the gastrointestinal tract and intravenous iodinated contrast material. Complete opacification of the small bowel and colon is essential, as the intestine occupies a large portion of the pelvis and the most common error in interpreting CT images is mistaking nonopacified intestinal loops for a pelvic mass. Patients of average habitus should imbibe 500 to 700 ml of a diluted barium solution before the examination. If the patient is reluctant to drink such a large amount of liquid, she may be given 40 to 50 ml diatrizoate meglumine (Gastrografin). Rectal contrast medium is sometimes administered via an enema. A tampon, which provides air density, may be inserted in the vagina to enhance the distinction between vagina and cervix and between paracervical and parametrial regions. Intravenous contrast media may also be used. In patients with suspected pelvic disease, transaxial images are obtained at 10-mm slice thicknesses. Thin or repeated sections are occasionally required to better delineate suspected abnormalities.

MRI has been a viable imaging technique since the early 1980s. Its advantages include its excellent tissue contrast, noninvasive nature, and complete lack of ionizing radiation. However, the examination takes some time, and children may be afraid of being placed in the machine. In addition, it may be difficult for the patient to remain in the same position for a long time, and young patients should not be made to suffer from claustrophobia. For all these reasons, sedatives may be used. Girls younger than 5 years should be sedated as a matter of routine; chloral hydrate (50 to 70 mg/kg) may be used.

Unfortunately, the physical principles on which MRI is based are considerably different from those used in radiographic and USG imaging. MRI is based on the interaction of tissue immersed in a static magnetic field with radiofrequency (RF) pulses that create perturbations of short duration on nuclei oriented by the static magnetic field. At cessation of the RF pulse, the nuclei restore the energy absorbed in the form of signals that are received by the same RF coil in reception phase. The MR signal is then amplified and converted from analog to digital to be processed by the computer. The latter reconstructs the image by localizing and interpreting the signal from each unit of volume. Some physical characteristics of the tissues and other variables controlled by the operator affect the signals emitted by the tissues. Specifically, the density of protons of hydrogen nuclei; the relaxation times, which express the time it takes protons to return to equilibrium after excitation; the velocity of blood flow; and the presence of paramagnetic substances (e.g., iron) that shorten the relaxion times all influence the formation of the image. The dependence of the signals on the relaxation times is particularly important. The latter reflect the water content and the dynamics of water in the tissues. There are two types of relaxation processes: T1, which expresses the interaction of the hydrogen nucleus with the surrounding molecular environment; and T2, which expresses the magnetic interaction among the protons. The images obtained can be T1 or T2 weighted by varying the pulse sequences used to accentuate contrasts among the various tissues with their different T1 and T2.

In MRI, the bladder serves as a reference for signal characterization within the pelvis. Cysts, which demonstrate a signal like that of urine are classified as simple (serous). Urine is isointense in T1 and hyperintense in T2 images, because the short T2 of the smooth muscles contrasts with the long T2 of the adjacent urine and perivesical fat. When reading the images, white signifies high signal intensity and black demonstrates low signal intensity. Solid formations present low signal intensities in both T1- and T2-weighted images. Fluid tissues with abundant free water (urine, stagnant blood) have low and high signal intensities in T1- and T2-weighted images, respectively. Proteinaceous liquids are distinguished by an intermediate signal in T1-weighted images and by a high signal in T2-weighted ones. Flowing blood is characterized by the absence of signals (black images). In T1-weighted images, white = elevated signal = short T1, whereas in T2-weighted images, white = elevated signal = long T2 and black = low signal = short T2.

Uterus. The neonatal uterus is relatively large as a result of residual stimulation from maternal hormones. Nussbaum[1] and Orsini et al.[2] reported a mean craniocaudal length of 3.4 cm (range, 2.5 to 4.6 cm) based on USG findings in 35 neonates in the first 7 days of life. In most cases the uterus is tubular or spade shaped, with the anteroposterior diameter of the cervix as long as or longer than that of the fundus. Up to the age of 7 years, the size of the uterus is not related to age, and the cervix is larger than the corpus, so that the organ has an inverse pear-shaped morphology (Fig. 28–1). The ratio between the anteroposterior diameters of the corpus and cervix is 1 (Fig. 28–2). Beginning at 7 years of age, the

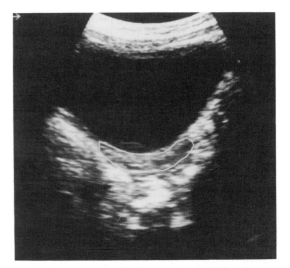

FIGURE 28–2 ••• Sagittal ultrasound scan of the uterus in a 5-year-old girl. The ratio between the anteroposterior diameters of the corpus and cervix is 1.

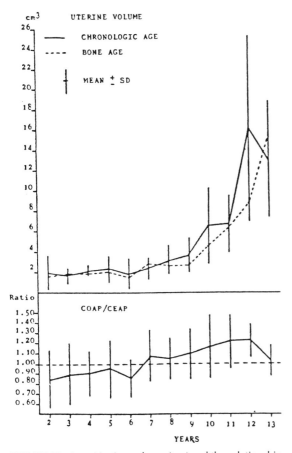

FIGURE 28–1 ••• Uterine volume *(top)* and the relationship between the anteroposterior diameters of the corpus (COAP) and the cervix (CEAP) *(bottom)*, as determined by ultrasonography, from ages 2 to 13. (From Orsini L, Salardi S, Pilu G, et al. Pelvic organs in premenarchal girls: Real-time ultrasonography. Radiology 1984; 153:113–116.)

diameter and the volume of the uterus increase in relation to age. The increase in total length and in the anteroposterior diameter of the corpus is more pronounced than the increase in the anteroposterior diameter of the cervix, so that the organ gradually acquires the typical pear-shaped morphology of the adult by the age of 12 to 13 years (Fig. 28–3).

Myometrium. Compared with the full bladder, the myometrium on USG possesses great echogenicity, producing dense echoes as a re-

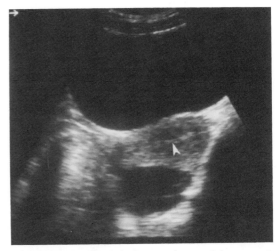

FIGURE 28–3 ••• Sagittal ultrasound scan of the uterus in a 13-year-old girl. The anteroposterior diameter of the corpus is more pronounced than that of the cervix. The endometrium appears as a linear cavity echo of high amplitude in the initial proliferative phase *(arrowhead)*. As a related finding, an ovarian cyst is seen in the pouch of Douglas.

sult of the abundance of muscular, fibrous, and vascular components. The myometrium may be traversed by thin, tortuous, anechoic formations that represent myometrial vessels. On CT, the best definition of the myometrium is obtained when intravenous contrast, which clearly differentiates this tissue from all other gynecologic structures, is used. On MRI scans the myometrium, like other smooth muscles, has a long T1 and short T2. In the adolescent with normal menses its thickness varies from 1.5 to 2 cm. Its appearance varies during the menstrual cycle, although this variance is less than that of the endometrium; it increases in thickness by 2.2% daily during the follicular phase and by 1.8% daily during the secretory phase.

Endometrium. On USG the endometrium appears as an elliptical shadow with distinct borders believed to represent the basalis myometrial junction; a longitudinal central line is evident that represents the interface of the anterior and posterior superficial endometrial layers (Figs. 28–4, 28–5). The endometrium is seen as a high signal layer in T2-weighted MR images because of the presence of tortuous vessels and abundant mucus. In the neonate the endometrial cavity is easily demonstrated by USG because of the stimulated endometrium and the mucus and secretions frequently present in the cavity (Fig. 28–6). Anatomic studies of neonatal uteri have shown that the cavity is often filled with blood, epithelial residues, and denuded stroma,[3] which is attributable to residual maternal hormonal stimulation. In normally menstruating adolescents, physiologic changes in the stratum basalis and stratum functionalis are reflected in the width

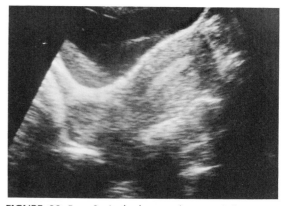

FIGURE 28–5 ••• Sagittal ultrasound scan of the uterus showing the secretory phase in the same case shown in Figure 28–4. The endometrium appears as a thickened echogenic area.

and degree of definition of the stripe on both USG and MRI scans.[4]

On both USG and MRI, a thin stripe is identified in the interface between the endometrium and myometrium. This stripe has a low signal intensity (short T2) on MRI (Fig. 28–7) and is echogenic on USG. The nature of this so-called junctional zone is still a mystery. It was visible on 29% of neonatal USG scans performed by Nussbaum et al.,[1] who also reported that the zone was 2 to 3 mm thick in postpubertal uteri. In adolescents with normal menses and who are taking oral contraceptives, the junctional zone becomes very difficult to identify.

Cervix. The cervix has echogenicity similar to that of the myometrium. Inside the cervix a mixed hypo- and hyperechoic stripe repre-

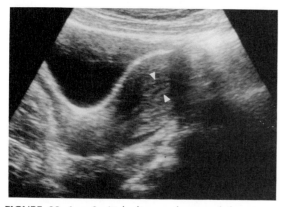

FIGURE 28–4 ••• Sagittal ultrasound scan of the uterus showing the endometrium in the proliferative phase. A three-striped elliptical shadow is seen (arrowheads).

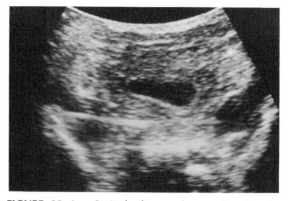

FIGURE 28–6 ••• Sagittal ultrasound scan showing the endometrial cavity in a neonate. The cavity is dilated and surrounded by stimulated endometrium, which appears as a thin, hyperechogenic line.

senting endocervical secretion is often seen. MRI of the cervix demonstrates a stripe of high intensity, corresponding to the endocervical glands and mucus, and an external zone with low signal intensity that represents the fibrous stroma and is continuous with the junctional zone of the corpus. A third layer, of undefined origin and with moderate signal intensity, has been described in continuation with the myometrium.

Ovaries. The ovaries are readily demonstrated by USG and MRI. It is sometimes difficult to recognize them because of their small size and the neonate's inability to maintain a full bladder for a sufficiently long time. Anatomic studies have demonstrated that neonatal ovaries vary from 0.5 to 1.5 cm in length and from 0.3 to 0.4 cm in thickness.[3] In prepubertal girls, the ovaries generally present a solid homogeneous morphology and are stable in size up to the age of 6 years (Fig. 28–8), after which time there is an age-related size increase, and microcystic aspects become increasingly frequent, although ultrasonographically homogeneous ovaries remain prevalent until the age of 11 years. At puberty the ovaries acquire their adult size and characteristics. Ovarian size may be calculated using the formula for ellipsoids, with a minimum ovarian size of 1 ml before puberty and a maximum of 6 ml in normally menstruating adolescents.[2, 5]

Vagina. On USG the vaginal canal is evident as a central linear echo created by the reflective

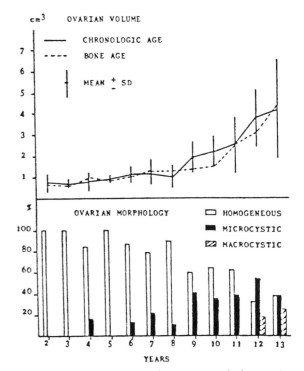

FIGURE 28–8 ••• Ovarian volume *(top)* and changes in ovarian morphology *(bottom)*, as determined by ultrasonography, from ages 2 to 13. (From Orsini L, Salardi S, Pilu G, et al. Pelvic organs in premenarchal girls: Real-time ultrasonography. Radiology 1984; 153:113–116. Reprinted with permission of the Radiological Society of North America.)

interface of the opposing walls of the organ and the presence of fluid in the canal. MRI clearly defines the vagina in T2-weighted images. The mucus in the lumen has a high signal intensity, contrasting with the low signal intensity of the muscular walls.

IMAGING OF CONGENITAL ABNORMALITIES

Hydrocolpos. Hydrocolpos is fluid accumulation in the vagina and possibly also the uterus (hydrometrocolpos). It is observed in neonates but may also occur late in childhood.[6] It is usually caused by a vaginal obstruction resulting from an imperforate hymen or a septum of varying thickness occluding the vaginal introitus.

Correct early diagnosis of hydrocolpos by USG makes laparotomy unnecessary. USG is not only safe but also reliable and specific in investigating both abdominal masses and the

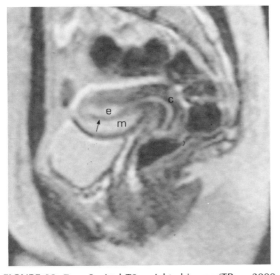

FIGURE 28–7 ••• Sagittal T2-weighted image (TR = 2000 ms; TE = 60 ms) demonstrating the uterine anatomy. c, Cervix; e, endometrium; m, myometrium. The arrow indicates the junctional zone.

urinary tract, and it is therefore strongly recommended before any radiologic examinations are performed. Plain radiographs of the abdomen are infrequently indicated when USG reveals a "cystic" hypogastric mass. However, if the vaginal fluid accumulation contains debris, the mass may appear "complex" or even "solid" and is thus diagnostically equivocal. The uterus may be slightly dilated by the vaginal fluid (Fig. 28–9). Cystography should be performed to exclude a refluxing megaureter and uterocele. Because obstruction of the lower urinary outlet occurs very rarely in females,[7] it is essential to differentiate ovarian tumors from hydrocolpos immediately after birth. With USG it is usually possible to ascertain the vaginal origin of the "cystic" mass with reasonable accuracy (Fig. 28–10). The association of such a mass with hydronephrosis and obstructive megaureter should be easy to recognize and is pathognomonic for hydrocolpos. On the other hand, it is unlikely that a complex or a solid mass is a hydrocolpos rather than a tumor. Barium enemas may be required to evaluate suspected intestinal involvement such as duplication or obstruction.

Imperforate Hymen. With an imperforate hymen, vaginal distention may be so great that a mass is clearly evident in the lower abdomen (Fig. 28–11).

Transverse Vaginal Septum. Low complete, or suprahymenal, septa may result in symptoms initially in early infancy (hydromucocolpos) or after the start of cyclic endometrial activity (similar to symptoms of an imperforate hymen) (Fig. 28–12A). High complete septa are less frequent and generally are located at

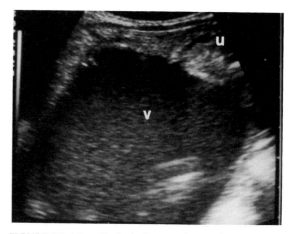

FIGURE 28–10 ••• Sagittal ultrasound scan demonstrating hydromucometrocolpos in the neonate shown in Fig. 28–9. The vagina (v) is very dilated and contains fine debris, and the endometrial cavity is slightly dilated. u, Uterus.

the junction of the mid and upper third of the vagina. USG is useful to demonstrate a normal cervix and for precise localization of the obstructive septum (Fig. 28–12B).

Cervical Agenesis. The pure form of cervical agenesis (Buttram and Gibbons' class IB)[8] is rare, and the clinical picture is always confused with that of a high complete vaginal septum. Differential diagnosis is fundamental and can be readily performed by USG (Fig. 28–13). The various surgical attempts to create a stable uterovaginal communication often entail or are complicated by the onset of ascending infection.

Agenesis of the Vagina and Uterus. This is the most frequent type of congenital absence of the vagina and is known as Mayer-Rokitansky-Küster-Hauser (MRKH) syndrome (Buttram and Gibbons' class IE) (Fig. 28–14). It is characterized by the following:

1. Normal external genitalia.
2. Absence of the vagina or of the upper and middle third of the urogenital sinus.
3. Absence of the uterus, which is transformed into two fibromuscular cords originating from the medial extremities of the salpinges and fused medially, resembling a double rudimentary uterus; on rare occasion endometrial tissue is present in one of the two horns, and menstrual blood accumulates.
4. Normal configuration of the salpinges.
5. Normal development and function of the ovaries.

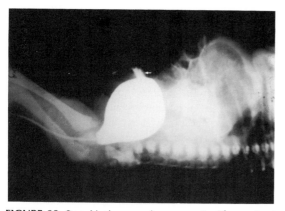

FIGURE 28–9 ••• Vaginogram in a neonate. The contrast medium opacifies the dilatation of the vagina and endocervix (arrow).

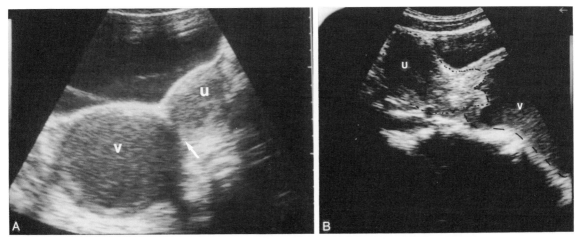

FIGURE 28–11 ••• Hematometrocolpos resulting from an imperforate hymen in a young adolescent. *A,* This sagittal sonogram of the pelvis shows a dilated uterine cavity (u) filled with echogenic debris (blood) and communicating via a wide endocervix *(arrow)* with the obstructed vagina (v), which is also filled with debris. *B,* Ultrasound image of the imperforate hymen. The cervix, with conserved morphology, projects into the large hematocolpos noted on the right. The uterus and the endometrial cavity are conserved. Black broken lines delineate these structures. u, Uterus; V, vagina.

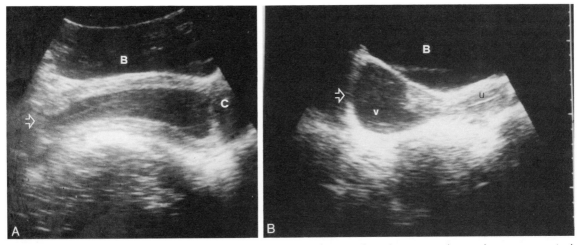

FIGURE 28–12 ••• Transverse vaginal septa. *A,* A small hematocolpos resulting from a suprahymenal transverse vaginal septum. This sagittal sonogram of the pelvis demonstrates a collection of fine debris (blood) under the bladder (B), delineated at the bottom by the suprahymenal septum *(arrow)* and at the top by the uterine cervix (C). *B,* Pelvic cyst in a 13-year-old girl. This sagittal ultrasound scan shows a normal cervix projecting into the dilated vagina (v) and containing fine debris (blood) that has accumulated as a result of the presence of a high complete transverse vaginal septum *(arrow)*. B, Bladder; u, uterus.

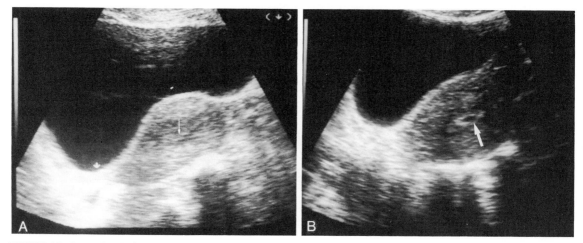

FIGURE 28–13 ••• Cervical agenesis. *A,* Longitudinal ultrasound scan of the uterus; the cervix is absent *(short arrow),* and the endometrium is thin *(long arrow). B,* Sonogram of the same patient 10 months later. Cavitation of the uterus is visible as an anechoic slit *(arrow)* surrounded by a hyperechoic halo (endometrium).

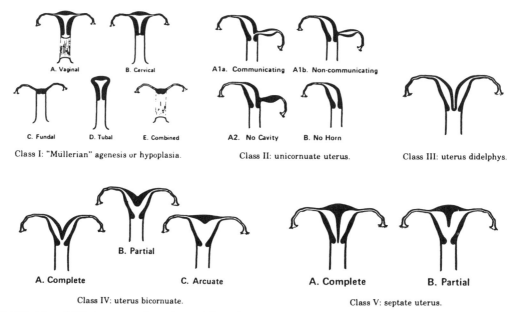

FIGURE 28–14 ••• Müllerian anomalies, classes I through V (From Buttram VC Jr, Gibbons WE. Mullerian anomalies: A proposed classification (an analysis of 144 cases). Fertil Steril 1979; 32:40–45. Reprinted with permission of the American Fertility Society.

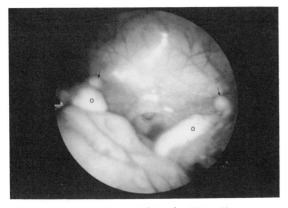

FIGURE 28–15 ••• Mayer-Rokitansky-Küster-Hauser syndrome. This laparoscopic image shows the absence of the uterus. Two small müllerian rudiments *(arrows)* are seen at the upper poles of the ovaries (O).

6. Presence of urinary tract anomalies in about 10% of cases.

7. Associated spinal malformations.

Laparoscopy has generally been considered necessary for definitive diagnosis of this anomaly (Fig. 28–15). However, USG findings are helpful when neither the uterus nor the uterine cavity can be visualized. Moreover, USG generally demonstrates the characteristics of müllerian rudiments and whether they are cavitary (Fig. 28–16).

In a study involving six girls with suspected MRKH syndrome,[9] it was noted that more precise information was obtained with MRI than with USG or laparoscopy (Fig. 28–17A). The greater diagnostic reliability of MRI compared with laparoscopy was due to the finding that the latter technique provided no information on subperitoneal structures. In fact, in MRKH syndrome, vaginal agenesis may be only partial; the cervix may be present, or there may be a fibrous, partially cavitary cord (Fig. 28–17B). The importance of such findings is not only theoretical, as this knowledge may be useful in creating a vagina using the McIndoe procedure.[10] Furthermore, laparoscopic assessment of cavitation of müllerian rudiments is only indirect and is based on their size, whereas MRI demonstrates cavitation easily by means of the high-intensity signal of the endometrial cavity on T2-weighted images (Fig. 28–17C). The clinical importance of these endometrial islands in the myometrium of müllerian rudiments is unclear; like the cavitary horns of unicornuate uteri, cavitary uterine rudiments should be routinely removed if they are large and cause cyclic pelvic pain. MRI provides equally good images of superficial and deep planes that are not affected by the patient's habitus and do not require a full bladder. In addition, MRI is more precise than USG in its ability to provide specific tissue characterization.

Unicornuate Uterus With Noncommunicating Cavitary Rudimentary Horn. This anomaly (Buttram and Gibbons' class IIA1b) may cause severe symptoms as a result of retained menstrual blood (Fig. 28–18). Retention does not always occur, because in most cases the endometrium of rudimentary horns undergoes only partial and attenuated cyclic modifications that do not determine true menstrual bleeding.[11] Because of the conserved menstrual function, the diagnosis may be delayed or confused with other diseases, particularly ovarian cysts and a "double" uterus with an imperforate hemivagina.

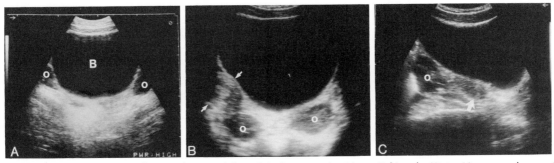

FIGURE 28–16 ••• Transverse ultrasound scans of the pelvis demonstrating Mayer-Rokitansky-Küster-Hauser syndrome. *A,* Two normal ovaries (O) can be visualized behind the full bladder (B); the uterus is absent. *B,* A cavitary müllerian rudiment *(arrows)* can be visualized at the center above the left ovary (O), with the endometrium appearing as a hyperechoic area. *C,* Longitudinal scan of the pelvis. A noncavitary müllerian rudiment *(arrow)* is visible below a micropolycystic ovary (O).

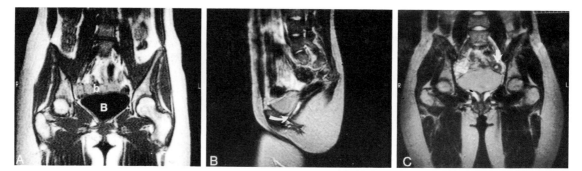

FIGURE 28–17 ••• Mayer-Rokitansky-Küster-Hauser syndrome. *A,* Coronal MRI scan (TR = 350 ms; TE = 20 ms). No uterine structure can be detected. The bowel (b) can be seen over the bladder (B). *B,* Medial sagittal scan (TR = 1510 ms; TE = 100 ms). A fibrous structure *(arrow)* appears between the rectum and the bladder. *C,* Coronal scan (TR = 1380 ms; TE = 100 ms) demonstrating a markedly lateralized cavitary müllerian rudiment *(arrow).* (From Fedele L, Dorta M, Brioschi D, et al. Magnetic resonance imaging in Mayer-Rokitansky-Küster-Hauser syndrome. Obstet Gynecol 1990; 76(4):593–596. Reprinted with permission from the American College of Obstetricians and Gynecologists.)

USG demonstrates the unicornuate uterus and its banana-shaped cavity.[12] Scanning the hemipelvis contralateral to the hemiuterus reveals the presence of a large, rounded rudimentary horn that has the same echogenicity as the myometrium and contains a thickened and hyperechoic zone resembling secretory endometrium (Fig. 28–19). MRI identifies the rudimentary horn lateral to the unicornuate uterus, and the high-signal-intensity central zone on T2-weighted images denotes cavitation (Fig. 28–20).[13]

Independently of menstrual retention, USG and MRI are both able to demonstrate subclasses IIA1b, IIA2, and IIB of a unicornuate uterus found in an adolescent—i.e., to detect the presence of a rudimentary horn (Fig. 28–

21) and establish whether it is cavitary (Fig. 28–22). Axial and paraxial scans oriented to contain the plane passing through the tubal ostium and internal uterine os allows simultaneous visualization of the entire endometrial cavity and the external profile of the uterus, thus clearly delineating the architecture of the organ. To visualize any endometrium inside the rudimentary horns, T2-weighted sequences are necessary to optimize the contrast between the different tissue layers. Unlike laparoscopy, USG and MRI do not reveal the presence of endometriosis, nor do they allow assessment of the fallopian tubes.

"Double" Uterus With an Obstructed Hemivagina. A "double" uterus—i.e., didelphic,

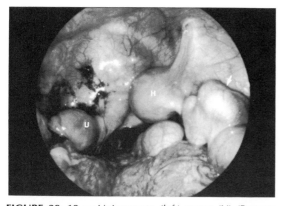

FIGURE 28–18 ••• Unicornuate *(left)* uterus (U) (Buttram and Gibbons' subclass AIb). This laparoscopic view reveals a large, dilated rudimentary horn (H) in communication with a large hematosalpinx *(arrow).* Free blood is present in the pouch of Douglas, and endometriosis can be identified on the bladder peritoneum.

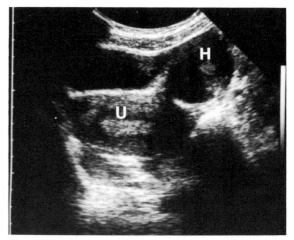

FIGURE 28–19 ••• Plain transverse sonogram of the pelvis with a partially full bladder shows a unicornuate uterus (U) with a large, round, cavitary rudimentary horn (H). Endometrium is seen as a hyperechoic area located centrally in the unicornuate uterus and cavitary horn.

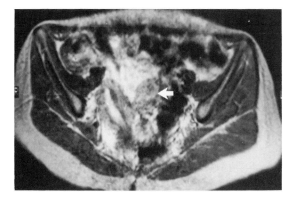

FIGURE 28–20 ••• MRI scan of the same unicornuate uterus shown in Figure 28–19 (T2-weighted image; TR = 2000 ms; TE = 100 ms). In the rudimentary horn, the central high signal zone *(arrow)* denotes cavitation. (From Fedele L, Dorta M, Brioschi D, et al. Magnetic resonance imaging of unicornuate uterus. Acta Obstet Gynecol Scand 1990; 69:511–513. Reprinted with permission of the Scandinavian Association of Obstetricians and Gynecologists.)

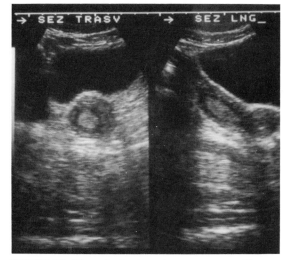

FIGURE 28–22 ••• A simple unicornuate uterus (Buttram and Gibbon's subclass B). *Left,* A transverse sonogram shows the uterus with a cylindric form. *Right,* On a longitudinal scan, the endometrium appears banana shaped.

bicornuate, or septate—is generally associated with a complete or partial vaginal septum, but occasionally a developmental abnormality of the urogenital sinus causes the formation of a complete vaginal diaphragm with an imperforate hemivagina. This müllerian anomaly is always associated with ipsilateral renal agene-

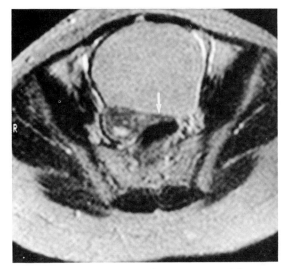

FIGURE 28–21 ••• MRI scan of a unicornuate *(right)* uterus with a small left rudimentary horn (TR = 1447 ms; TE = 50 ms). In the small rudimentary horn *(arrow)*, the high-signal central zone denoting cavitation is absent. (From Fedele L, Dorta M, Brioschi D, et al. Magnetic resonance imaging of unicornuate uterus. Acta Obstet Gynecol Scand 1990; 69:511–513. Reprinted with permission of the Scandinavian Association of Obstetricians and Gynecologists.)

sis. Three anatomic varieties of the anomaly have been described according to whether there is a communication between the two hemiuteri and whether the vaginal obstruction is complete or incomplete.[14]

In the noncommunicating type, the imperforate vagina and corresponding uterus constitute a cavity that is completely separate from the contralateral vagina and uterus; the only communication is with the peritoneal cavity through the corresponding salpinx. In the communicating form, the communication is between the two hemiuteri, generally at the level of the isthmus. In these first two varieties the imperforate vagina swells progressively with successive menstrual flows after menarche, and hematometra and hematosalpinx develop. In the type with incomplete vaginal obstruction, the septum is perforated at one or more points, preventing the formation of a true hematocolpos.

The clinical picture is characterized by a triad of symptoms (dysmenorrhea, pelvic mass, and ipsilateral renal agenesis), which, considering the usual age of presentation of the patient, is sufficiently pathognomonic.

In patients in whom hysterosalpingography can be performed, this may provide sufficiently characteristic images. Contrast medium, placed through the only demonstrable cervix, provides visualization of the hemiuterus contralateral to the pelvic mass; if there is an

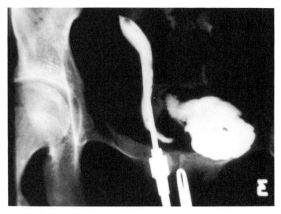

FIGURE 28–23 ••• Hysterosalpingography of a "double" communicating uterus with an obstructed right hemivagina. The contrast medium delineates a uterine horn above the cannulated cervix and the contralateral obstructed hemivagina. Opacification of the hemiuterus corresponding to the imperforate hemivagina is not possible because of the narrowness of the interisthmic communication.

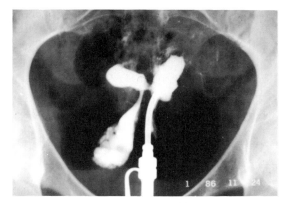

FIGURE 28–24 ••• Hysterosalpingography of a "double" communicating uterus with an obstructed right hemivagina. Three cavities are visualized (1) in a uterine horn directly above the cannulated cervix, (2) in a right horn communicating with the contralateral horn via a small isthmus, and (3) under the right uterine horn (obstructed hemivagina).

isthmic communication between the two hemiuteri, it may opacify the imperforate hemivagina (Fig. 28–23). Opacification of the hemiuterus, corresponding to the imperforate hemivagina, may occur if the interisthmic communication is wide (Fig. 28–24). Hysterosalpingography is useful in documenting the presence of an interisthmic communication between the two hemiuteri but shows only the internal profile of the uterus, whereas it is obviously equally essential to visualize the external morphology of the organ to classify the malformation precisely.

When a "double" uterus with imperforate hemivagina is suspected, USG is an excellent method of diagnosis (Fig. 28–25). The imperforate hemivagina caudal to the uterus appears as a sac delineated by a structure with echogenicity similar to that of the myometrium (vaginal wall) and containing hyperechoic fine debris or mixed hyper- and hypoechoic material. The nature of this material cannot be diagnosed by USG, but MRI has shown it to

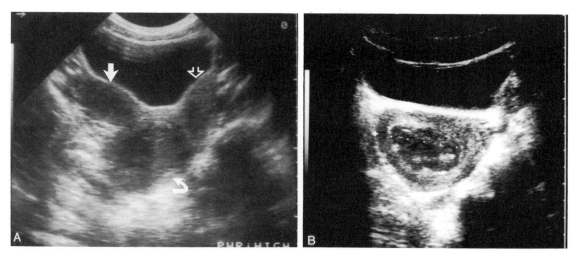

FIGURE 28–25 ••• "Double" uterus with an imperforate left hemivagina. *A*, A transverse sonogram of the pelvis shows a "double" uterus with a deep fundal notch. The right hemiuterus is of normal size *(open arrow)*; the left is dilated and contains debris (hematometra) *(solid arrow)*. A predominantly cystic mass (hematocolpos) is seen below the uterus *(curved arrow)*. *B*, A sonogram with a partially full bladder visualizes the hematocolpos more clearly *(calipers)*. The wall of the imperforate hemivagina circumscribes hyper- and hypoechoic material (blood and mucus, respectively).

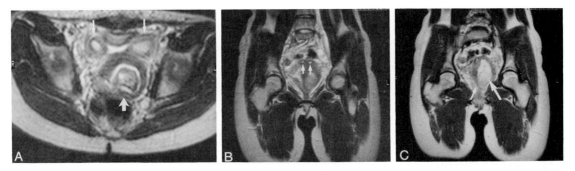

FIGURE 28–26 ••• MRI scan of a didelphic uterus with an imperforate left hemivagina. *A*, Transverse section (TR = 2000 ms; TE = 100 ms). Two distinct uterine bodies are visible *(small arrows)*, the left with a dilated endometrial cavity. Below the left hemiuterus is a vast saccular collection of high-signal-intensity fluid *(large arrow)*, consistent with a hematocolpos. *B*, Coronal section (TR = 2000 ms; TE = 100 ms). Two uterine cervices are seen with central high-intensity areas that delineate two cervical canals *(double arrows)*. Beneath them two vaginas can be detected, the left one dilated and containing a collection of blood. *C*, Coronal section (TR = 2000 ms; TE = 100 ms). The right hemivagina is normally patent *(small arrow)*, and the left one ends blindly *(large arrow)*. (From Fedele L, Dorta M, Brioschi D, et al. Magnetic resonance evaluation of gynecologic masses in adolescents. Adolesc Pediatr Gynecol 1990; 3:83–88.)

be blood alone or mixed with mucus and pus. Occasionally USG images of the two cervices and the normal vagina are poor. In contrast, MRI images are more panoramic and detailed (Fig. 28–26) and allow visualization of the two vaginas—one normal and the other transformed into an abundant saccular collection of fluid with high signal intensity consistent with blood. The two endometrial cavities are clearly identifiable, as is the presence of blood in cases of hematometra of the uterine body communicating with the imperforate hemivagina.

USG must be performed in the second half of the cycle. Fundal scanning performed parallel to the frontal planes of the uterus and with a half-full bladder is the only way to visualize the area surrounding the fundus and determine myometrial thickness and conformation of the endometrial cavity.[15] Once the orientation of the uterus is established, the organ is examined with MRI, using slices paralleling as much as possible the anatomic plane containing the tubal ostia and internal uterine os. These images are usually T2 weighted to obtain greater contrast resolution between peritoneal fat and the external contour of the uterus, but in some instances, T1-weighted slices are also obtained.[16]

Bicornuate and didelphic uteri are differentiated from partial and complete septate uteri according to the presence on USG and MRI images of a fundal indentation more than 10 mm deep and associated with an angle between the medial margins of the hemicavities of not less than 60 degrees (Figs. 28–27 through 28–29). These parameters are arbitrary but have

been found to be reliable in several studies.[15] The level of the lower apex of the myometrial septum in the cervical canal or uterine cavity is used to differentiate didelphic from bicornuate uteri and complete from partial septate uteri (Fig. 28–30).

The differential diagnosis of ovarian cysts and neoplasms must be considered when evacuating a pelvic mass in an adolescent who menstruates regularly. Pelvic examination may be misleading because of certain intrinsic difficulties at this age. The finding of renal agenesis is indicative, as are USG findings, including duplication of the uterine body. Another

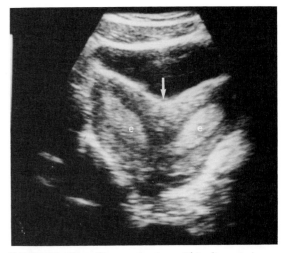

FIGURE 28–27 ••• Bicornuate uterus. This ultrasound scan shows a sagittal fundal notch larger than 10 mm *(arrow)*. The endometrial cavity is bifid. e, Endometrium.

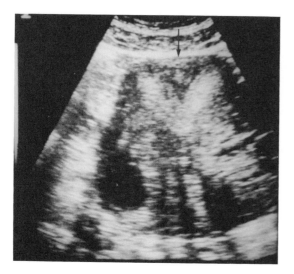

FIGURE 28–28 ••• Subseptate uterus. In this sonogram the peritoneal fundal profile of the uterus is regular *(arrow)*; the endometrial cavity is bifid.

FIGURE 28–29 ••• Bicornuate uterus. MRI reveals a deep peritoneal fundal notch. The two hemicavities are somewhat asymmetric, the left one slightly wider than the right. (From Fedele L, Dorta M, Brioschi D, et al. Magnetic resonance evaluation of double uteri. Obstet Gynecol, 1989; 74:844–847. Reprinted with permission from The American College of Obstetricians and Gynecologists.)

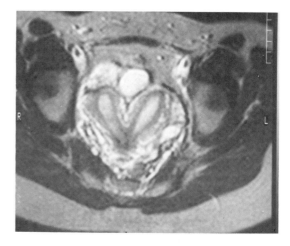

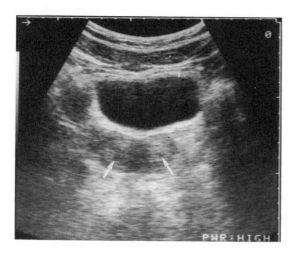

FIGURE 28–30 ••• Transverse ultrasound scan of the pelvis with a partially full bladder reveals two cervices. The two small anechoic areas surrounded by a hyperechogenic border are the two cervical canals *(arrows)* separated by a wide septum.

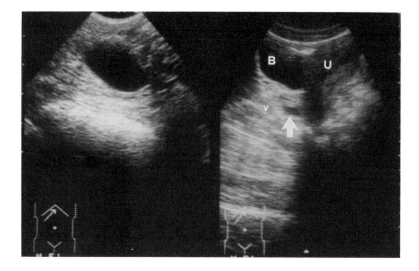

FIGURE 28–31 ••• Gartner's duct cyst. *Right,* Transabdominal ultrasound scan of the pelvis. A small anechoic mass is visible under the normal uterus (U). B, Bladder; v, vagina. *Left,* This transvaginal sonogram visualizes the anechoic formation better. Located in the vaginal wall, it has a diameter of 2 cm and thin, regular margins.

common diagnostic error arises from confusion of such masses with Gartner's duct cysts because of the characteristics of these masses and their location on the lateral wall of the vagina. Even exploratory puncture of the cyst mass does not resolve any doubts easily unless it yields a mucosanguineous fluid that is more characteristic of hematocolpos.

IMAGING OF BENIGN DISEASE

Hymenal Cysts. Hymenal cysts are occasionally found in the newborn. It is important for the diagnosis to establish with certainty whether the vaginal introitus is patent; if not, a hydromucocolpos is likely. USG may be helpful in differential diagnosis.

Vaginal Cysts. USG and MRI may be useful for differential diagnosis of an obstructed hemivagina by studying the cyst content and excluding a concomitant uterine malformation and renal agenesis. Sonographically, vaginal cysts appear as fluid-filled structures within the vagina (Fig. 28–31). Other vaginal cystic masses include paraurethral cysts, inclusion cysts, and paramesonephric (müllerian) duct cysts.

Benign Uterine Tumors. Benign uterine tumors are very rare in children and adolescents. Uterine leiomyomas are infrequent but may be large in adolescents (Fig. 28–32).

Ovarian Cysts. Non-neoplastic masses of the ovary, although benign, may cause serious general symptoms in children and adolescents because of the marked tendency toward tor-

sion of the adnexa and occasionally associated endocrine alterations.

Benign Cystic Teratoma. Formerly termed *dermoid tumor*, benign cystic teratoma is the most common benign ovarian neoplasm in children and adolescents, comprising 38.6% of all such lesions.[17] Approximately 50% are diagnosed incidentally during laparotomy or on radiographs of the pelvis (Fig. 28–33).

The USG appearance of teratomas depends on their internal composition.[18] They are most frequently noted to be a complex adnexal mass with echogenic internal components attributable to the fat and hair that are often present (Fig. 28–34). Some dermoids may be com-

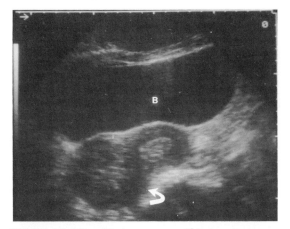

FIGURE 28–32 ••• Uterine myoma. This is a transverse ultrasound section of the uterus with a subserous fibroma. Typically this is seen as a large mass arising from the uterus with characteristically weak internal echoes and poor sound transmission *(arrow).* B, Bladder.

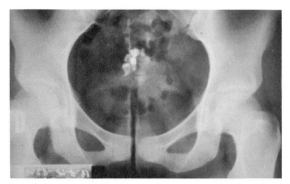

FIGURE 28–33 ••• Benign cystic teratoma. In this plain film of the pelvis, structured radio-opacities, representing calcified masses resembling teeth, can be seen in the right pelvis.

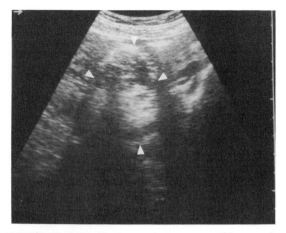

FIGURE 28–34 ••• Benign cystic teratoma. This transabdominal sonogram reveals a mixed formation, predominantly solid, with a hyperechoic area and poorly defined margins as a result of a posterior cone of shade *(arrowheads)*.

pletely solid and echogenic, and others may have cystic areas with or without internal septa (Fig. 28–35). Their echogenic structure explains how dermoids may sometimes be confused with the rest of the adnexa or mistaken for intestinal loops containing gas.

On MRI (Fig. 28–36) these lesions typically have a bright signal intensity on both T1- and T2-weighted images as a result of the sebaceous content.[19] Endometriomas and hemorrhagic cysts may also present with these findings. The hair, teeth, and debris found in benign cystic teratomas generate foci of very low signal intensity with both types of pulse sequences. However, lesions that are predominantly cystic may appear hypointense on T1-weighted images because of their primarily fluid, rather than lipid, contents, making them indistinguishable from other ovarian cystic masses.

Follicular and Lutein Cysts. Together with parovarian cysts, follicular and lutein cysts represent 35.9% of all ovarian lesions treated surgically in children and adolescents.[20] Manifestation of a functional cyst in children is not rare, as the follicular system of the developing ovary is hyperactive. Functional cysts have also been described in neonates as a consequence of disequilibrium of the maternal gonadotropins.

A functional cyst appears as a roundish transonic formation having thin margins with posterior intensification (Figs. 28–37, 28–38). MRI demonstrates follicular cysts as well circumscribed and smoothly marginated lesions with a thin wall. Because of their primarily

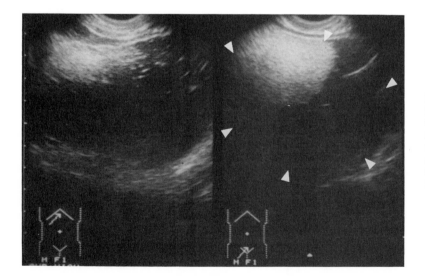

FIGURE 28–35 ••• Benign cystic teratoma. Transabdominal longitudinal *(left)* and transverse *(right)* ultrasound scans show a mixed mass, predominantly cystic *(arrowheads)*. Attached to the cyst wall is a bright, entangled echogenic area representing hair.

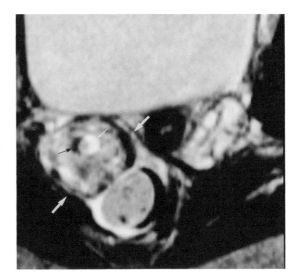

FIGURE 28–36 ••• MRI scan of the benign cystic teratoma shown in Figure 28–34 (TR = 2000 ms; TE = 25 ms). This coronal view of the pelvis reveals a mixed septate formation that is well encapsulated *(large arrows)*, with a central area of low signal intensity owing to bone formation *(black arrow)* and an area of high signal intensity resulting from fat *(small white arrow)* lateral to the uterine cervix.

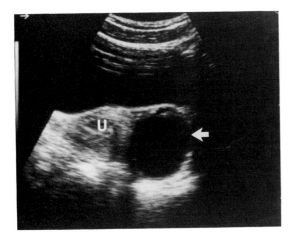

FIGURE 28–37 ••• Functional ovarian cyst in an adolescent. In this transverse sonogram of the pelvis, a transonic mass with regular wall *(arrow)* and smooth inner lining is visible lateral to the uterus (U).

FIGURE 28–38 ••• Multiseptate follicular cyst. This ultrasound image shows an ovary containing a transonic formation traversed by two thick, parallel septa. Three small follicles can be seen in the residual ovarian parenchyma.

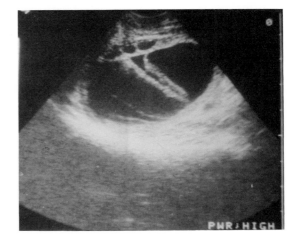

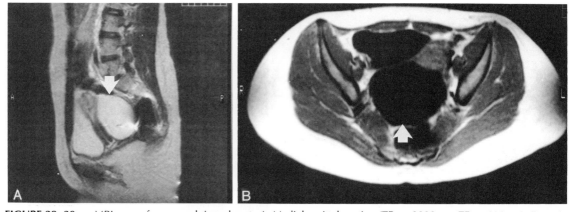

FIGURE 28–39 ••• MRI scan of a mesosalpingeal cyst. *A,* Medial sagittal section (TR = 2000 ms; TE = 100 ms). Posterior to the uterus and vagina, a cyst *(arrow)* with high-signal-intensity content occupies the entire pelvis. *B,* This transverse T1-weighted image of the cyst *(arrow)* shows a low signal intensity similar to that of the bladder, indicating a serous content (TR = 500 ms; TE = 20 ms). (From Fedele L, Dorta M, Brioschi D, et al. Magnetic resonance evaluation of gynecologic masses in adolescents. Adolesc Pediatr Gynecol 1990; 3:83–88.)

fluid contents, they have low and high signal intensity on T1- and T2-weighted images, respectively (Fig. 28–39).

When a lutein cyst is hemorrhagic, the sonogram is characterized by the presence of an internal echogenic area (Fig. 28–40). The cyst content generally becomes less echogenic when fibrinolysis begins in the coagulum. It must be remembered that in the newborn, ovarian cysts may present outside the pelvis, frequently in the upper abdomen. On MRI, if hemorrhage is present, the cysts may be bright on both T1- and T2-weighted sequences and may be indistinguishable from other hemorrhagic cysts, endometriomas, and dermoids (Fig. 28–41).

Endometriosis. Recent studies have demonstrated that endometriosis is not rare in adolescents, but is simply underestimated.[21] Early diagnosis allows prompt therapy and may avoid progression of the disease and consequent impaired fertility.

On USG, small endometriotic implants on the uterosacral ligaments or on the serous surface of the peritoneum and bowel are difficult to detect. Instead there is a spectrum of USG images of endometriomas according to the conformation and content.[22] When endometriomas become larger than 1 or 2 cm, they may be identified on USG as multiple cystic masses (Figs. 28–42, 28–43). Low-level echoes

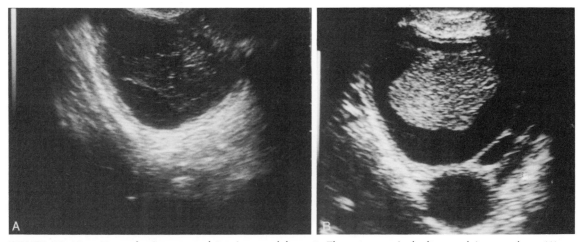

FIGURE 28–40 ••• Hemorrhagic corpora lutea in an adolescent. These transvaginal ultrasound images show *(A)* an irregularly shaped and echogenic trabecular structure surrounded by a sonolucent area of fluid and *(B)* a similar structure that is more echogenic and dense at the upper pole.

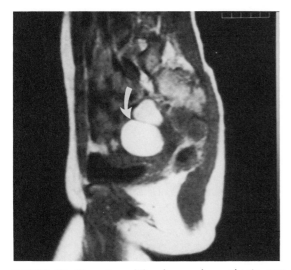

FIGURE 28–41 ••• A multilocular serohemorrhagic cyst *(arrow)* as shown by a medial sagittal MRI scan (TR = 550 ms; TE = 20 ms). (From Fedele L, Dorta M, Brioschi D, et al. Magnetic resonance imaging in Mayer-Rokitansky-Küster-Hauser Syndrome. Obstet Gynecol, 1990; 76:593–596. Reprinted with permission from The American College of Obstetricians and Gynecologists.)

are observed in some endometriomas as a result of the clotted blood that they contain.

MRI usually demonstrates endometriosis as a high-intensity image suggestive of blood on both T1- and T2-weighted scans (Fig. 28–44). Often, low-intensity regions are noted at the margins of the endometrioma. The lesions may have a hypointense fibrous capsule and be multilocular or multifocal; they may also be confused with benign teratomas, which are also

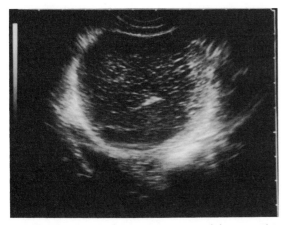

FIGURE 28–42 ••• Endometrioma in an adolescent. This transvaginal ultrasound scan demonstrates a cyst with rare, thin, internal echoes; part of the ovarian parenchyma is conserved.

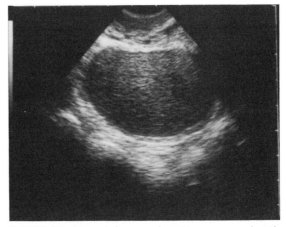

FIGURE 28–43 ••• A large endometrioma scanned with 6.5-MHz transvaginal probe. The uniformly echogenic thick blood content of the cyst is seen.

bright on both T1- and T2-weighted sequences. MRI has been reported to be sufficiently specific in identifying endometriotic ovarian cysts, but overall the best diagnostic tool for this disease is still endoscopy.[23]

As suggested by Zawin et al.,[24] MRI is probably more useful in monitoring treatment response than laparoscopy once the definite diagnosis of endometriosis is established.

Polycystic Ovary. In this condition the ovaries are usually enlarged to a volume of more than 10 ml. Multiple immature or atretic follicles are present along their periphery (Figs. 28–45, 28–46). However, as many as one third of adolescents with this disorder have normal-sized ovaries.[18] On MRI, low-signal-intensity cysts are revealed at the periphery of the gonads on T1-weighted images; typically, these become bright on T2-weighted images (Fig. 28–47). At the center of the ovaries, the signal intensity is low, probably because of fibrous luteinization.

Ovarian Torsion. Enlarged ovaries or those containing a neoformation may develop torsion involving the tube, ovary, or both. In the initial stages, only venous and lymphatic drainage is impaired, but the ovary increases markedly in volume in a few days and appears on USG as a solid mass, the result of vascular engorgement and stromal edema (Fig. 28–48). If the torsion is intermittent, ovarian enlargement may regress rapidly. In patients in whom torsion is associated with an ovarian mass, USG generally demonstrates a pelvic-abdominal mass with complex echoes (Fig. 28–49). In some individuals intraperitoneal fluid may be

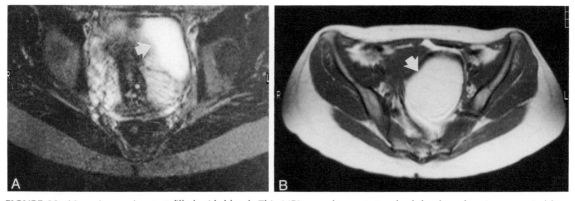

FIGURE 28–44 ••• An ovarian cyst filled with blood. This MRI scan demonstrates the left adnexal region occupied by a round structure *(arrow)* with clear outlines, no septation, and uniformly elevated signal intensity on T2-weighted sequences. *A,* Transverse section (TR = 2120 ms; TE = 100 ms). *B,* Transverse section (T1-weighted image) (TR = 500 ms; TE = 20 ms). (From Fedele L, Dorta M, Brioschi D, et al. Magnetic resonance evaluation of gynecologic masses in adolescents. Adolesc Pediatr Gynecol 1990; 3:83–88.)

evident as a result of hemorrhagic or exudative phenomena.[18] The differential diagnosis of ovarian enlargement should consider nongynecologic abdominal diseases, including mesenteric cysts and gastrointestinal duplication cysts. The former develop typically at the base of the mesentery and contain various septa. The latter derive from the distal small intestine and may or may not communicate with the intestinal lumen.

Disorders of Puberty. USG may be useful in the evaluation of a girl with known or suspected disorders of puberty and is performed in addition to a detailed history, physical examination, complete endocrine profile, chromosome analysis, and determination of bone age. Ovarian and uterine volume and USG characteristics are important indicators of pubertal change.[2, 5]

True precocious puberty is the result of premature maturation of the hypothalamic-pituitary-ovarian axis. In one study of 44 patients with this condition,[25] large-for-age or adult-size ovaries were detected on USG. This ovarian enlargement occurs early, whereas the uterus will vary from intermediate to adult size, depending on the duration of precocious puberty. USG has been used to monitor changes in ovarian and uterine size in patients treated with gonadotropin-releasing hormone (GnRH) analogues.

As noted in Chapter 5, precocious pseudopuberty includes a series of clinical conditions such as premature thelarche, premature adren-

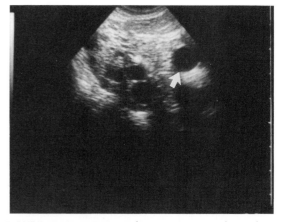

FIGURE 28–46 ••• Micropolycystic ovary as shown by a transvaginal ultrasound scan with 6.5-MHz probe. The ovary is normal in size with multiple discrete cysts <1 cm in diameter. There is a small hydatid cyst of Morgagni medial to the ovary but completely separate from it *(arrow).*

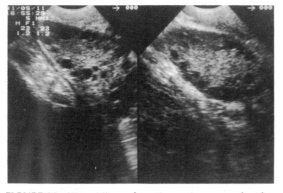

FIGURE 28–45 ••• Micropolycystic ovaries scanned with a 5-MHz probe. The ovaries are enlarged and round, with small follicles along their periphery.

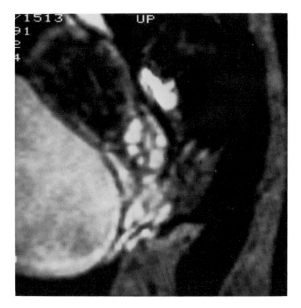

FIGURE 28–47 ••• MRI scan of a micropolycystic ovary (T2-weighted image) (TR = 2000; TE = 90). The follicles present as small cysts with high signal intensity at the ovarian periphery.

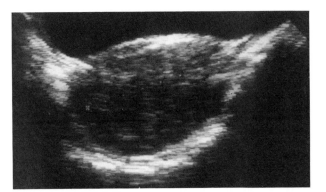

FIGURE 28–48 ••• Ovarian torsion. Ultrasound view; the ovary is seen as a large, dyshomogeneous solid mass *(calipers)* with a small hypoechoic space secondary to vascular engorgement and edema. B, Bladder. (Courtesy of Professor CA Dell'Agnola, University of Milan.)

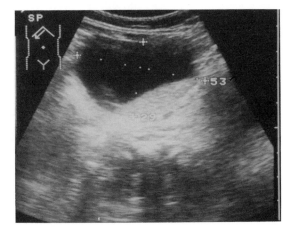

FIGURE 28–49 ••• Adnexal torsion secondary to an ovarian cyst in a 7-year-old girl. This transverse ultrasound scan of the pelvis shows the ovary *(calipers)* with an associated cyst in continuity with a uniformly hyperechoic structure that represents the ovarian parenchyma. (Courtesy of Professor CA Dell'Agnola, University of Milan.)

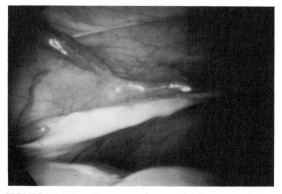

FIGURE 28–50 ••• Turner syndrome. This laparoscopic image shows a small left ovarian streak.

arche, congenital adrenal hyperplasia, and neurofibromatosis; it may also be caused by administration of estrogen compounds. Adrenal and ovarian tumors are rare causes of isosexual pseudopuberty that are detectable with USG.

Delayed puberty may sometimes be due to extragonadal causes such as juvenile hypothyroidism and cystic fibrosis. One study of five women with hypothyroidism demonstrated ovarian cysts 1 to 4 cm in diameter in all cases.[26] A transitory cyst larger than 3 cm was found in 43% of 13 patients with cystic fibrosis.[27] More often, delayed puberty is due to gonadal dysgenesis and its variants. In Turner syndrome, USG shows a wide range of ovarian findings, from absent to infantile to normal adult size (Figs. 28–50, 28–51). Normal ovaries can be predicted in Noonan's syndrome. USG has been used to monitor the effectiveness of

hormonal treatment in Turner syndrome by examining changes in uterine shape.[18]

Menometrorrhagia in the Adolescent. This pathophysiologic state is due to continuous, although variable, estrogenic stimulation of the endometrium, which at histology generally appears to be in the proliferative phase or is hyperplastic. Diagnosis is based on exclusion of other causes that may have the same clinical picture. USG is useful in excluding other concomitant pelvic diseases and is indispensable as a noninvasive study of the endometrium. It assesses endometrial thickness accurately (i.e., to within 1 mm of the measurement obtained at histopathologic examination). A diagnosis of endometrial hyperplasia must be established when endometrial thickness is >10 mm (Fig. 28–52). USG may also be useful in monitoring endometrial conditions after institution of hormonal treatment (Fig. 28–53).

Hydrosalpinx and Tubo-ovarian Abscesses. Pelvic inflammatory disease is a serious complication of sexually transmitted disease in adolescent girls. Generally the presenting symptom is acute lower abdominal and pelvic pain. Appendicitis is the first condition to be considered in the differential diagnosis. Initially the inflammatory fluid distends the fallopian tube, and USG identifies an anechoic adnexal mass, with the uterus presenting changes consistent with endometritis. However, Swayne et al.[28] described patients with an entirely normal pelvic sonogram. In the presence of a true tubo-ovarian abscess, USG reveals a pelvis completely filled with disorganized heterogeneous echoes mixed with solid and cystic areas (Fig. 28–54). In Fedele et al.'s

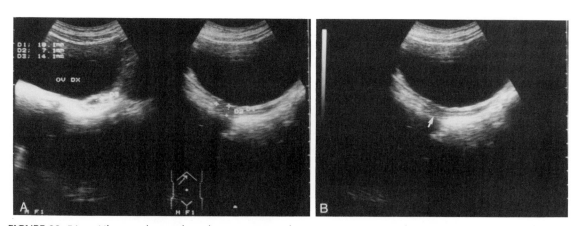

FIGURE 28–51 ••• Ultrasound scans from the same patient shown in Figure 28–50, demonstrating (A) a small, elongated ovary without evident follicular formation behind the bladder (calipers) and (B) a hypotrophic uterus (arrow).

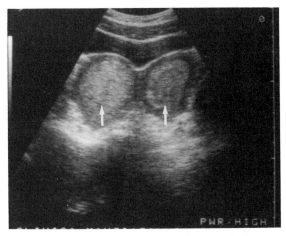

FIGURE 28–52 ••• Endometrial hyperplasia in a bicornuate uterus of a 13-year-old girl. A transverse ultrasound scan of the pelvis reveals two asymmetric, widely separated, enlarged uterine horns; thin myometrium; and hyperechogenic, markedly thickened (about 4 cm) endometrium *(arrows)*.

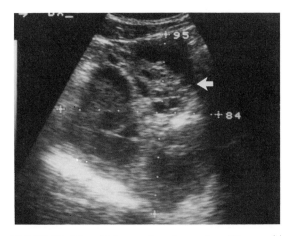

FIGURE 28–54 ••• Tubo-ovarian abscess in a 12-year-old girl. This transverse ultrasound scan of the pelvis shows a mixed mass with irregular outline *(calipers)* in which the ovary can be identified with follicular structures *(arrow)* and the dilated tube can be seen with thickened walls and fluid debris in the lumen.

series,[23] the contribution of MRI in the imaging of pelvic inflammatory disease was modest, although authors using T1-weighted images have reported that regions of low intensity may be noted along the uterine surface and within pelvic peritoneal recesses as a result of inflammatory fluid.[19] Laparoscopy allows a precise picture of the extent of the disease; a sample of intraperitoneal exudate may be obtained to plan appropriate therapy.

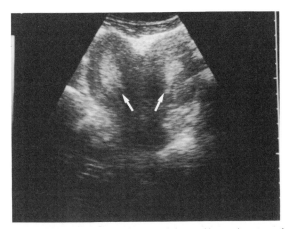

FIGURE 28–53 ••• Fundal scan of the malformed uterus of the same patient shown in Figure 28–52 after hormonal therapy. The notch of the external profile is evident. The myometrium is less thin, and the width of the endometrial cavity is normal *(arrows)*.

IMAGING OF MALIGNANT NEOPLASMS

Malignant tumors of the genital tract are infrequent in children and adolescents. Although all types of neoplasms found in adults have been reported, in this age group neoplasms usually consist of embryonal tumors or teratomas.

Vaginal Neoplasms. Vaginal neoplasms include two important lesions: mixed mesodermal tumor and clear-cell adenocarcinoma. The former, rhabdomyosarcoma, appears characteristically in infancy as a botryoid sarcoma; in the adolescent it originates from the vagina.

Clear-cell adenocarcinoma almost always derives from malignant transformation of vaginal adenosis. More than 500 cases have been reported in the literature, with an age range of 7 to 30 years and a peak incidence at 19 years of age.[17] On USG these tumors appear as solid, homogeneous masses filling the vaginal cavity (Fig. 28–55). On MRI, T2-weighted images have a high signal intensity, and correct tumor staging is theoretically possible.[29] In stage I, the signal intensity of the vaginal wall and the high signal intensity of the paravaginal fat are preserved. In stage II, the low-intensity vaginal wall is no longer recognized, and the interface between vaginal wall and fat is indistinct. In stage III, the normal low intensity of

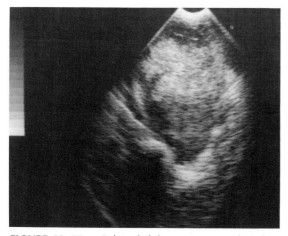

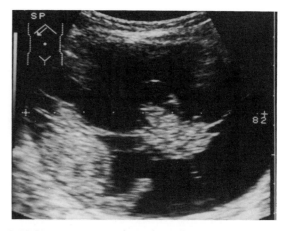

FIGURE 28–55 ••• Pelvic rhabdomyosarcoma. This ultrasound image demonstrates a solid homogeneous mass with an irregular outline. (Courtesy of Professor CA Dell'Agnola, University of Milan.)

FIGURE 28–57 ••• Sertoli-Leydig cell tumor in a 7-year-old girl. This ultrasound scan shows a cyst 8 cm in diameter containing irregular, wide, hyperechogenic areas connected by thickened septa. (Courtesy of Professor CA Dell'Agnola, University of Milan.)

the pelvic side wall muscles is disrupted, and in stage IV, T1-weighted scans demonstrate obliteration of the normal fat signals and planes, with extension into the bladder or rectum. Furthermore, MRI has clear advantages over other conventional imaging techniques in evaluating patients after radiotherapy or surgery, because it differentiates fibrotic tissue from grossly recurrent tumor.

Ovarian Cancers. Ovarian malignancies are rare in children and adolescents, representing only approximately 1% of all malignant tumors found in those between birth and 17 years of age.[20] Most ovarian tumors in children arise from germ cells, whereas in adult women, 80% to 90% have an epithelial origin.

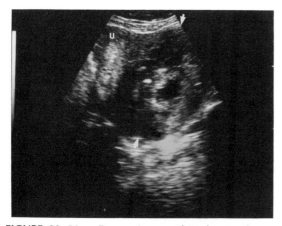

FIGURE 28–56 ••• Dysgerminoma. This ultrasound scan reveals a solid encapsulated mass (arrows) containing hypoechoic areas that represent hemorrhage and necrosis. U, Uterus.

Dysgerminoma. Dysgerminoma constitutes 16% of germ cell tumors and 11% of all ovarian tumors that occur in children and adolescents.[20] It usually presents as a large, solid, encapsulated mass with central hypoechoic areas caused by hemorrhage, necrosis, and cystic degeneration (Fig. 28–56).

Malignant Teratoma. Malignant transformation of an ovarian teratoma occurs in 1% of all ovarian neoplasms, most commonly in the first two decades of life.[30] In view of this, teratomas in children and adolescents should always be very carefully examined. Clinically, this tumor is characterized by rapid growth, weight loss, and abdominal-pelvic pain. USG characteristics resemble those of the benign type.

Sertoli-Leydig-Stromal Cell Tumors. These neoplasms contain Sertoli cells, Leydig cells, fibroblasts, or all three types of cells in varying proportions. Androgenic activity may be exhibited (hence the term *androblastoma*), but many of them have nonendocrine manifestations, and few are estrogenic or progestogenic. They vary in size from microscopic to large masses, but usually they have a diameter of between 5 and 15 cm. In general they are cystic and contain large, edematous papillae like those of serous papillary tumors (Fig. 28–57).

Granulosa and Thecal Cell Tumors. These are the most common ovarian tumors responsible for isosexual precocious puberty.[31] Diagnosis in children is based on the rapid development of secondary sex characteristics. In adolescents the effects of hormonal stimulation

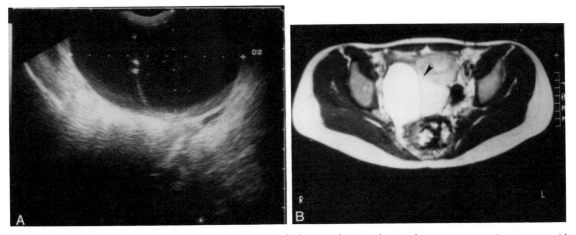

FIGURE 28–58 ••• Mucinous cystadenoma. *A*, A transvaginal ultrasound image shows a large, septate cystic structure with scanty internal echoes *(calipers)*. The septum is thickened and hyperechogenic. *B*, A transverse MRI scan (TR = 1585 ms; TE = 70 ms) showing the right hemipelvis, which contains a cystic structure with a maximum diameter of 10 cm *(arrowhead)* with thin walls and divided by a vertical septum into two cavities. The lateral cavity is larger and contains serous fluid; the medial one has a different signal, and its content is probably mucoid.

are less important and may include hypermenorrhea (75%), amenorrhea (25%), and ascites (20%). This delays diagnosis. The gross aspect is generally mixed (i.e., both solid and cystic), and the cyst may contain hemorrhagic fluid. The appearance on USG is nonspecific; these tumors have been reported as homogeneously solid or as solid with a central anechoic area.

Cystadenomas and Cystadenocarcinomas. Tumors of epithelial origin constitute 17% of all ovarian neoplasms diagnosed during the first two decades of life.[20] When papillary, they present as solid areas and vegetations inside the cystic cavity. Generally, the more solid and irregular its internal morphology, the more likely it is that a cystadenoma is malignant. In the presence of ascites, the tumor has probably spread beyond the capsule. Ascites is rarely associated with benign tumors such as ovarian fibroma (Meig's syndrome). Cystadenomas and cystadenocarcinomas cannot be differentiated by MRI.[19] Solid tumor nodules are associated with malignancy more often than not, but are also observed in benign mucinous cystadenomas (Fig. 28–58).

References

1. Nussbaum AR, Sanders RC, Jones MD. Neonatal uterine morphology as seen on real-time ultrasound. Radiology 1986; 160:641.
2. Orsini LF, Solardi S, Pilu G, et al. Pelvic organs in premenarchal girls: Real-time ultrasonography. Radiology 1984; 153:113.
3. Krantz KE, Atkinson JP. Gross anatomy. Ann NY Acad Sci 1967; 142:575.
4. McCarthy S, Tauber C, Gore J. Female pelvic anatomy: MR assessment of variations during the menstrual cycle and with use of contraceptives. Radiology 1986; 160:119.
5. Sample WF, Lippe BM, Gyepes MT. Gray-scale ultrasonography of the normal female pelvis. Radiology 1977; 125:477.
6. Dell'Agnola CA, Fedele L, Zamberletti D, et al. The management of hydrocolpos. Acta Eur Fertil 1984; 15:51.
7. Johnston JH. Female genital tract anomalies. In: Williams DI, Johnston JH (eds). Pediatric Urology. London: Butterworths, 1982. p 500.
8. Buttram VC Jr, Gibbons WE. Mullerian anomalies: A proposed classification. Fertil Steril 1979; 32:40.
9. Fedele L, Dorta M, Brioschi D, et al. Magnetic resonance imaging in Mayer-Rokitansky-Kuster-Hauser Syndrome. Obstet Gynecol 1990; 76:593.
10. McIndoe A. The treatment of congenital absence and obliterative conditions of the vagina. Br J Plast Surg 1950; 2:254.
11. Fedele L, Marchini M, Carinelli S, et al. Endometrium of cavitary rudimentary horn in unicornuate uteri. Obstet Gynecol 1990; 75:437.
12. Fedele L, Dorta M, Vercellini P, et al. Ultrasound in the diagnosis of subclasses of unicornuate uterus. Obstet Gynecol 1988; 71:274.
13. Fedele L, Dorta M, Brioschi D, et al. Magnetic resonance imaging of unicornuate uterus. Acta Obstet Gynecol Scand 1990; 69:511.
14. Rock JA, Jones HW. The double uterus associated with an obstructed hemivagina and ipsilateral renal agenesis. Am J Obstet Gynecol 1980; 138:339.
15. Fedele L, Ferrazzi E, Dorta M, et al. Ultrasonography in the differential diagnosis of "double" uteri. Fertil Steril 1988; 50:361.
16. Fedele L, Dorta M, Brioschi D, et al. Magnetic resonance evaluation of "double" uteri. Obstet Gynecol 1989; 74:844.
17. Kleinhaus S, Sheran M. Surgical gynecology. In:

Boley SJ, Cohen MI (eds). Surgery of the Adolescent. Orlando, FL: Grune & Stratton, 1986, p 89.

18. Fleischer AC, Shawker TH. The role of sonography in pediatric gynecology. Clin Obstet Gynecol 1987; 30:735.

19. Fishman-Javitt MC, Lovecchio JL, Syein HL. The ovary. In: Fishman-Javitt MC, Stein HL, Lovecchio JL (eds). Imaging of the Pelvis: MRI with Correlations to CT and Ultrasound. Boston: Little, Brown, 1990, p 109.

20. Breen J, Maxon WS. Ovarian tumors in childhood and adolescence. Clin Obstet Gynecol 1977; 20:923.

21. Vercellini P, Fedele L, Arcaini L, et al. Laparoscopy in the diagnosis of chronic pelvic pain in adolescent women. J Reprod Med 1989; 34:829.

22. Fleischer AC. Pelvic sonography. In: Fisher MR, Krieum ME (eds). Imaging of the Pelvis. Rockville MD: Aspen, 1989, p 151.

23. Fedele L, Dorta M, Brioschi D, et al. Magnetic resonance evaluation of gynecologic masses in adolescents. Adolesc Pediatr Gynecol 1990; 3:83.

24. Zawin M, McCartey S, Scoutt L, Comite F. Endometriosis: Appearance and detection at MR imaging. Radiology 1989; 171:693.

25. Lippe BM. Primary ovarian failure. In: Kaplan SA (ed). Clinical Pediatric and Adolescent Endocrinology. Philadelphia: WB Saunders, 1982, p 286.

26. Riddlesberger MM, Kuhn JP, Munschauer RW. The association of juvenile hypothyroidism and cystic ovaries. Radiology 1981; 139:77.

27. Showker T, Hubbard V, Reicher C, et al. Cystic ovaries in cystic fibrosis: An ultrasound and autopsy study. J Ultrasound Med 1983; 2:439.

28. Swayne LC, Love MB, Karasik SR. Pelvic inflammatory disease: Sonographic pathologic correlation. Radiology 1984; 151:751.

29. Stein HL, Lovecchio JL, Fishmen-Javitt MC. The vulva and vagina. In: Fishman-Javitt MC, Stein HL, Lovecchio JL (eds). Imaging of the Pelvis: MRI Correlations to CT and Ultrasound. Boston: Little, Brown, 1990, p 37.

30. Talerman J. Germ cell tumors of the ovary. In: Kurman RJ (eds). Blaunstein's Pathology of the Female Genital Tract. 3rd ed. New York: Springer-Verlag, 1989, p 660.

31. Thompson J, Dockerty M, Symmonds R, Hayles A. Ovarian and paraovarian tumors in infants and children. Am J Obstet Gynecol 1967; 97:1059.

CHAPTER 29

Delayed Consequences of Childhood Malignancies

DAVID MURAM

Modern therapy for childhood malignancies has resulted in an increase in disease-free intervals and improved cure rates. Although improvements in outcome are identified with all types of neoplasms, the increased survival rates for patients with non-Hodgkin's lymphoma, bone tumors, and rhabdomyosarcoma (sarcoma botryoides) are particularly striking.[1] It was estimated that in 1990, one of every 1000 20-year-olds was a survivor of childhood cancer.[2–4] This estimate is based on the incidence of the various malignancies occurring between birth and age 15 and an estimated overall cure rate of 60% (Table 29–1).[1, 3] Incidence and survival data from the National Cancer Institute's Surveillance, Epidemiology, and End Results (SEER) Program reveal that childhood cancer incidence rates remained relatively stable during the 1980s, with an overall incidence of 127 per 1 million children. For all forms of cancer combined, the 5-year relative survival rate was 57%. The 5-year relative survival rate exceeded 80% for fibrosarcomas, retinoblastomas, Hodgkin's disease, and gonadal and germ cell tumors (Figs. 29–1 through 29–3).[1] While the increasing number of pediatric cancer patients surviving the disease is gratifying, the lifelong sequelae that may occur following cure of childhood cancer must be considered. Most of these factors are relatively

minor, but in some patients severe disabilities are noted in terms of their ability to function physically, emotionally, or intellectually. Some complications are therapy specific, but many are general in nature and are related to the nature of the illness, its treatment, and fears related to potential recurrences.

As these children are cured of their malignancy, they are no longer treated by the oncologist but instead are referred back into the community health care system. Thus, the primary care physician becomes responsible for their care and therefore should be familiar with the various complications that are often encountered among survivors of childhood malignancies.

There are many variables that affect the long-term consequences of the cancer and its therapy: the primary malignancy, its location, the type of therapy provided, and the interval from therapy to the onset of possible complications. Often, the abnormality caused by the cancer therapy is obvious (e.g., when amputation is required to remove an osteosarcoma); in other cases, the abnormality may be subtle and its appearance so remote in time from cancer therapy that the physician may not recognize the connection unless specifically screening for it (e.g., hypothyroidism developing after irradiation for Hodgkin's disease). Special attention must be given to physical

TABLE 29–1 ••• KAPLAN-MEIER ESTIMATES OF SURVIVAL AND EVENT-FREE SURVIVAL OVER TIME

	Survival			Event-Free Survival		
	2-Year	*3-Year*	*5-Year*	*2-Year*	*3-Year*	*5-Year*
Non-T, non-B, noninfant ALL						
1976–80 (848 patients, 204/yr)	77 (1.5)	69 (2.0)	56 (1.8)	69 (1.7)	57 (3.8)	43 (1.8)
1980–81 (177 patients, 236/yr)	81 (3.1)	75 (3.2)	68 (3.7)	69 (3.6)	64 (3.7)	54 (3.9)
1981–86 (1504 patients, 336/yr)	87 (0.9)	80 (1.0)	73 (1.5)	75 (1.1)	69 (1.2)	56 (1.6)
1986–89 (1511 patients, 394/yr)	92 (1.1)	88 (2.3)	—	85 (1.5)	80 (2.7)	—
T-cell ALL						
1976–78 (61 patients, 27/yr)	54 (6.5)	48 (6.5)	39 (6.6)	48 (6.5)	41 (6.4)	34 (6.5)
1978–81 (71 patients, 28/yr)	59 (6.0)	49 (6.1)	47 (6.1)	49 (6.0)	46 (6.0)	45 (6.0)
1981–86 (283 patients, 57/yr)	87 (2.8)	58 (3.0)	50 (3.6)	54 (3.0)	49 (3.0)	43 (3.1)
1986–89 (300 patients, 78/yr)	75 (4.0)	60 (7.8)	—	64 (4.3)	56 (7.4)	—
Infant ALL						
1976–81 (31 patients, 6/yr)	54 (9)	36 (9)	24 (9)	27 (9)	19 (8)	13 (9)
1981–84 (32 patients, 9/yr)	44 (9)	34 (8)	31 (11)	22 (7)	16 (6)	13 (7)
1984–89 (83 patients, 20/yr)	45 (7)	36 (8)	—	30 (6)	28 (7)	—
ANLL						
1977–81 (195 patients, 52/yr)	37 (3.6)	27 (3.3)	24 (3.3)	26 (3.3)	21 (3.1)	18 (2.9)
1981–84 (266 patients, 89/yr)	41 (3.1)	34 (3.0)	28 (3.7)	34 (2.9)	25 (2.7)	23 (3.4)
1984–88 (293 patients, 72/yr)	48 (3.4)	37 (4.9)	—	39 (3.3)	32 (4.8)	—
Advanced lymphoblastic NHL						
1976–79 (41 patients, 15/yr)	73 (7)	63 (8)	57 (8)	71 (7)	58 (8)	53 (8)
1979–83 (77 patients, 19/yr)	67 (6)	59 (6)	52 (6)	55 (6)	49 (6)	45 (6)
1983–86 (53 patients, 20/yr)	76 (6)	64 (7)	64 (11)	66 (7)	60 (7)	58 (11)
1986–89 (130 patients, 34/yr)	73 (6)	73 (10)	—	75 (6)	69 (10)	—
Advanced DUL						
1979–81 (24 patients, 10/yr)	41 (10)	36 (10)	36 (13)	33 (10)	33 (10)	33 (10)
1981–86 (124 patients, 25/yr)	69 (4)	69 (5)	68 (7)	65 (4)	65 (5)	64 (7)
1986–89 (66 patients, 21/yr)	79 (11)	—	—	75 (12)	—	—
Advanced large-cell NHL						
1976–79 (18 patients, 7/yr)	56 (12)	56 (12)	56 (12)	56 (12)	56 (12)	56 (12)
1979–81 (32 patients, 13/yr)	72 (8)	72 (8)	68 (9)	63 (9)	63 (9)	63 (9)
1981–86 (28 patients, 6/yr)	68 (9)	68 (9)	—	54 (9)	54 (10)	54 (14)
1986–89 (61 patients, 19/yr)	77 (13)	—	—	67 (15)	—	—
Limited-stage NHL						
1976–79 (27 patients, 10/yr)	93 (5)	89 (6)	85 (7)	82 (7)	78 (8)	74 (9)
1979–83 (75 patients, 19/yr)	91 (3)	85 (4)	79 (5)	89 (4)	78 (8)	75 (5)
1983–87 (145 patients, 35/yr)	94 (2)	94 (2)	94 (5)	92 (2)	91 (3)	90 (6)
1987–89 (94 patients, 38/yr)	93 (10)	—	—	89 (15)	—	—
Osteosarcoma						
1982–84 (117 patients, 59/yr)	77 (4)	70 (5)	58 (7)	54 (5)	50 (5)	44 (6)
1984–86 (96 patients, 41/yr)	84 (4)	79 (6)	—	74 (5)	72 (6)	—
1986–89 (64 patients, 20/yr)	82 (11)	—	—	60 (14)	—	—
Neuroblastoma						
1981–84 (145 patients, 46/yr)	20 (3)	18 (3)	13 (3)	10 (3)	8 (2)	6 (3)
1984–87 (147 patients, 61/yr)	45 (4)	27 (4)	—	35 (4)	21 (4)	—
1987–89 (157 patients, 59/yr)	36 (10)	—	—	35 (9)	—	—

*Values represent percentages, with SE in parentheses. Annual accrual is month specific.

ALL, Acute lymphocytic leukemia; ANLL, acute nonlymphocytic leukemia; DUL, diffuse undifferentiated NHL; NHL, non-Hodgkin's lymphoma.

From The Pediatric Oncology Group. Progress against childhood cancer: The Pediatric Oncology Group experience. Pediatrics 1992; 89:597–600.

growth and development as well as sexual maturation of the child who has survived cancer.

The gynecologist may be asked to evaluate survivors of childhood cancer because of growth abnormality, delayed sexual maturation, or aberrant reproductive tract development. Because the gonads are particularly vulnerable to radiation and chemotherapeutic agents, impaired gonadal function is a fairly common complication of cancer therapy.[5, 6] The long-term effects of childhood malignancy on growth, sexual maturation, and reproductive function must be understood by the clinician.

GROWTH AND DEVELOPMENT

Therapy for cancer during childhood frequently affects the growth of bones and soft

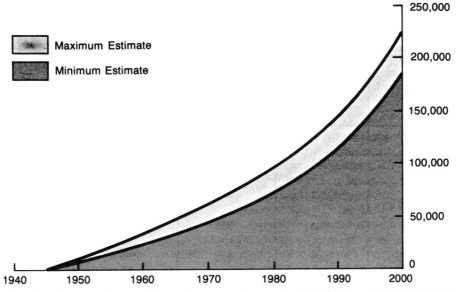

FIGURE 29–1 ••• Cumulative number of childhood cancer survivors in the United States, 1945–2000. (From Bleyer WA. The impact of childhood cancer on the United States and the world. CA 1990; 40:355–367.)

tissues. The determinants of growth operate through both local and central mechanisms. Sequelae involving the latter include growth hormone (GH) deficiency with subsequent diminished somatomedin production, thyroid hormone deficiency, gonadal dysfunction, malnutrition secondary to chronic illness, and psychological factors. Sequelae involving the former are predominantly due to radiation

therapy and its effects on bone and associated soft tissue and blood vessels.[7] These effects are dose related and are more pronounced in rapidly growing tissues. In general, the younger the patient and the higher the radiation dosage received, the more pronounced the long-term effects.[8]

Irradiation to bone may cause arrested chondrogenesis, deficient absorptive processes in

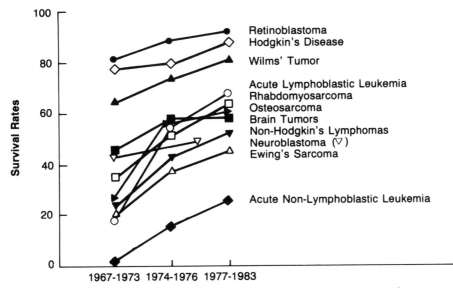

FIGURE 29–2 ••• Increased survival rates for individual types of childhood cancer. (From Bleyer WA. The impact of childhood cancer on the United States and the world. CA 1990; 40:355–367.)

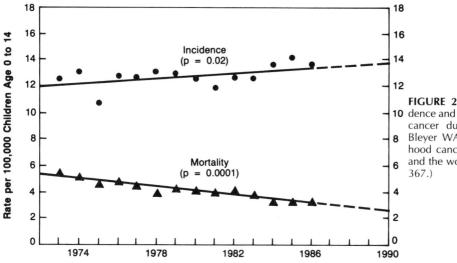

FIGURE 29–3 ••• Increasing incidence and declining mortality from cancer during childhood. (From Bleyer WA. The impact of childhood cancer on the United States and the world. CA 1990; 40:355–367.)

calcified bone and cartilage, and altered periosteal activity and bone modeling.[9] Radiographically, one may observe growth arrest lines and epiphyseal irregularities.[10] Decreased bone growth is also associated with decreased muscle and soft tissue mass.[11]

The spinal column is also affected by irradiation, and multiple abnormalities of the spine may affect final height.[12] These include impairment or irregularity of growth at the vertebral end plates, decreased vertebral body height, and changes in contour (Fig. 29–4).[10]

GH deficiency is a well-known complication causing growth abnormality in cancer survivors, particularly in children who received cranial irradiation. After external irradiation, the damage to the hypothalamic-pituitary axis is at the level of the hypothalamus, whereas patients who undergo pituitary ablation with interstitial radiotherapy or heavy particle beams sustain direct damage to the pituitary gland.[13]

In one study of 27 prepubertal and postpubertal children with brain tumors who had normal GH levels before therapy, impaired GH response to hypoglycemia was found in 10 of the children after chemotherapy and cranial irradiation (Fig. 29–5).[14] Although radiation doses were not reported, it is estimated that these patients received at least 3500 rad to the pituitary gland. When the radiation dose is lower, pituitary function is more likely to be unaffected. A study of 14 children with acute lymphocytic leukemia (ALL) who were treated with chemotherapy and cranial radiation therapy (2000 to 2500 rad) found only minor dysfunction of the hypothalamic-pituitary axis.[15] The relationship among radiation dose, pituitary damage, and subsequent GH deficiency was further supported by Shalet and Beardwell, who suggested that the total dose of radiation appears to be a more significant determinant of future pituitary function than the number of fractions and the dose given per each fraction.[16]

GH deficiency occurs primarily in children who have received cranial irradiation. Studies examining the effects of chemotherapy in children without cranial radiation show a normal GH response. Consequently, in children with ALL, height velocity was abnormally low after cranial radiation, whereas those receiving chemotherapy alone had a normal growth pattern.[17] However, a similar study of 12 patients noted no difference between irradiated and nonirradiated patients with respect to GH secretion or height. These patients, however, received total radiation dosages of 2400 rad, which is a lower dose than the 3500 rad reported to cause hypothalamic-pituitary dysfunction, which was noted to be associated with an abnormal GH response.[18] Low-dose total-body irradiation may also adversely affect growth. The majority of children who were treated with cyclophosphamide and single-fraction total-body irradiation (900 to 1000 rad) before a bone marrow transplant exhibited growth failure as a result of multiple endocrinopathies, including gonadal failure.[19]

The overall effects of therapy on growth pattern appear to be slight after chemotherapy, radiation therapy, or both, provided that total

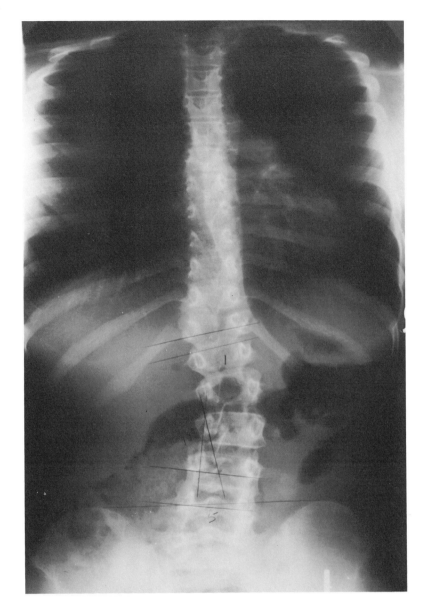

FIGURE 29–4 ••• Spinal column abnormalities caused by irradiation during childhood. Notice the decreased vertebral body height and changes in contour causing severe scoliosis.

radiation dose does not exceed 2500 rad. However, when radiation therapy is extended to include abdominal and gonadal radiation, children have shown an abnormal growth pattern.[20, 21] In one study, investigators concluded that any patient who receives a total irradiation dose of 2000 rad or more to the hypothalamic-pituitary axis is at risk of hypopituitarism, although the threshold dose may be lower. Furthermore, these patients are at increased risk of developing multiple deficiencies. A higher fraction size increases the risk of anterior pituitary failure.

Some investigators have shown that treatment with GH increases growth velocity in children who were adversely affected by the cranial irradiation.[22] However, other investigators found that such therapy failed to correct growth abnormalities after cranial irradiation but did benefit children in whom a surgical excision resulted in GH deficiency.[23] In fact, a study comparing patients with GH deficiency after CNS radiation therapy and normal subjects revealed no significant differences in height velocity, somatomedin activity, and bone age.[24] Thus, many physicians currently do not use GH therapy when treating these children.[24, 25]

Hypothyroidism, which may occur after radiation therapy to the head and neck region,

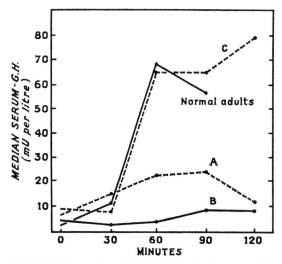

FIGURE 29–5 ••• Growth hormone levels during insulin-induced hypoglycemia. Group A and group B represent children treated for malignancy. Group C represents controls. (From Shalet SM, Morris-Jones PH, Beardwell CG, et al. Pituitary function after treatment of intracranial tumors in children. Lancet 1975; II:104–107.)

may also diminish linear growth during childhood. These children have reduced thyroxine (T_4) and/or elevated thyroid-stimulating hormone (TSH) levels. In a long-term follow-up study of patients who were treated with neck irradiation in childhood, more than half demonstrated some abnormality of T_4 or TSH or thyroid gland nodularity. Lymphangiography and an irradiation dose of 3000 rad or more increased the risk of patients to develop palpable thyroid nodules and to have thyroid hypofunction as demonstrated by elevated TSH levels. Thyroid hyperfunction may follow neck irradiation, with or without clinical signs of hyperthyroidism.[26, 27] Thyroid dysfunction may also interfere with the normal menstrual cycle.

Less is known about the effects, if any, of chemotherapy on thyroid function. In one study, 28 children were followed after treatment for Hodgkin's disease. Four received only chemotherapy, 15 received only radiation therapy (with an estimated thyroid dose of 4570 rad), and nine received chemotherapy combined with radiation (with an estimated thyroid dose of 4000 rad). None of the four children treated with chemotherapy alone developed hypothyroidism.[28] In comparison, 21 of the 24 children who received radiation therapy, with or without chemotherapy, developed thyroid dysfunction.

The physician who is following these survi-vors should measure and weigh the patients at regular intervals. Plotting these measurements on growth charts and growth velocity charts over time is essential to detect growth abnormalities. If patients appear to have growth failure, then referral to an endocrinologist is warranted for possible treatment with recombinant GH. If it is clear that poor growth is related only to local damage caused by the irradiation, intervention may not be necessary.

GONADAL FUNCTION

Cancer therapy can adversely affect gonadal function, both hormone production and the viability of germ cells. Variables that appear to be predictors of long-term effects include the sex of the patient, the nature of the therapy (radiation or chemotherapy), the dosage and duration of therapy, and, to a lesser degree, the age and sexual maturity of the patient. Amenorrhea and gonadal failure often follow fractionated total-body irradiation. Amenorrhea developed within 3 months of irradiation in all females, and gonadotropin levels were elevated in all patients.[21] The endocrine sequelae of total-body irradiation are often limited to gonadal failure and require estrogen replacement therapy.[21, 29] It has been estimated that the median lethal dose (LD_{50}) for the human oocyte does not exceed 400 rad.[29] After irradiation, 20% of prepubertal girls with leukemia had no follicle growth and 80% had incomplete follicular development. Another study showed a marked decrease in antral as well as primordial and primary follicles.[30]

It is currently a common practice to suspend the ovaries out of the planned radiation field (oophoropexy) of young female patients to decrease their exposure to the damaging effects of ionizing radiation and thus prevent the long-term sequela of ovarian failure. Future normal ovarian function is inversely related to the amount of radiation absorbed by the gonads, and the absorbed dose is dependent on distance from the radiation field. In one study, 71% of the patients undergoing ovarian transposition maintained ovarian function. Preservation of ovarian function was directly related to the estimated scatter dose to the ovaries. For patients whose calculated ovarian dose was 300 rad or less, only 11% had gonadal failure, compared with 60% of patients whose ovarian dose was more than 300 rad.[31] Lateral transposition of the ovaries reduces the radiation

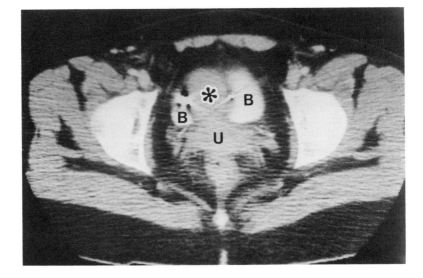

FIGURE 29–6 ••• Ovarian tissue *(asterisk)* can be identified indenting the bladder. Marker clips are seen laterally. B, bladder; U, uterus. (From Winer-Muram HT, Muram D, Salazar J, Thompson E. Ovariopexy—clinical and radiologic correlation. Adolesc Pediatr Gynecol 1988; 1:239–243.)

dose to the gonad, but for placement to be effective, the ovaries should be positioned above the iliac crest.[31] Patients who undergo ovarian transposition, however, are prone to develop symptomatic ovarian cysts, which may occur in up to 25% of patients secondary to vascular compromise.[31] In one study, computed tomographic (CT) scans were found to be of prognostic value in determining whether ovarian function was maintained after transposition. If the ovaries were identified on pelvic scans, ovarian function was likely to have been preserved (Figs. 29–6, 29–7).[32]

The gonads are very sensitive to irradiation damage, and radiation therapy to the ovary in doses ranging from 400 to 700 rad often causes ovarian failure. In one study, however, investigators reported that only 17 of 25 girls developed ovarian failure when both ovaries were exposed to doses ranging from 1200 to 5000 rad (mean, 3200 rad). They concluded that younger women are less susceptible to the deleterious effects of irradiation.[33] Puberty is usually, but not invariably, delayed by such treatment.[34]

Cancer chemotherapy, most notably alkylating agents, may cause menstrual irregularities or amenorrhea, loss of libido, menopausal symptoms, and possibly osteoporosis.[35, 36] The incidence of gonadal dysfunction after chemotherapy seems to be strikingly high and is 80% greater in women treated for Hodgkin's

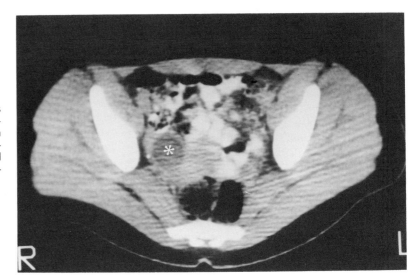

FIGURE 29–7 ••• A CT scan shows a functional ovarian cyst in a transposed ovary. (From Winer-Muram HT, Muram D, Salazar J, Thompson E. Ovariopexy—clinical and radiologic correlation. Adolesc Pediatr Gynecol 1988; 1:239–243.)

disease than in normal women.[15] Although lasting gonadal dysfunction may follow the use of a single chemotherapeutic agent, in general, chemotherapy-induced gonadal damage is related to the amount of cytotoxic agent administered.[37] Available data indicate that in subjects with abnormal gonadal function, the dysfunction is due to gonadal rather than hypothalamic-pituitary damage. Basal gonadotropin levels were elevated in 98% of affected individuals, and gonadotropin response to GnRH stimulation tests was consistent with primary gonadal dysfunction in 99% of patients with abnormal gonadal function.[37]

Although these symptoms of gonadal dysfunction are well known in postpubertal females, the effects of similar therapy during the prepubertal years are not as well documented. Numerous studies have been designed to assess the relationship of gonadal activity and chemotherapy-induced gonadal damage. Some have shown that prepubertal status affords some protection from chemotherapy-induced gonadal damage. Cyclophosphamide administered to prepubertal and pubertal females resulted in no gonadal dysfunction as measured by plasma levels of gonadotropins.[38, 39] One literature review of 30 studies evaluated gonadal function after either cyclophosphamide therapy for renal disease or combination chemotherapy for Hodgkin's disease or acute lymphocytic leukemia.[37] The data were stratified according to sex, illness, chemotherapeutic regimen and dose, and pubertal stage at the time of treatment. The likelihood of developing chemotherapy-induced damage was dependent on the chemotherapeutic regimen and the dose administered and was directly related to the degree of gonadal activity at the time of treatment.[37]

If chemotherapy-induced damage varies according to pubertal status, it might be assumed that it is related to gonadal activity at the time of treatment. Specifically, it would be expected that prepubertal children with inactive gametogenesis would have a lower incidence of chemotherapy-induced damage than would similarly treated adults and that adolescents who experience a progressive increase in gonadal activity would have an incidence of gonadal dysfunction intermediate between that of individuals treated prepubertally and those treated postpubertally.

In recent years, prevention of chemotherapy-induced gonadal damage has received significant attention. The basic premise is that artificial gonadal suppression may render the gonad more resistant to the deleterious effects of chemotherapy or irradiation therapy. The potential for preserving reproductive function through the suppression of ovarian activity by means of oral contraceptive therapy has shown some degree of success.[40] In one study, preservation of ovarian function was documented in five of five females treated for Hodgkin's disease concomitant with oral contraceptive treatment.[41] Other investigators reported that fertility rates were greater among women who had taken oral contraceptives during treatment of Hodgkin's disease than among those who did not take them.[42] However, in that particular study the patients taking oral contraceptives were younger than those who did not take oral contraceptives.[42]

Medroxyprogesterone acetate (Depo-Provera, or DMPA), a long-acting progestin, was also used to suppress gonadal function in males before treatment with chemotherapeutic agents.[43] A second group was not given MPA and was treated only with chemotherapy. In this particular study, there was no difference between the groups with respect to recovery of sperm cell production after chemotherapy. A DMPA-induced medical castration during intensive chemotherapy in male patients appears to be ineffective in protecting the testis against treatment-induced damage to spermatogenesis, at least if hormone treatment was provided simultaneously with chemotherapy.[43]

The hypothesis that the "downregulated" gonad is less vulnerable to the effects of cytotoxic chemotherapy has been investigated, with conflicting results reported. In one study, the investigators were able to demonstrate that treatment of rats with long-acting GnRH analogues resulted in diminution of histologically evident testicular damage secondary to chemotherapy.[44] A more recent study evaluated the protective effect of the GnRH agonist leuprolide acetate (Lupron). Animals were treated with cyclophosphamide in combination with Lupron, progesterone, or placebo. Both Lupron and progesterone were shown to protect the gonad from the negative effects of cyclophosphamide.[45] However, using GnRH agonists with chemotherapy, other investigators failed to preserve fertility in patients treated for Hodgkin's disease.[46]

Lifesaving therapy may mandate the use of agents that have toxic effects on the gonad. Because chemotherapy-induced gonadal damage is related to gonadal activity, further study is required to develop preventive strategies, and despite the conflicting data, it may be advisable to achieve gonadal quiescence to increase the resistance of the gonad to the side effects of therapy.

The natural history of gonadal dysfunction after chemotherapy has not been extensively characterized. Current evidence suggests that complete recovery of normal gonadal function generally does not occur.[37] In one study of female patients treated for Hodgkin's disease, 49% were amenorrheic, 34% had irregular menstrual cycles, and 17% had normal ovarian function soon after therapy.[35] However, during 16 months of continued observation, a progressive loss of ovarian function occurred in 30% of those who had had either normal or irregular menstrual cycles after treatment.[35] None of the women with amenorrhea regained normal ovarian function. Unfortunately, at the present time there are no medical means by which gonadal healing may be initiated or accelerated.[5, 35]

LATE CONSEQUENCES OF CURE

Survivors of childhood malignancies are at risk for developing a second malignancy, often 10 years or more after completion of therapy for the primary neoplasm. Although the exact risk has not been determined, it is estimated to be 3% to 12% for children diagnosed and treated before 1971. For children treated more recently, the incidence is estimated to be about 8%.[47–49] These rates represent an increased risk (i.e., 10 to 20 times greater) for these patients compared with the general population.

FERTILITY AND PREGNANCY OUTCOME

A potential mutagenic effect may be produced by chemotherapy or radiation therapy; these may adversely affect germ cells and, subsequently, the offspring of cancer survivors. The ultimate genetic effect, however, is determined by the sex and age of the exposed patient, because germ cells exist at different developmental stages in the two sexes and in the various stages of pubertal development. Oogonial mitosis is completed in fetal life; the ova are therefore less vulnerable than spermatogonia to point mutations, but more susceptible to nondisjunction. Offspring of treated females are at an increased risk for chromosomal aneuploidy, whereas the off-spring of treated males are more likely to sustain single-gene mutations or structural rearrangements than aneuploidy.[4]

The potential for chemotherapeutic agents to induce genetic abnormalities in offspring has not been determined. Radiation therapy, however, is known to produce germ cell effects. In humans, a gonadal dose of 200 rem (roentgen-equivalent–man) in childhood produces an increased genetic risk of about 1%. As the dose of radiation therapy increases up to 1000 rem, there is a linear increase in the genetic effects. Gonadal radiation therapy beyond 1000 rem usually produces sterility, while the risk of a genetic abnormality is approximately 1% to 5%, depending on the dosage.[4] Pregnancy outcome, however, is usually unaffected, and when compared with a control group, there is no significant increase in the rate of spontaneous abortions or abnormal offspring among survivors of childhood cancer treated with either chemotherapy or irradiation.[50, 51] However, in Holmes and Holmes' series,[50] the group treated with a combined modality did show a significantly higher incidence of spontaneous abortions or abnormal offspring.[50] In the series of Blatt et al., there was no increase in the rate of abortions. Follow-up study of children born to previously treated mothers showed no increase in the prevalence of congenital abnormalities.[51]

Infertility appears to be the major concern. In one study of 103 women who were treated for Hodgkin's disease with radiation and chemotherapy, the pregnancy rate was considerably lower than the expected rate adjusted for age.[52] The likelihood of becoming infertile was directly related to the radiation absorbed dose (rad) received by the gonads. Gonadal dysfunction after therapy commonly results in decreased fertility rates.[53] Recent advances currently permit some individuals with gonadal failure to conceive after receiving an egg or an embryo from a donor. After sequential administration of estrogen and progesterone, endometrial stimulation is synchronized with an ovum donor, and after fertilization, a preembryo is transferred on cycle days 16 to 21.[54]

NEOPLASMS IN THE OFFSPRING

Compared with the general population, offspring of survivors are at an increased risk for developing cancer.[55] Carcinomas in offspring of survivors may occur in two ways: the offspring may inherit the genes that caused the parent's cancer, or they may acquire new genetic abnormalities induced in parental germ cells by therapeutic agents.[55, 56] The first possibility, inheritance, is most likely in the offspring of children with genetic forms of embryonal tumors, such as retinoblastoma, Wilms' tumor, and neuroblastoma.[56–58]

PSYCHOSOCIAL ADJUSTMENT

In addition to the medical complications of therapy, many survivors suffer adverse psychological sequelae. Various studies have attempted to explore such issues, but the results have varied and at times have been controversial.[56–65]

Scholastic problems may arise as a result of absenteeism secondary to therapy, a decrease in intellectual performance after cranial irradiation, or social isolation of these children by their peers. A decrease in school performance may lead to dropout and its sequelae. Occasionally, physical impairment after amputation may require adjustments not only psychosocially, but also physically.

Special efforts must be made to allow these children to lead as normal a life as possible. Tutorial services should be provided in the hospital so that children can maintain their class standing. Counseling with parents and families may resolve conflicts that may have arisen after the diagnosis; fears of dying and cancer recurrence must also be dealt with during therapy. Counseling with peers who survived similar disease may also be beneficial. The combination of adolescence and cancer creates a high risk for emotional disturbances and negative psychosocial sequelae. Every effort must be made to permit survivors of childhood cancer to lead a normal and fulfilling life.

Finally, these survivors often worry about the impact of the treatment modalities on their future health, their reproductive ability, and their offspring. Intensive counseling is vital for cancer patients and must address these issues.

References

1. Young JL, Ries LG, Silverberg E, et al. Cancer incidence, survival, and mortality for children younger than age 15 years. Cancer 1986; 58(suppl):598–602.
2. Jenkin D, Berry M. Hodgkin's disease in children. Semin Oncol 1980; 7:202–211.
3. The Pediatric Oncology Group. Progress against childhood cancer: The Pediatric Oncology Group experience. Pediatrics 1992; 89:597–600.
4. Meadows AT, Silber J. Delayed consequences of therapy of childhood cancer. CA 1985; 35:271–286.
5. Sutcliffe SB. Cytotoxic chemotherapy and gonadal function in patients with Hodgkin's disease: Facts and thoughts. JAMA 1979; 242:1898–1899.
6. Chapman RM. Effect of cytotoxic therapy on sexuality and gonadal function. Semin Oncol 1989; 9:84–94.
7. Vaeth JM, Levitt SH, Jones MD, et al. Effects of radiation therapy in survivors of Wilms' tumor. Radiation 1962; 79:560–568.
8. Donaldson SS, Kaplan HS. Complications of treatment of Hodgkin's disease in children. Cancer Treat Rep 1982; 66:977–989.
9. Parker RG, Berry HC. Late effects of therapeutic irradiation on the skeleton and bone marrow. Cancer 1976; 37:1162–1171.
10. Riseborough EJ, Grabias SL, Burton RI et al. Skeletal alterations following irradiation for Wilm's tumor: With particular reference to scoliosis and kyphosis. J Bone Joint Surg 1976; 58:526–536.
11. Rubin P, Duthie RB, Young LW. The significance of scoliosis in postirradiated Wilms' tumor and neuroblastoma. Radiology 1962; 79:539–559.
12. Probert JC, Parker BR. The effects of radiation therapy on bone growth. Radiology 1975; 114:155–162.
13. Littley MD, Shalet SM, Beardwell CG. Radiation and hypothalamic-pituitary function. Clin Endocrinol Metab 1990; 4:147–175.
14. Shalet SM, Morris-Jones PH, Beardwell CG, et al. Pituitary function after treatment of intracranial tumors in children. Lancet 1975; 2:104–107.
15. Swift PGF, Kearney PJ, Dalton RG, et al. Growth and hormonal status of children treated for acute lymphoblastic leukemia. Arch Dis Child 1978; 53:890–894.
16. Shalet SM, Beardwell CG. Endocrine consequences of treatment of malignant disease in childhood: a review. J R Soc Med 1979; 72:39–41.
17. Wells RJ, Foster MB, D'Ercole AJ, et al. The impact of cranial irradiation on the growth of children with acute lymphocytic leukemia. Am J Dis Child 1983; 137:37–39.
18. Hakami N, Mohammad A, Meyer JW. Growth and growth hormone of children with acute lymphocytic leukemia following central nervous system prophylaxis with and without cranial irradiation. Am J Pediatr Hematol Oncol 1980; 2:311–316.
19. Leiper AD, Stanhope R, Lau T, et al. The effect of total body irradiation and bone marrow transplantation during childhood and adolescence on growth and endocrine function. Br J Haematol 1987; 67:419–426.
20. Robison LL, Nesbit ME Jr, Sather HN, et al. Height of children successfully treated for acute lymphoblastic leukemia: A report from the Late Effects Study Committee of Children's Cancer Study Group. Med Pediatr Oncol 1985; 13:14–21.
21. Littley MD, Shalet SM, Morgenstern GR, Deakin DP. Endocrine and reproductive dysfunction following fractionated total body irradiation in adults. Q J Med 1991; 78:265–274.
22. Romshe CA, Zipf WB, Miser A, et al. Evaluation of growth hormone release and human growth hormone treatment in children with cranial irradiation-associated short stature. J Pediatr 1984; 104:177–181.
23. Winter RJ, Green OC. Irradiation-induced growth hormone deficiency: Blunted growth response and accelerated skeletal maturation to growth hormone therapy. J Pediatr 1985; 106:609–612.
24. Shalet SM, Price DA, Breadwell CG, et al. Normal

growth despite abnormalities of growth hormone secretion in children treated for acute leukemia. J Pediatr 1979; 94:719–722.

25. Fisher JN, Aur RJA. Endocrine assessment in childhood acute lymphocytic leukemia. Cancer 1982; 49:145–151.

26. Kaplan MM, Garnick MB, Gelber R, et al. Risk factors for thyroid abnormalities after neck irradiation for childhood cancer. Am J Med 1983; 74:272–280.

27. Wasnich RD, Grumet CF, Payne RO, et al. Graves' ophthalmopathy following external neck irradiation for nonthyroidal neoplastic disease. J Clin Endocrinol Metab 1973; 37:703–713.

28. Devney RB, Sklar CA, Nesbit ME Jr, et al. Serial thyroid function measurements in children with Hodgkin's disease. J Pediatr 1984; 105:223–227.

29. Wallace WH, Shalet SM, Hendry JH, et al. Ovarian failure following abdominal irradiation in childhood: The radiosensitivity of the human oocyte. Br J Radiol 1989; 62:995–998.

30. Nicosia SV, Matus-Ridley M, Meadows AT. Gonadal effects of cancer therapy in girls. Cancer 1985; 55:2364–2372.

31. Chambers SK, Chambers JT, Kier R, Peschel RE. Sequelae of lateral ovarian transposition in irradiated cervical cancer patients. Int J Radiat Oncol Biol Phys 1991; 20:305–308.

32. Winer-Muram HT, Muram D, Salazar J, Thompson E. Ovariopexy—clinical and radiologic correlation. Adolesc Pediatr Gynecol 1988; 1:239–243.

33. Stillman RJ, Schinfeld JS, Schiff I. Ovarian failure in long-term survivors of childhood malignancy. Am J Obstet Gynecol 1981; 139:62–66.

34. Barrett A, Nichols J, Gibson B. Late effects of total body irradiation. Radiother Oncol 1987; 9:131–135.

35. Chapman RM, Sutcliffe SB, Malpas JS. Cytotoxic-induced ovarian failure in women with Hodgkin's disease. I. Hormone function. JAMA 1979; 242:1877–1881.

36. Chapman RM, Sutcliffe SB, Malpas JS. Cytotoxic-induced ovarian failure in women with Hodgkin's disease. II. Effects on sexual function. JAMA 1979; 242:1882–1884.

37. Rivkees SA, Crawford SD. The relationship of gonadal activity and chemotherapy-induced gonadal damage. JAMA 1988; 259:2123–2125.

38. Pennisi AJ, Grushkin CM, Lieberman E. Gonadal function in children with nephrosis treated with cyclophosphamide. Am J Dis Child 1975; 129:315–318.

39. Etteldorf JN, West CD, Pitcock JA, et al. Gonadal function, testicular histology, and meiosis following cyclophosphamide therapy in patients with nephrotic syndrome. J Pediatr 1976; 88:206–212.

40. Chapman RM, Sutcliffe SB. Protection of ovarian function by oral contraceptive use in women receiving chemotherapy for Hodgkin's disease. Blood 1981; 58:849–851.

41. King DJ, Ratcliffe MD, Dawson DD, et al. Fertility in young men and women after treatment for lymphoma: A study of a population. J Clin Pathol 1985; 38:1247–1251.

42. Siris ES, Leventhal BG, VCaitukaitis JL. Effects of childhood leukemia and chemotherapy on puberty and reproductive function in girls. N Engl J Med 1976; 294:1143–1146.

43. Fossa SD, Klepp O, Norman N. Lack of gonadal protection by medroxyprogesterone acetate-induced transient medical castration during chemotherapy for testicular cancer. Br J Urol 1988; 62:449–453.

44. Glode LM, Robinson J, Gould SF. Protection from cyclophosphamide induced testicular damage with analogue of gonadotropin-releasing hormone. Lancet 1981; 1:1132–1134.

45. Montz FJ, Wolff AJ, Gambone JC. Gonadal protection and fecundity rates in cyclophosphamide-treated rats. Cancer Res 1991; 51:124–126.

46. Waxman JH, Ahmed R, Smith D, et al. Failure to preserve fertility in patients with Hodgkin's disease. Cancer Chemother Pharmacol 1987; 19:159–162.

47. Tucker MA, Meadows AT, Boice JD Jr, et al. Cancer risk following treatment of childhood cancer. In: Boice JD, Fraumeni JF Jr (eds). Radiation Carcinogenesis: Epidemiology and Biological Significance. New York: Raven Press, 1984, pp 211–224.

48. Li FP. Second malignant tumors after cancer in childhood. Cancer 1977; 40:1899–1902.

49. Miké V, Meadows AT, D'Angio GJ. Incidence of second malignant neoplasms in children: Results of an international study. Lancet 1982; 2:1326–1331.

50. Holmes GE, Holmes FF. Pregnancy outcome of patients treated for Hodgkin's disease: A controlled study. Cancer 1978; 41:1317–1322.

51. Blatt J, Mulvihill JJ, Ziegler JL, et al. Pregnancy outcome following cancer chemotherapy. Am J Med 1980; 69:828–832.

52. Horning SJ, Hoppe RT, Kaplan HS, et al. Female reproductive potential after treatment for Hodgkin's disease. N Engl J Med 1981; 304:1377–1382.

53. Chapman RM. Reproductive potential after treatment for Hodgkin's disease. Letter. N Engl J Med 1981; 305:891.

54. Navot D, Laufer N, Kopolovic R, et al. Artifically induced endometrial cycles and establishment of pregnancies in the absence of ovaries. N Engl J Med 1986; 314:806–811.

55. Knudson AG Jr. Genetics and the child cured of cancer. In: van Eys J, Sullivan MP (eds). Status of the Curability of Childhood Cancers. New York: Raven Press, 1980, pp 295–305.

56. Knudson AG Jr. Genetics and the etiology of childhood cancer. Pediatr Res 1976; 10:513–517.

57. Lewis EB. Possible genetic consequences of irradiation of tumors in childhood. Radiology 1975; 114:147–153.

58. Mulvihill JJ, Connelly RR, Austin DF, et al. Cancer in offspring of long-term survivors of childhood and adolescent cancer. Lancet 1987; 2:813–817.

59. Greenberg HS, Kazak AE, Meadows AT. Psychologic function in 8-to-16-year-old cancer survivors and their parents. J Pediatr 1989; 114:488.

60. Lannering B, Marky I, Lundberg A, Olsson E. Long-term sequelae after pediatric brain tumor: Their effect on disability and quality of life. Med Pediatr Oncol 1990; 18:304–310.

61. Mulhern RK, Wasserman AL, Friedman AG, et al. Social competence and behavioral adjustment of children who are long-term survivors of cancer. Pediatrics 1989; 83:18.

62. Tebbi CK, Bromberg C, Piedmonte M. Long-term vocational adjustment of cancer patients diagnosed during adolescence. Cancer 1989; 63:213.

63. Carr-Gregg M, Hampson R. A new approach to the psychological care of adolescents with cancer. Med J Austr 1986; 145:580, 582–583.

64. Spirito A, Stark LJ, Cobiella C, et al. Social adjustment of children successfully treated for cancer. J Pediatr Psychol 1990; 15:359–371.

65. Wasserman AL, Thompson EI, Wilimas JA, et al. The psychological status of survivors of childhood/adolescent Hodgkin's disease. Am J Dis Child 1987; 141:626.

◯◯◯

CHAPTER 30

Sports-Related Problems in Reproductive Function

ROBERT W. REBAR

The notion that participation in sports in the adolescent years can affect reproductive function is commonly accepted. However, extrapolating data obtained from the study of elite adolescent and adult athletes engaged in endurance training to more typical teenagers may be more difficult. The elite athlete is defined here as one who trains for a competitive program; this individual must exercise strenuously over prolonged periods of time to accomplish certain goals. This chapter's focus initially will be on the impact of strenuous training on reproductive development and function. Integration of this information into the care of more commonly encountered gynecologic problems in adolescents then will be addressed.

REPRODUCTIVE DISORDERS ASSOCIATED WITH EXERCISE

Delayed Menarche

Malina and coworkers[1, 2] were the first to report an association between menarcheal delay and competition in track and field sports. In general, the more skilled the athlete, the later her age at menarche (Fig. 30–1). These investigators were extremely cautious in drawing any conclusions from their historically obtained data. They suggested that it was possible that the physical build associated with better performance in track and field events (i.e., increased height and longer limbs) might lead to a selection bias quite independent of any effect of exercise on pubertal development. One other historical study suggests that delayed menarche is associated with athletic success in running because it promotes tallness and thinness, characteristics that can be used to advantage in certain sports.[3] Furthermore, early sexual maturation may influence socialization away from physical activity within a given chronologic age group.

That endurance training itself does affect the pubertal process is supported by several subsequent studies. Frisch and colleagues[4] documented that intensive training of runners in the premenarcheal years delays menarche. In addition, both Frisch's group[5] and Warren[6] noted that menarche is delayed in serious ballet dancers who begin strenuous training before adolescence. Warren further noted that menarche is not delayed in serious musicians, who might be expected to suffer from a similar amount of mental stress.

Thus, it is probable that strenuous exercise before menarche contributes to a delay in menarche, but the mechanism remains unclear. It has been suggested that endurance

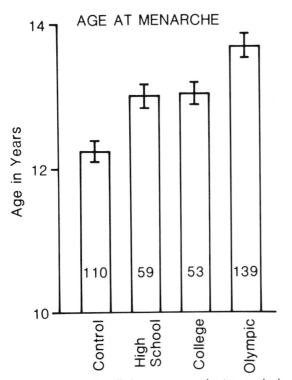

FIGURE 30–1 ••• Recalled age at menarche (± standard error) in nonathletes and in track and field athletes of varying competitive abilities. The Olympic athletes participated in the 1976 Olympic Games. The numbers in each bar refer to the number of athletes included in each group. (Data from Malina et al.[1, 2] Reprinted from Cumming DC, Rebar RW. Exercise and reproductive function in women: A review. Am J Ind Med 1983; 4:113. Copyright © 1983. Reprinted by permission of Wiley-Liss, a division of John Wiley and Sons, Inc.)

training promotes thinness and prohibits attainment of the "critical" percentage of body fat required for menarche.[7] However, body composition cannot be the only factor leading to menarcheal delay: ballet dancers exceeding the "critical" weight and percentage of body fat do not have onset of menses until they decrease their activity.[6] Thus, prospective studies of the effects of exertion on menarche still will be necessary to investigate the etiology of the delay in menarche.

Luteal Phase Defects

Suggestions that endurance training might lead to luteal phase abnormalities in elite athletes first appeared in the late 1970s. Perhaps the best of these early reports noted that four skilled teenage swimmers had shorter luteal phases than nonexercising girls.[8] Progesterone levels in the swimmers failed to increase despite a luteinizing hormone (LH) surge, suggesting nonluteinization of the follicle. The ratio of follicle-stimulating hormone (FSH) to LH was reduced in the swimmers, perhaps accounting for the luteal phase inadequacy. The data may suggest that a central mechanism may be responsible for the relative decrease in FSH, thus leading to inadequate follicular maturation. In a single case study of a 30-year-old woman runner, shorter luteal phases and lower midluteal progesterone levels were recorded during menstrual cycles in which the individual trained more extensively.[9] On the basis of basal body temperature changes, Prior et al.[10] reported that luteal phase defects developed in two women training for a marathon and resolved following the race. Based on additional basal body temperature data, Prior[11] suggested that luteal dysfunction may occur in as many as 50% of long-distance runners.

More recent studies have examined progesterone secretion in the luteal phase in greater detail. Schweiger and colleagues[12] reported that 14 of 18 endurance-trained athletes with cyclic gonadal function had reduced levels of circulating estradiol and progesterone during the luteal phase. Ellison and Lager[13] documented lower salivary progesterone levels in ovulatory recreational women runners.

Hoffman et al.[14] examined daily first morning urinary pregnanediol glucuronide (PDG) excretion during two successive menstrual cycles in a select group of elite eumenorrheic runners who ran 35 or more miles per week and had no previous history of menstrual irregularities.[14] PDG excretion in the nine runners differed from that in the seven age- and weight-matched control subjects in 14 of the 18 cycles examined. Each of the runners had at least one aberrant cycle, and in five runners, both cycles were altered. Compared with the cycles in the controls, those in the runners could be divided into three distinct groups: cycles in which the luteal phase was shortened (n = 7), cycles in which PDG excretion was decreased despite normal length (n = 7), and cycles in which both luteal phase length and PDG excretion were similar to those in controls (n = 4). Three runners who voluntarily reduced their training to 30 miles or less per week had increased PDG excretion in the very next menstrual cycle. Thus, these data indicate that luteal phase alterations are common even in eumenorrheic women engaged in endurance training.

More recently Beitins and colleagues[15] studied a group of athletic college women with normal menstrual cycles who were not participating in aerobic training but who wished to devote a summer to exercise training. During the first month the women ran 5 days per week, beginning at 4 miles per day during the first week and advancing by 1.5 miles during each successive week, reaching 10 miles per day by the fifth week. In addition to running, the subjects participated in 3.5 hours of moderate-intensity sports activities, including bicycling, tennis, and volleyball. During the second month, the running distance was held constant at 10 miles per day, with the subjects' heart rates corresponding to 70% to 80% of their maximum Vo_2. During the control month and the two exercise months, all subjects collected daily overnight urine samples for the determination of hormone excretion. Of the 28 participants, 18 women were identified who had a total of 20 cycles with urinary hormone excretion patterns consistent with an inadequate or short luteal phase. During the first exercise month, four women developed inadequate luteal phase cycles, and 10 women developed short luteal phase cycles. During the second exercise month, two developed inadequate luteal phase cycles, and four developed short luteal phase cycles. Two women had luteal phase defects in both exercise months. This study also indicates that initiation of strenuous endurance training in previously ovulating untrained women frequently leads to corpus luteum dysfunction. Because the midcycle LH surge was delayed in spite of increased estrogen secretion, the authors further suggested that exercise induces alterations in the neuroendocrine system.

It is true that almost all of the studies examining luteal function were conducted in women older than 18 years. However, it is highly probable that similar defects would develop in young adolescents engaged in endurance training.

Amenorrhea

Feicht and colleagues[16] first reported that long-distance runners are especially prone to amenorrhea. Using a questionnaire, they determined that 6% to 43% of collegiate runners were amenorrheic, with the incidence increasing directly with the training mileage (Fig. 30–2). Several other investigators subsequently

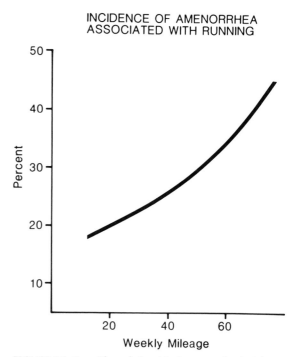

FIGURE 30–2 ••• The relationship between the incidence of amenorrhea (defined as fewer than three cycles in the preceding 12 months) and weekly running mileage of from 20 to 80 miles. (Adapted from Feicht et al.[16] Reprinted from Cumming DC, Rebar RW. Exercise and reproductive function in women: A review. Am J Ind Med 1983; 4:113. Copyright © 1983. Reprinted by permission of Wiley-Liss, a division of John Wiley and Sons, Inc.)

confirmed the observation that the incidence of amenorrhea is higher in runners than in the typical adult female population.[17–19] The incidence of amenorrhea also appears to be increased in ballet dancers[5, 6] and in swimmers and cyclists.[20] In view of the fact that adolescents as well as older women may be involved in endurance training, it is reasonable to conclude that the mechanisms involved in producing amenorrhea in athletes can occur in women of any age.

A Continuum of Reproductive Defects?

It is possible that endurance training can lead to luteal dysfunction first and later to amenorrhea in women who have already menstruated. In contrast, younger girls engaged in endurance training may experience delayed puberty. In other words, there may be a continuum of reproductive defects in susceptible women who engage in endurance training. What makes certain individuals susceptible and others relatively resistant is unclear, but a number of factors appear to play some role in the etiology of these disorders.

FACTORS INVOLVED IN EXERCISE-ASSOCIATED REPRODUCTIVE DYSFUNCTION

To date, most studies of reproductive dysfunction associated with exercise have been retrospective. Despite the limitations of such studies, it has been possible to identify a number of distinct factors that appear to be implicated in the etiology of exercise-associated reproductive dysfunction.

Specifically, several changes commonly occur during the course of an athletic training program. In association with regular aerobic exercise, women may lose weight,[18, 19] have changes in body composition,[18, 21] alter their diets,[18, 22] experience changes in several hormone secretion patterns,[18, 23, 24] and may be subject to physical and emotional stresses associated with their training programs.[5, 18]

Body Composition and Weight Loss

In a cross-sectional survey of women runners, Schwartz and colleagues[18] noted that amenorrheic runners had less body fat than eumenorrheic runners, who were, in turn, leaner than sedentary women (Fig. 30–3). In addition, it has been reported that ballet dancers with secondary amenorrhea are significantly leaner than those who are eumenorrheic.[5] Furthermore, women who became amenorrheic after beginning to run regularly also stated that they had lost more weight with the onset of exercise than those who remained eumenorrheic (Fig. 30–4).[18] As an estimate of thinness, total body water as a proportion of total weight decreases in women runners as the prevalence of amenorrhea increases.[20] Finally, it is currently recognized that young girls who voluntarily restrict their weights will delay pubertal progression and menarche.[25]

All of these observations are consistent with the hypothesis developed by Frisch and McArthur[7] that a minimum height for weight is required for the onset and continuation of regular menstrual cycles. However, if weight

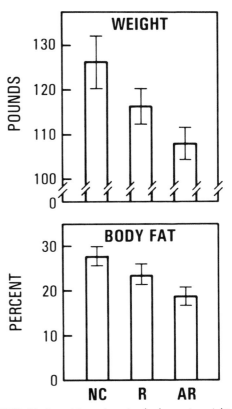

FIGURE 30–3 ••• Mean (± standard error) weight and percentage of body fat of women runners and nonrunners. Amenorrheic runners weighed significantly less (*P* < .01) and had less body fat (*P* < .05) than those in the other two groups. AR, Amenorrheic runners; NC, normal sedentary controls; R, eumenorrheic control runners. (Modified from Schwartz B, Cumming DC, Riordan E, et al. Exercise-associated amenorrhea: A distinct entity? Am J Obstet Gynecol 1981; 141:662.)

and body fat are the most important factors in the etiology of exercise-associated amenorrhea, then Warren's longitudinal observations[6] in amenorrheic ballet dancers defy explanation. She noted that young dancers failed to undergo menarche or had secondary amenorrhea despite weights and percentage body fat far exceeding the minimum quantities suggested by Frisch and McArthur.[7] Menarche or resumption of cyclic menses occurred only when injuries prevented exercise, not with any gain in weight or body fat. Thus, Warren's research indicates that other factors, perhaps commonly associated with weight loss and thinness, lead to exercise-associated amenorrhea. Her observations suggesting the importance of factors other than body fat should not be surprising in view of the fact that menarche is a late event in pubertal development.

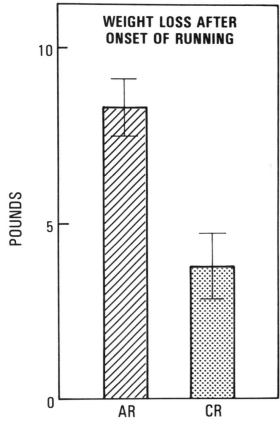

FIGURE 30–4 ••• Mean (± standard error) weight loss after the onset of running. The amenorrheic runners (AR) stated they had lost significantly more weight ($P < .05$) than did the eumenorrheic control runners (CR). (Modified from Schwartz B, Cumming DC, Riordan E, et al. Exercise-associated amenorrhea: A distinct entity? Am J Obstet Gynecol 1981; 141:662.)

Diet

Abundant evidence now indicates that individuals engaged in endurance training typically alter their diet. If anything, one would suspect this change to be more prominent in teens. Long-distance runners are more apt to eat less lean red meat and to be vegetarian than sedentary individuals. Prospective dietary histories confirm significant differences in diet between eumenorrheic and amenorrheic runners.[4, 18, 26]

How and why dietary changes may lead to amenorrhea is unclear. An inadequate supply of nutrients may trigger protective mechanisms to prevent pregnancy. It is possible that changes in diet also lead to changes in thyroid and steroid hormone metabolism.

Previous Menstrual Patterns and Obstetric History

Individuals developing amenorrhea with endurance training are more apt to have had irregular menses before beginning their training.[17, 18] More than half the women with past menses who developed amenorrhea with the onset of running had a history of previous menstrual irregularity.[18] In contrast, less than 15% of eumenorrheic runners had such a history. Amenorrhea also occurs more commonly in younger runners[27] and in those who are nulliparous.[17, 18]

The occurrence of a higher incidence of amenorrhea in younger runners suggests that menstrual dysfunction may occur in part because of relative immaturity of the hypothalamic-pituitary-ovarian axis or because of greater susceptibility in younger athletes. In view of the observation that pretraining menstrual irregularity is associated with beginning to run at an earlier age and with running sooner after menarche,[19] it is possible that some factor promoting premenstrual irregularity may inspire women to begin running.

Stress Associated With Exercise

Endurance training is commonly believed to be physically and mentally "stressful." The observation that menses may begin or resume in young ballet dancers during injury-imposed respites from training[6] supports this contention. So, too, does the observation that almost half of the first class of women recruits to the U.S. Military Academy were amenorrheic after just 6 months of classes and physical conditioning.[28]

In an effort to investigate the psychological stress of exercise, Schwartz et al.[18] utilized a number of psychometric assessment instruments to measure depression, hypochondriasis, psychasthenia, obsessive-compulsive tendencies, and recent stressful life events in eumenorrheic and amenorrheic runners and sedentary control subjects. No differences were identified among the three groups. However, when the runners were asked to evaluate subjectively the stress associated with running on a scale of 0 to 10 (with 10 being maximal), the amenorrheic runners reported significantly more stress than did the eumenorrheic runners, despite the fact that they did not run more or faster and did not engage in a greater number of competitive events.

Warren's observation[6] that menarche is delayed approximately 3 years in ballet dancers when compared with musicians preparing for professional careers suggested to her that the menarcheal delay in the dancers was not entirely related to stress. She pointed out that the goal-oriented life-styles of both groups provided similar stress.

Hormonal changes noted with exercise are more difficult to interpret but may well be indicative of stress. Because it is known that endogenous opiates within the hypothalamus inhibit gonadotropin-releasing hormone (GnRH) neurons and thus LH secretion and reproductive function,[29] it has been tempting to speculate a role for endorphins in exercise-associated amenorrhea. Carr et al.[30] reported that basal circulating levels of cortisol and opioid peptides increased with progressive aerobic training in women. The same investigators also reported that naloxone, an opioid antagonist given as an intravenous bolus, increased circulating LH pulses and levels in one of three amenorrheic runners tested.[31] However, Dixon and colleagues[32] failed to observe an increase in LH in any of seven amenorrheic runners, a finding confirmed by other investigators studying male runners.[33] Together, then, these data suggest that endogenous opiates in the CNS do not play a major role in the etiology of exercise-associated amenorrhea. The increases in opiates observed peripherally by Carr and coworkers[30] may not originate in the hypothalamus and may not directly affect hypothalamic-pituitary function.

It is well documented that both circulating cortisol levels[34, 35] and 24-hour urinary free cortisol secretion[34] are increased in both eumenorrheic and amenorrheic runners compared with sedentary control subjects (Fig. 30–5). Because increases in serum cortisol in response to exogenous corticotropin, the disappearance of exogenous cortisol from the circulation, and circulating corticoid-binding globulin concentrations are similar in runners and nonrunners,[34] it is reasonable to conclude that corticotropin secretion is increased in women. Furthermore, it would seem that increased corticotropin-releasing hormone (CRH) secretion results in increased corticotropin secretion. If this is true, then the data become more difficult to explain: both corticotropin and the opioid peptides are synthesized from a common precursor, and the release of corticotropin by exogenous CRH is associated with

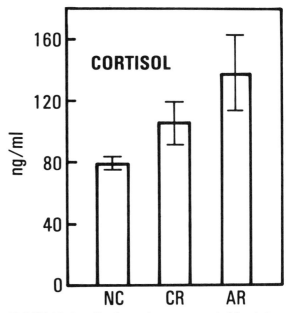

FIGURE 30–5 ••• Basal morning serum cortisol levels (± standard error) in women runners and nonrunners. Values in the normal sedentary controls (NC) were significantly lower than those in either the eumenorrheic control runners (CR) or the amenorrheic runners (AR). It is important to note that all values are in the normal range. (Data from Schwartz B, Cumming DC, Riordan E, et al. Exercise-induced amenorrhea: A distinct entity? Am J Obstet Gynecol 1981; 141:662.)

contemporaneous release of the opioid peptides.

How might CRH, corticotropin, and cortisol interact to affect reproductive function? Although any such relationship is poorly understood, it is possible to formulate a hypothesis linking the hypothalamic-pituitary-adrenal axis and reproductive function.

Administration of exogenous corticotropin or glucocorticoids can inhibit LH release and/or ovulation in experimental animals and humans.[36–40] Furthermore, intracerebral administration of CRH to rats[41, 42] and peripheral administration of CRH to monkeys[43] inhibit LH secretion. In ovariectomized rats, CRH can inhibit GnRH release into the portal circulation.[44] The inhibition of GnRH can be reversed by a CRH antagonist in the rat both in vitro[45] and in vivo,[46] suggesting that CRH-induced GnRH suppression is receptor mediated. In addition, the inhibition of LH can be reversed by naloxone in the rat[47, 48] and in the monkey,[49] indicating a relationship between CRH and endogenous opiates. That the effect of CRH on GnRH-LH secretion is direct is suggested by inhibition of LH secretion even in adrenalectomized animals.[41, 50]

Barbarino and colleagues have reported that exogenous CRH inhibits LH secretion during the midluteal phase of the menstrual cycle,[51] with the inhibition being blocked by naloxone.[52] However, Thomas et al.[53] have failed to document any decrease in LH in response to exogenous CRH in agonadal women. Hence, the effect of CRH on LH secretion in humans remains to be defined. In considering all of these studies together, however, it is tempting to postulate that stress, defined strictly as hypercortisolism, plays a major role in the pathophysiology of exercise-associated menstrual dysfunction. A reasonable hypothesis is that activation of the hypothalamic-pituitary-adrenal axis inhibits the hypothalamic-pituitary-ovarian axis.

Hormonal Changes Associated With Acute and Chronic Exercise

A defined series of hormonal changes occurs in both men and women exercising maximally for a short interval of time (Fig. 30–6).[24, 54–56] Cortisol levels are increased in the 2 hours before the onset of known exercise. Both LH and testosterone levels increase acutely in the 5 minutes before exercise begins. Because no other hormone increases acutely in anticipation of exercise, it would seem that the changes in LH and testosterone are specific. Moreover, in view of the abrupt and coincident secretion of both hormones, it is difficult to believe that testosterone secretion is stimulated by the increased LH secretion. It is possible that the increase in testosterone is due to adrenergic innervation of hilar cells in the ovary and Leydig cells in the testis. This possibility is supported by the observation that testosterone does not increase in anticipation of exercise in oophorectomized women.[56] Thus, the changes in testosterone that occur with exercise appear to be due to increased gonadal hormone secretion.

Virtually every pituitary peptide and gonadal and adrenal steroid hormone examined increases with exercise.[24, 54, 55] The differences in the time courses of the increases of cortisol and dehydroepiandrosterone (of adrenal origin) from that of testosterone again suggests separate adrenal and gonadal secretion. It is tempting to speculate that the dramatic increases in these hormones with exercise better allow an individual to respond to exercise. It

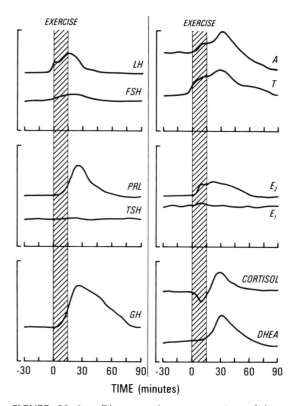

FIGURE 30–6 ••• Diagrammatic representation of hormonal changes observed before, during, and after symptom-limited incremental exercise on a bicycle ergometer in eumenorrheic untrained women. A, Androstenedione; DHEA, dehydroepiandrosterone; E_1, estrone; E_2, estradiol; FSH, follicle-stimulating hormone; GH, growth hormone; LH, luteinizing hormone; PRL, prolactin; T, testosterone; TSH, thyroid-stimulating hormone. (From Rebar RW, Effects of exercise on reproductive function in females. In: Givens JR (ed). The Hypothalamus. Chicago: Year Book Medical, 1984, pp 245–262.)

is also possible that repeated episodes of acute exercise, along with these associated hormonal changes, may precipitate menstrual dysfunction in susceptible individuals.

It has been suggested that the recurrent hyperprolactinemia associated with recurrent exercise may contribute to menstrual dysfunction.[57] However, no data support this hypothesis. In fact, it has been reported that amenorrheic runners subjected to acute exercise do not have any increase in serum prolactin levels, in contrast to the increases observed in eumenorrheic runners and in sedentary control women.[58] Thus, there are no data to support any role for prolactin in the etiology of exercise-associated amenorrhea.

Hypothalamic Dysfunction

The pulsatile secretion of LH is decreased in both eumenorrheic and amenorrheic runners compared with normal sedentary women.[23] These data suggest that diminished GnRH secretion in the hypothalamus is associated with endurance training. This observation also supports the notion that exercise-associated amenorrhea is a "hypothalamic" amenorrhea. That the hypothalamic dysfunction is minimal is suggested by the finding that temperature regulation is normal in amenorrheic adult runners,[32] in contrast to the profound abnormalities reported in women with anorexia nervosa and weight loss–associated amenorrhea.[59, 60]

A Multifactorial Etiology?

Together, the data suggest that the etiology of exercise-associated reproductive dysfunction is complex and ultimately involves hypothalamic dysfunction (Fig. 30–7). Although the hypothalamic dysfunction present in affected individuals may well result because of metabolic alterations in the periphery, a central cause for the amenorrhea cannot be excluded. Exercise-associated changes in reproductive function in women appear to result from the complex interaction of physical, hormonal, nutritional, psychological, and environmental factors. Weight loss, decreased body fat, and voluntary changes in diet may produce an effect by inducing changes in peripheral steroid and thyroid hormone metabolism. Altered feedback signals transmitted to the hypothalamic-pituitary unit might then contribute to reproductive dysfunction. Other factors, as noted in this chapter, may be important as

well. At present it seems overly simplistic to suggest that exercise-associated reproductive dysfunction has one single cause. In addition, it seems appropriate to regard exercise-associated amenorrhea as a form of hypothalamic amenorrhea that is related and similar to, yet distinct from, psychogenic amenorrhea, anorexia nervosa, and amenorrhea associated with malnutrition (Fig. 30–8). "Pure" forms of each of these forms of amenorrhea can be identified, while some individuals may suffer from "overlapping" forms.

OSTEOPOROSIS AS A CONSEQUENCE OF REPRODUCTIVE DYSFUNCTION

Bone mass increases in response to exercise but decreases in hypoestrogenic women. Thus, several studies have shown that spinal bone mineral density is increased in athletes who have normal menses but is decreased in those with exercise-associated amenorrhea.[61–64]

Although it is not yet clear precisely why there is this association between exercise-associated amenorrhea and decreased bone mass, several factors might play a role. The decrease could be due to delayed skeletal maturation, accelerated bone loss, or both. Individuals more likely to become amenorrheic generally begin endurance training at an earlier age than do others, so that bone mass may never become as great as in eumenorrheic athletes. In addition, dietary changes clearly

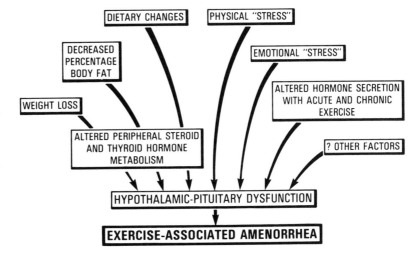

**FIGURE 30–7 ••• ** Diagrammatic representation of some of the factors involved in the pathophysiology of exercise-associated amenorrhea. (From Rebar RW. Effects of exercise on reproductive function in females. In: Givens JR (ed). The Hypothalamus. Chicago: Year Book Medical, 1984, pp 245–262.)

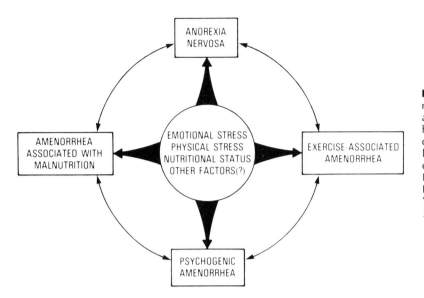

FIGURE 30–8 ••• Theoretical representation of the associations among various forms of functional hypothalamic amenorrhea. These disorders appear to be closely related. (From Rebar RW. The reproductive age: Chronic anovulation. In: Serra G (ed). Comprehensive Endocrinology. The Ovary. New York: Raven Press, 1983, pp 241–256.

exist in athletes, and calcium intake may be reduced relative to need in some athletes.

From the study of Drinkwater and colleagues,[65] it appears that the osteopenia in amenorrheic athletes is reversible. In seven amenorrheic athletes in whom menses returned (probably because of a decrease in the severity of the exercise), the bone mineral density in the lumbar spine increased by an average of 6.3% over 15.5 months compared with a decrease of 0.3% in seven regularly menstruating athletes. The return of ovarian function, if it occurs within several years of the onset of amenorrhea, seems to result in an increase in bone mass. It is not yet known whether bone loss is irreversible in women in whom amenorrhea persists for many years. It appears that the hypoestrogenic hypogonadism found in women with exercise-associated amenorrhea prevents the normally beneficial effects of exercise on bone mass.

Warren and colleagues have extended these observations in young ballet dancers.[66] In a survey of 75 professional dancers, the prevalence of scoliosis was 24%. Dancers with scoliosis were much more apt to have delayed menarche (to age 14 years or later). The incidence of fractures (61%) also rose with increasing age at menarche. The incidence of secondary amenorrhea was twice as high among dancers with stress fractures as among those who did not give such a history. Thus, their data, too, suggest that a delay in menarche and prolonged intervals of hypoestrogenic amenorrhea may predispose ballet dancers to scoliosis and stress fractures.

Together, these data indicate the importance of recognizing and treating young athletes with hypoestrogenism. It would seem prudent to encourage women who participate in endurance training not to train to the extent that menstrual function is impaired.

EVALUATION AND TREATMENT OF ATHLETES WITH REPRODUCTIVE DYSFUNCTION

Women who appear to be at particularly high risk of exercise-associated amenorrhea include runners, gymnasts, ballet dancers, cyclists, and lightweight rowers.[67] Regardless of the form of exercise, however, the athlete with menstrual dysfunction should be evaluated in the same way as any woman presenting with similar complaints. It is important to avoid the temptation to ascribe the reproductive dysfunction in an athlete to her exercise before evaluation. Thus, exercise-associated reproductive dysfunction must be regarded as a diagnosis of exclusion.

Delayed Puberty

Puberty is generally defined as "delayed" in the absence of development of any secondary sexual characteristics by age 13 or of menarche by age 16 or if 5 or more years pass after breast budding without the onset of menses.

When evaluating any teenager with delayed puberty, any possible serious cause must be excluded. It is particularly important in the young athlete to consider the age at onset and the type and intensity of endurance training. Anorexia nervosa and bulimia also warrant consideration. The history and physical examination, as always, are of paramount importance. Any evidence of a central neurologic disturbance, thyroid dysfunction, adrenal or pituitary disorders, or diabetes mellitus should be sought. An obstructed outflow tract should be apparent on pelvic examination and should be suspected if there is a history of intermittent abdominal pain and primary amenorrhea in a girl with normally developed secondary sexual characteristics.

Laboratory evaluation in the absence of an obvious cause should include measurement of circulating FSH and prolactin concentrations and evaluation of thyroid function. Radiographic estimation of bone age is generally indicated. A karyotype determination is warranted whenever genetic abnormalities are believed possible and in girls with elevated levels of FSH.

Girls with delayed puberty as a result of endurance training have no significant abnormalities. FSH concentrations are generally low to normal and are typical of those present in normal prepubertal children; the same is true of LH levels if they, too, are determined. Bone age may be delayed. It is important to ensure that the diet is adequate, and because of the risk of osteopenia, it is especially important that calcium ingestion be adequate. Reassurance, counseling, and a change in training patterns should allow resumption of pubertal development. It is important to follow affected individuals closely to be certain that a significant abnormality is not overlooked.

Secondary Amenorrhea or Oligomenorrhea

In general, exercise-associated amenorrhea is characterized by low to normal levels of circulating FSH, LH, and prolactin. Radiographic assessment of the sella turcica is indicated whenever both FSH and LH levels are less than 10 mlU/ml, even in the presence of normal serum prolactin levels, to rule out a pituitary adenoma.

Dietary adequacy must always be investigated in women engaged in endurance training. Individuals who begin such training programs without close professional supervision seem more apt to change their diets and suffer from unrecognized mineral deficiencies, especially of calcium and iron. As a consequence, a dietary history, complete blood cell count, and basic blood chemistry determinations are indicated in every woman presumed to have exercise-associated amenorrhea.

In view of the very real risk of osteopenia, calcium supplementation is warranted, and exogenous estrogen should be encouraged in women with exercise-associated amenorrhea. Low-dose oral contraceptives will maintain bone density in hypoestrogenic amenorrheic athletes and will provide contraception as well. For women who are not sexually active, cyclic estrogen and progestin may be provided as an alternative. There is no evidence that suppression of the hypothalamic-pituitary axis by exogenous steroids has any adverse effect on subsequent reproductive function. However, women must be informed that the amenorrhea that exists before ingestion of exogenous steroids still may be present when the steroids are discontinued. Thus, ovulation induction may be required when pregnancy is desired. Despite the advantages of therapy, many amenorrheic athletes refuse exogenous estrogen. Such individuals should have periodic estimates of spinal bone density to identify those with accelerated bone loss.

If exercise-associated menstrual dysfunction represents a continuum from luteal dysfunction to oligomenorrhea to euestrogenic amenorrhea and finally to hypoestrogenic amenorrhea, then athletes with oligomenorrhea and euestrogenic amenorrhea should be at increased risk of developing endometrial hyperplasia. However, these stages appear to be brief. Women seem either to progress to hypoestrogenic amenorrhea or to resume regular menses. To the present, there is no report of any woman with exercise-associated amenorrhea developing endometrial hyperplasia.

Despite the relative hypoestrogenism that exists in most amenorrheic athletes, complaints of signs and symptoms of estrogen deficiency are few. Thus, it is possible that the accelerated bone loss reported is due as much to dietary calcium inadequacy as to hypoestrogenism. It is difficult to believe that athletes so in tune with their bodies would fail to note the vaginal dryness, hot flushes, and emotional lability associated with hypoestrogenism.

Amenorrheic athletes who do not desire pregnancy and who refuse to use oral contraceptives should be advised to utilize some other form of contraception if they are sexually active. The majority of women with exercise-associated amenorrhea eventually resume menses, in many cases ovulating before any menstruation.

CONCLUSION

An understanding of the reproductive abnormalities that can accompany endurance training in women is necessary to counsel and treat women athletes appropriately. Although the etiology of these reproductive disorders is not understood, it is possible to make rational recommendations to amenorrheic women. It is important to reassure the patient that the disorder is not serious if it is treated appropriately. Failure to treat an amenorrheic athlete, however, may lead to permanent sequelae. It is also important to remember that accumulating data also indicate that relative hypogonadism may be found in male athletes, as well as in female athletes, who engage in endurance training.

References

1. Malina RM, Harper AB, Avent HH, Campbell DE. Age at menarche in athletes and non-athletes. Med Sci Sports 1973; 5:11.
2. Malina RM, Spirduso WW, Tate C, Baylor AM. Age at menarche and selected characteristics in athletes at different competitive levels and in different sports. Med Sci Sports 1978; 10:218.
3. Shangold MM, Kelly M, Berkeley AS, et al. The relationship between menarcheal age and adult height. South Med J 1989; 82:443.
4. Frisch RE, Gotz-Welbergen AV, McArthur JW, et al. Delayed menarche, irregular cycles and amenorrhea of college athletes in relation to the age of onset of training. JAMA 1981; 246:1559.
5. Frisch RE, Wyshak G, Vincent L. Delayed menarche and amenorrhea in ballet dancers. N Engl J Med 1980; 303:17.
6. Warren MP. The effects of exercise on pubertal progression and reproductive function in girls. J Clin Endocrinol Metab 1980; 51:1150.
7. Frisch RE, McArthur J. Menstrual cycles: Fatness as a determinant of minimum weight for height necessary for their maintenance or onset. Science 1974; 185:949.
8. Bonen A, Belcastro AN, Ling WY, Simpson AA. Profiles of selected hormones during menstrual cycles of teenage athletes. J Appl Physiol 1981; 50:545.
9. Shangold M, Freeman R, Thysen B, Gatz M. The relationship between long distance running, plasma progesterone and luteal phase length. Fertil Steril 1979; 31:130.
10. Prior JC, Ho Yuen B, Bowie L, et al. Reversible luteal phase defect and infertility associated with marathon running. Lancet 1982; 2:269.

11. Prior JC. Luteal phase defects and anovulation: Adaptive alterations occurring with conditioning exercise. Semin Reprod Endocrinol 1985; 3:27.
12. Schweiger U, Laessle R, Schweiger M, et al. Caloric intake, stress, and menstrual function in athletes. Fertil Steril 1988; 49:447.
13. Ellison PT, Lager C. Moderate recreational running is associated with lowered salivary progesterone profiles in women. Am J Obstet Gynecol 1986; 154:1000.
14. Hoffman D, Villanueva A, Mezrow G, et al. Luteal phase abnormalities in elite eumenorrheic runners. Abstract No. 220. Abstracts of the 35th Annual Meeting of the Society for Gynecologic Investigation, Baltimore, MD, March 17–20, 1988, p 169.
15. Beitins IZ, McArthur JW, Turnbull BA, et al. Exercise induces two types of luteal dysfunction: Confirmation by urinary free progesterone. J Clin Endocrinol Metab 1991; 72:1350.
16. Feicht CB, Johnson JS, Martin BJ, et al. Secondary amenorrhea in athletes. Lancet 1978; 2:1145.
17. Dale E, Gerlach DH, Whilhite AL. Menstrual dysfunction in distance runners. Obstet Gynecol 1979; 54:47.
18. Schwartz B, Cumming DC, Riordan E, et al. Exercise-associated amenorrhea: A distinct entity? Am J Obstet Gynecol 1981; 141:662.
19. Shangold MM, Levine HS. The effect of marathon training upon menstrual function. Am J Obstet Gynecol 1982; 143:862.
20. Feicht Sanborn C, Martin BJ, Wagner WW Jr. Is athletic amenorrhea specific to runners? Am J Obstet Gynecol 1982; 143:859.
21. Bullen BA, Skrinar GS, Beitins IZ, et al. Induction of menstrual disorders by strenuous exercise in untrained women. N Engl J Med 1985; 312:1349.
22. Loucks AB, Laughlin GA, Mortola JF, et al. Hypothalamic-pituitary-thyroidal function in eumenorrheic and amenorrheic athletes. J Clin Endocrinol Metab 1992; 75:514.
23. Cumming DC, Vickovic MM, Wall SR, Fluker MR. Defects in pulsatile LH release in normally menstruating runners. J Clin Endocrinol Metab 1985; 60:810.
24. Cumming DC, Rebar RW. Hormonal changes with acute exercise and with training in women. Semin Reprod Endocrinol 1985; 3:55.
25. Pugliese MT, Lifshitz F, Grad G, et al. Fear of obesity: A cause of short stature and delayed puberty. N Engl J Med 1983; 309:513.
26. Deuster PA, Kyle SB, Moser PB, et al. Nutritional intakes and status of highly trained amenorrheic and eumenorrheic women runners. Fertil Steril 1986; 46:636.
27. Baker ER, Mathur RS, Kirk RF, Williamson HO. Female runners and secondary amenorrhea: Correlation with age, parity, mileage, and plasma hormonal and sex-hormone-binding-globulin concentrations. Fertil Steril 1981; 36:183.
28. Anderson JL. Women's sports and fitness programs at the US Military Academy. Phys Sports Med 1979; 7:72.
29. Rasmussen DD, Gambacciani M, Swartz W, et al. Pulsatile gonadotropin-releasing hormone release from the human mediobasal hypothalamus in vitro: Opiate receptor-mediated suppression. Neuroendocrinology 1989; 49:150.
30. Carr DB, Bullen BA, Skrinar GS, et al. Physical conditioning facilitates the exercise-induced secretion of beta-endorphin and beta-lipotropin in women. N Engl J Med 1981; 305:560.
31. McArthur JW, Bullen BA, Beitins IZ, et al. Hypothalamic amenorrhea in runners of normal body composition. Endocr Res Commun 1980; 7:13.

32. Dixon G, Eurman P, Stern B, et al. Hypothalamic function in amenorrheic runners. Fertil Steril 1984; 42:377.

33. Rogol AD, Veldhuis JD, Williams FT, Johnson ML. Pulsatile secretion of gonadotropins and prolactin in endurance-trained men: Relation to the endogenous opiate system. J Androl 1984; 5:21.

34. Villanueva AL, Schlosser C, Hopper B, et al. Increased cortisol production in women runners. J Clin Endocrinol Metab 1986; 63:126.

35. Ding J-H, Sheckter CB, Drinkwater BL, et al. High serum cortisol levels in exercise-associated amenorrhea. Ann Intern Med 1988; 108:530.

36. Baldwin DM, Sawyer CH. Effects of dexamethasone on LH release and ovulation in the cyclic rat. Endocrinology 1974; 94:1397.

37. Liptrap RM. Effect of corticotropin and corticosteroids on oestrus, ovulation and oestrogen excretion in the sow. J Endocrinol 1970; 47:197.

38. Stoebel DP, Moberg GP. Effect of ACTH and cortisol on estrous behavior and the luteinizing hormone surge in cows. Fed Proc 1979; 38:1254.

39. Matteri RL, Watson JG, Moberg GP. Stress and acute adrenocorticotropin treatment suppresses LHRH-induced LH release in the ram. J Reprod Fertil 1984; 72:385.

40. Cunningham GR, Goldzieher JW, de LaPena A, Oliver M. The mechanism of ovulation inhibition by triamcinolone acetonide. J Clin Endocrinol Metab 1978; 46:8.

41. Rivier C, Vale W. Influence of corticotropin-releasing factor on reproductive functions in the rat. Endocrinology 1984; 114:914.

42. Ono N, Lumpkin MD, Samson WK, et al. Intrahypothalamic action of corticotropin-releasing factor (CRF) to inhibit growth hormone and LH release in the rat. Life Sci 1984; 35:1117.

43. Olster DH, Ferin M. Corticotropin-releasing hormone inhibits gonadotropin secretion in the ovariectomized rhesus monkey. J Clin Endocrinol Metab 1987; 65:262.

44. Petraglia F, Sutton S, Vale W, Plotsky P. Corticotropin-releasing factor decreases plasma luteinizing hormone levels in female rats by inhibiting gonadotropin-releasing hormone release into hypophysial-portal circulation. Endocrinology 1987; 120:1083.

45. Gambacciani M, Yen SSC, Rasmussen DD. GnRH release from the mediobasal hypothalamus: *In vitro* inhibition by corticotropin-releasing factor. Neuroendocrinology 1986; 43:533.

46. Rivier C, Rivier J, Vale W. Stress-induced inhibition of reproductive functions: Role of endogenous corticotropin-releasing factor. Science 1986; 231:607.

47. Petraglia F, Vale W, Rivier C. Opioids act centrally to modulate stress-induced decrease in luteinizing hormone in the rat. Endocrinology 1986; 119:2445.

48. Almeida OFX, Nikolarakis KE, Herz A. Evidence for the involvement of endogenous opioids in the inhibition of luteinizing hormone by corticotropin-releasing factor. Endocrinology 1988; 122:1034.

49. Gindoff PR, Ferin M. Endogenous opioid peptides modulate the effect of corticotropin-releasing factor on gonadotropin release in the primate. Endocrinology 1987; 121:837.

50. Xiao E, Luckhaus J, Niemann W, Ferin M. Acute inhibition of gonadotropin secretion by corticotropin-releasing hormone in the primate: Are the adrenal glands involved? Endocrinology 1989; 124:1632.

51. Barbarino A, DeMarinis L, Folli G, et al. Corticotropin-releasing hormone inhibition of gonadotropin secretion during the menstrual cycle. Metabolism 1989; 38:504.

52. Barbarino A, De Marinis L, Tofani A, et al. Corticotropin-releasing hormone inhibition of gonadotropin release and the effect of opioid blockade. J Clin Endocrinol Metab 1989; 68:523.

53. Thomas MA, Rebar RW, LaBarbera AR, et al. Dose-response effects of exogenous pulsatile human corticotropin-releasing hormone on ACTH, cortisol and gonadotropin concentrations in agonadal women. J Clin Endocrinol Metab 1991; 72:1249.

54. Cumming DC, Rebar RW. Exercise and reproductive function in women: A review. Am J Ind Med 1983; 4:113.

55. Cumming DC, Brunsting LA III, Strich G, et al. Reproductive hormone increases in response to acute exercise in men. Med Sci Sports Exerc 1986; 18:369.

56. Rebar RW, Benson M, Stern B, et al. Hormonal responses to acute exercise in oophorectomized and normal menstruating women. Abstract No. 977. Abstracts of the 67th Annual Meeting of The Endocrine Society, Baltimore, MD, 1985, p 245.

57. Baker ER. Menstrual dysfunction and hormonal status in athletic women: A review. Fertil Steril 1981; 36:691.

58. Bremer B, Cumming D, Stern B, et al. Hormonal responses to acute exercise in women with psychogenic hypothalamic amenorrhea (HA) and exercise-associated amenorrhea. Abstract No. 281. Abstracts of the 31st Annual Meeting of the Society for Gynecologic Investigation, San Francisco, CA, 1984, p 165.

59. Vigersky RA, Loriaux DL, Anderson AE, et al. Delayed pituitary hormone response to LRF and TRF in patients with anorexia nervosa and with secondary amenorrhea associated with simple weight loss. J Clin Endocrinol Metab 1976; 43:893.

60. Vigersky RA, Andersen AE, Thompson RH, Loriaux DL. Hypothalamic dysfunction in secondary amenorrhea associated with simple weight loss. N Engl J Med 1977; 297:1141.

61. Cann CE, Martin MC, Genant HK, Jaffe RB. Decreased spi al mineral content in amenorrheic women. JAMA 1984; 251:626.

62. Drinkwater BL, Nilson K, Chestnut CH III, et al. Bone mineral content of amenorrheic and eumenorrheic athletes. N Engl J Med 1984; 311:277.

63. Marcus R, Cann C, Madvig P, et al. Menstrual function and bone mass in elite women distance runners. Ann Intern Med 1985; 102:158.

64. Wolman RL. Bone mineral density levels in elite female athletes. Ann Rheum Dis 1990; 49:1013.

65. Drinkwater BL, Nilson K, Ott S, Chesnut CH III. Bone mineral density after resumption of menses in amenorrheic athletes. JAMA 1986; 256:380.

66. Warren MP, Brooks-Gunn J, Hamilton LH, et al. Scoliosis and fractures in young ballet dancers. Relation to delayed menarche and secondary amenorrhea. N Engl J Med 1986; 314:1348.

67. Wolman RL, Harries MG. Menstrual abnormalities in elite athletes. Clin Sports Med 1989; 1:95.

68. Rebar RW. Effects of exercise on reproductive function in females. In: Givens JR (ed). The Hypothalamus. Chicago: Year Book Medical, 1984, pp 245–262.

69. Rebar RW. The reproductive age: Chronic anovulation. In: Serra G (ed). Comprehensive Endocrinology. New York: Raven Press, 1983, pp 241–256.

CHAPTER 31

Reproductive Health Care Needs of the Developmentally Disabled

DAVID MURAM
THOMAS E. ELKINS

The field of developmental disabilities has seen significant change since the 1970s. Patients were previously kept in hospitals and chronic care institutions but are now integrated into the community (Tables 31–1 and 31–2). The presence of these former patients in the community has necessitated a major reorgani-

zation in the areas of rehabilitation and training services. This rehabilitation effort has extended beyond vocational training, attempting to incorporate means of addressing the social and emotional needs of these individuals. Placement of individuals within the community has resulted in a significant improvement in their quality of life. With the acquisition of new skills, the disabled individual can take advantage of previously unavailable education and employment opportunities. These changes enable such individuals to lead as normal a life as possible.

The health care system must also adjust to these changes. The care provided in an institution may be very different from that provided in the community. Previously, preventive care, routine examinations, immunizations, and treatment of minor illnesses were provided by most institutions, and contracts with hospitals provided acute care for serious illness; minimal involvement on the part of patients or their families was needed to provide adequate health care. However, as residents in the community they must seek their own care, participate in the decision making, and

TABLE 31–1 ••• PREVALENCE OF DISABILITY ACCORDING TO DEGREE OF LIMITATION FOR ADOLESCENTS 10 TO 18 YEARS OF AGE, UNITED STATES, 1984*

Degree of Limitation	% Distribution	Estimated Prevalence (thousands)
Unable to conduct major activity	0.5	165
Limited in kind or amount of major activity	3.7	1,185
Limited in other activities	2.0	629
Not limited	93.8	29,862

*Original tabulations from public use tapes, National Health Interview Survey.

From Newacheck PW. Adolescents with special health needs: Prevalence, severity and access to health services. Pediatrics 1989; 84:872–881.

TABLE 31–2 ••• PREVALENCE OF MENTAL RETARDATION IN URBAN AND RURAL AREAS

Area (reference no.)	Age (years)	Prevalence rates/1,000 population		Comments
		Urban	*Rural*	
England and Wales (2)	0–16	3.51	4.88	
	17–60+	3.20	5.61	
	Total*	6.71	10.49	
Onondaga County, NY (7)	0–17	36.8	33.4	
New York State (8)	5–15	2.9 (New York City) 3.7 (other cities)	2.3 (villages) 3.0 (rest of state)	Includes only severe mental retardation.
Wessex, England (16, 17)	15–19	3.54 (county boroughs)	3.84 (counties)	Includes only severe mental retardation.
Northeast Scotland (18)	0–80+	3.63 2.02	3.02 2.25	For mild mental retardation. For severe mental retardation.
Netherlands (25, 26)	19	34.2	26.7	Schooling as the criterion for mild mental retardation.
		52.1	62.4	Raven matrices as the criterion for mild mental retardation.
		56.6	66.8	ICD† code as the criterion for mild mental retardation.
		0.63	0.63	Men with severe mental retardation with diagnosis of Down syndrome.
		3.13	3.34	All men with severe mental retardation except those with Down syndrome.

*Totals are not age-adjusted.
†ICD, *International Classification of Diseases* (1948).
From Kiely M. The prevalence of mental retardation. Epidemiologic Reviews 1987; 9:194–218.

be partially responsible for compliance with prescribed treatment. Some communities may not be equipped to provide medical services that are as accessible or as comprehensive as needed, especially for individuals with complex conditions. A survey of community medical care for persons with mental retardation revealed that 89% of the study group had found a medical practitioner, and 90% were receiving adequate medical care.[1] However, preventive gynecologic care was notably incomplete, with 60% of the women having had no examination in the preceding 3 years.[2]

The health care needs of persons with developmental disabilities vary with the disability, so generalizations cannot be made (Table 31–3). Whereas some are only physically limited, others may be both physically and mentally disabled. Those with minor impairments have similar health care needs to people in the general population and thus do not require special consideration. However, highly sophisticated and specialized care is required by individuals at the other end of the spectrum. The health care delivery system must be sensitive and responsive to these dif-

ferent needs to be able to provide not only the basic level of care, but also the highly specialized services required by those with severe disabilities.

Furthermore, the health care needs of individuals with disabilities are constantly changing (Table 31–4). With improved medical technol-

TABLE 31–3 ••• LEADING CAUSES OF DISABILITY AMONG ADOLESCENTS 10 TO 18 YEARS OF AGE, UNITED STATES, 1984*

Main Cause of Disability	Estimated Prevalence (thousands)
Mental disorders	634
Diseases of the respiratory system	406
Diseases of the musculoskeletal system and connective tissue	295
Diseases of nervous system	115
Diseases of the ear and mastoid process	80

*Original tabulations from public use tapes, National Health Interview Survey.
From Newacheck PW. Adolescents with special health needs: Prevalence, severity and access to health services. Pediatrics 1989; 84:872–881.

TABLE 31–4 ••• REPRODUCTIVE HEALTH CARE NEEDS OF THE DEVELOPMENTALLY DISABLED

Accessibility to care
Care providers' ability to listen to family members
Coordination of professional services
Specific medical problems that interfere with the gynecologic examination
Communication with the patient
Obtaining an adequate cervical smear for cytologic examination
Menarche and subsequent menstrual hygiene

ogy and care, the life expectancy for people with disabilities currently is greater than ever before, as exemplified by a survey of persons with Down syndrome.[3] Many of these persons live a long life and therefore require different services and medical care. An even greater challenge to the community service system is presented by the older persons in this population who have multiple disabilities.

ACCESSIBILITY TO CARE

How health care is delivered is directly shaped by how it is financed. Many disabled persons rely on Medicaid to defray their health care costs (Table 31–5). The disincentives to the integration of these individuals into the "mainstream" are compounded by inefficient payment mechanisms.[4] Consideration of the special requirements of persons with disabilities must be taken into account. Otherwise the following can be expected:

1. Attempts to provide periodic examinations for prevention, screening, and health maintenance programs will be curtailed.
2. Choices among providers will be restricted.
3. The quality of health care services attained will be inferior to the modal quality of services in the community.
4. Health care will become increasingly crisis oriented.

Availability of medical and mental health services is essential to ensure delivery of appropriate care. Health care professionals are expected to be not only competent, but also understanding, sensitive, and empathetic. They should be skilled in listening to family members and care providers and willing to include them in the decision-making process. Above all, professional services delivered by various specialists and agencies must be well coordinated.

Like those in the general population, individuals with disabilities require the services of an identified primary health care provider who assumes longitudinal responsibility for their overall well-being, furnishes general medical and preventive care, and makes referrals to specialty care when needed. In such a setting, the person's health status is well known, an up-to-date and comprehensive medical record exists, and a long-term relationship can be developed with the patient and the family.

REPRODUCTIVE HEALTH CARE NEEDS

The reproductive health care needs of a disabled child or adolescent are not different from those of the general population. The disability, however, may create difficulties for the health care provider. Even young girls with disabilities may suffer from multiple health problems requiring consultation with multiple specialists and continuous medical attention. In one study, investigators found associated medical conditions in 80% of children with mental retardation.[5] Children with lower intelligence quotients had more complicated medical problems resulting in a more significant disability.

From a medical perspective, individuals with severe physical disabilities also have the following specific areas of concern that require constant monitoring and frequent intervention:

1. Seizure disorders are common and may be complex. Multidrug anticonvulsant therapy may be required for optimal management and may cause medication interactions, interfere with the menstrual cycle, and even impair the ability of the child to interact with others.
2. Multiple joint contractures, which often preclude ambulation, cause impaired sitting posture and make the conventional pelvic examination an impossibility.
3. Nutrition is often complicated by feeding difficulties. The presence of gastroesophageal reflux with vomiting further aggravates the situation.

An additional complication is the fact that many of these patients have only a limited ability to communicate. An alteration in be-

TABLE 31–5 ••• HEALTH CARE COVERAGE CHARACTERISTICS ACCORDING TO DISABILITY STATUS FOR ADOLESCENTS 10 TO 18 YEARS OF AGE, UNITED STATES, 1984*

Coverage Status of Adolescents With Known Coverage Status†	Distribution (%)		
	All Adolescents	**Adolescents With Disabilities**	**Adolescents Without Disabilities**
	100.0	100.0	100.0
Private only	74.0	64.6	74.7
Public only	10.0	18.6	9.4
Both private and public	1.9	3.0	1.8
None reported	14.1	13.8	14.1

*Original tabulations from public use tapes, National Health Interview Survey.
†Persons with unknown health care coverage status excluded.
From Newacheck PW. Adolescents with special health needs: Prevalence, severity and access to health services. Pediatrics 1989; 84:872–881.

attuned to this fact, particularly if they have known the person for some length of time, the severity of the problem may not be recognized and can result in a delay in providing the patient appropriate medical attention. This is a serious issue and should be addressed regularly in training and supervision.

THE GYNECOLOGIC EXAMINATION

The gynecologic examination of any adolescent girl may create significant anxiety. However, a girl with mental retardation may have only limited understanding of the examination and its purpose and may refuse to be examined (Table 31–6). Obtaining a cervical smear for cytologic examination may be an impossible task. However, these periodic examinations are required as part of the routine disease prevention care recommended for all patients (Table 31–7).

Patients with disabilities are sensitive to the physician's attitude. They tend to withdraw if the physician is hurried, brusque, or indiffer-

ent, but they react positively to a clinician who is kind, warm, and patient. The presence of the mother or the care provider in the examination room often provides a sense of security. Preexamination education is a key feature for a successful examination. The use of lifelike dolls and slide presentations that clarify the examination process have been helpful when performing pelvic examinations in difficult-to-examine patients (see Table 31–6).[6] The patient should be encouraged to help with the examination. This provides a sense of control and helps alleviate apprehension. Satisfactory palpation of the pelvic organs is usually accomplished by performing a rectal examination and should not cause pain. Samples for cytosmears may be obtained by inserting a cotton-tipped swab over a finger into the vagina and directing it toward the cervix. When the vagina requires evaluation, special instruments (e.g., vaginoscope, Huffman-Graves virginal speculum, etc.) may be required. As for any young patient, familiarizing her with the instrument before insertion usually decreases apprehension. Allowing her to touch the lubricated

TABLE 31–6 ••• ABILITY TO PERFORM PELVIC EXAMINATION IN 150 MENTALLY HANDICAPPED FEMALES

Complete pelvic exam	26
Bimanual/Cotton swab	91
Complete pelvic exam with sedation	
Chloral hydrate	0/8
Ketamine/Midazolam	21/25
Exam under general anesthesia	12

From Rosen DA, Rosen KR, Eklins TE, et al. Outpatient sedation: An essential addition to gynecologic care for persons with mental retardation. Am J Obstet Gynecol 1991; 164:825–828.

TABLE 31–7 ••• THE GYNECOLOGIC EXAMINATION

Physician should be sensitive, warm, and kind
Preexamination education
Use of lifelike dolls and a slide presentation
Encourage patient to help with the examination
Patient should have a sense of control over the examination process
Cytosmear with a cotton-tipped swab over a finger inserted into the vagina and directed toward the cervix
Bimanual (rectal) examination
Vaginoscopy if indicated
Periodic sonogram in lieu of pelvic examination
Sedation only if required

instrument is encouraged. She should notice that it feels slippery and cool. The instrument is then placed against the inner thigh, reminding the patient that it feels cool, slippery, and unusual. Only then is the instrument passed through the hymenal orifice. Vaginoscopy should not be attempted without sedation or general anesthesia if the aperture is too small for an instrument to be passed without discomfort or if the patient is uncooperative. Periodic sonograms may be substituted for routine pelvic assessment in selected patients, especially when a Pap smear is not required. Oral ketamine and midazolam (used alone or together) have been effective in providing enough sedation to allow outpatient pelvic examinations in more than 80% of patients who would otherwise have required general anesthesia for routine care (see Table 31–6).[7]

SEXUALITY

Although many physicians are familiar with the unusual medical requirements of the developmentally disabled, some are still uncomfortable dealing with issues of sexuality in this population. It is well accepted that every individual needs to develop his or her sexual feelings and be able to express these feelings freely. Because these disabled individuals currently live within the community, their sexuality is no longer a hidden phenomenon (Table 31–8; Figs. 31–1 and 31–2). Although the accepted sociosexual model is to find a partner, marry, and have children, many perceive the expression or acting out of these desires by a disabled person as abnormal. Lack of proper education has caused even those people who

TABLE 31–8 ••• PERCENTAGE OF MENTALLY RETARDED INDIVIDUALS WHO HAD EXPERIENCED VARIOUS SEXUAL ACTIVITIES MORE THAN TWO TIMES

Sexual Activity	% of Females	% of Males
Masturbation	30	60
Kissing a nonrelative of the opposite sex	60	70
Hugging and kissing for a long time	50	50
Going further than hugging and kissing	20	50

Modified from Ousley OY, Mesibov GB. Sexual attitudes and knowledge of high-functioning adolescents and adults with autism. J Autism Dev Disord 1991; 21:471–481.

approve of sexual expression to voice concerns that such sexual activity may result in an increase in handicapped children.

When these patients were cared for in an institutional setting, physicians and other health care professionals were responsible for all their needs. A high standard of behavior was expected from all patients, and any expression of sexuality was regarded as a potential public scandal that could damage the image of the institution. Sexual expression was regarded as a problem for which a solution must be found. The solution often was cessation of the behavior and, thus, suppression of sexual expression. This form of control cannot be practiced on patients residing within the community. The fact that disabled people are sexual individuals and have the right to express their feelings must be accepted. Instead of attempting to control this sexual behavior, these individuals must be helped to channel it into accepted social norms.

Like other parents, many parents of disabled children are uncomfortable discussing sexuality. Although they would very much like their child to be "like everyone else," many do not wish their child to receive sex education. The belief that ignorance makes the children innocent and therefore less likely to have sexual experiences in the future may be held by some parents. Many are convinced that the child has no interest in sexual expression and would have a sexual experience only because someone else would take advantage of their disability.

The concerns of parents vary as the child grows. Parents of a young girl with disabilities wish to learn how to prepare the girl for the physical changes that occur at puberty. As the child matures, the major concerns are menstruation, hygiene, dating, possible sexual activity, avoidance of sexual abuse, and contraception. Parents of older patients are more concerned with potential reproduction, and many request that their daughters be surgically sterilized (Table 31–9).

MENSTRUATION

For any girl, the first menstrual period is often a startling and frightening experience, and for a girl who is mentally disabled and not adequately prepared, it can be a traumatic

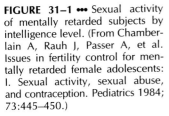

FIGURE 31–1 ••• Sexual activity of mentally retarded subjects by intelligence level. (From Chamberlain A, Rauh J, Passer A, et al. Issues in fertility control for mentally retarded female adolescents: I. Sexual activity, sexual abuse, and contraception. Pediatrics 1984; 73:445–450.)

event. This prompts many parents to seek medical advice as pubertal changes become apparent. Almost all patients with developmental disabilities are evaluated either just before menarche or immediately after initiation of the menstrual cycles (D. Muram, unpublished data). In some instances, menarche raises fears of initiation of sexual activity and, with it, the potential for unintended pregnancy. If the parents feel that the child's supervision is insufficient (e.g., the child is in school, special programs, etc.), they often request contraceptive advice. Older individuals are more likely to request contraception. Like all school-age children, individuals with developmental disabilities should be offered sex education programs appropriate for their level of understanding. Similarly, appropriate programs should be offered to the parents. Patients who are considered able to manage their own hygiene during menstruation should be provided with menstrual hygiene classes, and those who are sexually active should be given contraception.

Girls who are severely handicapped may not be able to provide proper perineal hygiene. In these girls, the menstrual blood may cause significant problems, and therefore they are often isolated from their normal environment during menstruation. Some who have had difficulty in mastering toilet control may decompensate at this time. Others who are not toilet trained have an added problem to cope with. Many parents become frustrated and request that a hysterectomy be performed to abolish the menstrual cycle. In some clinics, poor menstrual hygiene is a leading indication for hysterectomy in girls with severe disabilities.

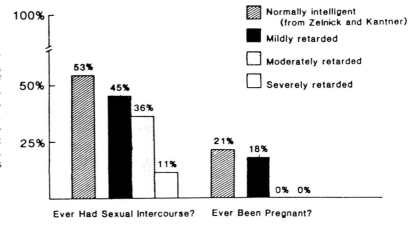

FIGURE 31–2 ••• Sexual activity of mentally retarded subjects ages 15 to 19 years, and a sample of 15- to 19-year-old females of normal intelligence. (From Chamberlain A, Rauh J, Passer A, et al. Issues in fertility control for mentally retarded female adolescents: I. Sexual activity, sexual abuse, and contraception. Pediatrics 1984; 73:445–450.)

TABLE 31–9 ●●● PARENT RESPONSE TO "EVER THOUGHT OF STERILIZATION?"

	No. of Parents Interviewed	Have you ever thought of sterilization for your daughter?			
		No	Yes, but decided against it	Yes, and still seeking	Yes, and obtained procedure
Mildly mentally retarded (MR)	33	24	3	6	0
Moderately MR	16	6	5	5	0
Severely MR	20	7	5	7	1
Total	69 (100%)	37 (54%)	13 (19%)	18 (26%)	1 (1%)

From Passer A, Rauh J, Chamberlain A, et al. Issues in fertility control for mentally retarded female adolescents: II. Parental attitudes toward sterilization. Pediatrics 1984; 73:451–454.

Anovulation and dysfunctional uterine bleeding are common in young adolescents after menarche, and adolescents with developmental disabilities are no exception. Many present with complaints of irregular and often heavy menstrual flow. Anovulatory cycles are common for the first year after menarche. Periods are often irregular, and the bleeding may be heavier than the flow in ovulatory cycles. Irregularity and heavy flow create additional difficulties for the patient and her family. The menstrual cycle may cause other problems as well. Some patients who suffer from epilepsy or emotional instability may notice a significant increase in the frequency of seizures or a marked impairment of social behavior. Some are sent home from school during menstruation. This disruption in special educational efforts may increase isolation. To address this problem, a nursing staff or social worker is employed to conduct home training sessions for menstrual hygiene. This behavior modification program is often successful when the parents are supportive and the patient is toilet trained. When properly prepared, many parents are willing to let the menstrual cycle establish its own pattern.

These problems may be alleviated by abolishing the menstrual cycle altogether, either medically or surgically. Menstrual control can often be achieved using medroxyprogesterone acetate (DMPA). Adequate menstrual control is usually achieved and hysterectomy is infrequently necessary. However, many centers perform a hysterectomy as initial therapy in developmentally disabled patients to abolish the menstrual cycle.[9] Because the long-term risks and benefits of hystrectomy and those of DMPA have not been established, a specific treatment modality should be selected jointly by the individual physician and the patient's family.

CONTRACEPTION

Despite recent developments, options for contraception in this population continue to be quite limited. Barrier methods, which are highly effective when used properly by a well-motivated patient, may be suited for certain mentally disabled individuals. In addition, condoms provide protection against sexually transmitted diseases. These methods are particularly suited for a patient who has infrequent sexual exposure. However, the use of barrier methods requires motivation and a supportive partner, and even among nondisabled adolescents, there is a tendency to use this method haphazardly. The relationship is sometimes casual, and the long-term consequences are not a deterrent to contraceptive failure.

Another consideration is the intrauterine contraceptive device (IUD). Once inserted, the IUD is quite effective, has a low failure rate, and requires no patient compliance. However, IUDs are probably not suitable for use in mentally disabled individuals, as these individuals may not recognize symptoms of the potential complications (e.g., pelvic inflammatory disease and ectopic pregnancy). Subsequent failure to seek early medical attention may prove to be fatal. Furthermore, the increased bleeding often seen with the IUD makes hygiene problems an even greater concern.[10]

Oral contraceptives (OCs) are highly effective, with a theoretic failure rate of less than 0.5%. The patient is required to take the medication on a daily basis, but in most instances the parents are supportive and can be trusted to ensure compliance. OCs are obviously not suitable for individuals who cannot swallow pills, for patients who live alone and therefore may be noncompliant, or for patients who experience severe side effects.

Long-term injectable contraceptives have

been developed and are in use throughout the world. The agent most commonly used is DMPA. It is a highly effective method of contraception, with a failure rate of 0.7 per 100 women-years for 12 months of use.[11] The medication has a low incidence of side effects, with the most common complaint being breakthrough bleeding, which may become quite disturbing. Concerns have been raised that long-term use of DMPA may result in bone loss and thus predispose these patients to develop osteoporosis.[12] Similarly, some physicians are concerned that DMPA, like other progestins, may adversely affect blood lipids.[13] It is recommended that a baseline lipid profile be obtained so that patients who are at higher risk may be provided with other contraceptive modalities. Even so, long-term injectable contraceptives are widely used by individuals with disabilities (Table 31–10).

Other injectable contraceptives using various combinations of estrogen and progestins are currently being tested in clinical trials, and levonorgestrel implants (Norplant) have recently been introduced into the market. Although the implant is effective for 5 years, breakthrough bleeding and the need for surgical insertion may limit its usefulness in a number of patients with developmental disabilities. For some, however, Norplant can provide long-term contraception with minimal reliance on patient compliance. (Contraception is discussed further in Chapter 18.)

STERILIZATION

The performance of sterilization for mentally disabled individuals must comply with appropriate constraints designed to protect the patient. Public Health Service regulations that govern sterilization programs supported in part by Federal Funding Agencies state that these programs shall not perform or arrange for the performance of a sterilization of any mentally incompetent individual or institutionalized individual.[14] Although other authorities feel that sterilization of the mentally handicapped is a decision for the courts,[15] successful litigation by the handicapped has made the practice of sterilization based on court order highly debatable.[16–18] Such limitations may be frustrating to a physician who wishes to perform a hysterectomy or tubal sterilization in a patient in whom such a procedure is reasonable or even essential. Each facility that cares for mentally handicapped patients must establish its own protocol, which must not only allow for the delivery of appropriate care, but must also take legal precedents into consideration and ensure "due process" and the rights of the disabled.[19] These obstacles do not exist when the patient is physically disabled but otherwise mentally competent. However, similar guidelines for the physically disabled are desirable.

SEXUAL ABUSE

Sexual exploitation is a major problem for this patient population and their families. Although the actual incidence of sexual abuse is unknown, it appears that sexual abuse of children is widespread. The National Center on Child Abuse and Neglect estimates the number of child victims to be more than 200,000 per year.[20]

Children of all ages, from infancy to young adulthood, have been victims of abuse, with the average reported age at first incident ranging between 8 and 11 years.[21, 22] One report suggests that younger children (ages 4 to 9) may be at higher risk because of a naïve and trusting approach to adults and a vulnerability to being misled regarding the meaning of various sexual activities.[23] Developmentally disa-

TABLE 31–10 ••• THE USE OF CONTRACEPTIVES BY INDIVIDUALS WITH MENTAL RETARDATION*

	Medroxyprogesterone Acetate (DMPA)	Oral Contraceptive Agents (OCA)	Intrauterine Device (IUD)	Total
Mildly mentally retarded (MR)	6	11	6	23
Moderately MR	9	3	1	13
Severely MR	13	5	0	18
Total	28	19	7	54

*Some subjects used more than one method.

From Chamberlain A, Rauh J, Passer A, et al. Issues in fertility control for mentally retarded female adolescents: I. Sexual activity, sexual abuse, and contraception. Pediatrics 1984; 73:445–450.

bled individuals are also victims of sexual abuse. Many parents believe that the severely retarded girl is at the greatest risk and that the assailant is often a stranger or another retarded individual. However, studies have shown that mildly retarded patients are at greatest risk, and assailants are more likely to be family members or persons well known to the victims.[24] Special effort is required for the development of effective prevention programs in the community if sexual exploitation of the disabled is to be controlled. In addition, there is a need for educational programs especially designed for the level of understanding of disabled individuals.

OTHER FAMILY MEMBERS

Although the crucial role of the family is beyond dispute, the needs of other family members are often forgotten. Most parents do well with their disabled children, but they require a variety of support mechanisms. They need training and advice concerning how to manage daily problems without creating a crisis. Common examples are mismanagement of masturbation through punitive measures and overprotection leading to isolation, low self-esteem, and depression. It is important to help these families learn to foster their children's success and achieve gratification from them. Most important, the parents need to participate in the decision-making process, and in fact, the family should provide the final decision regarding medical care for the disabled person. The physician's role is often limited to providing detailed information regarding the various treatment options and assisting the family in making the appropriate choice.

References

1. Minihan PM, Dean DH. Meeting the needs for health services of persons with mental retardation living in the community. Am J Public Health 1990; 80:1043–1048.
2. Crocker AC. Medical care in the community for adults with mental retardation. Editorial. Am J Public Health 1990; 89(9):1037–1038.
3. Thase ME. Longevity and mortality in Down's syndrome. J Ment Defic Res 1982; 26:177–179.
4. Master RJ. Medicaid after 20 years: Promise, problem, & potential. Ment Retard 1987; 25:211–214.
5. Smith DC, Decker HA, Herberg EN, Rupke LK. Medical needs of children in institutions for the mentally retarded. Am J Public Health 1969; 8:1376–1384.
6. Elkins TE, McNeeley SG, Rosen D, et al. A clinical observation of a program to accomplish pelvic exams in difficult-to-manage patients with mental retardation. Adolesc Pediatr Gynecol 1988; 1:195–198.
7. Rosen DA, Rosen KR, Elkins TE, et al. Outpatient sedation: An essential addition to gynecologic care for persons with mental retardation. Am J Obstet Gynecol 1991; 164:825–828.
8. Elkins TE, Gafford LS, Wilks CS, et al. A model clinic approach to the reproductive health concerns of the mentally handicapped. Obstet Gynecol 1986; 68:185–189.
9. Fraser IS, Holck S. Depo-medroxyprogesterone acetate. In: Mishell DR Jr (ed). Long Acting Steroid Contraception. New York: Raven Press, 1983.
10. American College of Obstetricians and Gynecologists. The intrauterine contraception device. ACOG technical bulletin no. 164, February, 1992.
11. Cundy T, Evans M, Roberts H, et al. Bone density in women receiving depo-medroxyprogesterone acetate for contraception. Br Med 1991; 303:13–16.
12. Sheth S, Malpani A. Vaginal hysterectomy for the management of menstruation in mentally retarded women. Int J Gynecol Obstet 1991; 35:319–321.
13. American College of Obstetricians and Gynecologists. Oral contraception. ACOG technical bulletin no. 106, July, 1987.
14. 42 OFR, §50.201–210, 1979.
15. Annas GJ. Sterilization of the mentally retarded: Is a decision for the courts. Hastings Center Rep 1981; August:18–19.
16. *Stump v Sparkman*, 435 US 349, 1978.
17. *Downs v Sawtelle*, 574 F2d 1(Cal 1978).
18. In re: Gloria Sue Lambert 1976.
19. Elkins TE, Hoyle D, Darnton T, et al. The use of a societally-based ethics/advisory committee to aid in decisions to sterilize mentally handicapped patients. Adolesc Pediatr Gynecol 1988; 1:190–194.
20. National Center on Child Abuse and Neglect (NCCAN). Child sexual abuse: Incest, assault and exploitation. Special Report. Washington, DC: HEW, Children's Bureau, August, 1978.
21. Kemp CE. Sexual abuse, another hidden pediatric problem. Pediatrics 1978; 62:382–389.
22. Kemp CE. Incest and other forms of sexual abuse. In: Kemp CE, Helfer RE (eds). The Battered Child. Chicago: University of Chicago Press, 1980.
23. Gelinas DJ. The persisting negative effects of incest. Psychiatry 1983; 46:312–332.
24. Chamberlain A, Rauh J, Passer A, et al. Issues in fertility control for mentally retarded female adolescents: I. Sexual activity, sexual abuse, and contraception. Pediatrics 1984; 73:445–450.
25. Passer A, Rauh J, Chamberlain, et al. Issues in fertility control for mentally retarded female adolescents II. Parental attitudes towards sterilization. Pediatrics 1984; 73:451–454.

CHAPTER 32

Treating Minors

STEVEN R. SMITH

The practice of pediatric and adolescent gynecology is increasingly influenced by the law. Legal issues arise from the formation of the physician-patient relationship and the consent to treatment, the obligations of confidentiality, the termination of treatment, and the payment for services. The emotionally charged and politically difficult questions of adolescent abortion rights and contraception have created a complex set of regulations in most states.[1, 2] Furthermore, the introduction of very broad reporting laws (including sexual abuse reporting statutes) have imposed new obligations on physicians.

It is therefore imperative that health care professionals treating children and adolescents be well versed in the legal principles affecting their patients and practice. The purpose of this chapter is to introduce the relevant basic legal principles, to describe some of the specific legal issues involving pediatric and adolescent patients, and to present some statutes that illustrate a number of states' approaches to these issues. Space will not permit us to detail all of the many legal issues involving obstetrics and gynecology, including professional liability, artificial insemination, in vitro fertilization, and genetic counseling; these are not unique to adolescents and are considered in texts in general obstetrics and gynecology.

In addition to understanding the general legal principles involved in adolescent obstetrics and gynecology, professionals should maintain a relationship with an organization or attorney who can keep them abreast of the laws affecting their treatment of patients. This is critical for three reasons. First, laws concerning pediatric and adolescent gynecologic care are changing rapidly and can be expected to continue to do so. Second, legal principles vary somewhat from state to state, and no general statement can describe the law in a given locale. Third, the law involving reproductive issues is a particularly complex tangle of overlapping and inconsistent state and federal statutes and constitutional provisions, federal and state court decisions, executive orders, and regulations.[3, 4]

BASIC LEGAL CONCEPTS

Several basic common law and constitutional concepts underlie virtually all of the current legal issues and principles concerning gynecologic care for minors. This section will briefly consider several of these legal concepts.*

State and Federal Law

State law has traditionally governed the regulation of medical care, the definition of the legal rights of minors, and the relationships

---

*All references to state and federal law are, of course, related to the United States' legal system. Although the broad, general legal principles described in this section have been accepted in other common law countries (e.g., Canada, Great Britain, and Australia), the specific rules regarding minors and obstetric and gynecologic care are not consistent and currently vary considerably even within common law countries.[5, 6]

between parents and minors. However, federal law has played an increasingly important role in these areas because of (1) United States Supreme Court interpretations of the provisions of the Constitution that limit state law (e.g., limit the ability of a state to prohibit abortions); (2) the increasing importance of federal funds in the delivery of health care services and the concomitant regulation of the provision of that care (e.g., Medicaid and federally funded family planning agencies); and (3) Congress's use of federal authority to control interstate commerce to regulate medical care (e.g., drugs and medical devices).[7] While this increasing federal role is important, state law still plays the dominant role in defining and regulating the provision of medical care to minors.*

The Parent-Child Relationship

Under common law, children are virtually the property of their parents and thereby subject to parental decisions, direction, and discipline.[8] Children are protected from their own immature judgment by their limited ability both to enter into contracts (except for necessities) and to consent to medical care (except under very limited circumstances). However, throughout this century the concept of parental ownership and control of children increasingly has come under legal attack. Although parents still have wide latitude in raising their children, minors are currently recognized as separate legal entities with their own rights and interests.[9] As a result of these changes, child abuse statutes limit the physical and mental abuse inflicted on children in the name of discipline, and mature minors, despite parental objection, may consent to medical procedures such as abortion.[10]

Minors

The law generally considers minors to be incapable of making binding legal decisions until the age of majority. States define this age differently, although it is usually between 18 and 21. The trend during the 1970s and 1980s, however, was to lower the age of consent to

18 and to permit some decisions to be made by those even younger.[11]

There have been some common exceptions to minors' inability to make legally binding decisions. The most common is the "emancipated minors" rule. Emancipated minors may make legally binding decisions, because they are viewed as formally free of the control and responsibility of their parents, usually as a result of marriage, military service, or (in some states) economic independence coupled with parental approval.[12] Some states also have recognized that "mature minors" may make legally binding decisions. The concept of the mature minor is not universally accepted and is somewhat unclear, but it generally refers to those who are able to understand and make complex decisions even though they have not reached the age of majority.[13] The legal tendency during the 1970s and 1980s, consistent with studies of the decision-making ability of older minors,[14, 15] was to give minors the legal authority to make legally binding decisions at an earlier age.[16, 17] In areas such as abortion, for example, the Supreme Court indicated a fairly broad authority for mature minors to make their own decisions. More recently, however, the trend seems to have reversed and currently may be toward expanding parental control over fundamental decisions, at least for adolescents under 18.[18]

Consent to Medical Care

Ordinarily, medical care may be provided only if the patient has given consent.[19] This is part of the general right of autonomy, the right of everyone to decide for themselves what will be done to their bodies.[20] When the treatment is important or invasive—surgery, for example—the patient must be informed of the risks and benefits and of alternative treatments and their consequences. The patient must give "informed consent."[21]

One exception is in an emergency in which no one is available to give consent. For example, when an adult is unconscious or when a minor has an emergency and there is no family available to give consent, treatment may be undertaken.* State statutes and court de-

---

*"Law" is used throughout this chapter to include constitutions, statutes, case law, and administrative regulations and directives.

*An additional exception to the requirement of *informed* consent is the so-called "therapeutic privilege." When providing information to a patient that would be quite harmful to the patient, that information may be withheld from the patient, although in many circumstances it should be revealed to others, such as the patient's family.[20]

cisions have provided additional exceptions to the usual minor consent rules.[22]

Confidentiality

Physicians have an obligation to respect patient confidentiality. Failure to maintain confidential information revealed during treatment may result in civil lawsuits based on negligence or invasion of privacy and may subject the physician to discipline by licensing agencies. Of course, there are exceptions to this requirement, such as when the patient has waived the right to secrecy or where the law specifically permits or requires the physician to release information about the patient.* There are many reasons for breaching confidentiality, ranging from the effort to obtain insurance (or other third-party) payment for services to the need to report a communicable disease under state law.[23] Any breach of confidentiality should be carefully considered by the physician.

Under the common law, it was assumed that parents were entitled to any important information about their children. This probably reflects current law, although because of individual state statutes and the constitutional privacy rights of minors, some exceptions may exist in the areas of psychiatric, obstetric, and gynecologic care. In many states, however, the right of minors and physicians to withhold information from parents is doubtful. The physician treating an adolescent patient may wish to reach a clear understanding about confidentiality, including any communication with the patient's parents, before treatment begins.[23] Where the treatment involves issues of sexuality or substance abuse, such an understanding is especially important.

THE PRIVACY RIGHTS OF MINORS

Fundamental Decisions Regarding Childbearing

In 1965, the Supreme Court, in *Griswold v. Connecticut,* first recognized a specific consti-

tutional right of privacy.[25] In *Griswold* the Court struck down a Connecticut statute prohibiting married couples from using contraceptives. The Court noted the private nature of the relationship between the couple and their physician, as well as the intimate relationship between husband and wife. The Court indicated that the constitutional right of privacy protects the right of the individual to make fundamentally important personal decisions without substantial government interference. Among the areas that the Court has identified as fundamentally important, and thus protected under the Constitution, are procreation decisions, marriage, childrearing, and family life.

Obviously much of the constitutional privacy doctrine directly affects obstetric and gynecologic care, because procreation and childrearing decisions are involved. After *Griswold* the Court recognized the constitutional right of unmarried persons to obtain contraceptives without governmental interference.[26] The Court stated if "the right of privacy means anything, it is the right of the *individual,* married or single, to be free from unwarranted governmental intrusion into matters so fundamentally affecting a person as the decision whether to bear or beget a child."[17]

In *Roe v. Wade* the Supreme Court struck down criminal abortion laws that outlawed abortions except to save the mother's life.[2] The Court noted that such laws interfered with a woman's right of privacy. However, it also held that the right of privacy is not absolute and may be limited if there is a compelling state interest. More recently, the Supreme Court has indicated that the right to have an abortion extends to minors,[12] that a minor cannot absolutely be required to have parental permission before undergoing an abortion,[27] that states may require parental notification before a minor receives an abortion,[28, 29] and that a minor has the right to at least some types of contraception without parental consent.[30] These decisions are obviously of direct concern in providing gynecologic services to adolescents, and they are discussed in detail subsequently in this chapter.

Controlling Personal Information

In addition to autonomy privacy, the right of privacy may include the right to withhold from others certain kinds of private informa-

---

*The obligation of maintaining confidentiality should not be confused with the existence of a physician-patient privilege.[24] The privilege permits physicians and patients to refuse to reveal, even to courts, the communications that occurred during treatment. Confidentiality is a broader obligation to maintain the secrets of the patient.

tion.[31, 32] The extent of this type of privacy is very poorly defined.[33] Thus far the Supreme Court has permitted states to collect very personal information, such as the names of women having abortions, as long as it ensures the confidentiality of such information.[18] The right to information privacy may play a future role in determining when a state may require the release of private information about abortions, contraceptives, or other personal matters.[34] The Court has already permitted states to pass laws that require that parents be notified that their minor child seeks to have an abortion.[28, 29] (This parental notification issue is considered in more detail later in this chapter.)

Limitations on the Right of Privacy

The nature and extent of the right of privacy are not certain. It is clear at this point, however, that privacy rights are not absolute. The state may interfere with the right of privacy in a number of ways, as described in this section.

Compelling State Interests. The right of privacy may be limited to protect a compelling state interest. For example, in *Roe v. Wade* the Supreme Court indicated that after the first trimester, the state may regulate abortions for the protection of the mother's health. After a fetus is "viable" (able to live outside the mother's body with or without artificial assistance), the state may regulate abortion, because at that time it has a compelling interest in the life of that fetus.[2] Relatively few legitimate compelling state interests can be identified.* The Court will permit a state to more broadly regulate abortion under a claim that the regulation does not unduly burden the right to choose an abortion. Thus, the Court has upheld 24-hour waiting periods for abortions, but has struck down "husband consent" laws.[1]

Conflicting Rights. Another potential limitation on minors' rights comes from the conflict between a minor's right of privacy to make procreation and childbearing decisions and the parents' childrearing privacy rights. Although the Supreme Court initially tended to favor the procreation decisions of the "mature minor" over the parents' childrearing rights,[27, 35] more recently it has seemed to place a higher constitutional value on parents' *childrearing*

rights than on the minors' *childbearing* rights.[28] Thus, a state cannot provide blanket authority for a parent to veto an adolescent's decision to have an abortion or to use contraceptives.[17] Nevertheless, the conflict may give the state some latitude in limiting a minor's obstetric and gynecologic care. Some states, for example, may require that parents be informed of the decision of a minor child to have an abortion.[28, 36, 37]

Promotion of Privacy Rights. Federal and state governments are not required to promote or encourage the exercise of privacy rights. For example, the federal government may refuse to fund abortions for women through the Medicaid system, even though it pays for other forms of obstetric care.[38] Furthermore, the Court has upheld federal regulations that prevent family planning centers from discussing the possibility of an abortion even when that part of the counseling center's activities was not paid for by federal funds.[39] The Court has only *permitted* such restrictions; neither the states nor the federal government is *required* to limit abortions or contraception. Indeed, in January 1993, President Clinton, by Presidential Order, removed the "gag rule" for federally funded clinics. Of course, it is possible that a future President could reinstate it. Furthermore, states are free to impose such rules.

State Action and Private Institutions. Private institutions, at least those not so involved with the government that they are thought of as quasipublic, have much greater latitude in prohibiting procedures such as abortions and sterilizations. This is because the constitutional right of privacy essentially applies to governmental action. Thus, private hospitals may be able to prohibit abortions or sterilizations if they choose to do so. However, the receipt of federal or state funds may be the basis for the regulation even of "private" hospitals.

Nonsubstantial Burdens on Privacy. To violate constitutional privacy, the government must significantly interfere with the ability of the individual to exercise privacy interests. An incidental or minor impediment is not considered an unconstitutional invasion, even though some particularly sensitive people might object to it. State recordkeeping of abortion information, for example, does not unconstitutionally burden the abortion decision.[27] On the other hand, a state law permitting only pharmacists to sell contraceptives does unconstitutionally burden the individual's right to make fundamental decisions concerning childbearing because it reduces access.[29] More recently, the

---

*Compelling interests may include the protection of human life, preventing violent overthrow of the government, and preserving democracy.[24]

Supreme Court has shown a willingness to accept limitations on abortion that are not an "undue" interference with abortion.[1]

The Court has upheld a state requirement that second-trimester abortions be performed in licensed hospitals (including outpatient hospitals),[40] but it has said that state statutes requiring all second-trimester abortions to be performed in general hospitals are unconstitutional.[35, 41] It has upheld 1- and 2 day waiting periods for abortions, very strong ("shock") abortion informed consent, and laws requiring that physicians report to the state the names of patients on whom they have performed abortions.[1] The Court has also permitted states to require parental notification[29] or consent[1] for abortion (with a judicial bypass, discussed subsequently), but it has struck down a state law requiring spousal (husband's) consent to abortion because that was an "undue interference" with a woman's abortion decision.[1] No clear line separates the insignificant from the impermissible burden, but the mere fact that a state regulation has some impact on obstetric or gynecologic care will not automatically invalidate it.

MINORS' CONSENT TO OBSTETRIC AND GYNECOLOGIC CARE

Consider Joan N., a 15-year-old living with her mother; her mother is not particularly supportive of Joan. Joan's father is seldom home but has been abusive to Joan and her mother from time to time. Joan has become pregnant, and at the prodding of a friend, she goes to see Dr. Snyder. She wants to have an abortion and to be given contraceptives to prevent future pregnancies. It also appears that she may have a sexually transmitted disease (STD). In this section we consider the following questions: May Dr. Snyder perform the abortion? Must Joan's parents consent to it? Must Dr. Snyder inform Joan's parents of the abortion or obtain their consent? May he provide advice regarding contraception, or prescribe a contraceptive? May he provide treatment for the STD? Should Dr. Snyder report the possible abuse by Joan's father?

To begin to answer these questions, we must look at the "minor consent" statutes, and then consider some constitutional questions.

Except in emergencies, as noted earlier, consent must be given before medical treatment. Unless the risks are minimal, some form of "informed" consent is necessary. Physicians providing medical care to minors without parental consent could be held liable in tort (negligence or battery) and run the risk of not being paid for their services.[12] Generally, parents must consent to treatment for their unemancipated children. However, some modifications of these general rules have been provided for adolescent obstetric and gynecologic care.[42] These have been made by statute in some states and by federal court decisions.[43] In addition to the care discussed in this section, emergency care generally can be provided to minors without parental consent, and life-saving care may be undertaken on the intervention of state social service agencies or courts.[9, 44, 45]

State Statutes

Some states allow adolescents to consent to some obstetric and gynecologic care, most often for treatment for venereal disease, pregnancy, and contraception. Several states, as part of the increased concern over child abuse, expressly allow the victims of abuse to consent to treatment for the abuse. Other changes have permitted adolescents to seek treatment without parental consent for drug or alcohol dependence. Not all states have such statutes, and where they do exist, an effort usually is made to limit their scope so that they do not apply to abortion.

These statutes often came about as a result of recognition during the 1970s and 1980s of the increased sexual activity and maturity of adolescents. The movement toward such statutes seems to have abated and may even have been reversed, as some states are considering modification or repeal. This may reflect both a change in public attitude and the fact that the courts have implemented some of the policies that the statutes promoted.

The following excerpts from a few statutes illustrate the approaches of several states.

California

34.5 Notwithstanding any other provision of the law, an unmarried minor may give consent to the furnishing of hospital, medical, and surgical care related to the prevention or treatment of pregnancy, and that consent shall not be subject to disaffirmance because of minority. The consent of the parent or parents of such minor shall not be necessary in order to authorize such hospital, medical, and surgical care.

This section shall not be construed to authorize a minor to be sterilized without the consent of his or her parent or guardian or to authorize an unemancipated minor to receive an abortion. . . .

[34.6 permits consent to all medical care by minors 15 or older who are living apart from parents, but permits the physician to inform parents of the treatment.]

34.7 Notwithstanding any other provision of law, a minor 12 years of age or older who may have come into contact with any infectious, contagious, or communicable disease may give consent to the furnishing of hospital, medical, and surgical care related to the diagnosis or treatment of such disease, if the disease or condition is one which is required by law . . . to be reported to the local health officer, or a related sexually transmitted disease. . . . Such consent shall not be subject to disaffirmance because of minority. The consent of the parent, parents, or legal guardian of such minor shall not be necessary to authorize hospital, medical, and surgical care related to such disease and such parent, parents, or legal guardian shall not be liable for payment for any care rendered pursuant to this section.

[34.8 and 34.9 permit minors who have been subjected to sexual assault to consent to treatment.

34.10 permits a minor 12 or older to consent to counseling related to drug or alcohol abuse, but requires efforts to include the parents in such treatment "if appropriate."][46]

Colorado

13-22-105 Except as otherwise provided . . . birth control procedures, supplies, and information may be furnished by physicians . . . to any minor who is pregnant, or a parent, or married, or who has the consent of his parent or legal guardian, or who has been referred for such services by another physician, a clergyman, a family planning clinic, a school or institution of higher education, or any agency or instrumentality of this state or any subdivision thereof, or who requests and is in need of birth control procedures, supplies, or information.

13-22-106 (1) Any physician licensed to practice in this state, upon consultation by a minor as a patient who indicates that he or she was the victim of a sexual assault, with the consent of such minor patient, may perform customary and necessary examinations to obtain evidence of the sexual assault and may prescribe for and treat the patient for any immediate condition caused by the sexual assault.

(2) (a) Prior to examining or treating a minor pursuant to subsection (1) of this section, a physician shall make a reasonable effort to notify the parent, parents, legal guardian, or any other person having custody of such minor of the sexual assault.[47]

Florida

381.382 (5) (a) Maternal health and contraceptive information and services of a nonsurgical nature may be rendered to any minor by persons licensed to practice medicine . . . as well as by the Department of Health and Rehabilitative Services through its family planning program, provided the minor:

    1. Is married;
    2. Is a parent;
    3. Is pregnant;
    4. Has the consent of a parent or legal guardian; or
    5. May, in the opinion of the physician, suffer probable health hazards if such services are not provided.

(b) Application of nonpermanent internal contraceptive devices shall not be deemed a surgical procedure.

[(6) Permits physicians to refuse to furnish contraceptives or services for "medical or religious reasons."][48]

Kentucky

214.185 (1) Any physician, upon consultation by a minor as a patient, with the consent of such minor may make a diagnostic examination for venereal disease, pregnancy [or alcohol or drug abuse], and may advise, prescribe for, and treat such minor regarding [these conditions], all without the consent of or notification to the parent, parents, or guardian of such minor patient, or to any person having custody of such minor patient. Treatment under this section does not include inducing of an abortion or performance of a sterilization operation.

[(2) permits those 16 and older to consent to mental health counseling.

(3) permits emancipated minors to consent to treatment.]

(6) The professional may inform the parent or legal guardian of the minor patient of any treatment given or needed where, in the judgment of the professional, informing the parent or guardian would benefit the health of the minor patient.

[(7) exempts parents from paying for most services for which they have not given consent.][49]

Texas

35.03 (a) A minor may consent to the furnishing of hospital, medical, surgical, and dental care by a licensed physician or dentist if the minor . . . [is an emancipated minor or]:

(3) consents to the diagnosis and treatment of any infectious, contagious, or communicable disease which is required by law or regulation adopted pursuant to law to be reported . . . and including all sexually transmitted diseases;

(4) is unmarried and pregnant, and consents to hospital, medical, or surgical treatment, other than abortion, related to her pregnancy; . . .

(6) seeks treatment for alcohol or drug addiction

(d) A licensed physician or dentist may, with or without the consent of a minor who is a patient, advise the parents, managing conservator, or guardian of the minor of the treatment given to or needed by the minor.

(e) A physician or dentist . . . shall not be liable for the examination and treatment of minors under this section except for his or its own acts of negligence.

[(f) permits a minor to consent to treatment for child abuse or for drug addiction. 35.04 also provides for treatment without consent in the event of child abuse.][50]

Dr. Snyder's treatment of Joan N., the case described at the beginning of this section, would be influenced directly by the minor consent statute in the state where treatment was provided. Most state statutes would permit Dr. Synder to provide treatment for the STD and to give advice regarding contraceptives and would not require that he notify Joan's parents of these actions. This is assuming, of course, that the contraception is not a permanent sterilization. These statutes would not, however, specifically permit a minor like Joan to consent to abortion. We will consider the issue of abortion in a subsequent section. First, however, we consider the question of Dr. Snyder's treatment of Joan if there is no statute permitting such treatment without parental consent.

Consent to Contraception

In *Carey v. Population Services*,[31] the Supreme Court held that the right of privacy includes the right of minors to have access to some contraceptives. It struck down a New York statute that limited access by minors younger than 16. Therefore, a state may not completely prohibit the use or availability of nonprescription contraceptives to minors.[51] This is an exception to the general requirement of parental consent. The issue of whether a state may require that parents be informed of

their child's use of contraceptives is another matter and is discussed later.

Informed consent regarding the use of intra-uterine contraceptive devices (IUDs) and other prescription drugs and Food and Drug Administration (FDA)-controlled devices should be obtained from the adolescent and, if required by state law, the parents. The constitutional right of a mature minor to prescription contraceptives without parental consent is not completely clear. However, it is likely that minors who can demonstrate "maturity" (competence) would not be required to have their parents' permission to use contraceptives. As always, practitioners must provide reasonable information about the benefits and risks of the proposed treatment and about contraceptive alternatives.[52]

Consent to Abortions

Since the *Roe v. Wade* decision, many states have tried to limit abortions by imposing a variety of fairly restrictive consent and other requirements. The federal courts have ruled many of these to be unconstitutional.[53] The states have then tried other approaches, resulting in something of a "cat-and-mouse" game.[54]

In *Planned Parenthood v. Danforth*,[28] the Court held that the right of privacy to decide to have an abortion extends to minors, and the state does not have the constitutional authority to delegate to a third party the decision of a "competent and mature minor" to have an abortion. In *Bellotti v. Baird*[17] the Court held that a state statute permitting a "judicial veto" of a mature minor's decision to have an abortion was unconstitutional. The statute allowed the state courts considerable latitude in deciding whether to consent to the abortion.[55] In 1983, the Court held unconstitutional an ordinance that provided that all minors younger than 15 were too immature to make abortion decisions.[35] However, in *Planned Parenthood Association of Kansas City v. Ashcroft*,[41] the Court upheld a state statute requiring all minors to obtain either parental or judicial consent for an abortion. This statute was constitutional, because the state courts were *required* to give consent to the abortion if the minor was mature enough to make the decision or if the abortion was in her best interest. This is known as a "judicial bypass" because it authorizes courts to bypass the usual family participation requirements. The Court believes that such provisions do not impose an "undue burden" on any right of a minor who wants or needs an abortion.

The Supreme Court has also recently upheld laws requiring preabortion, state-mandated graphic informed consent that includes information about the fetus.[1] Such laws, the Court held, do not unduly burden the abortion decision. It is likely that an increasing number of states will adopt such laws.[56] They probably will reduce and restrict—and are generally intended to do so—the availability of abortions to adolescents and the practice of obstetricians and gynecologists.[57] Professionals treating pregnant minors in states requiring parental or judicial consent may find it necessary to establish a method to assist them in obtaining judicial consent to abortion. This can be a daunting task for a minor to undertake alone.

The fact that a state is constitutionally *permitted* to require judicial or parental consent does not, of course, mean that it is *required* to pass such a law. However, it is likely that many states will move in this direction. That probably will mean that more states will require parental consent or a court order determining either (1) that the minor is sufficiently mature to make the decision, or (2) that the abortion is in the best interest of the minor. States will also probably require "shock" informed consent and provide waiting periods between the time of consent and the abortion.

Apart from special abortion informed consent statutes, the physician should remember that abortion is a significant medical procedure, and the informed consent of the minor is essential. Except in the most extraordinary circumstances, an abortion should not be done when the minor objects, and then should be done only with court approval.

Although the *Roe v. Wade* decision and subsequent cases have provided considerable protection for the right of adolescents to have an abortion, that right has been reduced considerably for minors. In 1992 the Supreme Court reaffirmed *Roe* but permitted considerable state regulation of abortion. Efforts in Congress to provide a national statutory abortion right have so far failed, and states have considerable latitude in formulating the abortion laws. As a result, inconsistent and shifting limits on abortion can be expected to occur. Because adolescents are a weak political force, they probably will be the focus of a great deal of regulation if *Roe* is abandoned.[58, 59]

Consent to Other Medical Procedures

There are a limited number of cases that address minor consent to other obstetric and gynecologic treatments. As noted earlier, many states have adopted statutes permitting treatment of a minor in a number of circumstances without parental consent. Furthermore, it is likely a court would order consent, even over parental objection, to treatment for contagious conditions such as venereal disease or when a condition is exceptionally harmful or life threatening.[9, 60] Thus, Dr. Snyder would probably be safe in treating Joan N.'s STD.

CONFIDENTIALITY AND THE RELEASE OF INFORMATION

The law may prohibit the release of certain information, require its release, or leave the release to the physician's discretion.[61] The usual obligation of a physician to maintain patient confidentiality is modified when a minor is involved so that parents have access to the information.[62] This is not an absolute right, and there are a number of instances in which the parents do not have a right to medical information about a child. This section addresses the release of information to parents.

State Statutes

Some states have defined by statute physicians' obligations regarding the release of obstetric and gynecologic information.[63, 64] These statutes vary considerably. Compare, for example, the Colorado[48] statute with sections of the Kentucky[49] and Texas[51] statutes, all excerpted earlier. Physicians are required to notify parents only in those states with a specific statute requiring such disclosure.[65, 66] Most states with specific statutory provisions on the release of contraception and abortion information either permit or require the release of information to parents.[5] The trend appears to be toward requiring its release and even requiring the physician to notify parents when a child requests an abortion or contraceptives.[6, 67]

In 1990, in *Ohio v. Center for Reproductive Health*[28] and *Hodgson v. Minnesota*,[29] the Court held that a state may constitutionally require the notification of one or even both parents when a minor seeks an abortion as long as the state also provides for a "judicial bypass." A bypass permits the minor to apply to a court to proceed with the abortion without parental notification if she is sufficiently mature to make the decision on her own or has been subject to abuse by her parents, or if it is in her best interest not to inform the parents.[29]

The judicial bypass exception is so complicated that it is unlikely that most minors would be able to negotiate it by themselves[68, 69] In some areas of the country there are organizations that will assist adolescents with the bypass procedures, and patients may known of these from their friends. However, physicians treating minors who may need or want to have an abortion should determine whether a parental consent or notification statute exists,[70] and whether they are permitted to assist the minor in completing the bypass. The initial studies suggest that courts overwhelmingly permit the bypass, but the adolescent patient is likely to need assistance in going through the court process.[71-73]

Returning to our hypothetical Dr. Snyder, it is apparent that he will face a difficult time providing abortion services to Joan N. As we have seen, Dr Snyder's obligations will depend on the state in which he is located. In a number of states he will be required to notify or obtain the consent of at least one parent. If there are good reasons not to have parental notification or consent, before proceeding, Dr. Snyder will need a court determination that Joan is sufficiently mature to make the abortion decision herself, or that it is in her best interest. The vast majority of such judicial bypass efforts are granted by courts, but Joan N. (and perhaps Dr. Snyder) will probably have to appear before a judge to receive judicial consent. The state may also require a "shock" informed consent and a 1- or 2-day waiting period between the consent and the abortion. Finally, in some states Dr. Snyder may be required to report to the state information about the abortion and about Joan N. It should also be noted that if Dr. Snyder is employed in some state or federally funded institutions, he may not be permitted to participate in the abortion or to directly refer Joan for an abortion.

A Practical Note

The purpose of parental notification rules is to encourage parents to counsel their pregnant or sexually active children and help them through a difficult time. In fact, notifying the parents may only increase some family problems. Some clinics have, therefore, steadfastly refused to inform parents of their children's treatment. It remains an open question whether such a position can be maintained in the face of specific state or federal laws requiring notification.[74]

The difficulty presented is illustrated by the Joan N. case described earlier. If Dr. Snyder tells Joan's parents about her desire to have an abortion or receive contraception, it is unlikely that Joan will receive parental counseling. Indeed, it is possible that such information will set off an abusive response by Joan's father. Requiring parental consent would be even more problematic. At the same time, seeking a judicial bypass would be extremely burdensome to Joan and to Dr. Snyder.

In jurisdictions requiring parental notification for certain types of obstetric and gynecologic care, the practitioner should inform minors at the beginning of treatment of this reporting requirement. This is another area where significant changes may be expected over the next several years, and particularly careful monitoring of changes in federal, state, and local law is important.[76]

Generally, even in states where parents have a right to their child's medical records, practitioners need not seek parents out to inform them of the therapy. That is not an option, of course, where the law specifies, as an increasing number of state abortion laws do, that parents *must* be notified before a treatment is undertaken.[28] Often parents do not know that their child is being treated. When the right of parents to information concerning the treatment of their child is unclear, practitioners may choose to refuse to release the information unless the parents obtain a court order or other judicial determination that the information must be released.

If the release of information to parents is optional, physicians usually should release confidential information about treatment only when the patient has consented to the release or when the release is clearly in the best interest of the minor. Ordinarily the minor should be told if the information is being released. Practitioners also may be asked to release information to an insurance company or other third parties for payment of services. In such instances, that information should be released only with the consent of the patient or a minor patient's parents.

In our hypothetical Joan N. case, it is very unlikely that Dr. Snyder will be able to avoid providing Joan N.'s parents with some very private information if he agrees to treat her. That is, unless Joan and Dr. Snyder are willing to go to court to receive judicial consent via judicial bypass, Joan's parents will probably be informed of the abortion.

MANDATORY REPORTING LAWS

In a number of circumstances practitioners are required by law to report certain diagnoses or findings to state authorities.[76] Reporting statutes vary from state to state, but obligations to report child abuse, neglect or sexual exploitation, and infectious venereal diseases are common. Some states require that records be kept or that reports be made to state authorities concerning abortions, certain prescription drugs, miscarriages, and infant deaths.

Child Abuse

All states require that child abuse be reported,[77] although statutes vary from state to state.[78] The Colorado statute, excerpts of which are reprinted below, is a fair representation of the scope of many state statutes.[79]

Colorado

19-3-303 As used [here], unless the context otherwise requires:

(1) (a) "Abuse" or "child abuse or neglect" means an act or omission in one of the following categories which threatens the health or welfare of a child:

(I) Any case in which a child exhibits evidence of skin bruising, bleeding, malnutrition, failure to thrive, burns, fracture of any bone, subdural hematoma, soft tissue swelling, or death, and either such condition or death is not justifiably explained; the history given concerning such condition is at variance with the degree or type of such condition or death; or the circumstances indicate that such condition may not be the product of an accidental occurrence;

(II) Any case in which a child is subjected to sexual assault or molestation, sexual exploitation, or prostitution;

(III) Any case in which a child is a child in need of services because the child's parents, legal guardian, or custodian fails to take the same actions to provide adequate food, clothing, shelter, medical care, or supervision that a prudent parent would take. . . .

(b) In all cases, those investigating reports of child abuse shall take into account accepted child-rearing practices of the culture in which the child participates. Nothing in this subsection (1) shall refer to acts which could be construed to be a reasonable exercise of parental discipline. . . .

19-3-304 (1) Any person specified in subsection (2) of this section who has reasonable cause to know or suspect that a child has been subjected to abuse or neglect or who has observed the child being subjected to circumstances or conditions which would reasonably result in abuse or neglect shall immediately report or cause a report to be made of such fact to the county department or local law enforcement agency.

(2) Persons required to report such abuse or neglect or circumstances or conditions shall include any [medical or mental health professional, school official, peace officer or film processor].

(3) In addition to those persons specifically required by this section to report known or suspect child abuse or neglect and circumstances or conditions which might reasonably result in child abuse or neglect, any other person may report known or suspected child abuse or neglect . . . to the local law enforcement agency or the county department.

(4) Any person who willfully violates the provisions of subsection (I) of this section:

(a) Commits a class 3 misdemeanor . . .

(b) Shall be liable for damages proximately caused thereby.[47]

Note the broad definition of abuse and neglect in the Colorado statute. A number of states currently require that emotional or mental abuse also be reported[75, 80]; sexual assault or molestation is specifically included. In addition, abuse must be reported when it is known or only suspected and in cases where conditions would reasonably be expected to result in abuse or neglect.[81]

Most states provide immunity against liability for those who report cases of suspected child abuse.[77, 78] Failure to report known or suspected abuse, neglect, or sexual exploitation is a criminal offense in most states and may also give rise to civil liability.[76, 82]

Claims of child abuse have recently been made against women who abuse a "child" (fetus) during pregnancy.[83] For example, women who continue to ingest illegal drugs during pregnancy, despite knowing that such conduct is seriously harming the fetus, may be seen as child abusers.[84, 85] Critics of this approach suggest that such prosecutions interfere with women's ability to control their own bodies.[86] It is not clear what direction the law will take, but some states are likely to consider the harmful use of illegal drugs (e.g., cocaine) by pregnant women to be child abuse.[85, 86] Those treating pregnant adolescents should be aware of legal developments in this area, as they may become responsible for reporting pregnant patients who are abusing their unborn children.

Venereal Disease

States commonly require that professionals report cases of venereal disease to a state or local board of health. The portion of the Iowa statute below is typical.

Iowa

140.4   Immediately after the first examination or treatment of any person infected with any venereal disease, the physician performing the same shall transmit to the Iowa department of health a report stating the name, age, sex, marital status, occupation of patient, name of the disease, probable source of infection, and duration of the disease; except, when a case occurs within the jurisdiction of a local health department, such a report shall be made directly to the local health department which shall immediately forward the same information to the Iowa department of health. Such reports shall be made in accordance with rules adopted by the state department of health. Such reports shall be confidential. Any person in good faith making a report of a venereal disease shall have immunity from any liability, civil or criminal, which might otherwise be incurred or imposed as a result of such report.[87]

As with child abuse–reporting statutes, failure to report cases may subject the professional to criminal prosecution. A report made in good faith is immune from liability.[78]

Dr. Snyder, in the case of Joan N., would almost surely be required by the laws of his state (regardless of where he practices) to make two kinds of reports to state agencies. First, if Joan N. told him of physical or sexual abuse by her father, Dr. Snyder must report this to a child protective services agency. The failure to do so is a criminal offense in most states. Second, Dr. Snyder would probably be required to report the STD to a health department.

OTHER LEGAL ISSUES

Payment for Services

Under common law, a minor cannot be held to contracts except for necessities, and a parent is obligated to provide the fundamentals of life. Thus, in most cases, a parent is required to pay for the minor's medical services, but if a minor legally contracts for necessary medical services, the minor can be held to that contract. It is not uncommon for states that permit minors to obtain medical treatment without parental consent to also release parents from financial responsibility for treatment to which they did not consent (e.g., see the Colorado, Kentucky, and Texas consent statutes reprinted earlier). Ordinarily the minor would be responsible for paying for such services.[60] Successfully securing payment, of course, may be difficult, even if it is legally due.

Involuntary Sterilization

Permanent sterilization of competent minors generally should not be undertaken unless it is necessary to save a life or is incidental to other essential treatment. Some states by statute specifically do not allow minors to consent to sterilization.[88]

A troublesome question has been whether it is appropriate for minors to be sterilized when parents or guardians consent. Sterilization is usually sought because profoundly incompetent female minors are unable to understand their own sexuality and the consequences of sexual contacts[89] and would be unable to care for any children they might bear. On the other hand, courts are reluctant to remove the fundamental right to procreation and are concerned about the potential for abuse.[90]

Courts currently permit some limited sterilization of profoundly incompetent minors after a process to determine that such a step is justified. This usually follows a formal hearing during which a guardian ad litem (for this legal process) is appointed for the minor. If she is judged to be permanently incompetent because of profound mental deficiency and it is determined that sterilization is in her best interest, the court may approve the procedure.* Even in the absence of express statutory

---

*Ordinarily a physician performing a sterilization pursuant to a court order can do so without incurring civil liability. When the court issuing the order does not have authority to do so, it is possible that the physician will be liable. This has led one expert to suggest some caution in implementing these orders.[60]

authority, some courts have utilized their "inherent" judicial authority to order sterilization.[91] These court-ordered sterilizations are appropriately limited to a narrow group of severely mentally retarded minors.[92]

PRACTITIONER PARTICIPATION IN THE LEGAL SYSTEM

It is important that practitioners treating pediatric and adolescent patients participate in the legal system to promote rational rules for the obstetric and gynecologic care of these patients. Sensible reform in the areas of minors' consent, parental notice of obstetric care, confidentiality of treatment, and involuntary sterilization depends on the participation of physicians who understand the medical issues and are willing to share their expertise with lawmakers.

CONCLUSION

In conclusion, current law would be more fair and compassionate if it were more realistic about the ability of older minors to consent to treatment. Adolescents 14 years of age and older—except for those who are not mentally competent—should be permitted to consent to most forms of medical treatment. Even without a general minor consent law, all states should adopt laws permitting minors to consent to treatment for pregnancy, contraception, abortion, and venereal disease. The Supreme Court's decisions, which apparently permit states to require that minors seeking abortions be judicially determined competent, are both unrealistic and likely to be a real burden to many minors.[29, 41] States should avoid adopting statutes requiring such determinations.[93]

The confidentiality of the adolescent-physician relationship should be respected. Minors seeking contraceptive advice, treatment for venereal disease, or abortions should be urged to confide in their families, and the majority do.[94] However, the decision of whether to involve parents should be left to the adolescent. Parental notification statutes are often based on a false idea of what families are like.

There is a significant price paid for required parental consent or notification. One study estimates that parental notice requirements might result in the approximately 125,000 minors who use family planning agencies to stop using effective methods of contraception. This would result in 33,000 additional pregnancies, leading to 14,000 abortions, 9000 out-of-wedlock births, 6000 forced marriages, and 4000 miscarriages. A parental notice requirement for abortions would mean that 42,000 minors would not have had legal abortions, the result of which would have been 19,000 illegal abortions, 18,000 unwanted births, and 5000 runaways. These figures are speculative, but they do indicate the magnitude of the problem presented by parental notification laws. Restricting the rights to abortion and contraception may injure the weakest members of society.[95, 96]

State reporting statutes can serve an important social function by eliminating and preventing disease and injury. It is essential, however, that the confidentiality of these reports be maintained. It is equally essential that the statutes be reasonably narrow and clear; some child abuse statutes are broad to the point of being vague, and such breadth may defeat the purpose of the statute. The law should recognize the ability of most "mature" minors to make treatment decisions and realistically face the fact that the lack of communication between some parents and their teenagers makes it difficult for these issues to be discussed openly.

References

1. *Planned Parenthood of Suutheastern Pennsylvania v Casey,* 112 S. CT. 2791 (1992)
2. *Roe v Wade,* 410 US 113 (1973).
3. Cohn SD. The evolving law of adolescent health care. NAACOGs Clin Issues Perinat Womens Health Nurs 1991; 2:201–208.
4. Silber TJ. Ethical and legal issues in adolescent pregnancy. Clin Perinatol 1987; 14:265–270.
5. Greydanus DE, Patel DR. Consent and confidentiality in adolescent health care. Pediatr Ann 1991; 20:80–84.
6. Czernecki MS. Constitution law: A minor's abortion right under a parental notice statute. Wayne Law Rev 1982; 28:1901–1928.
7. Hirt TC. Why the government is not required to subsidize abortion counseling and referral. Harvard Law Rev 1988; 101:1895–1915.
8. Ewald LS. Medical decision making for children: An analysis of competing interests. St. Louis Univ Law J 1982; 25:689–733.
9. Smith SR. Life and death decisions in the nursery: Standards and procedures for withholding lifesaving treatment from infants. NY Law School Law Rev 1982; 27:1125–1186.

10. Smith SR. Disabled newborns and the federal child abuse amendments: Tenuous protection. Hastings Law J 1986; 37:765–825.
11. Holder AR. Legal Issues in Pediatrics and Adolescent Medicine. New Haven, CT: Yale University Press, 1986.
12. Wright TE. A minor's right to consent to medical care. Howard Law J 1982; 25:525–544.
13. Sigman GS, O'Connor L. Exploration for physicians of the mature minor rule. J Pediatr 1991; 119:520–525.
14. Melton G. Children's participation in treatment planning: Psychological and legal issues. Prof Psychol 1981; 12:246–252.
15. Ambuel B, Rappaport J. Development trends in adolescents' psychological and legal competencies to consent to abortion. Law & Human Behav 1992; 16:129–154.
16. American Academy of Pediatrics. A model act providing for consent of minors to health services. Pediatrics 1973; 51:293–299.
17. *Bellotti v Baird* (Bellotti II), 443 US 622 (1979).
18. Melton GB. Judicial notice of "facts" about child development. In: Melton GB (ed). Reforming the Law: Impact of Child Development Research. New York: Guilford Press, 1987.
19. *Schloendorff v Society of New York Hospital*, 211 NY 125, 105 NE 92 (1914).
20. *Canterbury v Spence*, 464 F2d 772 (DC Cir 1972).
21. Rozovsky FA. Consent to Treatment: A Practical Guide. 2nd ed. Boston: Little, Brown, 1990.
22. Capron AM. The competency of children as self-deciders in biomedical interventions. In: Gaylin W, Macklin R (eds). Who Speaks for the Child: The Problems of Proxy Consent. New York: Plenum, 1981, pp 57–114.
23. Smith SR. Medical and psychotherapy privileges and confidentiality: On giving with one hand and removing with the other. Ky Law J 1987; 75:473–557.
24. Kelly KP. Abandoning the compelling interest test in free exercise cases. Catholic Univ Law Rev 1991; 40:929–965.
25. *Griswold v Connecticut, 381 US 479 (1965)*.
26. *Eisenstadt v Baird*, 405 US 438 (1972).
27. *Planned Parenthood of Missouri v Danforth*, 428 US 52 (1975).
28. *Ohio v Akron Center for Reproductive Health*, 497 US 502 (1990).
29. *Hodgson v Minnesota*, 497 US417 (1990).
30. *Carey v Population Services*, 431 US 678 (1977).
31. *Nixon v Administrator of General Services*, 433 US 425 (1977).
32. *Whalen v Roe*, 429 US 589 (1977).
33. Leigh LJ. Informational privacy: Constitutional challenges to the collection and dissemination of personal information by government agencies. Hastings Constitutional Law Q 1976; 3:229–259.
34. Smith SR. Constitutional privacy in psychotherapy. George Washington Law Rev 1980; 49:1–60.
35. *Akron v Akron Center for Reproductive Health*, 462 US 416 (1983).
36. *H. L. v Matheson*, 450 US 398 (1981).
37. Moore SA. Constitutional law: Right of privacy. *H. L. v Matheson*. Cincinnati Law Rev 1981; 50:867–881.
38. *Harris v McRoe*, 448 US 297 (1980).
39. *Rust v Sullivan*, 111 SCt 1759 (1991).
40. *Simopoulos v Virginia*, 462 US 506 (1983).
41. *Planned Parenthood of Kansas City v Ashcroft*, 462 US 476 (1983).
42. Holder AR. Disclosure and consent problems in pediatrics. Law Med Health Care 1988; 16:219–228.
43. Holder A. Minors' rights to consent to medical care. JAMA 1987; 257:3400–3402.
44. Rice MM. Medicolegal issues in pediatric and adolescent emergencies. Emerg Med Clin North Am 1991; 9:677–695.
45. Pieranunzi VR, Freitas LG. Informed consent with children and adolescents. Child Adolesc Psychiatr Ment Health Nurs 1992; 5:21–27.
46. California Civil Code (sections as cited in text) (Deering 1991).
47. Colorado Revised Statutes (sections as cited in text) (1990).
48. Florida Statutes (sections as cited in text) (1990).
49. Kentucky Revised Statutes (sections as cited in text) (Baldwin 1991).
50. Texas Family Code Annotated (sections as cited in text) (1991).
51. Brown RT, Cromer BA, Fischer R. Adolescent sexuality and issues in contraception. Obstet Gynecol Clin North Am 1992; 19:177–191.
52. Elkins TE, McNeeley SG, Tabb T. A new era in contraceptive counseling for early adolescents. J Adolesc Health Care 1986; 7:405–408.
53. Wildey LS. Legal issues in the management of the pregnant adolescent. Pediatr Health Care 1992; 6:93–111.
54. Melton GB. Legal regulation of adolescent abortion. Am Psychologist 1987; 42:79–83.
55. Stuhlberg, SF. When is a pregnant minor mature? When is an abortion in her best interest? Univ Cincinnati Law Rev 1992; 60:907–961.
56. Cates W Jr, Gold J, Selik RM. Regulation of abortion services: For better or worse? N Engl J Med 1979; 301:720–723.
57. Benshoof J. The chastity act: Government manipulation of abortion information and the First Amendment. Harvard Law Rev 1988; 101:1916–1937.
58. Interdivisional Committee on Adolescent Abortion. Adolescent abortion. Am Psychologist 1987; 42:73–76.
59. Scott ES. Legal and ethical issues in counseling pregnant adolescents. In: Melton GB (ed). Adolescent Abortion: Psychological and Legal Issues. Lincoln, NE: University of Nebraska Press, 1986, pp 116–137.
60. Clark HH, Jr. Children and the Constitution. Univ Illinois Law Rev 1992; 1–40.
61. Eaddy JA, Graber GC. Confidentiality and the family physician. Am Fam Physician 1982; 25:141–145.
62. Smith SR, Meyer RG. Law, Behavior, and Mental Health: Policy and Practice. New York: New York University Press, 1987.
63. Embree MG, Dobson TA. Parental involvement in adolescent abortion decisions: a legal and psychological critique. Law Inequality 1991; 10:53–79.
64. American Academy of Pediatrics Committee on Adolescence. Contraception and adolescents. Pediatrics 1990; 86:134–138.
65. English A. Adolescent health care: Barriers to access—consent, confidentiality, and payment. Clearinghouse Rev 1986; 20:481–490.
66. Thompson HA. Consent requirements for treatment of minors. Tex Med 1989; 85:56–59.
67. Marcararage LT. Limiting minors' abortion rights. Ohio Nor Univ Law Rev 1991; 18:169–178.
68. Crosby ML, English A. Mandatory parental involvement/judicial bypass laws: Do they promote adolescents' health? J Adolesc Health 1991; 12:143–147.

69. Worthington EL Jr., Larson DB, Lyons JS, et al. Mandatory parental involvement prior to adolescent abortion. J Adolesc Health 1991; 12:138–142.

70. Comment: The viability of parental abortion notification and consent statutes: Assessing fact and fiction. Am Univ Law Rev 1989; 38:881–918.

71. Rogers JL, Boruch RF, Stoms GB, DeMoya D. Impact of the Minnesota parental notification law on abortion and birth. Am J Public Health 1991; 81:294–298.

72. Ehrlich JS, Sabino JA. A minor's right to abortion—the unconstitutionality of parental participation in bypass hearings. N Engl Law Rev 1991; 25:1185–1209.

73. Council on Ethical and Judicial Affairs, American Medical Association. Mandatory parental consent to abortion. JAMA 1993; 269:82–86.

74. Bridge B. Parent versus child: *H. L. v Matheson* and the new abortion litigation. Wisc Law Rev 1982; 1982:75–116.

75. Rhodes AM. Legal issues related to adolescent pregnancy: Current concepts. Semin Adolesc Med 1986; 2:181–190.

76. Smith SR, Meyer RG. Child abuse reporting laws and psychotherapy: A time for reconsideration. Int J Law Psychiatry 1984; 7:351–366.

77. Fraser BG. A glance at the past, a gaze at the present, a glimpse at the future: A critical analysis of the development of child abuse reporting statutes. Chicago-Kent Law Rev 1978; 54:641–686.

78. Besharov DJ. The legal aspects or reporting known and suspected child abuse and neglect. Villanova Law Rev 1978; 23:458–520.

79. Savage D. The physician's duty to report the battered child syndrome. J Fam Pract 1979; 9:429–440.

80. Murphy GK. Are you complying with reporting statutes? Postgrad Med 1983; 73:283–287.

81. Guyer MJ. Child abuse and neglect statutes: Legal and clinical implications. Am J Orthopsychiatry 1982; 52:73–81.

82. Smith SR. Mental health malpractice in the 1990s. Houston Law Rev 1991; 28:209–283.

83. Landwirth J. Fetal abuse and neglect: An emerging controversy. Pediatrics 1987; 79:508–514.

84. Comment: Prosecution of mothers of drug-exposed babies: Constitutional and criminal theory. Univ Pa Law Rev 1990; 139:505–539.

85. Roberts DE. Punishing drug addicts who have babies: Women of color, equality, and the right of privacy. Harvard Law Rev 1991; 104:1419–1482.

86. Note: The prosecution of maternal fetal abuse: Is this the answer? Univ Ill Law Rev 1991; 1991:533–580.

87. Iowa Code Annotated (sections as cited in text) (1989).

88. Marcus J. Sterilization and competency. Denver Univ Law Rev 1991; 68:106–118.

89. Bambrick M, Roberts GE. The sterilization of people with mental handicaps: The view of parents. J Ment Res 1991; 35:353–363.

90. Burnett BA. Voluntary sterilization for persons with mental disabilities: The need for legislation. Syracuse Law Rev 1981; 32:913–955.

91. Lachance D. *In re Grady:* The mentally retarded individual's right to choose sterilization. Am J Law Med 1981; 6:559–590.

92. *Mental and Physical Disability Law Reporter* monitors changes in the law regarding sterilization of the mentally retarded. Washington, DC: American Bar Association.

93. Lundberg S, Plotnick RD. Effects of state welfare, abortion and family planning policies on premarital childbearing among white adolescents. Fam Plann Perspect 1990; 22:246–291.

94. Torres A, Forrest JD, Eisman S. Telling parents: clinical policies and adolescents' use of family planning and abortion services. Fam Plann Perspect 1980; 12:284–292.

95. Berger LR. Abortions in America: The effects of restrictive funding. N Engl J Med 1978; 298:1474–1477.

96. Harrison LK, Naylor KL. The laws that affect abortion in the United States and their impact on women's health. Nurse Pract 1991; 16:53–59.

CHAPTER 33

Puberty Aberrancy in the Third World

GEETA N. PANDYA

In the Third World, a plethora of female adolescent problems has been manifested in recent years, largely because age-old inhibitions against seeking medical care for young girls are rapidly disappearing. In the past, such problems as abnormal genitalia and menstrual irregularities were kept hidden by family members because of a rigid pattern of arranged marriages in which the family's primary concern remained the possibility of not finding a mate for the girl in question. Only if all family members were in agreement would they venture a consultation with the family physician; this, of course, was done under oath of complete secrecy. However, that was usually as far as the family was willing to go; the suffering patient would continue to be denied the services of a trained specialist. Consequently, specialists in large communities currently are having to deal with the after-effects of long-time pubertal neglect. When going through the history of many postadolescent cases, the origin of the problem can often be pinpointed to a period in the patient's pubertal or prepubertal age. Since the 1970s, the enhanced awareness of availability of specialized centers in large cities has reduced the neglect and mismanagement of pediatric and adolescent problems. This in turn has led to a reduction in female reproductive iatrogenic abnormalities.

Tuberculosis (TB) is responsible for a large percentage of chronic disease in India. Apart from TB, other conditions seen with increasing incidence include malnutrition associated with chronic gastrointestinal conditions caused by amebiasis and resultant anemia, chronic renal disease, cardiac problems from childhood rheumatic fever, and congenital abnormalities.

Menstrual disturbances occur because of hematologic conditions such as thalassemia and purpura. These chronic conditions affect young girls before the prepubertal phase and become even more evident at puberty. These conditions may produce a variety of menstrual irregularities such as primary amenorrhea resulting from delayed puberty, polymenorrhea, and menorrhagia, as well as secondary amenorrhea. Because the basic problem in thalassemia and purpura is anemia resulting from hemoglobinopathy, it becomes especially difficult to manage polymenorrhea and menorrhagia in this patient population.

Case Study: Anemia Associated With Helminths

A 17-year-old female from Adhikari, India, presented as a very thin, weak, short adolescent with no secondary sex characteristics, with primary amenorrhea, and with the body habitus of a child of 10. On general examination, the girl had characteristic findings associated with anemia. She was found to be infested with worms and had a hemoglobin level of 6 gm/dl. After being treated for helminths and anemia, her growth and general condition improved, with resulting menarche and cyclic menses, confirming that the patient's delayed puberty was caused by anemia and malnutrition (Fig. 33–1).

GENITAL TUBERCULOSIS

Information concerning the extent and magnitude of TB in Third World countries is

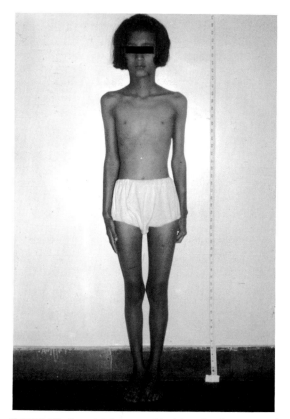

FIGURE 33–1 ••• Adolescent with delayed puberty caused by anemia and malnutrition.

TABLE 33–1 ••• TYPES OF GENITAL TB INFECTION

1. *Primary*. Very rarely, genital tuberculosis is of primary origin.
2. *Secondary*. Genital tuberculosis is nearly always secondary to pulmonary or extrapulmonary lesions such as lymph nodes, intestines, urinary tract, gonads, and joints.

difficult to gauge, but TB is known to be a significant factor contributing to gynecologic problems. Statistics regarding incidence, morbidity, and mortality rates are available only at government or municipal hospitals or at institutes where TB is treated. Since the 1940s, the incidence of TB has been described by many authors and depends on the particular case load and the type of institution and location (urban or rural) where the data were collected.[1]

In 1990 it was estimated that 1.7 billion people, or one third of the world population, have been infected with the tubercle bacillus.[1] However, such infection is responsible for 0.76%[2] to 9.8%[3] of all gynecologic admissions among infertile women. A patient with TB may be seen by a pediatrician or, in the case of an adult, by a chest physician or general or orthopedic surgeon, gynecologist, neurologist, or nephrologist. Thus, practitioners in associated disciplines may be able to document the incidence and type of TB.[1]

The incidence of TB among adolescents is

extremely difficult to determine, because young girls at puberty are usually seen by general practitioners or gynecologists with inadequate statistical reporting techniques. Most of the time, parents do not like to acknowledge any past history, and repeated interrogation may be necessary to find out whether the girl ever suffered from TB. Invariably, the physician must determine indirectly whether the girl has had episodes of repeated fever, cough, and coldlike symptoms or was ever prescribed 3 to 6 months of continuous medication. The prevalence of infection with pulmonary TB increases with age from 2.1% to 16.5% in the pediatric age group and to about 50% in those above age 15.[4] The incidence of genital TB in children is fairly high (Table 33–1). When pulmonary TB is treated, it remains in a dormant state, often until puberty, when the primary infection of the lung or intestines, which has been silent for a long time, tends to flare up and manifest as a genital infection. It also can present as a new infection spread via the blood stream from a different primary source. The result is genital TB occurring as a secondary infection with the primary focus lying elsewhere and the infection spreading in the early stages of the disease (frequently in adolescence or early maturity). Thus, in most cases, the primary infection not only has healed but also is "inconspicuous." Even so, genital TB can be associated with impaired fertility (Table 33–2).[4]

The pathophysiology of the disease must

TABLE 33–2 ••• ROUTE OF INFECTION OF GENITAL TB

1. *Blood stream*—the most common mode (although the primary extragenital focus is somewhere else, usually the lungs).
2. *Lymphatic spread*—possible from tuberculosis involving the mesenteric lymph nodes and/or peritoneum.
3. *Direct spread*—possible through peritonitis, although direct adhesion of a tuberculous lesion with the genital tract forms an important means of direct spread.

be understood. Bacteriologically, in approximately 95% of all cases, genital TB is caused by a human bacilli *(Mycobacterium tuberculosis)* rather than a bovine type.

Primary Amenorrhea

Case Studies

Patient M.P. presented at 16 years of age. The patient's mother was particularly worried about her primary amenorrhea, because she herself had begun menarche at age 13. Physical findings included a tall, thin, cachectic-appearing adolescent with Tanner stage IV breasts (Fig. 33–2A). She had long, thin fingers with clubbing of the nails (Fig. 33–2B). A lower gastrointestinal series revealed typical findings of tuberculosis of the cecum (Fig. 33–2C). She was put on antituberculosis therapy; during the third month of treatment she attained menarche.

Patient K., age 17, was an obese young woman who had developed tuberculous meningitis at age 15. She then developed secondary hypopituitarism and was placed on thyroid and corticosteroid replacement. On psychiatric evaluation, the patient's intelligence quotient (IQ) was found to be low, and her parents were not eager for her to continue sex steroid replacement, allowing her to menstruate cyclically.

Although a debated topic, many scientists are of the opinion that primary infection of the reproductive organs does not occur. Tuberculosis of the vulva or the vagina without any infection in the upper genital tract has been reported.[5] However, such a lesion appears to occur in association with a primary infection elsewhere in the body. Coitus is the most common method of transmission of primary infection.[5]

Sites of Lesions

1. *Tubercular salpingitis.* The tuberculous bacilli has a high affinity for the fallopian tubes.[6] In 90% of the cases, both tubes are affected.[6] From the fallopian tubes, the infection spreads to other pelvic organs.

2. *Corpus uteri.* In 50% of these cases, TB manifests itself as tubercular endometritis.[7] Contiguous spread occurs from the affected tubes. Only in very rare cases is the uterus infected without any significant infection in the tubes.[7]

3. *Cervix.* The infection coming down from the fallopian tubes to the uterus affects the cervix in about 5% of cases.[8]

4. *Vagina and vulva.* Infection of the vagina or vulva sometimes can be traced to tubercular cervicitis.

5. *Ovaries.* In about 20% of patients, the ovaries are affected secondary to infection involving the fallopian tubes.[9]

6. *Unusual presentations.* Patients with TB can present with infertility, nonspecific menstrual disturbances, pain, or abdominal distention.[10] The infection appears to occur via hematogenous spread from a distant focus, with the fallopian tubes being most commonly involved.[10] Other complications associated with

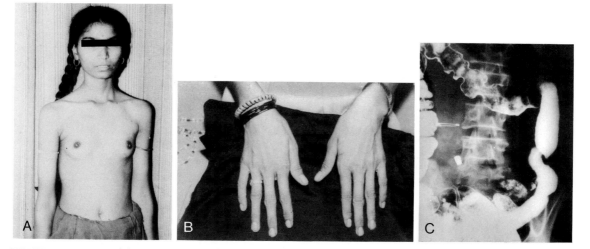

FIGURE 33–2 ••• *A,* Adolescent with genital tuberculosis with primary amenorrhea. *B,* Long, thin fingers with clubbing. *C,* Barium enema showing changes in cecal area secondary to tuberculosis.

TB include abdominal pregnancy 10 years after treatment for pelvic TB.[11] Characteristic endoscopic findings have been identified.[12]

Diagnosis in Adolescents

In adolescent girls, diagnosis of TB is not a simple matter, as certain investigative procedures (e.g., vaginal examination with a speculum or sampling of the endometrium for confirmation) are often not possible. Therefore, whenever a young woman presents with menstrual irregularities, a detailed history of past illnesses, as well as a family history—especially when looking for a history of TB, treated or untreated—becomes essential. This must be followed by a general investigation to rule out other chronic illnesses. Genital TB is suspected when menstrual irregularities are associated with one or more of the following symptoms: weakness, general malaise, evening increase in temperature, repeated history of cough, repeated urinary infection, persistent high sedimentation rate, and/or leukopenia. In 69% of cases, a past history of extragenital TB is documented;[13] in 20%, a family history of TB is present.[14]

Generally, the investigations for confirmation of genital TB consist of histopathologic and bacteriologic examinations of endometrial scrapings and/or menstrual blood. A hysterosalpingogram identifying a typical tuberculous pattern and sometimes an ultrasonogram noting a tubo-ovarian mass provide confirmation of genital TB. Diagnostic tests are somewhat problematic in adolescent girls, except for ultrasonography, because according to cultural norms, virginity must be preserved unless an extreme condition prevails (e.g., therapeutic curettage required for treatment of severe menorrhagia).

Pediatric TB, when suspected, is easily diagnosed and cured. Adolescent girls at puberty (when various hormonal changes occur) are at a higher risk in countries where TB is widely prevalent.

Pathology of Tuberculous Fallopian Tubes

The classic gross description of TB-affected tubes is that of a long, thin, beaded, obstructed tube or a short, thick, pocketed tube with associated hydrosalpinx (Fig. 33–3). Many times these young girls go undiagnosed at

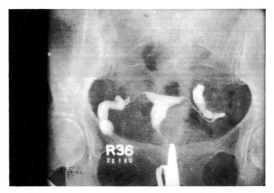

FIGURE 33–3 ••• A, Hysterosalpingogram showing hydrosalpinx with tuberculous involvement.

puberty. As time goes by, they mature and marry; the damage done at the time of pubertal infection may then present itself as infertility.

Tubercular Salpingitis. In a few cases, the mucosa of the tubes (endosalpingitis) are first affected and are followed by an infection in the remainder of the tube.

Adhesion Formation. The tubes thicken with dense "plastic" adhesions around the tubes. The distal ostia may be adherent or open, and fimbria may be destroyed. Tubercles may be visible on the surface.

Tuberculous Pyosalpinx. Fallopian tubes are enlarged as a result of accumulation of caseous material, which causes distention. The walls become thick and hard, surrounding adhesions are dense, and the distal ostium is occluded. Tubercles are seen on the surface of the pyosalpinx.

Miliary Form. The surfaces of the tubes are covered with tubercles. Microscopically, the endosalpinx and the subserous segments have tubercles with giant cells, a characteristic of tuberculosis. In advanced cases, caseation may occur, a condition that can result in a tubo-ovarian mass or ovarian abscess.

Menstrual Aberration Resulting From Tuberculosis

Frequently a young girl with TB begins menarche spontaneously and may subsequently develop secondary amenorrhea. In other cases, onset of menarche is delayed.

In cases of primary amenorrhea, the condition is usually diagnosed relatively early, as the patient is usually taken to a physician because she has not started menstruating. Primary amenorrhea stemming from generalized or chronic disease is not an unknown entity; it is quite common to see the initiation of menstruation after 2 or 3 months of antituberculosis treatment.

In cases of secondary amenorrhea, the patient may cease menstruating after a few periods. This may be succeeded by menorrhagia, often with a flow so heavy that curettage becomes necessary to stop the abnormal uterine bleeding. If intense curettage is not performed and the tissue not sent for histopathologic examination, there is a chance that the correct diagnosis will not be made, thereby preventing the patient from receiving appropriate treatment. Indeed, this may lead to uterine synechiae resulting in secondary amenorrhea (Fig. 33–4). It appears that if the patient was married early, curettage is more readily performed whenever there is menorrhagia or oligomenorrhea as a result of TB infection. This is done to "rule out suspected pregnancy." Before the availability of laparoscopy, the diagnosis of endometrial TB was established by histopathologic investigation of the endometrium. With diagnostic laparoscopy the clinician is able to identify the fine tubercles on the tubes and note any characteristics of the tubes that are typical of TB. Many times, in cases of secondary amenorrhea or oligomenorrhea associated with infertility, hysterosalpingography will identify the typical picture of TB. TB affecting the meninges (TB meningitis) may lead to disturbance of the hypothalamic-pituitary axis, sometimes resulting in hypopituitarism. Genital TB per se leading to menorrhagia, oligomenorrhea, or secondary amenorrhea is seen in association with

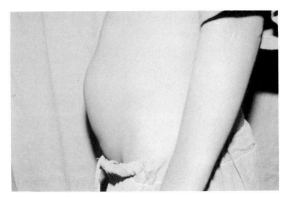

FIGURE 33–5 ▪▪▪ Abdominal distention associated with secondary amenorrhea in a patient with a large, caseating, tubo-ovarian abscess.

tuberculous salpingo-oophoritis or tuberculous endometritis, as well as a caseating tubo-ovarian mass.

In the Third World it is very common for patients to go unevaluated for long periods of time owing to lack of adequate medical facilities. Examples of such cases are described here.

Secondary Amenorrhea

Case Studies

Patient D., age 15, presented with abdominal distention and secondary amenorrhea (Fig. 33–5). Menarche occurred at 12½ years. Her menses were initially regular, but at age 14, one episode of very heavy menses occurred. Gradually her cycles became oligomenorrheic, and ultimately, secondary amenorrhea of 6 months duration developed. At laparotomy, a large caseating tubo-ovarian mass was noted (Fig. 33–6).

Patient P., age 19, had been married for 2 years and presented with a chief complaint of primary infertility and oligomenorrhea. Since 4 to 5 years of age, a cyclic scanty flow for 1 to 1½ days had been the pattern. Menarche occurred at age 12, with initially regular cycles gradually becoming "scanty." Hysterosalpingography showed a septate uterus with occluded fallopian tubes (Fig. 33–7). A diagnosis of Asherman's syndrome secondary to tuberculous endometritis was established. (The condition had probably developed several years previously.) On inquiry, the patient reported a history of intermittent fever between the ages of 13 and 15, a condition that was neither evaluated nor treated.

Patient S. was a 19-year-old girl who became amenorrheic and hirsute over an 11-month period. She presented with rapid onset of hirsutism, and

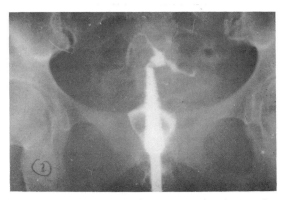

FIGURE 33–4 ▪▪▪ Hysterosalpingogram showing uterine synechiae.

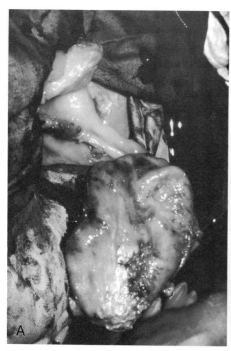

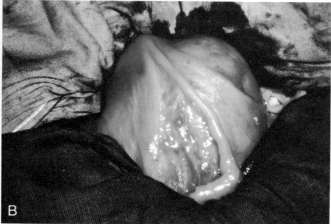

FIGURE 33–6 ••• A & B, Tubo-ovarian mass with caseation.

there was clinical evidence of an androgen-producing tumor. Arrhenoblastoma was detected (Fig. 33–8).

FEMALE CIRCUMCISION

Female circumcision is a ritual particular to certain cults in India and Nigeria (Fig. 33–9). In Nigeria, the Edo tribe has been known to have the highest proportion of circumcised females (76.7%), followed by the Ibos (61%).[15] The age at circumcision is usually infancy, with only 5.9% being circumcised as adults.[15] Statistics regarding morbidity and mortality from this procedure are difficult to compile.

Two types of circumcision are performed. Shaving of the clitoris, practiced by certain sects of Muslims in India, is done when a girl is 8 years of age. In complete excision of the clitoris, the sutured skin covers the urethra and upper part of the introitus, which is narrowed.

Obstetric sequelae of female circumcision have been reported, with the most apparent problems being increased maternal morbidity and fetal loss. No apparent long-term compli-

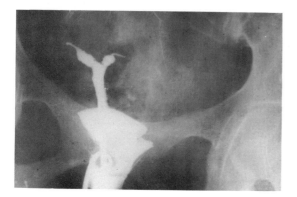

FIGURE 33–7 ••• Hysterosalpingogram showing double uterus with occluded fallopian tubes.

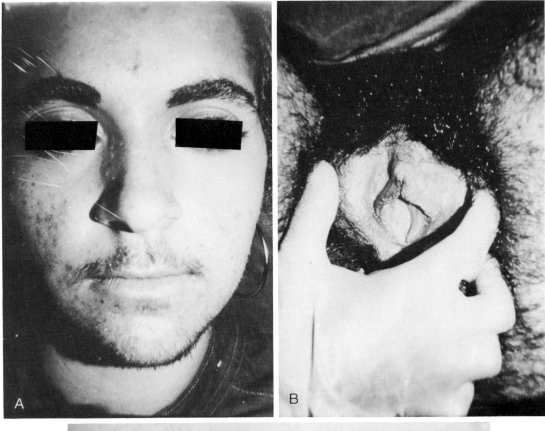

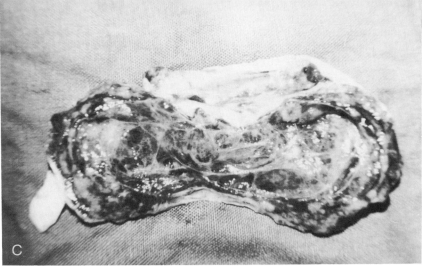

FIGURE 33–8 ••• *A*, Face of 19-year-old female showing acne and hirsutism. *B*, Vulva of the same patient showing excessive hair and an enlarged clitoris (the changes occurred over an 11-month period). *C*, Gross appearance of arrhenoblastoma from the same patient.

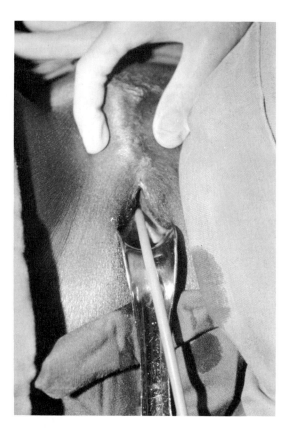

FIGURE 33–9 ••• Typical appearance of a circumcised female.

cations were noted in the series reported by DeSilva.[16]

Two types of complications, immediate and delayed, have been noted by El-Dareer.[17] Immediate complications were noted in 25% of patients and included difficulty with urination, wound infection, and bleeding. Delayed complications include urinary tract infection, chronic pelvic infection, and "tight circumcision."

GENITAL MUTILATION

Female genital mutilation presents a significant hazard to a woman's emotional and psychological health.[18] Female circumcision is included in the concern regarding genital mutilation. More than 25% of women subjected to severe forms of circumcision such as "pharonic rituals" suffer serious physical complications (Fig. 33–10).[18]

Figure 33–11A shows a 15-year-old girl who was attacked by a water buffalo and suffered complete perineal and partial vaginal tear. Plastic surgery restored normal genital func-

tion (Fig. 33–11B). Five months later, she married and after 1 year delivered a child by cesarean section.

CASTRATION

Indian culture is permeated with many religious cults. Among these are a group of eunuchs known as Hijras, who used to serve as harem-guards in the Indian Royal Palaces.[19] They are feminized in outward appearance by the use of female attire, makeup, jewelry, and the swinging gait of a dancing girl. The individuals who join this cult are usually born with ambiguous genitalia or are normal adult men who have chosen castration, often because of homosexual tendencies. Figures 33–12 through 33–14 are representative of these castrated males who act as females.

CASE STUDIES

Pubertal Aberration

Two sisters, aged 18 and 19, complained of hirsutism and acne along with primary amenorrhea.

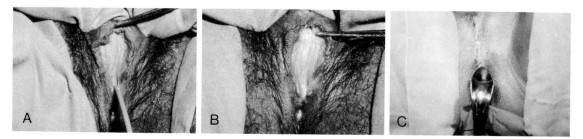

FIGURE 33–10 ••• *A through C, Genital mutilation in a patient subjected to extensive circumcision.*

Figure 33–15 shows the outward appearance of the genitalia of these "females." They were found to have male external genitalia; both had testicles, and one had an undescended testicle and perineal hypospadias. They had one older sister and six brothers. At birth, both patients had had undescended testicles and a slightly enlarged, clitoral type penis, and thus they were reared as girls. Their hirsutism was diagnosed as normal male hair growth along with pubertal acne. They underwent plastic surgery for hypospadias, and were reidentified as boys.

A 19-year-old recently married woman presented with ambiguous genitalia (Fig. 33–16). She had Tanner stage I breast development and had recently undergone surgery for removal of bilateral undescended testicles from the lower inguinal region. She had perineal hypospadias and was unaware of being a male. She was the third wife of an Arab man and professed to be having anal coitus.

47,XXY/46,XY Mosaic With Ovotestes

An 18-year-old girl with well-developed breasts, primary amenorrhea, a vaginal dimple, and a tall, thin appearance was determined upon laparoscopy to have ovotestes. Diagnostic laparoscopy con-firmed an absent uterus with gonads. The fimbria of the fallopian tubes showed an abnormality. She was noted to have 46 XX,XY chromosomes. When removed, the gonads showed tissue of 40% testicular origin and 60% ovarian origin (Pandya G. Unpublished data) (Fig. 33–17).

Iatrogenic Trauma to the Penis

A young monk during his training period performed the ritual of rolling his penis on a stick (Fig. 33–18). This is done in an effort to stretch and destroy nerve endings and elastic tissue, preventing an erection and eliminating sexual desire.

Past and Future Perspectives

As age-old inhibitions against seeking medical care for young girls break down, many unique problems relating to abnormal genitalia and menstrual irregularities that previously remained hidden are being identified at regional medical centers throughout India and other underdeveloped countries. The reluctance of parents to seek medical care in the past was largely due to their fears of being unable to effect the customary "arranged marriage" for their daughter.

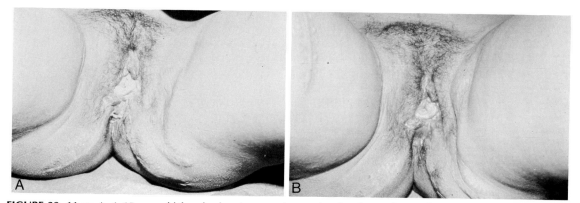

FIGURE 33–11 ••• *A, A 15-year-old female showing complete perineal and partial vaginal tear from the horn of a water buffalo. B, The perineal area of the same patient after surgical reconstruction.*

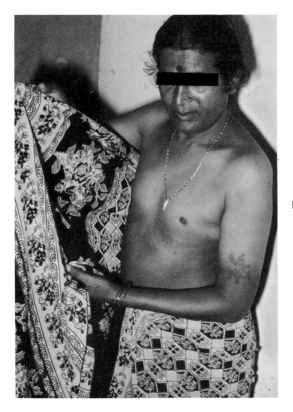

FIGURE 33–12 ••• A castrated Indian male known as a Hijras.

FIGURE 33–13 ••• Eunuch showing no breasts or genitalia.

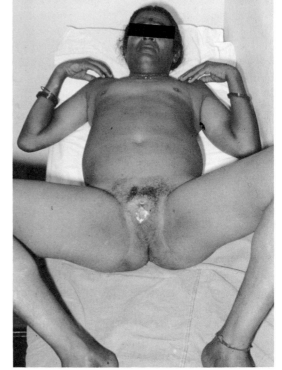

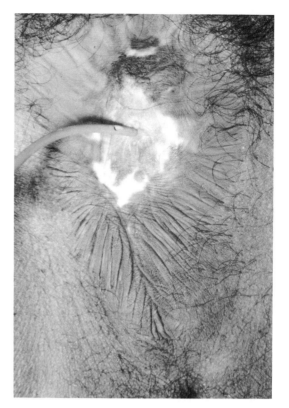

FIGURE 33–14 ••• Castrated male showing scar tissue with a small opening for a catheter for passage of urine.

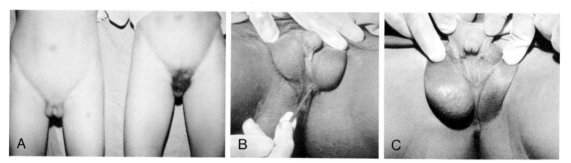

FIGURE 33–15 ••• A, Siblings reared as females showing male external genitalia. B and C, Their genital appearance is similar.

FIGURE 33–16 ••• A 19-year-old married woman showing ambiguous genitalia. She had Tanner stage I breast development and undescended testes.

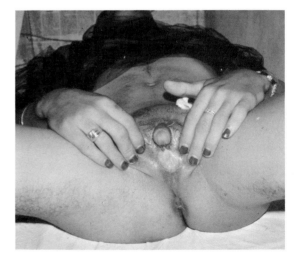

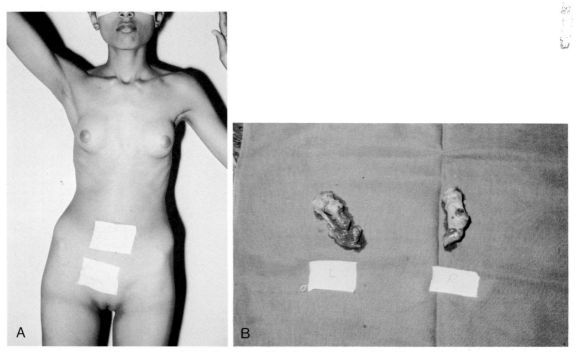

FIGURE 33–17 ••• *A*, An 18-year-old female showing tall height and well-developed breasts. *B*, Gross appearance of the gonads: 40% testicular and 60% ovarian.

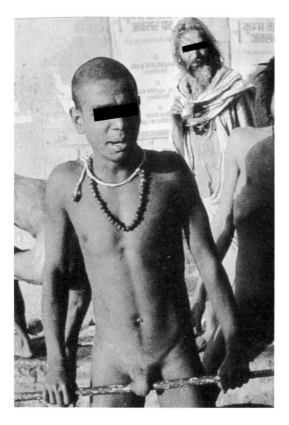

FIGURE 33–18 ••• Young monk showing ritualistic genital trauma from rolling his penis onto a stick.

TB continues to be responsible for a significant degree of chronic disease in India. It can manifest as exclusively genital TB with associated pubertal aberration and possible impaired fertility. Many unique problems have been presented.

The rituals associated with female circumcision in India and Africa remain a challenge for the pediatric/adolescent gynecologist caring for such patients. Genital mutilation, with its associated emotional and psychological sequelae, is currently being identified more often as these patients are evaluated.

Appropriate means of evaluation and treatment, including the psychosocial aspects of these disease processes, are of paramount importance in the management of this patient population.

References

1. Kochi A. Government intervention programs in HIV tuberculosis infection. Outline of guidelines for national tuberculosis control programs in view of the HIV epidemic. Bull Int Union Tuberc Lung Dis 1991; 66(1):33–36.
2. Bhaskara Rao KJ. Clinical aspect of genital tuberculosis in the female. J Obstet Gynecol India 1959; 10:26–31.
3. Malkani P, Banerji A. The role of tuberculosis in pathogenesis of sub-acute and chronic adnexitis. J Obstet Gynaecol India 1959; 10:32–42.
4. Oosthuizen A, Wessels P, Herfer J. Tuberculosis of the female genital tract in patients attending an infertility clinic. S Afr Med J 1990; 77(11):562–564.
5. Naik R, Srinivas C, Balachandran C, et al. Esthiomene resulting from cutaneous tuberculosis of external genitalia. Genitourin Med 1987; 63(2):133–136.
6. Tang L, Cho H, Wong T. Atypical presentation of female genital tract tuberculosis. Eur J Obstet Gynecol Reprod Biol 1984; 17(4):355–363.
7. Tripathy S, Tripathy S. Endometrial tuberculosis. J Indian Med Assoc 1987; 85(5):136–140.
8. Kumar N, Kapila K, Verma K. Cervical tuberculosis—case report. Aust NZ J Obstet Gynaecol 1989; 29(3pt 1):270–272.
9. Kalogirou D, Mantzavinos T, Zourlas P, Deligiorgi E. Primary adenocarcinoma of the fallopian tube with tuberculosis. Short communication. Eur J Gynaecol Oncol 1989; 10(5):307–309.
10. Carter J. Unusual presentations of genital tract tuberculosis. Int J Gynecol Obstet 1990; 33(2):171–176.
11. Durukan T, Urman B, Yarali H, et al. An abdominal pregnancy ten years after treatment for pelvic tuberculosis. Am J Obstet Gynecol 1990; 163(2):594–595.
12. Merchant R. Endoscopy in the diagnosis of genital tuberculosis. J Reprod Med 1989; 34(7):468–470.
13. Shah Hansa M. Genital tuberculosis—a study of 30 cases. J Obstet Gynecol Naecol India 1963; 13:374–381.
14. Stalworthy J. Genital tuberculosis in females. J Obstet Gynecol Naecol Br Emp 1952; 59:729–749.
15. Odujinrin O, Akitoye C, Oyediran A. A study of female circumcision in Nigeria. West Afr J Med 1989; 8(3):183–192.
16. DeSilva S. Obstetrical sequelae of female circumcision. Eur J Obstet Gynecol Naecol Reprod Biol 1989; 32(3):233–240.
17. El-Dareer A. Complications of female circumcision in the Sudan. Trop Doct 1983; 13(3):131–133.
18. Cutner LP. Female genital mutilation. Obstet Gynecol Surv 1985; 40(7):437–443.
19. Mukherjee J. Castration—a means of induction into the Hijras group of the Eunuch community in India. A critical study of 20 cases. Am J Forens Med Pathol 1980; 1(1):61–65.

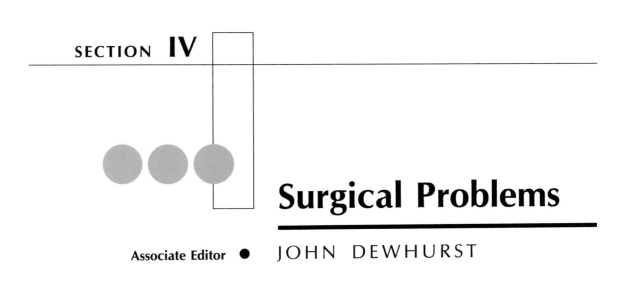

Surgical Problems

Associate Editor ● JOHN DEWHURST

○○○

CHAPTER 34

Genital Trauma

MARY E. RIMSZA

In this era of increasing awareness and concern about sexual abuse, genital trauma has become an important topic in pediatric and adolescent gynecology. Knowledge of the presentation, differential diagnosis, and management of genital trauma in children and adolescents is important for clinicians dealing with patients in this age group.

INCIDENCE

The incidence of genital trauma in children and adolescents is difficult to assess. Much of the literature on genital trauma consists of anecdotal case reports[1-5] or has been drawn from biased population samples, such as children who were evaluated for suspected sexual abuse.[6-11] A more accurate estimate of the true incidence of genital trauma would require a study of an unbiased population group, such as all children and adolescents presenting to an emergency department or a pediatric clinic.

ACCIDENTAL GENITAL INJURIES

Children and adolescents do occasionally sustain accidental injuries to the external genitalia. The most common form of accidental genital injury is a blunt injury caused by a fall across a dull object, such as a bicycle bar. The vagina, urethra, and hymenal areas are usually spared in these falls because of the protection

provided by the overlying labia. However, the external genitalia of the child are less protected against injury than those of the adult.[12] With most blunt injuries caused by a fall, the most prominent bruising will be on the surface that sustained most of the impact (i.e., the labia majora, mons pubis, and buttocks) (Table 34–1). Bruising, abrasions, and hematomas are the most typical injuries seen; lacerations are uncommon unless the child falls on a sharp object. The less superficial areas, including the urethra, the hymenal area, and the vagina, are usually not as prominently injured by blunt trauma. However, small tears, abrasions, and bruises can occur in these protected areas as well. The typical history given in cases involving blunt trauma is that the patient sustained a "straddle-type injury," meaning that they fell with the legs abducted onto a bar, fence, or bike. (Bicycle seats and center support bars are especially notorious sources of these injuries.)

Figure 34–1 demonstrates the kind of straddle injury that can occur following blunt trauma. This 8-year-old girl was brought to the pediatric clinic for evaluation after falling on

TABLE 34–1 ▪▪▪ EVALUATION AND TREATMENT OF STRADDLE INJURIES

Active bleeding
Ability to urinate
Extent of lesions
Decision regarding examination under anesthesia
Analgesics
Cold compresses

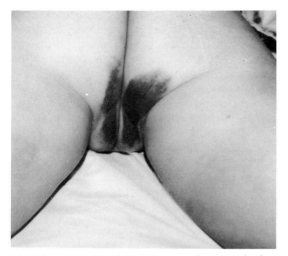

FIGURE 34–1 ••• Labial bruising extending onto the buttocks secondary to a straddle injury.

the edge of the bathtub as she was attempting to get out of the tub. She sustained a straddle-type injury with prominent bruising on the buttock. Figure 34–1 demonstrates the extensive bruising on the external aspect of the labia majora and extending onto the buttocks. There was also a small, clinically insignificant tear of the posterior fourchette, but no vaginal or hymenal injuries were noted. These traumatic lesions are consistent with the history provided. The photograph was taken approximately 8 hours after the injury. It is important to remember that bruises may not be present on external surfaces immediately after the injury, so a repeat examination at 24 hours is often helpful to determine whether the pattern of injury is compatible with the history.

West et al.[13] reported a series of 13 children who had sustained accidental vulvar injuries. Eight of the children had a straddle injury, three had a penetrating injury, and one had a stretch injury. The children with straddle injuries often had linear bruising like that demonstrated in Figure 34–1, usually located anteriorly over the labia.[13] Straddle injuries cause crushing of the soft tissue overlying bone or tendon and are also more likely to be anterior, perhaps because children are more likely to fall forward and have less superficial fat over the mons pubis compared with the buttocks.

With more severe accidental injuries, vulvar hematomas or lacerations may occur. The vulvar area and perineum are extremely vascular. Bleeding under the perineal skin results in a rounded, tense, tender swelling that varies in color from red to purple (Fig. 34–2). These children are usually examined soon after the injury because of the associated pain. Often the hymen and the vaginal area will be difficult to visualize because of swelling and tenderness in the vulvar area. Dysuria and local swelling may lead to urinary retention, and in some cases, it may be necessary to place a suprapubic catheter. If deeper injury is suspected, an examination under general anesthesia may be required. If so, consideration should be given to placement of a suprapubic catheter while the patient is anesthetized. Usually, however, bleeding is self-limited.

Treatment of vulvar hematomas is primarily expectant. Ice packs applied with pressure may be helpful in controlling the bleeding and limiting the size of the hematoma. Such cold compresses are of no value, however, after the first 24 hours. Muram recommends incision for a hematoma that is very large and/or continues to grow despite conservative therapy.[12] The clotted blood can be removed and the bleeding points indentified and ligated. If the source of the bleeding cannot be identified, the hematoma cavity can be packed with gauze and a firm pressure dressing applied; the pack can then be removed after 24 hours.[12]

Vulvar lacerations do not usually bleed excessively, but it should be remembered that even minor periurethral injuries can cause urethral spasm that may lead to urinary retention. Therefore, before any child with vulvar injuries is discharged home, it should be determined whether the child is able to void. Because injuries may extend into the urethra and bladder, examination of the urine for blood is also necessary. In West et al.'s series of 13 patients with accidental vulvar injuries, one child had hematuria.[13] Perineal abrasions and

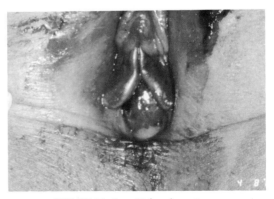

FIGURE 34–2 ••• Vulvar hematoma.

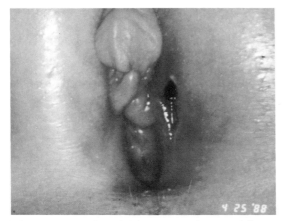

FIGURE 34–3 ••• Superficial tear secondary to a fall onto a stick.

tears may cause dysuria even in patients with no direct injury to the urethra. In these cases, an analgesic agent such as pyridium may be helpful for 2 to 3 days until these superficial abrasions are healed. Sitz baths may help relieve local pain, and increasing fluid intake may also be useful. If pain is persistent or severe, the possibility of a pelvic fracture should be considered.

Accidental vaginal injuries usually occur as the result of a penetrating injury. These internal injuries can be due to falls, especially if the child or adolescent falls on a pointed or sharp object such as a fence post (Fig. 34–3). Hymenal injuries are uncommon but may occur. The hymenal ring may be torn by penetrating injuries, but the bleeding that follows these hymenal injuries is usually minimal and requires no treatment. However, whenever the history or external genital examination suggests a penetrating injury, the possiblity of other serious injuries to the upper vagina and intrapelvic viscera must be ruled out. This will require both an examination under general anesthesia and appropriate repair.

Vaginal lacerations are often superficial and limited to the mucosal tissues. If suturing is necessary, a fine absorbable suture material should be used. Care should be taken to identify all bleeding points so that complete hemostasis can be achieved. If this is not done, a vaginal wall hematoma may develop. Such a hematoma can dissect into the submucosal tissue, causing intense pain. On examination of the vagina, a dark blue swelling of the vaginal wall will be noted.

If there is evidence that the upper vagina has been penetrated by a sharp object, the physician must rule out an extension of the tear into the broad ligament and the peritoneal cavity. An exploratory laparotomy is usually necessary in these cases. Examination of the urinary tract and bowel will be required to rule out injuries to these areas.

In rare instances, a large retroperitoneal hematoma may develop when a penetrating vaginal injury tears a major vessel above the pelvic floor. This can lead to a massive hemorrhage into the retroperitoneal space. The child may present in shock because of the amount of blood lost. These patients will require close observation and fluid replacement. Large hematomas may compress the ureters, leading to urinary retention. Large retroperitoneal hematomas will usually stop bleeding spontaneously as pressure increases. Exploratory laparotomy is rarely necessary to identify and control bleeding.[12]

Perineal injuries may extend to the anus and rectum. Black et al.[4] reviewed 16 cases of anorectal trauma in children seen in an emergency department setting. Most of the injuries were due to sexual abuse, but one child sustained a rectovaginal tear from a straddle injury. This was an 8-year-old girl who fell astraddle a baton, sustaining a rectovaginal tear that extended through the anal sphincter and distal rectal mucosa and across the perineum into the distal posterior vagina.[4] Similar injuries can also occur with severe motor vehicle trauma. Figure 34–4 demonstrates persistent scarring of the posterior fourchette suffered by a 3-year-old girl after a complete tear extending from the introitus through the rectal mucosa. She had fallen under a moving car, and tire marks were visible on her abdomen at the time of the initial injury. This photo-

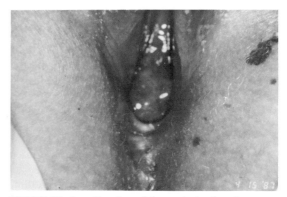

FIGURE 34–4 ••• Scarring of the posterior fourchette secondary to accidental trauma.

graph was taken 1 year after the injuries had been repaired. There have been other reports of anorectal injuries from "impalement" onto vacuum cleaner handles or fence posts.[14]

SPORTS INJURIES

Although a traditional argument against women's participation in sports has been the concern for injury of the genitalia and reproductive organs, such injuries are rare. The genital area statistically has the lowest incidence of injuries in women athletes,[15] and women's reproductive organs are obviously much better protected from injury than those of males who participate in sports. Garrick and Requa prospectively studied sports injuries in adolescent girls who participated in high school athletics over a 2-year period. There were 870 participant seasons in nine girls sports and 192 reported injuries. There were no injuries involving the breasts or genitalia. Gymnastics and softball had the highest injury rates.[16] Although vulvar hematomas and straddle injuries may occur in noncontact sports such as gymnastics, they are not common. Caine et al. conducted a prospective study of 50 highly competitive female gymnasts over a period of 1 year.[17] During this period, the 50 gymnasts amassed more than 40,000 hours of training and sustained 147 injuries, but no genital or groin injuries were reported.[17]

Bicycle-related genital injuries are also uncommon. In a retrospective study of 520 children between the ages of 1 and 18 who presented to an emergency department because of bicycle-related injuries, Selbst et al.[18] noted that only 4% of the patients sustained primary injuries to the genital area.

SEX-RELATED TRAUMA

Sexual activity is a common cause of genital injury in the adolescent. Vaginal lacerations may result from normal coital activity as well as from sexual assault.[19–21] Minor, sometimes microscopic, trauma to the vagina probably occurs frequently with vaginal intercourse. Such trauma most often involves the lower, posterior portion of the vagina. Norvell et al. conducted colposcopic examinations of the vulvovaginal area in 18 women within 6 hours of vaginal intercourse.[22] These patients were selected so that all other possible sources of

vaginal trauma were minimized; none of them were pregnant, bleeding or having menses, using any barrier contraceptive method, or having symptoms of vaginitis. These women were examined on two occasions. The first examination was performed after abstaining from vaginal intercourse for at least 72 hours. The second examination was done within 6 hours of vaginal intercourse. The examination was performed with the aid of a colposcope at $16 \times$ magnification. The introitus, hymen, and distal 2 cm of the vagina were inspected with both white light and a green filter. After the initial examination, the same area was stained with Lugol's solution diluted 1:6 with normal saline. The hymen, introitus, and distal vagina were again inspected both grossly and with the aid of a colposcope. After intercourse, 11 of the 18 women had positive findings consisting of microabrasions, telangiectasias, and broken blood vessels with small areas of fresh blood. The most common finding was telangiectasias, which were seen in 7 of the 11 patients with positive findings, whereas only two women had positive findings at the time of the first examination when they had abstained from intercourse for at least 72 hours. There were no cases in which the use of Lugol's solution aided in gross visualization of the microtrauma.[22]

Lauber and Souma used toluidine blue dye to aid in the identification of genital trauma after intercourse. Toluidine blue was used because it is a nuclear stain, and because normal vulvar skin contains no nuclei, it will not bind this dye. However, if there is a laceration to the vulva, deeper dermis that contains nuclei may pick up the stain. Two groups of patients (44 women total) were examined. The first group was evaluated within 48 hours of a sexual assault and the second group within 48 hours of consensual vaginal intercourse. A 1% solution of toluidine blue was applied to the posterior fourchette before examination. Ten (40%) of the 22 women who had been sexually assaulted had toluidine-positive lacerations of the fourchette. Only 2 of the 10 had visible lacerations before the application of the toluidine blue. In the second group of 22 women who were examined after consensual intercourse, only two had toluidine blue–positive staining. Both of these women were nulliparous and admitted to dry or painful intercourse.[23]

McCauley et al. reported on the use of toluidine blue staining in the detection of perineal lacerations in the pediatric and adolescent age group. Application of toluidine blue increased the detection rate of posterior four-chette tears from 4% to 28% in 25 sexually abused adolescent patients and from 16.5% to 33% in 25 sexually abused preadolescent patients ranging in age from 6 months to 10 years. Toluidine blue dye was also applied to the perineal area of 25 adolescent girls who had engaged in voluntary coitus within 48 hours of the medical examination. No posterior fourchette lacerations were noted in this group before the application of the dye, but 28% of these adolescents had visible lacerations after application of toluidine. This indicates that in adolescents, posterior fourchette lacerations are not diagnostic of sexual abuse, since lacerations were equally common in the sexually abused adolescent and the sexually active control group. A control group of 25 children who ranged in age from 1 to 7 years were also examined after application of toluidine blue. None of the girls in this control group had any lacerations noted either before or after application of the dye.[20]

The first large study on the use of colposcopy to identify genital trauma, particularly hymenal injuries, after sexual assault was done by Teixeira,[9] who conducted genital examinations in 500 patients who gave a history of sexual assault. The patients ranged in age from 4 to 51 years, and most were postpubertal. Colposcopic examinations were useful to clarify the hymenal injuries in 59 (11.8%) of the cases. This technique was most useful in examining children who had been assaulted and in diagnosing incomplete tears and fimbriated hymens. The most common location for hymenal tears or "ruptures" was in the posterior region of the hymen. These tears were often symmetric, which was helpful in distinguishing them from congenital notches. Forty-one patients had hymenal tears of recent origin. An attempt was made to determine the time period for healing of these hymenal tears. Unfortunately, only a few patients returned for follow-up colposcopic examinations; in these patients, the fastest healing period was 9 days, and the longest was 24 days. Other authors have reported healing periods ranging from 6 to 30 days.[9]

In Teixeira's study, vulvar coitus was noted to be associated with lesions on the posterior fourchette, as well as "partial ruptures" of the hymen.[9] These partial ruptures consisted of tears that did not completely transact the hymenal membrane and were only visualized with the aid of the colposcope.[9] This again emphasizes the importance of careful examination of the posterior fourchette for signs of trauma in suspected sexual abuse cases.

Some posterior fourchette tears may lead to labial and posterior fourchette adhesions. McCann et al. reported on six girls, ranging in age from 4 to 9 years, who had been sexually abused by their father, grandfather, and uncle.[24] All of the girls had labial adhesions/scars ranging in size from 2 to 10 mm.

Upper vaginal lacerations account for 75% of the genital injuries that require surgical repair. These injuries may occur as a result of penile impact or foreign bodies inserted into the vagina. Figure 34–5 demonstrates a large vaginal-hymenal tear caused by sexual abuse. This 12-year-old gave a history of incest involving vaginal penetration since the age of 8. There was also a history of vaginal bleeding after vaginal penetration. She had not received medical care for this injury. Lacerations can also be secondary to "home" abortions. Upper vaginal lacerations usually range in size from 3 to 5 cm and are primarily located posteriorly in the area of the right fornix.[19, 21, 25] It has been postulated that the right fornix is more often involved because it is larger than the left, since the cervix is often tilted toward the left fornix.[25] The primary clinical presentation is vaginal bleeding (80%) and pain (10%). In a series of 37 patients age 5 to 57 years who had coital injuries of the vagina, Wilson and Swartz noted that 19 had severe vaginal lacerations that required surgical repair. Seventeen had profuse vaginal bleeding, but only four complained of vaginal and lower abdominal pain. Ten of these patients required transfusions. The posterior cul-de-sac could be visualized through the vaginal wound in three

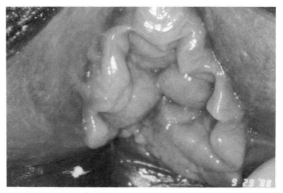

FIGURE 34–5 ••• Vaginal-hymenal tear secondary to sexual abuse. Note the disruption of the hymen at the lower margin of the photograph.

patients, and the peritoneum was ruptured in two.[25]

Deaths from exsanguination owing to vaginal lacerations have been reported.[19] Rarely, other pelvic organs are also injured, and the bowel, omentum, or fallopian tubes may eviscerate through the laceration.[19] Immediate management of these tears consists of control of hemorrhage, treatment of shock (if present), and repair of the injuries. Temporary control of the bleeding may be obtained by moist vaginal packings, which will tamponade the bleeding until more definitive repair can be accomplished.[19] Further examination is indicated to determine whether there are associated rectal injuries. Methylene blue or radiopaque contrast media may be instilled into the bladder to check for associated injuries. The bowel is usually not injured when the vaginal laceration is due to penetration of the vagina by a blunt object.[19] It has been estimated that approximately 1% of reported rape victims suffer genital injuries severe enough to require laceration repair.[21] Nulliparous women and women with abnormal vaginal anatomy resulting from either congenital anomalies or surgery may be at greater risk for vaginal lacerations.[19]

GENITAL LESIONS/INJURIES CONFUSED WITH TRAUMA

There are a number of genital conditions that may be confused with trauma. These include dermatologic conditions, congenital anomalies, infections, and normal variations in genital appearance (Table 34–2).[2, 26–30] The most common dermatologic condition confused with genital trauma is lichen sclerosus et atrophicus. This disease occurs most often in the vulvar and perianal areas of postmenopausal women. The etiology is unknown, although some researchers feel it may represent an autoimmune phenomenon.[27, 30] The initial lesions consist of ivory-colored macules that

coalesce to form homogeneous white atrophic plaques. The affected skin is sharply demarcated from the surrounding normal skin. Because this atrophic skin is fragile and easily traumatized, petechiae, bruises, and hemorrhage are noted after minimal pressure.[30] These children usually present for evaluation of possible sexual abuse because of the vulvar bleeding and/or the unusual appearance of the vulvar skin.

Chronic dermatitis involving the vulvar area can also be mistaken for trauma. If the skin is pruritic, self-induced excoriations may be mistaken for trauma, and in some cases the chronic changes associated with eczema, seborrhea, and psoriasis may be mistaken for scarring. Vulvar hemangiomas (Fig. 34–6) have also been confused with traumatic lesions of the external genitalia.[2]

With the advent of hymenal colposcopy, many genital lesions that previously went unrecognized have been reported. These lesions were first noted in a group of children who were examined because of suspected sexual abuse, and there was a tendency to attribute the findings to trauma. Fortunately, new studies have determined the incidence of a number of these findings in a normal population of girls who were carefully selected for nonabuse.[26] Periurethral bands are one common example of a normal variant that can be confused with trauma. These bands extend from the urethral meatus, creating a false pocket on either side of the urethra (Fig. 34–7). The periurethral pits created by these bands can be distinguished from traumatic penetrating wounds by their location adjacent to the urethra, their symmetry, and the lack of bruising or bleeding. Figure 34–3 shows a penetrating

TABLE 34–2 ••• GENITAL LESIONS CONFUSED WITH TRAUMA

Lichen sclerosus
Chronic dermatitis
Urethral prolapse
Urethral caruncles
Other bullous and ulcerative lesions

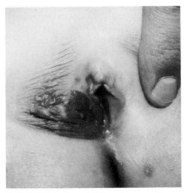

FIGURE 34–6 ••• Vulvar hemangioma.

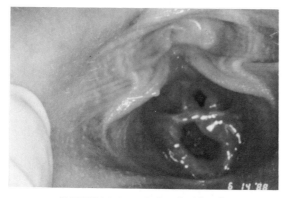

FIGURE 34–7 ••• Periurethral bands.

wound adjacent to the labia minora that has a similar appearance to these periurethral pits. McCann noted that these periurethral bands can be found in 50% of nonabused children with the aid of colposcopy.[26] Other anatomic variations that can be confused with trauma include congenital pits of the perineal body,[2] epispadias,[3] and perineal grooves.[31]

Urethral abnormalities may also be confused with genital trauma. Urethral prolapse and periurethral caruncles have been misdiagnosed as genital trauma.[2] Both of these conditions may initially present as vaginal bleeding, which can add to the diagnostic confusion.[29]

References

1. Baker RB. Seat belt injury masquerading as sexual abuse. Pediatrics 1986; 77:436.
2. Bays J, Jenny C. Genital and anal conditions confused with child sexual abuse trauma. Am J Dis Child 1990; 144:1319.
3. Reinhart MA. Sexual abuse of battered young children. Pediatr Emerg Care 1987; 3:36.
4. Black CT, Pokorny WJ, McGill CW, Harberg FJ. Ano-rectal trauma in children. J Pediatr Surg 1982; 17:501.
5. Finkel MA. Anogenital trauma in sexually abused children. Pediatrics 1989; 84:317.
6. Rimsza ME, Niggemann EH. Medical evaluation of sexually abused children: A review of 311 cases. Pediatrics 1982; 69:8.
7. Muram D. Child sexual abuse: Relationship between sexual acts and genital findings. Child Abuse Negl 1989; 13:211.
8. Paul DM. The medical examination in sexual offenses against children. Med Sci Law 1977; 17:251.
9. Teixeira WRG. Hymenal colposcopic examination in sexual offenses. Am J Forens Med Pathol 1981; 2:209.
10. Lindblad F, Ormstad K, Elinder G. Child sexual abuse: Physical examination. Acta Paediatr Scand 1989; 78:935.
11. Cartwright PS. The Sexual Assault Study Group. Factors that correlate with injury sustained by survivors of sexual assault. Obstet Gynecol 1987; 70:44.
12. Muram D. Genital tract injuries in the prepubertal child. Pediatr Ann 1986; 15:616.
13. West R, Davies A, Fenton T. Accidental vulval injuries in childhood. Br Med J 1989; 298:1002.
14. Fox PF. Impalement injuries of the perineum. Am J Surg 1951; 82:511.
15. Roy S, Irvin R. Sports Medicine. Englewood Cliffs, NJ: Prentice-Hall, 1983.
16. Garrick JG, Requa RK. Girls sports injuries in high school athletics. JAMA 1978; 239:2245.
17. Caine D, Cochrane B, Caine C, Zemper E. An epidemiologic investigation of injuries affecting young competitive female gymnasts. Am Sports Med 1989; 17:811.
18. Selbst SM, Alexander D, Ruddy R. Bicycle-related injuries. Am J Dis Child 1987; 141:140.
19. Elam AL, Ray VG. Sexually related trauma: A review. Ann Emerg Med 1986; 15:576.
20. McCauley J, Gorman RL, Guzinski G. Toluidine blue in the detection of perineal lacerations in pediatric and adolescent sexual abuse victims. Pediatrics 1986; 78:1039.
21. Geist RF. Sexually related trauma. Emerg Med Clin North Am 1988; 6:439.
22. Norvell MK, Benrubi GI, Thompson RJ. Investigation of microtrauma after sexual intercourse. 1984; 29:269.
23. Lauber AA, Souma ML. Use of toluidine blue for documentation of traumatic intercourse. Obstet Gynecol 1982; 60:644.
24. McCann J, Voris J, Simon M. Labial adhesions and posterior fourchette injuries in childhood sexual abuse. Am J Dis Child 1988; 142:659.
25. Wilson F, Swartz DP. Coital injuries of the vagina. Obstet Gynecol 1972; 39:182.
26. McCann J, Wells R, Simon MD, Voris J. Genital findings in prepubertal girls selected for nonabuse: A descriptive study. Pediatrics 1990; 86:428.
27. Handfield-Jones SE, Hinde FRJ, Kennedy CTC. Lichen sclerosis et atrophicus in children misdiagnosed as sexual abuse. Br Med J 1987; 294:1404.
28. McCann J, Voris J, Simon M, Wells R. Perianal findings in prepubertal children selected for nonabuse: A descriptive study. Child Abuse Negl 1989; 13:179.
29. Esposito JM. Circular prolapse of the urethra in children: A cause of vaginal bleeding. Obstet Gynecol 1968; 31:363.
30. Jenny C, Kirby P, Fuquay D. Genital lichen sclerosis mistaken for child sexual abuse. Pediatrics 1981; 83:597.
31. Shaw A, DeWitt GW. Picture of the month: Perineal groove. Am J Dis Child 1977; 131:921.

CHAPTER 35

○○○ # Sexual Developmental Anomalies and Their Reconstruction: Upper and Lower Tracts

D. KEITH EDMONDS

The development of the genital tract is a complex process that involves tissue differentiation and the development of the fallopian tubes, uterus, cervix, and vagina, all of which develop from the wolffian or paramesonephric ducts, and subsequent union of this embryologic process with the vulva, which develops from the cloaca. Congenital abnormalities of this system are more common than usually appreciated. However, a detailed knowledge of the embryology of this process is paramount to an ability to provide an accurate anatomic diagnosis and subsequent management of these disorders. The reader is referred to Chapters 1 and 2 before considering the management outlined in this chapter. Only by understanding the anatomic malformations and the psychological and sexual implications of the anomaly can the physician expect a successful outcome from his management. Surgery alone is inadequate in managing these patients, and a team of trained individuals whose skills involve psychosexual counseling, psychological support,

and social support is necessary for a successful long-term outcome.

EMBRYOLOGY

Sexual differentiation occurs as the end point of a number of maxims. The default state is that of the female form, and thus the development of the gonad into an ovary or a testis is fundamental to subsequent development. Failure of the development of a testis or failure of its function in producing testosterone will mean female phenotypic development. Conversely, the presence of androgen in a chromosomally normal female (i.e., 46,XX) will influence the external genitalia, as conversion of testosterone by 5α-reductase to dihydrotestosterone leads to masculinization of the cloaca. In the normal female, the ovary and müllerian ducts develop separately and independently. The cephalic portion of the müllerian duct develops into the fallopian tube, and the caudal end becomes the uterus after fusion of the müllerian bulbs on either side. These migrate to the midline, and fusion occurs at this point, leading to the development of the vaginal plate at the site of the cervix. Subsequent development of the vagina is considered in further detail in Chapter 1, but extension of the vaginal plate toward the normal developing female vulva eventually leads to a canalization process and creation of the vagina.

UPPER TRACT ANOMALIES

Uterus

Classification

There have been numerous classification systems used for uterine abnormalities.[1-3] All of these systems are descriptive and their necessity is obvious when comparing the management of different anomalies. Some of the classification systems have had a greater emphasis on the embryologic aspects of development; others have been based on obstetric performance, and still others on hysterosalpingographic findings. However, the classification system of Buttram and Gibbons[4] appears to be the most enduring. This system, shown in Fig. 35–1, describes six classes of müllerian anomalies but fails to take into account communicating uteri; a new classification for this type of uterus is noted in Fig. 35–2. This is a subclassification of Buttram and Gibbons' classes III and IV.[5, 6] Thus the classification system is complex, but using these two systems in combination provides some standardization of uterine anomalies.

Incidence

The incidence of uterine anomalies is really unknown. A large number of estimates exist, but discovery of uterine abnormalities depends on the diligence of the investigator and the techniques being used in the study population. In obstetric patients, the incidence of abnormalities ranges from 1 in 7[7] to 1 in 625,[3] but in an infertile population, the incidence of uterine abnormalities increases from between 1 in 100[8] to 1 in 20.[9] In patients who have recurrent abortions, the incidence of abnormal uteri is approximately 12%.[10, 11] The exact incidence of uterine malformations is almost certainly grossly underestimated, as the majority of patients do not have any disordered reproductive function and therefore never present with problems leading to consideration of a uterine abnormality.

Genetics

The genetic aspects of uterine anomaly presentation probably reflect failure of the developmental process at various stages. The apposition of the müllerian bulbs during their migration from the lateral pelvic side walls to the midline must be controlled at the level of various genes that determine not only such movement, but also subsequent uterine union and dissolution of the septum between the two müllerian systems. This involves the release of cellular components that induce this change. Failure of any part of this system will result in the septum being maintained at any level, and thus any variation from complete fusion to complete duplication of the system (bicornuate uterus with a double vagina) may occur, hence the classification seen earlier.

The exact location of the genes involved in müllerian development remains unknown and may be on an autosome or a sex chromosome. It is likely that the anomalies are acquired by a polygenic multifactorial inheritance giving a recurrence risk of between 1% and 5%.[12]

Associated Abnormalities

The association between müllerian abnormalities and abnormalities of other organ systems is well known, but the literature often omits any reference to this association. Renal abnormalities in patients with a didelphic uterus occur in about 9% to 12.5% of cases,[13, 14] but multiple malformation syndromes are also associated with incomplete müllerian fusion. Associations exist with hand-foot dysplasia,[15] Meckle syndrome,[16] and Rudiger syndrome,[17] and therefore extragenital malformations must alert the physician to the possible association with uterine abnormalities.

Presentation

Uterine abnormalities are usually asymptomatic, but often the condition is diagnosed after recurrent abortions, primary infertility, menstrual disorders, or exposure to diethylstilbestrol. Recurrent pregnancy wastage and primary infertility will not be considered here,

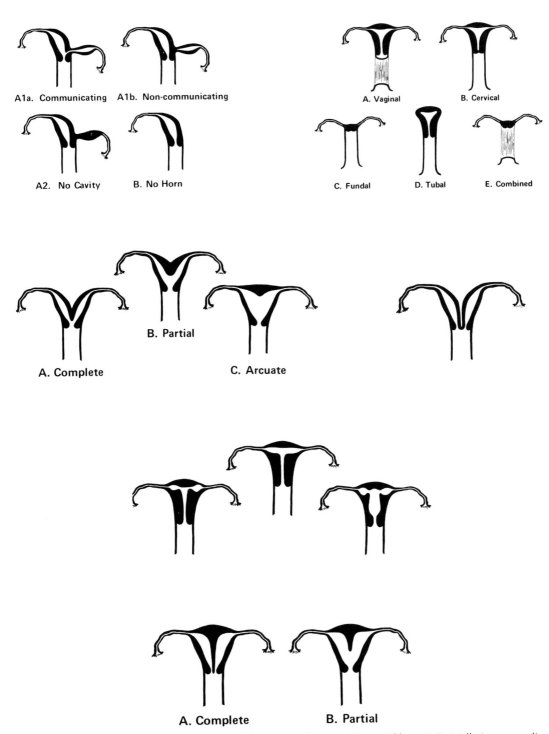

FIGURE 35–1 ••• Classification of uterine abnormalities. (From Buttram VC Jr, Gibbons WE. Mullerian anomalies: A proposed classification (an analysis of 144 cases). Fertil Steril 1979; 32:40–6. Reproduced with permission of the publisher, The American Fertility Society.)

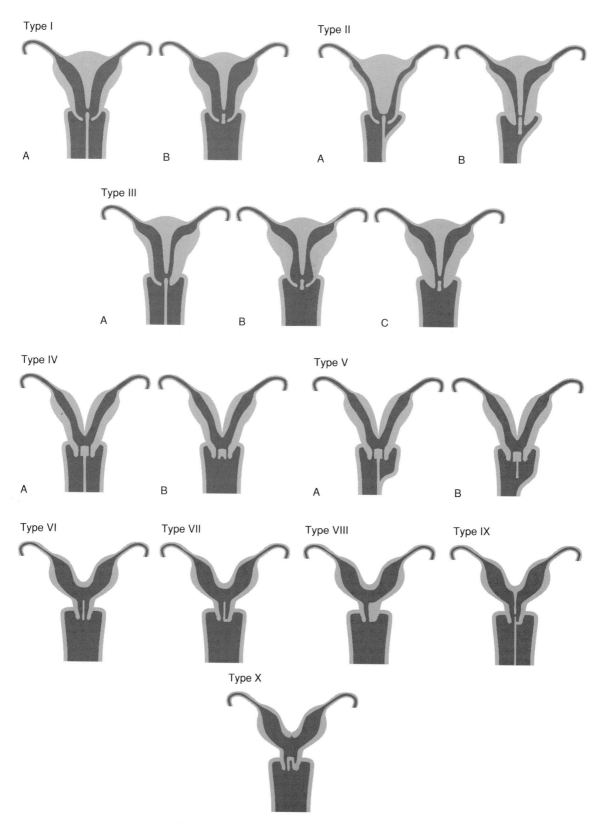

Type I A B

Type II A B

Type III A B C

Type IV A B

Type V A B

Type VI

Type VII

Type VIII

Type IX

Type X

FIGURE 35–2 ••• Classification of communicating uteri.

as they are rarely dealt with by clinicians with an interest in pediatric and adolescent gynecology. Menstrual disorders may well present in patients with uterine anomalies. Oligomenorrhea was found in 56% of patients with mild uterine abnormalities,[18] and it has been suggested that this may be the result of an abnormality in steroid receptor development in the malformed uterus.

Dysmenorrhea may also present as a uterine abnormality in patients with a rudimentary horn. This is secondary, as it begins before the onset of menses and persists throughout menstruation.

A wide variety of anomalies have been described in patients who present after exposure to diethylstilbestrol (DES).[19] Women exposed to DES were found to have a uterine abnormality in 41.6% of cases; these included hypoplasia, constriction, T-shaped hypoplastic abnormalities, and uni- and bicornuate abnormalities. Pregnancy outcome in women with these abnormalities is impaired, with pregnancy wastage estimated at between 37% and 60%.[19, 20] It is important to counsel such women regarding their reproductive performance in the future, although this is unlikely to be a major problem for the pediatric and adolescent gynecologist.

Diagnosis

The diagnosis of uterine anomalies may be made in a number of ways. It may be established at the time of curettage, although this is grossly inaccurate. Second, hysterosalpingography has long been the cornerstone of diagnosis of these abnormalities, although it is important to stress the experience of the radiologist or gynecologist in providing the correct interpretation of the hysterogram. Even with this technique it is often difficult to differentiate between a bicornuate and a septate uterus, and laparoscopy may be necessary to determine the uterine abnormality. At the time of laparoscopy, a septate uterus is indistinguishable from a normal one when viewed exteriorly, but a bicornuate uterus has a midline separation that may vary in depth. Because the management of the two anomalies is very different, the appropriate diagnosis must be established.

Diagnosis of uterine anomalies using ultrasound has been well described. In a study comparing real-time ultrasound with hysterosalpingography and surgical diagnosis of uterine abnormalities,[21] ultrasound was as accurate as hysterosalpingography in demonstrating the anomaly and provided a more complete assessment of the uterine cavity. Assessment was enhanced by using saline in the uterine cavity during the ultrasound examination. Thus hysterosalpingography and its associated discomfort may not be necessary to assess uterine shape.

Hysteroscopy. The use of hysteroscopy in the diagnosis of uterine abnormalities has become more popular. It provides an excellent view of the internal anatomy of the uterus, thus allowing direct assessment of any septum that may exist.

Surgical Management

Surgical management of uterine anomalies is unusual during adolescence, as the manifestations are usually related to reproductive ability. The presence of uterine abnormalities as a cause of dysmenorrhea is the only reason for treatment.[22]

Rudimentary Uterine Horn. A rudimentary uterine horn (Fig. 35–3) causing dysmenorrhea in an adolescent may require surgical removal. This procedure is relatively straightforward, and the remaining unicornuate uterus does not impair subsequent fertility. Relief of dysmenorrhea may be marked.

Metroplasty. Three basic procedures have been described for treatment of the bicornuate and septate uterus. Strassman's operation advocates a transverse incision on the superior aspect of the fundus; this is extended inferiorly until both uterine horns are exposed on their inner surface. The septum is then excised and the uterine horns reunited, as shown in Figure 35–4.

In the Jones metroplasty, a wedge-shaped incision is made, removing the uterine septum with the wedge (Fig. 35–5) and reuniting the uterus. However, this operation has not become popular because of the difficulty in identifying the line of incision, thereby resulting in a considerable reduction in intrauterine space.

The third procedure is that described by Tompkins (Fig. 35–6), which involves a vertical incision in the fundus of the uterus down the center of the septum until the cavity is reached. This is relatively bloodless, and the cavities can then be exposed through lateral incisions and the uterus reunited. Strassman's

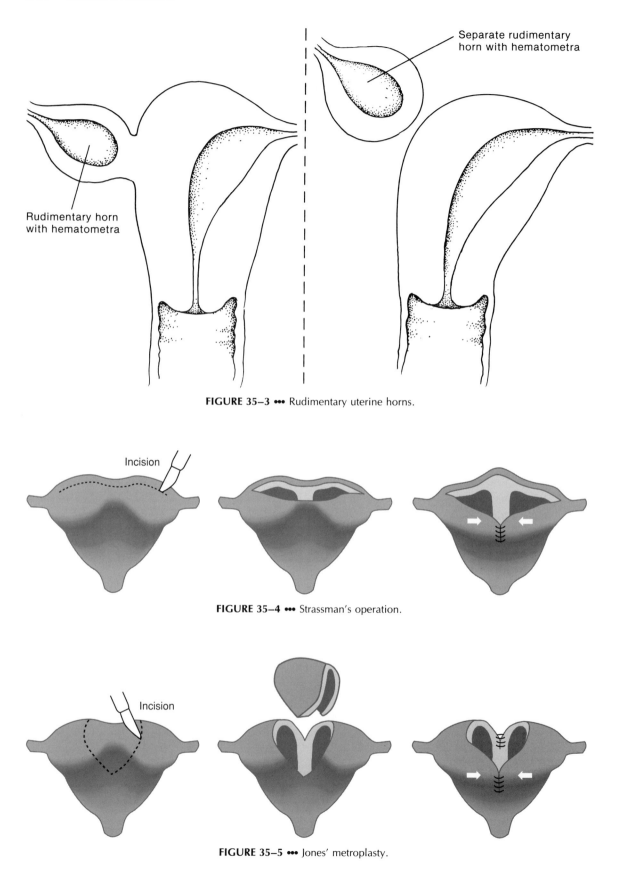

FIGURE 35–3 ••• Rudimentary uterine horns.

Separate rudimentary horn with hematometra

Rudimentary horn with hematometra

Incision

FIGURE 35–4 ••• Strassman's operation.

Incision

FIGURE 35–5 ••• Jones' metroplasty.

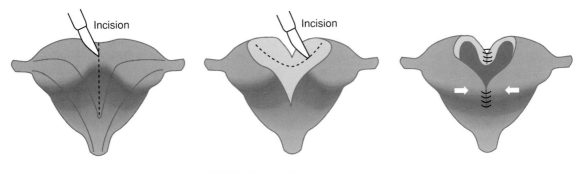

FIGURE 35–6 ••• Tompkins' metroplasty.

procedure is the most feasible operation for a bicornuate uterus and the Tompkins open laparotomy for the septate uterus.

Hysteroscopic Metroplasty. The ability of the hysteroscope to visualize the uterine cavity allows its use as an operating instrument to incise the uterine septum. This may be done either with an operating resectoscope[23] or with a laser.[24] The septum is incised from below, and as it is removed, it retracts, leaving the cavity united. Resectoscopic scissors[24] have also been used to divide the septum in the midline and then allow it to retract. The hysteroscopic approach to metroplasty is useful if the septum is no more than 1 cm thick.

Cervix

Congenital absence of the cervix, an extremely rare condition, consists of a functional uterus with failure of development of the uterine cervix. The true diagnosis of cervical atresia requires absence of the vagina, as embryologically the upper part of the vagina cannot develop without the development of the cervix. In the literature there are many reports of an absent cervix in conjunction with an existing vagina. In one series, a normal vagina was present in 75% of cases.[25] It would therefore seem that there is some debate in the use of the term *absent cervix* to mean aplasia or agenesis of the cervix. Complete absence would seem to indicate a hypoplastic or rudimentary cervix, whereas the term *cervical atresia* should be used to mean total absence of the cervix.

The incidence of this condition is unknown, with a total of only 58 cases described.[25, 26]

Because the treatment for this condition traditionally has been hysterectomy, it may well be that it is underreported. These patients primarily present with cyclical abdominal pain in the absence of menstruation, usually between the ages of 13 and 17 years, although one patient is reported to have presented at age 31.[25, 26]

A number of other malformations have been described in association with cervical atresia; the extragenital anomalies are similar to those associated with an absent vagina and primarily relate to the renal tract (e.g., renal agenesis, hypoplasia, and duplication of the collecting system).[27]

The diagnosis is often difficult to establish. In most cases diagnosis is made at laparotomy with discovery of a hematometra but with no definitive cervix and the vagina and transverse vaginal septum absent. Currently, preoperative ultrasonography can delineate the absence or presence of a cervix and can easily demonstrate the upper transverse vaginal septum and the open cervix. An absent cervix produces an image of an echogenic uterus without a cervix or vagina. One report[28] describes the use of magnetic resonance imaging (MRI) in the diagnosis of cervical atresia concomitant with vaginal agenesis. Again, both ultrasound and MRI can be used to assess the anomaly before a surgical procedure is performed.

Management

When cervical atresia is present in conjunction with a functioning endometrium, surgical treatment is of paramount importance, as the hematometra must be drained and the development of pelvic endometriosis must be avoided. A number of authors have advocated hysterectomy with ovarian conservation as the primary procedure[26, 29]; the possibility of pregnancy is remote, and success from procedures to preserve the uterus has been negligible. Rock et al.[29] advocate hysterectomy as the absolute treatment of choice. However, this has been disputed by a number of authors, [27, 30] and adaptation of techniques for preserving a functional uterus and creating a persistent fistula from the endometrial cavity into the neovagina has been described. The procedure is performed by a combined abdominal and vaginal approach. The neovagina may be created in a number of ways.

A Pfannenstiel incision is made abdominally to expose the hematometra and absent cervix. The absence of the cervix results in the two uterine arteries lying essentially in apposition, and great care must be taken to identify them before creating the fistula. The bladder is reflected inferiorly and the upper part of the vagina exposed from above. This is then incised to create a vaginal orifice. The uterus is incised longitudinally on its anterior surface and the incision extended between the uterine arteries to create the fistulous space. A stent is then placed from the fundus of the uterus through the fistulous aperture into the vagina. A number of different stents have been used; I prefer a No. 14 Foley catheter. The stent is sutured in place with a slowly dissolving suture material, and the uterus is reconstructed over the stent. The paracervical fascia is brought to lie anteriorly so that the fistulous space is covered, thereby preventing trauma to the bladder base. The upper part of the vagina is sutured to the lower part of the uterus, taking great care to avoid the major vessels. The abdomen is then closed in the traditional manner. The catheter remains in place for 6 to 8 weeks and is usually expelled spontaneously as the suture dissolves. Menstruation may occur through the fistulous space before the catheter's removal, with the blood escaping through the cavity in the catheter. This operation has been performed 11 times in patients with congenital absence of the cervix, and regular menstruation has been achieved in nine cases.[31] The remaining two patients required subsequent hysterectomy.

Outcome

Conservation of the uterus in any woman provides a major psychological boost, and the described cases of pregnancy following this procedure justify an attempt at preservation. The first two cases of pregnancy[32, 33] were reported some time ago, but in 1990 a third case was reported of spontaneous pregnancy and delivery by cesarean section.[34] Another report[35] describes the successful use of zygote intrafallopian tube transfer (ZIFT) in a patient with congenital cervical atresia following a fistulous drainage procedure. Thus, the newer assisted reproduction techniques may further enhance the ability of these women to conceive, as their ovaries are totally normal.

LOWER TRACT ANOMALIES

Vagina

Developmental abnormalities of the vagina may be classified into two groups: those disorders in which there is congenital absence of the vagina with or without the presence of a functional uterus, and disorders that are obstructive in nature, being anomalies of either vertical or transverse fusion.

Congenital Absence of the Vagina

Incidence. The incidence of vaginal malformation has been variously estimated at between 1 in 4000 and 1 in 20,000 female births.[36, 37] This is difficult to ascertain because of its low frequency of presentation. However, as a cause of primary amenorrhea, it is second only to gonadal dysgenesis.[38]

Etiology. The etiology of this condition remains speculative. In its most common presentation (i.e., the presence of remnants of the müllerian duct and an absent vagina), it is known as the Mayer-Rokitansky-Küster-Hauser syndrome. These individuals lack a vagina and have either complete absence of the uterus, an extremely rudimentary uterus, or rudimentary uterine horns lying on the lateral pelvic side wall. There are two aspects of the etiology that are interesting to comment on:

1. Whether there is any familial trait involved in the mechanism of vaginal absence remains to be clarified, but congenital absence has been described in 46,XX siblings[39] and in one set of monozygotic twins.[40]
2. It is more likely that the inheritance of this disorder is a polygenic multifactorial one. The suggestion that this condition was a female

limited autosomal dominant trait[41] was the impetus for beginning a study to determine whether probands would in fact manifest the same abnormalities. This study[42] failed to report affected relatives and thereby disproved the previous theory. The polygenic multifactorial inheritance theory is a much more likely one, as the recurrence risk in first-degree relatives with these abnormalities is reported to be between 1% and 5%. The additive affect of several genes interacting with genetic and environmental factors and therefore leading to this mode of inheritance is the most likely etiology.

Associated Anomalies. Vaginal atresia is associated with urinary tract defects in 40% of cases when all urinary tract abnormalities are considered. Some 15% of patients with the Mayer-Rokitansky-Küster-Hauser syndrome suffer major defects of the urinary tract, including absence of a kidney or the presence of a pelvic kidney. In view of this high incidence of renal tract abnormalities, all patients diagnosed as having absence of the vagina should undergo an abdominal ultrasound to determine whether two kidneys are present. If the ultrasound fails to delineate a normal urinary system, an intravenous pyelogram should be performed as the final definitive procedure.

Skeletal abnormalities are also commonly found in patients with Mayer-Rokitansky-Küster-Hauser syndrome (i.e., some 12% of cases).[43] Two thirds of the abnormalities involve the spine, and limb and rib abnormalities account for the majority of the remainder. The vertebral abnormalities include wedge vertebrae, rudimentary vertebral bodies, and supernumerary and asymmetric vertebrae. There is an association with the Klippel-Feil syndrome (congenital fusion of the cervical spine, short neck, low posterior hair line, and painless limitations of cervical movement) although the incidence is low.[44]

A number of other abnormalities have been described in association with vaginal atresia, although their low incidence rates suggest that they are incidental rather than associated.

Ovarian Function. Studies that have been performed on patients with congenital absence of the cervix have failed to demonstrate any abnormalities in endocrine function. Endocrinologically, the menstrual cycle is of normal length, and hypothalamic control of gonadotropin release is also normal.[45] One report describes successful stimulation and retrieval of oocytes from a patient with the Mayer-Rokitansky-Küster-Hauser syndrome with a view to fertilization of these oocytes and subsequent surrogacy.[46]

Diagnosis. Congenital absence of the vagina is usually not suspected until puberty, when primary amenorrhea occurs. Secondary sexual characteristics develop normally and at the appropriate time, as ovarian function is normal; as a result, detection of the absent vagina may be delayed, as the clinician may not associate the presence of secondary sexual characteristics with vaginal absence. The diagnosis is confirmed by clinical examination, which reveals a vaginal dimple in an otherwise normal vulva. Ultrasound examination of the pelvis can determine the presence of a rudimentary uterus, an absent uterus, or small, nonfunctional uterine horns on the lateral pelvic side wall. A case of functional anlage has been described with the two hemiuteri lying on the lateral pelvic side walls but the uterus absent.[47] Fibroids have been described in the rudimentary uterus[48]; if they enlarge, excision may be necessary.

Examination under anesthesia and using laparoscopy is unnecessary to establish the diagnosis.

Management. The history of attempts to form a vagina spans from ancient times to the present.[49] The Romans discussed management of the absent vagina, and Celsus described the operation for the creation of a new vagina.[49] Soranus, a Greek, described this operation around 100 A.D.[49] During the next 1500 years there were several references to the operation in Muslim literature, primarily by Avicenna (980–1037).[49] The first recorded case of absence of the vagina and uterus is often attributed to Matteo Realdo Columbo, but the description is vague at best. By the nineteenth century, a number of surgeons had attempted a vaginoplasty, including Dorsey (1783–1818) and Dupuytren (1717–1835).[49] The use of split-thickness skin grafting was pioneered by Robert Abbe,[50] and although his first case was a failure, he persevered to develop a successful operation. Around the turn of the century a number of surgeons, including Baldwin,[51] described success using transposed intestine, but the greater complexity and morbidity of this procedure require that it be used only for the most difficult cases. The first description of a simple nonsurgical technique was by Frank,[52] who used glass dilators to create a satisfactory vagina for coitus. New grafting techniques,[53] tissue expanders,[54] and endoscopic procedures currently are being used for this purpose.

Psychological Aspects. The psychological impact of an absent vagina is immense both to the girl and to her parents. The initial interlude of shock is followed by a prolonged period of depression when many patients question their femininity and view themselves as human freaks. They have serious doubts as to their ability to maintain a heterosexual relationship, even though they have been told that sexual intercourse will almost certainly be possible. The most difficult aspect they have to cope with is the problem of their sterility, and often they never come totally to terms with this difficulty. They resent the fact that they are not able to try to conceive, and thus their situation is completely different from infertile couples who fail in their attempts to conceive, despite their best efforts.

The parents feel guilty and responsible for their daughter's abnormality. They often inquire as to whether difficulties during the pregnancy may have predisposed to the problem, but they should be reassured that there is no evidence for this. They also need reassurance as to their daughter's ability to have a normal sex life.

Cultural problems may arise that make management difficult. In some ethnic groups, the ability to procreate is fundamental to marriage and social acceptance, and the absence of a vagina and its associated sterility can mean total isolation. These patients and their parents can be almost impossible to console, refusing to accept the situation and in some cases contemplating suicide.

It is not surprising that the patients and their parents often request immediate surgery to return them to "normal." However, this is a major mistake unless adequate psychological and physical preparation is carried out. A recommended minimum of 6 months of preparation time is required before any attempts at vaginal surgery are pursued; ideally, a heterosexual relationship should be established. It is extremely important that these patients and their parents have adequate psychological support before embarking on any therapy.

During this period of adjustment, counseling can be extremely difficult. These teenagers may be reactionary because of normal adolescence, and the impact of this major congenital abnormality on their sexuality can be immense. Management of their loss of self-esteem and inevitable depression requires counseling with properly trained personnel who are familiar with the problems of patients with an absent vagina. Unfortunately, few psychologists have this expertise, and their inability to understand these difficulties makes counseling sometimes inadequate or inappropriate. It is important that gynecologists involved in the care of these patients have meaningful discussions with the counselors so that they are fully conversant with the situation and able to manage these patients appropriately.

A second problem involves psychosexual counseling and the difficulties associated with sexual behavior in the absence of a vagina. The counseling of these girls involves reestablishment of the belief that a sex life will be possible, and they must be advised and reassured that they have a normally functioning clitoris and therefore are quite capable of orgasm. However, a very careful choice of words is necessary, and the word "artificial" must be avoided when referring to the vagina. It is important that these girls understand the normality of their created vagina and the fact that they will experience the same feelings as females with a normally formed vagina. Equally difficult is the understanding that their vagina will feel normal to their partners, and therefore counseling should involve the heterosexual partner so that he also understands the difficulties associated with a neovagina.

The fear of failure both sexually and reproductively may take years or even a lifetime to overcome. Thus psychological counseling must begin before any attempt to form a vagina, and the best results accrue from therapy carried out during a stable relationship. Girls who are appropriately managed can achieve a completely normal sex life comparable to that of the normal population.[55]

Frank's Procedure. This is the technique of choice in all cases of congenital absence of the vagina and of a functional uterus. This nonsurgical technique involves the repeated use of graduated vaginal dilators over a period of 6 to 12 weeks (Fig. 35–7) It is important for the patient to become familiar with her own anatomy, and in most cases, these girls have never explored their anatomy because they have never menstruated, and therefore it has never been necessary. They are completely unfamiliar with the position of their vagina in relationship to the vulva and need to be taught digital exploration before the use of the dilator. Once they are familiar with this, the tip of the smallest dilator is placed in the appropriate

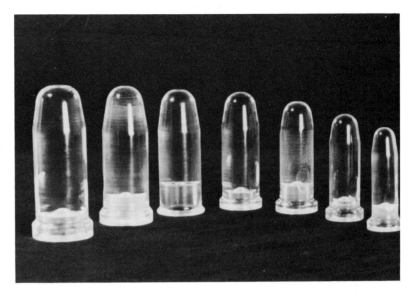

FIGURE 35–7 ••• Frank's dilators.

position on the dimple of the vagina with the patient pressing steadily in the direction of the normal vagina (i.e., 30 degrees posteriorly). This is done for 20 minutes, three times a day, and the pressure should not cause any pain. Occasionally a lubricant may be used to facilitate the insertion of the vaginal dilator and make it more comfortable. It is extremely important that instruction be given by personnel who are totally familiar with the technique and in an atmosphere of commitment. Close supervision is necessary for the first 3 to 4 days, and by doing this, patients are able to progress through the first three sizes of dilators within 4 to 5 days of commencement. A modified bicycle seat has been recommended to facilitate the procedure (Fig. 35–8). The patient should then be seen regularly, at least every 2 weeks, to ensure that she is continuing the use of the dilator. Sexual intercourse may be attempted at any stage during therapy, and patients are encouraged to involve themselves with their partners in sexual discovery. The results are usually very gratifying; over 6 to 8 weeks the girls progress to a No. 5 dilator, which is adequate for most sexual practices. In the largest series reported so far,[55] 78 patients were subjected to this dilator regimen, and 80% were sexually functional within 3 months of commencing therapy. By applying good psychological management and encouraging the use of dilators, this can be a highly successful and perhaps the most appropriate form of therapy for patients with the Mayer-Rokitansky-Küster-Hauser syndrome. For girls who fail to achieve a functional vagina with this

technique, surgery is required. The two most common types of vulvovaginoplasty are the McIndoe split-thickness skin graft technique and the amnion vaginoplasty.

McIndoe Vaginoplasty. This technique was first described in 1938 by McIndoe and Banister,[56] although split-thickness skin grafts had been used previously by Abbe.[50] As in the amnion vaginoplasty, the initial part of the procedure is to place the patient in the lithotomy position and make a transverse incision in the middle of the vaginal dimple. A neovaginal space is created digitally in the connective tissue lying between the bladder and the rectum (Fig. 35–9). It is imperative that digital exploration be performed with the fingers moving in a lateral and posterior direction. No exploration should be performed in the direction of the bladder or the rectum, as damage to these structures is extremely easy. As the peritoneum of the pouch of Douglas is approached, a median raphe is encountered; it is imperative that this be divided so that subsequent retraction of the vagina does not occur in the midline. When a neovaginal space of adequate depth is achieved, hemostasis must be obtained. A soft vaginal mold (stent) of foam rubber is then made and individualized for each patient. This use of a soft mold rather than a solid mold is known as the Counsellor and Flor modification of the McIndoe technique.[57] A split-thickness skin graft is then obtained from a donor site using an electrodermatome (Fig. 35–10). The vaginal mold is then covered with a condom and the skin graft placed skin side down over the mold and

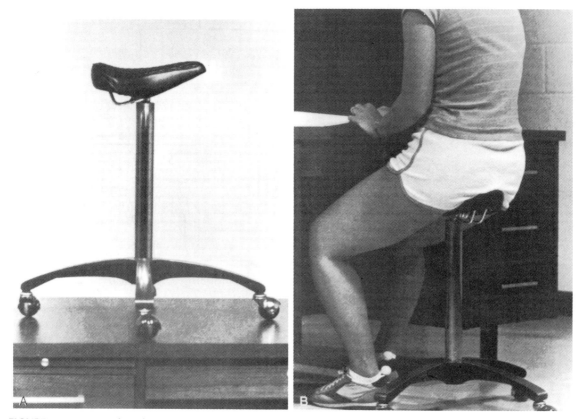

FIGURE 35–8 ••• *A,* A bicycle seat stool. *B,* The patient sits on the stool, leaning forward slightly with the dilator held in place by a light girdle, for at least 2 hours each day. (From Ingram JM. The bicycle seat stool in the treatment of vaginal agenesis and stenosis: A preliminary report. Am J Obstet Gynecol 1981;140:867–871.)

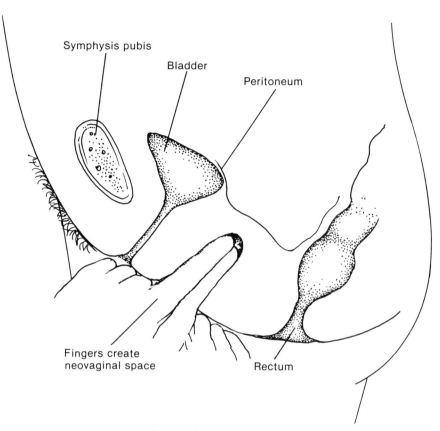

Symphysis pubis

Bladder

Peritoneum

Fingers create
neovaginal space

Rectum

FIGURE 35–9 ••• Digital creation of the neovaginal space.

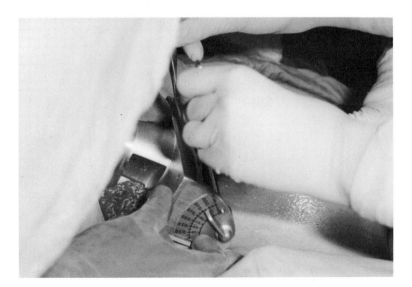

FIGURE 35–10 ••• Split-thickness
skin graft.

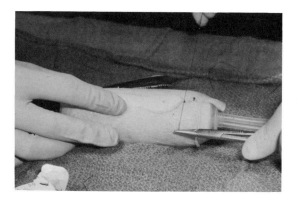

FIGURE 35–11 ••• Vaginal mold.

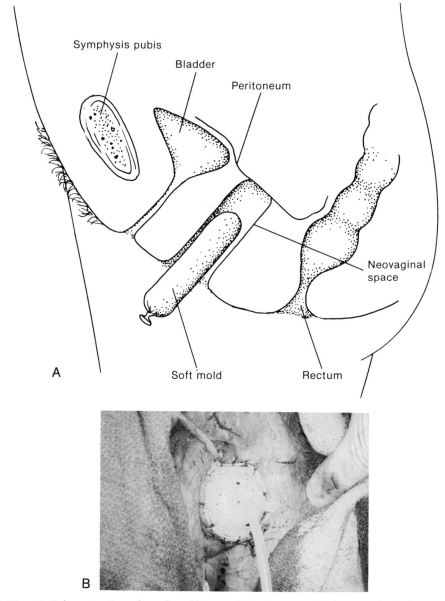

Symphysis pubis

Bladder

Peritoneum

Neovaginal space

A

Soft mold

Rectum

B

FIGURE 35–12 ••• *A,* Schematic view of a soft mold inserted into the neovaginal space. *B,* At the completion of the procedure, the mold is shown within the neovagina.

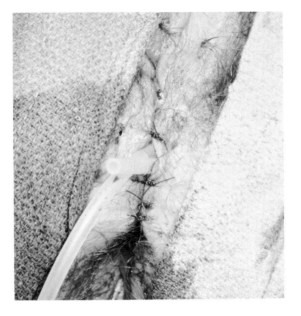

FIGURE 35–13 ••• Neovagina showing interrupted silk sutures placed between the labia to hold the mold in place.

sutured to fit (Fig. 35–11). The mold is then inserted in the neovagina (Fig. 35–12) and interrupted silk sutures are placed between the labia to hold the mold in place (Fig. 35–13). An indwelling catheter should be placed in the urethra to prevent pressure and allow free urinary drainage. The mold is removed 7 days later under general anesthesia and the vaginal cavity irrigated. A second soft rubber mold is then placed in situ, and the patient is taught to remove the mold and douche daily, with the mold remaining in place for 6 weeks (Fig. 35–14). Following this, she is taught to use vaginal dilators until the healing process is complete, usually 3 months.

The results of the McIndoe vaginoplasty seem very satisfactory. About 85% to 95% of all procedures result in a sexually functional vagina.[58–60] Before the introduction of the soft mold technique, some serious complications existed because of the pressure and associated necrosis produced by the solid mold. However, the introduction of the soft mold eradicated these complications, and 75% of patients can expect a 100% graft take. To avoid infection, antibiotics are routinely used during the perioperative and postoperative periods.

Amnion Vaginoplasty. In this technique, amnion is substituted for the skin graft. The disadvantage of the McIndoe procedure is the anatomic scar remaining at the skin graft site. If this is to be avoided, a different epithelial-

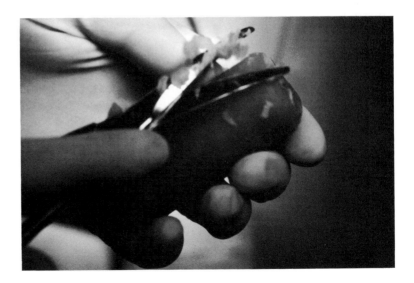

FIGURE 35–14 ••• Soft rubber mold placed in situ.

izing promoter must be used. The use of amnion was first described in 1934[61] and subsequently has been reported by a number of authors.[62, 63] The technique involves the creation of the neovaginal space as previously described and the insertion of a soft vaginal mold covered with amnion obtained from a donor at the time of elective cesarean section. The mesenchymal surface of the amnion is placed against the new vaginal surface to promote epithelialization. The amnion mold is replaced after 7 days and a new amnion cover inserted for another week. Thereafter, patients are encouraged to frequently use dilators to maintain the neovaginal passage.

Again, a high degree of success in terms of sexual function has been achieved with this technique (i.e., about 85% for published series).[60, 61] However, 25% of patients report dyspareunia owing to scarring of the upper margin of the vagina that involves the peritoneum. Similar instances of dyspareunia have been reported in nearly all series of vaginoplasty, and it seems to occur regardless of technique. The artificial vagina created in this way acquires the characteristics of normal vaginal epithelium, although there is no increase in estrogen receptors at the new site.[64] The artificial vagina is susceptible to malignant change, and intraepithelial neoplasia[65] and squamous cell carcinoma[66, 67] have been described. Girls who are sexually active following vaginoplasty should be viewed by their health screeners as having a risk of malignant change equal to that of those with a functional cervix. It is therefore recommended that a vault smear, similar to a Pap smear, be obtained on a regular basis (i.e., every 3 years).

Prolapse of the neovagina following Frank's procedure has been described.[68] This may be managed by sacrocolpopexy in the manner used for a recurrent enterocele, as this prolapse is actually an enterocele. Condylomata acuminata have also been described in the neovagina.[69]

Other Operative Procedures

Use of Bowel. Earlier in this century the use of bowel as a substitute for the vagina was extremely popular. The introduction of skin grafting techniques has made this procedure less frequently performed, but it is still necessary in cases in which inadequate space exists between the rectum and the urethra to create an adequate neovagina using traditional techniques. Various parts of the ileum and colon have been used, although the cecum or sigmoid colon is used most commonly.

A segment of the bowel to be used is dissected free with its vascular pedicle and, after creation of the neovaginal space, is transected and swung on its pedicle to lie in apposition to the vulva at one end. It is then sutured in place along with the upper cut edge. A reanastomosis of the remaining bowel is then performed, concluding the procedure. A number of authors have reported success,[70] but all accept the complication of excessive mucous discharge in a considerable number of patients. Functionally, however, this is an extremely useful technique in a number of circumstances.

Davydov Operation. The procedure described by Davydov and Zhvitiashvili[71] involves the use of pelvic peritoneum to line the neovaginal space (Fig. 35–15). The neovaginal space is created in the traditional way (see Fig. 35–9) and the peritoneum identified. An abdominal incision is then made, and the peritoneum is dissected from its interstitial pelvic tissue, then pulled down through the neovagina (Fig. 35–16), sutured to the introitus, and the upper portion closed over a peritoneal lining to the neovagina (Fig. 35–17). Dilators must be used subsequently to avoid constriction.

Williams Vulvovaginoplasty. This procedure, first described in 1964,[72] is still useful for those cases when dissection of a neovagina is impossible. The technique involves the creation of a vulvar pouch from the labia majora (Fig. 35–18), which allows a normal sex life and orgasm. However, it also involves surgical mutilation of a previously normal vulva, with the consequent psychological disadvantages. The operation has been reported to be very successful.[73]

The Flap Vaginoplasty. This procedure has two forms. The first is a simple flap technique,[74] as shown in Figure 35–19, in which two flaps of skin are mobilized from the labia through incisions and swung on their base into the neovaginal space, a tubular structure having previously been created by the union of the anterior and posterior surfaces of the flaps.

The second technique involves the use of a donor site in the scapular region with mobilization of this donor skin flap and its vascular supply. This is then formed into a skin-lined tube and transferred to the neovagina, with the vascular supply being anastomosed to the major vessels in the inguinal region.[75]

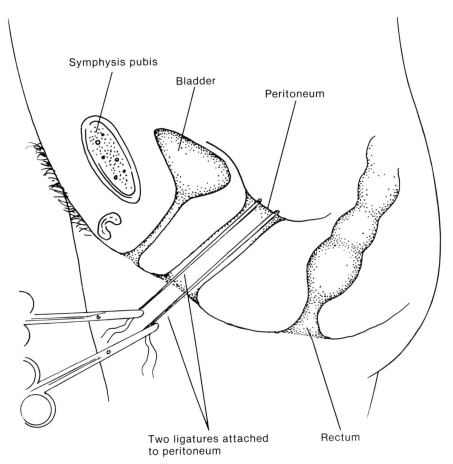

FIGURE 35–15 ••• The use of peritoneum in the Davydov operation.

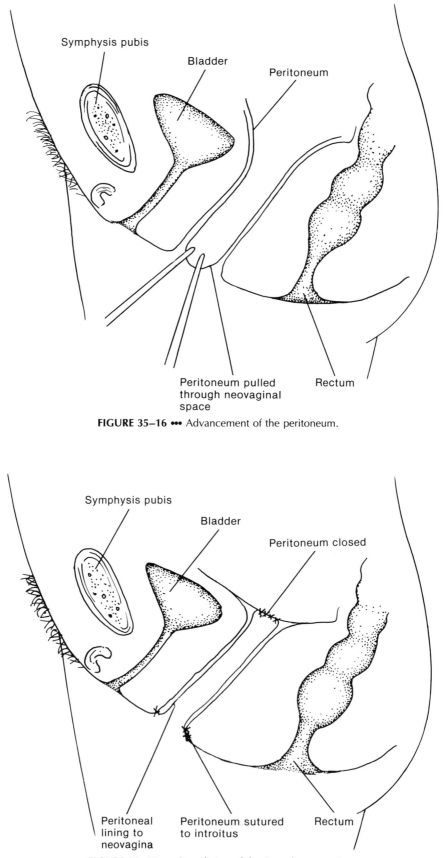

FIGURE 35–16 ••• Advancement of the peritoneum.

FIGURE 35–17 ••• Completion of the Davydov operation.

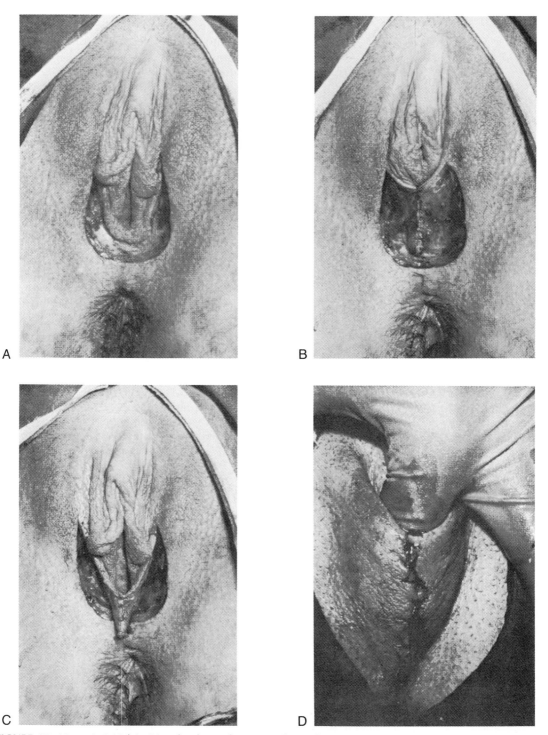

FIGURE 35–18 ●●● *A*, Initial incision for the performance of a Williams vulvovaginoplasty. (The anterior limbs of this incision are more medial than is desirable.) *B*, After freeing and undercutting the deeper tissues, the inner skin layer is being brought together to form a tube that will be the new vagina. *C*, Suturing the inner skin layer has almost been completed. *D*, The outer skin layer has been brought together over the inner, and two fingers are inserted into the introitus of the new vagina. A satisfactory functional result occurred in this case. (From Edmonds DK. Dewhurst's Practical Paediatric and Adolescent Gynaecology. 2nd ed. London: Butterworth & Co (Publishers) Ltd, 1989, p 42.)

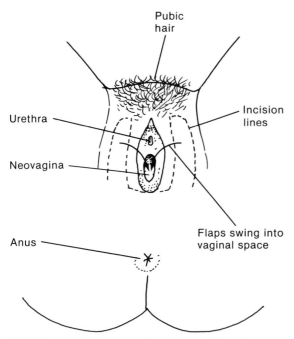

Pubic
hair

Urethra

Neovagina

Anus

Incision
lines

Flaps swing into
vaginal space

FIGURE 35–19 ••• Incisions for creation of the flap vaginoplasty.

Tissue Expansion Techniques. Use of subcutaneous balloons to increase and stretch the surface of the skin in the vulvar region has resulted in a modified flap vaginoplasty.[54] This procedure requires placement of subcutaneous balloons in the region of the vulva. These are gradually increased in size by the introduction of fluid into the balloons over a 3-month period. This then allows a large area of skin to be used as a flap to create a vagina as described in the flap vaginoplasty. This procedure, although it provides for an increased amount of skin, causes considerable discomfort to patients during the time of the tissue expansion.

The Vecchetti Technique. A modification of Frank's procedure, the Vecchetti technique involves the use of a sphere placed in the blind vagina. Two wires attached to it are guided through the potential neovaginal space to exit on the anterior vaginal wall. An apparatus is then strapped to the anterior vaginal wall to which the wires are attached, and pressure is increased daily on the ball, leading to continuous stretching of the blind vaginal pouch. After 2 to 3 months, the skin is stretched sufficiently, and the apparatus and ball are removed, leaving a functional vagina behind. This elaborate technique has become popular in Europe but is less popular elsewhere.

Obstructive Disorders

Obstructive disorders of the vagina may be divided into disorders of longitudinal or transverse fusion.

Disorders of Longitudinal Fusion. As the two müllerian ducts fuse, a single vagina usually results, but if this is incomplete, then a duplex system may be created with a double vagina. This double vaginal system may have a variety of anomalies associated with it.

Septate Vagina. In this condition the vagina is duplicated but may be asymptomatic, in which case no therapy is required. However, on occasion dyspareunia owing to narrowing of the vagina may require removal of the vaginal septum. This excision is a relatively simple operation but necessitates removal of the septum in its entirety. Because it is rather thick, care must be taken to ensure that adequate pedicles are taken and good hemostasis is maintained. Following excision, the tissue margins retract, resulting in an excellent functional vagina.

Imperforate Unilateral Vagina. Outflow obstruction of menstrual flow may result if blood collects in the blind vagina. This may cause severe dysmenorrhea and the development of a cystic swelling that bulges into the side of the patent vagina and may be sufficiently large to be palpable abdominally. This imperforate unilateral vagina is treated by excising the septum between the two vaginas, thereby allowing one to drain into the other. The incision should be large enough to excise the complete septum, as failure to create an adequate ostium will result in contraction and sealing of the sinus and subsequent retention of menstrual fluid, which may become infected.

Disorders of Transverse Fusion. These obstructive disorders may result from incomplete canalization of the vagina at any of four levels: the imperforate hymen, the high vaginal septum, the middle vaginal septum, and the lower vaginal septum. All of these disorders give rise to a hematocolpos, and patients present with cyclic abdominal pain. The hematocolpos may be so large that it is palpable abdominally.

Imperforate Hymen. This is typically seen in 14- to 16-year-old girls with normal secondary sexual development who have not menstruated. The intermittent lower abdominal pain is due to accumulation of blood in the vagina; if the hematocolpos reaches sufficient size, it may exert pressure on the urinary tract, leading to urinary retention. Vulvar examination reveals a tense, bulging, bluish membrane at the introitus; this blue coloration is due to the presence of retained menstrual fluid. The diagnosis is straightforward, and treatment involves a stellate incision of the membrane and removal of any redundant segments. No additional surgery is required, and any swabbing or irrigation of the vagina should be resisted. Once treatment is complete, the retained blood drains within a few days. No further treatment is necessary and sexual function is normal.

Transverse Vaginal Septum. Most of these occur at the junction of the middle and upper two thirds of the vagina (Fig. 35–20).[76] Before any attempt at surgical treatment, the amount of vagina present must be determined either clinically or with the aid of ultrasound or magnetic resonance imaging (MRI). It is extremely important to perform an intravenous pyelogram to exclude renal abnormalities, especially a pelvic kidney, and the urologic situation must be clearly defined before any surgical procedure is performed. In general, the less residual vagina that is present, the

more difficult the surgery becomes, and success may be hampered by the presence of endometriosis[77] and concurrent hematosalpinges.

In those cases where the transverse vaginal septum is in the lower and middle third of the vagina, dissection may be performed from below through a transverse incision in the blind part of the vagina. After the initial incision, dissection should be performed along the track of the absent vagina into the hematocolpos above. This is probably best accomplished by blunt dissection until the hematocolpos is reached, when it is incised and the retained menstrual blood released. The vaginal septum must then be excised with scissors, and the upper and lower parts of the vagina are re-anastomosed (Fig. 35–21). The importance of complete excision of the septum cannot be overemphasized, as failure to do so will result in a vaginal stenotic ring owing to the creation of a fibrous band. This makes subsequent sexual function difficult and painful.

In cases where the transverse septum is high and there is difficulty delineating the presence of the hematocolpos, an approach from both

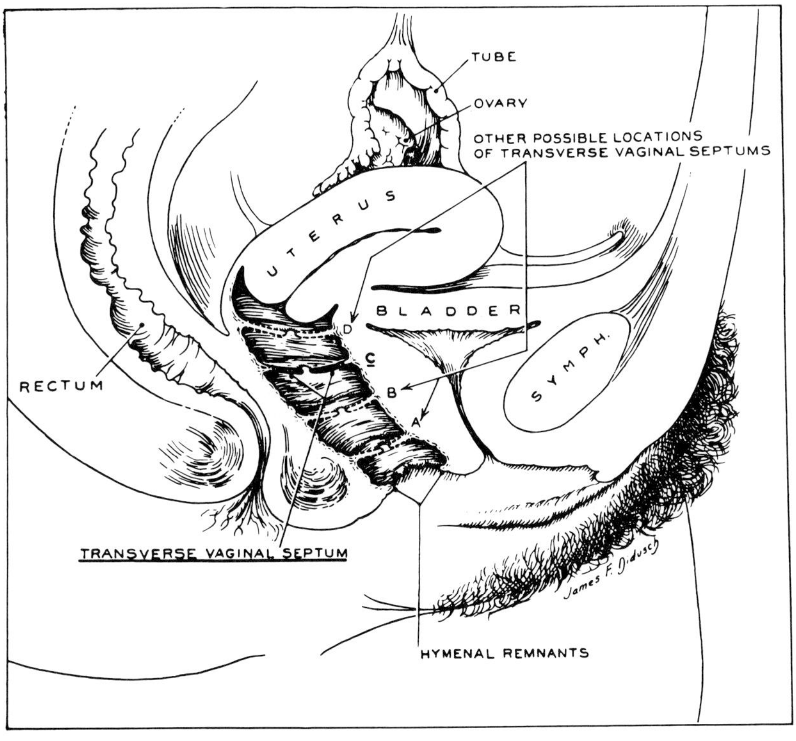

FIGURE 35–20 ••• Sketch of a congenital transverse vaginal septum showing the possible locations of the vagina. (From Bowman JA, Scott RB. Transverse vaginal septum. Report of four cases. Obstet Gynecol 1954; 3:444. Reprinted with permission from The American College of Obstetricians and Gynecologists.)

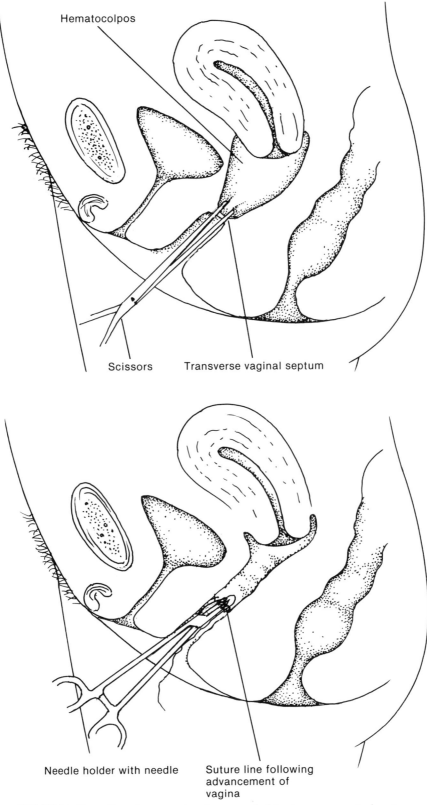

Hematocolpos

Scissors   Transverse vaginal septum

Needle holder with needle   Suture line following
                              advancement of
                              vagina

FIGURE 35–21 ••• Operative procedure for removal of the transverse vaginal septum.

the vagina and the abdomen may be required. The abdomen is opened and the hematometra hematocolpos identified. The hematocolpos is then incised and the menstrual blood aspirated. With another surgeon operating through the vagina, a probe can then be passed from above to meet the upper vagina from below. The septum may then be incised and removed either from above or below, but the anastomosis of the upper vagina to the lower is usually best performed from above. The drainage incision in the vagina is then closed, completing the operation. A mold is usually left in place and removed 1 week later.

In those cases where a large portion of the vagina is absent, drainage of the hematocolpos may be necessary following removal of the septum and the anastomotic procedure, or the creation of a neovagina may be delayed by 1 week to reduce the risk of infection. A mold is usually left in situ for 3 to 4 months to ensure that the upper vagina does not contract and that there is a drainage channel through the middle to allow passage of menstrual blood. The prospects for fertility after these procedures are difficult to assess. In patients with an imperforate hymen, the fertility potential is probably normal, but those with a transverse vaginal septum may be less fortunate, as they present later and the incidence of endometriosis and adhesions is much greater, thereby adversely affecting fertility. An overall pregnancy rate of 47% is reported.[76] In cases of lower third obstruction, all patients conceived; 43% of middle third obstruction cases conceived, but only 25% of upper third obstruction patients conceived. Thus, prompt diagnosis and treatment are necessary to preserve reproductive capacity in these patients.

Vulva

Problems that arise in the vulva in pediatric and adolescent patients are those associated with intersex and the androgenization of the female vulva during development. This section will consider female intersex induced by congenital adrenal hyperplasia, endogenous and exogenous androgen production, incomplete androgen insensitivity, and 5 α-reductase deficiency.

Congenital Adrenal Hyperplasia

The endocrine problems produced by congenital adrenal hyperplasia are considered in Chapter 6, but the end result is excess production of androgen, which is converted peripherally to dihydrotestosterone in the perineal region, resulting in cloacal virilization. The degree of virilization depends on the dose of androgen exposure, and thus there is a wide range of physical changes, with increasing masculinization. There are two aspects of the cloaca that deserve attention: those related to the vulva per se and those related to clitoral or phallic growth. The urogenital sinus in its normal development allows the urethra to exit in the mid-vulvar position between the clitoris and the vaginal opening. As masculinization increases, the urethra may become enclosed and open at the base of the phallus, almost like a hypospadias (Fig. 35–22). More commonly, as the vulva becomes occluded by labial fusion, the urethra opens high on the anterior vaginal wall (Fig. 35–23). The increasing severity of androgenization is associated with increased thickening of the lower vagina, which may open into the urethra in severe cases. A vagina is always present in congenital adrenal hyperplasia, and drainage of the uterus at the time of menstruation through this vagina is always possible. The genetic aspects of the various types of congenital adrenal hyperplasia are considered in Chapter 6.

Prenatal Diagnosis. Prenatal diagnosis of congenital adrenal hyperplasia is possible, and women who are known to be at risk may undergo either chorionic villus sampling (CVS) or amniocentesis to diagnose the condition. The use of CVS is preferred, as the direct DNA probe for congenital adrenal hyperplasia can be used and intrauterine treatment of the fetus commenced. This is performed by administering steroids (dexamethasone) to the mother, which are then transferred across the placenta to suppress adrenocorticotropic hormone (ACTH) release, preventing adrenal hyperplasia and excessive androgen production in utero.

Diagnosis. In the child born with an intersex problem, it is extremely important to establish the diagnosis as quickly as possible. The most important and appropriate endocrinologic assessment techniques are addressed in Chapter 5. A pelvic ultrasound is advised to determine the presence of a normal uterus and vagina, which makes the diagnosis of congenital adrenal hyperplasia most likely. Chromosomal studies can be obtained very quickly on blood, and a sample should be drawn for the measurement of serum 17α-hydroxyprogesterone; these two serum tests should be performed

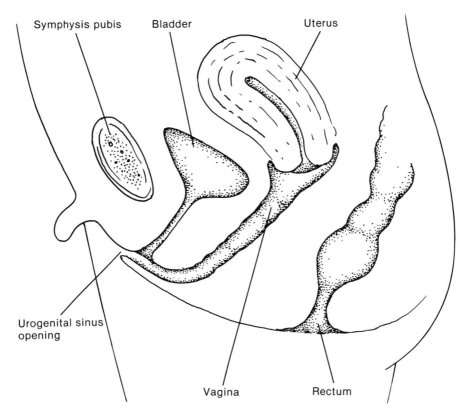

Symphysis pubis

Bladder

Uterus

Urogenital sinus opening

Vagina

Rectum

FIGURE 35–22 ••• Urogenital sinus opening in mild and moderate congenital adrenal hyperplasia.

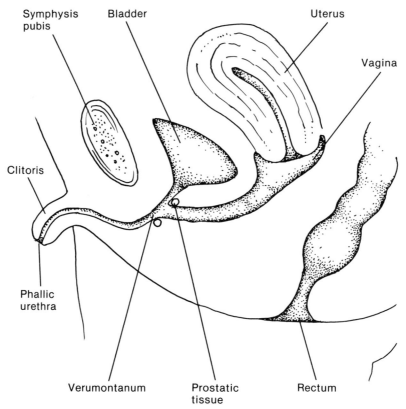

Symphysis pubis

Bladder

Uterus

Vagina

Clitoris

Phallic urethra

Verumontanum

Prostatic tissue

Rectum

FIGURE 35–23 ••• Severe congenital adrenal hyperplasia with clitoral hypertrophy and the vagina entering into the urethra.

simultaneously. Thus, within 2 or 3 days of life a diagnosis of both gender and sex of rearing can be established. The most common abnormality is 21-hydroxylase deficiency, and associated mineralocorticoid therapy and management of water and sodium intake must be considered. There are two forms of congenital adrenal hyperplasia: the salt-losing and the non–salt-losing forms. The former causes the most severe virilizing problems, which in themselves lead to long-term difficulties of management in the adolescent years.

Surgical Management. Once the diagnosis of congenital adrenal hyperplasia has been confirmed, the child must be reared as a female, regardless of the degree of masculinization of the external genitalia. This masculinization can always be corrected surgically. The ovaries are normal and function at puberty for the initiation of normal female fertility. Having established that the child is female, any enlargement of the clitoris and excessive fusion of the labial folds must be addressed. If the degree of clitoral enlargement is sufficient to cause parental distress, then a reduction clitoroplasty should be undertaken, with the labial folds divided at the same time to expose the vaginal opening, thereby giving the vulva a more normal female appearance. A reduction clitoroplasty is best performed during the neonatal period, as the parents will be anxious to take a child home with no visible evidence of masculinity, thereby avoiding mental anguish. The procedure is shown in Figure 35–24.

A V-shaped incision is made and the skin over the anterior wall reflected downward and excised, revealing the body of the phallus. The principle behind the reduction clitoroplasty is to maintain the neurovascular bundle supplying the glans of the clitoris with its sensory and vascular supply, thereby maintaining its function. Two lateral incisions must be made along the corpora to allow dissection of the connective tissue on the lateral walls. Dissection is then carried dorsally, identifying the vascular bundle lying on the dorsal surface of the phallus and thereby separating the body of the phallus from the vascular bundle. When this has been achieved, the corpora is transected at its base and just below the level of the glans. Two major arteries are always present at its base, and these must be suitably ligated. Hemostasis is extremely important; once it has been achieved, the glans of the phallus is then sutured with interrupted absorbable sutures to its base and the skin closed over the new clitoris. Bruising is reasonably common after this procedure, but the anatomic outcome is excellent. It is difficult to ascertain whether this procedure has resulted in improved sexual function when compared with a total clitoridectomy; studies are as yet unpublished. A vulvoplasty, if performed at the same time, is done in the manner shown in Figure 35–25. It is imperative that the urethra be identified and catheterized before any procedure is performed, as damage to the urethra can easily occur. After catheterizing the patient, an instrument is placed behind the vulvar skin and opened to stretch the fused labia, thereby identifying the line of fusion. Incision is then made in the midline and the cut edges of the labia sutured as illustrated. The vagina is always visible behind this, but the necessity for further introital surgery should be decided when puberty has passed and adult maturation has been achieved.

When the patient presents in adolescence and the vulva must be reconstructed, the procedure may be approached in a slightly different way if the degree of masculinization is much greater. In this case a flap vaginoplasty is required. This may be carried out in one of two ways: as described in Figure 35–25 or, if the degree of masculinization is greater, as described in Figure 35–26. In the latter procedure a perineal flap is created by incisions, as shown in the diagram, and the skin reflected posteriorly, revealing the posterior vaginal wall. As can be seen, before any incisions are made, the urethra must be catheterized. The posterior vaginal wall must be dissected away from the interstitial tissue, and an instrument is often required to identify the vaginal orifice. Having identified this, the vagina is then incised longitudinally, and the lateral walls are sutured. The defect in the posterior wall is repaired by insertion of the flap of vulvar skin. This procedure allows opening of the introitus with minimal subsequent scarring and contraction (Fig. 35–27).

The outcome of these surgical procedures is generally very good, although successful sexual function is more likely in the non–salt-losing form than the salt-losing type. Menstruation generally is delayed slightly beyond the norm.[78] Fertility rates in patients with congenital adrenal hyperplasia are also related to (1) compliance with therapy, which influences the onset of menstruation and subsequent normal hypothalamic-pituitary-ovarian function, and (2) the degree of androgenization. In the larg-

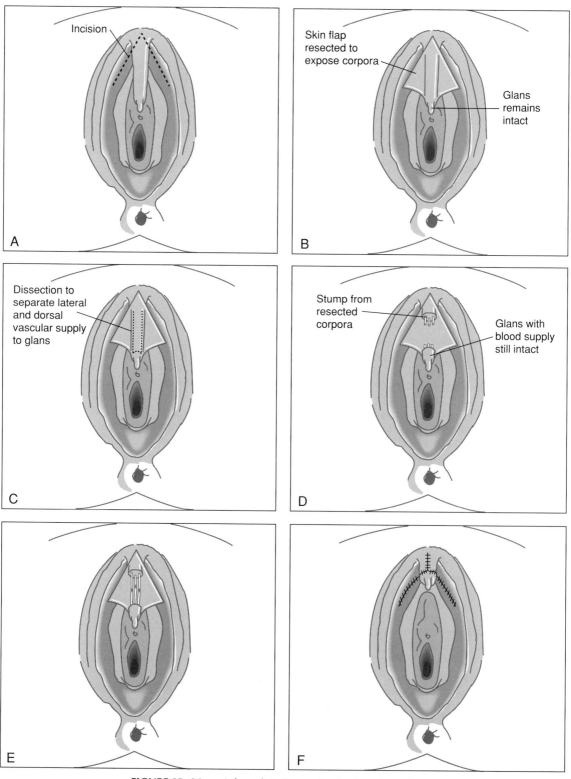

FIGURE 35–24 ••• *A through E, Stages of reduction clitoroplasty.*

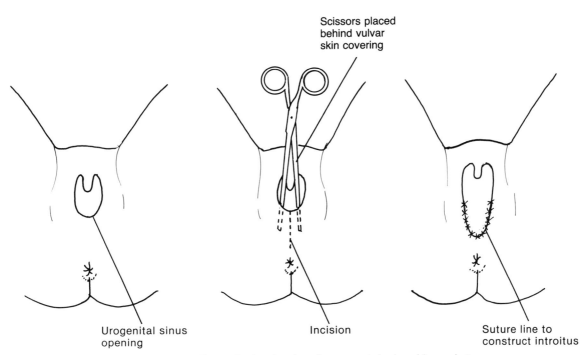

FIGURE 35–25 ••• The cut-back vulvoplasty for congenital adrenal hyperplasia.

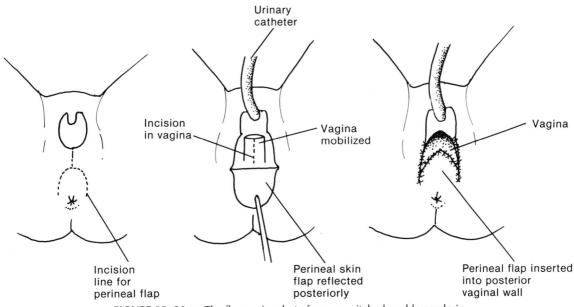

FIGURE 35–26 ••• The flap vaginoplasty for congenital adrenal hyperplasia.

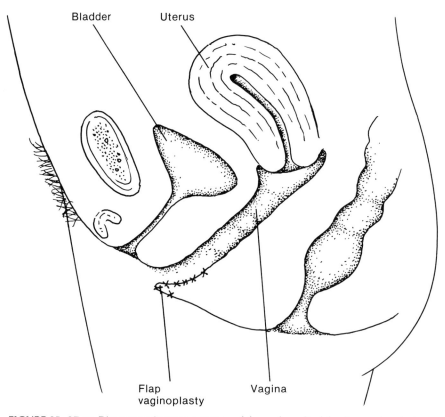

Bladder   Uterus

Flap
vaginoplasty   Vagina

FIGURE 35–27 ••• Diagrammatic representation of the end result of the flap vaginoplasty.

est review reported thus far,[79] 80 women were assessed with respect to fertility. In those patients with simple virilization, satisfactory surgical correction was achieved in 73%, but 56% of those in the salt-losing group had an inadequate introitus. In 15 of 25 patients with the simple virilizing form, 25 pregnancies resulted in 20 normal children; only 1 of 15 women with the salt-losing form became pregnant. Thus, achieving adequate medical control and using good surgical technique to ensure normal sexual function are imperative.

Endogenous Androgen Production

Androgenization of the vulva has been described in various circumstances. The most common conditions are adrenal adenomas, luteomas, and virilization in pregnancy associated with polycystic ovarian disease. These are extremely rare phenomena, and the degree of androgenization depends on the dose of androgen. Surgical management is similar to that described for congenital adrenal hyperplasia.

Exogenous Androgen Production

This is also a rare situation, with seemingly no reasons for its occurrence. However, one case of a female infant with virilization following administration of danazol to the mother has been described.[80] Again, surgical management is as described for congenital adrenal hyperplasia.

Incomplete Androgen Insensitivity

This condition, although extremely rare, covers a wide spectrum of disorders ranging from gynecomastia with azoospermia to the presence of a pseudovagina (Table 35–1). The most common presentation is a male neonate with perineoscrotal hypospadias and associated cryptorchidism. The testes are small but contain normal Leydig cells. Endocrinologically, these individuals undergo normal postpubertal development, with high levels of testosterone, and are similar to 46,XY females. Psychosexually, most subjects behave in a male manner.

TABLE 35–1 ••• CLINICAL FEATURES OF ANDROGEN RESISTANCE SYNDROMES

Feature	5α-Reductase Deficiency	Androgen Receptor Disorders				
		Complete Testicular Feminization	Incomplete Testicular Feminization	Reifenstein's Syndrome	Infertile Male Syndrome	Undervirilized Male Syndrome
Inheritance	Autosomal recessive	X-linked recessive	X-linked recessive	X-linked recessive	X-linked recessive	X-linked recessive
Hormonal profile	Normal male androgen and estrogen production	Increased androgen and estrogen (usually)	Increased androgen and estrogen (usually)	Increased androgen and estrogen (usually)	Increased androgen and estrogen (usually)	Increased androgen and estrogen (usually)
Phenotypic features						
Spermatogenesis	Decreased	Absent	Absent	Absent	Absent or decreased	Normal or decreased
Müllerian derivatives	Absent	Absent	Absent	Absent	Absent	Absent
Wolffian derivatives (epididymis, vas deferens, seminal vesicle)	Male	Absent	Male	Male	Male	Male
Urogenital sinus derivatives (prostate and urethra)	Female	Female	Female	Underdeveloped male	Male	Male
External genitalia (penis and scrotum)	Female (may virilize at puberty)	Female	Posterior fusion and clitoromegaly	Perineoscrotal hypospadias	Male	Male
Breasts	Male	Female	Female	Gynecomastia	Gynecomastia in some	Gynecomastia

From Griffin JE. Androgen resistance—the clinical and molecular spectrum. N Engl J Med 1992; 326(9):611–618. Reprinted, by permission of The New England Journal of Medicine.

This is almost certainly because these individuals show a quantitative defect in androgen receptors, and this incomplete androgen insensitivity leads to varying degrees of masculinization. There may also be difficulty in assessing the gender role; because they are psychosexually male and androgen receptors exist in the brain to influence psychological sex, the choice is between a male role with a microphallus that may not be reconstructible and a female role with removal of the gonads and subsequent perineal reduction. The latter is most commonly chosen, because creation of a vagina is almost always feasible, whereas building and construction of a penis are extremely difficult. Vaginoplasty may be performed in a manner similar to that described for the absent vagina, although creation of labial folds is very difficult, as the perineum in these patients is generally flat.[81]

5α-Reductase Deficiency

In this rare condition, children are born with a markedly bifid scrotum that appears similar to the labia, but the phallus is enlarged, and there is a urogenital sinus with a blind vaginal pouch. The testes are usually found in the abdomen but may also be located in the inguinal canal or in the scrotum. There are no müllerian structures present, and the wolffian ducts are normally developed. It is important to establish this diagnosis soon after birth, because at puberty, rising levels of testosterone will cause rapid virilization, with deepening of the voice and phallus growth. Failure to remove the gonads before puberty will result in testicular descent and even ejaculation from the urethral orifice. This is a familial condition and is almost certainly an autosomal recessive disorder specifically found in males. Surgical management may involve reduction clitoroplasty and subsequent development of a vagina as described earlier for vaginoplasty.

CONCLUSION

Successful management of congenital anomalies of the genital tract demands both intense psychological support and a high degree of surgical skill. All patients should be referred to specialized centers where such expertise is available. Otherwise, results may be less than optimal, with traumatic results for the patient.

References

1. Jarcho J. Malformations of the uterus. Am J Surg 1946; 71:106.
2. Jones WS. Obstetric significance of female genital anomalies. Obstet Gynecol 1957; 10:113.
3. Semmens JP. Congenital anomalies of female genital tract. Obstet Gynecol 1962; 19:328.
4. Buttram VC, Gibbons WE. Mullerian anomalies: A proposed classification. Fertil Steril 1979; 32:90.
5. Toaff ME, Lev-Toaff AS, Toaff R. Communicating uteri: Review and classification with introduction of two previously unreported types. Fertil Steril 1984; 41:661.
6. Fedele L, Vercellini P, Marchini M, et al. Communication uteri; description and classification of a new type. Int J Fertil 1988; 33:168.
7. Bennett MJ, Berry JVJ. Preterm labour and congenital malformations of the uterus. Ultrasound Med Biol 1979; 5:83.
8. Strassman EO. Fertility and unification of double uterus. Fertil Steril 1966; 17:165.
9. Sanfilippo JS, Yussman MA, Smith O. HSG in the evaluation of infertility. A six year review. Fertil Steril 1978; 30:636.
10. Sandler SW. Spontaneous abortion in perspective. S Afr Med J 1977; 52:1115.
11. Stray-Petersen B, Stray-Petersen S. Etiologic factors and subsequent reproductive performance in 195 couples with a prior history of habitual abortion. Am J Obstet Gynecol 1984; 148:140.
12. Elias S, Simpson JL, Carson SA, et al. Genetic studies in incomplete mullerian fusion. Obstet Gynecol 1984; 63:276.
13. Gurin J, Lester E. Associated anomalies of mullerian and wolffian duct structures. South Med J 1981; 74:805.
14. Rock JA, Zacur HA. The clinical management of repeated early pregnancy wastage. Fertil Steril 1983; 39:123.
15. Stern AM, Gall JC, Perry BL, et al. The hand-foot-uterus syndrome. J Pediatr 1970; 77:109.
16. Winter JSD, Kohn G, Mellman WJ, Wagner S. A familial syndrome of renal, genital and middle ear anomalies. J Pediatr 1968; 71:88.
17. Rudiger RA, Schmidt W, Loose DA, Passarge E. Severe developmental failure with coarse facial features, distal limb hypoplasia, thickened palmar creases, bifid uvula and ureteral stenosis. J Pediatr 1971; 79:977.
18. Sorenson SS. Minor mullerian anomalies and oligomenorrhoea in infertile women. Am J Obstet Gynecol 1981; 140:636.
19. Kaufman RH, Binder GL, Gray PM, Adam E. Upper genital tract changes associated with exposure in utero to diethylstilboestrol. Am J Obstet Gynecol 1977; 128:51.
20. Kaufman RH, Irwin JF. DES exposure and reproductive performance. In: Bennett MJ, Edmonds DK (eds). Spontaneous and Recurrent Abortion. Oxford: Blackwell,   .
21. Malini S, Valdes C, Malinaki LR. Sonographic diagnosis and classification of anomalies of the genital tract. J Ultrasound Med 1984; 3:397.
22. Sanfilippo JS. Strassman operation for the correction of a class II anomaly in an adolescent. J Adolesc Health 1991; 12:63.

23. Daly DC, Maier D, Soto-Albors C. Hysteroscopic metroplasty: Six years experience. Obstet Gynecol 1989; 73:201.

24. Candiani GB, Vercellini P, Fedele L, et al. Argon laser versus microscissors for hysteroscopic incision of uterine septa. Am J Obstet Gynecol 1991; 164:87.

25. Jacob JH, Griffin WT. Surgical reconstruction of the congenitally atretic cervix: Two cases. Obstet Gynecol Surv 1989; 44:556.

26. Regan L, Dewhurst J. Atresia of the cervix. Pediatr Adolesc Gynecol 1985; 3:83.

27. Farber M. Congenital atresia of the uterine cervix. Semin Reprod Endocrinol 1986; 4:33.

28. Markham SM, Parmley TH, Murphy AA, et al. Cervical agenesis combined with vaginal agenesis diagnosed by MRI. Fertil Steril 1987; 48:143.

29. Rock JA, Schlaff WD, Zacur HA, Jones HW. The clinical management of congenital absence of the uterine cervix. Int J Gynaecol Obstet 1984; 22:231.

30. Edmonds DK. Congenital malformations of the vagina and their management. Semin Reprod Endocrinol 1988; 6:91.

31. Edmonds DK (ed). Practical Paediatric and Adolescent Gynaecology. London: Butterworths, 1988, p 37.

32. Zarou GS, Espesito JM, Zarou DM. Pregnancy following surgical correction of congenital atresia of the cervix. Int J Obstet Gynecol 1973; 11:143.

33. Singh J, Devi YL. Pregnancy following surgical correction of non fused mullerian bulbs and absent vagina. Obstet Gynecol 1983; 61:267

34. Hampton HL, Meeks GR, Bates W, Wiser WL. Pregnancy after successful vaginoplasty and cervical stenting for partial atresia of the cervix. Obstet Gynecol 1990; 76:900.

35. Thijssen RFA, Hollanders JMG, Willemsen WNP, et al. Successful pregnancy after ZIFT in a patient with congenital cervical atresia. Obstet Gynecol 1990; 76:902.

36. Bryan AL, Nigro JA, Counsellor VS. One hundred cases of congenital absence of the vagina. Surg Gynecol Obstet 1949; 88:79.

37. Evans TN, Poland ML, Boving RL. Vaginal malformations. Am J Obstet Gynecol 1981; 141:910.

38. Reindollar RH, Byrd JR, McDonough PG. Delayed sexual development: A study of 252 patients. Am J Obstet Gynecol 1981; 140:371.

39. Jones HW, Mermut S. Familial occurrence of congenital absence of the vagina. Obstet Gynecol 1974; 42:38.

40. Lischke JH, Curtis CH, Lamb EJ. Discordance of vaginal agenesis in monozygotic twins. Obstet Gynecol 1973; 41:920.

41. Shokeir MHK. Aplasia of the mullerian system: Evidence of possible sex limited autosomal dominant inheritance. Birth Defects 1978; 14:147.

42. Carson SA, Simpson JL, Malinak LR, et al. Heritable aspects of uterine anomalies II: Genetic analysis of mullerian aplasia. Fertil Steril 1983; 40:86.

43. Griffin JE, Edwards C, Madden JD. Congenital absence of vagina. Ann Intern Med 1976; 85:224.

44. Willemson WNP. Combination of Mayer-Rokitansky-Kuster and Klippel-Feil Syndromes. A case report and review of literature. Eur J Obstet Gynecol Reprod Biol 1982; 13:229.

45. Shane JM, Wilson EA, Schiff I, Naftolin F. A preliminary report on gonadotrophin release in the Rokitansky syndrome. Am J Obstet Gynecol 1977; 127:326.

46. Egarter CH, Huber J. Successful stimulation and retrieval of oocytes in a patient with Mayer-Rokitansky-Kuster syndrome. Lancet 1988; i:1283.

47. Rock JA, Baramki TA, Parmley TH, Jones HW. A functioning unilateral uterine anlage with mullerian duct agenesis. Int J Gynaecol Obstet 1980; 18:99.

48. Farber M, Stein A, Adashi E. Rokitansky-Kuster-Hauser syndrome and leiomyoma uteri. Obstet Gynecol 1978; 51:70S.

49. Goldwyn RM. History of attempts to form a vagina. Plast Reconstr Surg 1977; 59:319.

50. Abbe R. New method of creating a vagina in a case of congenital absence. Med Rec 1898; 54:836.

51. Baldwin JF. The formation of an artificial vagina by intestinal transplantation. Ann Surg 1904; 40:398.

52. Frank RT. The formation of an artificial vagina without operation. Am J Obstet Gynecol 1938; 35:1053.

53. Lilford RJ, Johnson N, Batchelor A. A new operation for vaginal agenesis: Construction of a neovagina from a rectus abdominous musculo-cutaneous flap. Br J Obstet Gynaecol 1989; 96:1089.

54. Lilford RJ, Sharpe DT, Thomas DFM. Use of tissue expansion techniques to create skin flaps for vaginoplasty. Br J Obstet Gynaecol 1988; 95:402.

55. Edmonds DK, Rose GL. Non-surgical technique to create a neovagina in the Rokitansky syndrome. In press.

56. McIndoe AH, Banister JB. An operation for the cure of congenital absence of the vagina. J Obstet Gynaecol Br Commonw 1938; 45:490.

57. Counsellor VS, Flor FS. Congenital absence of the vagina. Surg Clin North Am 1957; 37:1107.

58. McIndoe AH. Discussion on treatment of congenital absence of the vagina with emphasis on long term results. Proc R Soc Med 1959; 52:952.

59. Cali RH, Pratt JH. Congenital absence of the vagina. Am J Obstet Gynecol 1968; 100:752.

60. Rock JA, Reeves LA, Retto H, et al. Success following vaginal creation for mullerian agenesis. Fertil Steril 1983; 39:809.

61. Brindeau A. Creation d'une vagin artificiel à l'aide des membranes ovulaire d'un oeuf à terme. Gynecol Obstet 1934; 29:385.

62. Dhall K. Amnion graft for the treatment of congenital absence of the vagina. Br J Obstet Gynaecol 1984; 91:279.

63. Morton KE, Dewhurst CJ. Human amnion in the treatment of vaginal malformations. Br J Obstet Gynaecol 1986; 93:50.

64. Smith MR. Vaginal aplasia: Therapeutic options. Am J Obstet Gynecol 1983; 146:488.

65. Lathrop JC, Ree HJ, McDuff HC. Intraepithelial neoplasia of the neovagina. Obstet Gynecol 1985; 65:91S.

66. Hopkins MP, Morley GW. Squamous cell carcinoma of the neovagina. Obstet Gynecol 1987; 69:525.

67. Baltzer J, Zander J. Primary squamous cell carcinoma of the neovagina. Gynecol Oncol 1989; 35:99.

68. Peters WA, Uhlir JK. Prolapse of the neovagina created by self dilatation. Obstet Gynecol 1990; 76:904.

69. Buscema J, Rosensheim NB, Shah K. Condylomata acuminata arising in a neovagina. Obstet Gynecol 1987; 69:528.

70. Burger RA, Riedmiller H, Knapstein PG, et al. Ileocecal vaginal construction. Am J Obstet Gynecol 1989; 161:162.

71. Davydov SN, Zhvitiashvili OD. Formation of vagina from peritoneum of Douglas pouch. Acta Chir Plast 1974; 16:35.
72. Williams EA. Congenital absence of the vagina; a simple operation for its relief. J Obstet Gynaecol Br Commonw 1964; 71:511.
73. Williams EA. Uterovaginal agenesis. Ann R Col Surg Eng 1976; 58:266.
74. Morton KE, Davies D, Dewhurst CJ. The use of the fasciocutaneous flap in vaginal reconstruction. Br J Obstet Gynaecol 1986; 93:970.
75. Johnson N, Lilford RJ, Batchelor A. The free flap vaginoplasty; a new surgical procedure for the treatment of vaginal agenesis. Br J Obstet Gynaecol 1991; 98:184.
76. Rock JA, Zacur HA, Dlugi AM. Pregnancy success following surgical correction of imperforate hymen and complete transverse vaginal septum. Gynecology 1982; 59:448.
77. Sanfilippo JS, Wakim NG, Schikler KN, Yussman MA. Endometriosis in association with uterine abnormalities. Am J Obstet Gynecol 1986; 154:39.
78. Grant D, Muram D, Dewhurst CJ. Menstrual and fertility patterns in patients with congenital adrenal hyperplasia. Pediatr Adolesc Gynecol 1983; 1:97.
79. Mulkaikal RM, Migeon CJ, Rock JA. Fertility rates in female patients with congenital adrenal hyperplasia due to 21-hydroxylase deficiency. N Engl J Med 1987; 316:178.
80. Duck SC, Katayama KP. Danazol may cause female pseudohermaphroditism. Fertil Steril 1981; 35:230.
81. Rock JA, Jones HW. Construction of a neovagina for patients with a flat perineum. Am J Obstet Gynecol 1989; 160:845.

CHAPTER 36

Urologic Problems

DIANE FRANCOEUR

ANTHONY CASALE

ALAN RETIK

Children and adolescents evaluated by the primary care specialist often have complaints that are related to both the urinary tract and the reproductive organs. Pediatric patients evaluated for perineal pruritus and pain may in fact be dysfunctional voiders, and the clinician must be aware of those specific genitourinary conditions seen in either children or adolescents. This chapter will review the most common urologic abnormalities encountered in this age group.

Whenever a child has a urinary tract problem, obtaining a careful history is paramount. The major abnormality, its severity, and associated circumstances must be defined. Information should be obtained regarding voiding pattern; day and night frequency; quality of stream; urgency or stress phenomena; day and night wetting; and previous infection, treatment, and evaluation. The physical examination should include assessment of the abdomen and external genitalia; a brief neurologic examination that includes assessment of reflexes, perineal sensation, and sphincter tone; and inspection of the lower back for evidence of sacral dimpling or cutaneous anomalies suggestive of a spinal abnormality.

Compared with childhood, adolescence is a unique period with respect to genitourinary function. Urinary tract abnormalities in the adolescent essentially fall into two broad categories: abnormalities of childhood that have failed to resolve and abnormalities related to the onset of sexual activity. When sexual activity is initiated, an increase in the incidence of urinary tract infections is not uncommon.

Many genitourinary congenital anomalies are first detected in adolescence primarily because of their association with menstrual abnormalities that become symptomatic with menarche. Overall, the structure and function of the adolescent urinary tract does not differ significantly from those of the adult.

Knowledge of lower and upper urinary tract infections (UTIs), voiding dysfunction, enuresis, incontinence, vesicoureteral reflux, hematuria, and some other specific conditions such as pelvic pain, sexual abuse, urologic manifestation of sexually transmitted diseases (STDs), and understanding the child with special needs should be part of the armamentarium of the clinician providing care to this age group.

URINARY TRACT INFECTION

Asymptomatic Bacteriuria

The prevalence of asymptomatic bacteriuria in childhood is influenced by age, sex, and the method of diagnosis. In a 3-year prospective study conducted in Sweden of infants less than 1 year old, 0.9% of girls were found to have asymptomatic bacteriuria.[1] During the preschool and school years, screening studies revealed a bacteriuria prevalence of 0.7% to 1.9% in girls.[2] In this age group, the risk of developing acute upper UTI with untreated bacteriuria is low unless there is a change in bacterial strain associated with antibiotic treatment.[3] Asymptomatic bacteriuria is usually associated with low-virulence bacterial strains that lack the ability to adhere to the uroepithelium, resulting in a number of nonspecific symptoms.[4, 5] Because asymptomatic bacteriuria in children may be a marker for the presence of underlying renal abnormality, it is recommended that young children with asymptomatic bacteriuria be investigated and appropriately managed.[6]

Clinical Presentation (Table 36–1)

Cystitis

In very young patients, the classic signs and symptoms of cystitis are often absent, and such infants are usually evaluated for irritability, poor feeding, failure to grow, vomiting or abdominal distention. Fever may be absent in the neonate but is usually present in older infants and children. In the latter, symptoms such as unsuccessful toilet training (at an age when the child should be toilet trained), primary or secondary enuresis, incontinence, urgency, frequency, and dysuria are the more common symptoms of acute, chronic, or recurrent UTI. Approximately 10% of girls will experience recurrence, and dysfunctional voiding patterns are common.

Adolescents with cystitis present with the same symptoms as adults; however, clinical presentation may be more intense, and hemorrhagic cystitis is more common. Most girls complain of an initial onset of low back pain that does not lateralize and may be associated with irritable bladder symptoms. Within 24 hours, dysuria becomes severe, and infection is often accompanied by nausea and low-grade fever. The variability in the severity of symptoms is striking, ranging from mild discomfort to a virtually bedridden state.

Bacterial vaginitis, especially contact vaginitis (related to bubble bath or soaps), is an important differential diagnosis in children thought to have UTI. Vaginal discharge can lead to contamination of voided urine specimens with white blood cells, and the symptoms of vaginitis in children may be identical to those of UTI.

Pyelonephritis

Patients with pyelonephritis usually are quite ill, with a high, spiking fever; flank pain; nausea; chills; vomiting; and myalgia; they often require hospitalization. Lower tract symptoms are preceded by upper tract symptoms by hours or days. Unlike in patients with cystitis, leukocytosis with a marked left shift is usually present. However, these symptoms are not always obvious in young infants, who usually present with nonspecific findings.

Vesicoureteral reflux is the single most common risk factor in the etiology of pyelonephritis. Obstruction of any kind and severe malformation of the urinary tract are also obvious predisposing factors. Inefficient emptying of urine owing to a dilated or obstructed urinary tract compromises renal defenses and allows bacteria to multiply and initiate infection. The significance of pyelonephritis in children is that it may lead to renal scarring in 25% to 30% of patients.[7] The acute inflammatory response is the most important step in the subsequent development of renal scarring. When the bacteria are phagocytized, they simultaneously release toxins that directly affect the renal tubular epithelium, and associated ischemia may result in permanent renal scarring.[8] A clear association between the number of episodes of pyelonephritis and the incidence of renal scarring has been reported by Jordal[8];

TABLE 36–1 ••• SYMPTOMS OF UTI

	Cystitis	Pyelonephritis
Very young children	Irritability, poor feeding, failure to grow, vomiting or distended abdomen.	Nonspecific findings associated with high fever.
Young children	Failure to be toilet-trained, enuresis, incontinence, urgency, frequency, dysuria.	High fever, abdominal or flank pain, nausea, vomiting, symptoms of cystitis may or may not be present.
Older children	Urinary frequency, dysuria, enuresis, low back pain, low-grade fever.	

studies have demonstrated that aggressive early antibiotic treatment may prevent or diminish renal scarring.

Diagnosis

The only reliable method of diagnosing UTI is urine culture. Although urinalysis may be helpful in providing criteria for initiating treatment, the association of inflammatory cells in urine is reliable, at best, only 70% of the time.

The method of collection varies with the age of the child. A U collecting bag applied to the perineum is associated with a high level of contamination and is only reliable when the culture is negative or if a single organism is isolated. The amount of bacteria thought to be significant was established in 1956 by Kass, who demonstrated that more than 95% of children with UTI had cultures growing 10^5 colonies/ml.[9a]

Bacteriology

The majority of UTIs are caused by Enterobacteriaceae spp. These gram-negative organisms are most often represented by *Escherichia coli*, which is present in 60% to 80% of cases. The most common gram-positive organisms identified are *Staphylococcus* and *Enterococcus*. The majority of uncomplicated UTIs are caused by a single organism. Lactobacilli, corynebacteria, and streptococci rarely cause UTI and should be considered contaminants unless the specimen was obtained by way of suprapubic aspiration or catheterization. Stamey has demonstrated that in the majority of UTIs, responsible bacteria originate in the gut, are present in the flora of the vaginal vestibule, and surround the urethral meatus.[10a] They gain access to the bladder by ascending the relatively short female urethra. Sexual intercourse may cause minor trauma to the urethra and lead to bacterial invasion. As the female urogenital tract becomes more accustomed to sexual activity, the frequency of infection decreases.

Evaluation

Current standards of care dictate evaluation of the child after the first documented UTI. Epidemiologic studies[9] have revealed that reinfection occurs within 18 months in up to 40% to 60% of all children. All patients with evidence of upper UTI should have a complete radiographic evaluation, including an upper and lower urinary tract examination, after the initial infection.

Radiologic Studies

The evaluation required is related to the age of the patient. The upper and lower urinary tract should be evaluated in children. A voiding cystourethrogram (VCUG) to detect the presence of vesicoureteral reflux and to determine the size, shape, and function of the bladder is useful and should be performed whenever the child is asymptomatic and the urine is sterile. Prophylactic antibiotics should be prescribed before and after the examination to prevent reinfection. Radiologic evaluation has shown the presence of reflux in 35% of patients.[10] In younger girls, the upper urinary tract is best evaluated with a renal ultrasound. In children, sonography has been found to be as sensitive as an intravenous pyelogram (IVP) for the detection of significant renal abnormalities except for uncomplicated duplication anomalies and focal scarring.[11]

Since the early 1980s there has been a drastic reduction in the use of IVPs. The contrast agent concentrates less in the infant than in the older patient, and thus the IVP often results in a washed-out image hidden by a sea of intestinal gas. However, older adolescent girls with recurrent infection may be best served by an IVP rather than ultrasonography, and cystoscopic evaluation often replaces or augments VCUG evaluation and facilitates determination of the presence of renal stones or neoplasms.[12]

Nuclear examinations also are used in evaluation of the urinary tract. A number of centers utilize the radioactive isotope for a nuclear cystogram to test for reflux. In the absence of reflux, hydronephrosis is best evaluated by diuretic renography using mercuroacetylglycylglycine (MAG III). It provides quantitative assessment of renal function and drainage of the dilated collecting system. Dimercaptosuccinic acid (DMSA), also known as succimer, is a radionuclide agent that is fixed by renal tubules with only minimal excretion and provides optimal visualization of the renal parenchyma. It is useful to demonstrate renal scarring and to establish the location of acute pyelonephritis.

Treatment

Uncomplicated UTI

Agents that are successful in the treatment of acute, uncomplicated lower UTI are sulfon-amides, such as trimethoprim-sulfamethoxa-zole (TMP-SMX)[13]; nitrofurantoin; trimetho-prim; and cephalosporins. Ampicillin and amoxicillin are often administered but are not the best choice, as high intestinal levels of these medications result in development of resistant bacteria in the gastrointestinal tract, which then become the reinfecting bacteria.[14] This problem can be corrected with the use of the combination of amoxicillin and clavulanate potassium (Augmentin), which inhibits the β-lactamase–resistant enzymes.[15] Unfortunately, this combination is more expensive than other medications. The fluoroquinolones, a new class of oral antibacterials, have a wide spectrum of activity covering most gram-positive and gram-negative organisms, including *Pseudomonas* and *Proteus* spp. Fluoroquinolone studies in animals, however, have demonstrated toxicity to developing cartilage, and therefore their use is best avoided in children and growing ado-lescents.[15]

Duration of Treatment. There is controversy about the ideal duration of treatment. Several randomized controlled studies have reported on the efficacy of single-dose verses short-course (3 to 5 days) antibiotic treatment in children.[16, 17] The advantages with the former are obvious: lower cost, better compliance, and fewer side effects. Because it is not always easy to distinguish lower UTI from pyelone-phritis, most pediatric urologists still recom-mend treatment for 7 to 10 days because of the higher risk of anatomic anomalies. After the first UTI the child should remain on pro-phylactic antibiotics until the radiologic eval-uation is obtained, usually within 2 to 3 weeks. Short-term treatment has also been associated with an increased recurrence of UTI, even though the first treatment was initially effec-tive, in 93.5% of patients.[16]

Pyelonephritis

Treatment must be initiated as soon as the diagnosis is established, as the degree of renal damage is influenced by the rapidity of effec-tive therapy.[18] Oral medications can be initi-ated in the older child who is not toxic and compliant, provided there is close follow-up.

TMP-SMX or cephalosporins are effective in most cases.

In the younger or toxic child, immediate parenteral therapy should be initiated. After appropriate cultures are obtained, combina-tion therapy that includes broad-spectrum antibiotics such as aminoglycosides or cepha-losporins should be prescribed until the sensi-tivity is known. Parenteral treatment should be continued until the child is afebrile for 48 to 72 hours and full-dose oral therapy has been administered for 10 to 14 days. Control cul-tures should be obtained, and the child should be maintained on low-dose prophylaxis until radiologic evaluation is completed.

Prophylaxis

Long-term antibiotic prophylaxis is recom-mended in children with reflux, recurrent UTI, or dysfunctional voiding problems. Girls with recurrent UTI should remain on prophylaxis until their underlying urologic problem is cor-rected. Such patients usually require cultures every 3 months to assess the efficacy of the prophylaxis. Antimicrobials of choice are ni-trofurantoin or TMP-SMX in one half to one third of the daily dose.[19]

Sexually active adolescents with postcoital cystitis represent a special category of patients. Cultures should be obtained, and these pa-tients should be treated and kept either on low-dose prophylaxis or postcoital antibiotics for several months. Immediate postcoital void-ing may reduce recurrent infections. Urethral manipulation in young girls is rarely, if ever, necessary. In the absence of significant abnor-malities that necessitate further diagnostic evaluation, the role of dilatation and urethrot-omy is minimal.

REFLUX

Incidence

Vesicoureteral reflux (VUR) is the retro-grade flow of urine from the bladder into the ureters and kidneys. Its prevalence in healthy children is unknown but is estimated at 1%.[20] In a group of patients with UTI, reflux oc-curred in 70% of those younger than 1 year of age; in 25% at 4 years of age; in 15% at 12 years of age; and in 5.2% of adults. VUR is less common in black children.[20]

Diagnosis

Virtually all children present with UTI, and a number have signs of cystitis or pyelonephritis. Reflux is found in 90% of children with UTIs when their fever exceeds 38.5°C.[21] With the widespread use of ultrasound in pregnancy, severe reflux may even be detected in utero and usually presents as bilateral hydronephrosis.

Evaluation

The diagnosis of reflux is accurately established by the use of a VCUG (Figs. 36–1, 36–2). Reflux may occur either during bladder filling or during voiding. The dynamic VCUG is preferably obtained when the child is awake, as this allows a better demarcation of the bladder outline and of the bladder neck and urethral anatomy and also gives an approximation of bladder capacity.

Ultrasonography is also a safe, accurate, and noninvasive study to assess the integrity of the upper urinary tract. Radioisotopic renal scanning is a useful adjunct to assess renal scarring, growth, and function.

Classification

The grading system used by the International Reflux Study Group offers a standard classification, allowing more accurate comparison of treatment modalities. Reflux is graded from I through V according to severity (Fig. 36–3).

Etiology

The anatomy of the normal ureterovesical junction is characterized by oblique entry of the ureter into the bladder and adequate length of the intramural ureter, especially in the submucosal segment. With bladder filling, the ureteral lumen is flattened between the bladder mucosa and the detrusor, creating a valve that prevents reflux. In the vast majority of children with reflux, the cause of reflux is congenital maldevelopment of this ureterovesical junction. In children with severe bladder dysfunction, a normal valve mechanism may be overwhelmed by high pressure, leading to reflux. Acute cystitis may produce a transient reflux on the VCUG. VUR in the setting of a normal bladder and without infection is a benign condition. Reflux and infection, however, often lead to renal scarring.

Clinical Aspects

Renal scars caused by reflux and infection usually develop during the first 5 years of life. Reflux may affect renal growth, and its effect is directly proportional to the presence of an abnormal kidney on the contralateral side, recurrent UTI, and grade of the reflux.[22] Scar

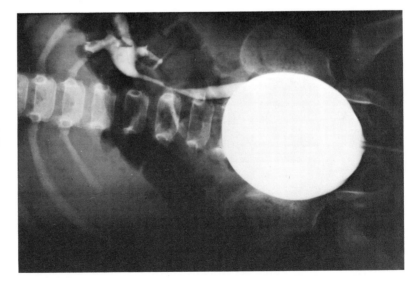

FIGURE 36–1 ••• A voiding cystouretogram revealing grade III vesicoureteral reflux.

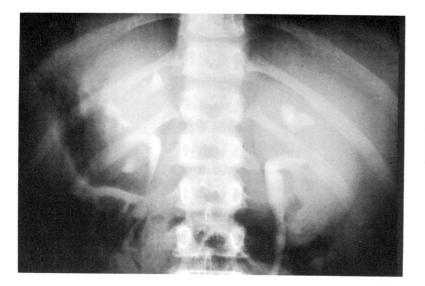

FIGURE 36–2 ••• An intravenous pyelogram showing a small left kidney and narrow parenchyma from recurrent pyelonephritis.

formation occurs predominantly at the renal poles and is associated with hypertrophy of the remaining normal parenchyma. Reflux occurs in conjunction with a neuropathic bladder in 15% to 60% of patients.[23] VUR can occasionally occur secondary to UTI and then usually resolves spontaneously with treatment of the infection. The most common urodynamic abnormality in patients with reflux is uninhibited bladder contractions. Taylor demonstrated that as many as 75% of girls with reflux had evidence of uninhibited bladder contractions.[22a] Most low-grade reflux in these patients resolves spontaneously with improved bladder function.

Treatment

Medical Management

The main goal in management of reflux is the prevention of ascending UTI and renal

scarring. Low-grade reflux has a natural tendency to resolve spontaneously over time. Skoog demonstrated in a large retrospective study that reflux resolves in 90% of patients with grade I, in 80% with grade II, in 50% with grade III, in 10% with grade IV, and in essentially none with grade V (Table 36–2).[23a] Most spontaneous resolutions occur within the first few years after diagnosis, and the rate of reflux resolution remains constant both during and after childhood, approximately 10% to 15% per year.[10, 24] Puberty is not associated with either an increase or a decrease in resolution rate of reflux. However, surgical treatment in older adolescents is technically more difficult and more painful. Thirty percent to 50% of children with reflux have renal scarring on initial evaluation, and the absence of renal scarring is associated with the ability to maintain sterile urine with prophylactic antibiotics.[25]

Reflux nephropathy is the most common

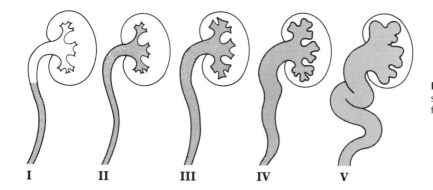

FIGURE 36–3 ••• International scale for grading vesicoureteral reflux.

I II III IV V

TABLE 36–2 ••• SPONTANEOUS RESOLUTION OF REFLUX

Grade	% of Cases that Resolve
Grade I:	90%
Grade II:	80%
Grade III:	50%
Grade IV:	10%
Grade V:	none

disorder leading to hypertension in children and is related to the intensity of parenchymal damage resulting in renal insufficiency. It may develop in as many as 10% to 20% of children with reflux and renal scarring.[10, 24] Reflux is present in 30% to 40% of children who experience renal failure before 16 years of age. Medical management must emphasize prevention of UTI with the use of daily antibiotic prophylaxis, frequent voiding, and avoidance of constipation. The chemoprophylaxis should be prescribed at bedtime, as it is during this time that the child retains urine longest and infection is most likely to develop. The best choices for chemoprophylaxis are TMP-SMX and nitrofurantoin. These patients should undergo a urine culture every 3 to 4 months and radiographic evaluation of the upper urinary tract annually until the reflux disappears.

Surgical Management

Ureteral reimplantation is highly successful in more than 95% of children. Various techniques have been described, but the basis for the procedure remains the development of an adequate length of submucosal ureter allowing a valvelike flap.

Indications for surgery are (1) persistent or recurrent infection despite antibiotic prophylaxis, (2) noncompliance with medical treatment, (3) development of new scarring or failure of renal growth, or (4) persistent significant reflux in adolescent girls.

VOIDING DYSFUNCTION AND DAYTIME INCONTINENCE

Most children with minor voiding disturbances do not have underlying anatomic disease and therefore do not need invasive urologic investigation. Although wetting problems are "benign," the ridicule, disgrace, humilia-tion, and low self-esteem that some of these children suffer can place these problems in a "malignant" category.[26]

Evolution of Normal Urinary Control

In the infant, a simple reflex governs bladder emptying. When urine distends the bladder sufficiently, it stimulates the reflex arc, and contraction occurs. Simultaneously, reflex relaxation of the external sphincter occurs, allowing the bladder to empty. While the bladder fills, the sphincter tightens to maintain continence. In infancy, there is no conscious or voluntary mediation of this voiding reflex.

The development of an adult pattern of voiding or urinary control is dependent on three separate events.[27] First, the capacity of the bladder must increase to act as a reservoir. Second, voluntary control over the external sphincter must be gained, allowing initiation and termination of micturition. This step is usually mastered by 3 years of age and is first acquired in the daytime. Third, direct voluntary control over the voiding reflex must develop to initiate or inhibit bladder contraction. By approximately 4 years of age, the adult pattern, in which no involuntary or uninhibited detrusor contractions occur during bladder filling, is usually acquired.

Non-neurogenic Voiding Dysfunction in Children

The underlying problem in the great majority of children with voiding dysfunction is an unstable bladder in which detrusor contraction occurs at a time when these children have not yet acquired the ability to voluntarily inhibit the infantile voiding reflex.[28] This is not a pathologic or neurologic disorder, but rather is a delay in CNS maturation. Because these contractions are involuntary and nonsuppressible, a child attempting to maintain continence must constrict the sphincter to stay dry. This results in dyssynergia between the bladder and the sphincter, leading to high intravesical pressure. The external sphincter then acts as an outflow obstruction, causing high intravesical pressure that may damage the bladder, leading to trabeculation, diverticula, reflux, and upper urinary tract damage.

Children with uninhibited bladder contractions and weak sphincters present with urgency, frequency, and urge incontinence. Those with contractions and a strong sphincter maintain continence despite urgency and frequency. Trabeculation, saccules, diverticula, and abnormalities of the ureteric orifices occur in both groups and tend to persist long after the symptoms of dysfunction cease. Reflux may occur in as many as 50% of this patient population. UTI is also common, especially when large residual urine volume is present. In such children, the most important diagnostic aid is the description of the voiding pattern.

Little girls often report "tricks" that they use to stay dry (Fig. 36–4). The most pathognomonic sign is Vincent's curtsey, so named because the child squats and, with her heel, compresses the perineum to obstruct the urethra and thereby prevent leakage. Other girls will cross their legs or dance around. Children trying to hold in urine when they have strong bladder contractions can sometimes complain of abdominal pain, as the pain is related to a bladder trying to empty against an outflow tract obstruction.

Sexual abuse can have significant effects on the voiding pattern. Little girls that have been abused can return to an immature pattern of voiding (i.e., either enuresis or daytime wetting). They can also develop voiding dysfunction when they hold urine as much as they can, either to avoid going to the bathroom and undressing or to try to regain some control over their body.

At the severe end of the voiding dysfunction spectrum are children with day and night wetting, recurrent UTI, constipation, encopresis, and urinary tract abnormalities such as trabeculated bladder, residual urine, vesicoureteral reflux, and upper tract damage. Their bladders strongly resemble the true neurogenic bladder.

Daytime Wetting

Daytime wetting that persists into childhood is never normal and suggests an organic or possibly neurologic etiology. This problem warrants a thorough evaluation.[29] It may otherwise be episodic and associated only with recurrent UTIs. In adolescent girls with borderline continence from underlying neurologic disorders, intermittent continence may be related to periurethral changes precipitated cyclically by the menstrual cycle.

A complete urologic evaluation should be performed, including a cystogram and cystoscopy to evaluate the anatomy of the lower urinary tract. The upper urinary tract should be assessed by IVP or ultrasonography. Finally, a full urodynamic evaluation, including a cystometrogram with electromyography, is recommended.

Neurogenic dysfunction of the bladder is often due to forms of spinal dysraphism. The more overt types of spinal abnormalities, including myelomeningocele and sacral agenesis, are usually discovered early in childhood. Occult types of spinal dysraphism such as lipoma

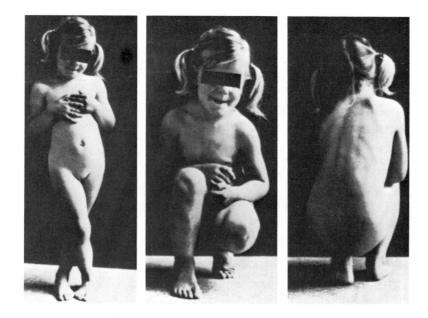

FIGURE 36–4 ••• Example of different postures assumed by children trying to avoid urination. The two photographs on the right show Vincent's curtsey. Note the heel placed to compress the perineum.

of the cord, tethered cord, neurenteric cyst, diastematomyelia, and dermal sinus tract may present in the adolescent.[30] These lesions alter the sacral nerve roots, and the first sign of neurologic dysfunction usually is bladder dysfunction. Patients may also complain of weakness, pain, and numbness of the lower extremities. Physical examination reveals that up to 90% have a skin lesion (e.g., discoloration, a hairy patch, a small fat pad, or sinus tract) over the base of the spine just above the lateral cleft.[30] Spinal radiographs, computed tomographic (CT) or magnetic resonance imaging (MRI) scans, and, occasionally, myelography are necessary to establish the diagnosis of lower spinal cord lesions.

Treatment

The primary goal is resolution of the incontinence by eliminating the uninhibited bladder contraction. The basis of treatment is combined therapy that includes anticholinergic medication, reduction of fluid intake, and control of voiding and constipation.

Anticholinergic medications are used to decrease or eliminate the intensity of the bladder contraction and increase functional bladder capacity. The most commonly used medication is oxybutynin chloride (Ditropan), a moderately potent anticholinergic with strong smooth-muscle antispasmodic activity. Oxybutynin is also known to have analgesic properties, which may decrease bladder sensation and, therefore, urgency. Children can thus increase their bladder capacity and decrease the frequency and intensity of uninhibited bladder contractions. The usual dosage in children is 2.5 to 5 mg two to three times a day; common side effects are mouth dryness and flushing.

Voiding frequency and control of constipation are the two most common variables; these are readily changeable and are perhaps the most important variables in effecting a change in the susceptibility to infection. Frequency and complete bladder emptying play a critical role in the elimination of bacteria. Establishing a voiding schedule in the young child is extremely difficult and sometimes provokes conflicts in the parent-child relationship. However, children should respect the schedule, even though they do not feel the urge to void. Treatment of constipation to eliminate possible compression by a large fecaloma may necessi-

tate intensive therapy with laxatives and stool softeners.[31]

Acute urinary retention in the adolescent is unusual. Urinary retention may be caused by painful voiding from urethritis, vaginitis, trauma, or, more often, psychogenic causes.[30] Herpetic lesions should always be sought with these symptoms. Hysteria of this type can be a result of family, school, or social problems, in which case the patient should undergo psychological evaluation and treatment. The urinary tract is best managed with either intermittent or short-term catheterization, which is basically a stop-gap measure until the underlying psychological cause of the disorder is resolved.[30]

Some adolescents have deep-seated psychological fears of either the "bathroom" or the act of voiding or defecating. These children may have a history of being severely punished by their parents for either wetting or fecal soiling and usually have other manifestations of psychological disturbances. The family situation usually is problematic, and social counseling is most important.[30]

NOCTURNAL ENURESIS

Enuresis is defined as the involuntary voiding of urine beyond the age of anticipated control. The diagnosis of primary enuresis is reserved for those who have never been dry for extended periods; secondary enuresis applies to those who have been dry for at least 6 months before developing enuresis. Nocturnal enuresis involves only nighttime wetting with normal daytime continence and voiding.

The reported prevalence of nocturnal enuresis (Table 36–3) is approximately 15% to 20% of the 5-year-old patient population.[32] Of these, 15% to 20% will achieve nocturnal urinary continence each year; thus, by the age of 15, only 1% to 2% of these adolescents remain enuretic.[32] Secondary enuresis accounts for approximately 20% to 25% of the enuretic population and occurs more frequently in lower socioeconomic populations, in larger

TABLE 36–3 ••• FACTS ABOUT ENURESIS

Prevalence at 5 years of age: 15% to 20%
Patients achieving control each year: 15% to 20%
Patients with associated diurnal enuresis: 15% to 20%
Patients with secondary enuresis: 20% to 25%

families, and in children from discordant families.

Enuresis causes enormous stress and anxiety for the adolescent patient. It is an embarrassing symptom that affects normal development, social confidence, and the ability to develop a positive self-image. Adolescents may secretly believe that there is a relationship between the bladder and sexual functioning that can alter future fertility and may be too embarrassed to seek medical attention.

Etiology

Many causes have been theorized for enuresis. The theory of delayed functional maturation remains the most popular and is supported by a high incidence of a positive family history of enuresis. When both parents have enuresis, 77% of their children are likely to be enuretic; when only one parent is enuretic, 44% are likely to be; when neither parent is enuretic, only 15% of children have bedwetting.[33] The neurophysiologic defect may be related to an abnormality in pelvic floor activity, altering the urethral guarding reflex. This abnormality may be explained by an inadequate central inhibition or by a defect in recognition of adequate bladder filling.

Lovibond argued that enuresis is more likely to be the result of a deficient learning pattern; the basis for this affirmation is that conditioning therapy can be operant and is independent of neurophysiologic maturation.[33a] Mackeith postulated that complete maturation is attained by the age of 5 and that an intense episode of stress occurring between the second and fourth year of life could prevent emergence of the behavioral skills necessary for nocturnal urinary control.[33b]

Enuretic children have been noted to have significantly lower increases in mean serum antidiuretic hormone (ADH) levels when compared with controls.[34] Higher mean nocturnal urinary excretion rates were also observed. No differences in total diurnal urinary volume, osmolality, or water reabsorption were found. Even though there may be a physiologic explanation for some of these cases, it is not known why these children do not wake up to empty their bladder.[34] The pattern of ADH secretion after these children stop bedwetting has not been studied. Notably, enuresis is independent of sleep stage. However, it has been noted consistently that children with nocturnal enuresis are usually very deep sleepers and difficult to awaken.

Although a higher proportion of enuretic children are maladjusted and exhibit behavioral symptoms when compared with nonenuretic children, only a minority have any underlying psychopathology.[35] However, some studies have demonstrated that the enuretic child tends to be more immature and less secure and have less ambition. Children who seek help for enuresis are under more stress and have more behavioral symptoms than those who do not.[35]

An uncommon but important cause of secondary enuresis is UTI. The increased incidence of bacteriuria in the enuretic population may be related to an unstable bladder and associated with a voiding disorder.

Evaluation

After obtaining a careful history, with emphasis on the parent's and child's motivation, the enuresis can be categorized as complicated or uncomplicated.

The vast majority of children with only nighttime wetting, normal physical examination, and normal urine cultures have uncomplicated enuresis. The incidence of associated urinary tract anomalies is so low that it does not justify further investigation. Therefore, whenever underlying pathology is suspected, enuretic children should undergo a VCUG, ultrasound, and spinal radiographs as basic investigation.

Treatment

Individual therapy must be determined with the child and the parents whenever all manifest interest and motivation in being cured. Therapy is rarely necessary before the age of 5 or 6 years. Unfortunately, some families lack the necessary motivation and skills required for a behavioral modification program. Others refuse any medication. Physicians tend to prescribe methods that have been shown to be of limited efficacy, such as fluid restriction, rewards, and reassurance or drug therapy alone.

Behavioral Modification Therapy

The behavioral modification approach requires greater commitment and involvement of the parents, the child, and the physician. The greatest factor to conditioning therapy consists of a signal alarm device that is triggered when the child begins to void. Use of this treatment is limited by the difficulty in awakening the child, as many are deep sleepers. The initial cure rate after 4 to 6 months of treatment averages 60%.[36] Success depends on a cooperative and motivated child, and therefore treatment is inappropriate before 7 to 8 years of age. Results are not as good if there is associated behavioral (psychological) disturbances. Some children fail to awake to the alarm, whereas others are frightened and stressed by it. Adjunctive measures may be a reward after a predetermined number of dry nights. The child is also encouraged to keep a record of progress by placing stickers on a calendar for every dry night. Relapse occurs in 20% to 30% of the children, but this can also be expected with treatment.[37] Transistorized alarm modifications (e.g., Wet-stop, Mytene) use a small sensor that is attached to the child's underwear with an alarm attached to the wrist or pajama.

Pharmacologic Therapy

There appears to be no benefit from the use of sedatives, stimulants, or sympathomimetic agents. Imipramine (Tofranil) is the most widely used tricyclic antidepressant. Its action is a combination of multiple effects such as an antidepressant effect, alterations in arousal and sleep mechanism, and anticholinergic effects. It is usually not used before adolescence, and success rates approach 50%.[37] The recommended dose is 0.9 to 1.5 mg/kg/day, given 1 to 2 hours before bedtime, for 3 to 6 months. After that period of time, the child should be weaned by reducing the dose and then the frequency (every 2 to 3 nights over 3 to 4 weeks). Side effects include daytime sedation, anxiety, insomnia, dry mouth, nausea, and adverse personality changes. Overdose can preclude fatal cardiac arrhythmias, hypotension, respiratory distress, and convulsions. The use of this drug has decreased dramatically, and because of its side effects and dangers, it should be used only in select circumstances with proper warnings and precautions.

DDAVP (1-deamino-[8-D-arginine]-vasopressin) is an analogue of arginine vasopressin (AVP) and produces a marked increase in antidiuretic activity when compared with AVP. It also has a longer duration, is readily absorbed by the nasal mucosa, and does not affect endogenous secretion of AVP. The commercially available spray delivers a dose of 10 μg of DDAVP per spray. DDAVP is considerably more expensive than imipramine, and its effects are usually immediate, so it can be used on a prn basis. The proposed mechanism of action is reduction in nocturnal urine output to a volume smaller than the bladder capacity of the enuretic child.[34]

DDAVP is particularly effective in a subgroup of enuretic patients who do not manifest the normal circadian rhythm of vasopressive excretion. Response varies from a 60% reduction in wetting to up to a 50% cure rate.[37] The initial recommended dose is 20 μg (one spray in each nostril) at bedtime. In nonresponders and partial responders, the dosage can be increased to 40 μg/day. Relapse rates after discontinuation are high. The optimal duration is unknown, but it is rare for treatment to extend beyond 6 months, and it is preferable to taper the dose when discontinuation is planned. Side effects are rare but include transient headache, nausea, mild abdominal cramps, and vulvar pain; they appear to be dose related.

Other Treatment

Anticholinergics such as oxybutynin reduce or abolish uninhibited bladder contractions and may be particularly beneficial in patients who have daytime frequency or enuresis associated with an unstable bladder. Prophylactic antibiotherapy may be added to this regimen in girls with recurrent UTI until they have better control of their bladder. This regimen is effective in 80% of children.[37]

Other "Suspected" Voiding Dysfunctions

True stress incontinence is rare in neurologically normal children, and urodynamic studies are generally normal. Bladder emptying before exertion may be helpful. The daytime urinary frequency syndrome is characterized by the onset of daytime-only urgency and frequency in a previously toilet-trained child.[27] Bladder emptying may occur as often as every 20 minutes without any infection or anomaly. Affected children are usually young, and a previous history of enuresis is present in as many as 40%. The etiology is unknown, but stressful situations are usually noticed. Left untreated, symptoms usually disappear after 2 days to 16 months; the recurrence rate is approximately 3%.

The "lazy bladder" syndrome applies to "busy" girls who hold their urine as much as they can and do not empty their bladder for periods of 8 to 12 hours or longer. The bladder enlarges, and the emptying capacity is often insufficient, with a fair amount of residual urine. Urinary retention develops, reflecting bladder decompensation without obstruction. Investigation is mandatory to identify an underlying neuropathy, but results are usually normal. Treatment consists of patient education, scheduled voiding, and, occasionally, catheterization.

If wetting occurs in a dribbling fashion when the child stands up or just after voiding, pooling of urine into the vagina must be suspected. Unless labial adhesions are present, the problem can be solved by having the child void while standing with her knees far apart over the commode. However, continuous dribbling should raise the suspicion of a more complicated problem such as an ectopic ureter.

HEMATURIA

Hematuria is a common presenting symptom in neonates and children, but its implications in children are very different from those in adults, as neoplasia is a rare cause of hematuria in children (Table 36–4). Stress hematuria is a special situation encountered in adolescents and may be associated with sports. This condition must be seriously evaluated even though results are usually negative and the etiology unknown.

In children presenting to the emergency department with gross hematuria, Ingelfinger and coworkers found that 49% had associated UTI.[37a] Microscopic hematuria is even more common. A screening of school-aged children revealed that 34% had microscopic hematuria.[38]

The initial evaluation of hematuria in children should include a urine culture and studies to localize the bleeding if the culture is negative. Urinalysis of a freshly voided specimen demonstrating proteinuria, oval fat bodies, or granular casts is strongly suggestive of renal parenchymal disease. However, when gross hematuria is present in the absence of UTI or

TABLE 36–4 ••• ETIOLOGY OF GROSS HEMATURIA IN 150 CHILDREN

	Number (%)
Readily Apparent Causes	
Documented urinary tract infection	39 (26)
Perineal irritation	16 (11)
Meatal stenosis with ulcer	11 (7)
Trauma	10 (7)
Coagulopathy	5 (3)
Stones	3 (2)
Other Causes	
Suspected urinary tract infection	35 (23)
Unknown	13 (9)
Recurrent gross hematuria	7 (5)
Acute nephritis	6 (4)
Ureteropelvic junction obstruction	2 (1)
Cystitis cystica	1 (<1)
Epididymitis	1 (<1)
Tumor	1 (<1)

renal parenchymal damage, a complete urologic evaluation is necessary to rule out neoplasms, urolithiasis, a foreign body, or an anatomic cause for the hematuria such as horseshoe kidney or cystic renal damage. In every unexplained case of hematuria, the possibility of sexual abuse must also be ruled out.

Urinary Calculi

Urinary stones or calculi are quite rare in adolescents and children. The exact incidence is unknown but is reported to be 3 to 6 per 100,000 in the United Kingdom.[38] In children younger than 16 years of age, the vast majority of the stones are composed of a mixture of elements, with the most common element (61%) being struvite, followed by ammonium urate and calcium oxalate.[38] The etiology is unknown except for associated inborn errors of metabolism, but these usually present earlier in childhood. Calculi may also be associated with anatomic obstructive abnormalities and recurrent infection. Stone disease should be treated surgically if there is evidence of obstruction, pain, or associated infection.

Urinary Tract Malignancies

Urinary tract malignancies are quite rare in childhood and adolescence. In the kidney, Wilms' tumor and renal cell adenocarcinoma are commonly considered. In the bladder, transitional cell carcinoma and sarcoma have been reported. These tumors will usually present as recurrent painless hematuria, abdominal pain, recurrent UTI, or an abdominal mass.

A renal tumor is suggested by palpation of a mass in the flank. The most common differential diagnoses of a renal mass include multicystic renal dysplasia, hydronephrosis, Wilms' tumor, simple cyst, or abscess. Such masses can be quite large and often compress the bladder in such a way that difficulty with urination is the first presenting symptom. The contralateral kidney should be assessed, as 40% of anomalies have been reported in the contralateral side.

Trauma

Trauma is the leading cause of death in children.[38] Renal trauma, like other types of trauma, is classified as blunt or penetrating. Blunt trauma is more common in children and is usually associated with other significant injuries. Renal injuries are more common than splenic or hepatic injuries associated with rapid deceleration or severe flexion involving the renal pedicle. Because the adventitia of the renal artery is more elastic than the intima, a tear may occur, leading to subintimal dissection and post-traumatic thrombosis of the renal artery. Preexisting renal abnormalities such as hydronephrosis or abnormal position increase the potential for renal damage.

Physical findings such as abdominal tenderness, flank mass, ecchymosis or hematoma over the flank, or fractured ribs can be important markers for potential renal injury. Hematuria is usually the first and the most reliable indicator for injury. Blood at the urethral meatus may suggest severe urethral injury.

There is controversy with respect to the amount of hematuria considered indicative of severe renal injury.[38] Stalker et al. reported that more than 50 red blood cells per high power field (RBC/HPF) are significant, while Lieu and coworkers agreed that 20 RBC/HPF are significant.[38, 38a, 38b] Complications of renal trauma can be early or late. The former include delayed bleeding, infection, abscess, sepsis, urinary fistula, or extravasation and urinoma; the latter include strictures, hydronephrosis, and hypertension.

In infants and young children, the full bladder sits more cephalad and is primarily an abdominal organ not protected by the bony pelvis. Blunt lower abdominal trauma, with or without pelvic fracture, may cause bladder rupture. When rupture occurs, it is noted in either the peritoneal or extraperitoneal space; 90% of bladder ruptures are extraperitoneal. Diagnosis is established with cystography.

Usually straddle-type injuries affect the anterior urethra. In this instance, the urethra is compressed against the ischial rami. When injury is significant, the patient may present with blood at the meatus or difficulty in voiding, leading to a distended bladder.

ANOMALIES OF THE URINARY TRACT

Anomalies of the urogenital tract are among the most common anomalies of all organ systems. It has been estimated that almost 10% of the population have a symptomatic urogenital anomaly. A complete understanding of the embryologic development of the urinary tract is a prerequisite for the evaluation and management of a child with a congenital genitourinary malformation.

Renal Agenesis

Absence of a kidney results from failure of induction of the metanephric blastema by the ureteral bud. The clinical incidence found on IVP during autopsies is between 1 in 1500 and 1 in 100. There is a slight male predominance, and the condition most often occurs on the left side.[39]

In most cases there are many associated anomalies (e.g., absence of the ipsilateral ureter). Anomalies of the contralateral kidney (e.g., malrotation and ectopia) may be encountered in 15% of patients. The genital tract is by far the most common system involved in associated anomalies.[39] Such anomalies usually involve the uterus and vagina and are represented by either a unicornuate or a bicornuate uterus with rudimentary or absence of the ipsilateral fallopian tube.[39]

The diagnosis is confirmed on excretory urography, which identifies the absence of a kidney with a compensatory contralateral kidney. Ultrasonography may be helpful in screening parents or siblings. Bilateral agenesis (Potter's syndrome) occurs in 1 in every 4000 births; 40% of these infants are stillborn and the remainder often succomb secondary to pulmonary hypoplasia. Complete duplication of the vagina, cervix, and uterus with imperforate hemivagina is a rare condition caused by combined müllerian and mesonephric duct abnormalities. The syndrome is always associated with unilateral renal agenesis on the side of vaginal obstruction.

Associated Anomalies

Malrotation or abnormal rotation is associated with an ectopic or fused kidney. The condition is usually an incidental finding and may be either unilateral or bilateral. Most patients are symptomatic unless there is an obstruction caused by an anomalous accessory vessel.

Failure of the kidney to complete its ascent, or renal ectopia, can be secondary to a number of factors, including an abnormality of the ureteral bud, a teratogen, or a vascular anomaly. The incidence of renal ectopy is higher at autopsy (1 in 500 to 1 in 1290) than in clinical studies, suggesting that many cases remain unrecognized.[39] The most commonly encountered position is at the sacrum immediately below the aortic bifurcation.

Of this class of renal anomalies, most are identified during childhood. UTIs are a common presentation occurring in 30% of children. Pelvic kidneys may be difficult to visualize, but excretory urography and ultrasound confirm the location of the anomaly. The contralateral kidney may be abnormal in 50% of patients, and 10% have contralateral renal agenesis.[38] Associated VUR may be present in 70% of patients. Associated anomalies of the genitalia include cardiovascular and skeletal anomalies. Although many patients remain asymptomatic, surgical intervention may be necessary, primarily because of the increased incidence of ureteropelvic junction obstruction and high-grade VUR.

Horseshoe kidney is the most common type of renal fusion defect, with an incidence of 1 in 400. The isthmus joining the kidney may consist of renal parenchyma or fibrous tissue. There is a 3.5% incidence of associated congenital malformations in several syndromes such as Turner's syndrome or trisomy 18.[38]

Urethral Prolapse

Urethral prolapse occurs most often in black girls less than 10 years old. These patients

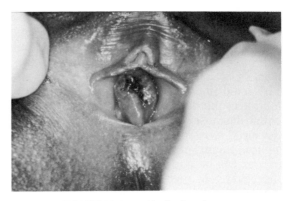

FIGURE 36–5 ••• Urethral prolapse.

usually present with dysuria and vaginal spotting; frank hematuria is not common. On physical examination, a rather typical-appearing, everted, hemorrhagic, doughnut-shaped mass is seen superior to, but often obscuring, the hymenal ring.

Some researchers have advocated surgical excision by excising the prolapsed epithelium at the 12 o'clock position and securing the edge with a suture (Fig. 36–5).[38] Nonsurgical approaches (e.g., application of an antimicrobial ointment or a conjugated estrogen cream in association with sitz baths) are effective and should be the initial treatment. Excision is reserved for persistent or recurrent cases.

OTHER ABNORMALITIES RELATED TO THE URINARY TRACT

Sexually Transmitted Diseases

Urethritis, or inflammation of the urethra, is manifested as urethral discharge, burning, or pain on initiation of urination. The symptoms of urethritis in adolescents are similar to those in adults. In children, additional symptoms include urethral discharge, meatal inflammation (e.g., erythema, edema), pyuria, and urethral tenderness. The most common cause of urethritis is infection with *Chlamydia trachomatis, Neisseria gonorrhoeae, Mycoplasma* spp., *Trichomonas vaginalis,* herpes simplex virus, or coliform bacteria.

Dysuria occurs in 20% of women with chlamydial or gonococcal infection; the erroneous diagnosis of UTI is often made based on this symptom. Urinalysis may often show pyuria with a nonsignificant growth on culture.[9] Pyuria (10 white blood cells per high power field) in the absence of significant bacteria is the hallmark sign of underlying urethritis. Treatment, of course, is based on identifying the underlying source of infection.

Abnormalities in Adolescents With Special Needs

Upper and lower urogenital tract dysfunction often occurs in children and adolescents with neurologic handicaps. Patients with special needs include those with CNS lesions (e.g., cerebral palsy, mental retardation) and those with spinal cord lesions from either congenital anomalies (spina bifida, myelomeningocele, or sacral agenesis) or acquired lesions (trauma, neoplasms.)

The major concerns of the child or adolescent with these abnormalities are management of bladder control and bowel and sexual functions. A program of early urologic surveillance (radiographic and urodynamic) should therefore be instituted in newborns with spinal disorders and should continue during childhood and adolescence.

Those patients who exhibit high intravesical pressures should be identified and treated as soon as possible to prevent irreversible lower and upper urinary tract damage. A program of intermittent catheterization, along with anticholinergic medications, may be needed to reduce the chronically elevated intravesical pressure. This will resolve or improve reflux and hydronephrosis in the majority of cases. Clean intermittent self-catheterization can be accomplished in children as young as 4 to 6 years of age and be successfully performed if taught by a supportive multidisciplinary team. This approach has virtually revolutionized the care of these patients. Anticholinergic agents, as well as imipramine, can be helpful. In patients with high pressure in the bladder refractory to intermittent catheterization, or in very young infants, a cutaneous vesicostomy can be performed to temporarily relieve upper urinary tract pressure and prevent reflux.[30]

References

1. Jordal U. The natural history of bacteriuria in childhood. Infect Dis Clin North Am 1987; 1:713.
2. Lindbergh U, Bjure J, Haugstredt S, et al. Asymptomatic bacteriuria in school girls: Relation between residual urine volume and recurrence. Acta Pediatr Scand 1975; 64:437.
3. Lindbergh V, Claesson I, Harisen LA, et al. Asymptomatic bacteriuria in school girls: VIII. Clinical course during a three-year follow-up. J Pediatr 1978; 92:194.
4. Kallenius GS, Svensson SB, Hultbey H, et al. Occurrence of P-fimbriated *E. coli* in urinary tract infection. Lancet 1981; 2:1369.
5. Savage DC, Wilson MI, McHardy M, et al. Covert bacteriuria of childhood. Arch Dis Child 1973; 48(1):8–20.
6. Siegel SR, Siegel B, Sokoloff BZ, et al. Urinary infection in infants and preschool children. Am J Dis Child 1980; 134:369.
7. Rushton HG, Massoud M. Dimercaptosuccinic acid renal scintigraphy for the evaluation of pyelonephritis and scarring. J Urol 1992; 148:1726.
8. Jordal U. Host risk factors in pyelonephritis. In: Rushton HG, Erlich RM (eds). Dialogues in Pediatric Urology. Vol 13. Pearl River, NY: William J. Miller Associates, 1990.
9. Kunin CM, Deutscher R, Paquin A Jr. Urinary tract infection in school children: An epidemiologic, clinical and laboratory study. Medicine 1964; 4:91.
9a. Kass EH. Asymptomatic infections of the urinary tract. Trans Assoc Am Phys 1956; 69:56–60.
10. Smellie JM, Edwards D, Hunter N, et al. Vesicoureteric reflex and renal scarring. Kidney Int 1975; (suppl 4):65.
10a. Stamey TA, Sexton CC. The role of vaginal colonization with enterobacteriaceae in recurrent urinary infections. J Urol 1975; 113:214–217.
11. Johnson CE, DeBaz EP, Shurin PA, et al. Renal ultrasound evaluation of urinary tract infections in children. Pediatrics 1986; 78, 871–878.
12. Berdon WE. Contemporary imaging approach to pediatric urology problems. Radiol Clin North Am 1991; 29(3):605–618.
13. Rajkumar S, Saxena Y, Rajaggral V, et al. Trimethoprim in pediatric urinary tract infection. Child Nephrol Urol 1988–89; 9:77.
14. Roberto U, D'Eufenua P, Martino F, et al. Amoxicillin and clavulanic acid in the treatment of urinary tract infection in children. J Int Med Res 1989; 17:168.
15. Ball P. Ciprofloxacin: An overview of adverse experiences. J Anti Chem 1986; 18(suppl D):187.
16. Madrigal G, Ohio CM, Mohs E, et al. Single dose antibiotic therapy is not as effective as conventional regimens for management of acute urinary tract infections in children. Pediatr Infect Dis J 1988; 7:316.
17. Bailey R. Review of published studies on single dose therapy of urinary tract infections. Infection 1990; Suppl 18(2):53.
18. Ransley PG, Risdon RA. Reflux nephropathy: Effects of antimicrobial therapy on the evolution of the early pyelonephritic scar. Kidney Int 1981; 20:733.
19. Smellie JM, Normand ICS, Kaz G. Children with urinary infection: A comparison of those with and those without vesicoureteric reflux. Kidney Int 1981; 20:717.
20. Baker R, Moxted W, Majlath J, et al. Relation of age, sex and infection to reflux and data indicating high spontaneous cure rate in pediatric patients. J Urol 1966; 95:27.
21. Woodard JR, Holden S. The prognostic significance of fever in childhood urinary infections: Observations in 350 consecutive patients. Clin Pediatr 1976; 15:1051.

22. Hannerz K, Wikstad I, Celsi G, et al. Influence of vesicoureteral reflux and urinary tract infection and renal growth in children with upper urinary tract duplication. Acta Radiol 1989; 30:391.

22a. Taylor CM. Unstable bladder activity and the rate of resolution of vesico-ureteric reflux. Contrib Nephrol 1984; 39:238.

23. Sidi AA, Perry W, Gonzalez R. Vesicoureteral reflux in children with myelodysplasia: Natural history and results of treatment. J Urol 1986; 136:239.

23a. Skoog SJ, Belman AB, Majd M. A nonsurgical approach to the management of primary vesicoureteral reflux. J Urol 1987; 138:1205.

24. Smellie JM, Edwards D, Hunter N, et al. Vesicoureteric reflux and renal scarring. Kidney Int 1975 (suppl 4):65.

25. Olbing H, Claesson I, Ebel KD, et al. Renal scars and parenchymal thinning in children with vesicoureteral reflux: A 5-year report of the international reflux study in children. J Urol 1992; 148:1653.

26. Himsl KK, Hurwitz RS. Pediatric urinary incontinence. Urol Clin North Am 1991; 18(2):283.

27. Nash DFE. The development of micturition control with special reference to enuresis. Ann Radiol Coll Surg Engl 1949; 5:318.

28. Koff SA. Relationship between dysfunctional voiding and reflux. J Urol 1992; 148:1703.

29. Koff SA. Evaluation and management of voiding disorders in children. Urol Clin North Am 1988; 15(4):769.

30. Reshef E, Casale AJ, Sanfilippo JS. Age specific urinary tract problems: Young adult female. In: Buchsbaum HJ, Schmidt JD (eds). Gynecologic and Obstetric Urology. 3rd ed. Philadelphia: WB Saunders, 1993.

31. van Gool JD, Hjalmas K, Tamminen-Mobius T, Olbing H. Historical clues to the complex of dysfunctional voiding, urinary tract infection and vesicoureteral reflux. J Urol 1992; 148:1699.

32. Miller JFW. Children who wet the bed in bladder control and enuresis. In: Kolvin I, Mackeith RC, Meadow SR (eds). Bladder Control and Enuresis. London: Medical Books Ltd, 1973.

33. Bakwin H. The genetics of enuresis. In: Kolvin RC, Mackeith SR (eds). Bladder Control and Enuresis. London: Medical Books Ltd, 1973.

33a. Lovibond SH, Coote MA. Enuresis. In: Costello CG (ed). Symptoms of Psychopathology. New York: John Wiley, 1970.

33b. Mackeith RC. Is maturation delay a frequent factor in the origins of primary nocturnal enuresis? Dev Med Child Neurol 1972; 14:217.

34. Norgaard JP, Rittig S. Recent studies of the pathophysiology of nocturnal enuresis. In: Meadow SR (ed). Desmopressin in Nocturnal Enuresis. Proceeding of an International Symposium. Conwell, Sutton, Coldfield, England: Horus Medical, 1989.

35. Moffatt MEK. Nocturnal enuresis: Psychologic implications of treatment and non-treatment. J Pediatr 1989; 114(suppl):697.

36. Turner RK. Conditioning treatment of nocturnal enuresis present status. In: Kolvin I, Mackeith RC, Meadow SR (eds). Bladder Control and Enuresis. London: Medical Books Ltd, 1973.

37. Walsh PC, Retik AB, Stamey TA, Vaughan ED Jr. Campbell's Urology. 6th ed. Philadelphia: WB Saunders, 1992.

37a. Ingelfinger JR, Davis AE, Grupe WE. Frequency and etiology of gross hematuria in a general pediatric setting. Pediatrics 1977; 59:557.

38. Kelalis PP, King LR, Belman AB. Clinical Pediatric Urology. 3rd ed. Philadelphia: WB Saunders, 1992.

38a. Stalker HP, Kaufman RA, Stedje K. The significance of hematuria in children after blunt abdominal trauma. AJR 1990; 154:569.

38b. Lieu TA, Fleischer GR, Mahboubi S, Schwatz JS. Hematuria and clinical findings as indication for intravenous pyelography in pediatric blunt renal trauma. Pediatrics 1988; 82:216.

39. Anderson KA, McAninich JW. Uterus didelphys with left hematocolpos and ipsilateral renal agenesis. J Urol 1982; 127:550–553.

CHAPTER 37

Breast Disorders

PATRICIA S. SIMMONS

It is common in medical practice to apply principles to the care of children and adolescents that have been derived from experience with adult patients. This is not surprising, as many pathologic entities are more common in adults and many of the studies in the medical literature have been derived from adult populations, for humanitarian as well as practical reasons. The ethics as well as the technical aspects of research in minors are necessarily complex and limit data generation. However, caution should be taken when applying principles and lessons derived from adult medicine to the young. Nowhere is this more true than in physiologic and pathologic conditions of the female breast. This chapter on normal and abnormal aspects of the breast in female children and adolescents represents a synthesis of the relevant pediatric and adolescent medical literature and the impressions of physicians who frequently deal with these issues. Specific topics will include congenital anomalies of the breast, normal and abnormal development, and breast masses in the child and adolescent.

In addition, the issue of the adolescent breast self-examination will be explored, with discussions of the value and potential hazards of this health maintenance practice. One of the most important developments in breast disease has been the advent of imaging techniques in the pediatric and adolescent population. While mammograms are the mainstay of evaluation of the adult female breast, this modality has less value in the young. The role of other forms of breast imaging, as well as mammography, in the pediatric and adolescent patient will be explored.

EXAMINATION OF THE BREAST IN THE CHILD AND ADOLESCENT

Infant and Young Child

Examination of the breast should begin in the neonatal period. The physician should examine the infant for the presence of normal breast buds and to rule out a congenital anomaly. Examination of the breast is part of the gestational age assessment, as the amount of tissue varies with maturation. Polymastia may be detectable in the newborn but may not be recognized until the child is older. Examination of the infant with the parent present provides an opportunity to educate the family about normal breast appearance and any related concerns. Well-child examinations and general medical evaluations through childhood provide the physician with an opportunity to monitor the normal stages of breast development and to detect any developmental or structural abnormality. Simple inspection and palpation of the juvenile breast should not be emotionally traumatic, as it can be readily accomplished during anterior chest inspection and auscultation. Just as in adults, it is imperative to respect the child's or the adolescent's modesty.

Pubertal Girl

Examination of the pubertal girl should include Tanner staging of the breast and the pubic hair.[1] Reassuring the patient of her normality and some discussion of normal pubertal progression are appropriate and encouraged. Many young girls question their own normalcy, including their degree or lack of breast development. Breasts should be checked for asymmetry as well as for masses, congenital anomalies, developmental abnormalities, and nipple discharge.

Adolescent

Breast examination should be performed as part of routine health care for and general examination of the adolescent female. Tanner staging should be accomplished along with visual inspection and palpation of the breasts to exclude abnormality. The technique for examination of the adolescent breast is not dissimilar to that for adults. Later this chapter will review the subject of the adolescent breast self-examination. If self-examination is to be taught, this point in the patient's visit is an appropriate time to do so. Most adolescents prefer to have their breasts examined with parents out of the room and should be given that option. This provides an opportunity to explain normal development to the adolescent, address any abnormalities, and review any concerns the patient has. The physician, working together with the adolescent, must determine who should be present during the breast examination, considering the parent, accompanying person, and/or a chaperone.

INFANCY AND EARLY CHILDHOOD

The presence of palpable and often visible breast tissue in the term newborn infant is normal and expected. Premature infants are less likely to have neonatal breast buds, a fact that has been incorporated into the assessment of gestational age system defined by Dubowitz and Dubowitz.[2] The amount of breast tissue present in the normal newborn varies and may be associated with milk production ("witch's milk"). The presence of breast tissue in the newborn has been attributed to maternal hormone stimulation, but there is reason to believe that another mechanism may be involved, as breast buds may persist for months, long after the direct effect of maternal hormones

should be gone.[3] In fact, the natural history of neonatal breast development is incompletely understood. Persistence of neonatal breast buds through 10 months of age has been documented in normal infants by McKiernan and Hull.[4] However, persistence of breast tissue in normal female children through the first 2 years of life has been observed. This observation is complicated by the fact that the presence of breasts in this age group also occurs in an abnormal condition, precocious puberty. Defining the normal amount of breast tissue present through early life is important, as it may help in understanding when it is appropriate to be concerned about the presence of breast tissue in young children and embark on an evaluation to rule out true, incomplete, or pseudoprecocious puberty (see Chapter 5). Currently a study in progress is looking at normal degrees of breast tissue during the first 2 years of life, as well as possible modifying factors. For the present, in the individual patient, it can be useful to document breast tissue on well-child evaluations, as new appearance versus persistence may be pertinent in distinguishing an abnormality from normal physiology.

Congenital Anomalies of the Breast

The most common congenital anomaly of the breast is polythelia (Fig. 37–1). In this condition, accessory nipples and areolae may appear anywhere along the milk ridge from the axilla to the groin. Most commonly an incomplete nipple/areola appears a few centimeters inferior to the breast on one or both

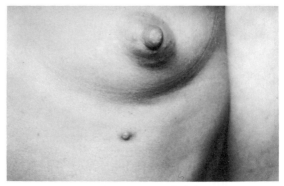

FIGURE 37–1 ••• Polythelia.

sides. Polymastia (i.e., accessory breast tissue) is less common and may become a significant problem at puberty or during pregnancy and lactation. Sometimes surgical excision of the extramammary tissue is indicated.

Congenital amastia is extremely rare (Fig. 37–2). Occasionally concern will arise because of what appears to be poor nipple/areolar development in a child with hypopigmentation. However, at puberty development of the breasts can be expected to occur.

Mastitis

Mastitis in the newborn presents as erythema, tenderness, and sometimes swelling of the affected breast; it is usually unilateral but may also be bilateral. The underlying mechanism may involve obstruction of a mammary duct. Treatment with warm compresses is generally effective, but if there is engorgement in the newborn's breast, the physician may express some milk to relieve pressure, increase comfort, and hasten resolution. Antibiotics are not usually necessary, but these infants must be watched carefully for signs of infection in the breast. If infection is suspected, antibiotic therapy, as well as close observation and local care, may be indicated. Mastitis, although uncommon, also occurs in older infants and children. Management includes warm compresses to the affected breast, antibiotics, and monitoring for signs of systemic infection.

BREAST ENLARGMENT AND MASSES IN THE PREPUBERTAL AGED CHILD

Unilateral Breast Masses

The presence of a breast mass in a young child provokes anxiety in parents and often in physicians (Fig. 37–3). Fortunately, breast malignancy is extremely rare in this age group, and most of these masses are benign. A variety of types of masses have been identified in children's breasts, including hemangioma, lipoma, papilloma, lymphangioma, benign cyst, fibrosis, localized mastitis, hematoma, fat necrosis, and other benign tumors (Table 37–1). Of these, breast hemangioma is probably the most common, and the diagnosis is usually obvious on inspection. A breast hemangioma

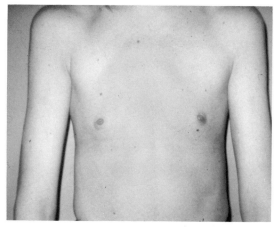

FIGURE 37–2 ••• Congenital amastia.

is most often found superior and lateral to the areola and is soft, freely movable, nontender, and of the consistency of hemangiomas that occur elsewhere on the body. A superficial vascular pattern on the breast may be apparent. These are actually hemangiomas of the connective tissue superficial to the breast parenchyma. Breast hemangiomas in children are best left alone and observed only. Surgical excision is not necessary and in fact can destroy the underlying breast bud and lead to iatrogenic unilateral amastia. The hemangioma may persist for years and becomes less apparent with pubertal breast development.

Cysts are rare in this age group and more likely to occur in the pubertal or adult female. Transillumination, ultrasonography, and transdermal aspiration may be useful in the diagnosis just as in older patients, but again, care should be taken to avoid trauma, and follow-up is very important.

A mass lesion underlying the area of the breast but not truly in the breast may also mimic a breast mass. This differentiation tends to be more difficult in the pubertal child or adolescent with more breast tissue. However, specific imaging techniques may help localize a mass and suggest its etiology.

When breast development is asynchronous at thelarche, the first breast bud may be mistaken for a neoplasm. Either precocious or normal puberty may present with a unilateral breast bud as its first sign. Development of the second breast or other secondary sex characteristics may not be apparent for up to 6 months. Again, biopsy should be avoided.

Malignancy of the breast is extremely rare in children, and although case reports exist, it

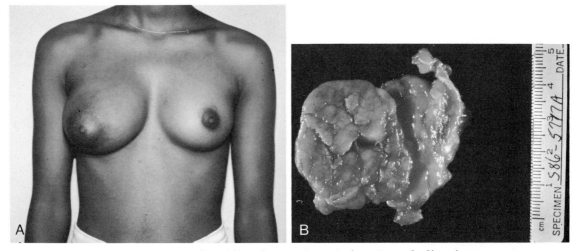

FIGURE 37–3 ••• *A,* Unilateral fibroadenoma. *B,* Surgical specimen of a fibroadenoma.

is difficult to determine its incidence or prevalence. Only 17 cases of primary carcinoma of the breast have been reported in children 15 years old or younger.[5]

When the clinical assessment suggests a benign process leading to development of a mass in the breast, observation is preferred over surgical excision or biopsy for most children. However, when malignancy or infection refractory to medical management alone is suspected, surgery must be undertaken and extreme care exhibited to protect the breast bud.

TABLE 37–1 ••• DIFFERENTIAL DIAGNOSIS OF BREAST ENLARGEMENT IN PREPUBERTAL AGE GIRLS

Unilateral
  Hemangioma
  Lipoma
  Papilloma
  Lymphangioma
  Cyst
  Fibrosis
  Mastitis
  Hematoma
  Fat necrosis
  Tumors of adjacent structures
  Thelarche
  Breast cancer (extremely rare)
Bilateral
  Premature thelarche
  Precocious puberty
    True precocious puberty
    Exogenous estrogen exposure
    Endogenous estrogen hyperproduction (usually an ovarian source)
    Hypothyroidism ("overlap syndrome")

Early Breast Development

The normal breast buds present in newborn infants of both sexes resolve over the early weeks and months of life. Breast development before age 8 in females is considered abnormal. Bilateral breast enlargement may result from premature thelarche or precocious puberty. Differentiation of these two conditions is important, as the former represents a self-limited process without significant underlying pathology or sequelae, and the latter represents a progressive process that may have a serious underlying cause and adverse sequelae.

Premature Thelarche and Precocious Puberty

By definition, premature thelarche is isolated breast development before age 8 in females; it was first described in 1946 and named in 1965.[6] Its prevalence is calculated to be 2%.[7] This common cause of breast development in young girls represents an incomplete, transient, and benign form of precocious puberty. The most common age for presentation is 15 months, and most girls are younger than 2 years. There is another peak of incidence in children between 6 and 8 years, but this is less common. Patients with premature thelarche are characterized by isolated bilateral breast development. They have normal growth and no other clinical signs of estrogen or androgen effect (i.e., no sex hair, axillary sweat, acne, virilization, gross vaginal mucosa estrogenization, or menses). Their growth velocity is normal. This is not a familial condition, and it is not associated with central nervous system gross pathology or other symptoms or findings. The past medical history is usually unremarkable, although some data suggest that premature infants may be at risk for developing premature thelarche.[8] Others have failed to show this association.[9] It is important to obtain a thorough history to rule out exogenous estrogen exposure. Presently, the most common form of exogenous estrogen ingestion may be the oral contraceptive. Estrogen-containing creams and other preparations may also result in breast development, as well as other hormonal effects. Pseudoprecocious puberty has also been linked to meat treated or contaminated with sex steroids.[10]

If the patient meets the clinical criteria for premature thelarche, certain studies are recommended to exclude precocious puberty, as breast development may be the first sign of precocity. Radiographic imaging to determine bone age is recommended. In premature thelarche, the bone age should be within two standard deviations of the chronologic age. Bone age may be advanced in precocious puberty, and delayed bone age may result from hypothyroidism. An assessment of estrogen is also recommended. This can be obtained either through venous sampling for estradiol levels or with a vaginal maturation index. The vaginal maturation index is obtained atraumatically by swabbing the vaginal wall with a saline-moistened urethral swab, taking care to avoid touching the hymen.[11] Contact with the hymen can cause pain and can falsely elevate the percentage of superficial cells, leading to an overestimation of estrogen effect. Often, multiple serum estradiol levels are necessary to detect or rule out hyperestrogenemia. Mild elevations of estradiol have been described in premature thelarche[12, 13]; higher elevations suggest another diagnosis. Table 37–2 shows the results of vaginal maturation index and serum estradiol for normal girls and for those with premature thelarche and precocious puberty. Assessment of thyroid function is also appropriate. Serum total thyroxine and thyroid-stimulating hormone levels should be normal and are assessed in order to exclude the "overlap syndrome." Sexual precocity can occur with severe hypothyroidism, although this is rare. Patients with hypothyroidism associated with breast development should have low serum thyroxine levels, elevated thyroid-stimulating hormone levels, short stature and/or decreased growth velocity, and delayed bone age.

Random or basal levels of luteinizing hormone (LH) and follicle-stimulating hormone (FSH) are not useful in diagnosing premature thelarche. Levels of these hormones should be in the prepubertal normal range, but similar levels may also be seen in precocious puberty and hence do not rule out the latter diagnostic possibility. Provocative testing with gonadotropin-releasing hormone is used to document LH and FSH elevations of precocious puberty. Assessment of serum prolactin also does not contribute to the diagnosis. Basal levels of both prolactin and thyrotropin-releasing hormone–stimulated prolactin are normal in premature thelarche and precocious puberty.

In general, other than bone age, imaging studies are not necessary to make the diagnosis

TABLE 37–2 ••• HORMONAL ACTIVITY IN NORMAL PREPUBERTAL GIRLS COMPARED WITH THAT IN GIRLS WITH PREMATURE THELARCHE AND PRECOCIOUS PUBERTY

	Normal	Premature Thelarche	Precocious Puberty
Serum estradiol[9] (pg/ml)	4 ± 0.6	5.5 ± 0.32	38 ± 9
VMI[12]	60–90/10–20/0–3	60/30/5–10	20/50/30
Bone age	Normal	Normal	Usually advanced
Serum prolactin	Normal	Normal	Normal
Stimulated prolactin	Normal	Normal	Elevated*
Serum LH	Normal	Normal	Normal or elevated
Stimulated LH	Normal	Normal	Elevated
Serum FSH	Normal	Normal or elevated	Normal or elevated
Stimulated FSH	Normal	Elevated	Elevated

*Greater than 2 S.D. above the mean.

FSH, Follicle-stimulating hormone; LH, Luteinizing hormone; VMI, Vaginal maturation index, expressed as a percentage of basal/intermediate/superficial cells.

of premature thelarche. Brain imaging using computerized tomography or nuclear magnetic resonance is indicated in patients with suspected precocious puberty or central nervous system abnormality. Pelvic ultrasound may also be useful if the diagnosis of premature thelarche is questionable. The ultrasound should show a normal prepubertal uterus as compared with the estrogen-stimulated uterus of larger size and different proportions expected in either normal or precocious pubertal females. Pelvic ultrasound is useful if an ovarian etiology is suspected (i.e., hormonally active ovarian cyst or tumor leading to pseudo-precocious puberty). One author has described a difference in the appearance of ovarian cysts in girls with premature thelarche compared with that of cysts in girls with precocious puberty. In premature thelarche, cysts are isolated or nonexistent, whereas in precocious or normal puberty, multiple cysts are seen.[14] This observation has not been applied to a large number of patients, and its clinical utility is not established.

The prognosis for patients with premature thelarche is excellent. If the child is younger than 2 years, the breast tissue regresses. In the older child, breast development may regress or persist.[15] In either case, normal puberty occurs at the appropriate age.

The mechanism of premature thelarche is intriguing. A number of theories have been put forward, including increased breast sensitivity to estrogen, transient estrogen-secreting follicular cysts of the ovaries, increased estrogen from adrenal precursors, increased dietary estrogen, and transient partial activation of the hypothalamic-pituitary-ovarian axis with excessive follicle-stimulating hormone secretion. This last theory appears most likely and is supported by a number of studies.[13, 14, 16–18]

It is important to differentiate premature thelarche from precocious puberty in girls who present with early breast development. Premature thelarche is a transient and benign condition that is diagnosed by exclusion. Precocious puberty is progressive and may have a serious underlying origin and sequelae. Clinically, these conditions may be distinguished by examination of growth, bone age, vaginal maturation index and/or serum estradiol level, course, presence of other hormonal effects, and clinical or laboratory exclusion of primary hypothyroidism. The laboratory findings in normal young girls are compared with those in girls with premature thelarche and precocious puberty in Table 37–2. When precocious puberty is suspected from clinical and/or laboratory findings, further evaluation is indicated to look for an underlying cause. The particular studies indicated depend on the results of the initial clinical assessment. In isosexual precocity, brain imaging using computerized tomography (coronal views) or nuclear magnetic resonance should be performed to rule out a central nervous system mass lesion. Signs of virilization mandate evaluation for excessive androgen production, which is nearly always of adrenal or ovarian origin. Patients suspected of having precocious puberty should be appropriately evaluated and have close follow-up (see Chapter 5). Although most cases of isosexual precocious puberty in girls are idiopathic, the psychological manifestations of early pubertal development, as well as the potential for short stature from prematurely fused epiphyses, mandate careful follow-up by a physician familiar with this condition. In addition, malignant or benign tumors, more often of the ovary than of the adrenal, may present as precocious puberty and require surgical intervention for diagnosis and therapy.

THE BREAST AT PUBERTY

Thelarche is defined as the onset of breast development in the female. The normal age range for thelarche is 8 to 14 years, with a mean age of 11 years. Thelarche is usually the first sign of puberty and is followed within 6 months by pubarche and within 2 to 4 years by menarche. It is not uncommon for asynchronous breast development to occur, in which case the second breast may not begin to develop until up to 6 months after the first. Appearance of sex hair before thelarche is also normal and not uncommon. The stages of breast development have been described by Marshall and Tanner, who provide an excellent classification system that is of great use in evaluating pubertal progress.[1] The Tanner staging criteria are presented in Chapter 2. Absence of breast development at age 13 years is of concern and at 14 years is abnormal and should be evaluated. Family history is pertinent to predicting the expected age of thelarche in girls.

When delayed thelarche is diagnosed, the initial evaluation should be directed toward determining whether this is an isolated abnormality or is associated with other delays and abnormalities in puberty. Specifically, height, growth velocity, presence of sex hair, body habitus, and virilization should be assessed. In addition, associated congenital anomalies, particularly those of the cardiovascular and genitourinary systems, should be sought. Stigmata of syndromes, particularly Turner's syndrome or other forms of gonadal dysgenesis and karyotypic abnormalities, must be sought. This initial evaluation should lead to a more extensive and directed evaluation for disorders of puberty. Referral to a pediatric endocrinologist is recommended. For a more extensive discussion of delayed puberty, the reader is referred to Chapter 5.

ABNORMALITIES OF THE ADOLESCENT FEMALE BREAST

Congenital anomalies of the breast, as described in the section on infancy and childhood, may first be recognized in the adolescent. This is a time when the patient is usually quite aware of her anatomy, particularly secondary sex characteristics. It is important to address the psychological as well as physical aspects of developmental or congenital abnormalities of the breast.

Anatomic Abnormalities

Asymmetry of the breast is common and may be clinically detectable in most patients (Fig. 37–4). Most often the larger breast is associated with the handedness of the patient. Following examination to exclude any pathologic explanation for the asymmetry (e.g., a breast mass or unilateral hypoplasia), most adolescents simply need reassurance if the

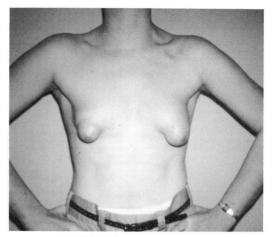

FIGURE 37–5 ••• Tuberous breasts.

asymmetry is apparent to them. Improvement may occur with maturation. When the degree of asymmetry and the patient's body image are of great concern, instruction to improve cosmetic appearance is appropriate. For many, the use of padded brassieres and swimming suits with padded brassieres is adequate to achieve a desired result. Others may require a breast prosthesis in the form of a foam insert. Patients with significant asymmetry should be followed through puberty, and once breast development is complete (Tanner stage 5), surgery may be a consideration. Either unilateral reductive mammoplasty or augmentative mammoplasty may be preferred. Some of the prostheses used in augmentation mammoplasty can be inserted relatively early and, using a valve device, enlarged to correspond to the growth of the nonoperative breast. This is particularly useful in managing patients with unilateral breast hypoplasia or aplasia. Bilateral breast hypoplasia, with normal maturation but insufficient final breast volume, may also be amenable to bilateral augmentative mammoplasty. These patients should be allowed to achieve adequate maturation before surgery is undertaken so that natural growth can be optimized.

Another developmental abnormality is tuberous breast deformity (Fig. 37–5). These patients have a small breast volume and appear to have a protuberant and overdeveloped areola. Depending on the severity of the deformity and patient perception, plastic surgery may be indicated. These patients are not readily staged using the Tanner system, so other criteria may be applied in determining the

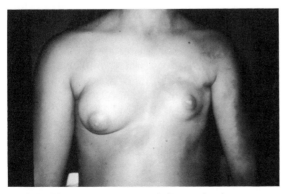

FIGURE 37–4 ••• Asymmetric breast development.

optimal time for surgery (i.e., course, pubertal staging, menarche, growth, bone age).

Inverted nipples may occur, and diagnosis can be made once the breasts are Tanner stage 5. Although this can be a cosmetic problem, surgical correction may prevent the ability to breast-feed.

Breast Atrophy

Breast size and shape are controlled by a number of variables, including genetic factors. Because breasts are largely composed of fatty tissue, there is an association between breast size and weight. Significant weight loss may result in decreased breast volume. Breast atrophy may also result from other causes, including hypoestrogenism and virilization syndromes. When systemic disease results in breast atrophy, it is because of associated weight loss, catabolic state, and/or hypoestrogenism. However, in scleroderma, there may be localized changes leading to atrophy of the breast.

Juvenile or Virginal Hypertrophy

The terms *virginal hypertrophy* and *juvenile hypertrophy* are used synonymously and refer to pathologic overgrowth of the breast (Fig. 37–6). This condition may involve one or both breasts and may be familial. Deciding when breasts are too large is subjective. However, some patients with juvenile or virginal hypertrophy develop such severe enlargement that

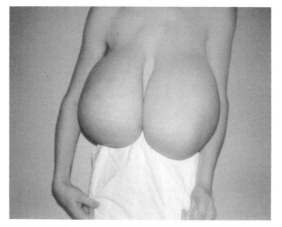

FIGURE 37–6 ••• Breast hypertrophy.

they suffer adverse physical as well as psychological consequences. Massive and rapid enlargement of the breasts may result in pain, hypovascularization, tissue necrosis, and even rupture of the skin. Even without these serious physical consequences, the psychosocial aspects of massive breast enlargement can be significant, and these patients often require sympathetic and expert psychological intervention. Of 24 patients with juvenile hypertrophy who underwent reductive mammoplasty in one published series, 10 had more than 500 gm of breast tissue excised.[19]

Clinically, virginal or juvenile hypertrophy is a subjective diagnosis, but there are distinct histologic changes in the breasts of these patients. Interestingly, the histopathologic findings are similar to those seen in gynecomastia of males. Some patients have benefited from medical treatment with danazol,[20] but experience is limited. Reductive mammoplasty can be an important therapeutic modality for these patients to prevent or treat the physical or psychological consequences of massive breast enlargement.

Breast Pain

Breast pain (mastalgia or mastodynia) may occur in the adolescent. Causes include puberty, estrogen therapy, trauma, hypertrophy, infection, and mammary dysplasia. Sometimes breast pain is the result of physical activity, particularly running, which results in discomfort from friction and jarring. Oral contraceptives, especially higher dose preparations, have led to stimulation of breast growth and associated pain. Sometimes it is necessary to discontinue or decrease the dose of estrogen being administered. Symptomatic relief of breast pain may be provided with analgesics, nonsteroidal antiinflammatory medications, and supportive measures. Well-fitting brassieres that provide good support can be useful. Nonspecific breast pain has been treated with oral vitamin E preparations, but there are few data to demonstrate the efficacy of this therapy; some have even noted improvement in mastalgia when vitamin E was discontinued. Danazol and avoidance of caffeine and dairy products have had some success in reducing the pain associated with mammary dysplasia.

Mastitis and Breast Abscess

Although mastitis is most common in lactating females, this bacterial infection can also occur in nonlactating individuals, including adolescents. Breast trauma may result in infection. Plucking of areolar hair or sexual activity involving the breasts may lead to infection. These patients present with erythematous, tender, warm induration of the breast. Fluctuance or failure of mastitis to resolve on medical management suggests an associated abscess. Systemic signs of infection may indicate the need for study, including blood cultures. The patient should be evaluated for pregnancy. When an abscess is suspected, breast ultrasound may be useful for diagnosis and has been used to guide therapeutic needle aspiration. Treatment of mastitis consists of warm compresses, supportive measures, and antibiotics. When outpatient antibiotic therapy is indicated, amoxicillin–clavulanate potassium (Augmentin), 500 mg orally tid for 10 days, provides good coverage of the most likely bacterial pathogens. Surgical drainage may be necessary if an abscess is present.

Galactorrhea and Nipple Discharge

When a patient presents with a breast discharge, galactorrhea (production of breast milk) can be confirmed with a Sudan stain of the discharge for fat. The differential diagnosis of milk production includes pregnancy, lactation, hyperprolactinemia, hypothyroidism, and benign galactorrhea. Other causes of idiopathic nipple discharge include pus-producing infection; intraductal papillomatosis, which usually produces a bloody serous fluid; breast cyst; and secretions from areolar glands.

BREAST MASSES IN ADOLESCENTS

The detection of a breast mass by an adolescent or her physician provokes significant anxiety. Single or multiple fibroadenomata are the most common mass lesions of the breast. Fibrocystic disease is the second most common etiology and includes cysts, sclerosing adenosis, parenchymal fibrosis, and duct ectasia. Proliferative breast disease may also present as one or more masses and includes the diagnoses of papillomatosis and intraductal papillomata. Other causes of breast masses include hemangioma, intramammary lymph node, fat necrosis, abscess, localized mastitis, hematoma, and malignant neoplasm. Relative frequencies of breast disease treated surgically are listed in Table 37–3.

A variety of benign tumors may involve the breast of the adolescent female. Neoplasms and cysts originating from the breast tissue itself, as well as from anatomically related tissues such as lymph nodes, may occur.

Fibroadenoma

Fibroadenomas account for more than half of breast masses occurring in adolescent females. In surgical series, up to 95% of breast masses have been fibroadenomas. Clinically, this benign neoplasm is well-defined, nontender, mobile, and most often found in the upper outer quadrants of the breasts. Although most often solitary, 10% to 15% may be multiple. When followed through one or more menstrual cycles, they may remain constant in size or increase mildly to moderately. Occasionally

TABLE 37–3 ••• INCIDENCE OF VARIOUS CAUSES OF BREAST DISEASE BASED ON SURGICAL DIAGNOSES

	No.	Age (yr)	Fibroadenoma (%)	Fibrocystic or Proliferative Disease (%)	Infection (%)	Malignancy (%)
Goldstein and Miler[21]	51	8–20	81	12	1	0
Ligon et al.[22]	249	11–30	67	15		2
Bower et al.[23]	134	0–16	76	3	7	1
Stone et al.[24]	143	11–20	72	6	3	1
Gogas et al.[25]	63	10–20	67	14	8	5
Daniel and Mathews[26]	95	12–21	94	2	2	0
Turbey et al.[27]	42	12–18	71		19	0
Simmons and Wold[19]	185	11–17	54	24	1	2

Totals do not equal 100%, because not all diagnoses are reported here.

these tumors will grow extremely large (>500 gm) and are then termed *giant fibroadenomas*. In this case, they can result in changes of the overlying skin, including a prominent venous pattern, pressure necrosis, and even ulceration. When the mass is large or growing, surgical excision is recommended to rule out the possibility of malignancy and to prevent significant cosmetic consequences of the fibroadenoma replacing and compressing breast tissue. Adolescents with a fibroadenoma tend to have very good recovery of breast size and shape after surgery, as the previously compressed breast tissue tends to fill in the defect with time. For that reason, breast prostheses are generally not recommended after excision of a fibroadenoma.

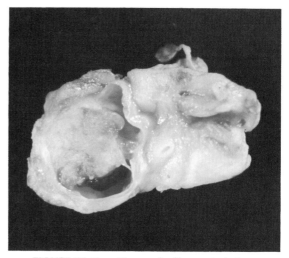

FIGURE 37–7 ••• Biopsy of a fibrocystic lesion.

Cystosarcoma Phylloides

A less common condition that is sometimes confused with fibroadenoma is cystosarcoma phylloides. Like fibroadenoma, this tumor tends to be firm, nontender, and well defined; it is usually slow growing. When cystosarcoma is suspected or cannot be differentiated from a fibroadenoma, excision is indicated. Although most cystosarcoma phylloides are benign, some may be malignant and may metastasize. Malignant phylloides tumors vary in their biologic behavior, and this behavior cannot be predicted reliably by histology.

Fibrocystic and Proliferative Disease

Fibrocystic and proliferative disease may also manifest as a breast mass in adolescents. After fibroadenoma, these are the most common surgical diagnoses in adolescent breast disease (Fig. 37–7). Clinically, these patients may present with an otherwise asymptomatic breast mass, but they often complain of pain or tenderness of the breast, particularly premenstrually. Disease may be focal or diffuse and bilateral. Following these patients through one or two menstrual cycles often demonstrates resolution of the mass. If a cystic mass is suspected and persists, fine-needle aspiration (FNA) is useful. Aspiration is discussed further in the section on evaluation of breast masses in adolescents. The proliferative disease of intraductal papilloma or papillomatosis may be

associated with a bloody discharge from the nipple. Although usually benign, these proliferative diseases may be premalignant.

Breast Malignancy in Adolescent Females

Most experience with breast malignancy is with adult women who have breast carcinoma. Only 0.2% of patients with carcinoma of the breast are younger than 25 years.[28] The incidence of primary carcinoma of the breast in children and adolescents has not been reported, and medical knowledge of this condition consists of only a small number of case reports. Therefore, when considering an adolescent with a breast mass, it is important to keep in perspective the very low incidence of breast malignancy in this population and not to translate experience from the adult population directly to the younger female.

Risk factors for breast carcinoma (based predominantly on studies in adults) include chest radiation[29] and chronic anovulation.[30] The issue of whether unopposed estrogen therapy may increase the risk of breast cancer is the subject of a number of studies and remains unresolved.[31-34] Breast cancer has been reported in two women in their twenties who received chest radiation as children.[29] Even if there is an increased risk with unopposed therapy, the latency period for breast cancer after unopposed estrogen is 15 to 20 years, so presentation during adolescence is not likely. However, controversial data in postmenopausal women on the protective effect of progestin added to estrogen therapy[35] may be applicable to young patients requiring estrogen therapy to reduce the risk of endometrial or breast carcinoma later in life.

In the rare child or adolescent with breast carcinoma, the condition tends to present as an asymptomatic nodule adjacent to, but discreet from, the nipple (Fig. 37–8).[36] Only 17 cases of breast carcinoma have been reported in patients 15 years old or younger.[5] The natural history of these tumors is not well defined because of their rarity. Both disseminating carcinoma and carcinomas in the young that seemed less aggressive than expected have been reported.[37]

Malignant phylloides tumors have been reported in adolescents. Although these neoplasms are usually benign, they may be malignant and may disseminate via hematogenous spread, most often to the lungs. Because this neoplasm is rare in the young, little is known about its natural history. Its biologic behavior cannot be reliably predicted from its histologic appearance. Malignant cystosarcoma phylloides are treated aggressively with surgery, radiation, chemotherapy, and sometimes hormonal manipulation.

Malignancies of the breast in adolescents are more likely to be something other than carcinoma. Rhabdomyosarcoma, lymphoma, neuroblastoma, acute leukemia, and other primary and metastatic neoplasms have been reported. In the Mayo Clinic experience of four patients with malignancies of the breast, none were primary carcinoma. The breast mass was the presenting complaint and the source of tissue diagnosis in three of the four patients. In the fourth patient, the breast mass occurred 3 years after metastatic rhabdomyosarcoma had been diagnosed.[19]

The presentation of malignancies other than carcinoma in the breast of the adolescent can be dramatic. The mass is usually nontender, fixed, and associated with overlying skin changes, including prominent vascularity, dimpling, and/or ulceration. In addition, there may be other clinical features suggestive of malignancy, including constitutional symptoms (i.e., fever, weight loss, malaise), lymphadenopathy, hepatosplenomegaly, or masses elsewhere. However, these associated findings and mass characteristics are not universally present in breast malignancy, and thus an enlarging mass should provoke concern and consideration for biopsy.

Intraductal papilloma or papillomatosis of the breast is rare in the young. This benign condition may be premalignant. The variant of juvenile papillomatosis has been reported to be linked with a high risk of breast carcinoma in the patient's family.[38] These masses may be associated with a bloody discharge from the nipple, which is often the presenting complaint. Patients with papilloma or papillomatosis should be carefully followed for malignancy.

Most breast disease in adolescence does not require surgery, as it is benign and self-limited. However, in cases of abscess, hypertrophy or mass resulting in destruction of breast architecture, or suspected malignancy, surgery is indicated.

Although malignancy of the breast is rare in adolescents and is less likely to be carcinoma than another malignant neoplasm, it does occur and should influence the evaluation and management of breast masses and the health maintenance practices and education for this population.

EVALUATION OF BREAST MASSES IN ADOLESCENT FEMALES

A careful history and physical examination by an experienced clinician will generally lead to the correct diagnosis of a breast mass in an adolescent female. When the diagnosis is questionable or the extent of the disease requires

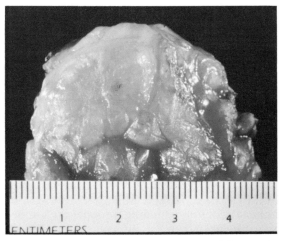

**FIGURE 37–8 ••• ** Breast carcinoma in an adolescent female.

better definition, imaging techniques can be extremely useful. When coupled with the clinical examination, nearly all patients can be diagnosed without or before operative intervention. Key features of the clinical evaluation are listed in Table 37–4.

History

The evaluation of the adolescent female with a breast mass should include a history for previous or intercurrent malignancy, as malignant breast disease may be metastatic or represent a second primary. Other risk factors for breast cancer include chest radiation, and, in adults at least, chronic anovulation. The association between unopposed estrogen therapy and breast cancer is not entirely resolved, at least for adult females. A history of constitutional symptoms is suggestive of malignancy or infection. These may include weight loss, fever, sweats, pain elsewhere, malaise, nausea, or anorexia. The menstrual history should be obtained and the possibility of pregnancy explored. Any history of trauma should be elic-

ited, as trauma may lead to mastitis, breast abscess, hematoma, or fat necrosis. Occasionally the history of trauma is a "red herring" and has just called attention to a preexisting mass. Areolar hair follicle disruption may lead to mastitis or abscess formation. A history concerning hair plucking, sexual activity involving the areola, or other areolar trauma should be obtained. With respect to the mass itself, it is important to ask about duration, size change, and any precipitating factors. A history of nipple discharge raises the possibility of galactorrhea, lactation, malignancy, papillomatosis, or infection. Family history is important in that patients with close relatives, especially the mother or sister, with breast carcinoma are at greater risk and may develop the disease earlier in life than the relative did.[39]

Physical Examination

The physical examination should be a complete, general evaluation. The breasts should be inspected visually for asymmetry, mass effect, and overlying skin changes. Dimpling of the skin, a prominent venous pattern, and ulceration are worrisome and raise the likelihood of malignancy. Pressure should be applied to the breast to elicit any nipple discharge. A clear or mucoid discharge from the nipple can be studied with a Sudan stain for fat to identify milk. The presence of breast milk (galactorrhea) may suggest pregnancy, lactation, hypothyroidism, hyperprolactinemia, or benign galactorrhea. Although conditions resulting in galactorrhea would not be expected to result in a breast mass, with the exception of mastitis in a lactating female, it is important to rule out an intercurrent condition if galactorrhea is present. A serosanguineous nipple discharge may be found in breast infection, inflammation, papillomatosis, or malignancy. Examination of the mass itself provides much useful information about its etiology. Palpation to distinguish a cystic from a solid lesion may be augmented by transillumination of the mass. The location of the mass in the breast may also give a clue as to its etiology. The most common breast mass, the fibroadenoma, is usually located in the upper outer breast quadrant. Most breast abscesses appear under or extending from the area under the areola. It can be difficult to localize in what structure a mass palpated during breast examination actually exists. For instance, a

---

TABLE 37–4 ••• CLINICAL EVALUATION OF BREAST MASSES IN ADOLESCENT FEMALES

History
  Previous breast disease
  Previous or intercurrent malignancy
  Chest radiation
  Unopposed estrogen
  Chronic anovulation
  Constitutional symptoms
  Menstrual history
  Pregnancy
  Trauma
  Mass history
    Duration
    Size change
    Precipitating factors
  Nipple discharge
  Family history
Physical Examination
  Complete, general
  Visual breast inspection
  Expressible nipple discharge
  Mass characteristics
    Location
    Consistency
    Mobility
    Cystic/fluctuance
    Tenderness
    Warmth
  Lymph nodes
  Hepatosplenomegaly
  Signs of malignancy

mass lesion of an underlying rib or the anterior chest wall may appear to be a breast mass.

Imaging techniques as well as palpation may be necessary to define the structure of origin. Most benign breast masses will be well defined, discreet, and mobile. Fibroadenomas, in particular, may seem encapsulated. Tenderness of the mass should also be assessed by history and physical examination. Most fibroadenomas are nontender, as are most malignancies. Mastitis, with or without abscess formation, is likely to be tender, as are areas that have been recently traumatized. Warmth and erythema also suggest mastitis. Palpation of fluctuance suggests abscess or cyst.

Examination of the lymph nodes is very important and should not be limited to the axillae, as malignancies of the breast may be associated with lymphatic spread elsewhere, including to the supraclavicular area. The abdomen should be palpated for hepatosplenomegaly, and the patient should be examined for any signs of malignancy elsewhere, including mass lesions.

When a cystic lesion of the breast is suspected, consideration should be given to diagnostic aspiration. This can usually be accomplished atraumatically in the office setting. A simple cyst, most likely associated with fibrocystic disease, should diminish with aspiration. When aspiration does not result in disappearance of the cyst or when other findings suggest malignancy, the aspirated breast fluid should be sent for cytologic analysis. Sometimes these cysts are complex or multiple, and simple aspiration does not result in complete resolution. Persistence or recurrence of a mass after aspiration or obtaining fluid that is bloody or cytologically abnormal mandates excisional biopsy because of the risk of malignancy.

Fine needle aspiration (FNA) of a breast mass has not been adequately studied in adolescents to determine its value. At the present, it is not usually recommended, because if the mass is worrisome and the results of FNA are negative, biopsy is indicated. If the results of FNA are positive, surgical excision is indicated for most malignant breast masses in adolescents. In a patient with known malignancy who develops a breast mass, FNA may be useful in establishing the nature of the mass if surgery is not indicated or possible. However, a negative biopsy result should not be considered definitive.

Growing experience in using imaging techniques in young patients is encouraging. These techniques have been applied in the evaluation of children and adolescents with a breast mass, with clinically useful results.

Other diagnostic studies may be indicated if malignancy is suspected; these should be tailored to the individual patient.

IMAGING IN THE ADOLESCENT WITH A BREAST MASS

Imaging of the adolescent with a breast mass varies from that of the mature woman because of the extremely uncommon occurrence of breast malignancy in this younger population.[40] The need to diagnose or exclude malignancy is not as imperative as in older women. If a breast mass appears clinically benign by examination and history, the clinician may elect to follow the patient closely but conservatively without imaging studies. Imaging studies are indicated in the diagnostic work up of a breast mass that is persistent, growing, painful, fixed, hard, associated with overlying skin changes, or otherwise clinically worrisome. Even in the adolescent with a breast mass and a positive family history of breast cancer, imaging should be based on the clinical examination because of the rare occurrence of breast carcinoma in this age group.

Various imaging modalities may be helpful in the diagnostic evaluation of breast masses. These include mammography, ultrasonography, plain radiography, and computed tomography (CT).

Mammography

The type and order of imaging employed depends on the clinical presentation. Mammography is routinely used as the initial imaging choice in most adult women. It has proven very useful in the detection of clinically occult lesions and has helped characterize palpable masses. Because breast malignancies are rare in adolescents, there is no reason to perform breast screening in this age group. Mammography is also of limited value in adolescents presenting with a breast mass. The developing breast is usually dense on mammograms,[41] and a discrete mass in an adolescent may be obscured on mammography by this surrounding dense, normal tissue. Breast tissue in developing adolescents is composed primarily of dense fibroglandular tissue with a minimal component of fatty tissue (Fig. 37–9). Fatty tissue supplies low-density contrast to the denser fibroglandular tissue. During a woman's lifetime, the proportion of adipose tissue increases, making mammography a useful imaging modality for mature women.

Adolescents with breast masses in whom mammography may be helpful include those with large breasts that are difficult to examine and image using other modalities, patients with diffuse breast disease, and patients at high risk for developing breast cancer or breast metastasis. This last group includes those patients who have undergone high-dose chest irradiation as therapy for a previous malignancy and those with a known malignancy.[19]

If a mass can be visualized mammographically, it is evaluated using the same criteria used in adults. Signs of benignity include a well-defined border, round or oval shape, and homogeneous density. Signs suggesting malignancy include an irregular, poorly defined bor-

der that fades into the surrounding normal breast tissue, a stellate or spiculated shape, and clusters of punctate, irregular calcifications. Secondary signs of malignancy include skin thickening and retraction, architectural distortion of the parenchyma, and enlarged regional lymph nodes.

State-of-the-art mammography using high-resolution film/screen combination delivers a mean glandular dose of 200 mrad to each breast for a two-view study. This is a low level of exposure, equivalent to the amount of background radiation to the breast received by women living in the upper elevations of Colorado for a year.

Ultrasonography

Breast sonography is valuable in determining the cystic or solid nature of a palpable mass. Unlike in mammography, the density of the developing breast does not affect the sen-

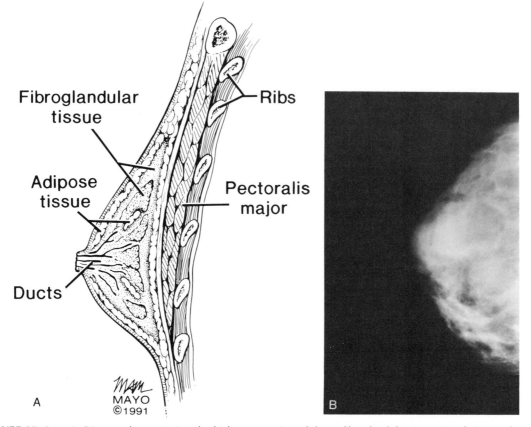

FIGURE 37–9 ••• *A*, Diagram demonstrating the higher proportion of dense fibroglandular tissue in relation to the scant adipose tissue in the adolescent breast. *B*, Mammogram demonstrating the diffusely dense breast of the adolescent.

sitivity of ultrasound in identifying masses. The sonographic characteristics of a simple cystic mass are smooth, sharp margins; absence of internal echoes; and posterior acoustic enhancement (i.e., increased echoes beneath the mass) (Fig. 37–10).[42] Cysts may be multiple in number, round or lobular in shape, and/or contain internal septations. Complex cystic masses meet some but not all of the criteria for simple cysts. They may be partly solid and partly cystic or contain internal echoes (Fig. 37–11). The differential diagnosis of complex cystic masses includes a cyst with internal debris, pus, or blood; intracystic papilloma; hematoma; and abscess.

If the mass meets the criteria of a cyst, whether simple or complex, aspiration may be helpful. Percutaneous aspiration can be performed under ultrasound guidance. The needle can be visualized and guided accurately into the cyst, and the cyst can be imaged as it is evacuated.[42] Ultrasound is also helpful in defining the extent of breast abscess.

Fibroadenomas, the most common breast mass in adolescents, often have a typical sonographic appearance. They tend to be hypoechoic and homogeneous, with smooth margins (Fig. 37–12).[43] They are usually 2 to 3 cm in size and are multiple in 10% to 15% of patients (Fig. 37–13). Some fibroadenomas seen on ultrasound may not be detected on mammograms because of the normally increased density of the adolescent's breast. The diagnosis of fibroadenoma can be suggested but not definitively made on the sonographic appearance. There is significant overlap between the sonographic appearances of benign and malignant solid masses.

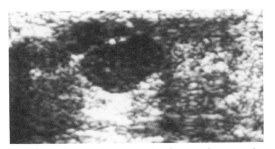

FIGURE 37–11 ••• Ultrasonogram of a complex cyst. There are multiple internal echoes, thought to represent a focal area of fat necrosis.

Plain Radiography and Computed Tomography

Breast masses may, in fact, represent chest wall lesions, particularly in thin adolescents. When the mass is found to be fixed to the chest wall on clinical examination, chest radiographs or high-resolution rib films may be of benefit in identifying rib lesions. These lesions may be benign (e.g., an enchondroma or healing rib fracture), infectious (e.g., osteomyelitis), or malignant. Thin-section, high-resolution computed tomography (CT) is helpful in evaluating bony rib lesions as well as the overlying soft tissue (Fig. 37–14). Calcifications within the soft tissue may represent myositis ossificans from previous trauma. Extension of the CT through the chest and abdomen may reveal the full extent of an inflammatory or other lesion in a patient with a malignant-appearing process. Biopsy can also be attempted under CT or fluoroscopic guidance.

Comparison of Breast Imaging Techniques and Their Clinical Application

Management of breast masses in adolescents is conservative and is based on clinical diagnosis and careful follow-up.[40, 44] Imaging studies are not routinely indicated but may be of assistance in diagnosis and management. Mammography is less useful than in adult women because of the nature of the dense fibroglandular tissue in adolescents and the low risk of breast malignancy. Mammography plays a role in those individuals who have a mass and are at high risk for primary malignancy or metastasis. Ultrasonography is perhaps the most

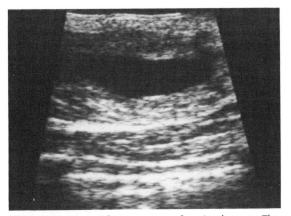

FIGURE 37–10 ••• Ultrasonogram of a simple cyst. The wall is smooth, with no internal echoes and enhancement of the posterior echoes.

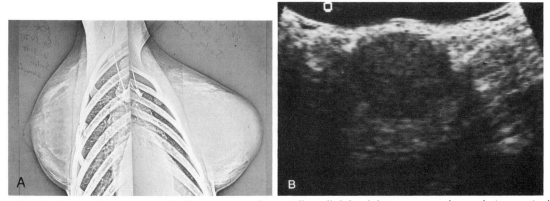

FIGURE 37–12 ••• *A,* Fibroadenoma. *B,* Ultrasonogram of a partially well-defined, homogeneous, hypoechoic mass in the subareolar region. At surgery this was found to be a fibroadenoma.

useful imaging modality in adolescent breast disease. It is easy to perform and sensitive and avoids radiation exposure. It is used most commonly to confirm the cystic or solid nature of a mass. A chest wall mass is better evaluated with plain films, CT, or magnetic resonance imaging (MRI).

TEACHING THE ADOLESCENT THE BREAST SELF-EXAMINATION

The advent of routine breast self-examination has been important in the health of adult women. In well-intentioned efforts to improve the health quality of adolescents, many clinicians have advocated and practiced teaching the breast self-examination to their adolescent female patients. There are many reasons, in addition to detecting breast cancer, for advocation of this practice. Proponents cite teaching the adolescent this technique as an opportunity to teach her about her own body, increase her level of comfort with her body, enhance her perception of the examiner as contributing to her health care, and provide a basis for discussion of a number of puberty and sexuality-related issues. Although efforts to improve adolescent self-knowledge and health maintenance are admirable, data do not currently exist to support the utility of the breast self-examination in this population. There are no data to show that adolescents who have been taught or who practice breast self-examination detect breast tumors, including malignancy, more frequently or earlier. In a review of the reports on malignant tumors of the adolescent breast, there is no information to show that these tumors were detected by patients practicing breast self-examination. Breast self-examination in adults is designed primarily to detect breast carcinoma, and carcinoma is uncommon in the adolescent. Physicians must also consider any potential negative outcome of the breast self-examination in adolescents. Goldbloom has warned of the potential for increased anxiety, unnecessary physician visits, and increased unnecessary surgery if the breast self-examination is taught to such a low-risk population.[45] Because there are no long-term studies, the compliance during the higher risk adult years in women who were taught the breast self-examination during adolescence cannot be reliably predicted. Certainly, patients seen during adolescence may not receive ongoing care and may not have another opportunity to be taught the technique and benefits of breast self-examination in her

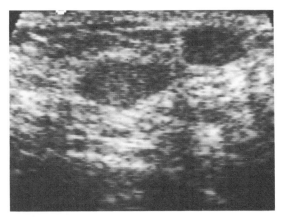

FIGURE 37–13 ••• Ultrasonogram demonstrating multiple fibroadenomas.

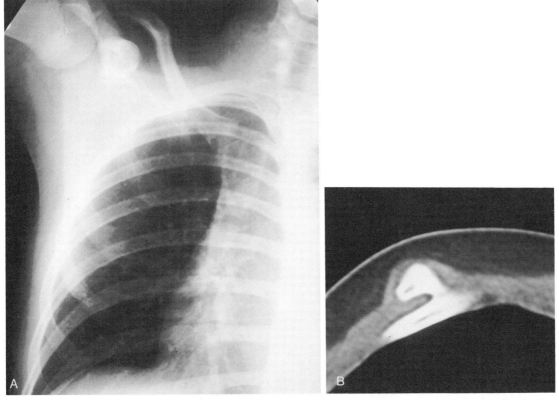

FIGURE 37–14 ••• *A,* Radiograph demonstrating a subtle irregularity and increased density in the anterior fourth rib. *B,* Thin-section computed tomographic scan through the fourth rib demonstrates a small bony protuberance of the anterior rib. This is an enchondroma, which is a benign bony lesion.

higher risk, later years. It is also not known whether patients taught the breast self-examination during adolescence will maintain compliance or, after 20 years of detecting no disease, will discontinue the practice before they enter their higher risk years.

At present, there are no sufficient data to establish the validity of teaching the breast self-examination to the general population of adolescent females. The major impact this practice has had on the adult population should motivate clinicians to study its applicability to the adolescent and establish recommendations.

There are high-risk patients to whom the breast self-examination should be taught. Patients with a strong family history of breast carcinoma should be taught the breast self-examination in their adolescent years, as they have a risk of developing carcinoma earlier in life than their affected relative did.[39] Patients with a previous breast malignancy or a malignancy that may metastasize to the breast should also be taught the breast self-examination. Other high-risk patients include those with breast papillomatosis, a history of radiation to the chest, or a history of unopposed estrogen.

References

1. Marshall WA, Tanner JM. Variations in pattern of pubertal changes in girls. Arch Dis Child 1969; 44:291.
2. Dubowitz L, Dubowitz V. Gestational age of the newborn. Reading, MA: Addison-Wesley, 1977.
3. McKiernan JF, Hull D. Prolactin, maternal oestrogens, and breast development in the newborn. Arch Dis Child 1981; 56:770.
4. McKiernan JF, Hull D. Breast development in the newborn. Arch Dis Child 1981; 56:525–529.
5. Sutow WW, Fernbach DJ, Vietti TJ. Clinical Pediatric Oncology. 3rd ed. St. Louis: CV Mosby, 1984.
6. Speroff L, Glass RH, Kase NG. Clinical Gynecologic Endocrinology and Infertility. 4th ed. Baltimore: Williams & Wilkins, 1988.
7. VanWinter JT, Noller KL, Zimmerman D, Melton LJ III. Natural history of premature thelarche in Olmsted County, Minnesota, 1940–1984. J Pediatr 1990; 116(2):278–280.
8. Nelson KG. Premature thelarche in children born prematurely. J Pediatr 1983; 103(5):756.

9. D'Ambrosio F, Angiolillo M, Flauto U, et al. La mortalità perinatale e neonatale in Lombardia. Notizie Sanità 1981; 32:7.

10. Sa'enz de Rodriguez CA, Bongiovanni AM, Conde de Borrego L. An epidemic of precocious development in Puerto Rican children. J Pediatr 1985; 107(3):393–396.

11. Emans Herriott SJ, Goldstein DP. Pediatric and Adolescent Gynecology. 3rd ed. Boston: Little, Brown, 1990.

12. Radfar N, Ansusingha K, Kenny FM. Circulating bound and free estradiol and estrone during normal growth and development and in premature thelarche and isosexual precocity. J Pediatr 1976; 89(5):719.

13. Ilicki A, Prager Lewin R, Kauli R, et al. Premature thelarche—natural history and sex hormone secretion in 68 girls. Acta Paediatr Scand 1984; 73:756.

14. Stanhope R, Abdulwahid NA, Adams J, Brook CGD. Studies of gonadotrophin pulsatility and pelvic ultrasound examinations distinguish between isolated premature thelarche and central precocious puberty. Eur J Pediatr 1986; 145:190.

15. Pasquino AM, Tebaldi L, Cioschi L, et al. Premature thelarche: A follow up study of 40 girls. Arch Dis Child 1985; 60:1180.

16. Beck W, Stubbe P. Pulsatile secretion of luteinizing hormone and sleep-related gonadotropin rhythms in girls with premature thelarche. Eur J Pediatr 1984; 141:168.

17. Pescovitz OH, Hench KD, Barnes KM, et al. Premature thelarche and central precocious puberty: The relationship between clinical presentation and the gonadotropin response to luteinizing hormone-releasing hormone. J Clin Endocrinol Metab 1988; 67(1):474.

18. Forest MG. Sexual maturation of the hypothalamus: Pathophysiological aspects and clinical implications. Acta Neurochir 1985; 75(104):23–42.

19. Simmons PS, Wold LE. Surgically treated breast disease in adolescent females: A retrospective review of 185 cases. Adol Pediatr Gynecol 1989; 2:95.

20. Taylor PJ, Cumming DC, Corenblum B. Successful treatment of D-penicillamine-induced breast gigantism with danazol. Br Med J 1981; 282:362.

21. Goldstein D, Miler V. Breast masses in adolescent females. Clin Pediatr 1982; 21:17.

22. Ligon R, Stevenson D, Diner W, et al. Breast masses in young women. Am J Surg 1980; 140:770.

23. Bower R, Bell M, Ternberg J. Management of breast lesions in children and adolescents. J Pediatr Surg 1976; 11:337.

24. Stone A, Shenker I, McCarthy K. Adolescent breast masses. Am J Surg 1977; 134:275.

25. Gogas J, Sechas M, Skalkeas G. Surgical management of diseases of the adolescent female breast. Am J Surg 1979; 137:634.

26. Daniel WA, Mathews MD. Tumors of the breast in adolescent females. Pediatrics 1968; 41(4):743.

27. Turbey W, Buntain W, Dudgeon D. The surgical management of pediatric breast masses. Pediatrics 1975; 56:736.

28. Haagensen CD. Diseases of the Breast. 2nd ed. Philadelphia: WB Saunders, 1971.

29. Ivins JC, Taylor WF, Wold LE. Elective whole-lung irradiation in osteosarcoma treatment: Appearance of bilateral breast cancer in two long-term survivors. Skeletal Radiol 1987; 16:133.

30. Coulam C, Annegers J, Kranz J. Chronic anovulation syndrome and associated neoplasia. Obstet Gynecol 1983; 61:403–407.

31. Korenman SG. The endocrinology of breast cancer. Cancer 1980; 46:876–878.

32. Hulka BS. Hormone-replacement and the risk of breast cancer. CA 1990; 40(5):289–296.

33. Dupont WD, Page DL. Menopausal estrogen replacement therapy and breast cancer. Arch Intern Med 1991; 151:67–72.

34. Steinberg KK, Thacker SB, Smith SJ, et al. A meta-analysis of the effect of estrogen replacement therapy on the risk of breast cancer. JAMA 1991; 265(15):1985–1990.

35. Gambrell RD, Maier R, Sanders B. Decreased incidence of breast cancer in postmenopausal estrogen-progestogen users. Obstet Gynecol 1983; 62:435–443.

36. Capraro VJ, Gallego MB. Breast disorders. Pediatr Ann 1975; 47:82.

37. McDevitt RW, Stewart FW. Breast carcinoma in children. JAMA 1966; 195:144.

38. Rosen PP, Kimmel M. Juvenile papillomatosis of the breast: A follow-up study of 41 patients having biopsies before 1979. Am J Clin Pathol 1990; 93:599–603.

39. Lynch HT, Guirgis H, Brodkey F, et al. Early age of onset in familial breast cancer. Arch Surg 1976; 111:126.

40. Ferguson CM, Powell RW. Breast masses in young women. Arch Surg 1989; 124:1338–1341.

41. Hart BL, Steinbock RT, Mettler FA, et al. Age and race related changes in mammographic parenchymal patterns. Cancer 1989; 63:2537–2539.

42. Hackeloer BJ, Duda V, Lanth G. Ultrasound Mammography. New York: Springer-Verlag, 1989.

43. Fornage BD, Lorigan JG, Andry E. Fibroadenoma of the breast: Sonographic appearance. Radiology 1989; 172:671–675.

44. Diehl T, Kaplan DW. Breast masses in adolescent females. J Adolesc Health Care 1985; 6:353–357.

45. Goldbloom R. Self-examination by adolescents. Pediatrics 1985; 76(1):126.

CHAPTER 38

○○○ # Oncologic Problems

MICHAEL L. HICKS

M. STEVEN PIVER

Recent advances in the management of childhood gynecologic malignancies have resulted in improved survival, less radical surgery, and in some instances, greater preservation of fertility compared with the 1970s. Malignancies specific to the pediatric and adolescent patient include pelvic rhabdomyosarcoma, diethylstilbestrol (DES)-related adenocarcinoma of the vagina and cervix, and germ cell and juvenile granulosa cell tumors of the ovary.

RHABDOMYOSARCOMAS

Sarcomas of gynecologic origin in the pediatric population are primarily rhabdomyosarcomas (RMS). These tumors represent the most common soft tissue neoplasms in children, accounting for 4% to 8% of all malignant diseases in children under 15, and they are the seventh leading cause of death among children.[1, 2] Genital and urinary tract RMS accounts for 20% of the cases in children and is the most common malignancy of the lower genital tract in young girls.[3, 4]

RMS originates from primitive or incompletely differentiated mesenchyme of the urogenital ridge.[5] There are five types: pleomorphic, embryonal, botryoid, alveolar, and undifferentiated. The embryonal variant, botryoid sarcoma, represents the most common subtype of RMS presenting as a genital lesion.

Primary lesions of RMS can originate from the vagina, cervix, vulva, perineum, or uterus. All of the various sites of origin have different peaks of incidence during childhood; the lower genital lesions of the perineum, vulva, and vagina occur early in childhood, usually before the age of 2, and cervical or uterine lesions occur more frequently in the adolescent age group.

The clinical presentation in the pediatric or adolescent patient with RMS can be with an enlarging vulvar, perineal, or vaginal lesion or a large polypoid mass protruding from the introitus of the vagina and resembling a bunch of grapes (Fig. 38–1). These lesions are usually clinically visible, but occasionally the only symptom the patient may present with is unexplained vaginal bleeding or, on examination, an abdominopelvic mass.

Before the 1970s, prognosis for those with this rare malignancy was extremely dismal. Initial approaches were individualized, but it wasn't until 1950 that Shackman reported the first successful use of a total pelvic exenteration in a patient with RMS, followed by 2.5-year disease-free interval.[6] This report marked the beginning of the use of radical pelvic surgery for the treatment of RMS. However, even with ultraradical surgery, the survival rate before 1970 rarely exceeded 20%.[7] Attempts were made to improve survival using radiation alone or in combination with radical pelvic surgery, but this was successful only when there was microscopic disease limited to the margins of the resected lesion.[7–11]

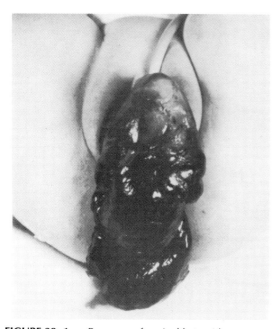

FIGURE 38–1 ••• Response of vaginal botryoid sarcoma to preoperative combination therapy. This is a large hemorrhagic mass staged as nonresectable vaginal tumor (stage IIB). (From Kumar APM, Wrenn EL, Fleming ID, et al. Combined therapy to prevent complete pelvic exenteration for rhabdomyosarcoma of the vagina or uterus. Cancer 1976; 37:120.)

The onset of multimodality therapy began in the mid 1970s; this combined radical surgery, radiotherapy, and adjuvant chemotherapy and was noted to improve survival significantly (Table 38–1).[12–18] Later, the Intergroup Rhabdomyosarcoma Study Group evaluated the response to chemotherapy and radiotherapy in early stages of RMS (stages I and II) and the response to chemotherapy alone in advanced stages of RMS (stages III and IV) (Table 38–2). The authors concluded the following:

1. Combined vincristine, actinomycin D, and cyclophosphamide (VAC) therapy was an effective adjuvant for stage I disease with or without radiotherapy, resulting in 92% survival with no evidence of disease at 2 years in both groups.
2. VAC given over 2 years or vincristine and actinomycin D (VA) therapy given over 1 year, both with localized radiotherapy, were equally effective in patients with stage II disease (microscopic residual disease after surgery), with 85% of patients having no evidence of disease at 2 years.
3. Of patients with gross residual disease

after surgery (stage III) or metastatic disease at the time of diagnosis (stage IV), 81% to 82% responded favorably to chemotherapy.[19]

Although survival improved with multimodality therapy, young patients with RMS still underwent radical surgery requiring the removal of the uterus, fallopian tubes, ovaries, vagina, and rectum and occasionally a portion of the vulva (Figs. 38–2, 38–3). With the development of successful multimodality therapy and improvement in the survival rate, new approaches were explored in an attempt to avoid radical pelvic surgery and thereby preserve the bladder, rectum, and reproductive organs of these young children.

The introduction of preoperative chemotherapy with VAC was initially reported by Kumar and associates, who were able to obtain complete regression of tumor when preoperative chemotherapy with VAC was followed by localized resection of vaginal RMS, with preservation of the bladder and rectum.[20] Later, Voute and associates reported their experience with 24 patients; 7 patients (29%) experienced complete remission after chemotherapy alone, requiring no surgical intervention, and 10 patients (42%) had no evidence of disease after preoperative chemotherapy and limited pelvic surgery, again showing the chemosensitivity of these tumors.[21]

If complete regression of tumor is not obtained after VAC chemotherapy, with or without limited resection of the genital lesion, radical pelvic surgery may still be avoided. Flamant and colleagues reported that 15 of 17 young girls were cured of RMS of the vagina and vulva after treatment with incomplete excision followed by localized brachytherapy (intracavitary application or interstitial) and 18 months of alternating VAC and vincristine and adriamycin therapy. Twelve of the pubescent or postpubescent girls were followed for long-term sequellae; 11 had normal puberty, 11 had normal menses, and two eventually had a total of three healthy children.[22]

Currently, treatment for RMS should begin with tissue confirmation and staging to rule out systemic disease; this should include a chest radiograph and a bone marrow aspiration. Primary therapy should consist initially of combination chemotherapy with VAC, and the response to chemotherapy should be monitored closely (Table 38–3). After rapid tumor regression with chemotherapy, conservative surgery can be attempted without compromising survival. In this way, most young children

TABLE 38–1 ••• SURVIVAL RATES UTILIZING MULTIMODALITY THERAPY FOR RHABDOMYOSARCOMA

Authors	No. of Patients	Treatment Regimen	Survival Rate
Grosfeld et al.[13]	5	Surgery, RT, VAC	5/5 (100%)
Pratt et al.[17]	20	Surgery, RT, VAC	9/20 (45%)
Kilman et al.[15]	31	Surgery, RT, VA	28/31 (90%)
Piver et al.[16]	3	Surgery, RT, VA, VC	3/3 (100%)
Rivard et al.[18]	9	Surgery, RT, VAC	5/9 (56%)
Donaldson et al.[12]	19	Surgery, RT, VAC	14/19 (74%)
Heyn et al.[14]	28	Surgery, RT, VA	24/28 (86%)

RT, Radiation therapy; VA, vincristine, actinomycin D; VAC, vincristine, actinomycin D, cyclophosphamide.
From Hicks ML, Piver MS. Conservative surgery plus adjuvant therapy for vulvovaginal rhabdomyosarcoma, DES/clear cell adenocarcinoma of the vagina and unilateral germ cell tumors of the ovary. Obstet Gynecol Clin North Am. 1992; 19(1):219.

with the diagnosis of RMS will be able to experience preservation of the function of the rectum, bladder, vagina, and ovaries, thereby allowing conservation of reproductive function.

CLEAR-CELL ADENOCARCINOMA OF THE VAGINA/CERVIX

Primary adenocarcinoma of the vagina or cervix has been infrequently reported in the pediatric age group.[23–26] In 1971, Herbst and associates reported eight cases of adenocarcinoma of the vagina, six in adolescents (ages 9 to 15).[27] This single report of vaginal adenocarcinoma exceeded the total of all documented cases in the world literature before 1945. More significantly, this report was the first to show the association of vaginal clear cell adenocarcinoma with intrauterine exposure to DES, which became commercially available in 1938 and was primarily used in pregnant patients at high risk for spontaneous abortion. Four months after the original report by Herbst, Roswell Park Cancer Institute reported five additional cases of adenocarcinoma of the vagina in daughters exposed to DES or other synthetic estrogens in utero.[28] After these two reports linking DES exposure to

TABLE 38–2 ••• STAGING CLASSIFICATION SYSTEM FOR RHABDOMYOSARCOMA AFTER SURGERY FOR PRIMARY LESION

Stage I	Local disease only
Stage II	Microscopic residual disease in regional lymphatic or positive margins after surgery
Stage III	Gross residual disease after surgery
Stage IV	Distant metastasis

clear-cell adenocarcinoma of the vagina, the use of DES was banned by the Food and Drug Administration in 1971, and a registry was established to centralize and study epidemiologic, clinical, and pathologic findings of patients developing adenocarcinoma of the vagina or cervix.

Herbst and Anderson have summarized their most recent findings from the Registry for Research on Hormonal Transplacental Carcinogenesis, which are as follows:[29]

1. Currently there are 547 reported cases of clear-cell adenocarcinoma of the vagina and cervix.
2. Of these patients, 60% were exposed to DES or similar synthetic estrogens in utero.
3. Patient age ranges from 7 to 34, with a median age of 19.
4. Sixty percent of the primary lesions are vaginal, and 40% are cervical.
5. Cervical lesions are located primarily on the exocervix, and vaginal lesions are mainly located on the upper third of the anterior vaginal wall.
6. Ninety percent were in early stages (stage I and stage II) at the time of diagnosis.
7. The risk of developing adenocarcinoma of the cervix or vagina in an exposed female from birth to 34 years of age is approximately 0.1% (or one case per 1000 women exposed), implying that these tumors are extremely rare among DES-exposed females and that DES is not a complete carcinogen.[29]

Treatment for early stage clear-cell adenocarcinoma of the vagina and cervix has traditionally been with radical pelvic surgery (radical hysterectomy, pelvic lymphadenectomy, partial or total vaginectomy, and replacement of the vagina with a split-thickness skin graft). Radiation therapy (whole-pelvis radiotherapy and vaginal brachytherapy) has been used for more advanced stages, large bulky lesions, and

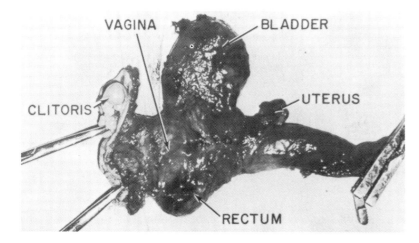

FIGURE 38–2 ••• Specimen from a total pelvic exenteration in a 10-month-old patient with rhabdomyosarcoma of the vagina. A tumor involving the clitoris can be seen. (From Piver MS, Barlow JJ, Wang JJ, Shah NK. Combined radical surgery, radiation therapy and chemotherapy in infants with vulvovaginal embryonal rhabdomyosarcoma. Obstet Gynecol 1973; 42(4):524. Reprinted with permission from the American College of Obstetricians and Gynecologists.)

in cases with extension to the lymphatic systems.[30–32]

The majority of cases (90% or more) of clear-cell adenocarcinoma of the vagina and cervix present as stage I or stage II disease, and the survival rate usually exceeds 90% (Fig. 38–4). To date, treatment has become more conservative. Wharton and colleagues reported on five patients with stage I or II clear-cell adenocarcinoma of the vagina or cervix who were treated entirely with transvaginal cone or interstitial irradiation. Four of the five were reported to be living without any evidence of disease 2 to 8 years after completion of therapy. In the one nonsurvivor, death was related to pulmonary embolism and not to progression of disease.[33] Senekjian and associates reported on 219 cases of stage I vaginal clear-cell adenocarcinoma; 176 had radical therapy, and 43 had only localized therapy (wide local excision and/or local irradiation). The 5- and 10-year survival rates were equivalent in the two groups. In addition, a subgroup of patients receiving localized irradiation had a recurrence experience equal to that of the conventional therapy group (radical therapy), which was more favorable than that of patients undergoing local excision alone.[34] The authors concluded that to preserve reproductive function in the young patient, the combination of wide local excision with retroperitoneal pelvic lymphadenectomy to rule out lymph node metastasis, followed by local radiation, is an effective treatment modality for small (<2 cm) vaginal clear-cell adenocarcinomas.

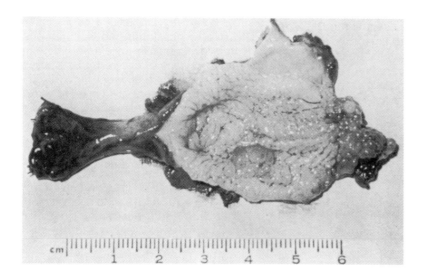

FIGURE 38–3 ••• Specimen from a hysterectomy and total vaginectomy in an 11-month-old patient with rhabdomyosarcoma of the vagina and cervix. The entire vagina was involved with grape-like lesions of rhabdomyosarcoma. (From Piver MS, Barlow JJ, Wang JJ, Shah NK. Combined radical surgery, radiation therapy and chemotherapy in infants with vulvovaginal embryonal rhabdomyosarcoma. Obstet Gynecol 1973; 42(4):525. Reprinted with permission from the American College of Obstetricians and Gynecologists.)

TABLE 38–3 ••• VAC CHEMOTHERAPY REGIMEN FOR VULVOVAGINAL RHABDOMYOSARCOMA

Drug	Dosage
Vincristine	2 mg/m^2 IV weekly × 12 courses
Actinomycin D	0.015 mg/kg/day IV × 5 courses at 12-week intervals
Cyclophosphamide	2.5 mg/kg/day PO daily × 90 weeks, beginning on the 7th week.

From Hicks ML, Piver MS. Conservative surgery plus adjuvant therapy for vulvovaginal rhabdomyosarcoma, DES/clear cell adenocarcinoma of the vagina and unilateral germ cell tumors of the ovary. Obstet Gynecol Clin North Am. 1992; 19(1):219.

TABLE 38–4 ••• GERM CELL TUMORS OF THE OVARY

Dysgerminoma
Nondysgerminoma tumors
   Endodermal sinus tumors
   Embryonal carcinoma
   Immature teratoma
   Choriocarcinoma
   Mixed germ cell tumors (any combination of dysgerminoma and nondysgerminoma)

From Hicks ML, Piver MS. Conservative surgery plus adjuvant therapy for vulvovaginal rhabdomyosarcoma, DES/clear cell adenocarcinoma of the vagina and unilateral germ cell tumors of the ovary. Obstet Gynecol Clin North Am. 1992; 19(1):219.

OVARIAN GERM CELL TUMORS

Malignant germ cell tumors represent a segment of human solid tumors in which there has been a significant improvement in survival with the introduction of combination chemotherapy. Although these tumors are rare, 60% to 70% of childhood gynecologic malignancies originate in the ovaries.

With regard to therapy, these tumors can be divided into two classifications: pure dysgerminomas and nondysgerminomas (Table 38–4).

Dysgerminomas

Of all the germ cell tumors of the ovaries, dysgerminomas are the most common. Dysgerminomas are the female homologue of the seminoma of the testes. Microscopically, these tumors show sheets of polygonal cells with clear cytoplasm in a fibrous stroma infiltrated with lymphocytes (Fig. 38–5). They represent approximately 3% to 5% of all ovarian malignancies and occur primarily before the age of 30 (median age at occurrence, 17 years).

Dysgerminomas are usually unilateral but can be bilateral in approximately 15% of cases, in contrast to all other germ cell tumors of the ovaries, which are bilateral in only 1% of patients.[35–38] Although almost all patients with dysgerminomas have normal sexual development, rare instances of dysgerminomas have been associated with phenotypic females with dysgenetic gonads in such disorders as pure gonadal dysgenesis, testicular feminization, Turner syndrome, and hermaphroditism.[39–43]

Tumor markers for dysgerminomas are usually absent. However, levels of human chorionic gonadotropin (hCG) have been noted to be elevated in isolated cases in which these

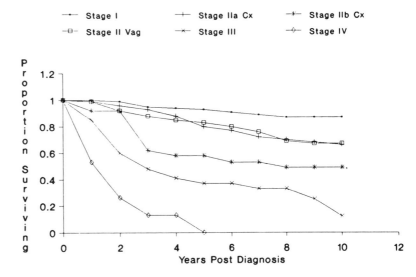

FIGURE 38–4 ••• Survival for each International Federation of Gynecology and Obstetrics stage for vaginal and cervical clear-cell adenocarcinoma over a span of 10 years. Stage I, n = 323; stage II, n = 79; stage IIA, n = 70; stage IIB, n = 26; stage III, n = 34; stage IV, n = 9. (From Herbst AL, Anderson D. Clear cell adenocarcinoma of the vagina and cervix secondary to intrauterine exposure to diethylstilbestrol. Semin Surg Oncol 1990; 6:345. Copyright © 1990. Reprinted by permission of Wiley-Liss, a division of John Wiley and Sons, Inc.)

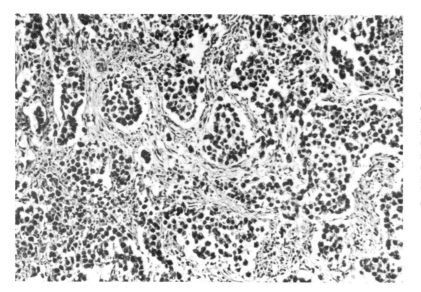

FIGURE 38–5 ••• Dysgerminoma composed of islands of tumor cells surrounded by connective tissue stroma containing lymphocytes. (From Talerman A. Germ cell tumors of the ovary. In: Kurman RJ (ed). Blaustein's Pathology of the Female Genital Tract. 3rd ed. New York: Springer-Verlag, 1987, p 663.)

tumors may contain syncytial giant cells that produce histochemically detectable amounts of hCG. hCG production may rarely result in precocious puberty, and virilization may also occur, although infrequently, when dysgerminomas are admixed with gonadoblastomas owing to hormonal stimulation by the surrounding stroma. Lactic dehydrogenase (LDH) levels, especially fractions of LDH 1, 2, and 3 have been noted to be elevated in many cases of dysgerminoma.[39, 44–47]

Treatment of suspected dysgerminomas begins with complete exploration of the abdomen and pelvis followed by unilateral salpingo-oophorectomy. A frozen section should be obtained at the time of laparotomy to confirm the diagnosis. Dysgerminomas have a higher propensity than other ovarian malignancies to spread to the retroperitoneal regional lymph nodes.[12, 35, 36, 48–59] Therefore, appropriate surgical staging should be done using paraaortic and ipsilateral pelvic lymphadenectomy, pelvic and paracolic washings, diaphragmatic sampling, and omentectomy to determine the extent of disease. At the time of laparotomy, the surgeon must keep in mind the possibility of contralateral ovarian involvement. If the contralateral ovary is grossly negative, then a biopsy can be performed to rule out occult microscopic involvement; if the result is negative, the ovary should be left in situ.[55] If there is bilateral ovarian involvement (gross and microscopic), after bilateral salpingo-oophorectomy, the uterus can be preserved for future childbearing via assisted reproductive technol-

ogies. In more advanced stages of disease (stages II through IV), cytoreduction should be performed. This has been shown to improve the response to adjuvant chemotherapy; if the remaining ovary is not involved, preservation of the contralateral ovary and uterus should be accomplished.

Adjuvant therapy after conservative surgery with unilateral salpingo-oophorectomy has been a controversial issue with regard to preservation of fertility in these young patients. It has been shown that a near-100% cure rate can be achieved with postoperative radiation to the pelvis and abdomen, but this leads to loss of fertility.[12, 36, 51, 54, 56] Gordon et al. reported a 92% 10-year actual survival rate for patients who underwent conservative surgery with unilateral salpingo-oophorectomy without adjuvant postoperative radiotherapy.[53] However, with this conservative treatment, there was a 17% recurrence rate and a 6% mortality rate in these young children, which brings into question its validity. The high recurrence rates can be partially explained by inadequate surgical staging.

Adjuvant ipsilateral hemipelvic and paraaortic lymph node radiation, with shielding of the contralateral ovary and uterus, after conservative surgery with unilateral salpingo-oophorectomy has been reported by DePalo and associates. In this series of 13 patients with stage I dysgerminoma, there have been no reported relapses, with a median follow-up of 77 months.[60]

According to a report by Gershenson and

colleagues, five patients with dysgerminoma underwent conservative surgery (unilateral salpingo-oophorectomy), followed by adjuvant chemotherapy with bleomycin, etoposide, and cisplatin (BEP). With a median follow-up time of 22.4 months, there were no recurrences, indicating that adjuvant chemotherapy may be just as effective as adjuvant radiotherapy.[61]

Combination chemotherapy has also been shown to be effective in the treatment of the more advanced stages (II through IV) of dysgerminoma. Gershenson and colleagues reported seven cases of advanced stages of dysgerminoma and two cases of recurrent dysgerminoma treated with BEP, resulting in complete remission of disease in all instances with a median follow-up time of 22.4 months.[61] Williams et al., reporting for the Gynecologic Oncology Group, used two consecutive protocols, cisplatin-vinblastine-bleomycin (PVB) and BEP, in the treatment of metastatic dysgerminoma. Of 18 evaluable patients with stage III or IV disease (most with large residual disease), 17 were disease free at a median follow-up of 26 months.[62]

The 1990s will probably witness the abandonment of radiotherapy in the treatment for dysgerminomas. Cisplatin-based chemotherapy, particularly the BEP regimen (Table 38–5) seems to be equally as effective as radiotherapy in the treatment of dysgerminomas, but with the distinct advantage of preservation of ovarian function and fertility.

Endodermal Sinus Tumor

Endodermal sinus tumors of the ovary represent approximately 5% of all malignant ovarian tumors and are the second most common germ cell tumor. They are usually exclusively unilateral.

These tumors were originally thought to be of mesonephric origin but later were found to originate from extraembryonic germ cells.[63–65] The median age at the time of presentation is 19 years.[66, 67] Histologically, endodermal sinus

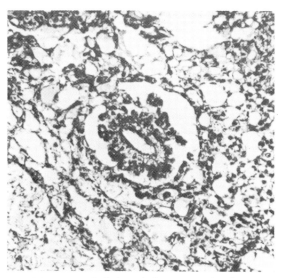

FIGURE 38–6 ••• Endodermal sinus tumor showing a typical perivascular formation (Schiller-Duval body). (From Talerman A. Germ cell tumors of the ovary. In: Kurman RJ (ed). Blaustein's Pathology of the Female Genital Tract. 3rd ed. New York: Springer-Verlag, 1987, p 673.)

tumors are noted to have papillary projections with a peripheral lining of neoplastic cells associated with blood vessels (Schiller-Duval bodies) (Fig. 38–6).

Endodermal sinus tumors produce a very specific tumor marker, α-fetoprotein (α-FP), which is present in virtually 100% of all cases of endodermal sinus tumors.[67] This tumor marker gives the clinician a parameter to follow during the course of therapy.

Endodermal sinus tumors usually present with abdominal pain, fever, vaginal bleeding, or an abdominal pelvic mass. Treatment should begin with surgical exploration, unilateral salpingo-oophorectomy, and frozen section for tissue confirmation, followed by appropriate staging as discussed earlier. Cytoreductive surgery should be performed for more advanced stages of the disease. The most frequent stage at the time of laparotomy is stage I.[66, 67] Several researchers analyzing the management of endodermal sinus tumors reported 2-year survival rates of 25%, 18%, and 9% with the use of conservative surgery (unilateral salpingo-oophorectomy) alone in stage I patients and a 100% mortality rate with adjuvant radiotherapy, indicating, unlike dysgerminomas, the radioresistance of endodermal sinus tumors.[66–68]

Improvement in survival rates for endodermal sinus tumors was not accomplished until

TABLE 38–5 ••• BEP COMBINATION CHEMOTHERAPY REGIMEN

Drug	Dosage
Cisplatin	20 mg/m², days 1–5
Etoposide	100 mg/m², days 1–5
Bleomycin	20 U/m²/wk

the institution of VAC combination chemotherapy. Kurman and Norris and Gershenson and associates reported 75% and 92% 2-year survival rates, respectively, for stage I endodermal sinus tumor after postoperative administration of VAC.[66, 67] In a follow-up study, Gershenson and colleagues reported a 94% sustained remission rate in stage I endodermal sinus tumor patients with a median follow-up of 100 months[69]; however, that same year, the Gynecologic Oncology Group reported only a 50% sustained remission rate for such patients.[70]

Subsequent to the development of VAC chemotherapy, the cisplatin-based PVB regimen has been shown to achieve a 74% complete remission rate in nonseminomatous testicular carcinomas.[71] In an effort to improve remission rates in ovarian germ cell tumors, investigators began to evaluate the effectiveness of PVB. For stage I endodermal sinus tumors treated with PVB, the sustained remission rate was 100% in the 11 reported series,[72–82] compared with a 72% complete remission rate in the collective series reporting the use of VAC.

With more advanced stages of endodermal sinus tumor (II through IV), remission rates were even more dismal. Gershenson and colleagues reported a 30% complete remission rate with VAC chemotherapy, with the Gynecologic Oncology Group reporting a 56% sustained remission rate. In an attempt to improve remission rates in the advanced stage group, PVB was evaluated, with a collective series noting a remission rate of 68%. However, although PVB seemed to be slightly more efficacious for advanced stages of endodermal sinus tumor, it was also clearly more toxic than VAC chemotherapy. Myelosuppression, nephrotoxicity, neurotoxicity, and pulmonary fibrosis have been reported, and deaths have been attributed to PVB therapy.

In an attempt to achieve a more active and less toxic combination of chemotherapy, Williams and associates compared PVB and BEP in the treatment of disseminated germ cell tumors.[83] The authors concluded that BEP was superior in inducing remission, with 83% of patients reported as disease free after BEP therapy, compared with 74% after therapy with PVB. Also, the BEP group had significantly less toxicity. Gershenson and colleagues in 1990 reported a 100% sustained remission rate when BEP was used as primary therapy for patients in all stages of endodermal sinus tumor, with minimal toxicity.[61] In 1990, Hicks

TABLE 38–6 ••• GYNECOLOGIC ONCOLOGY GROUP REGIMENS FOR NONDYSGERMINOMATOUS GERM CELL TUMORS OF THE OVARY

Protocol	Dosage
Protocol 44	
Vincristine	1.5 mg/m²*, days 1 and 15
Actinomycin D	350 ugm/m², days 1–5
Cyclophosphamide	150 mg/m², days 1–5
Protocol 78	
Cisplatin	20 mg/m², days 1–5
Etoposide	100 mg/m², days 1–5
Bleomycin	20 U/m²/wk†

*Maximum dose, 2.0 mg.
†Maximum dose, 30 U.
From Hicks ML, Piver MS. Conservative surgery plus adjuvant therapy for vulvovaginal rhabdomyosarcoma, DES/clear cell adenocarcinoma of the vagina and unilateral germ cell tumors of the ovary. Obstet Gynecol Clin North Am. 1992; 19(1):219.

et al. reported dose intensification with BEP induction followed by VAC maintenance chemotherapy in stage III endodermal sinus tumor patients, resulting in complete resolution of disease, as documented by second-look laparotomy, and minimal toxicity.[84] The Gynecologic Oncology Group, comparing VAC and BEP in the treatment of nondysgerminomatous germ cell tumors, reported that BEP was clearly more effective in producing a complete remission as documented by second-look laparotomy with a remission rate of 76% and 96%, respectively, with the two protocols (Tables 38–6, 38–7).[85]

Adjuvant chemotherapy is absolutely necessary in the treatment of all stages of endodermal sinus tumor. Therapy using BEP for

TABLE 38–7 ••• NONDYSGERMINOMATOUS GERM CELL TUMORS OF THE OVARY TREATED WITH GYNECOLOGIC ONCOLOGY GROUP PROTOCOLS

	Protocol 44	Protocol 78
Number of evaluable cases	100	52
Stage		
I	76	35
II	8	4
III	16	13
Cell type		
Immature teratoma	50	19
Endodermal sinus tumor	30	16
Mixed germ cell tumor	20	15
Choriocarcinoma	0	2

From Hicks ML, Piver MS. Conservative surgery plus adjuvant therapy for vulvovaginal rhabdomyosarcoma, DES/clear cell adenocarcinoma of the vagina and unilateral germ cell tumors of the ovary. Obstet Gynecol Clin North Am. 1992; 19(1):219.

endodermal sinus tumors has shown excellent progression-free survival rates compared with all other regimens of chemotherapy (VAC or PVB). Therefore, to achieve complete remission and preservation of fertility in young girls with the diagnosis of endodermal sinus tumor, conservative surgery in early stages of the disease or conservative surgery and cytoreductive surgery in more advanced stages of disease should be followed by BEP chemotherapy.

Embryonal Carcinoma

Embryonal carcinoma of the ovary is analogous to embryonal carcinoma of the testes (Fig. 38–7). This is a very rare tumor, and until the report by Kurman and Norris[86] classifying these tumors as a separate entity, they were routinely confused with choriocarcinoma and endodermal sinus tumors of the ovary. Embryonal carcinoma of the ovaries are rarely found in a pure form but usually exist as part of a mixed germ cell tumor. The median age at presentation is 13, and the tumor primarily presents as a stage I lesion and is usually exclusively unilateral. Embryonal carcinomas have totipotential cells capable of extraembryonic or embryonic differentiation. Sixty percent of embryonal carcinomas produce hormonal manifestations consistent with precocious puberty in premenarchal girls, abnormal vaginal bleeding in postmenarchal women, and a positive pregnancy test.[86] All pure embryonal carcinomas produce hCG, and occasionally α-FP levels are elevated.

Treatment for suspected embryonal carci-

noma of the ovary should begin with exploration of the abdomen, appropriate staging, unilateral salpingo-oophorectomy, and cytoreduction in advanced stages as described for other germ cell tumors.

Reports evaluating the efficacy of adjuvant chemotherapy for embryonal carcinomas are limited because of the rarity of the tumor. Williams and associates have reported sustained remissions after therapy with etoposide and cisplatin with or without bleomycin for advanced stages of testicular embryonal carcinomas.[83, 87]

Currently, embryonal carcinomas of the ovary should be treated essentially the same as endodermal sinus tumors of the ovary (i.e., with BEP combination chemotherapy).

Immature Teratomas

Immature teratomas represent the third most common germ cell tumor of the ovary, accounting for approximately 15% of all germ cell tumors and 1% of all teratomas. These tumors are composed of elements from all three germ cell layers (ectoderm, mesoderm, and endoderm) (Fig. 38–8). Immature teratomas are usually exclusively unilateral, and the median age at presentation is 19 years.[88–90] This neoplasm is usually without evidence of tumor marker production, although Gershenson et al. have reported elevated levels of α-FP in 5 of 16 (31%) immature teratoma cases.[89] These tumors usually present primarily as stage I lesions.[89, 91]

Treatment of patients with suspected immature teratomas also begins with surgical exploration, unilateral salpingo-oophorectomy, appropriate staging, and, in advanced stages of disease, cytoreduction. Norris and associates noted a clear relationship between the grade of immature teratomas and ultimate survival. The authors noted that in patients treated with conservative surgery (i.e., unilateral salpingo-oophorectomy only), individuals with a grade I lesion had a 93% survival rate, compared with a 33% survival rate for those with grade III lesions (Table 38–8). For all stage I disease, the survival rate was reported as 76%, compared with 38% for advanced stage disease (stages II and III).[90] Gallion and colleagues noted an 83% 2-year disease-free survival rate in patients with grade I immature teratoma lesions, compared with a 33% rate in patients with grade III lesions; the 2-year

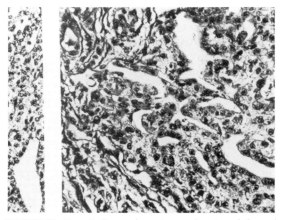

FIGURE 38–7 ••• Embryonal carcinoma forming clefts and spaces. (From Talerman A. Gonadoblastoma associated with embryonal carcinoma. Obstet Gynecol 1974; 43:138.)

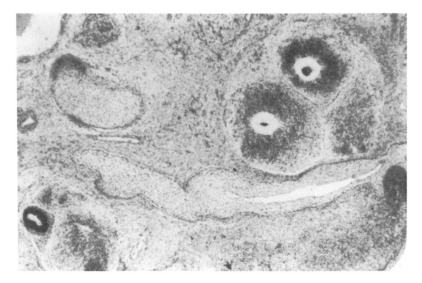

FIGURE 38–8 ••• Immature neural elements evident along with squamous epithelium and cartilage. (From DiSaia PJ, Creasman WT. Germ cell, stromal and other ovarian tumors. In: Clinical Gynecologic Oncology. 3rd ed. St. Louis: CV Mosby, 1989, p 433.)

disease-free survival rate was 63% for stage I disease, compared with 30% for stage III lesions.[88] Both of these studies indicate the importance of adequate exploration and sampling of all lesions in the abdomen and pelvis, as prognosis is related to the grade of the most advanced lesion in the abdominal cavity.

Adjuvant chemotherapy is necessary to ensure complete remission and improve survival. In 1986 Gershenson and associates treated 21 patients with VAC; 18 of 21 (85%) (all stages) had sustained remission. Of stage I patients, 91% treated with VAC had sustained remission, versus 9% treated with surgery alone; for advanced stages, an 80% remission rate was noted in the chemotherapy-treated group versus 0% in the non–chemotherapy-treated group.[89] Slayton and colleagues reported a 100% sustained remission rate in stage I immature teratomas treated with VAC and a 58% sustained remission rate for advanced stages of disease so treated.[70]

Until recently, VAC chemotherapy was

thought to be the best adjuvant therapy, especially in stage I disease. However, the Gynecologic Oncology Group compared the effectiveness of VAC chemotherapy (protocol 48) with BEP chemotherapy (protocol 78), and their results demonstrated BEP to be far superior, with a 96% complete remission rate, compared with a 76% complete remission rate using VAC chemotherapy (see Tables 38–6, 38–7).[85] Gershenson reported complete remission with BEP chemotherapy in two cases of stage I and one case of recurrent immature teratoma with a 22.4-month median follow-up time, again indicating the superior activity of the BEP regimen.[61]

Mixed Germ Cell Tumors

Mixed germ cell tumors have more than one malignant germ cell component. These tumors present primarily as stage I lesions, and the mean age at presentation is 16 years.[92, 93] These tumors are usually unilateral and often produce hCG and α-FP and occasionally LDH. Most often mixed germ cell tumors are composed of dysgerminomas and endodermal sinus tumors, but any combination of germ cell tumors may be present. Treatment of mixed germ cell tumors begins with exploration of the abdomen, unilateral salpingo-oophorectomy (with contralateral ovarian biopsy in the presence of dysgerminoma), appropriate staging, and cytoreduction in advanced stages of disease. Survival after surgery alone has been poor, indicating the need for adjuvant che-

TABLE 38–8 ••• SURVIVAL RATES FOR STAGE I IMMATURE TERATOMA ACCORDING TO GRADE

Grade	No. of Patients	No. Survived
I	14	13 (93%)
II	30	11 (55%)
III	6	2 (33%)

From Hicks ML, Piver MS. Conservative surgery plus adjuvant therapy for vulvovaginal rhabdomyosarcoma, DES/clear cell adenocarcinoma of the vagina and unilateral germ cell tumors of the ovary. Obstet Gynecol Clin North Am. 1992; 19(1):219.

motherapy.[68, 92, 93] Gershenson and associates and Slayton and colleagues reported 75% and 83% remission rates, respectively, with VAC chemotherapy in stage I disease, but for advanced stages, the remission rates were 33% and 22%, respectively.[69, 70] PVB has been infrequently used in the treatment of mixed germ cell tumors but has shown some activity in early and advanced stage mixed germ cell tumors.[72, 74, 78, 80, 81] The report by Williams and associates represents the largest series of patients with mixed germ cell tumors treated by two different comparative protocols. As stated earlier, protocol 78, which included BEP, was far superior in producing complete remission than protocol 44, which incorporated the VAC chemotherapy regimen.[85] Thus BEP appears to be the most effective regimen in this subcategory of germ cell tumors.

Nongestational Ovarian Choriocarcinoma

Pure ovarian choriocarcinomas are extremely rare tumors (Fig. 38–9). These neo-

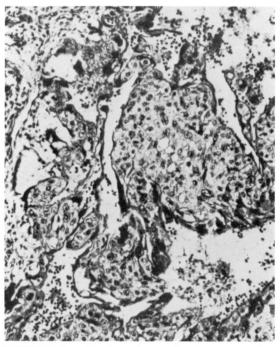

FIGURE 38–9 ••• Choriocarcinoma showing a cytotrophoblast composed of medium-sized cells situated centrally and a syncytiotrophoblast composed of very large multinucleated cells situated peripherally. (From Talerman A. Germ cell tumors of the ovary. In: Kurman RJ (ed). Blaustein's Pathology of the Female Genital Tract. 3rd ed. New York: Springer-Verlag, 1987, p 685.)

plasms are usually a component of mixed germ cell tumors. They are primarily unilateral and are associated with elevated hCG levels.

Treatment, as with all germ cell tumors, begins with surgical exploration and appropriate staging, followed by unilateral salpingo-oophorectomy. Experience with adjuvant chemotherapy has been limited because of the rarity of this tumor. Methotrexate, actinomycin D, and chlorambucil have been successful in achieving long-term remission.[94] PVB has also been shown to have some activity in the treatment of ovarian choriocarcinoma. The Gynecologic Oncology Group has also noted that BEP is an effective adjuvant for nongestational ovarian choriocarcinoma.[85]

JUVENILE GRANULOSA CELL TUMORS

Juvenile granulosa cell tumors (JGCTs) account for approximately 5% of all ovarian tumors in children (Fig. 38–10). More than 80% of these tumors occur in the first two decades of life; 5% are diagnosed in the prepubescent period. Eighty percent of patients with JGCT present with isosexual precocity, but in the postpubertal period, menstrual irregularities (i.e., dysfunctional uterine bleeding) may be the only presenting sign.[95–101] In addition to hormonal abnormalities, the patient with JGCT may present with signs of peritonitis, ascites, or an abdominopelvic mass.

JGCT differs from adult granulosa cell tumor in its recurrence pattern, age at onset, and histologic characteristics (Table 38–9).[95] These tumors occur bilaterally only very infrequently, and in most cases the tumor is confined to the ovary at the time of laparotomy (stage IA).

Treatment of JGCT begins with exploration of the abdomen and appropriate staging (pelvic and right and left paracolic washings; diaphragmatic sampling; omentectomy; and pelvic and paraaortic lymph node sampling). Because the majority of these lesions are unilateral, conservative surgery (unilateral salpingo-oophorectomy only) is usually all that is necessary, but in the presence of advanced disease, cytoreductive surgery should be performed.

After limited surgery (unilateral salpingo-oophorectomy only), disease confined entirely to the ovary (stage IA) requires no further therapy, with survival rates ranging from 80%

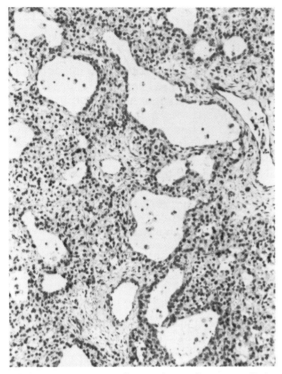

FIGURE 38–10 ••• Juvenile granulosa cell tumor. Follicles of varying sizes and shapes are separated by cellular areas. (From Young RH, Dickersin GR, Scully RE. Juvenile granulosa cell tumor of the ovary. A clinicopathological analysis of 125 cases. Am J Surg Pathol 1984; 8:575–596.)

TABLE 38–10 ••• SURVIVAL RATES FOR STAGE I JUVENILE GRANULOSA CELL TUMORS OF THE OVARY TREATED WITH SURGERY ALONE

	Number	%	Median Follow-up
Zaloudek and Norris[102]	24/26	92	19 yr
Lack et al.[103]	10/10	100	21 yr
Young et al.[95]	87/95	92	5 yr
Vassal et al.[104]	4/5	80	6 yr
Total	125/136	92	

results in terms of sustained clinical remissions.[95, 102–104] For advanced and recurrent adult granulosa cell tumors, the PVB regimen has been shown to be of some therapeutic efficacy in improving survival.[105] However, PVB is also associated with severe hematologic and neurologic toxicity, and treatment-related deaths have been reported. Because JGCT is a rare tumor, the small numbers of advanced JGCT cases do not permit adequate evaluation of chemotherapeutic agents in the treatment of this disease process.

to 100% (Table 38–10). Survival rates of less than 100% can be explained by the fact that patients were sometimes inadequately staged, and therefore, some cases represent more advanced stages of disease.

For more advanced stages of JGCT, no effective modality of therapy has been determined. Radiotherapy and various combinations of chemotherapy have yielded poor

TABLE 38–9 ••• DIFFERENCES BETWEEN ADULT AND JUVENILE GRANULOSA CELL TUMORS

	Adult	Juvenile
Age	Infrequently prepubertal Presents at >30 years of age	Primarily prepubertal Presents at <30 years of age
Microscopic findings	Call-Exner bodies common No mucin Pale nuclei and grooved No luteinization	No Call-Exner bodies Irregular follicles Dark nuclei and nongrooved Luteinization present
Recurrence	Late	Early

References

1. Bartholomew TH, Gonzales ET, Starling KA, et al. Changing concepts in management of pelvic rhabdomyosarcoma in children. Urology 1979; 13:613.
2. Sutow WW, Sullivan MP, Ried HL, et al. Prognosis in childhood rhabdomyosarcoma. Cancer 1970; 25:1384–1390.
3. Maurer HM. The Intergroup Rhabdomyosarcoma Study: Update, November 1978. Natl Cancer Inst Monogr 1981; 56:61–68.
4. Maurer HM. The Intergroup Rhabdomyosarcoma Study (NIH): Objectives and clinical staging classification. J Pediatr Surg 1975; 10:977–978.
5. Dehner LP. Soft tissue sarcomas of childhood: The differential diagnostic dilemma of the small blue cell. Natl Cancer Inst Monogr 1981; 56:43.
6. Shackman R. Sarcoma botryoids of the genital tract in female children. Br J Surg 1950; 38:26–30.
7. Hilgers RD, Malkasian GD, Soule EH. Embryonal rhabdomyosarcoma (botryoid type) of the vagina. A clinicopathologic review. Am J Obstet Gynecol 1970; 107:484–501.
8. Hilgers RD. Pelvic exenteration for vaginal embryonal rhabdomyosarcoma. A review. Obstet Gynecol 1975; 45:175–180.
9. Cassady JR, Sagerman RH, Tretter P, et al. Radiation therapy for rhabdomyosarcoma. Radiology 1968; 91:116–120.
10. Edland RW. Embryonal rhabdomyosarcoma. Am J Roentgenol Rad Ther Nucl Med 1965; 93:671–685.
11. McNeer GP, Cantin J, Chu F, et al. Effectiveness of radiation therapy in the management of sarcomas of the soft somatic tissues. Cancer 1968; 22:391–397.
12. Donaldson SS, Castro JR, Wilbur JR, et al. Rhabdomyosarcoma of head and neck in children. Com-

bination treatment by surgery, irradiation, and chemotherapy. Cancer 1973; 31:26–35.

13. Grosfeld JL, Smith JP, Chatworthy HW. Pelvic rhabdomyosarcoma in infants and children. J Urol 1972; 107:673–675.

14. Heyn RM, Holland R, Newton WA, et al. The role of combined chemotherapy in the treatment of rhabdomyosarcoma in children. Cancer 1974; 34:2128–2142.

15. Kilman JW, Clatworthy HW, Newton WA, et al. Reasonable surgery for rhabdomyosarcoma. A study of 67 cases. Ann Surg 1973; 178:346–351.

16. Piver MS, Barlow JJ, Wang JJ, et al. Combined radical surgery, radiation therapy and chemotherapy in infants with vulvovaginal embryonal rhabdomyosarcoma. Obstet Gynecol 1973; 42:522–526.

17. Pratt CB, Hustu HO, Fleming ID, et al. Coordinated treatment of childhood rhabdomyosarcoma with surgery, radiotherapy and combination chemotherapy. Cancer Res 1972; 32:606–610.

18. Rivard G, Ortega J, Hittle R, et al. Intensive chemotherapy as primary treatment for rhabdomyosarcoma of the pelvis. Cancer 1975; 36:1593–1597.

19. Maurer HM, Moon T, Donaldson M, et al. The Intergroup Rhabdomyosarcoma Study. A preliminary report. Cancer 1977; 40:2015–2026.

20. Kumar APM, Wrenn EL, Fleming ID, et al. Combined therapy to prevent complete pelvic exenteration for rhabdomyosarcoma of the vagina or uterus. Cancer 1976; 37:118–122.

21. Voute PA, Vos A, deKraker J, Behrendt H. Rhabdomyosarcomas: Chemotherapy and limited supplementary treatment program to avoid mutilation. Natl Cancer Inst Monogr 1981; 56:121–125.

22. Flamant F, Gerbaulet A, Nihoul-Fekete C, et al. Long term sequelae of conservative treatment by surgery, brachytherapy, and chemotherapy for vulvar and vaginal rhabdomyosarcoma in children. J Clin Oncol 1990; 8:1847–1853.

23. Nix HG, Wright HL. Mesonephric adenocarcinoma of the vagina. Am J Obstet Gynecol 1967; 99:893–899.

24. Novak E, Woodruff JD, Novak ER. Probable mesonephric origin of certain female genital tumors. Am J Obstet Gynecol 1954; 68:1222–1242.

25. Scannel RC. Primary adenocarcinoma of the vagina. Am J Obstet Gynecol 1939; 38:331–333.

26. Studdiford WE. Vaginal lesions of adenomatous origin. Am J Obstet Gynecol 1957; 73:641–656.

27. Herbst AL, Ulefelder H, Poskanzer DC. Adenocarcinoma of the vagina. Association of maternal stilbestrol therapy with tumor appearance in young women. N Engl J Med 1971; 284:878–881.

28. Greenwald P, Barlow JJ, Nasca PC, et al. Vaginal cancer after maternal treatment with synthetic estrogens. N Engl J Med 1971; 285:390–392.

29. Herbst AL, Anderson D. Clear cell adenocarcinoma of the vagina and cervix secondary to intrauterine exposure to diethylstilbestrol. Semin Surg Oncol 1990; 6:343–346.

30. Herbst AL, Kurman RJ, Scully RE, et al. Clear cell adenocarcinoma of the genital tract in young females. Registry report. N Engl J Med 1972; 287:1259–1264.

31. Herbst AL, Norusis MJ, Rosenow PJ, et al. An analysis of 346 cases of clear cell adenocarcinoma of the vagina and cervix with emphasis on recurrence and survival. Gynecol Oncol 1979; 7:111–122.

32. Robboy SJ, Herbst AL, Scully RE. Clear cell adenocarcinoma of the vagina and cervix in young fe-

males. Analysis of 37 tumors that persisted or recurred after primary therapy. Cancer 1974; 34:606–614.

33. Wharton JT, Rutledge FN, Gallagher HS, Fletcher G. Treatment of clear cell adenocarcinoma in young females. Obstet Gynecol 1975; 45:365–368.

34. Senekjian EK, Frey KW, Anderson D, et al. Local therapy in stage I clear cell adenocarcinoma of the vagina. Cancer 1987; 60:1319–1324.

35. Asadourian LA, Taylor HB. Dysgerminoma. An analysis of 105 cases. Obstet Gynecol 1969; 33:370–379.

36. DePalo G, Pilotti S, Kenda R, et al. Natural history of dysgerminoma. Am J Obstet Gynecol 1982; 143:799–807.

37. Gershenson DM, Wharton JT. Malignant germ cell tumors of the ovary. In: Alberts D, Surwit E (eds). Ovarian Cancer. Martinus Nijhoff, Norwell, MA: Kluwer Publishing, 1985, pp 227–269.

38. Santesson L. Clinical and pathological survey of ovarian tumors treated at the Radium-Hemmet. 1. Dysgerminoma. Acta Radiologica (Stockholm) 1947; 28:643–668.

39. Hart WR, Burkons DM. Germ cell neoplasms arising in gonadoblastomas. Cancer 1979; 43:669–678.

40. Schellhas HH, Trujillo JM, Rutledge FN. Germ cell tumors associated with XY gonadal dysgenesis. Am J Obstet Gynecol 1971; 109:1197–1204.

41. Schwartz IS, Cohen CJ, Deligdisch L. Dysgerminoma of the ovary associated with true hermaphroditism. Obstet Gynecol 1980; 56:102–106.

42. Talerman A, Jarabak J, Amarose AP. Gonadoblastoma and dysgerminoma in a true hermaphrodite with a 46,XX karyotype. Am J Obstet Gynecol 1981; 140:475–477.

43. Teter J, Bozkowski K. Occurrence of tumors in dysgenetic gonads. Cancer 1967; 20:1301–1310.

44. Friedman M, White RG, Nissenbaum MM, et al. Serum lactic dehydrogenase—a possible tumor marker for an ovarian dysgerminoma: A literature review and report of a case. Obstet Gynecol Surv 1984; 39:247–265.

45. Lippert MC, Javadpour N. Lactic dehydrogenase in the monitoring and prognosis of testicular cancer. Cancer 1981; 48:2274–2278.

46. Sheiko MC, Hart WR. Ovarian Germinoma (dysgerminoma) with elevated serum lactic dehydrogenase: Case report and review of literature. Cancer 1982; 49:994–998.

47. Zondag HA. Enzyme activity in dysgerminoma and seminomas. A study of lactic dehydrogenase isoenzymes in malignant diseases. The 1963 Fiske essay. RI Med J 1964; 47:273–281.

48. Afridi MA, Vongtama V, Tsukada Y, et al. Dysgerminoma of the ovary. Radiation therapy for recurrence and metastases. Am J Obstet Gynecol 1976; 126:180–194.

49. Boyes DA, Pankratz E, Galliford BW, et al. Experience with dysgerminomas at the Cancer Control Agency of British Columbia. Gynecol Oncol 1978; 6:123–129.

50. Burkons DM, Hart WR. Ovarian germinomas (dysgerminomas). Obstet Gynecol 1978; 51:221–224.

51. Buskirk SJ, Schray MF, Podratz KC, et al. Ovarian dysgerminoma: A retrospective analysis of results of treatment, sites of treatment failure and radiosensitivity. Mayo Clin Proc 1987; 62:1149–1157.

52. Freel JH, Cassir JF, Pierce VK, et al. Dysgerminoma of the ovary. Cancer 1979; 43:798–805.

53. Gordon A, Lipton D, Woodruff D. Dysgerminoma: A review of 158 cases from the Emil Novak Ovarian Tumor Registry. Obstet Gynecol 1981; 58:497–504.

54. Krepart G, Smith JP, Rutledge F, et al. The treatment for dysgerminoma of the ovary. Cancer 1978; 41:986–990.

55. Kurman RJ, Norris HJ. Malignant germ cell tumors of the ovary. Hum Pathol 1977; 8:551–564.

56. Lucraft HH. A review of thirty-three cases of ovarian dysgerminoma emphasizing the role of radiotherapy. Clin Radiol 1979; 30:585–589.

57. Mueller CW, Topkins P, Lapp WA. Dysgerminoma of the ovary. An analysis of 427 cases. Am J Obstet Gynecol 1950; 60:153–159.

58. Pedowit P, Felmus LB, Grayzel DM. Dysgerminoma of the ovary. Prognosis and treatment. Am J Obstet Gynecol 1955; 70:1284–1297.

59. Talerman A, Huyzinga WT, Kuipers T. Dysgerminoma clinicopathologic study of 22 cases. Obstet Gynecol 1973; 41:137–147.

60. DePalo G, Lattuada A, Kenda R, et al. Germ cell tumors of the ovary: The experience of the National Cancer Institute of Milan. I. Dysgerminoma. Int J Radiat Oncol Biol Phys 1987; 13:853–860.

61. Gershenson DM, Morris M, Cangir A, et al. Treatment of malignant germ cell tumors of the ovary with bleomycin, etoposide, and cisplatin. J Clin Oncol 1990; 8:715–720.

62. Williams SD, Blessing J, Hatch K, et al. Chemotherapy of advanced ovarian dysgerminomas: Trials of the Gynecologic Oncology Group. Abstract. Proc Am Soc Clin Oncol 1990; 9:155.

63. Schiller W. Mesonephroma ovarii. Am J Cancer 1939; 35:1–21.

64. Teilum G. Gonocytoma: Homologous ovarian and testicular tumors, with discussion of "Mesonephroma Ovarii" (Schiller W. Am J Cancer 1939). Acta Pathol Microbiol Scand 1946; 23:242.

65. Teilum G. Endodermal sinus tumors of the ovary and testes, comparative morphogenesis of the so-called mesonephroma ovarii (Schiller) and extra embryonic (yolk-sac allantoic) structure of the rat's placenta. Cancer 1959; 12:1092–1105.

66. Gershenson DM, DelJunco G, Herson J, et al. Endodermal sinus tumor of the ovary. The M.D. Anderson experience. Obstet Gynecol 1983; 61:194–202.

67. Kurman RJ, Norris HJ. Endodermal sinus tumor of the ovary. A clinical and pathologic analysis of 71 cases. Cancer 1976; 38:2404–2419.

68. Jimerson GK, Woodruff JD. Ovarian extraembryonal teratoma II. Endodermal sinus tumor mixed with other germ cell tumors. Am J Obstet Gynecol 1977; 127:302–304.

69. Gershenson DM, Copeland LJ, Kavanagh JJ, et al. Treatment of malignant nondysgerminomatous germ cell tumors of the ovary with vincristine, dactinomycin and cyclophosphamide. Cancer 1985; 56:2756–2761.

70. Slayton RE, Park RC, Silverberg SG, et al. Vincristine, dactinomycin and cyclophosphamide in the treatment of malignant germ cell tumors of the ovary. A Gynecologic Oncology Group Study (a final report). Cancer 1985; 56:243–248.

71. Einhorn LH, Donohue J. Cis-diaminedichloroplatinum, vinblastine, and bleomycin combination chemotherapy in disseminated testicular cancer. Ann Intern Med 1977; 87:293–298.

72. Carlson RW, Sikic BI, Turbow MM, et al. Cisplatin,

73. vinblastine and bleomycin (PVB) therapy for ovarian germ cell tumors. J Clin Oncol 1987; 1:645–651.

73. Davis TE, Loprinzi CL, Buchler DA. Combination chemotherapy with cisplatin, vinblastine, and bleomycin for endodermal sinus tumor of the ovary. Gynecol Oncol 1984; 19:46–52.

74. Gershenson DM, Kavanagh JJ, Copeland LJ, et al. Treatment of malignant nondysgerminomatous germ cell tumors of the ovary with vinblastine, bleomycin and cisplatin. Cancer 1986; 57:1731–1737.

75. Julian CG, Barrett JM, Richardson RL, et al. Bleomycin, vinblastine and cisplatin in the treatment of advanced endodermal sinus tumor. Obstet Gynecol 1979; 56:396–401.

76. Lockey JL, Baker JJ, Prince NA, et al. Cisplatin, vinblastine and bleomycin for endodermal sinus tumor of the ovary. Ann Intern Med 1981; 94:56–57.

77. Sawada M, Okudaira Y, Matsui Y, et al. Cisplatin, vinblastine and bleomycin therapy of yolk sac (endodermal sinus) tumor of the ovary. Gynecol Oncol 1985; 20:162–169.

78. Schwartz PE. Combination chemotherapy in the management of ovarian germ cell malignancies. Obstet Gynecol 1984; 64:564–572.

79. Sessa C, Bonazzi C, Landoni F, et al. Cisplatin, vinblastine and bleomycin combination chemotherapy in endodermal sinus tumor of the ovary. Obstet Gynecol 1987; 70:220–224.

80. Taylor MH, DePetrillo AD, Turner AR. Vinblastine, bleomycin and cisplatin in malignant germ cell tumors of the ovary. Cancer 1984; 56:1341–1349.

81. Vriesendorp R, Aalders JG, Sleijfer DT, et al. Treatment of malignant germ cell tumors of the ovary with cisplatin, vinblastine, and bleomycin (PVB). Cancer Treat Rep 1984; 68:779–781.

82. Wiltshaw E, Stuart-Harris R, Barker GH, et al. Chemotherapy of endodermal sinus tumor (yolk-sac tumor) of the ovary. Preliminary communication. J R Soc Med 1982; 75:888–892.

83. Williams SD, Birch R, Einhorn EH, et al. Treatment of disseminated germ-cell tumors with cisplatin, bleomycin, and either vinblastine or etoposide. N Engl J Med 1987; 316:1435–1440.

84. Hicks ML, Maxwell SL, Kim W. Management of advanced endodermal sinus tumor of the ovary with preservation of reproductive function. Henry Ford Hosp Med J 1990; 38:76–78.

85. Williams SD, Blessing JA, Slayton R, et al. Ovarian germ cell tumors: Adjuvant trials of the Gynecologic Oncology Group. In: Salmon S (ed). Proceedings of the Sixth International Conference on the Adjuvant Therapy of Cancer. 1990, pp 501–503.

86. Kurman RJ, Norris HJ. Embryonal carcinoma of the ovary. A clinicopathologic entity distinct from endodermal sinus tumor resembling embryonal carcinoma of the adult testis. Cancer 1976; 38:2420–2433.

87. Williams SD, Einhorn LH, Greco A, et al. VP-16-213 salvage therapy for refractory germinal neoplasms. Cancer 1980; 46:2154–2158.

88. Gallion H, VanNagell JR, Donaldson ES, et al. Immature teratoma of the ovary. Am J Obstet Gynecol 1983; 146:361.

89. Gershenson DM, DelJunco G, Silva EG, et al. Immature teratoma of the ovary. Obstet Gynecol 1986; 68:624.

90. Norris HJ, Zerkin HJ, Benson WL. Immature (malignant) teratoma of the ovary. Cancer 1976; 37:2359.

91. Perrone T, Steeper TA, Dehner LP. Alpha-fetoprotein localization in pure ovarian teratoma. An im-

munohistochemical study of 12 cases. Am J Clin Pathol 1987; 88:713.

92. Gershenson DM, DelJunco G, Copeland LJ, et al. Mixed germ cell tumors of the ovary. Obstet Gynecol 1984; 64:200–206.

93. Kurman RJ, Norris HJ. Malignant mixed germ cell tumors of the ovary. Obstet Gynecol 1976; 48:459–589.

94. Wider JA, Marshall JR, Bardin CW, et al. Sustained remissions after chemotherapy for a primary ovarian cancer containing choriocarcinoma. N Engl J Med 1969; 280:1439.

95. Young RH, Dickersin GR, Scully RE. Juvenile granulosa cell tumor of the ovary. A clinicopathological analysis of 125 cases. Am J Surg Pathol 1984; 8:575–596.

96. Morris JM, Scully RE. Endocrine Pathology of the Ovary. St. Louis: CV Mosby, 1958.

97. Scully RE. Ovarian tumors with endocrine manifestations. In: DeGroot LJ (ed). Endocrinology. Vol 3. New York: Grune & Stratton, 1979.

98. Scully RE. Ovarian tumors. A review. Am J Pathol 1977; 87:686–720.

99. Scully RE. Sex cord stromal, lipid cell and germ cell tumors. In: Sciarra JJ (ed). Gynecology and Obstetrics. Vol 4: Gynecologic Oncology. Hagerstown, MD: Harper & Row, 1980.

100. Scully RE. The ovary. In: Wolfe HJ (ed). Endocrine Pathology. New York: Springer-Verlag, 1986.

101. Scully RE. Tumors of the ovary and maldeveloped gonads. In: Atlas of Tumor Pathology. 2nd ser. Fasc. 16. Washington, DC: Armed Forces Institute of Pathology, 1979.

102. Zaloudek C, Norris HJ. Granulosa tumors of the ovary in children. A clinical and pathologic study of 32 cases. Am J Surg Pathol 1982; 6:513–522.

103. Lack EE, Perez-Atayde AR, Murthy ASK, et al. Granulosa theca cell tumors in premenarchal girls: A clinical and pathologic study of ten cases. Cancer 1981; 48:1846–1854.

104. Vassal G, Flamant F, Caillaud JM, et al. Juvenile granulosa cell tumor of the ovary in children: A clinical study of 15 cases. J Clin Oncol 1988; 6:990–995.

105. Colombo N, Sessa C, Landoni F, et al. Cisplatin, vinblastine and bleomycin combination chemotherapy in metastatic granulosa cell tumor of the ovary. Obstet Gynecol 1986; 67:265–268.

CHAPTER 39

Surgically Correctable Congenital Anomalies: Diagnosis and Management

STEVEN S. ROTHENBERG
WILLIAM J. POKORNY

Since the 1970s the increasing use of ultrasound in routine obstetric care, along with advances in imaging technology and expertise, has resulted in a marked increase in the antenatal diagnosis of congenital anomalies.[1–25] In fact, nearly one third of newborns with major congenital defects are currently diagnosed prenatally.[7, 13, 14] This has dramatically altered the management of these high-risk patients and contributed to the development of perinatal medicine.

Antenatal diagnosis has proved important for the following reasons:

1. It helps define the anomalies, enabling consideration of termination of high-risk pregnancies.

2. It allows the family and physician to prepare for the birth of a child with special needs.

3. Both the mother and the newborn infant with serious birth defects should be referred to a tertiary care medical center with a Level III nursery and personnel trained to deal with the specific needs of that newborn. The postnatal and preoperative care of these newborns is simplified when they are delivered at a tertiary care facility.

4. The timing and type of delivery may be determined by the specific anomaly of the fetus.

5. An experienced neonatal and surgical team, as well as appropriate resources, can be mobilized to the operating room for the planned delivery.

Current indications for obtaining prenatal ultrasounds and indications for which anomalies should be suspected are listed in Table 39–1.[14, 21, 26]

Because obstetricians are diagnosing major congenital anomalies prenatally, they must be familiar with the various anomalies, their treatment, and their prognosis. The obstetrician is now the referring physician and must be aware of the resources available for the care of both

TABLE 39–1 ➤➤➤ INDICATIONS FOR PRENATAL ULTRASOUND

Absolute
   Large or small uterus for gestational age
   Maternal diabetes mellitus
   Elevated serum α-fetoprotein levels
   History of previous birth defects
   Poly- or oligohydramnios
   Evidence of intrauterine growth retardation
   Suspected fetal demise
   Amniocentesis
   Rh sensitization
   Exposure to teratogens
Relative
   Determination of gestation dates
   Monitoring of fetal development
   Placental and fetal position
   Suspicion of multiple gestation
   Maternal age (>35)

the family and the infant at various local medical centers. Many centers are developing a team approach to these problems. This team should include a perinatologist, a geneticist, a pediatrician, and a pediatric surgeon.[14]

During the 4-year period from July 1985 to June 1989, antenatal ultrasonography was performed on 66% of neonates with major anomalies who underwent surgical correction at Texas Children's Hospital; 35% of these were diagnostic. The most commonly diagnosed problem, abdominal wall defects, was diagnosed prenatally in 61% of neonates born with these defects. Congenital diaphragmatic hernia and intestinal obstruction were also diagnosed with a high frequency (40%). A prenatal diagnosis resulted in a prenatal consultation and/or a change in the delivery site in nearly half of the cases. During this 4-year period there was a marked increase in both the number of antenatal ultrasounds performed and the accuracy of the diagnosis. During the academic year 1985 to 1986, 50% of the newborns seen by pediatric surgeons for major congenital anomalies had had prenatal ultrasounds, but only 20% of these were diagnostic. During the academic year 1988 to 1989, 85% of newborns operated on for major congenital anomalies had had prenatal ultrasounds, and nearly 40% of these were diagnostic. With continuing advances in ultrasound technology and user expertise, these numbers are likely to continue to increase.

This chapter will focus on the major anatomic defects that may be diagnosed by antenatal ultrasound and for which surgical intervention in the early neonatal period (or, in

some instances, in utero) may be indicated. These include abdominal wall defects (omphalocele and gastroschisis), congenital diaphragmatic hernias, bowel obstructions and atresias, tumors and cysts, and urogenital anomalies. A number of neural tube and cardiac defects are also evident in utero but are beyond the scope of this discussion. Treatment options range from close prenatal and postnatal observation to prenatal referral to a tertiary care facility with specialized support systems, including a Level III nursery, neonatologists, and pediatric surgeons. In rare cases, referral for consideration of fetal surgery may be appropriate. Many of these decisions will be based on the quality and quantity of information obtained by the initial obstetric evaluation.

ABDOMINAL WALL DEFECTS

Omphalocele and gastroschisis are the two main types of abdominal wall defects discovered in utero.[10, 12, 27–31] The high rate of discovery is due to mass screening of maternal serum for α-fetoprotein, levels of which are elevated in the presence of neural tube and abdominal wall defects.[21] Differentiation between the two processes by antenatal ultrasound is important, as the associated problems and prognosis for the two defects differ greatly. Overall, omphalocele occurs in 1 of every 5000 live births, with a similar incidence in adolescent pregnancies.[21] During early fetal development, the midgut migrates into the umbilical cord and returns to the abdominal cavity during the 10th to 12th week. The defect results from a failure of the midgut to return to the abdominal cavity during this period. The abdominal contents extrude through the defect and are covered by the amniotic membrane, an extension of the peritoneal sac (Fig. 39–1).

Omphalocele has a high association (40% to 70%) with other major congenital anomalies, especially neural tube defects and cardiac abnormalities.[9, 27, 32, 33] A study from Guy's Hospital in London, England, reported that 8 of 17 fetuses with omphalocele had congenital heart disease evident on fetal echocardiography.[10] Intensive prenatal screening to detect other defects is extremely important, not only to determine fetal viability, but also to help predict the postnatal needs of the fetus. This screening should include extensive ultrasound evaluation and amniocentesis. A number of studies have correlated omphalocele size

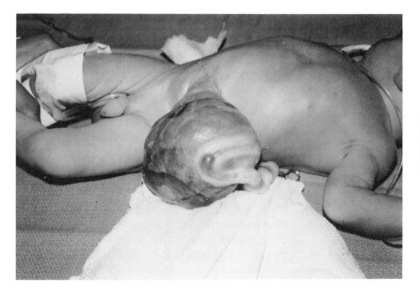

FIGURE 39–1 ••• A newborn infant with the majority of the small intestine contained in the omphalocele sac; note the relatively small ventral wall defect.

greater than 5 cm with eventual poor outcome, but these are inconclusive.[34, 35] In general, otherwise normal neonates with omphaloceles containing only bowel have improved survival over those with extrusion of the liver or other organs. On the other hand, Nyberg et al. showed a correlation between abnormal karyotype and an omphalocele containing bowel only.[36] Abnormal chromosomes were present in 10 of 13 infants with omphalocele that contained bowel only, compared with 3 of 23 with omphalocele containing liver. An association was also present between abnormal karyotype and abnormal amniotic fluid volume. Eight of 11 fetuses that had abnormal amniotic volume also had chromosomal abnormalities, whereas only 5 of 19 with normal volumes had such abnormalities. Karyotype is also important, as trisomy 18 and trisomy 13 are both highly associated with omphalocele. Measurement of acetylcholinesterase levels in the amniotic fluid helps to discover evidence of associated neural tube defects.[27]

Once the diagnosis has been established, plans for postnatal care should be made. In most cases, this should include determination of a time for delivery in a tertiary care facility that provides immediate neonatal intensive care and subsequent surgical repair. There is no good evidence to suggest that a cesarean section is beneficial unless fetal distress occurs at the time of delivery. Although the overall survival rate of neonates with omphalocele is only 70% because of associated anomalies, survival and life expectancy of infants without other anomalies is excellent.

Gastroschisis is an abdominal wall defect that occurs to the right of the intact umbilical cord. It is thought to result from a weakness in the wall at the site of a previous right umbilical vein.[30] The bowel herniates through this defect and directly contacts the amniotic fluid (Fig. 39–2). Gastroschisis has a much lower incidence of associated anomalies (10% to 20%), but because the bowel is exposed to amniotic fluid, an intense serositis, which is described as a thick rind with shortening of the bowel, can potentially develop. Associated atresias occur in 10% to 15% of patients secondary to vascular compromise of the herniated bowel caused by torsion or impingement of the mesenteric blood supply as it traverses through the defect.[37] Some have suggested that exposure of the bowel to the amniotic fluid causes problems with the bowel and have advocated early cesarean section to decrease the time during which the intestine is in contact with the amniotic fluid.[31, 38–41] However, three large reviews have found no benefit to early cesarean section over vaginal delivery in the degree of bowel injury or in the long-term outcome of these infants.[28, 42, 43] Nearly 95% of infants with gastroschisis survive with a normal life expectancy.

The important perinatal considerations in the care of neonates with omphalocele and gastroschisis include nontraumatic sterile care of the intestine, gastrointestinal decompression with an orogastric tube, prevention of hypothermia, and early surgical repair. Prevention of hypothermia requires a warm environment and prevention of evaporative water loss from

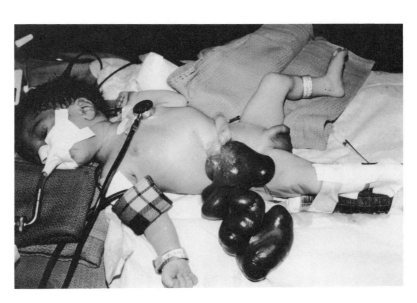

FIGURE 39–2 ••• A newborn with gastroschisis; note the lack of peritoneal covering. The small intestine is covered by a thick "rind" that makes assessment of the intestine impossible.

the exposed gut. Evaporative loss can be effectively decreased by placing the lower half of the infant, including the sterile wrapped intestine, in a clear plastic bag closed at the mid torso (Fig. 39–3). The bag creates a closed space in which the relative humidity rapidly reaches 100%, thereby minimizing evaporative loss. Transport to an appropriate center before delivery is much safer than transfer after delivery when ventilatory support, hypothermia, fluid and electrolyte management, and the interval of time until surgery is performed all become critical factors.

CONGENITAL DIAPHRAGMATIC HERNIA

Congenital diaphragmatic hernia (CDH) is one of the most difficult, as well as one of the most exciting, areas of perinatology and neonatal surgery. The defect occurs in 1 of every 2000 live births, with a similar incidence in adolescent pregnancies.[44, 45] It results from a failure of proper closure of the diaphragm during the 8th to 11th week of gestation. This posterolateral defect occurs on the left in nearly 90% of cases and is associated with herniation of abdominal contents into the thoracic cavity and compression of the lung (Fig. 39–4). This occurs during a critical stage of lung bud development and results in severe pulmonary hypoplasia on the affected side. The contralateral side is also affected but to a lesser degree. At birth this may result in severe

respiratory distress, pulmonary hypertension, and a persistence of the fetal circulation. Although surgical repair of the defect is usually indicated in the early postnatal period, the major problems in management are those associated with pulmonary hypertension, which is not usually improved by the repair alone.[46] This has led to a search for other methods to assist in sustaining the infant during the early postnatal period when conventional medical therapy (standard ventilation, fluid resuscitation, and pulmonary vasodilators) fails.[47, 48] Researchers are investigating fetal surgery to allow improved in utero lung development and prevent the late sequelae[49] (as is discussed below).

The survival rate for neonates with CDH has been reported as 50%. Evidence of the stomach or liver within the chest, polyhydramnios, associated anomalies, and early antenatal diagnosis have been shown to be associated with a significantly worse prognosis. Nevertheless, experience with improved ventilatory techniques, high-frequency ventilation, and extracorporeal membrane oxygenation (ECMO) have shown promising early results, with survival rates of 85% to 90%. ECMO provides adequate arterial oxygenation for up to 10 to 14 days, during which the infant's hypoplastic lung can adapt and pulmonary hypertension diminish.

Because of the major respiratory and circulatory problems associated with this defect, early consultation with a neonatologist and pediatric surgeon is essential. The infant should be delivered at a tertiary care facility

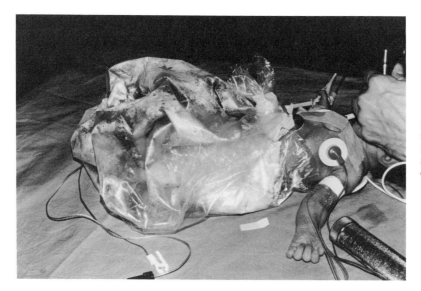

FIGURE 39–3 ••• Infant with gastroschisis. The legs and abdomen, including the extruding intestine, are in a cellophane bag to prevent evaporative losses and heat loss.

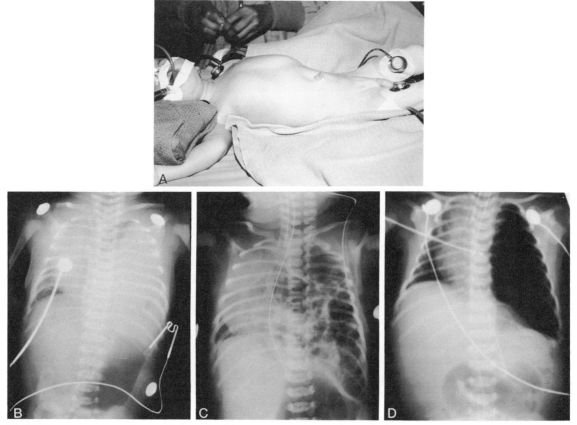

FIGURE 39–4 ••• *A,* A newborn with a scaphoid abdomen typical of congenital diaphragmatic hernia (CDH). *B,* Immediate postnatal chest radiograph of an infant with CDH. Before insufflation of the malpositioned intestine, the chest on the side of the hernia appears opacified. *C,* The same infant after 15 to 20 minutes. Swallowed air now fills the loops of small intestine that were present in the left side of the chest. *D,* Chest radiograph after diaphragm repair. Note the lack of normal lung on the left.

that has significant experience in the management of these infants. The infant is likely to require emergent respiratory resuscitation after delivery and often surgery in the first 24 hours. If the diagnosis is made antenatally, the neonate can be paralyzed and intubated in the delivery room. This prevents gaseous distention of the intrathoracic stomach and intestine. An orogastric tube is used to keep the gastrointestinal tract decompressed. By keeping the infant adequately oxygenated and the pH in the normal to alkalotic range, the development of pulmonary hypertension can be decreased. Pulmonary vasodilators may also be helpful. From January 1988 to October 1992, the survival rate for infants with diaphragmatic hernias treated at Texas Children's Hospital by conventional techniques has been nearly 80%.

As mentioned previously, the role of fetal surgery in treatment of this particular anomaly is still experimental, and although early clinical results have been poor, experimental work is encouraging.[49] There may be some adolescent and adult patients whose prognosis, based on ultrasound findings, is so poor that fetal intervention may be warranted. Further work in this area is indicated before surgery becomes a significant option.

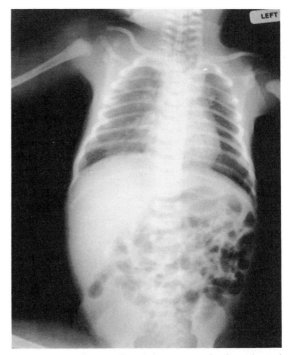

FIGURE 39–5 ••• An infant with type C tracheal esophageal fistula (esophageal atresia with distal tracheal esophageal fistula). Note the orogastric tube curled in the upper pouch.

ESOPHAGEAL ATRESIA

Esophageal atresia with or without tracheoesophageal fistula occurs in 1 in every 3000 to 5000 births. It should be suspected in patients with polyhydramnios and in whom the stomach cannot be identified on ultrasound.[50, 51] However, the diagnosis is very difficult to make by antenatal ultrasound. Esophageal atresia is also highly associated with other anomalies and is part of the vertebral, anal, cardiac, tracheoesophageal, renal, and limb (VACTERL) association. Patients in whom esophageal atresia is suspected require antenatal karyotyping and echocardiography, as well as a thorough survey to check for other anomalies. Antenatal obstetric management need not be changed, but there must be recognition that the infant with esophageal atresia and/or fistula is at high risk for aspiration and respiratory compromise after birth.[7] After delivery the diagnosis must be considered when the neonate cannot handle oral secretions or first feedings. The diagnosis is then confirmed by the inability to pass a nasogastric tube into the stomach (Fig. 39–5). The upper pouch should be kept aspirated with a short sump tube (e.g., a Replogle tube) to prevent aspiration and dilatation of the upper esophageal pouch and compression of the immature trachea. Nearly 90% of infants with esophageal atresia have a tracheoesophageal fistula between the lower trachea and the distal esophagus (Fig. 39–6). If a fistula is present, special care must be taken to prevent gastric distention and reflux of gastric fluid into the tracheobronchial tree. This is best accomplished by avoiding excessive assisted ventilatory pressure, particularly with a bag and mask. Early division and closure of the tracheoesophageal fistula and primary anastomosis of the esophagus is the treatment of choice. However, if there will be an excessive delay before primary repair can be undertaken or if gastric distention occurs, a decompressing gastrostomy should be performed. To prevent gastroesophageal reflux, it is best to keep the infant prone with the head of the bed elevated.

The mortality rate for infants with esophageal atresia with or without a fistula is about 10%. Death is rarely the result of the esophageal anomaly but is due to other anomalies, including cardiac and chromosomal anomalies.

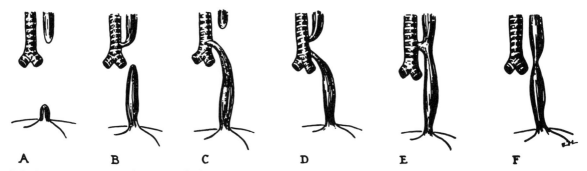

FIGURE 39–6 ••• Types of congenital abnormalities of the esophagus. *A,* Esophageal atresia. There is no esophageal communication with the trachea. In such circumstances the lower esophageal end is very apt to be quite short. *B,* Esophageal atresia, with the upper segment communicating with the trachea. *C,* Esophageal atresia, with the lower segment communicating with the back of the trachea. More than 90% of all esophageal malformations fall into this category. *D,* Esophageal atresia, with both segments communicating with the trachea. *E,* The esophagus has no disruption of its continuity, but a tracheoesophageal fistula is present. *F,* Esophageal stenosis. (From Gross RE. The Surgery of Infancy and Childhood. Philadelphia: WB Saunders, 1964; p 76.)

Infants without other anomalies typically have normal growth and development.

BOWEL OBSTRUCTION

Evidence of bowel obstruction has been detected with increasing frequency in the antenatal period.[3, 6, 8, 50, 52–61] Evidence of polyhydramnios is often the heralding sign and warrants further investigation. Intestinal atresias (duodenal atresia being the most common), meconium ileus, imperforate anus, malrotation, intestinal duplications, and even Hirschsprung's disease have been diagnosed or suggested antenatally. Although these defects cause few problems in utero and often only minimal difficulties in the immediate postdelivery period, prenatal diagnosis has been shown to improve overall outcome and mortality.[62]

Duodenal atresia is caused by a failure of recanalization of the primitive duodenum during the first trimester after a period of exuberant endothelial growth, which results in a solid cordlike duodenum (Fig. 39–7). In contrast, other intestinal atresias are thought to be secondary to an in utero vascular accident resulting in transient ischemia with localized scarring and stenosis or to frank infarction with the loss of continuity and atresia. These infants present with total obstruction and must undergo decompression immediately to prevent respiratory compromise from abdominal distention and intestinal perforation. Surgical correction should be carried out shortly after birth. The consulting obstetrician should be aware that duodenal atresia is often associated with other malformations and chromosomal abnormalities, including Down syndrome, which is present in nearly 30% of infants with duodenal atresia. This well-known association allows the perinatologist to check for other manifestations that may affect outcome and

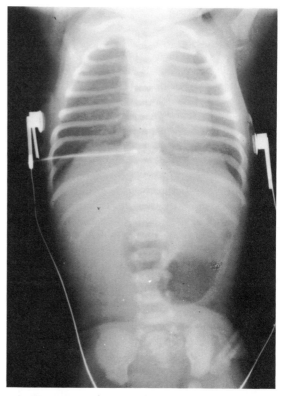

FIGURE 39–7 ••• Classic double-bubble sign. Differential diagnosis includes duodenal atresia, duodenal web, and annular pancreas.

fetal viability, including cardiac and vertebral anomalies, nonimmune hydrops, and cystic hygromas. Therefore, karyotyping and echocardiography are indicated. Arrangements for prenatal transport to an appropriate referral center should be made, as this has been shown to improve overall fetal outcome and survival.

More distal obstructions, denoted by evidence of dilated loops of bowel on ultrasound, should act as a warning of the possibility of a number of other pathologic conditions such as meconium ileus, malrotation, or imperforate anus. Meconium ileus, which is nearly always a manifestation of cystic fibrosis, may present on ultrasound as increased echogenicity of the markedly dilated ileum filled with thick, abnormal meconium.[58] If perforation has occurred with resultant meconium peritonitis, peritoneal wall calcifications may be seen.[59] Malrotation, Hirschsprung's disease, and imperforate anus may present on antenatal ultrasound simply as dilated loops of bowel. Although these exact diagnoses cannot usually be made antenatally, arrangements should be made for immediate postnatal decompression and appropriate evaluation, usually at a tertiary referral center.

TUMORS AND CYSTS

Antenatal diagnosis of fetal tumors and cysts is occurring with increasing frequency.[7, 12, 63] Mass lesions are being found more commonly on routine ultrasound, and their significance in utero is still being delineated. Reports of prenatally diagnosed neuroblastomas, Wilms' tumors, hepatoblastomas, teratomas, and other solid tumors have shown good correlation with neonatal evaluation and surgical findings.[64–70] However, with rare exceptions, these findings have little impact on the antenatal care or delivery of the fetus. One exception is sacrococcygeal teratoma (Fig. 39–8), in which case the large size of the tumor may be an indication for cesarean section.[71] Other than evidence of a mass or lesion, associated findings can include nonimmune hydrops and polyhydramnios and should warrant further antenatal investigation.[67] Suspicion of any mass or lesion warrants consultation with a pediatric surgeon to plan a full neonatal evaluation.

Cystic hydroma, normally thought to be a relatively benign condition when present in the neonate, has been shown to be associated with chromosomal abnormalities and a high mor-

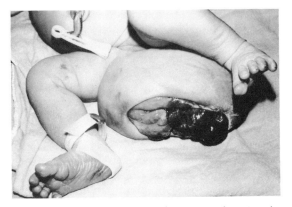

FIGURE 39–8 ••• Sacrococcygeal teratoma obscuring the perineum and perineal structures. It arises from the coccyx, which must be included in the resection.

tality rate when diagnosed in utero before 30 weeks of gestation. Diagnosis after this time is usually associated with a benign course and requires only elective resection in the newborn period. However, there are reported cases of large cervical teratomas causing airway obstruction in the immediate postnatal period.[72, 73] These obstructing tumors may be associated with polyhydramnios, as they are also likely to obstruct the esophagus. Large cervical tumors with polyhydramnios may be an indication for elective cesarean section with planned surgical intervention available immediately in the delivery suite to provide an airway, if necessary.

OVARIAN CYST

Antenatal diagnosis of ovarian cyst, although relatively rare, is a well-documented occurrence.[74–88] These are functional cysts and are usually follicular and benign in nature.[75, 76, 89–94] In general, they are of little prenatal significance and should not alter routine obstetric care. An association between large ovarian cysts and torsion has encouraged some to pursue an aggressive interventional approach. There are reports of in utero aspiration, but the associated risks do not seem appropriate for this relatively benign condition.

Management of these cysts after delivery is somewhat controversial. Observation alone is usually recommended for simple cysts less than 2 to 3 cm in diameter with no evidence of cystic debris. Evidence of debris within the cyst is suggestive of torsion or neoplasia and therefore warrants exploration.[74, 76, 81, 94, 95] For cysts more than 4 to 5 cm in diameter, previous recommendations for adolescents and adults called for exploration with planned cystectomy to preserve the ovary, if technically possible.[81] However, more recent reports have documented regression of even the larger cysts with long-term follow-up.[75] Other clinicians have aspirated the cysts percutaneously, performing excision only if the cyst recurs.[93, 96, 97] These larger cysts must be dealt with on a case-by-case basis and require close follow-up and a concern for the development of ovarian torsion.

Other cystic lesions discovered on antenatal ultrasound include mesenteric cysts, omental cysts, hepatic cysts, renal cysts, and choledochal cysts.[50, 70, 98, 99] Differential diagnosis of these lesions in utero can be extremely difficult. However, prenatal recognition and observation are all that is required. The cysts rarely cause problems in utero and therefore should not affect antenatal care. Nevertheless, early postpartum evaluation is indicated, and the pediatrician and pediatric surgeon should be notified early so that the appropriate evaluation and treatment can be arranged. Except for choledochal cysts, which may be associated with biliary obstruction, these lesions tend to be benign and cause problems only when their size causes symptoms of obstruction.[99]

URINARY TRACT ANOMALIES

Anomalies of the urinary tract are often heralded by the presence of oligohydramnios.[100–102] Obstruction can often be detected by the presence of hydronephrosis, and the site of obstruction can often be determined by the site and degree of dilatation of the urinary collecting system.[103, 104] Complete obstructions result in a loss of renal parenchyma and possible renal failure.

Abnormalities of the urinary tract were some of the first lesions to be detected by fetal ultrasound. Hydronephrosis or cystic lesions of the kidney can often be detected as early as 16 weeks of gestation with routine prenatal ultrasound. Urinary tract obstruction, renal dysfunction, or dysplasia will also result in oligohydramnios, which can alert the examiner to more closely define the urinary collecting system. Obstructing lesions may occur at either the ureteropelvic junction, ureterovesicle junction, or in the urethra itself (i.e., posterior

urethral valves). This may result in unilateral or bilateral dilatation of part or all of the collecting system. Ureteropelvic junction obstruction is a relatively rare anomaly and is almost always unilateral. It may be secondary to fibrous bands, valves, or an unusual ureteral insertion.[105] Ultrasound typically shows a normal amount of amniotic fluid, as the contralateral side is unaffected. Also, the affected kidney will be hydronephrotic. There are no strict criteria to define hydronephrosis in utero, but Harrison et al. have suggested a rough estimate of abnormal size: mild dilatation will be demonstrated as an enlarged renal pelvis, branching infundibula, and calices; severe dilatation will be demonstrated as a large unilocular fluid collection.[101] If the obstruction is thought to be unilateral and there is a normal amount of amniotic fluid, then no fetal intervention is indicated. If there is marked oligohydramnios and unilateral hydronephrosis, the clinician must consider contralateral renal agenesis, in which case fetal intervention may be indicated in an effort to save the remaining kidney. Routine obstetric care otherwise should not be altered.

Posterior urethral valves, a more common problem, can result in dilatation of the entire collecting system. These can occur secondary to an exaggeration of the development of the urethrovaginal folds or possibly secondary to abnormal canalization of the urogenital membrane. This results in obstruction of the bladder outflow tract. Diagnosis is made by identification of dilatation of the lower urinary tract (i.e., dilated bladder, hydroureter, and hydronephrosis). The degree of associated oligohydramnios is an indicator of the degree of obstruction and is a relative prognostic indicator. Absent or mild oligohydramnios is associated with absent or minimal renal dysfunction, whereas severe oligohydramnios suggests a poor prognosis.[107] Both unilateral and bilateral obstruction are associated with a 10% to 20% incidence of other anomalies, and therefore, a careful screening of the entire fetus should be accomplished.

A fetus with bilateral obstruction can be considered for fetal intervention and drainage. Glick et al. identified six prognostic criteria based on urinalysis via an ultrasound-guided bladder tap: severe oligohydramnios, cystic kidneys, Na >100 mg/ml, Cl >90 mg/ml osmolarity, >210 mOsm, and urinary output less than 2 ml/hr are poor prognostic indicators.[105] If the results indicate a poor prognosis, then fetal termination may be indicated. If the results indicate a good prognosis, then fetal intervention (i.e., drainage either by decompression with catheters or by operative suprapubic vesicostomy) should be considered. These decisions must be made by an experienced perinatal and fetal surgery team, and these patients should be referred as soon as the diagnosis of bilateral obstructive uropathy is established.

Other abnormalities that may be detected antenatally include solitary or multiple renal cysts, renal agenesis, or tumors. Solitary cysts are of little consequence and should be followed with postpartum ultrasound. Infantile polycystic disease has a variable prognosis that depends on the degree of collecting duct dilatation and loss of renal parenchyma. Cases diagnosed in utero are usually severe and are commonly associated with fetal or infant death.[107] Therefore, cases diagnosed before viability may be considered for fetal termination. If the fetus goes to term, massively enlarged kidneys may cause soft tissue dystonia, and a cesarean section may be required. Bilateral multicystic kidneys have a similarly poor prognosis and are usually fatal. Fetal karyotyping should be done and fetal termination considered in severe bilateral cases. On the other hand, the prognosis for infants with a unilateral multicystic kidney is excellent. Solid renal tumors have been sporadically reported. These tend to have little effect on normal fetal development, but neonatal evaluation, including ultrasound, should be performed in the early postpartum period.

FETAL SURGERY

The rapid advances in prenatal diagnosis since the 1970s has resulted in a better understanding of the natural history of many congenital anomalies. This understanding of both the development and pathophysiology of these diseases has led to a large body of research directed at fetal intervention in an attempt to change the course of these diseases. The vast majority of work in this area has been pioneered by Michael Harrison and his group at University of California, San Francisco. Significant advances have been made in three primary areas of fetal surgery. The first, and in some ways the most important advances, are in maternal and fetal monitoring preoperatively, intraoperatively, and postoperatively.[107–112] The greatest obstacle to human fetal surgery remains the irritability of the uterus and the high spontaneous abortion rate after any degree of uterine manipulation, unlike in sheep, the most widely used animal model for fetal research, who are much more tolerant of uterine manipulation.[111, 113] Some of the methods found to decrease irritability include a preoperative dose of indomethacin, the use of halothane for general anesthesia to promote uterine relaxation, and the use of methylphenidate hydrochloride (Ritalin) or indomethacin infusion postoperatively to act as a tocolytic.[114] Other advances have included the development of a fetal transcutaneous pulse oximeter and electrocardiography to allow for monitoring both intraoperatively and postoperatively.[111, 114]

The second area of major advancement has been in the management of congenital hydronephrosis.[57, 115–120] It has previously been shown that fetuses with marked hydronephrosis can have many severe deficits, including renal dysgenesis and poor function, as well as pulmonary hypoplasia secondary to oligohydramnios.[105, 121] Harrison et al. hypothesized that intrauterine decompression could prevent this serious sequelae. Initial attempts at decompression used simple vesicoamniotic shunts, a high rate of catheter occlusion and infection led these researchers to favor surgical vesicostomy.[117, 118] Guidelines for selection of fetuses appropriate for fetal intervention have been suggested by Glick et al., as previously mentioned, and the surgery has achieved a moderate degree of success.[105]

The third major area of advancement has been in the area of fetal surgery for congenital diaphragmatic hernia.[109, 122–127] As discussed previously, the diaphragmatic defect may result in severe and potentially fatal pulmonary hypoplasia. The theory behind fetal intervention is that in utero repair at an early stage will allow for more normal pulmonary development and prevent the fatal irreversible disease that occurs in the most severe cases. Harrison's aggressive approach to this is also fueled by the fact that the mortality rate for conventionally treated congenital diaphragmatic hernia remains as high as 75%, despite advances in ECMO, pharmacologic manipulation, and ventilatory support.[46, 109, 111] In an animal model Harrison et al. have shown that the pulmonary hypoplasia is caused by pulmonary compression and that the process is reversible by prenatal repair.[49, 126]

The surgery itself is performed through a hysterotomy with just the left fetal arm and a portion of the fetal torso extruded. A subcostal incision is used to enter the abdomen and reduce the bowel. A Gore-Tex patch is then placed to repair the diaphragmatic defect. Three of the first six fetuses undergoing this procedure died intraoperatively, one died shortly after birth, and two died of nonpulmonary complications at a few weeks of age.[123] Although the possibilities for this type of fetal intervention are exciting, the exact effect on the disease process is unclear, and the technical challenges remain formidable.

References

1. Barkin SZ, Pretorius DH, Beckett MK, et al. Severe polyhydramnios: Incidence of anomalies. AJR 1987; 148:155.
2. Benacerraf BR, Cnann A, Gelman R, et al. Can sonographers reliably identify anatomic features associated with Down's syndrome in fetuses? Radiology 1989; 173:377.
3. Bergmans MGM, Merkus JMWM, Baars AM. Obstetrical and neonatological aspects of a child with atresia of the small bowel. J Perinat Med 1984; 12:325.
4. Bidwell JK, Nelson A. Prenatal ultrasonic diagnosis of congenital duplication of the stomach. J Ultrasound Med 1986; 5:589.
5. Brock DJH, Bedgood D, Barron L, Hayward C. Prospective prenatal diagnosis of cystic fibrosis. Lancet 1985; I:1175.
6. Cacciari A. Gastrointestinal tract anomalies: Neonatal surgical problems. Fetal Ther 1986; 1:101.
7. Canty TG, Leopold GR, Wolf DA. Maternal ultrasonography for the antenatal diagnosis of surgically significant neonatal anomalies. Ann Surg 1981; 194:353.
8. Carrera JM. Prenatal diagnosis of gastrointestinal tract obstructions. Fetal Ther 1986; 1:96.
9. Cobellis G, Iannoto P, Stabile M, et al. Prenatal ultrasound diagnosis of macroglossia in the Wiedemann-Beckwith syndrome. Prenat Diagn 1988; 8:79.
10. Crawford DC, Chapman MG, Allan LD. Echocardiography in the investigation of anterior abdominal wall defects in the fetus. Br J Obstet Gynecol 1985; 92:1034.
11. DiSessa TG, Emerson DC, Felker RE, et al. Anomalous systemic and pulmonary venous pathways diagnosed in utero by ultrasound. J Ultrasound Med 1990; 9:311.
12. Dibbins AW, Curci MR, McCrann DJ Jr. Prenatal diagnosis of congenital anomalies requiring surgical correction. Implications for the future. Am J Surg 1985; 149:528.
13. Gauderer MW, Jassani MN, Izant RJ Jr. Ultrasonic antenatal diagnosis: Will it change the spectrum of neonatal surgery? J Pediatr Surg 1984; 19:404.
14. Grisoni ER, Gauderer MWL, Wolfson RN, Izant RJ Jr. Antenatal ultrasonography: The experience in a high risk perinatal center. J Pediatr Surg 1986; 21:358.
15. Leonhardt A, Schmidt W, Wille L. Fetal and neo-
natal ascites: A report of 15 cases and a review of the literature. Klin Padiatr 1987; 199:9.
16. McLaughlin JF, Marks WM, Jones G. Prospective management of exstrophy of the cloaca and myelocystocele following prenatal ultrasound recognition of neural tube defects in identical twins. Am J Med Genet 1984; 19:721.
17. Pijlman BM, deKoning WB, Wladimiroff JW, Stewart PA. Detection of fetal structural malformations by ultrasound in insulin-dependent pregnant women. Ultrasound Med Biol 1989; 15:541.
18. Purkiss S, Brereton RJ, Wright VM. Surgical emergencies after prenatal treatment for intra-abdominal abnormality. Lancet 1988; 1:289.
19. Rieth KG, Comite F, Shawker TH, Cutler GB Jr. Pituitary and ovarian abnormalities demonstrated by CT and ultrasound in children with features of the McCune-Albright syndrome. Radiology 1984; 153:389.
20. Tepper R, Schoenfeld A, Ovadia J. Ultrasonic assessment of fetal colon by comparing ratios of colon circumference to abdominal circumference in normal pregnancy and two abnormal cases. Fetal Ther 1987; 2:123.
21. Touloukian RJ, Hobbins JC. Maternal ultrasonography in the antenatal diagnosis of surgically correctable fetal abnormalities. J Pediatr Surg 1980; 15:373.
22. Lanjham MR, Krammel TM, Bartlett RH. Mortality with ECMO following repair of congenital diaphragmatic hernia in 93 infants. J Pediatr Surg 1987; 12:1150.
23. Albright SG, Katz VL. Alpha-fetoprotein findings in a case of cystic adenomatoid malformation of the lung. Clin Genet 1989; 35:75.
24. Jouppila P, Kirkinen P. Ultrasonic and clinical aspects in the diagnosis and prognosis of congenital gastrointestinal anomalies. Ultrasound Med Biol 1984; 10:465.
25. Shkolnik A. Applications of ultrasound in the neonatal abdomen. Radiol Clin North Am 1985; 23:141.
26. Satoh Y. Ultrasonic diagnosis of perinatal and infant diseases. Rinsho Hoshasen 1984; 29:1315.
27. Ardinger HH, Williamson RA, Grant S. Association of neural tube defects with omphalocele in chromosomally normal fetuses. Am J Med Genet 1987; 27:135.
28. Carpenter MW, Curci MR, Dibbins AW, Hadow JE. Perinatal management of ventral wall defects. Obstet Gynecol 1984; 64:646.
29. Hertzberg BS, Bowie JD. Fetal gastrointestinal abnormalities. Radiol Clin North Am 1990; 28:101.
30. Hoyme HE, Jones MC, Jones KL. Gastroschisis: Abdominal wall disruption secondary to early gestational interruption of the omphalomesenteric artery. Semin Perinat 1983; 7:294.
31. Lenke RR. Congenital defects of the abdominal wall. Am J Obstet Gynecol 1987; 158:1015.
32. Hughes MD, Nyberg DA, Mack LA, Pretorius DH. Fetal omphalocele: Prenatal ultrasound detection of concurrent anomalies and other predictors of outcome. Radiology 1989; 173:371.
33. Grundy H, Walton S, Burlbaw J, et al. Beckwith-Wiedemann syndrome: Prenatal ultrasound diagnosis using standard kidney to abdominal circumference ratio. Am J Perinatol 1985; 2:236.
34. Knight PJ, Sommer A, Clatworthy HW. Omphalocele: A prognostic classification. J Pediatr Surg 1981; 16:599.

35. Mayer T, Black R, Matlak ME, et al. Gastroschisis and omphalocele. Ann Surg 1980; 192:783.
36. Nyberg DA, Fitzsimmons J, Mack LA, et al. Chromosomal abnormalities in fetuses with omphalocele: The significance of omphalocele contents. J Ultrasound Med 1989; 8:299–308.
37. Louw JH. Jejunoileal atresia and stenosis. J Pediatr Surg 1966; 1:8.
38. Lenke RR, Hatch EI Jr. Fetal gastroschisis: A preliminary report advocating the use of cesarean section. Obstet Gynecol 1986; 67:395.
39. Haller JA Jr, Kehrer BH, Shaker IJ, et al. Studies of the pathophysiology of gastroschisis in fetal sheep. J Pediatr Surg 1974; 9:627.
40. Glick PL, Harrison MR, Adzickins NS, et al. The missing link in the pathogenesis of gastroschisis. J Pediatr Surg 1985; 20:406.
41. Bond SJ, Harrison MR, Filly RA, et al. Severity of intestinal damage in gastroschisis: Correlation with prenatal sonographic findings. J Pediatr Surg 1988; 23:520.
42. Kirk EP, Wah RM. Obstetric management of the fetus with omphalocele or gastroschisis: A review and report of one hundred twelve cases. Am J Obstet Gynecol 1983; 146:512.
43. Moretti M, Khoury A, Rodriguez J, et al. The effect of mode of delivery on the perinatal outcome in fetuses with abdominal wall defects. Am J Obstet Gynecol 1990; 163:833.
44. David TJ, Illingworth CA. Diaphragmatic hernia in the southwest of England. J Med Genet 1976; 13:253.
45. Puri P, Gorman F. Lethal nonpulmonary anomalies associated with congenital diaphragmatic hernia: Implications for early intrauterine surgery. J Pediatr Surg 1984; 19:29.
46. Harrison MR, Bjordal RI, Langmark R, Knutrud O. Congenital diaphragmatic hernia: The hidden mortality. J Pediatr Surg 1978; 13:227.
47. Howell CG, Hatley KM, Boed RF, et al. Recent experience with diaphragmatic hernia and ECMO. Am Surg 1990; 211:793.
48. Heiss K, Manning P, Oldham KT, et al. Reversal of mortality for congenital diaphragmatic hernia with ECMO. Am Surg 1989; 209:225.
49. Harrison MR, Bressack MA, Churg AM, et al. Correction of congenital diaphragmatic hernia in utero. II. Simulated correction permits fetal lung growth with survival at birth. Surgery 1980; 88:260.
50. Farrant P. The antenatal diagnosis of oesophageal atresia by ultrasound. Br J Radiol 1980; 53:1202.
51. Pretorius DH, Gosink BB, Clautice-Engle T, et al. Sonographic evaluation of the fetal stomach: Significance of nonvisualization. AJR 1988; 151:987.
52. Bahgat O, Lev-Gur M, Divon MY. Prenatal ultrasound diagnosis of intestinal obstruction: A case report. Am J Perinatol 1989; 6:324.
53. Blott M, Greenough A, Gamsu HR, et al. Antenatal factors associated with obstruction of the gastrointestinal tract by meconium. Br Med J 1988; 296:250.
54. Jassani MN, Gauderer MWL, Fanaroff AA, et al. A perinatal approach to the diagnosis and management of gastrointestinal malformations. Obstet Gynecol 1982; 59:33.
55. Imai A, Kawabata I, Tamaya T. Antenatal evaluation of upper gastrointestinal dilatation complicated by non-immune hydrops fetalis and polyhydramnios. J Med 1989; 20:399.
56. Kjoller M, Holm-Nielsen G, Meiland H, et al. Prenatal obstruction of the ileum diagnosed by ultrasound. Prenat Diagn 1985; 5:427.
57. Langer JC, Adzick NS, Filey RA, et al. Gastrointestinal tract obstruction in the fetus. Arch Surg 1989; 124:1183.
58. Van Dam LJ, deGroot CJ, Hazebrook FW, Wladimiroff JW. Case report. Intrauterine demonstration of bowel duplication by ultrasound. Eur J Obstet Gynecol Reprod Biol 1984; 18:229.
59. Clair MR, Rosenberg ER, Ram PC, Bowie JD. Prenatal sonographic diagnosis of meconium peritonitis. Prenat Diagn 1983; 3:65.
60. Denholm TA, Crow HC, Edwards WH, et al. Prenatal sonographic appearance of meconium ileus in twins. AJR 1984; 143:371.
61. Finkel LI, Slovis TL. Meconium peritonitis, intraperitoneal calcifications and cystic fibrosis. Pediatr Radiol 1982; 12:92.
62. Romero R, Ghidini A, Costigan K, et al. Prenatal diagnosis of duodenal atresia: Does it make any difference? Obstet Gynecol 1988; 71:739.
63. Helin I, Persson PH. Intra-abdominal cysts detected at prenatal ultrasound screening. Helv Paediatr Acta 1985; 40:55.
64. Forman HP, Leonidas JC, Berdon WE, et al. Congenital neuroblastoma: Evaluation with multimodality imaging. Radiology 1990; 175:365.
65. Graham D, Winn K, Dex W, Sanders RC. Prenatal diagnosis of cystic adenomatoid malformation of the lung. J Ultrasound Med 1982; 1:9.
66. Gross SJ, Benzie RJ, Sermer M, et al. Sacrococcygeal teratoma: Prenatal diagnosis and management. Am J Obstet Gynecol 1987; 156:393.
67. Kazzi NJ, Chang CH, Roberts EC, Shankaran S. Fetal hepatoblastoma presenting as nonimmune hydrops. Am J Perinatol 1989; 6:278.
68. Kurjak A, Zalud I, Jurkovic D, et al. Ultrasound diagnosis and evaluation of fetal tumors. J Perinat Med 1989; 17:173.
69. Teele RL, Share JC. The abdominal mass in the neonate. Semin Roentgenol 1988; 23:175.
70. Wu A, Siegel MJ. Sonography of pelvic masses in children: Diagnostic predictability. AJR 1987; 148:1191.
71. Johnson JW, Porter J Jr, Kellner KR, et al. Abdominal rescue after incomplete delivery secondary to large fetal sacrococcygeal teratoma. Obstet Gynecol 1988; 71:981.
72. Holinger LD, Birnholz JC, Bruce DR, et al. Management of an infant with prenatal ultrasound diagnosis of upper airway obstruction. Int J Pediatr Otorhinolaryngol 1985; 10:263.
73. Holinger LD, Birnholz JC. Management of infants with prenatal ultrasound diagnosis of airway obstruction by teratoma. Ann Otol Rhinol Laryngol 1987; 96:61.
74. Alrabeeah A, Galliani CA, Giacomantonio M, et al. Neonatal ovarian torsion: Report of three cases and review of the literature. Pediatr Pathol 1988; 18:143–149.
75. Amodio J, Abramson S, Berdon W, et al. Postnatal resolution of large ovarian cysts detected in utero. Pediatr Radiol 1987; 17:467.
76. Battin J, Colle M, Audebert A, Nehme K. Benign tumors of the ovary and follicular cysts in children and adolescents. Ann Pediatr 1987; 34:55.
77. Bergqvist C, Esscher T, Lindgren PG, et al. Cystic ovaries in a pre-term newborn infant. Z Kinderchir 1984; 39:403.
78. Eggermont E, Lecoutere D, Devlieger H, et al. Ovarian cysts in newborn infants. Am J Dis Child 1988; 142:702.

79. Fleischer AC, Shawker TH. The role of sonography in pediatric gynecology. Clin Obstet Gynecol 1987; 30:735.

80. Giacoia GP, Wood BP. Ovarian cyst of the newborn. Am J Dis Child 1987; 141:1005.

81. Grapin C, Montagne JP, Sirinelli D, et al. Diagnosis of ovarian cysts in the perinatal period and therapeutic implications (20 cases). Ann Radiol 1987; 30:497.

82. Ikeda K, Suita S, Nakano H. Management of ovarian cyst detected antenatally. J Pediatr Surg 1988; 23:432.

83. Kirkinen P, Jouppila P. Perinatal aspects of pregnancy complicated by fetal ovarian cysts. J Perinat Med 1985; 13:245.

84. Liapi C, Evain-Brion D. Diagnosis of ovarian follicular cysts from birth to puberty: A report of twenty cases. Acta Paediatr Scand 1987; 76:91.

85. McKeever PA, Andrews H. Fetal ovarian cysts: A report of five cases. J Pediatr Surg 1988; 23:354.

86. Nussbaum AR, Sanders RC, Hartman DS, Dudgeon DL. Neonatal ovarian cysts: Sonographic-pathologic correlation. Radiology 1988; 168:817.

87. Suita S, Ikeda K, Koyanagi T, Nakana H. Neonatal ovarian cyst diagnosed antenatally: Report of two patients. J Clin Ultrasound 1984; 12:517.

88. Weintraub Z. Fetal ovarian cysts. A report of five cases. J Pediatr Surg 1988; 23:1228.

89. Portuondo JA, Gimenez B, Rivera JM, et al. Clinical and pathologic evaluation of 342 benign ovarian tumors. Int J Gynaecol Obstet 1984; 22:263.

90. Shawis RN, El-Gohary A, Cook RC. Ovarian cysts and tumors in childhood. Ann R Coll Surg Engl 1985; 67:17.

91. Scheye T, Rodier JF, Vanneuville G, et al. Benign cysts of the ovary. Homogeneous experience in 22 cases observed in 10 years. Chir Pediatr 1986; 27:185.

92. Zachariou Z, Roth H, Boos R, et al. Three years experience with large ovarian cysts diagnosed in utero. J Pediatr Surg 1989; 24:478.

93. Ohagan DB, Pudifin J, Mickel RE, Wittenberg DF. Antenatal detection of a fetal ovarian cyst by real-time ultrasound. A case report. S Afr Med J 1985; 67:471.

94. Sandler MA, Smith SJ, Pope SG, Madrazo BL. Prenatal diagnosis of septated ovarian cysts. J Clin Ultrasound 1985; 13:55.

95. Graif M, Itzchak Y. Sonographic evaluation of ovarian torsion in childhood and adolescence. AJR 1988; 150:647.

96. Eggermont E, Lecoutere D, Devlieger H, et al. Ovarian cysts in newborn infants. Am J Dis Child 1988; 40:481.

97. Debeugny P, Huillet P, Cussac L, et al. The non-operative treatment of ovarian cysts in the newborn. Chir Pediatr 1989; 30:30.

98. Elrad H, Mayden KL, Ahart S, et al. Prenatal ultrasound diagnosis of choledochal cyst. J Ultrasound Med 1985; 4:553.

99. Howell CG, Templeton JM, Weiner S, et al. Antenatal diagnosis and early surgery for choledochal cyst. J Pediatr Surg 1983; 18:387.

100. Turnock RR, Shaws R. Management of fetal urinary tract anomalies detected by prenatal ultrasound. Arch Dis Child 1984; 59:962.

101. Harrison MR, Golbus MS, Filley RA, et al. Fetal surgery for congenital hydronephrosis. N Engl J Med 1982; 306:59.

102. Farrant P. Ultrasound diagnosis of fetal urinary obstruction. In: Lubec G (ed). Non-invasive Diagnosis of Kidney Disease. Basel: Karger, 1983.

103. Barss VA, Benacercaf BR, Frigoletto FD. Second trimester oligohydramnios: A predictor of poor fetal outcome. Obstet Gynecol 1984; 64:608.

104. Drake DP, Stevens PS, Ecksten HB. Hydronephrosis secondary to ureteropelvic junction obstruction in children: A review of 14 years experience. J Urol 1978; 119:649.

105. Glick PL, Harrison MR, Golbus MS, et al. Management of the fetus with congenital hydronephrosis. II: Prognostic criteria and selection for treatment. J Pediatr Surg 1985; 20:376.

106. Beck AD. The effect of intrauterine urinary obstruction upon the development of the fetal kidney. J Urol 1971; 105:784.

107. Harrison MR. Fetal surgery. West J Med 1990; 153:648.

108. Longaker MT, Golbus MS, Filly RA, et al. Maternal outcome after open fetal surgery: A review of the first 17 human cases. JAMA 1991; 265:737.

109. Evans MI, Drugan A, Manning FA, Harrison MR. Fetal surgery in the 1990's. Am J Dis Child 1989; 143:1431.

110. Langer JC, Harrison MR. Adzick NS, et al. Perinatal management of the fetus with an abdominal wall defect. Fetal Ther 1987; 2:216.

111. Adzick NS, Harrison MR, Glick PL, et al. Fetal surgery in the primate. III. Maternal outcome after fetal surgery. J Pediatr Surg 1986; 21:477.

112. Harrison MR, Adzick NS. The fetus as a patient: Surgical considerations. Ann Surg 1991; 213:279.

113. Adzick NS, Harrison MR. Flake AW. Experimental studies on prenatal treatment of congenital anomalies. Br J Hosp Med 1985; 34:154.

114. Longaker MT, Adzick NS, Harrison MR. Update on the status of fetal surgery. Unpublished data.

115. Crombleholme TM, Harrison MR, Longaker MT, Langer JC. Prenatal diagnosis and management of bilateral hydronephrosis. Pediatr Nephrol 1988; 2:334.

116. Crombleholme TM, Harrison MR, Golbus MS, et al. Fetal intervention in obstructive uropathy: Prognostic indicators and efficacy of intervention. Am J Obstet Gynecol 1990; 162:1239.

117. Crombleholme TM, Harrison MR, Langer JC, et al. Early experience with open fetal surgery for congenital hydronephrosis. J Pediatr Surg 1988; 23:1114.

118. Harrison MR, Golbus MS, Filly RA, et al. Fetal hydronephrosis: Selection and surgical repair. J Pediatr Surg 1987; 22:556.

119. Flake AW, Harrison MR, Sauer L, et al. Ureteropelvic junction obstruction in the fetus. J Pediatr Surg 1986; 21:1058.

120. Nakayama DK, Harrison MR, deLorimier AA. Prognosis of posterior urethral valves presenting at birth. J Pediatr Surg 1986; 21:43.

121. Adzick NS, Harrison MR, Flake AW, Laberge JM. Development of a fetal renal function test using endogenous creatinine clearance. J Pediatr Surg 1985; 20:602.

122. Harrison MR, Adzick NS, Longaker MT, et al. Successful repair in utero of a fetal diaphragmatic hernia after removal of herniated viscera from the left thorax. N Engl J Med 1990; 322:1582.

123. Harrison MR, Langer JC, Adzick NS, et al. Correction of congenital diaphragmatic hernia in utero, V. Initial clinical experience. J Pediatr Surg 1990; 25:47.

124. Langer JC, Harrison MR, Adzick NS. Congenital diaphragmatic hernia: Current controversies in prenatal and postnatal management. Fetal Ther 1987; 2:209.

125. Harrison MR, Adzick NS, Nakayama DK, de-Lorimier AA. Fetal diaphragmatic hernia: Pathophysiology, natural history, and outcome. Clin Obstet Gynecol 1986; 29:490.

126. Adzick NS, Outwater KM, Harrison MR, et al. Correction of congenital diaphragmatic hernia in utero. IV. An early gestational fetal lamb model for pulmonary vascular morphometric analysis. J Pediatr Surg 1985; 20:673.

127. Adzick NS, Harrison MR, Glick PL, et al. Diaphragmatic hernia in the fetus: Prenatal diagnosis and outcome in 94 cases. J Pediatr Surg 1985; 20:357.

CHAPTER 40

Rectovaginal Fistulae and Associated Anomalies

JOHN DEWHURST

On rare occasions the gynecologist may be consulted regarding any of a variety of anomalies that affect both the lower bowel and the genital tract. A number of these defects can be treated simply, whereas others require one or more major surgical procedures and the cooperation of a surgical team with expertise in the pediatric patient, complemented by considerable ingenuity. Guidelines for the gynecologist unexpectedly confronted with one of these abnormalities are of utmost importance. Outcomes of reconstructive surgery have been previously reported.[1–7] An International Classification was proposed by Stephens and Smith[7] and modified in 1985.[8]

It is not always possible to determine how such defects arise, since all malformations are, by definition, "abnormal," but in general terms, they derive from errors in division of the primitive cloaca, exteriorization of the vagina onto the vestibule, and posterior migration of the anal opening.

EMBRYOLOGY

In the very early embryo (4 weeks; 4 mm in size) the allantois and primitive gut come together to form a common cavity, the cloaca, which at this point has no external opening. By 6 weeks (16 mm), this cavity has been divided by the urorectal septum, shortly after which the cloacal membrane breaks down. As development proceeds, the anus moves backward with the formation of the perineum, while the phallic and pelvic portions of the urogenital sinus flatten out to bring the vaginal introitus to the vestibule. An arrest in development may occur at any stage. If this happens early, the individual will be left with a primitive cloaca into which the bladder, genital tract, and bowel open. Arrest soon after this stage (i.e., after formation of the urorectal septum) may leave the bowel opening into the upper vagina as a high rectovaginal fistula, while subsequent arrest may result in a fistula entering low into the vagina or vestibule or to a more normally formed anal opening situated in front of the usual site, sometimes immediately alongside the vagina. This is a very simplistic explanation of these anomalies; other abnormalities, far more bizarre (e.g., when an accessory phallic urethra is found in association with a cloaca), defy explanation.

THE LOW RECTOVAGINAL FISTULA AND PERINEAL ANUS

These are the simplest of the anogenital anomalies. The bowel may open at some point

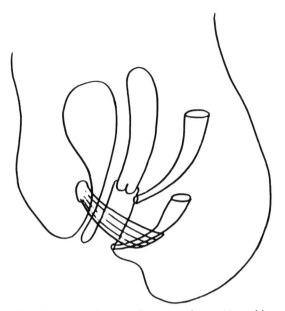

FIGURE 40–1 ••• Diagram illustrating the position of low and high rectovaginal fistulae relative to the levator sling. Contraction of the sling can control egress of fecal matter from a low fistula, but not from a high one.

on the perineum in front of its usual situation, at the fourchette, or into the lowest part of the vagina. The important point to understand about all these abnormalities is that the bowel passes through the levator sling, contraction of which can produce an effective sphincteric action and close the opening (Fig. 40-1). Despite this, the normal process of defecation may be interfered with by the size of the external opening, which is frequently contracted (Fig. 40–2). This leads to a condition

that was referred to many years ago as the *syndrome of rectal inertia*. Because of the greater resistance to defecation, the rectum becomes filled with more and more impacted fecal matter, and soon, the rectal reflex is lost. This impacted fecal matter may extend into the descending or even the transverse colon. There is much straining at stool, but despite this the child still soils her clothes, as fluid fecal matter from a high level flows past the solid rectal masses.

In most instances, an abnormality is evident at birth. Sometimes absence of the anal opening is noticed, and the labia have to be parted to allow the fistula to be identified with a probe (Fig. 40–3). If the child is older and no treatment has been given, it may be possible to palpate the feces-filled colon on abdominal examination.

TREATMENT

In most cases, treatment should be instituted early to avoid the rectal inertia syndrome. Management can be approached in two ways:

1. The anal opening may be left where it lies, closely adjacent to the vagina, but the contracted opening enlarged by a "cut back" or by anal dilatation (Fig. 40–4).[9]

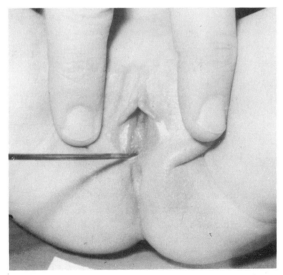

FIGURE 40–3 ••• A low rectovaginal fistula in a newborn. The anus is absent from its normal site, but the abnormal opening can be identified by a probe. (Dewhurst J. Surgery to repair disorders of development. In: Nichols D (ed). Gynecologic Obstetric Surgery. St. Louis, Mosby Year-Book, 1993.)

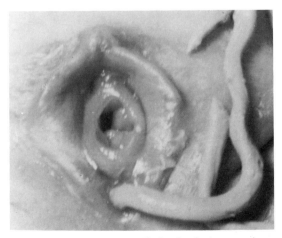

FIGURE 40–2 ••• A rectovestibular fistula in a newborn. Note the contraction of the abnormal opening.

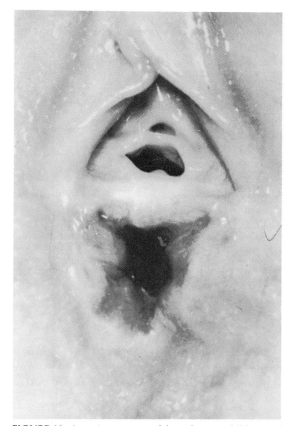

FIGURE 40–4 ••• Appearance of the vulva in a child treated by a "cut back." The anus, although immediately adjacent to the vagina, functioned well, and vaginal soiling did not occur. (Dewhurst J. Surgery to repair disorders of development. In: Nichols D (ed). Gynecologic and Obstetric Surgery. St. Louis, Mosby Year-Book, 1993.)

2. Some form of pull-through procedure may be carried out, an option currently preferred by many pediatric surgeons in all but the most superficial abnormalities. The fistulous opening is dissected off the vagina and the bowel pulled through to the normal position, taking infinite care not to damage sphincteric action in the process. This is a difficult and delicate maneuver.

The gynecologist is not, as a rule, involved in early management but may be consulted later, especially if a cut back or dilatation has been performed. In most cases of an anteriorly placed anus, good bowel control can be expected from a cut back procedure carried out early in life. A surgeon asked to see a pediatric patient whose anal opening lies close to the vaginal introitus, or even just within it, may fear the risk of genital tract infection as a result of vaginal soiling with fecal matter or of

dyspareunia that will be experienced in later life. A perineorrhaphy may be contemplated to build up a thicker septum between the two openings. However, this procedure is neither necessary nor advisable, since neither vaginal soiling nor dyspareunia is likely to occur; moreover, the surgical procedure involved may compromise rectal continence, which must be avoided at all costs. This need for preservation of sphincteric control makes cesarean section desirable in later life when the patient conceives.

These recommendations should be discussed with the parents when they are counseled about their daughter's future. They must understand that sexual life and fertility are unlikely to be affected.

When a pull-through procedure has been carried out, the process of dissecting the bowel off the vagina and closing the ostium may lead to vaginal contraction at that point. This is a more likely problem with the high rectovaginal fistula and is discussed later.

The most formidable gynecologic problem associated with a rectovestibular fistula or perineal anus is the coexistence of congenital absence of the vagina. The customary procedure for dealing with vaginal absence, which involves the use of a mold after a space has been dissected between bladder and bowel (McIndoe procedure), is not applicable in this situation, as the use of a mold would almost certainly lead to pressure necrosis of the immediately adjacent rectum and anus and development of an additional fistula. A successful alternative is to mobilize an isolated loop of cecum between the bowel and bladder, which requires no molds.[10] However, this operation is a surgical tour de force and should be attempted only by the most experienced surgeons.

HIGH RECTOVAGINAL FISTULA

When the abnormal rectal opening is situated in the upper or middle vagina, it lies above the levator sling, the contraction of which cannot prevent the flow of fecal matter entering the vagina (see Fig. 40–1). These are much more serious anomalies and inevitably require major surgery. In most instances a preliminary colostomy is necessary initially, with a pull-through procedure delayed for a short time until the child is well enough. Freeman and Bulut[11] performed immediate sigmoid loop colostomy in 18 patients with high fistulae; this was followed with a sacroperineal or abdominosacroperineal pull-through operation at the age of 1 to 14 days in seven patients, at 15 to 40 days in another seven, and not until 60 to 120 days in the remainder. Longer delays may be necessary.

Cases managed in this fashion are unlikely to involve the gynecologist at first but may do so subsequently. Many patients with a congenital rectovaginal defect, whether major or minor, have associated genital tract anomalies that may also require subsequent intervention. Fleming and colleagues[12] identified uterine anomalies in 18 of 51 female adolescents whose upper genital tract had been examined. In eight of these, the uterus was bicornuate; in an additional eight, there was a didelphic uterus; and in two, a hypoplastic uterus was diagnosed. Vaginal anomalies, in addition to the fistula, were present in 22 out of 71 girls; in 13 there was a septate vagina; in five the vagina was absent; and distal vaginal stenosis, absence of the lower one third of the vagina, an imperforate hymen, and a bifid hymen each occurred once. Abnormalities of the urinary tract were also frequent and included bladder exstrophy, unilateral renal agenesis, hydronephrosis, and ectopic and malformed kidneys. A number of these associated genital tract developmental abnormalities (e.g., a bicornuate uterus or didelphic uterus) require no treatment, and others (e.g., hymenal abnormalities or a septate vagina) can be treated without difficulty. However, congenital absence of the vagina along with a vestibular fistula or perineal anus is a formidable problem, as discussed earlier.

An acquired defect that may result from dissection of the fistula from the vagina and closure of the opening is vaginal narrowing at the surgical site. Constriction of this type may lead to dyspareunia in later life, but no attempt should be made to correct this surgically during childhood or adolescence. Division of the constricting fibrous tissue may need to be carried out widely to restore normal vaginal capacity; in the child this is exceedingly difficult. More importantly, a vaginal mold must be worn until epithelialization is complete, and thereafter, a mold must be inserted and removed from the vagina several times each day or else the vagina will contract. The younger, less mature patient may not be able to cooperate with this regimen, and thus intervention must be postponed until emotional maturity has been reached.

CLOACAL AND OTHER GROSS ABNORMALITIES

The high rectovaginal fistula usually occurs when development in this area is abnormal; in its earliest expression the child may be born with a cloaca, a single opening into which bladder, genital tract, and bowel all open (Fig. 40–5). As in high fistula cases, an immediate colostomy is generally required, after which an attempt may be made to determine the best way to manage the genitourinary aspects of the case. Again, other malformations affecting the uterus and upper renal tracts may coexist; one of the most serious, which may defeat all attempts to establish urinary control, is sacral agenesis, which is a rare accompaniment. Such patients may have difficulty establishing urinary control. Despite the dismal prognosis for many of these patients, a degree of success is often achieved by the pediatric surgeon such that a gynecologist may later be consulted when the patient reaches adolescence or adulthood. The variations seen are so considerable that management is beyond the scope of this

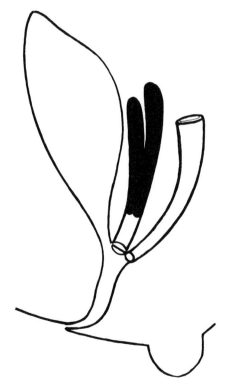

FIGURE 40–5 ••• Diagram of the appearances found in a newborn girl with a cloaca. Note that the bladder, genital tract, and bowel all share the same opening; note also the double uterus and bifid short vagina.

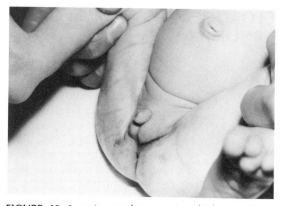

FIGURE 40-6 ••• A complex case in which a newborn female with a cloaca had, in addition, a second filiform urethra that extended to the tip of an enlarged phallus.

discussion.[13–15] Pregnancy has occasionally been achieved.[16]

A most curious form of anomaly rarely described in the literature is a cloaca or urogenital sinus defect associated with an enlarged phallus with a second filiform urethra running down from the tip.[17–20] No convincing explanation for this enlargement of the phallus has been advanced, and it does not seem to be related to the more common forms of phallic enlargement, such as congenital adrenal hyperplasia, androgen stimulation in utero, or true hermaphroditism. Several cases have been reported in the literature, although even among these, great variation is found (Fig. 40–6).

References

1. Stephens FD. Congenital Malformation of the Rectum, Anus, and Genitourinary Tracts. London: Churchill Livingstone, 1963.
2. Stephens FD, Smith ED. Anorectal Malformations in Children. Chicago: Year Book, 1971.
3. Nixon HH, Puri P. The results of treatment of anorectal anomalies. J Pediatr Surg 1977; 12:27–37.
4. Smith EI, Tunel WP, Williams GR. Clinical evaluation of the surgical treatment of anorectal malformation. Ann Surg 1978; 187:583–592.
5. de Vries PA. The surgery of anorectal anomalies. Curr Probl Surg 1984; 21(5):1–75.
6. Iwai N, Yanagihara J, Tokiwa K, et al. Results of surgical correction of anorectal malformation. Ann Surg 1984; 207:219–222.
7. Stephens FD, Smith ED. Anorectal Anomalies (Proposed International Classification). Chicago: Year Book, 1971.
8. Stephens FD, Smith ED. Classification identification and assessment of surgical treatment of anorectal anomalies. Report of a workshop meeting, Racine, WI, March 1984. Cited in de Vries PA, Cox KL. Surgery of anorectal anomalies. Surg Clin North Am 1985; 65(5):1139–1169.
9. Dewhurst CJ. Gynaecological Disorders of Infants and Children. London: Cassell, 1963.
10. Morton K, Dewhurst J. The use of bowel to create a vagina. Pediatr Adolesc Gynecol 1984; 2:51–61.
11. Freeman NV, Bulut M. High anorectal anomalies treated by early (neonatal) operation. J Pediatr Surg 1986; 21:218–220.
12. Fleming SE, Hall R, Gysler M, McLorie GA. Imperforate anus in females: Frequency of genital tract involvement, incidence of anomalies and functional outcome. J Pediatr Surg 1986; 21:146–150.
13. Escobar LF. Urorectal septum malformation sequence. Am J Dis Child 1987; 141:1021–1031.
14. Hendren WH. Urogenital sinus and anorectal malformation: Experience of 22 cases. J Pediatr Surg 1980; 15:628–634.
15. Nakayama DK, Snyder HW, Schnaufer L, et al. Posterior sagittal exposure for reconstructive surgery for cloacal anomalies. J Pediatr Surg 1987; 22:588–592.
16. Water EG. Cloacal dysgenesis: Related anomalies and pregnancies. Obstet Gynecol 1982; 59:398–402.
17. Belis JA, Hrabovsky EE. Idiopathic female intersex with clitoromegaly and urethral duplication. J Urol 1979; 122:805–809.
18. Belinger MF, Duckett JW. Accessory phallic urethra in the female patient. J Urol 1982; 127:1159–1163.
19. Hurwitz RS, Fitzpatrick TJ. Vaginal urethra, clitoral hypertrophy and accessory phallic urethra. J Urol 1982; 127:1165–1170.
20. Gale DH, Stocker JT. Cloacal dysgenesis with urethral vaginal outlet and anal agenesis and functioning internal genitourinary excretion. Pediatr Pathol 1987; 7:475–466.

CHAPTER 41

◯◯◯ # Chronic Pelvic Pain: Medical and Surgical Approach

JOSEPH S. SANFILIPPO

Chronic pelvic pain in the adolescent gynecologic patient continues to be a clinical challenge. By definition, chronic pelvic pain is 6 or more months of persistent lower abdominal pain.[1] The typical scenario involves distraught parents making multiple visits to a clinic or physician's office with their child in a frantic effort to identify the underlying origin of the pain. At the same time, the adolescent may use chronic pelvic pain as a means of attracting attention, which makes it imperative that the physician assess interaction between the patient and her parents and siblings, who might contribute to a psychological cause of the pelvic pain.

Initial evaluation requires a thorough history and physical examination. The former should include specific information regarding any gastrointestinal problem such as spastic colon or regional enteritis. When evaluating the genitourinary system, the clinician should look for evidence of recurring cystitis or a gynecologic disorder (e.g., persistent vaginal discharge) that may lead to upper and lower reproductive tract infections. The patient should be questioned about the possible presence of dysmenorrhea. The presence of abnormal uterine bleeding is important in the overall assessment of pelvic pain, because the discomfort may be secondary to menstrual aberration, often including passage of clots. In addition, endomyometritis may be associated with pelvic pain and abnormal uterine bleeding. This infectious/inflammatory problem is primarily asso-

ciated with gestation. The pattern of pubertal development and any problems associated with obstruction to the outflow tract, which may result in pelvic pain, also must be determined. Childhood diseases rarely cause pelvic pain; however, any infection such as mumps oophoritis also must be ruled out during the history (Table 41–1).[2]

A general physical examination must be performed, as well as a pelvic examination to determine whether the pelvic area is tender or if there are any masses. A rectovaginal examination also is helpful if endometriosis is suspected; nodular areas along the uterosacral ligaments and cul-de-sac regions or cul-de-sac masses, as with abscess formation, although rare in the adolescent, may be discovered. Thus the essential aspects of pelvic pain assessment include (1) ruling out any significant pelvic abnormality, (2) emphasizing the importance of a thorough history, and (3) performing a careful pelvic examination, including rectovaginal assessment.

The necessary laboratory tests are determined by the symptoms and pelvic findings. It may be necessary to assess the gastrointestinal (GI) tract radiologically (upper GI, small bowel follow-through) and obtain a barium enema and gall bladder series if the pelvic pain is associated with specific GI symptoms; in addition, sigmoidoscopy may be indicated if there is evidence of lower GI tract symptoms such as hematochezia.

Diagnostic laparoscopy is an integral part of

TABLE 41–1 ••• PERIPHERAL CAUSES OF CHRONIC PELVIC PAIN

Gynecologic	Genitourinary
Noncyclic	Recurrent or relapsing cystourethritis
Adhesions	Urethral syndrome
Endometriosis	Interstitial cystitis
Salpingo-oophoritis	Ureteral diverticuli or polyps
Acute	Carcinoma of the bladder
Subacute	Ureteral obstruction
Ovarian remnant syndrome	Pelvic kidney
Pelvic congestion syndrome (varicosities)	Neurologic
Ovarian neoplasms	Nerve entrapment syndrome
Pelvic relaxation	Neuroma
Cyclic	Musculoskeletal
Primary dysmenorrhea	Low back pain syndrome
Secondary dysmenorrhea	Congenital anomalies
Imperforate hymen	Scoliosis and kyphosis
Transverse vaginal septum	Spondylolysis
Cervical stenosis	Spondylolisthesis
Uterine anomalies (congenital malformation—	Spinal injuries
bicornuate uterus, blind uterine horn)	Inflammation
Intrauterine synechiae (Asherman's syndrome)	Tumors
Endometrial polyps	Osteoporosis
Uterine leiomyoma	Degenerative changes
Adenomyosis	Coccyodynia
Pelvic congestion syndrome (varicosities)	Myofascial syndrome
Gastrointestinal	Systemic
Irritable bowel syndrome	Acute intermittent porphyria
Ulcerative colitis	Abdominal migraine
Granulomatous colitis (Crohn's disease)	Systemic lupus erythematosis
Carcinoma	Lymphoma
Infectious diarrhea	Neurofibromatosis
Recurrent partial small bowel obstruction	
Diverticulitis	
Hernia	
Abdominal angina	
Recurrent appendiceal colic	

Adapted from Rapkin AJ, Reading AE. Chronic pelvic pain. Curr Probl Obstet Gynecol Fertil 1991; XIV(4):110.

the assessment of pelvic pain in this age group. Goldstein and coworkers[3] used laparoscopy to examine 109 adolescent girls between the ages of 10½ and 19 years who had unexplained chronic pelvic pain. Of interest is the finding that the youngest documented patient to have endometriosis was 10.8 years of age; she had reached menarche 5 months earlier.[3]

PSYCHOLOGICAL ASPECTS

The psychological aspects of chronic pelvic pain have been evaluated by Gross and coworkers[4] in a multidisciplinary study of 25 gynecologic patients. Although each patient had a normal pelvic examination, psychiatric assessment determined that the most frequent diagnosis was "significant pathology with borderline syndrome, and hysterical character disorder." A significant incidence of early childhood family dysfunction and incest also was noted. Psychological testing corroborated the high incidence of psychopathology.

Differences between organic and psychogenic functional pelvic pain have been found.[1] Organic pain frequently is sharp and "crampy," waking the patient at night with intermittent radiation, whereas psychogenic pain usually is absent during sleep. Some authors suggest that women with chronic pelvic pain are psychiatrically disturbed. The onset of pelvic pain can be linked to a stressful event or "life crisis."[1]

Treatment of chronic pelvic pain often involves reassuring the patient that there is no pelvic abnormality. The adolescent must be apprised of the role of stress in her pain experience, and she must be allowed the proper forum to express anger or frustration.

ACUTE ABDOMINAL PAIN

Acute abdominal pain in the adolescent is often a clinical challenge. Particular attention should be paid to signs of acute appendicitis and torsion of an adnexa, the latter occurring more commonly on the right and usually characterized by sudden onset of pain radiating down the involved extremity. Mittelschmerz also must be considered in the differential diagnosis; this typically is characterized by acute abdominal pain at mid cycle. The discomfort associated with mittelschmerz is ephemeral and is associated with leakage of fluid from the ovary at the time of ovulation and resultant peritoneal irritation. A ruptured corpus luteum also may be observed; these patients present with acute abdominal pain and evidence of intraabdominal hemorrhage. Dysmenorrhea, either primary or secondary, also must be considered. Acute abdominal pain as a result of cystitis is common in the pediatric or adolescent patient and may be associated with trauma to the urethra, including contusion to the urethral meatus, which provides a pathway for bacteria to enter the bladder and produce cystitis. Infection of the reproductive organs also must be considered when the adolescent with abdominal pain is assessed.

Establishing the diagnosis of acute pelvic inflammatory disease (PID) in the adolescent may require diagnostic laparoscopy. Kleinhaus and coworkers[5] diagnosed acute PID endoscopically in 28 of 50 patients; preoperative diagnosis was correct in 15 of 32 patients. The term *chronic PID* frequently is misleading and should not be determined solely by physical examination.

ENDOMETRIOSIS

Endometriosis is not considered a common disorder in teenagers. Clinical presentation and treatment of endometriosis are similar for both adolescents and adults. Although endometriosis has been a recognized disorder for years,[6, 7] its exact occurrence in adolescents is difficult to discern. However, the prevalence of this disorder in young women may not differ greatly from that in older women. Ranney[8] has suggested that between 4% and 17% of all menstruating women have pelvic endometriosis. The incidence depends in part on the patient population. In the adolescent age group, Meigs[9] reported a 6% incidence at laparoscopy, whereas Goldstein et al.[3] reported that 47% of adolescents referred for chronic pelvic pain had documented endometriosis.[10]

Development

Fallon[11] believes the development of endometriosis requires 5 or more years of menstrual cycles with premenstrual ovulation. The mean interval between menarche and diagnosis of endometriosis has been calculated at 4.5 years,[3] but as previously mentioned, Goldstein and colleagues[3] reported endometriosis in a 10.8-year-old who had had menarche only 5 months earlier. Thus, controversy continues regarding the length of time between menarche and actual development of endometriosis. Although onset of menses is thought by many to precede the development of endometriosis, Whitehouse[12] reported endometriosis in a 22-year-old female with primary amenorrhea. Similarly, Seitz[13] reported endometriomas in a 21-year-old with primary amenorrhea. Although older teens are more likely to seek gynecologic care than younger adolescents, clinicians must also realize that the disease can and does exist in the preteen and younger teenager.

The exact mechanism of development of endometriosis definitely continues to be a challenge to our understanding of its pathophysiology. Current theories of origin apply to both adults and adolescents. These include Sampson's theory of retrograde menstruation,[14] Meyer's theory of totipotential cells undergoing metaplasia,[15] hematogenous dissemination,[16] and lymphatic spread.[16] No one theory provides the total answer.

A genetic or familial tendency for development of endometriosis has been demonstrated. A polygenic multifactorial mode of inheritance for endometriosis has been reported by Simpson et al.,[17] who found a 6.9% rate of endometriosis in first-degree relatives of women with the disease, compared with only 1% in the control population. Thus, endometriosis should be especially suspected in symptomatic adolescents who have a family history of the disease.

The major distinction between adolescents and adults in the development of endometriosis is its association with anomalies of the reproductive system. Several müllerian developmental defects associated with the reproductive tract and development of endometriosis have been reported, including imperforate hymen, vaginal septum, hematocolpos, hematometra, uterine anomalies, and associated urinary tract abnormalities such as unilateral renal agenesis.[18] Obstruction of the outflow tract appears to be associated with the formation of endometriosis. Examples of reproductive tract anomalies that may cause endometriosis are presented in Figure 41–1. In a series reported by Schifrin and coworkers, 6 of 15 patients (40%) under age 20 with endometriosis had a genital tract anomaly.[18] Goldstein and coworkers[3] found congenital abnormalities of the reproductive tract in 11% of 74 teenagers with endometriosis. The American Fertility Society has provided the definitive classification system for müllerian anomalies, shown in Figure 41–2.

The clinical course of endometriosis associated with a reproductive tract abnormality appears to be different from that in which endometriosis is not associated with outflow obstruction.[19] In the former, once a patent outflow tract is established, reversal of extensive pelvic cavity endometriosis results.[19]

Endometriosis has been reported to be associated with mature ovarian teratomas and gliomatosis peritonei in a 10-year-old patient.[20] Endometriosis also has been associated with "smooth muscle metaplasia,"[21] hemangiomas,[22] leiomyomas, and adenomyosis of the gastrointestinal tract.[23] In addition, metastatic endometriosis in abdominal scars has been reported.[24] Endometriosis associated with these disorders is likely to be incidental and not specifically related to the disorder per se.

Endometriosis may well represent an immunologic abnormality. Ectopic implantation of endometrial cells under normal circumstances would not occur, but an alteration in immune function theoretically could result in implantation in the form of endometriosis; as noted previously, there may be a genetically transmitted link to such immunologic abnormalities.[25] Alteration in humoral immunity normally is manifested by beta lymphocytes producing humoral (antibody) immunity. Startseva[26] has reported that increased T-cell reactivity occurs in women with either endometriosis or adenomyosis. It appears that the complement component (C3), when identified using immunofluorescent techniques, results in immunoglobulin G (IgG) deposits in the uterine endometrium of women with endometriosis with a resultant reduction in total complement levels.[25] All of this is enhanced by an increase in total immunoglobulin levels as complement is consumed. Cell-mediated immunity (T-lymphocyte related) may also be a factor in endometriosis. As noted earlier, this theory initially was suggested by Startseva[26] in his observation that, in endometriosis patients, a reduction in T-cell immunity occurs simultaneously with increased B-cell reactivity. Furthermore, Badawy and associates[27] identified an increase in the number of T and B cells, as well as in T-helper cells in patients with endometriosis. The T-suppressor ratio in the peripheral blood and peritoneal fluid of patients with endometriosis is decreased. Interleukins also appear to be in disarray, with higher levels of interleukin-1 (IL-1) as has been previously reported.[28] Fibronectin also seems to be in increasing quantity in both of these substances and may be integrally involved in adhesion formation, which commonly is seen with endometriosis.[25, 29] Natural killer cells also are associated primarily with prevention of endometriosis.[30] However, if there is some disturbance in their antigen-eliminating capabilities, this, too, may play a role in the development of endometriosis in the adolescent as well as in the adult.

Clinical Presentation

The characteristic symptom associated with endometriosis in the adolescent is pelvic pain, primarily in the form of dysmenorrhea. It appears to be refractory to medical therapies, especially nonsteroidal antiinflammatory agents (NSAIDs) and ovulation suppression. Chatman and Ward[31] noted that the most common complaint in this age group was dysmenorrhea (78% of patients) followed by bowel symptoms (37%), abnormal bleeding (35%), and dyspareunia (14%). The presenting signs and symptoms of endometriosis are listed in Table 41–2.

Diagnosis

A careful history of symptoms characteristic of endometriosis is helpful in diagnosing this disorder, as well as in distinguishing it from other possible causes of pelvic pain. Pelvic examination in an adolescent may be difficult; a rectal examination may be the only means to evaluate the pelvis for tenderness, nodularity, a retrodisplaced uterus, or an adnexal mass. Anomalies of the hymen, vagina, and cervix can be detected during pelvic examination, and a search should be made for these and other congenital abnormalities that are more likely to cause adolescent endometriosis. An analgesic or even general anesthesia may

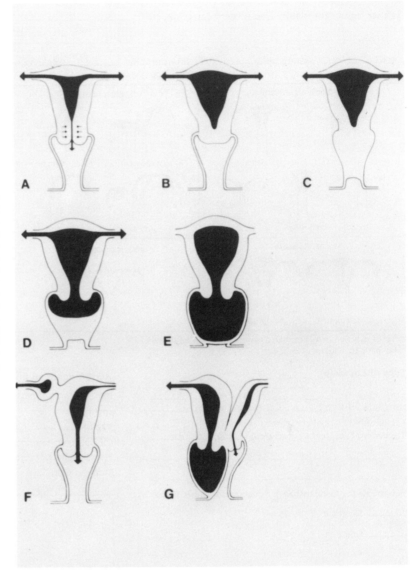

FIGURE 41–1 ••• Anomalies of the reproductive tract that could result in adolescent endometriosis. *A,* Cervical stenosis. *B,* Cervical agenesis. *C,* Vaginal agenesis. *D,* Transverse vaginal septum. *E,* Imperforate hymen. *F,* Rudimentary uterine horn. *G,* Unilateral vaginal obstruction. (From Sanfilippo JSS. Endometriosis in adolescents. In: Wilson EA (ed). Endometriosis. New York: Alan R. Liss, 1987, p 165. © Copyright 1987. Reprinted by permission of Wiley-Liss, a division of John Wiley and Sons, Inc.)

be required for adequate examination of the pelvis.

Ultrasonography may be helpful, particularly in adolescents difficult to examine or when documenting the presence or size of adnexal masses. It can also be used to monitor the size of ovarian cysts in response to therapy. However, endometriomas cannot be distinguished definitively from other pelvic masses by ultrasound, and a persistent mass requires surgical evaluation.

Preoperative assessment of patients presenting with chronic pelvic pain also should include a complete blood cell count, urinalysis, and cervical cytologic examination. Cervical cultures for gonorrhea and chlamydia can be performed to identify those patients with acute or chronic inflammatory processes.

As previously mentioned, diagnostic laparoscopy is an integral part of the assessment of pelvic pain and the diagnosis of endometriosis in adolescents. Early endometriosis usually does not appear as characteristic blue-black or whitish lesions; hemorrhagic or polypoid areas have been noted (Figs. 41–3, 41–4). Therefore, the clinician must be aware that early endometriosis may present with a hemorrhagic or polypoid appearance.

When there is evidence of endometriosis at laparoscopy, the American Fertility Society

Patient's Name _____ Date _____ Chart # _____

Age _____ G _____ P _____ Sp Ab _____ VTP _____ Ectopic _____ Infertile Yes _____ No _____

Other Significant History (i.e. surgery, infection, etc.) _____

_____

HSG _____ Sonography _____ Photography _____ Laparoscopy _____ Laparotomy _____

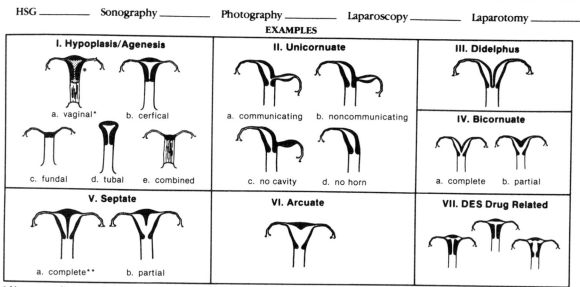

EXAMPLES

I. Hypoplasis/Agenesis
a. vaginal*   b. cerfical
c. fundal   d. tubal   e. combined

II. Unicornuate
a. communicating   b. noncommunicating
c. no cavity   d. no horn

III. Didelphus

IV. Bicornuate
a. complete   b. partial

V. Septate
a. complete**   b. partial

VI. Arcuate

VII. DES Drug Related

* Uterus may be normal or take a variety of abnormal forms.
** May have two distinct cervices

Type of Anomaly

Class I _____   Class V _____
Class II _____   Class VI _____
Class III _____   Class VII _____
Class IV _____

Treatment (Surgical Procedures): _____

_____

_____

Prognosis for Conception & Subsequent Viable Infant*

_____ Excellent (> 75%)

_____ Good   (50-75%)

_____ Fair   (25%-50%)

_____ Poor   (< 25%)

*Based upon physician's judgment.

Recommended Followup Treatment: _____

_____

_____

Additional Findings: _____

_____

_____

Vagina: _____
Cervix: _____

Tubes: Right _____ Left _____
Kidneys: Right _____ Left _____

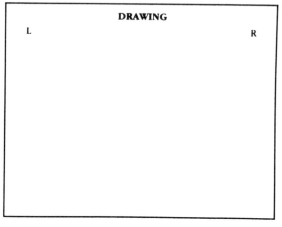

DRAWING

L   R

Property of
The American Fertility Society

For additional supply write to:
The American Fertility Society
2140 11th Avenue, South
Suite 200
Birmingham, Alabama 35205

FIGURE 41–2 ●●● The American Fertility Society classification of müllerian anomalies. (From The American Fertility Society classifications of adnexal adhesions, distal tubal occlusion, tubal occlusion secondary to tubal ligation, tubal pregnancies, Mullerian anomalies and intrauterine adhesions. Fertil Steril 1988; 49:944–955. Reproduced with permission of the publisher, The American Fertility Society.)

TABLE 41–2 ••• SYMPTOMS OF ENDOMETRIOSIS

Progressive pelvic pain just before and/or during
   menstruation
Dyspareunia
Dyschezia
Premenstrual bleeding
Suprapubic pain, dysuria, and cyclic hematuria
Infertility

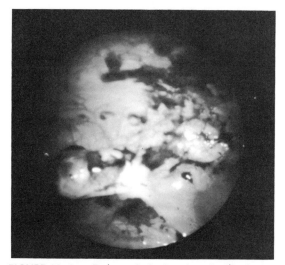

FIGURE 41–4 ••• Endometriosis, American Fertility Society stage IV. This is indicative of extensive endometriosis in association with retrograde menstruation secondary to outflow tract obstruction.

Revised Classification (Fig. 41–5) should be used to stage the extent of the endometriosis.[32] Thus, the typical presentation of dysmenorrhea refractory to nonsteroidal antiinflammatory agents and oral contraceptive therapy should alert the clinician to the possibility of endometriosis. Bowel symptoms—rectal pressure, dyschezia, and urgency, especially during the late luteal and menstrual phases—may clearly be indicative of endometriosis. The high percentage of young patients with bowel symptoms (21% to 37%) is somewhat surprising, but emphasizes how endometriosis can progress symptomatically, even in adolescents.[33]

Dyspareunia is another common form of pelvic pain associated with endometriosis that teenagers may experience but be reluctant to report. The dyspareunia is likely related to the presence of tender endometriotic implants in the cul-de-sac.

Preoperative pelvic findings in teenagers with endometriosis are similar to those in older patients. Chatman and Ward[31] found that tenderness in the cul-de-sac could be elicited in 78% of adolescents with documented endometriosis and nodularity with tenderness in

36%. Adnexal masses were present in 11% of teenagers. On the other hand, the pelvic examination is often well within normal limits, as noted by Goldstein and coworkers.[3] These authors emphasized that the examination should be performed during menses or the late luteal phase to enhance the pelvic findings.

Treatment for an adolescent who has no immediate interest in fertility centers primarily on control of pain. When pelvic pain is encountered in an adolescent, NSAIDs should be prescribed with the initial onset of pain or immediately before anticipated dysmenorrhea and continued on a regular basis until the dysmenorrhea has completely subsided. All antiprostaglandins basically inhibit prostaglandin synthesis and/or inhibit prostaglandin binding to its receptors to alleviate dysmenorrhea. For the adolescent with cyclical pelvic pain who does not respond to nonsteroidal antiprostaglandins, the next step is to suppress ovulation with an oral contraceptive. A low-dose (35 μg) estrogen preparation should be prescribed in the usual cyclic manner. Failure of these primary measures to alleviate symptoms indicates a need for further evaluation.

Diagnosis of endometriosis primarily involves operative assessment of the pelvic organs. Before scheduling any surgical intervention, the physician should counsel the patient and parent (or guardian) about the possible need for intraoperative therapeutic alterna-

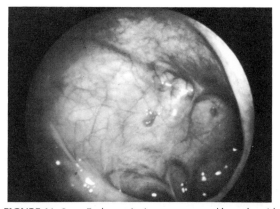

FIGURE 41–3 ••• Endometriosis as represented by polypoid structures (American Fertility Society stage I).

Patient's Name _____ Date _____

Stage I (Minimal) · 1-5
Stage II (Mild) · 6-15
Stage III (Moderate) · 16-40
Stage IV (Severe) · >40
Total _____

Laparoscopy _____ Laparotomy _____ Photography _____
Recommended Treatment _____
_____

Prognosis _____

PERITONEUM	**ENDOMETRIOSIS**	<1cm	1-3cm	>3cm
	Superficial	1	2	4
	Deep	2	4	6
OVARY	R Superficial	1	2	4
	Deep	4	16	20
	L Superficial	1	2	4
	Deep	4	16	20

	POSTERIOR CULDESAC OBLITERATION	Partial		Complete
		4		40

	ADHESIONS	<1/3 Enclosure	1/3-2/3 Enclosure	>2/3 Enclosure
OVARY	R Filmy	1	2	4
	Dense	4	8	16
	L Filmy	1	2	4
	Dense	4	8	16
TUBE	R Filmy	1	2	4
	Dense	4*	8*	16
	L Filmy	1	2	4
	Dense	4*	8*	16

*If the fimbriated end of the fallopian tube is completely enclosed, change the point assignment to 16.

Additional Endometriosis: _____
_____
_____

Associated Pathology: _____
_____
_____

To Be Used with Normal
Tubes and Ovaries

L   R

To Be Used with Abnormal
Tubes and/or Ovaries

L   R

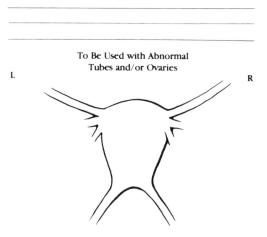

For additional supply write to: The American Fertility Society, 2140 11th Avenue South,
Suite 200, Birmingham, Alabama 35205-2800

FIGURE 41–5 ••• *See legend on opposite page*

tives such as laparoscopic fulguration or laser vaporization of the endometrial foci. Improvement in symptoms is greater when fulguration or vaporization of implants and lysis of adhesions are performed during laparoscopy. Rarely, conservative surgery (laparotomy) may be necessary during the same procedure. Persistent endometriomas should be excised and as much functional ovarian tissue as possible preserved.

The patient should be evaluated carefully for congenital anomalies of the reproductive tract that may obstruct menstrual outflow. The cervix should be probed and/or dilated to assure patency of the cervical canal and to alleviate any element of stenosis. It is important that the clinician correct müllerian tract outflow obstruction and retrograde menstruation promptly to prevent or reverse endometriosis. Vaginal splinting or continued dilatations may be required to maintain a patent outflow tract. If these initial measures are unsuccessful, removal of the involved müllerian structures should be considered. A didelphic or rudimentary horn–containing uterus with unilateral obstruction also can be surgically corrected by lateral anastomosis of the obstructed horn to the unobstructed horn (Strassman's procedure). Pregnancy outcome in relation to various müllerian anomalies is shown in Table 41–3.[34, 35]

Postoperative management of the adolescent patient with endometriosis is a unique challenge. In addition to pain control, a major concern is preservation of subsequent fertility. Patients interested in fertility usually are advised to attempt pregnancy as soon as possible. For most teenagers, however, pregnancy in the immediate postoperative period is not an alternative. In these young women, the issue is how to preserve fertility by preventing further progression of endometriosis. No well-designed prospective studies have been conducted with respect to treatment of endometriosis in adolescents. Postoperative management of these patients is based on knowledge of endometriosis, which is inadequate; use of medical therapy, some actions of which are theoretical; and clinical experience, which is anecdotal.

After laparoscopic or conservative surgery,

TABLE 41–3 ••• PREGNANCY OUTCOME IN RELATION TO VARIOUS MÜLLERIAN ANOMALIES

Type of Reproductive Tract Anomaly	Pregnancy (Preg) Outcome
Vertical fusion septum defects	50% term preg
Congenital absence of cervix	One preg in 20 reported cases
Lateral fusion defects	
Obstructive	64%–85% term preg in normal horn
Rudimentary horn (75% do not communicate with normal hemiuterus)	
Uterine duplication with unilateral vaginal obstruction	
Nonobstructive	Intrauterine growth retardation
Asymmetric: uterus unicollis	Overall fetal wastage 31%
Symmetric:	Increase in spontaneous abortion
Didelphic	Malpresentation
Bicornuate	Premature labor
Septate	Postpartum hemorrhage
	Term pregnancy before surgery:
	Septate 15%
	Bicornuate 10%
	Didelphic 57%
	Term pregnancy after surgery
	Septate >80%
	Bicornuate (rarely surgically corrected)
	Didelphic 75%

Reprinted by permission of Elsevier Science Publishing Co., Inc., from Strassman procedure for correction of a Class II mullerian anomaly in an adolescent; by JS Sanfilippo, JOURNAL OF ADOLESCENT HEALTH CARE, Vol. No. 12, pp. 63 and 65. Copyright 1991 by The Society of Adolescent Medicine.

a form of medical therapy is often advised to prevent progression or to treat recurrence of endometriosis. The choice of medical regimens includes oral contraceptives, danazol (Danocrine), medroxyprogesterone acetate (Depo-Provera), and gonadotropin-releasing hormone (GnRH) agonists (nafarelin acetate [Synarel] or leuprolide acetate [Lupron]). Which oral contraceptive to choose remains a point of controversy; often a progestin-dominant oral contraceptive is advocated for suppression of endometrial growth and reduction of menstrual reflux.

FIGURE 41–5 ••• The American Fertility Society revised classification of endometriosis. (From The American Fertility Society revised classification of endometriosis: 1985. Fertil Steril 1985; 43:351–352. Reproduced with permission of the publisher, The American Fertility Society.)

In summary, evaluation of pelvic pain in the adolescent requires a systematic approach. The patient with recurrent lower abdominal pain, especially of a cyclic nature, who has a normal pelvic examination is best treated initially with NSAIDs and/or oral contraceptive therapy. If these medications fail to alleviate the symptoms, consideration should be given to diagnostic laparoscopy with intraoperative resection of the foci of endometriosis using either laser vaporization or fulguration. Depending on the postoperative symptoms and reevaluation, ovulation suppression with any of several medical modalities of treatment is in order.

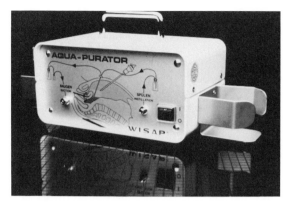

FIGURE 41–6 ••• Aquapurator. (Courtesy of Wisap, Tomball, TX.)

OPERATIVE LAPAROSCOPY

The origin of endoscopy may be traced to a description in the Babylonian Talmud.[36] Development of a light source and optic lens systems by Stein[37] provided the ability to endoscopically evaluate structures such as the bladder mucosa. Currently, operative endoscopy incorporates ingenious instrumentation such as the Verres needle, as originally described in 1924; devices for insufflation; and instrumentation for accomplishing hemostasis.[36]

Patient Positioning and Instrumentation

Patient positioning is a critical aspect of operative laparoscopy in both adolescents and adults; both the Trendelenburg and Fowler positions are used. Frequently, the use of Allen universal stirrups prevents trauma to the nerves of the lower extremities. This is especially important with prolonged endoscopic surgical procedures. Endotracheal intubation seems to be critically important with this type of endoscopic procedure.

Instrumentation can be basic or quite extensive. Basic equipment includes an electronic insufflator; a means of accomplishing hemostasis (bipolar coagulation, endocoagulator systems, or use of laser in a defocused mode); a suction irrigation apparatus such as the Aquapurator (Fig. 41–6) or Cabot irrigation system (Fig. 41–7) for removal of blood and debris, aquadissection, and identification of actively bleeding areas; atraumatic grasping forceps and bipolar forceps; hook scissors (Fig. 41–8);

and tooth forceps and other 3- or 5-mm instrumentation. Large grasping forceps (10-mm instrumentation—spoon and claw forceps) (Fig. 41–9), as well as sutures, are often very useful to the endoscopic surgeon, especially when attempting to resect large masses. Multipronged atraumatic ovarian forceps and the ovarian basket are quite helpful in stabilizing the ovary during surgical procedures involving the adnexa (Fig. 41–10).

Other means of accomplishing hemostasis include the use of Endoloops, a slip-knot suture device placed around the structures to be extirpated. Suturing with intracorporeal or extracorporeal knot tying also is of great benefit in reapproximating structures as well as achieving hemostasis (Fig. 41–11). Both 3- and 5-mm needle holders facilitate both extracorporeal and intracorporeal suturing techniques. Pelviscopic surgical procedures often include a combination of sharp and blunt dis-

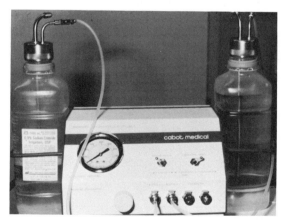

FIGURE 41–7 ••• Cabot irrigator. (Courtesy of Cabot Medical, Langhorne, PA.)

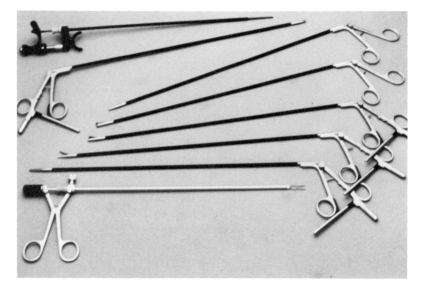

FIGURE 41–8 ••• Basic instruments for operative laparoscopy.

section complemented by use of a laser for resection and vaporization of abnormal tissue.

Operative laparoscopy is performed in pediatric patients with intraabdominal testes to occlude the cephalad-derived blood supply and provide the primary blood supply from the testicular vessel in preparation for subsequent orchiopexy, ideally before 2 years of age. When approached in this manner, spermatogenesis and androgen production may well be preserved (see below). Procedures in the adolescent include resection of ectopic pregnancy, removal of ovarian cysts, adhesiolysis, and correction of selected benign neoplastic processes. Endometriosis can be treated endoscopically, with excellent results. Endoscopic surgery also has been used in this age group for ovarian biopsy when deemed clinically necessary.

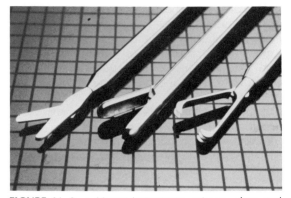

FIGURE 41–9 ••• 10-mm instruments: scissors, claw, and spoon forceps.

The surgeon should be well versed in the use of the traditional 10-mm trocar and sleeve, as well as in open laparoscopic techniques (e.g., Hasson cannula, which includes a blunt trocar and adjustable cone, the latter to aid in maintaining the pneumoperitoneum) (Fig. 41–12). This becomes especially important in the pediatric patient, as well as in the adolescent with suspected multiple abdominal adhesions and potential bowel trauma. The importance of sharp instrumentation cannot be overemphasized as most traumatic injury to the bowel, bladder, and other vital structures appears to be associated with dull instrumentation.[38]

Ectopic Pregnancy

Ectopic gestations do occur in adolescents,[39] and an endoscopic approach appears to be most worthwhile. Early diagnosis can be made with the use of serum human chorionic gonadotropin (hCG) if the clinician is aware that, in general, when the serum hCG level is 2500 mIU/ml (first or second International Standards), a sac in the uterus usually can be identified with a vaginal probe.[40] At 5000 mIU/ml, a fetal pole can be identified; at 15,000 mIU/ml, fetal cardiac activity is perceptible (Fig. 41–13).[41] Early diagnosis cannot be overemphasized, as it allows the clinician to correct the problem before rupture and avoid the potential adverse sequelae of ectopic gestation.

The technique includes use of double punctures and clear identification of the ectopic

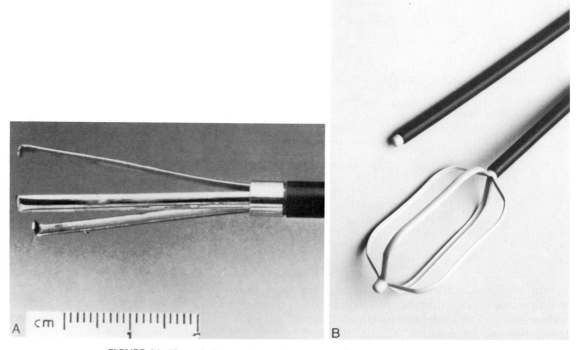

FIGURE 41–10 ••• A, Atraumatic ovarian grasping forceps. B, Ovarian basket.

gestation. The ampulla of the fallopian tube is the site of ectopic gestation in more than 90% of ectopic pregnancies.[41] Coagulation on the antimesenteric border using a laser, bipolar endocoagulator, or needle unipolar system appears to provide appropriate hemostasis. Endoscopic scissors are often necessary to incise the fallopian tube over the ectopic pregnancy. A suction irrigation system is then introduced

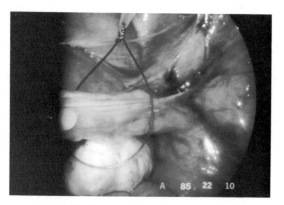

FIGURE 41–11 ••• Endoloop and its application.

to "float out" the products of conception. Hydrostatic pressure appears to be instrumental in separating the implantation bed from the fallopian tube mucosa. Meticulous hemostasis is mandatory. The patient should then be followed with serial determinations of serum hCG beginning on the fourth postoperative day[42] and continuing until the serum hCG level is negative. On occasion, this may require 30 to 40 days postoperative. If an increase or significant plateau in hCG is noted, then consideration should be given to the use of methotrexate or repeat surgical intervention.

DeCherney and coworkers[43] noted that 56% of the time, a conservative approach to an ectopic gestation and preservation of the fallopian tubes results in an intrauterine gestation. The incidence of subsequent ectopic gestation does not appear to be increased with a linear salpingostomy, also a conservative approach. The American Fertility Society Classification of Tubal Pregnancy should be incorporated into the permanent record to allow the clinician to review his or her own statistics, as well as determine prognosis for each individual case (Fig. 41–14).[44] Segmental resection of the involved fallopian tube may become necessary for a number of reasons, including

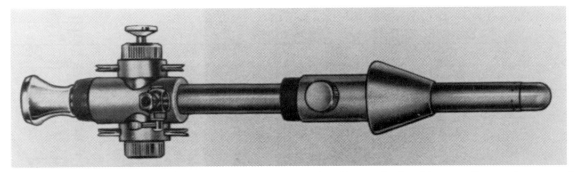

FIGURE 41–12 ••• Open laparoscopy cannula. A blunt trocar with a sleeve and adjustable cone allows maintenance of pneumoperitoneum.

an inability to accomplish hemostasis with more conservative approaches. If this is deemed necessary, then either a coagulation system or Endoloops can be used effectively to resect the ectopic gestation.

Currently, several medical therapies are being evaluated in terms of efficacy for initial treatment of ectopic pregnancy. These include methotrexate, the antiprogesterone RU-486, and prostaglandin $F_2\alpha$.[45–47] These are easily delivered via hysteroscopic or fluoroscopic means or under ultrasound guidance.

Ovarian Surgery

Ovarian surgery may be indicated for adolescents with a neoplasm (e.g., a benign teratoma [dermoid], which appears to be the most common ovarian neoplasm in the adolescent patient).[48] The patient should be properly screened preoperatively with ultrasound, and with tests to determine the presence of the tumor marker CA-125 when an adnexal mass is identified.[49] If a cystic structure is identified and CA-125 tests are normal, then in many cases an endoscopic approach is feasible. If there is a significant elevation in CA-125, then the underlying pathophysiology of the neoplastic process should be determined. This should be complemented carefully by ultrasonographic findings (i.e., if a solid mass is noted, then the clinician must carefully discern whether an endoscopic approach is warranted). If a decision is made to proceed with resection of the ovarian cyst, every effort should be made to preserve normal ovarian tissue. Principles similar to those used for

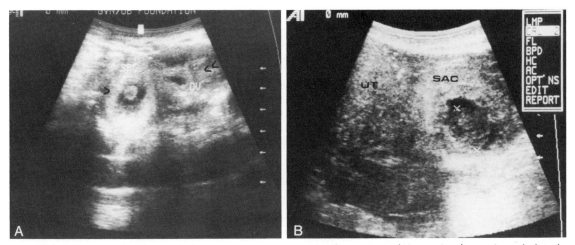

FIGURE 41–13 ••• *A*, Ultrasonogram of an ectopic pregnancy equivalent to 5 weeks' gestational age. Acoustic imaging 5200, 7.5-MHz, endovaginal probe. OV, Ovary; SAC, gestational sac; <, sac; <<, ovary. *B*, Ultrasonogram of ectopic pregnancy at 7.8 weeks gestational age. Acoustic imaging 5200, 7.5-MHz, endovaginal probe. SAC, Gestational sac; UT, uterus.

Patient's Name _____ Date _____ Chart # _____

Age _____ G _____ P _____ Sp Ab _____ VTP _____ Ectopic _____ Infertile Yes _____ No _____

Other Significant History (i.e. surgery, infection, etc.) _____

_____

HSG _____ Sonography _____ Photography _____ Laparoscopy _____ Laparotomy _____

TUBAL PREGNANCY

	Right	Left	Contralateral Tube & Ovary
Infundibular	_____	_____	Normal _____ Absent _____
Ampullary	_____	_____	Abnormal _____
Isthmic	_____	_____	_____
Interstitial	_____	_____	_____
Size (cm)	_____	_____	_____

Treatment (Surgical Procedures):

Laparoscopy _____
  No Surgery _____
  Surgery _____
    Expression
    Linear Salpingostomy _____
      Sharp Dissection _____
      Laser _____
      Cautery _____

Laparotomy _____
  Linear Salpingostomy _____
    1° Closure _____
    2° Closure _____
  Segmental Resection _____
    1° Anastomosis _____
    2° Anastomosis Planned Yes _____ No _____

Other: _____
_____
_____
_____
_____

Prognosis for Conception & Subsequent Viable Infant*

_____ Excellent (> 75%)

_____ Good (50-75%)

_____ Fair (25%-50%)

_____ Poor (< 25%)

* Physician's judgment based upon adnexa with least amount of pathology.

Recommended Followup Treatment: _____
_____
_____

Additional Findings: _____
_____
_____
_____
_____

DRAWING

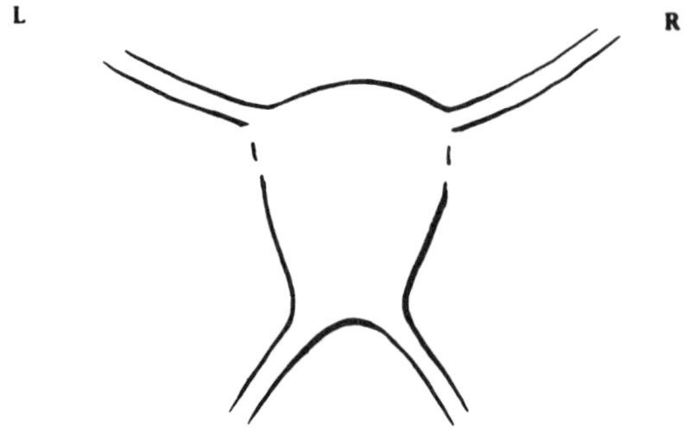

L   R

For additional supply write to:
The American Fertility Society
2140 11th Avenue, South
Suite 200
Birmingham, Alabama 35205

Property of
The American Fertility Society

FIGURE 41–14 ••• The American Fertility Society classification of tubal pregnancies. (From The American Fertility Society classifications of adnexal adhesions, distal tubal occlusion, tubal occlusion secondary to tubal ligation, tubal pregnancies, Mullerian anomalies and intrauterine adhesions. Fertil Steril 1988; 49:944–955. Reproduced with permission of the publisher, The American Fertility Society.)

resection of the ectopic pregnancy apply. Aquadissection can be useful in separating the cyst wall from the ovarian tissue per se, and reapproximation of the ovary may be necessary using endoscopic suturing. Meticulous hemostasis remains mandatory, especially before reapproximating the incised edges of the ovary. If the surgeon decides to resect the dermoid, a small incision should be made into the ovarian cyst and suction irrigation immediately applied. The suction apparatus will then allow the sebaceous hair material and calcified contents to be removed with minimal spillage. Ultimately, the entire cyst wall, as well as the contents of the teratoma, should be removed. A 10-mm spoon or claw forceps often proves helpful. Copious amounts of irrigation are important to remove all potential chemical peritonitis-producing material. Oophorectomy is rare in the adolescent female, but patients with a Y-bearing chromosome (e.g., male pseudohermaphrodites) should have their gonads extirpated to prevent malignant potential. Oophorectomy is accomplished by any of a number of means. Bipolar coagulation with an incision using laparoscopic scissors is appropriate. Use of Endoloops around the ovary also is instrumental in establishing hemostasis. Endoclips also can be applied over the vascular structures. The use of the Endo GIA allows placement of two rows of staples with incision of the tissue between them (Fig. 41–15). This enables the clinician to completely excise an adnexa. Again, careful hemostasis is mandatory.

Acute Pelvic Inflammatory Disease

Endoscopic treatment of acute pelvic inflammatory disease in adolescents has been re-

ported by Reich and McGlynn.[50] The rationale is that excision of fibrinous exudate, which is associated with sequestration of bacterial inoculum, may well improve the prognosis. Laparoscopic drainage of pelvic abscesses also has been advocated.[51] Significant cost savings can result from an endoscopic approach when compared with prolonged hospitalization and expensive antibiotic therapy.

The goals of managing acute tubo-ovarian abscess are prevention of infertility and pelvic pain in association with sequelae of pelvic adhesions and hydrosalpinx. Laparoscopic treatment is effective and economical.[51] Accuracy of diagnosis is virtually 100%, and the probability of preservation of future fertility is increased. The combination of laparoscopic surgery and antibiotics may well prove the most efficacious means of therapy.

The economic impact of gynecologic endoscopy has been addressed by a number of authors.[52, 53] An endoscopic approach results in a reduction in operative time and morbidity, as well as in total hospital stay and recovery time. The therapeutic effects are quite comparable to those of laparotomy, and the overall effect is significant total direct cost savings to the patient, hospital, and third-party payers. The procedure is primarily an outpatient one, with the adolescent recovering quickly and usually returning to work or school within 1 week. Thus, the clinician should consider the possibility of an endoscopic approach to correct benign pelvic abnormalities in pediatric and adolescent patients.

Torsion of an Adnexa

An endoscopic approach enables removal of a torsed fallopian tube and/or ovary. The typical presentation is unilateral abdominal pain, more often located on the right because of the anatomic suspension of the tube and ovary. When an ovary has a cystic structure, it is predisposed to torsion.[54] The endoscopic surgical principles are similar to those used when performing a laparotomy. If the decision is to proceed with adnexectomy, an Endoloop may be placed around the torsed structure to prevent embolization; and the involved organ can then be extirpated. This procedure can be done either on an outpatient basis or with a short hospital stay (less than 24 hours). The potential

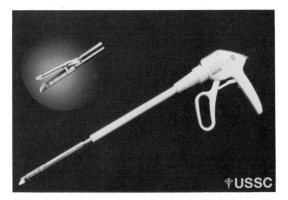

FIGURE 41–15 ••• Endo GIA stapler. (Courtesy of U.S. Surgical Corp., Norwalk, CT.)

for de novo adhesion formation appears to be less with an initial endoscopic approach.[55]

A conservative approach to adnexal torsion has been reported.[56, 57] Wagaman and Williams noted bilateral adnexal torsion secondary to dermoid cysts.[56] Untwisting of the twisted adnexa resulted in reestablishment of the blood supply. In the report by Vancaille and coworkers,[57] there was subsequent evidence of active ovarian follicle formation when the adnexa was untwisted.

Shun has reported unilateral ovarian loss in childhood, an indication for contralateral oophoropexy.[58] In a 35-year retrospective chart review of 51 children, a total of 53 associated ovarian lesions required surgical intervention. Twenty-one of the ovarian lesions were the result of torsion. Five of the "torsed ovaries" were subsequently noted to be normal on microscopic assessment. Spontaneous castration occurred in three children. It was Shun's opinion that in one of these cases, spontaneous castration could have been prevented by contralateral oophoropexy. In one patient with acute torsion, the process was aborted by immediate intervention in the form of ovarian cystectomy. Shun thus concluded that contralateral oophoropexy at the time of ipsilateral oophorectomy is recommended to prevent torsion of the remaining adnexa and, thus, castration. Whether ovarian torsion is a repetitive event is a challenging question. Davis and Feins have reported subsequent asynchronous torsion of normal adnexa in children.[59] In their series, patients who had previously had ovarian torsion appeared to be at increased risk for subsequent torsion of the remaining adnexa. Torsion in an abnormal adnexa is due to excessive mobility, the result of a congenitally long ligamentous support. Oophoropexy, or shortening of the ligaments supporting the remaining "normal" ovary, is recommended. The clinician should always consider the possibility of adnexal torsion when evaluating a female with abdominal pain. Preoperative ultrasonography appears to be helpful in establishing the diagnosis. The clinician must be aware of the fact that torsion of an adnexa is not a phenomenon restricted to the adolescent and adult, but has been reported in the premenarchal girl.[60]

Isolated necrosis of the tubal fimbria has also been reported in a prepubertal girl; hemorrhagic necrosis of the fimbria was the presumptive etiology.[61] A total of four cases of tubal torsion independent of the ovary have been reported as of 1990. The clinical presentation mimics acute appendicitis, and the right side is the more frequent location. Endometriosis and perimenarchal tubal torsion have also been noted in a case report.[62] These authors observed tubal torsion with associated endometriosis in a perimenarchal female, and they emphasized the importance of considering both entities in the pediatric patient who presents with unilateral pelvic pain.

In a series reported in the pediatric literature, one problem with adnexal torsion appears to be delay in diagnosis.[63] An average of 5.2 days between the first symptom and actual hospitalization was reported. Furthermore, on the average, 30.2 hours passed between consultation and surgical intervention. Nausea and vomiting appear to be prominent symptoms, occurring in 84% of the 19 consecutive reported cases. The age range was 3 to 19 years (mean, 9.6 years). The primary location was on the right side. Again, ultrasound appeared to be instrumental in making a preoperative diagnosis.

Adnexal torsion can result in partial calcification of the adnexal mass.[64] Calcification was associated with torsion and resultant amputation of the right ovary. The "detached ovary" resulted in a cystic mass containing necrotic material and solid partially calcified segments.

Ovarian neoplasms have been reported in association with adnexal torsion.[65] Ovarian torsion is primarily associated with benign ovarian neoplasms; however, malignant ovarian neoplasms also can be involved. Over a 10-year period, Sommerville and coworkers noted that benign ovarian neoplasms had a 12.9-fold increased risk of undergoing adnexal torsion when compared with malignant neoplasms (95% confidence interval, 10.22 to 15.9).[65] Serous cystadenoma was the neoplasm most frequently associated with torsion.

Endoscopic Assessment With Vaginal Agenesis

Diagnostic laparoscopy has often been advocated in assessment of pelvic organs when a patient presents with vaginal agenesis. However, laparoscopy should be preceded by ultrasound and/or other high-resolution radiologic assessment such as magnetic resonance imaging (MRI). An MRI scan will provide details of any uterine musculature, as well as discern whether there is a fibrotic vaginal canal to

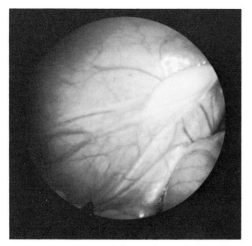

FIGURE 41–16 ••• Intraabdominal testicle in a 22-month-old male.

assist in preoperative planning. A word of caution must be clearly conveyed regarding absence of the uterus and adnexa at laparoscopy and subsequent cyclic menses. In a case report by Joshi and Sotrel, a patient was placed on conjugated estrogen and progestins and was noted to have cyclic menses indicative of minimal functional endometrial tissue capable of responding to exogenous estrogen-progestins.[66] In general, current thinking is that radiologic assessment alone is probably the only test indicated for uterine agenesis (e.g., Mayer Rokitansky-Küster-Hauser syndrome).[67]

Intraabdominal Testes

In the case of a male (often an infant) presenting with absence of palpable testicles, the initial assessment primarily involves administration of hCG and monitoring for testosterone production, specifically as an indication of testicular tissue. Radiologic imaging, in the form of either ultrasound or MRI, should be performed to identify the location of the testes. As noted above, if there is evidence of an intraabdominal location, an endoscopic approach can be used. Subsequently, an orchiopexy is often performed within 6 months. If this procedure is performed before 2 years of age, both spermatogenesis and androgen production may be preserved.[68] Occlusion of the cephalad blood supply allows establishment of one "primary" and exclusive blood supply from the testicular artery. The initial endoscopic approach for establishment of one testicular blood supply can be achieved without an initial laparotomy (Fig. 41–16).

Fetal Ovarian Cysts

The clinician should be cognizant of prenatal diagnosis of fetal ovarian cysts. With the in-

FIGURE 41–17 ••• Ultrasonogram identifying a fetal ovarian cyst at 27.1 weeks' gestational age. Note the thick-walled fetal bladder and the thin-walled ovarian cyst. Acoustic imaging 5200, 7.5-MHz, endovaginal probe. B, Bladder; C, cyst.

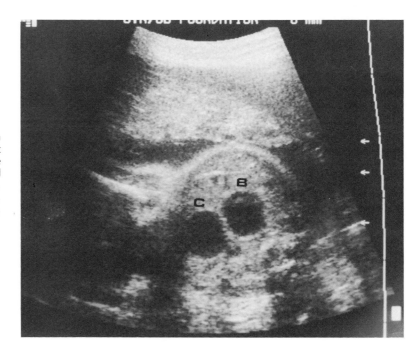

creasing sophistication and resolution of ultra-sonography, incidental findings of ovarian cysts continue to be reported.[69] Rizzo and colleagues reported 14 fetal ovarian cysts, primarily during the second and third trimesters of gestation. A conservative approach appears to be the most feasible when congenital ovarian cysts are diagnosed. The prognosis appears to be excellent, but the clinician must be aware that the cysts may increase or decrease in size or even spontaneously disappear. Torsion and rupture of the ovarian cyst have been reported; these carry increased risk to the fetus.[69]

Ideally, when a congenital fetal ovarian cyst is identified, serial ultrasonographic reevaluation should be carried out. If there is evidence of torsion or rupture, serious consideration should be given to prompt cesarean section (Fig. 41–17).[70]

References

1. Glinter K. Chronic pelvic pain. J Am Osteopath Assoc 1974; 74:335–341.
2. Cramer D, Welch W, Cassell S, et al. Mumps, menarche, menopause and ovarian cancer. Am J Obstet Gynecol 1983; 147:1–6.
3. Goldstein D, DeCholnoky C, Leventhal J, et al. New insights into the old problem of chronic pelvic pain. J Pediatr Surg 1979; 14:675–680.
4. Gross R, Doerr H, Caldirola D, et al. Borderline symptom and incest in chronic pelvic pain patients. Int J Psychiatr Med 1980; 10:79–96.
5. Kleinhaus S, Hein K, Sheran M, et al. Laparoscopy for diagnosis and treatment of abdominal pain in adolescent girls. Arch Surg 1977; 112:1178–1179.
6. Ebers G. The Papyrus Ebers—I. Bell E, Lewin B, Munksgaard E, trans. Copenhagen: Jnar-Munksgaard, 1937.
7. von Rokitansky J. Ueber Uterusdausen-Neubildung in uterus and ovarian sarcoma. Ztschrdkk Gesellsch Aertweinezy 1860; 37:377.
8. Ranney B. Etiology, prevention and inhibition of endometriosis. Clin Obstet Gynecol 1980; 23:875.
9. Meigs J. Endometriosis. Ann Surg 1948; 127:795.
10. Goldstein D, DeCholnoky C, Emans SJ. Adolescent endometriosis. J Adolesc Health Care 1980; 1:37.
11. Fallon J. Endometriosis in youth. JAMA 1946; 131:1405.
12. Whitehouse H. Endometrioma invading the bladder removed from a patient who had never menstruated. Proc R Soc Med 1925; 19:15.
13. Seitz L. Uber genese, klinik und therapie der endometriosis. (heterotopein der uterus-schleimhaut). Arch Gynaekol 1932; 149:529.
14. Sampson J. The development of the implantation theory for the origin of peritoneal endometriosis. Am J Obstet Gynecol 1940; 141:549.
15. Meyer R. Ueber endometrium in der tube sowie uber die hieraus ent stehenden wirkichen un vermeintlichen folgen. Zentralbl Gynaekol 1927; 51:1482–1491.
16. Haney A. Endometriosis: Pathogenesis and patho-physiology. In: Wilson E (ed). Endometriosis. New York: Alan R. Liss, 1987.
17. Simpson J, Elias S, Malinak L, Buttram V. Heriditable aspects of endometriosis. I. Genetic studies. Am J Obstet Gynecol 1981; 37:327.
18. Schifrin B, Erez S, Moore J. Teenage endometriosis. Am J Obstet Gynecol 1973; 116:973.
19. Sanfilippo J, Wakim N, Schikler K, Yussman M. Endometriosis in association with a uterine anomaly. Am J Obstet Gynecol 1986; 154:39.
20. Bässler R, Theele C, Labach H. Nodular and tumor-like gliomatosis peritonei with endometriosis caused by a mature ovarian teratoma. Pathol Res Pract 1982; 175:392.
21. Pueblitz-Peredo S, Luevano-Flores E, Rincon-Taracena R. Uterus-like mass of the ovary: Endometriosis or congenital malformation. Arch Pathol Lab Med 1985; 109:361.
22. Acosta A, Kaplan A, Kaufman R. Gynecologic cancer in children. Am J Obstet Gynecol 1972; 112:944.
23. Bush W, Hall D, Ward B. Adenomyosis of the gastric antrum in children. Pediatr Radiol 1974; 111:179.
24. Huffman J. Endometriosis in young teenage girls. Pediatr Ann 1981; 10:44.
25. Dmowski WP, Braun D, Gebel H. Endometriosis: Genetic and immunologic aspects. Prog Clin Biol Res 1990; 323:99–122.
26. Startseva N. Clinico-immunological aspects in genital endometriosis. Akush Ginekol (Mosk) 1980; 3:23.
27. Badawy SZ, Cuenca V, Stitzel A, Tice D. Immune rosettes of T and B lymphocytes in infertile women with endometriosis. J Reprod Med 1987; 32:194.
28. Fakih H, Baggett B, Holtz G, et al. Interleukin-1: A possible role in fertility associated with endometriosis. Fertil Steril 1987; 47:213.
29. Kauma S, Clark M, White C, Halme J. Production of fibronectin by peritoneal macrophages and concentration of fibronectin in peritoneal fluid from patients with or without endometriosis. Obstet Gynecol 1988; 72:13.
30. Reshef E, Prasthofer EF, Tilden AB. Natural killer cell activity in endometriosis and pelvic adhesions. Abstract no. 093. Proc 44th Annual Meeting, The American Fertility Society, Atlanta, Oct 10–13, 1988.
31. Chatman D, Ward A. Endometriosis in adolescents. J Reprod Med 1982; 27:156.
32. The American Fertility Society. Revised classification of endometriosis. Fertil Steril 1985; 43:351.
33. Sanfilippo J, Yussman M. Gynecologic problems of adolescence. In: Lavery J, Sanfilippo J (eds). Pediatric and Adolescent Gynecology. New York: Springer-Verlag, 1985.
34. Jones H. Reproductive impairment and the malformed uterus. Fertil Steril 1981; 36:137.
35. Sanfilippo J. Strassman procedure for correction of a class II müllerian anomaly in an adolescent. J Adolesc Health Care 1991; 12:63–66.
36. Semm K. History. In: Sanfilippo JS, Levine RL (eds). Operative Gynecologic Endoscopy. New York: Springer-Verlag, 1990.
37. Stein S. Das Photo-endoskop. Klin Wochenschr, Part 3, 1874.
38. Kolmorgen K, Seiden Schnur G, Panzer W. Analysis of 35,013 gynecologic laparoscopies (East German survey) 1986; 108(6):365–370.
39. Ammerman S, Schafer M, Synder D. Ectopic pregnancy in adolescents: A clinical review for pediatricians. J Pediatr 1990; 117(5):677.
40. Fossum G, Davajan V, Kletzky O. Early detection of

pregnancy with transvaginal ultrasound. Fertil Steril 1988; 49:788.

41. Nichols D. Tubal and Peritoneal Factors. Precis IV 1990. The American College of Obstetricians and Gynecologists, Washington, DC, p 199.

42. Reich H, De Caprio J, McGlynn F, et al. Peritoneal trophoblastic tissue implants after laparoscopic treatment of tubal ectopic pregnancy. Fertil Steril 1989; 52:337–339.

43. DeCherney A, Maheux R, Naftolin F. Salpingostomy for ectopic pregnancy in the sole patent oviduct: Reproductive outcome. Fertil Steril 1982; 37:619–622.

44. The American Fertility Society. Classification of ectopic pregnancy. Fertil Steril 1985; 49:944.

45. Stovall T, Ling F, Gray L. Single-dose methotrexate for treatment of ectopic pregnancy. Obstet Gynecol 1991; 77:749–753.

46. Vervest H, Haspels A. Preliminary results with the antiprogestational compound RU-486 (mifepristone) for interruption of early pregnancy. Fertil Steril 1985; 44:627–632.

47. Lindblom B, Hahlin M, Lundorff P, Thorburn J. Treatment of tubal pregnancy by laparoscope-guided injection of prostaglandin $F_2\alpha$. Fertil Steril 1990; 54(3):404.

48. Huffman J, Dewhurst J, Capraro V. The Gynecology of Childhood and Adolescence. 2nd ed. Philadelphia: WB Saunders, 1981.

49. Luxman D, David M. Postmenopausal adnexal mass: Correlation between ultrasound and pathologic findings. Obstet Gynecol 1991; 77:726.

50. Reich H, McGlynn F. Laparoscopic treatment of tuboovarian and pelvic abscess. J Reprod Med 1987; 32:747.

51. Reich H. Endoscopic management of tuboovarian abscess in pelvic inflammatory disease. In: Sanfilippo J, Levine R, (eds). Operative Gynecologic Endoscopy. New York: Springer-Verlag, 1990.

52. Levine R. Economic impact of pelviscopic surgery. J Reprod Med 1985; 30:655.

53. Method M, Keith L. Economic impact of gynecologic endoscopy. In: Sanfilippo J, Levine R (eds). Operative Gynecologic Endoscopy. New York: Springer-Verlag, 1990.

54. Merritt D. Torsion of the uterine adnexa: A review. Adolesc Pediatr Gynecol 1991; 4(1):3–13.

55. Operative Laparoscopy Study Group. Postoperative adhesion development after operative laparoscopy: Evaluation at early second-look procedures. Fertil Steril 1991; 55:700–704.

56. Wagaman R, Williams RS. Conservative therapy for adnexal torsion. A case report. J Reprod Med 1990; 35(8):833–834.

57. Vancaille T, Schmidt E. Recovery of ovarian function after laparoscopic treatment of acute adnexal torsion. J Reprod Med 1987; 32:561.

58. Shun A. Unilateral childhood ovarian loss: An indication for contralateral oophoropexy? Aust NZ J 1990; 60(10):791–794.

59. Davis A, Feins N. Subsequent asynchronous development of normal adnexa in children. J Pediatr Surg 1990; 25(6):689.

60. Isenberg J, Silech R. Isolated torsion of the normal fallopian tube in premenarcheal girls. Surg Gynecol Obstet 1991; 70(4):353.

61. Clickstein I, Lancet M, Rozenman D, Missen F. Isolated necrosis of the tubal fimbriae in a prepubertal girl. Z Kinderchir 1989; 44(3):172–173.

62. Peng G, Parmley TD, Genadry R. Endometriosis and perimenarcheal tubal torsion: A case report. J Reprod Med 1980; 34(11):934–936.

63. Spigland N, Ducharme J, Wazabk S. Adnexal torsion in children. J Pediatr Surg 1989; 24(1):974–976.

64. Corrarin O, Rutledge J. Ovarian torsion and amputation resulting in partially calcified pedunculated cystic mass. Pediatr Radiol 1989; 19(6–7):395–399.

65. Sommerville M, Grimes D, Koonigs P, Campbell K. Ovarian neoplasms and the risk of adnexal torsion. Am J Obstet Gynecol 1991; 164(2):577–578.

66. Joshi N, Sotrel G. Diagnostic laparoscopy in apparent uterine agenesis. J Adolesc Health 1988; 9(5):403–406.

67. Fedele L, Dorta M, Brioschi D, et al. Magnetic resonance imaging in Mayer-Rokitansky-Kuster-Hauser Syndrome. Obstet Gynecol 1990; 76:593–596.

68. Castilho LN. Laparoscopy for the nonpalpable testis: How to interpret the endoscopic findings. J Urol 1990; 144(5):1215–1218.

69. Rizzo N, Gabrielli S, Perolo A, et al. Prenatal diagnosis and management of fetal ovarian cysts. Prenat Diagn 1989; 9(2):97–103.

70. Meizner I, Levy A, Katz M, et al. Fetal ovarian cysts: Prenatal ultrasonographic detection and postnatal evaluation and treatment. Am J Obstet Gynecol 1991; 164(3):874–878.

CHAPTER 42

Future Perspectives

LEO PLOUFFE, Jr.

PAUL G. McDONOUGH

The major developments in pediatric and adolescent gynecology that will be emerging during the next decade are intriguing and exciting. Looking back at the past decade, few would have accurately predicted most of the major advancements seen thus far (e.g., polymerase chain reaction [PCR] and laparoscopic cholecystectomy). When the 1990s are over, these predictions may seem primitive, and it will be to the credit of our society and profession if we go beyond them, as all will reap the benefits.

PUBLIC HEALTH

Demographic Trends

The current worldwide demographic data are of great concern to many. The U.S. Census Bureau estimates that the population of individuals younger than 18 in the United States will increase from 64 million to 66 million by the year 2000, decreasing to 63 million by the year 2010.[1]

While this age group represents a relatively stable number of individuals, the actual percentage of the total population represented by children and teenagers will decrease from the current 25% to 22% by 2010. This age group truly represents the future of America, and it is therefore critical for our society to devise health care measures to keep this segment of the population in good health.

By contrast, third world countries are still facing dramatic increases in their overall population, and the percentage of individuals younger than 18 years is constantly on the rise. Barring any major epidemics or famine, these countries face mounting medical crises that not only affect the health of their youth, but also threaten the future security of their societies.

Health Care Access

Health care access remains a major problem for American society. An estimated 30 million Americans are without health care insurance coverage. Equally staggering are the numbers of children and adolescents who live in families that are below the poverty level or homeless (estimated to be between 500,000 and 2 million).[2] The controversy over the latest U.S. Census report highlights the difficulty in gaining an appropriate estimate of individuals living in these deprived socioeconomic conditions.

In those countries where government-sponsored health maintenance programs exist, problems are still pervasive. The health care systems of Canada, Great Britain, and Australia, to name but a few, are all under stress and are likely to undergo dramatic changes in the years to come. These systems have been slightly more responsive to the needs of the young, but the increased numbers of elderly individuals within these societies are placing a greater burden on the system, often at the expense of health care for children and teen-agers.

Even when health care programs are available, they are grossly underutilized. Teenage pregnancy provides a good model to study this behavioral pattern. Most states have adjusted their Medicaid program by broadening eligibility criteria and streamlining the application process. However, many eligible teenagers fail to seek available medical care, and many parents fail to bring their children in for regular health care visits. These represent sociocultural barriers that must be overcome.

At a time when local, state, and federal budgets are being cut, it is difficult to paint an optimistic picture in this area. There is no doubt about the will of the American people to deal with the situation. In terms of youth health care, three areas must be specifically addressed. The challenge is great, but the solutions are within our grasp.

First, the financial barriers must be overcome. Much emphasis has been placed on the need for reform of the medical care system finances, while too little attention has been paid to socioeconomic conditions. It is obvious that our efforts must concentrate on prevention, not on the delivery of expensive tertiary care. However, medical practice is too often driven by a response to emergencies.

Perhaps the best illustration of the current situation was given in a series of broadcasts on National Public Radio in the fall of 1991 that reported on children's health care in New York City. A pediatric trauma surgeon commented on the enormous number and complexity of cases and their amazing success figures. The cost estimates to provide this acute care were staggering. Meanwhile, the coordinator of the neighborhood pediatric outreach program decried the lack of funding for basic necessities such as vaccinations and routine health maintenance. His final statement was dramatic and touching: "Sometimes, I feel like telling the parents to shoot their child in the foot so they can get access to acute care medicine and get all their medical needs taken care of."

Change, therefore, must focus not only on the delivery of medical care, but also, most importantly, on our neighborhoods and life conditions. This is by no means a new concept. Victories over major diseases have come from public health measures coordinated through social changes, not through the provision of sophisticated tertiary care procedures. These thoughts are best expressed by Rosen in his essay on the relationship between health care delivery and society.[3]

Second, we must broaden our definition of health care providers and place them in environments where children and adolescents interact. This should start with effective day-care centers and follow all the way through to college. A good model for the role of educators in health care has been presented recently by Graves et al.[4] Unfortunately, many of the current budget cuts have been targeted at these institutions. It is imperative that medical professionals speak up against such measures and strengthen their key role in preventive health care medicine.

Last, but far from least, our programs must be accessible to children and adolescents. The sociocultural environment must be considered and facts presented in a relevant fashion. Language barriers and life circumstances must be dealt with. Many efforts in this area have been plagued by vocal opposition from special political interest groups. Unfortunately, these groups present no realistic alternatives. Once more, medical professionals must speak up to help guide the future not only of our health care system, but also of the social fabric of our society.

Issues of health care access must be dealt with immediately. The root of these difficulties lies deep in social, cultural, and economic problems. The Carnegie Corporation of New York has reviewed these issues and formulated specific recommendations to deal with them.[5] Violence in the home also plays a major role in this dilemma.[6a–6c, 7] All of these elements must be addressed along with reforms of the medical care system if true improvement in the health status of children and adolescents is to be seen.

Health Screening

The efficacy of universal newborn screening for metabolic genetic disorders is well established in many countries (Table 42–1). In the United States, all state health departments screen for phenylketonuria and hypothyroidism.[8] Many routinely screen for other disorders, including congenital adrenal hyperplasia, homocystinuria, galactosemia, maple syrup urine disease, and tyrosinemia.[9]

All of the current newborn metabolic tests rely on biochemical assays. Recent developments and preliminary results obtained with

TABLE 42–1 ⚬⚬⚬ CURRENT AND FUTURE TECHNIQUES IN NEWBORN SCREENING

First-trimester fetal cell sampling on maternal serum to identify a fetus at risk
  Molecular testing with polymerase chain reaction
Cord blood sampling for hemoglobinopathies
Dried blood spot sampling from a heel prick
  Biochemical/endocrine testing
    Hypothyroidism
    21-hydroxylase deficiency
    Phenylketonuria
    Maple syrup urine disease
    Homocystinuria
    Galactosemia
    Tyrosinemia
  Molecular testing/polymerase chain reaction
    21-hydroxylase deficiency
    Cystic fibrosis
    Sickle cell disease
    X-linked mental retardation

polymerase chain reaction (PCR) make it feasible to perform these tests on stored clots of blood dried on paper. This is the current sampling technique used for newborn screening, and therefore many of the current biochemical assays should soon be replaced by PCR technology (JA Phillips, personal communication). Care must be taken to fully establish the merit of DNA technology in this context, as false-positive and false-negative results can occur with these molecular techniques, just as with biochemical assays. Appropriate follow-up on these newborn screening tests is required. One report highlights the potential life threat from failure to follow through on newborn screening for congenital adrenal hyperplasia and hemoglobinopathies.[10]

Congenital hypothyroidism was the first endocrine disease targeted in mass screening programs. Aronson et al. have highlighted the benefits of such screening by displaying a normal growth pattern in children with congenital hypothyroidism treated from birth.[11] Another study has established that these children have normal performance in school compared with control individuals.[12] This highlights the merits of newborn screening for a potentially devastating condition. The efficacy of such a program, however, relies on effective treatment of the affected individual, and this is a key element of screening.

Problems with the availability of treatment and the effectiveness of early intervention are probably best highlighted by studies on newborn screening for cystic fibrosis. Hammond et al. reported on a biochemical assay with a sensitivity of 88%.[13] However, only 6.1% of the infants with a positive first test turned out to be truly affected with cystic fibrosis. Testing without the availability of effective treatment renders such a program futile and extremely cost inefficient at present.[7]

Many other endocrine disorders are likely targets for newborn screening in the coming decade. The full merit of screening for 21-hydroxylase deficiency (21-OH def) is still under scrutiny.[14] Many states have already established this part of their armamentarium, while many others are still debating the issue. The screen detects the salt-wasting form and is obviously of greatest use in affected males, as females are most often detected because of ambiguous genitalia.

Valentino et al. have reported on a newborn assay system that allows screening for both 21- and 11β-hydroxylase deficiencies.[15] This was based on a radioimmunoassay performed on the standard microfilter paper used for newborn screening. Although this study was limited to a small sample, this approach may prove useful for broader screening of adrenal enzyme deficiencies.

X-linked mental retardation is the most common identified form of mental retardation. It primarily affects males, but up to one third of carrier females demonstrate some degree of mental retardation. Although cytogenetic studies have long shown a "fragile" site on the long arm of the X chromosome, there has been no universally effective method for the detection of affected or carrier individuals. Molecular techniques currently permit accurate diagnosis through both DNA Southern analysis and PCR.[16, 17] This holds great promise for those at risk. More importantly, the underlying molecular mechanism for this disorder may be shared by many other disease processes. This is the beginning of a new era for molecular diagnosis.

A truly futuristic development is that of maternal sampling for fetal screening. Already this technique has been reported for fetal sexing.[18] It is most likely that by the year 2000, a single sample of maternal blood can be used to perform a broad battery of molecular tests and identify the fetuses at risk for any of the above disorders. Potentially, such screening procedures may be performed during the early part of the first trimester, which may afford the opportunity for in utero treatment.

Routine comprehensive medical care for children and adolescents is too seldom practiced. Guidelines have long existed, but few children have been the beneficiaries of these screening tests. Relatively recent guidelines for teenagers[19] may lead to improved health in this segment of the population.

Child Physical and Sexual Abuse Prevention

Child physical and sexual abuse has long been a problem in American society; the 1980s brought an increasing awareness of this plight. It is estimated that in the United States, between 100,000 and 500,000 children are sexually molested each year.[20] It is difficult to determine whether the number of cases is increasing or simply more cases are being reported. The 1990 President's Commission on Child Health declared child abuse a national emergency.[21]

While sexual abuse is by no means confined to specific socioeconomic strata of society, there are certain predisposing conditions. Substance abuse is one such element,[22] and there is a great need to establish effective screening and prevention programs to deal with this problem. These efforts can easily be misdirected if they fail to address true issues,[23, 24] but they can be very effective when appropriately designed.[25]

Sharma and Sunderland have reported a 30-fold increase in reported cases of sexual abuse.[26] The number of cases involving serious injuries did not increase; instead, instances of minor injuries accounted for the dramatic rise in reported incidents. Not all of the reported incidents, however, were confirmed to be sexual abuse. The authors point out the heavy burden that such reports impose on child health services. The ultimate result may be an overall decrease in preventive and health maintenance services to children because of the resources that are absorbed in the investigation of abuse cases.

One way to curtail inappropriate referrals for suspected abuse is to educate health care workers about findings associated with gynecologic problems compared with those arising from sexual abuse. This is a difficult area and always a subject of intense debate. Nonetheless, classification systems such as the one proposed by Muram are a step in the right direction.[27] This is discussed in Chapter 23.

One major change in the investigation of such cases is the advent of molecular probes for forensic use. After a somewhat shaky start

TABLE 42–2 ▪▪▪ DEVELOPMENTS IN MOLECULAR TECHNOLOGY FOR FORENSIC APPLICATION

Standards for sample collection and chain of evidence
Standardization of molecular probes for Southern blotting
Development of standard primers for polymerase chain reaction
Quality control programs
National Registry of Bar Codes for various ethnic and racial groups
National Registry of Individual Molecular Bar Codes

because of unscrupulous data interpretation, this technology, greatly enhanced by PCR, is finding its place among major crime-solving techniques.[28] Most states have established one or more forensic molecular laboratories, with quality control standards set by the Federal Bureau of Investigation (FBI). Plans are under way to establish a national registry of molecular bar codes, analogous to the ones that currently exist for fingerprints. This should greatly facilitate the tracking of suspects, particularly repeat offenders.

Major inroads will be accomplished in this area in coming years. Child abuse protocols should be established within every hospital and social service agency. Public awareness of this problem will continue to increase as medical professionals improve their ability to correctly recognize the signs and symptoms of sexual abuse. Finally, the judicial system will likely establish appropriate and stringent guidelines for the effective use of molecular technology in the area of criminal investigation (Table 42–2).

Sexual Issues: Education, Sexually Transmitted Diseases, and Teenage Pregnancy

Sexual activity in the teenage years is widespread. For example, one survey conducted in a blue-collar midwestern junior high school revealed that the percentage of sexually active teenagers progressed from almost 30% at age 12 to 90% by age 16.[29] As stated by Grant and Demetriou, "The problem is not that teens are sexually active but rather that they have little preparation and guidance in developing responsible sexual behavior."[30] These authors also summarize the various psychological and social factors at play in teenage sexuality.

Sex education is a source of major debate.

It is part of the curriculum in many grade schools and high schools, but the effectiveness of such programs has not been demonstrated, and current evidence is not encouraging. Stout and Rivara found little evidence of any benefit of sex education in the schools.[31] Perhaps a better approach would be to educate parents and facilitate communication about sexual issues at home.[32] Unfortunately, with so many children in single-parent families or having no parental figure, this seems impractical.[33]

In many sex education programs, emphasis is placed on the risk, and sometimes the prevention, of sexually transmitted diseases. Such programs stress the risks of sexual activity, rather than the positive effects of the healthy expression of sexuality. An illustration of this is provided by the failure of programs designed to encourage condom use because of the acquired immunodeficiency syndrome (AIDS) epidemic.[34]

Teenage sexuality carries with it the risk for teenage pregnancy, which is recognized as a major problem, particularly in the United States.[35, 36] Prevention is acknowledged to be the most effective approach in dealing with this problem, but how this is best achieved is a matter of great debate.[37]

Issues that appear relevant to adults may not be viewed in the same light by adolescents.[38] Similar problems occur when dealing with menstrual physiology.[39] Physicians themselves have progressed little in their attitudes toward sex and their ability to discuss these concerns with their patients. These attitudes become obvious during medical school but appear to reflect lifelong social mores.[40]

Once again, little progress will occur in the area of teenage sex education until society deals with the issues. It may be that separate programs will evolve to deal with human sexuality and behavior and with prevention of communicable diseases. These efforts will have to be driven by the medical profession and supported by local, state, and federal funding agencies with broad public approval. In this way education will occur in the home, at school, and through the media.

Many clinicians are particularly excited by the development of computer-assisted education programs.[41] These may be able to compete with music videos and arcade games for the attention of teenagers.

Finally, to achieve these goals, the political system will have to be freed from misdirected lobbying (Table 42–3). At the same time, society will have to rethink many of its social

TABLE 42–3 ▪▪▪ AREAS FOR EFFECTIVE INTERVENTION IN TEENAGE SEXUALITY EDUCATION

Issues of sexuality, reproductive physiology, and sexually transmitted disease
Home/community
  Programs to encourage and facilitate parent-child communication
  Family programs for sexuality education in instances where there is no family unit
School
  Effective biology teaching programs emphasizing reproductive physiology
  Community-supported programs that encourage open communication about sexual issues (e.g., how to say "no" to sex)
  Health care resources to provide needed counseling and contraceptive services
  Computer-assisted education program
Community/society
  Support for family and school programs, as outlined above
  Efforts to foster a mature and responsible approach to sexuality

standards. It seems difficult to talk about sexual responsibility and maturity to an audience of teenagers who idolize musical artists whose music videos emphasize sexual stereotypes. If changes are not effected, sex education may become the responsibility of those who dare to talk openly and seriously about sex in public, such as Dr. Ruth Westheimer.

Nutrition and Exercise

Malnutrition in children and teenagers has truly become a universal problem. There are incredible discrepancies not only among countries, but also among social units within the same country. Some die young from undernutrition, while others suffer for years from overeating disorders. Some strive every minute to obtain the barest amount of food and escape famine, while others starve themselves or eat and then induce vomiting to obtain the "ideal" body image.

The role of nutrition in health is gaining increasing recognition, particularly as related to individuals with special needs (e.g., children suffering from an inborn error of metabolism, such as phenylketonuria).[42] Nutrition not only is extremely relevant during the childhood years, but also is critical for good health status during the reproductive years and beyond. It is well accepted that postmenopausal osteoporosis is profoundly affected by the total bone mass of the individual, the implication being that good nutrition in the form of adequate calcium intake must occur many years before menopause. Similarly, coronary artery disease starts early in life in response to the nutritional status of the individual.

Nutritional deficiencies tend to be highly prevalent in the adolescent years. Chan found that children had adequate dietary calcium intake up to age 11, but this fell to less than 15% of the recommended level in the teenage years.[43] Furthermore, lower dietary calcium intake was reflected in lower bone density levels. Another study found that close to 70% of teenage ballet dancers were taking less than 70% of the USDA recommended daily essential nutrients.[44]

However, the link between nutrition, calcium intake, ovulatory status, and bone mass still must be clarified. One study has established a link among nutritional status, body weight, and the incidence of stress fractures in ballet dancers.[45] Other studies suggest that ovulatory disorders can independently compromise bone mass.[46]

Many of the key answers to these nutritional issues will be provided during the next decade. Once this information is obtained, the huge challenge of modifying the nutritional habits of children and teenagers can be met.

Several models have been proposed to achieve these goals (Table 42–4). Some advocate a family-oriented approach.[47] Others have proposed the involvement of role models or teachers, such as high school coaches and trainers, in nutritional education.[4] Both of these approaches are highly attractive and likely to succeed. This is particularly true in

TABLE 42–4 ••• MODELS TO ADDRESS
NUTRITIONAL DEFICIENCIES

Recognition of its high prevalence in children
  and adolescents
Family-oriented approach
  Food stamps/subsidies
  Community help agencies
  Community kitchens
School-based models
  Funded meals
  Year-round school-based programs
  Education: Teachers, coaches, trainers
  Targeted programs: Coaches, trainers
Government programs
  Effective food quality monitoring
  Effective food labeling
  Subsidy programs

view of the dramatic changes taking place in society.

The role of government in nutritional programs cannot be minimized. It appears that the necessary infrastructure is present to ensure good state-administered nutritional programs,[48] and broad nutritional guidelines have also been well defined.[49] Yet all levels of government, in many countries, have targeted school- or institution-based nutrition programs for budget cuts. This seems extremely short sighted and may have a devastating impact on the future health of all nations.

DIAGNOSTIC AND THERAPEUTIC METHODS

Laboratory Assays

Whereas the 1970s was the decade of radio-immunoassays, the 1980s was the advent of multiple immunometric assays and many non-radioisotopic techniques. The 1990s should see not only the proliferation of these techniques, but also a simplification of the process such that many laboratory tests can be performed on saliva or urine samples by patients themselves or in the physician's office.

Immunometric procedures have greatly reduced inter- and intra-assay variation and broadened the effective range of operation of assay systems.[50] However, this progress must be viewed with some degree of skepticism. The highly sensitive thyroid-stimulating hormone (hsTSH) assay is a good case in point. Initial reports on this system suggested that it would completely supplant the traditional TSH assay and obliterate the need for the thyrotropin-releasing hormone (TRH) stimulation test in the diagnosis and management of patients with thyroid disorders. However, many commercially available assay kits have fallen short of these expectations.[51] Many of the assay systems present major deficiencies either in the lower or upper range and therefore are at best equal, and in some cases even inferior, to traditional TSH assays. Of major concern is the introduction of these assay systems in clinical practice without full understanding and awareness on the part of clinicians.

Androgen assays are also rapidly evolving and are of particular importance in the diagnosis and management of adolescents and pre-adolescents with conditions ranging from premature adrenarche to hirsutism or ovulatory disorders. The free testosterone assay has thus far been based on a computation combining total testosterone and binding proteins or a testosterone dialysate. The development of a direct free testosterone immunometric assay holds great promise,[52] as this system is far less costly and seems to have good characteristics and reliability. Thus the determination of free testosterone may soon become part of the routine assessment of this patient population.

The prodigious development of molecular biology and its direct clinical application is provoking a major revolution in the laboratory, with two primary areas evolving over the next decade: endocrine testing and microbiologic techniques. Both of these have found direct clinical applications, and their utilization should be broadened in the years to come.

In the arena of endocrine diseases, dynamic testing will be supplanted by direct molecular diagnosis of disorders. The well-defined genetics of congenital adrenal hyperplasia is an excellent example of an area that should soon lend itself entirely to molecular diagnosis.[53] In addition, concerted efforts aimed at the molecular basis of most endocrine disorders should yield more and more information. The molecular approach to the diagnosis of these conditions will span from the embryonic period to adult life. Technically, we should expect a rapid proliferation of the application of PCR, as well as nonradioisotopic techniques.

In the microbiologic arena, most culture techniques will likely be abandoned. The laboratory will become molecular, with the use of specific probes to identify the various bacteria.[54] Cultures, however, may persist as a way to identify various pathogens. Hopefully, the next decade will see the development of appropriate management for human papilloma virus (HPV) infection. The progression of HPV in adolescents and children seems to follow a different course from that in the adult. It is hoped that a knowledge of viral integration sites will shed light on the mechanism of virus-genome interaction and the prediction of malignant transformation.

An already obvious application of molecular techniques is in the area of ambiguous genitalia and gonadal dysgenesis. Identification of the putative testicular determining factor sex-determining region (SRY) has led to a tremendous amount of activity in this field.[55–57] Patients with true hermaphroditism and a 46,XX complement still elude our understanding.[57] It is quite possible that more than one gene is involved in testicular differentiation; the next

few years should see the resolution of this complex problem.

It must also be recognized that the area of the Y chromosome thought to be responsible for oncogenesis in individuals with dysgenetic gonads is different from the SRY locus. Until we achieve precise localization of this oncogenic gene, we must rely on Y centromeric probes to detect the presence of Y material in these patients.[58] This technique should become ever more utilized in the coming years, and hopefully clinicians will become aware of its existence and its importance in clinical practice. Soon the entire human Y chromosome will be sequenced and cloned in Yac vectors. Currently, any single or multiple target sequences can be amplified with PCR in parallel or in series.

Imaging Techniques

The beginning of the 1990s saw the advent of color Doppler ultrasound. There is a great deal of enthusiasm at present for this new technology, and its full place in clinical practice will likely be established soon. The safety of the technique seems well established except during early pregnancy. The exact role of color Doppler ultrasound in pediatric and adolescent gynecology must still be defined. Current data suggest that it will facilitate identification of the gonads by following the pelvic vessels as well as discerning the uterus through detection of the uterine vessels. However, this constitutes a relatively minor contribution of this extremely expensive technology.

Some work suggests that color Doppler ultrasound may be of assistance in identifying endometrial polyps and distinguishing them from endometrial leiomyomas. This may prove useful for the adolescent with dysfunctional uterine bleeding. Its greatest promise probably lies in the interpretation of ovarian cysts. Current work aims at distinguishing benign from malignant ovarian lesions, and it appears that color Doppler may provide additional information and facilitate this distinction. This would permit and facilitate the selection of long-term management of ovarian cysts in adolescents.

At present only preliminary data exist on color Doppler in the evaluation of müllerian anomalies. However, it may be that it will facilitate identification of the anatomic structures and permit better resolution of complex anomalies.

The technique of hysterovaginosonography has been reported.[59] According to the data, this approach facilitates the delineation of uterine anatomy as well as pelvic anatomy. Whether it can be utilized in the pediatric or adolescent age group merits further study.

Ultrasound contrast media are currently under study and should become available commercially soon.[60] This will greatly enhance the versatility of ultrasound and may be of practical use in the adolescent patient.

Digital imaging has greatly reduced the radiation levels utilized for radiologic procedures.[61] It also permits higher resolution and may redefine the role of computed tomographic (CT) scanning in the evaluation of the female pelvis.

Perhaps more promising is the advent of microprobes initially designed for intravascular ultrasound purposes. These probes, measuring <1 cm in diameter, could potentially be introduced in the vagina and permit vaginal scanning in the pediatric and early adolescent age group. Whether these will demonstrate improvement over transvaginal probes applied to the perineum remains to be determined.

Both CT scanning and magnetic resonance imaging (MRI) have been studied for their role in the diagnosis of müllerian anomalies. The currently available data seem to favor MRI as the method of choice, provided the quality of the MRI unit is appropriate and the physicians involved in the evaluation are familiar with these anomalies.

The increasing role of ultrasonography and other imaging techniques in the operative suite cannot be overemphasized.[62] New intraoperative probes will soon make their appearance on the market and greatly modify the approach to numerous conditions. Within a few years, microultrasound probes may be introduced, through a laparoscopic trocar and high-frequency scanning used to obtain high-resolution images of cysts and determine their malignant potential. These techniques are summarized in Table 42–5.

Endoscopic Diagnostic and Therapeutic Applications

The rapid proliferation of endoscopic techniques and equipment is unlikely to be halted in the next decade, but the technology will likely undergo further refinement. Its precise

TABLE 42–5 ••• RECENT AND FUTURE DEVELOPMENTS IN IMAGING TECHNIQUES

Ultrasound
  High-resolution/high-frequency probes
  Vaginosonography
  Hysterovaginosonography
  Microprobes/semiinvasive techniques
  Color Doppler imaging
  Ultrasound contrast media
Radiology
  Digital imaging (lower radiation levels)
Computed tomographic imaging
  Digital reading (lower radiation levels and faster
    imaging times)
  Higher resolution
Magnetic resonance imaging
  Higher resolution
  Quicker
  Contrast media (gadolinium, etc.)

role and eventual place in the pediatric and adolescent arena should be decided.

In terms of equipment, the advent of improved fiberoptic endoscopes holds great promise for the pediatric and adolescent age group. These fibers, measuring from a few millimeters to 1 cm in diameter, can be directly inserted in the vagina, bladder, or urogenital sinus and provide a high-quality image that no doubt will further improve in coming years. From a laparoscopic perspective, the fibers can be passed through a Veress needle and the procedure potentially accomplished under local anesthesia or at least intravenous sedation, thereby making it a relatively noninvasive diagnostic technique.

Currently available automatic stapling and cutting devices should be refined in the coming years and become more widely available, especially if the current enthusiasm for endoscopic procedures expands from general surgeons to pediatric surgeons. These instruments will be of great assistance in laparoscopic as well as vaginal surgical procedures.

Currently available tissue expanders are of great assistance in the management of many problems, including developmental asymmetry of the female breast.[63, 64] These prosthetic devices open exciting new vistas in terms of reconstructive surgery, and their use in pediatrics is rapidly gaining acceptance.[65] They have great potential in the management of congenital anomalies of the vagina.

Medical Therapeutics

Whereas surgical therapy dramatically changed during the 1980s, an even more dra-

TABLE 42–6 ▪▪▪ CURRENT AND FUTURE APPROACHES TO GENE THERAPY

Embryo selection
Healthy gene transfer
  Early introduction of a healthy gene into an embryo
  Transfer of cells expressing the healthy gene
    Bone marrow transplantation
  Delivery to cell machinery
    Retroviral carriers
    Soluble gene transfer systems
Gene therapy
  Site-targeted mutation of the diseased gene
  DNA repair

matic revolution in medical therapy will be seen during the 1990s. This will be the era of new hormones, recombinant molecules, and molecular therapy.

Gonadotropin-releasing hormone (GnRH) antagonists will definitely make their clinical debut in the coming years. This should prove of great interest, not only in the management of premature pubertal development but also for treatment of growth disorders, endometriosis, androgen excess, and anovulation.

Many of the hormonal preparations currently in use will be replaced by genetically engineered products. One has only to consider the current place of recombinant insulin and growth hormone to realize the extent of development in this area. This is an irreversible evolution, and hopefully, increased competition will also mean lower prices for many of these products. Some age-old questions will also be resolved, including the optimal treatment regimens for individuals with short stature and for those with gonadal dysgenesis.

The greatest revolution will occur in the area of gene therapy.[66–68] Such a therapeutic approach could be used from the moment of conception onward and may even involve gamete manipulation.[69] It could be applied to any disease process for which we know the genetic basis, including such diverse disorders as adenosine deaminase deficiency, Duchenne's muscular dystrophy, the thalassemias, and hypercholesterolemia.[70–73] The promise is also great for cancer treatment.[74]

Most current efforts are targeted at the introduction of a healthy gene in diseased individuals (Table 42–6). Later efforts may actually target gene repair, but this is not likely to occur soon. The problems of gene therapy are multiple[75] and involve the introduction of the healthy gene in the body, its delivery to the appropriate cells, and its incorporation in the cell machinery. The most commonly employed model at present uses retroviral carriers.[76] Bone marrow transplantation has also been considered to introduce the gene in the body.[77] A promising new system consists of a soluble DNA carrier that can be targeted to specific receptors, such as hepatocytes.[78]

There is no doubt that this area of medical therapy will be highly successful. Many endocrine disorders appear to be good candidates for such treatment (e.g., growth hormone deficiency and congenital adrenal hyperplasia). Eventually, embryonic diagnosis and therapy may be available for such disorders as Tay-Sachs disease and cystic fibrosis.

There is a need for major developments in the field of teenage contraception. Many methods are currently available,[79] and the 1990s may see further delineation of the role of implantable contraceptives (Norplant), "safe" intrauterine devices, and female condoms for this age group. Many new progestin preparations are being used in Europe and introduced in the United States, but the full potential of these agents must still be defined, particularly in terms of their impact on lipid profiles and long-term health consequences.

References

1. Bureau of the Census. Statistical abstract of the United States—1990. 110th ed., Washington, DC: US Dept of Commerce, 1990, p 16.
2. Health care needs of homeless and runaway youths. Council on Scientific Affairs. JAMA 1989; 262:1358.
3. Rosen G. Health, history and the social sciences. In: Rosen G. From Medical Police to Social Medicine: Essays on the History of Health Care. New York: Science History Publications, 1974, p 37.
4. Graves KL, Farthing MC, Smith SA, Turchi JM. Nutrition training, attitudes, knowledge, recommendations, responsibility, and resource utilization of high school coaches and trainers. J Am Diet Assoc 1991; 91:321.
5. Hechinger FM. Fateful choices: Healthy youth for the 21st century. New York: Carnegie Council on Adolescent Development, Carnegie Corporation of New York, 1992.
6a. Bijur PE, Kurzon M, Overpeck MD, Scheidt PC. Parental alcohol use, problem drinking, and children's injuries. JAMA 1992; 267:3166.
6b. AMA Council on Scientific Affairs. Violence against women: Relevance for medical practitioners. JAMA 1992; 267:3184.
6c. AMA Council on Ethical and Judicial Affairs. Physicans and domestic violence: Ethical considerations. JAMA 1992; 267:3190.
7. Flitcraft AH. Violence, values and gender. JAMA 1992; 267:3194.
8. Holtzman NA. What drives neonatal screening programs? Editorial. N Engl J Med 1991; 325:802.

9. National screening status report. Infant Screening 1991; 14:5.

10. Listernick R, Frisone L, Silverman BL. Delayed diagnosis of infants with abnormal neonatal screens. JAMA 1992; 267:1095.

11. Aronson R, Ehrlich RM, Bailey JD, Rovet JF. Growth in children with congenital hypothyroidism detected by neonatal screening. J Pediatr 1990; 116:33.

12. Elementary school performance of children with congenital hypothyroidism. New England Congenital Hypothyroidism Collaborative. J Pediatr 1990; 116:27.

13. Hammond KB, Abman SH, Sokol RJ, Accurso FJ. Efficacy of statewide neonatal screening for cystic fibrosis by assay of trypsinogen concentration. N Engl J Med 1991; 325:769.

14. Tsuji A, Maeda M, Arakawa H. Recent progress in neonatal mass screening for congenital hypothyroidism and adrenal hyperplasia using enzyme immunoassays. Adv Clin Chem 1990; 28:109.

15. Valentino R, Tommaselli AP, Rossi R, et al. A pilot study for neonatal screening of congenital adrenal hyperplasia due to 21-hydroxylase and 11-beta-hydroxylase deficiency in Campania region. J Endocrinol Invest 1990; 13:221.

16. Rousseau F, Heitz D, Biancalana V, et al. Direct diagnosis by DNA analysis of the fragile X syndrome of mental retardation. N Engl J Med 1991; 325:1673.

17. Pergolizzi RG, Erster SH, Goonewardena P, Brown WT. Detection of full fragile X mutation. Lancet 1992; 339(8788):271.

18. Lo YM, Patel P, Wainscoat JS, et al. Prenatal sex determination by DNA amplification from maternal peripheral blood. Lancet 1989; 2(8676):1363.

19. Cromer BA, Seifert McLean C, Heald FP. A critical review of comprehensive health screening in adolescents. J Adolesc Health 1992; 13(suppl):1S.

20. Fuller AK. Child molestation and pedophilia. An overview for the physician. JAMA 1989; 261:602.

21. Krugman RD. Child abuse and neglect: Critical first steps in response to a national emergency. The report of the US Advisory Board on Child Abuse and Neglect. Am J Dis Child 1991; 145:513.

22. Murphy JM, Jellinek M, Quinn D, et al. Substance abuse and serious child mistreatment: Prevalence, risk, and outcome in a court sample. Child Abuse Negl 1991; 15:197.

23. Budin LE, Johnson CF. Sex abuse prevention programs: Offenders' attitudes about their efficacy. Child Abuse Negl 1989; 13:77.

24. Kleemeier C, Webb C, Hazzard A, Pohl J. Child sexual abuse prevention: Evaluation of a teacher training model. Child Abuse Negl 1988; 12:555.

25. Hazzard A, Webb C, Kleemeier C, et al. Child sexual abuse prevention: Evaluation and one-year follow-up. Child Abuse Negl 1991; 15:123.

26. Sharma A, Sunderland R. Increasing medical burden of child abuse. Arch Dis Child 1988; 63:172.

27. Muram D. Child sexual abuse—genital findings in prepubertal girls. I. The unaided medical examination. Am J Obstet Gynecol 1989; 160:328.

28. Plouffe L. The molecular ID card: A powerful forensic tool for today or tomorrow? Adolesc Pediatr Gynecol 1990; 3:49.

29. Orr DP, Wilbrandt ML, Brack CJ, et al. Reported sexual behaviors and self-esteem among young adolescents. Am J Dis Child 1989; 143:86.

30. Grant LM, Demetriou E. Adolescent sexuality. Pediatr Clin North Am 1988; 35:1271.

31. Stout JW, Rivara FP. Schools and sex education: Does it work? Pediatrics 1989; 83:375.

32. Huston RL, Martin LJ, Foulds DM. Effect of a program to facilitate parent-child communication about sex. Clin Pediatr (Phila) 1990; 29:626.

33. Curtis HA, Lawrence CJ, Tripp JH. Teenage sexual intercourse and pregnancy. Arch Dis Child 1988; 63:373.

34. Kegeles SM, Adler NE, Irwin CE Jr. Sexually active adolescents and condoms: Changes over one year in knowledge, attitudes, and use. Am J Public Health 1988; 78:460.

35. Davis S. Pregnancy in adolescents. Pediatr Clin North Am 1989; 36:665.

36. McAnarney ER, Hendee WR. Adolescent pregnancy and its consequences. JAMA 1989; 262:74–77.

37. McAnarney ER, Hendee WR. The prevention of adolescent pregnancy JAMA 1989; 262:78–82.

38. Kegeles SM, Adler NE, Irwin CE Jr. Adolescents and condoms. Associations of beliefs with intentions to use. Am J Dis Child 1989; 143:911.

39. Cumming DC, Cumming CE, Kieren DK. Menstrual mythology and sources of information about menstruation. Am J Obstet Gynecol 1991; 164:472.

40. Fisher WA, Grenier G, Watters WW, et al. Students' sexual knowledge, attitudes toward sex, and willingness to treat sexual concerns. J Med Educ 1988; 63:379.

41. Paperny DM, Starn JR. Adolescent pregnancy prevention by health education computer games: Computer-assisted instruction of knowledge and attitudes. Pediatrics 1989; 83:742.

42. Reilly C, Barrett JE, Patterson CM, et al. Trace element nutrition status and dietary intake of children with phenylketonuria. Am J Clin Nutr 1990; 52:159.

43. Chan GM. Dietary calcium and bone mineral status of children and adolescents. Am J Dis Child 1991; 145:631.

44. Benson JE, Geiger CJ, Eiserman PA, Wardlaw GM. Relationship between nutrient intake, body mass index, menstrual function, and ballet injury. J Am Diet Assoc 1989; 89:58.

45. Frusztajer NT, Dhuper S, Warren MP, et al. Nutrition and the incidence of stress fractures in ballet dancers. Am J Clin Nutr 1990; 51:779.

46. Prior JC, Vigna YM, Schechter MT, Burgess AE. Spinal bone loss and ovulatory disturbances. N Engl J Med 1990; 323:1221.

47. Nicklas TA, Johnson CC, Arbeit ML, et al. A dynamic family approach for the prevention of cardiovascular disease. J Am Diet Assoc 1988; 88:1438.

48. Thompson EB, Bellamy MM, Kaufman M, Jarka E. Capacity of state health agencies to meet nutrition objectives in maternal and child health. J Am Diet Assoc 1990; 90:1423.

49. Nutrition management of adolescent pregnancy: Technical support paper. J Am Diet Assoc 1989; 89:105.

50. Tijssen P, Adam A. Enzyme-linked immunosorbent assays and developments in techniques using latex beads. Curr Opin Immunol 1991; 3:233.

51. Hay ID, Klee GG. Thyroid dysfunction. Endocrinol Metab Clin North Am 1991; 17:473.

52. Green PJ. Free testosterone determination by ultrafiltration, and comparison with dialysis. Clin Chem 1982; 28:1237.

53. Reindollar RH, Gray MR. The molecular basis of 21-hydroxylase deficiency. Semin Reprod Endocrinol 1991; 9:34.

54. Diamandis EP. Analytical methodology for immunoassays and DNA hybridization assays—current status and selected systems—critical review. Clin Chim Acta 1990; 194:19.

55. Berta P, Hawkins JR, Sinclair AH, et al. Genetic evidence equating SRY and the testis-determining factor. Nature 1990; 348(6300):448.

56. Plouffe L. The search for the testicular determining factor (TDF): The saga continues. Adolesc Pediatr Gynecol 1990; 4:218.

57. Shulman LP. Testis determining factor—the role of SRY. Adolesc Pediatr Gynecol 1991; 4:213.

58. Tho SPT, Behzadian A. Detection and amplification of Y sequences. Semin Reprod Endocrinol 1991; 9:46.

59. Hoetzinger H. Hysterosonography and hysterography in benign and malignant diseases of the uterus. A comparative in vitro study. J Ultrasound Med 1991; 10:259.

60. Hilpert PL, Mattrey RF, Mitten RM, Peterson T. IV injection of air-filled human albumin microspheres to enhance arterial Doppler signal: A preliminary study in rabbits. AJR 1989; 153:613.

61. Haendle J, Marhoff P. Current methods of digital imaging in conventional X-ray diagnostics. Eur J Radiol 1990; 10:218.

62. McGahan JP, Gerscovich E. Intraoperative and interventional ultrasound. Curr Opin Radiol 1990; 2:213.

63. Cohen M, Marschall M. Tissue expansion. An alternative technique in reconstructive surgery. Surg Annu 1990; 22:343.

64. Rintala AE, Nordstrom RE. Treatment of severe developmental asymmetry of the female breast. Scand J Plast Reconstr Surg Hand Surg 1989; 23:231.

65. Paletta C, Campbell E, Shehadi SI. Tissue expanders in children. J Pediatr Surg 1991; 26:22.

66. Fleischman RA. Human gene therapy. Am J Med Sci 1991; 301:353.

67. Green ED, Waterston RH. The human genome project. Prospects and implications for clinical medicine. JAMA 1991; 266:1966.

68. Karson EM. Prospects for gene therapy. Biol Reprod 1990; 42:39.

69. Gordon JW. Micromanipulation of embryos and germ cells: An approach to gene therapy? Am J Med Genet 1990; 35:206.

70. Hirschhorn R. Adenosine deaminase deficiency. Immunodefic Rev 1990; 2:175.

71. Ray PN, Klamut HJ, Worton RG. The DMD gene promoter: A potential role in gene therapy. Adv Exp Med Biol 1990; 280:107.

72. Gale RP. Prospects for correction of thalassemia by genetic engineering. Prog Clin Biol Res 1989; 309:141.

73. Wilson JM, Chowdhury JR. Prospects for gene therapy of familial hypercholesterolemia. Mol Biol Med 1990; 7:223.

74. Rosenberg SA. Immunotherapy and gene therapy of cancer. Cancer Res 1991; 51(18 suppl):5074s.

75. Hesdorffer C, Markowitz D, Ward M, Bank A. Somatic gene therapy. Hematol Oncol Clin North Am 1991; 5:423.

76. Cornetta K, Wieder R, Anderson WF. Gene transfer into primates and prospects for gene therapy in humans. Prog Nucleic Acid Res Mol Biol 1989; 36:311.

77. Lehn PM. Gene therapy using bone marrow transplantation: A 1990 update. Bone Marrow Transplant 1990; 5:287.

78. Wu GY, Wu CH. Delivery systems for gene therapy. Biotherapy 1991; 3:87.

79. Greydanus DE, Lonchamp D. Contraception in the adolescent. Preparation for the 1990s. Med Clin North Am 1990; 74:1205.

Appendices

BARBARA R. HOSTETLER

Growth Charts

**BOYS: BIRTH TO 36 MONTHS
PHYSICAL GROWTH
NCHS PERCENTILES***

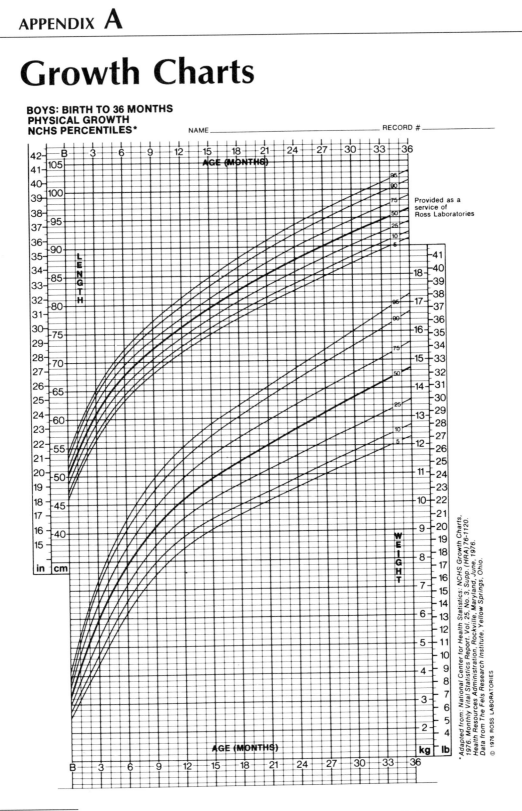

From Summitt RL. Comprehensive Pediatrics. St. Louis: C. V. Mosby, 1990, pp. 14–22. Modified from National Center for Health Statistics: NCHS growth charts, 1976; Monthly vital statistics report, vol 25, no 3, suppl (HRA) 76-1120, Health Resources Administration, Rockville, MD, June 1976; Data from The Fels Research Institute, Yellow Springs, OH. Published by Ross Laboratories, Columbus, OH, 1976.

GIRLS: BIRTH TO 36 MONTHS
PHYSICAL GROWTH
NCHS PERCENTILES*

NAME _____ RECORD # _____

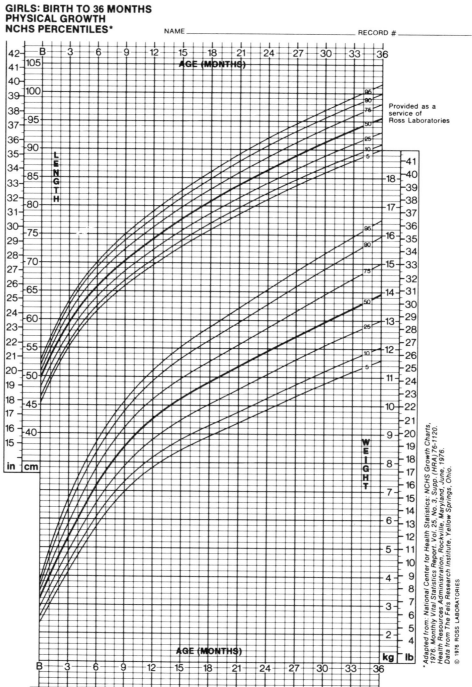

Provided as a
service of
Ross Laboratories

* Adapted from: National Center for Health Statistics: NCHS Growth Charts,
1976. Monthly Vital Statistics Report, Vol. 25, No. 3, Supp. (HRA) 76-1120.
Health Resources Administration. Rockville, Maryland, June, 1976.
Data from The Fels Research Institute, Yellow Springs, Ohio.

© 1976 ROSS LABORATORIES

**BOYS: 2 TO 18 YEARS
PHYSICAL GROWTH
NCHS PERCENTILES***

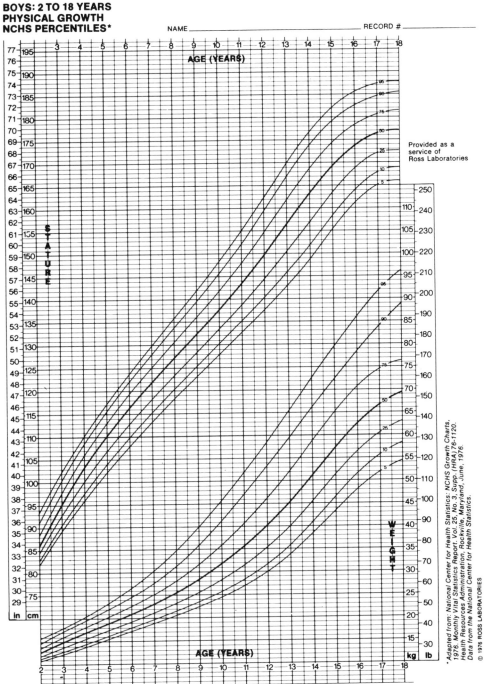

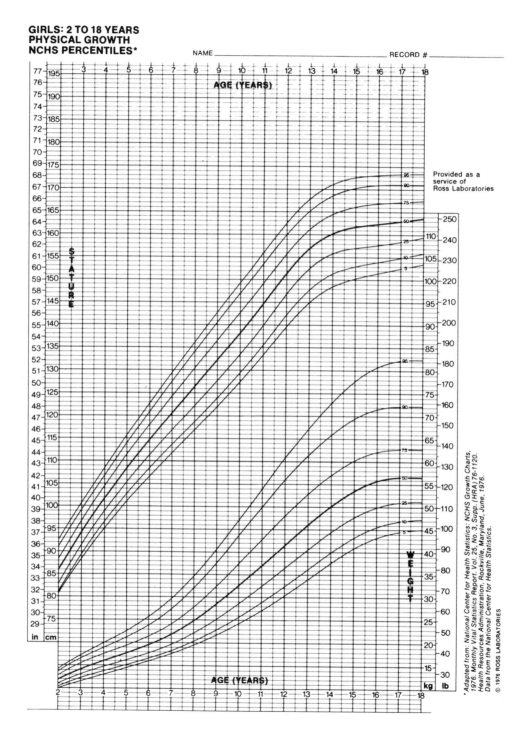

GIRLS: 2 TO 18 YEARS
PHYSICAL GROWTH
NCHS PERCENTILES*

* Adapted from: National Center for Health Statistics: NCHS Growth Charts, 1976. Monthly Vital Statistics Report. Vol. 25, No. 3, Supp. (HRA) 76-1120. Health Resources Administration, Rockville, Maryland, June, 1976. Data from the National Center for Health Statistics.

© 1976 ROSS LABORATORIES

Provided as a service of Ross Laboratories

Name.. Date of Birth.......................... Reg. No....................

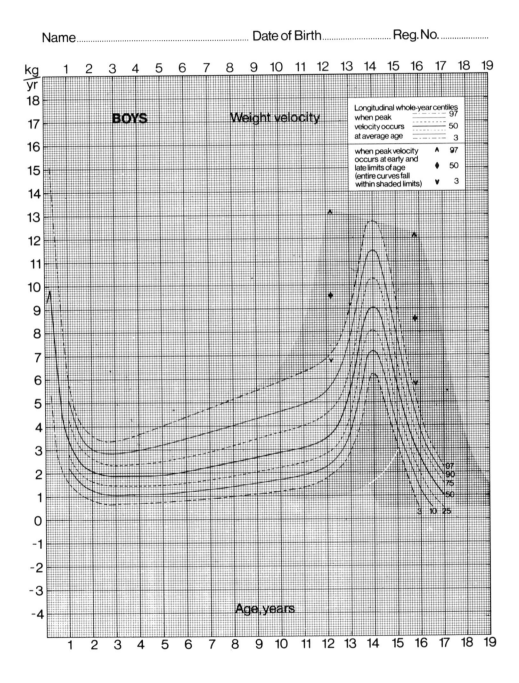

Name.. Date of Birth.......................... Reg. No. ....

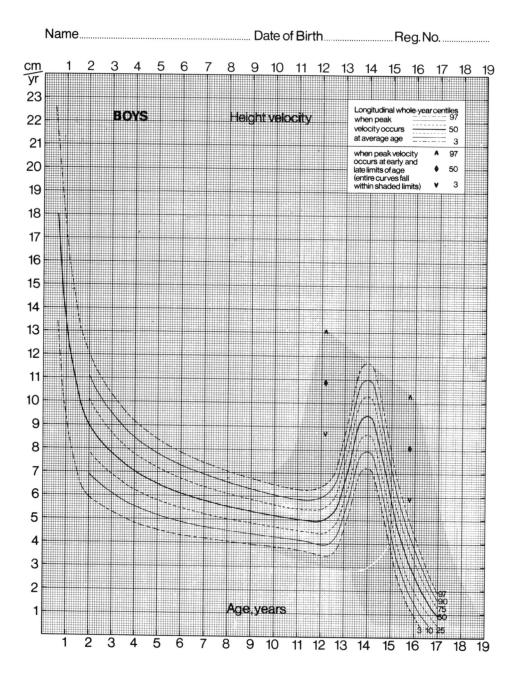

Name.. Date of Birth........................... Reg. No. ....

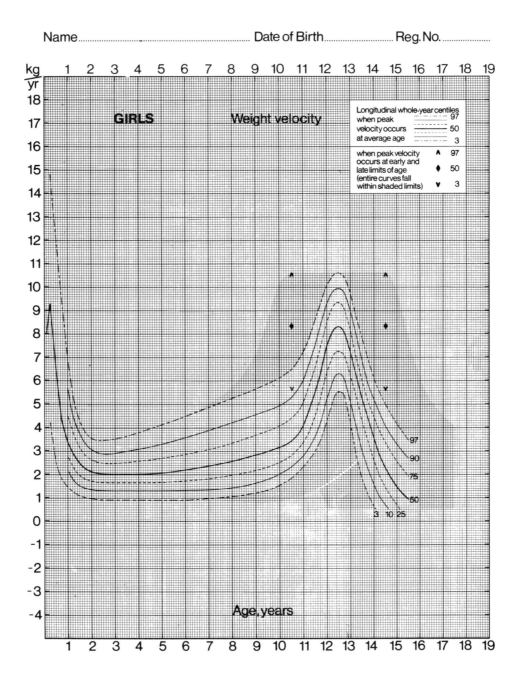

Name.. Date of Birth.......................... Reg.No....................

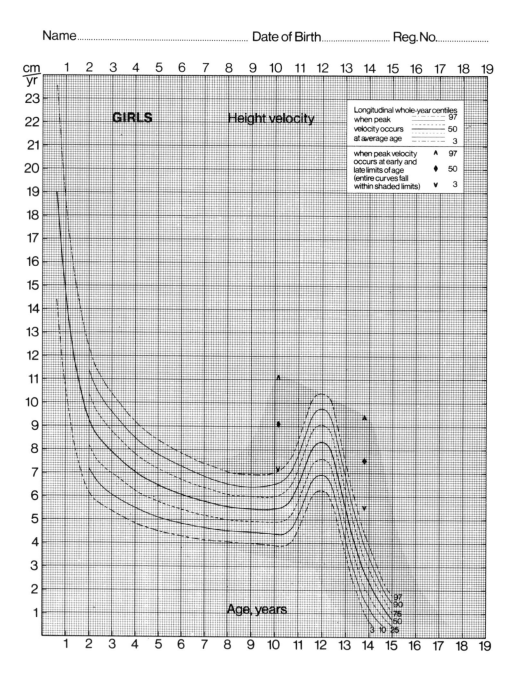

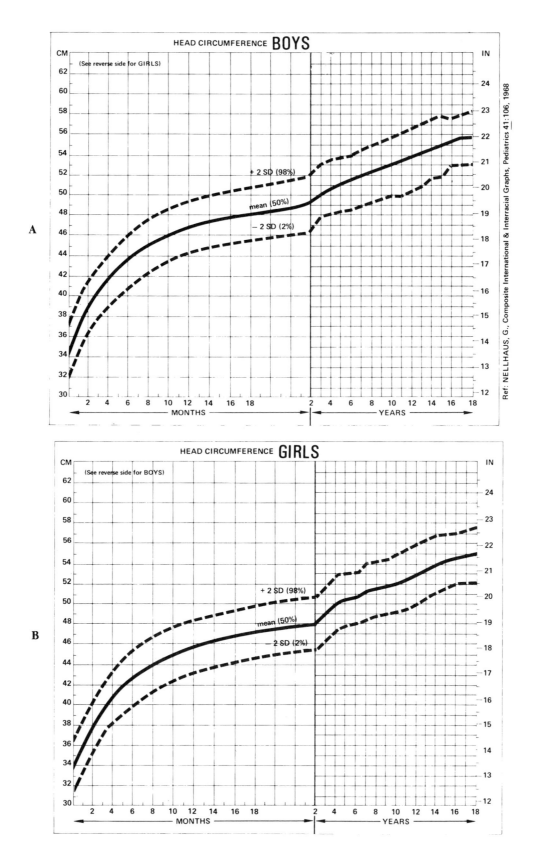

Tanner Staging

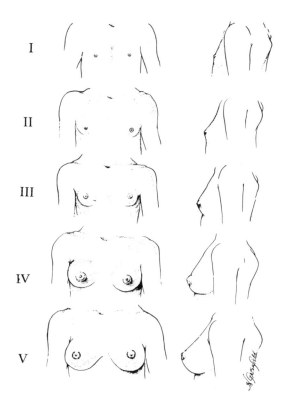

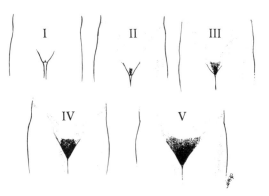

Both Sexes: Pubic Hair

Stage I   Preadolescent. The vellus over the pubes is not further developed than that over the abdominal wall; that is, no pubic hair.

Stage II   Sparse growth of long, slightly pigmented downy hair, straight or curled, chiefly at the base of the penis or along the labia.

Stage III   Considerably darker, coarser, and more curled. The hair spreads sparsely over the junction of the pubes.

Stage IV   Hair now adult in type, but area covered is still considerably smaller than in the adult. No spread to the medial surface of the thighs.

Stage V   Adult in quantity and type with distribution of the horizontal (or classically "feminine") pattern. Spread to medial surface of thighs but not up linea alba or elsewhere above the base of the inverse triangle (spread up linea alba occurs late and is Stage VI).

Girls: Breast Development

Stage I   Preadolescent. Elevation of papilla only.

Stage II   Breast bud stage. Elevation of breast and papilla as small mound. Enlargement of areolar diameter.

Stage III   Further enlargement and elevation of breast and areola with no separation of their contours.

Stage IV   Projection of areola and papilla to form a secondary mound above the level of the breast.

Stage V   Mature stage. Projection of papilla only caused by recession of the areola to the general contour of the breast.

Figures adapted from Marshall WA, Tanner JM. Variations in patterns of pubertal changes in girls. Arch Dis Child 1969; 44:291. Reprinted from Ross GT, Vande Wiele RL, Frantz AG. The normal ovary. In: Williams RH (ed). Textbook of Endocrinology. 6th ed. Philadelphia: W.B. Saunders, 1981, p 362.

Normal Laboratory Values

Test	Specimen	Reference Range		Factor	Reference Range International
Androstenedione	Serum		*ng/dl*	× 0.0349	*nmol/L*
		Child:	8–50		3–18
		Adult, M:	75–205		26–72
		Adult, F:	85–275		30–96
Creatinine clearance	Serum or plasma and urine	Newborn: 40–65 ml/min/1.73 m²			
		<40 yr., M: 97–137			
		F: 88–128			
		Decreases 6.5 ml/min/decade			
Dehydroepian-drosterone (DHEA)	Serum		*ng/ml*	× 3.467	*nmol/L*
		Cord:	5.6–20.0		19.4–69.3
		Child:	1.0–3.0		3.5–10.4
		Adult, M:	1.7–4.2		5.9–14.6
		Adult, F:	2.0–5.2		6.9–18.0
		Pregnancy:	0.5–12.5		1.7–43.3
	Urine, 24-hr		*mg/ml*	× 3.467	*μmol/d*
		Child, 0–1 yr:	<0.1		<0.35
		10–15 yr:	<0.4		<1.4
		Adult, M:	0–2.3		0–8.0
		Adult, F:	0–1.2		0–4.2
Dehydroepian-drosterone sulfate (DHEAS)	Serum or plasma (heparin or EDTA)		*μg/ml*	× 2.608	*μmol/L*
		Newborn,	<300		<780
		1–4 d:	<20		<52
		Child:	0.60–2.54		1.6–6.6
		Adult, M:	1.99–3.34		5.2–8.7
		Adult, F:			
		Premenopausal:	0.82–3.38		2.1–8.8
		Pregnancy, term:	0.23–1.17		0.6–3.0

Test	Specimen	Reference Range			Factor	Reference Range International	
Dihydrotestos-terone (DHT)	Serum		*ng/dl*		× 0.03443	*nmol/L*	
		Prepubertal:	<3.5			<0.12	
		Pubertal:	M	F		M	F
		stage I:	<10	<10		<0.34	<0.34
		II:	<20	<15		<0.7	<0.5
		III:	<35	<25		<1.2	<0.86
		IV–V:	<75	<25		<2.6	<0.86
		Adult:	<30–85	4–22		1.03–2.92	0.14–0.76

Table continued on following page

Modified from Behrman RE, Vaughan VC. Nelson Textbook of Pediatrics. 13th ed. Philadelphia: W.B. Saunders, 1987, pp 1537–1558.

Test	Specimen	Reference Range		Factor	Reference Range International
Estradiol	Serum or plasma (heparin or EDTA)		*pg/ml*	×3.671	*pmol/L*
		M. pubertal:			
		stage I:	2–8		7–29
		II:	11		40
		III:	>20		>73
		Adult, M:	8–36		29–132
		F, pubertal:			
		stage I:	0–23		0–84
		II:	0–66		0–242
		III:	0–105		0–385
		IV:	20–300		73–1101
		Follicular:	10–90		37–330
		Midcycle:	100–500		367–1835
		Luteal:	50–240		184–881
	Urine 24-hr		*µg/d*	× 3.671	*nmol/d*
		Adult, M:	0–6		0–22
		Adult, F:			
		Follicular:	0–3		0–11
		Ovulatory peak:	4–14		15–51
		Luteal:	4–10		15–37
Estrogens, Total	Serum		*pg/ml*	× 1	*ng/L*
		Child:	<30		<30
		M:	40–115		40–115
		F, cycle days			
		1–10 d:	61–394		61–394
		11–20 d:	122–437		122–437
		21–30 d:	156–350		156–350
		Prepubertal:	≤40		≤40
	Urine, 24-hr		*µg/d*	× 1	*µg/d*
		Child:	<10		<10
		Adult, M:	5–25		5–25
		Adult, F:			
		Preovulation:	5–25		5–25
		Ovulation:	28–100		28–100
		Luteal peak:	22–80		22–80
		Pregnancy:	<45,000		<45,000
		Postmenopausal:	<10		<10
Follicle stimulating hormone (FSH)	Serum or plasma (heparin)		*mU/ml* (IRP-2-hMG)	× 1	*IU/L*
		Birth–1 yr, M:	<1–12		<1–12
		F:	<1–20		<1–20
		1–8 yr, M:	<1–6		<1–6
		F:	<1–4		<1–4
		9–10 yr, M:	<1–10		<1–10
		F:	2–8		2–8
		11–12 yr, M:	2–12		2–12
		F:	3–11		3–11
		13–14 yr, M:	3–15		3–15
		F:	3–15		3–15
		Adult, M:	4–25		4–25
		Adult, F:			
		Premenopausal:	4–30		4–30
		Midcycle peak:	10–90		10–90
		Pregnancy:	Low to undetectable		Low to undetectable

Test	Specimen	Reference Range		Factor	Reference Range International
Growth hormone (hGH, somato-tropin)	Serum of plasma (EDTA, hep-arin)	Cord:	*ng/ml* 10–50	× 1	*μg/L* 10–50
	Fasting, at rest	Newborn:	10–40		10–40
		Child:	<5		<5
		Adult, M:	<5		<5
		Adult, F:	<8		<8
Hematocrit (HCT, Hct)	Whole blood (EDTA)	% of packed red cells (V red cells/V whole blood × 100)		Volume fraction (V red cells/V whole blood)	
Calculated from MCV and RBC (electronic dis-placement or laser)	1 d (cap):	48–69		× 0.01	0.48–0.69
	2 d:	48–75			0.48–0.75
	3 d:	44–72			0.44–0.72
	2 mo:	28–42			0.28–0.42
	6–12 yr:	35–45			0.35–0.45
	12–18 yr, M:	37–49			0.37–0.49
	F:	36–46			0.36–0.46
	18–49 yr, M:	41–53			0.41–0.53
	F:	36–46			0.36–0.46
17-Hydroxy-progesterone (17-OHP)	Serum	M,	*ng/ml*	× 3.026	*nmol/l*
		Pubertal stage I:	0.1–0.3		0.3–0.9
		Adult:	0.2–1.8		0.6–5.4
		F,			
		Pubertal stage I:	0.2–0.5		0.6–1.5
		Follicular:	0.2–0.8		0.6–2.4
		Luteal:	0.8–3.0		2.4–9.0
		Postmenopausal:	0.04–0.5		0.12–1.5
Luteinizing hor-mone (LH)	Serum or plasma (heparin)	Child:	*m/U/ml* 1–6	× 1	*IU/L* 1–6
		M, 10–13 yr:	4–12		4–12
		12–14 yr:	6–12		6–12
		12–17 yr:	6–16		6–16
		15–18 yr:	7–19		7–19
		F, 8–12 yr:	2–12		2–12
		9–14 yr:	2–14		2–14
		12–18 yr:	3–29		3–29
		Adult, M:	6–23		6–23
		Adult, F,			
		Follicular phase:	5–30		5–30
		Midcycle:	75–150		75–150
		Luteal:	3–40		3–40
		Postmenopausal	30–200		30–200

Table continued on following page

Test	Specimen	Reference Range		Factor	Reference Range International
Progesterone	Serum		*ng/ml*	× 3.18	*nmol/L*
		M,			
		Pubertal stage I:	0.11–0.26		0.35–0.83
		Adult:	0.12–0.3		0.38–1
		F,			
		Pubertal stage I:	0–0.3		0–1
		II:	0–0.46		0–1.5
		III:	0–0.6		0–2
		IV:	0.05–13.0		0.16–41
		Follicular:	0.02–0.9		0.06–2.9
		Luteal:	6.0–30.0		19–95
Prolactin (PRL)	Serum		*ng/ml*	× 1	*μg/ml*
		Adult, M:	<20		<20
		Adult, F,			
		Follicular phase:	<23		<23
		Luteal phase:	5–40		5–40
		Pregnancy,			
		1st trimester:	<80		<80
		2nd trimester:	<160		<160
		3rd trimester:	<400		<400
		Newborn: >10-fold adult levels			>10-fold adult levels

Temperature Conversion

C	F	C	F	C	F	C	F
0	32.0	37.2	99	39.2	102.6	41.2	106.2
20	68.0	37.4	99.3	39.4	102.9	41.4	106.5
30	86.0	37.6	99.7	39.6	103.3	41.6	106.9
31	87.8	37.8	100.1	39.8	103.7	41.8	107.2
32	89.6	38.0	100.4	40.0	104	42	107.6
33	91.4	38.2	100.8	40.2	104.4	43	109.4
34	93.2	38.4	101.2	40.4	104.7	44	111.2
35	95.0	38.6	101.5	40.6	105.1	100	212
36	96.8	38.8	101.8	40.8	105.4		
37	98.6	39.0	102.2	41.0	105.8		

*To convert Celsius (centigrade) readings to Fahrenheit, multiply by 1.8 and add 32. To convert Fahrenheit readings to Celsius, subtract 32 and divide by 1.8.

From Behrman RE, Vaughan VC. Nelson Textbook of Pediatrics. 13th ed. Philadelphia: W.B. Saunders, 1987, p 1560.

Commonly Used Medications

Drug	How Supplied	Dose and Route	Remarks
Acetaminophen (Panadol, Tempra, Tylenol, and others)	Tabs: 325, 500 mg Chewable Tabs: 80 mg Caplets: 160 mg Drops: 80 mg/0.8 ml Elixir: 160 mg/5 ml Syrup: 160 mg/5 ml	*Usual Dose:* 10–15 mg/kg/dose Q4h **Max. dose:** 5 doses/d *Alternative:* 0–3 mo: 40 mg/dose 4–11 mo: 80 mg/dose 12–24 mo: 120 mg/dose 4–5 yr: 240 mg/dose 6–8 yr: 320 mg/dose 9–10 yr: 400 mg/dose 11–12 yr: 480 mg/dose Adult: 325–650 mg Q4h **Max. dose:** 65 mg/kg/d	T 1/2: 1–3 h. **Contraindicated** in patients with G6PD deficiency. Overdose may cause hepatotoxicity, often delayed. Some preparations contain alcohol.
Acyclovir (Zovirax)	Capsules: 200 mg Inj: 500 mg/10 ml Ointment: 5% (15 gm)	*Herpes Simplex Virus:* Newborns: 30 mg/kg/d admin. Q8h IV Children (<12 yrs): 750 mg/M^2/d admin. Q8h IV; give over 1 hour. *Genital HSV:* 200 mg PO Q4h × 5 doses/d. Treat 10 d for first genital HSV infection, 5 d for recurrences. Topical Use: Apply oint. 5–6 ×/d Suppression: 200 mg PO QID for **max. dose** 6 months *Varicella Zoster:* 1500 mg/M^2/d admin. Q8h IV	Can cause renal impairment; adequate hydration essential to prevent renal tubular crystallization. Encephalopathic reactions have been reported. Dose alterations necessary in preterm infants and in patients with reduced creatinine clearance. May cause nausea, vomiting, diarrhea, headache, dizziness, arthralgia, fatigue, rash, insomnia, fever.
Amoxicillin (Amcill, Amoxil, Larotid, Trimox, Wymox, Utimox)	Drops: 50 mg/ml (15, 30 ml) Susp: 125, 250 mg/5 ml (80, 100, 150, 200 ml) Caps: 250, 500 mg Chewable Tabs: 125 mg	*Child:* 20–40 mg/kg/d admin. Q8h PO *Adult:* 250–500 mg/dose Q8h PO *Gonorrhea* (acute uncomplicated): ≤45 kg: 50 mg/kg/single PO dose with 25 mg/kg probenecid (**Max. dose:** 1 g probenecid) >45 kg: 3 gm as single PO dose with 1 gm probenecid	Renal elimination. Achieves serum levels about twice those achieved with equal dose of ampicillin. Fewer GI effects, but otherwise similar to ampicillin. Side effects: rash and diarrhea.
Amoxicillin-Clavulanic Acid (Augmentin)	Tabs: 125, 250 mg Chewable Tabs: 125, 250 mg Susp: 125, 250 mg/5 ml (31.25, 62.5 mg clavulanate) (75, 150 ml)	*Child:* 20–40 mg/kg/d as amoxicillin admin. Q8h PO *Adult:* 250–500 mg/dose Q8h PO **Max. dose:** 1.5 gm/d	Beta lactamase inhibitor extends the activity of amoxicillin to include beta-lactamase–producing strains of *H. influenzae, B. catarrhalis,* some *S. aureus.* Causes diarrhea more than amoxicillin.

*Modified from Greene MG. Drug doses. In: Johns Hopkins The Harriet Lane Handbook. 12th ed. St. Louis: C.V. Mosby, 1991.

†Suspensions are not commercially available; must be extemporaneously compounded by a pharmacist.

Drug	How Supplied	Dose and Route	Remarks
Ampicillin (Omnipen, Polycillin, Principen)	Drops: 100 mg/ml (20 ml) Susp: 125, 250 mg/5 ml (80, 100, 150, 200 ml) 500 mg/5 ml (100 ml) Caps: 250, 500 mg Injection: 125, 250, 500 mg; 1, 2 gm	*Neonate:* <7 days: 50–150 mg/kg/d admin. Q8h–12h >7 days: 75–200 mg/kg/d admin. Q6–8h IM or IV *Child:* Mild-moderate infections: 50–100 mg/kg/d admin. Q4–6h PO, IM or IV **Max. dose:** 2–4 gm/d Severe infections: 200–400 mg/kg/d admin. Q4–6h IM or IV (**Max. dose:** 10–12 gm/d) Uncomplicated gonorrhea: See Chapter 15.*	Use higher doses to treat CNS disease. Same side effects as penicillin, with cross-reactivity. Rash commonly seen at 5–10 days. May cause interstitial nephritis.
Aspirin (ASA, various trade names)	Tabs: 65, 75, 200, 300, 325, 500, 600, 650 mg Chewable Tabs: 65, 81 mg Caps: 325 mg Supp: 60, 120, 130, 195, 300, 325, 650, and 1.2 gm.	*Antipyretic:* 10–15 mg/kg/dose Q4h up to total 60–80 mg/kg/d (**Max. dose:** 3.6 gm/d) *Antirheumatic:* 60–100 mg/kg/d PO admin. Q4h *Kawasaki Disease:* 80–100 mg/kg/d PO admin. QID during febrile phase until defervesces × 36h then decrease to 5–10 mg/kg/d PO Q AM	Use with caution in platelet and bleeding disorders. Follow serum levels used as antirheumatic or with Kawasaki disease. May cause GI upset, allergic reactions, and liver toxicity. See Chapter 19 for management of overdose. **Therapeutic levels: 20–100 mg/L antipyretic/analgesic; 10–30 mg/dL antiinflammatory.**
Cefaclor (Ceclor) (2nd generation)	Caps: 250, 500 mg Susp: 125, 250 mg/5 ml (75 ml, 150 ml)	*Infant and Child:* 40 mg/kg/d admin. Q8h PO **Max. dose:** 2 gm/d *Adult:* 250–500 mg/dose Q8h PO **Max. dose:** 4 gm/d	Not recommended for infants <1 month old. Use with **caution** in patients with penicillin allergy or renal impairment. May cause positive Coombs or false positive test for urinary glucose.
Ciprofloxacin (Cipro)	Tabs: 250, 500, 750 mg	*Adults:* 250–750 mg/dose Q12h PO **Max. dose:** 2 gm/d	Like other quinolones, ciprofloxacin causes cartilage arthropathy in experimental animals. **Its use in children <16–18 y is *not* recommended.**
Clindamycin (Cleocin)	Caps: 75, 150, 300 mg Oral Liquid: 75 mg/5ml (100 ml) Injection: 150 mg/ml	*Neonates:* Preterm: 15 mg/kg/d admin. Q8h IV/IM Term: 20 mg/kg/d admin. Q6h IV/IM *Children:* 10–25 mg/kg/d admin. Q6–8h PO; 15–40 mg/kg/d admin. Q6–8h IM or IV *Adults:* 150–450 mg Q6h PO; 600–2700 mg/d admin. Q6–12h IM or IV **Max. dose:** 4 gm/d IV; 2 gm/d PO	Not indicated in meningitis. Use with caution in hepatic or renal insufficiency. Pseudomembranous colitis may occur up to several weeks after cessation of therapy but generally is uncommon in pediatric patients. May cause diarrhea, rash, Stevens-Johnson syndrome, granulocytopenia, thrombocytopenia, or sterile abscess at injection site.
Clotrimazole (Lotrimin, Mycelex)	Cream: 1% (15, 30, 45, 90 gm) Solution: 1% (10, 30 ml) Vaginal Tabs: 100, 500 mg Vaginal Cream: 1% (45, 90 gm) Oral Troche: 10 mg	*Topical:* apply to skin BID *Vaginal Candidiasis:* 1 tab per vaginal daily × 7 d *Thrush:* Dissolve one troche in the mouth 5 times/d	May cause erythema, blistering, or urticaria where applied.
Codeine (Various brands)	Tabs: 15, 30, 60 mg Inj: 15, 30, 60 mg/ml Oral Sol'n: 15 mg/5 ml Combination product with acetaminophen: Elixir: Acet 120 mg and codeine 12 mg/5 ml Tabs: (all contain 300 mg acetaminophen per tab) Tylenol #1–7.5 mg Codeine Tylenol #2–15 mg Codeine Tylenol #3–30 mg Codeine Tylenol #4–60 mg Codeine	*Analgesic:* Children: 0.5–1.0 mg/kg/dose Q4–6h IM, SC or PO Adults: 30–60 mg/dose Q4–6h IM, SC or PO *Antitussive:* Children (2–6 yrs): 1 mg/kg/d admin. QID; **Max. dose:** 30 mg/d Children (6–12 yrs): 5–10 mg/dose Q4–6h; **Max. dose:** 60 mg/d Adults: 15–30 mg/dose Q4–6; **Max. dose:** 120 mg/d	Side effects include CNS and respiratory depression, constipation, cramping. May be habit forming. For analgesia, use with acetaminophen orally. **Do not use in children <2 yr. Do not administer by IV route.**

Table continued on following page

Drug	How Supplied	Dose and Route	Remarks
Co-trimoxazole (Trimethoprim-sulfamethoxazole) (Bactrim, Septra, TMP-SMX)	Tabs (reg. strength): 80 mg TMP/400 mg SMX Tabs (double strength): 160 mg TMP/800 mg SMX Susp: 40 mg TMP/200 mg SMX per 5 ml Inj: 16 mg TMP/ml and 80 mg SMX/ml	**Doses based on TMP component.** *Minor infections:* (PO or IV): Child: 8–10 mg/kg/d admin. Q12h Adult (>40 kg): 160 mg/dose/Q12h *UTI prophylaxis:* 2 mg/kg/d QD *Severe infections and Pneumocystis carinii pneumonitis* (PO or IV): 20 mg/kg/d admin. Q6–8h *Pneumocystis prophylaxis:* 10 mg/kg/d/Q12h	Do not use in infants <2 months old. Available as a fixed combination of 5 mg of sulfamethoxazole to each 1 mg of trimethoprim. May cause kernicterus in newborns, blood dyscrasias, crystalluria, glossitis, renal or hepatic injury, GI irritation, allergy, or hemolysis in G6PD. Reduce dose in renal impairment.
Doxycycline (Vibramycin and other brand names)	Caps: 50, 100 mg Tabs: 50, 100 mg Syrup: 50 mg/5 ml (30 ml) Susp: 25 mg/5 ml (60 ml) Injection: 100, 200 mg	*Initial:* ≤45 kg: 5 mg/kg/d admin. BID PO or IV × 1 d to max. of 200 mg/d >45 kg: 200 mg/d admin. BID PO or IV × 1 d *Maintenance:* <45 kg: 2.5–5 mg/kg/d admin. QD-BID PO or IV >45 kg: 100–200 mg/d admin. QD-BID PO or IV **Max. adult dose:** 300 mg/d PID: see Chapter 15, p 249.*	Use with **caution** in hepatic and renal disease. May cause increased intracranial pressure. **Do not use in children <8 yr;** may result in tooth enamel hypoplasia and discoloration. May cause GI symptoms, photosensitivity, hemolytic anemia, hypersensitivity reactions. Infuse over 1–4 h IV. Avoid direct sunlight. See Tetracycline. Avoid use in pregnancy.
Erythromycin Preparations (Erythrocin, E-Mycin, EryPed, Pediamycin, and others)	*Erythromycin:* Caps: 125, 250 mg Tabs: 250, 333, 500 mg Topical Sol'n: 1.5%, 2% (60 ml) Ophth. Oint.: 0.5% (3.75 gm) *E. Ethyl Succinate (EES):* Susp: 200, 400 mg/5 ml (60, 100, 200 ml) Drops: 100 mg/2.5 ml (50 ml) Tabs: 200, 400 mg *Erythro, Lactobionate:* Inj: 500, 1000 mg *Erythromycin Estolate:* Tabs: 500 mg Chewable tabs: 125, 250 mg Drops: 100 mg/ml (10 ml) Caps: 125, 250 mg Susp: 125, 250 mg/5 ml *Erythromycin Stearate:* Tabs: 125, 250, 500 mg *Erythromycin Gluceptate:* Inj: 250, 500, 1000 mg	*Oral:* Children: 30–50 mg/kg/d admin. Q6–8h. **Max. dose:** 2 gm/d Adults: 1–4 gm/d admin. Q6h **Max. dose:** 4 gm/d *Parenteral:* Children: 20–50 mg/kg/d admin. Q6h IV or as continuous infusion. Adults: 15–20 mg/kg/d admin. Q6 IV or as continuous infusion. **Max. dose:** 4 gm/d *Rheumatic Fever Prophylaxis:* 500 mg/d admin. Q12h PO *Endocarditis Prophylaxis:* 20 mg/kg (**Max. dose:** 1 gm) PO 1h before **and** 10 mg/kg. (**Max. dose:** 4 gm) PO 6h after procedure *Ophthalmic:* Apply 0.5 inch ribbon to affected eye BID-QID *Pertussis:* Use estolate salt 50 mg/kg/d PO admin. Q6h	Avoid IM route (pain, necrosis). GI side effects common (nausea, vomiting, abdominal cramps). Give doses after meals. Use with **caution** in liver disease. Estolate may cause cholestatic jaundice, although hepatotoxicity is uncommon (2% of reported cases). May produce elevated digoxin, theophylline, carbamazepine, cyclosporine, methyl-prednisolone levels. Oral therapy should replace IV as soon as possible. Because of different absorption characteristics, higher oral doses of EES are needed to achieve therapeutic effects. **Note:** formulations other than the estolate have a high incidence of relapse in the treatment of pertussis.
Erythromycin Ethylsuccinate and Sulfisoxazole Acetyl (Pediazole)	Susp: 200 mg erythro and 600 mg sulfa/5 ml (100, 150, 200 ml)	*Otitis Media:* 50 mg/kg/d (as erythro) and 150 mg/kg/d (as sulfa) admin. Q6h PO **Max. dose:** 6 gm sulfisoxazole/d	See adverse effects of erythromycin and sulfisoxazole. **Not recommended in infants <2 months old.**
Fludrocortisone Acetate (Florinef, 9a-Fluoro-hydrocortisone)	Tabs: 0.1 mg	*Infants:* 0.1–0.2 mg/d QD PO *Children and Adults:* 0.05–0.1 mg/d QD PO Titrate dose to suppress plasma renin activity to normal levels	Preferably administered in conjunction with cortisone or hydrocortisone. Has primarily mineralocorticoid activity. If BP rises, decrease dose to 0.05 mg/24 h. 0.1 mg 9a-fluorocortisol = 1 mg DOCA. See Chapter 15, p 247.*

Drug	How Supplied	Dose and Route	Remarks
Gentamicin (Garamycin and others)	Inj: 10, 40 mg/ml Ophth. Oint.: 0.3% (3.5 gm) Drops: 0.3% (5 ml) Topical Ointment: 0.1% Intrathecal Inj: 2 mg/ml	*Parenteral* (IM or IV): Neonates*: <7 days: <28 wks: 2.5 mg/kg/dose Qd 28–34 wks: 2.5 mg/kg/dose Q18h Term: 2.5 mg/kg/dose Q12h >7 days: <28 wks: 2.5 mg/kg/dose 18h 28–34 wks: 2.5 mg/kg/dose Q12h Term: 2.5 mg/kg/dose/Q8h Children: 6–7.5 mg/kg/d admin. Q8h Adults: 3–5 mg/kg/d admin. Q8h **Max. dose:** 300 mg/d *Intrathecal/Intraventricular:* >3 mos: 1–2 mg daily Adults: 4–8 mg daily *Ophth. Oint:* apply Q6–8h *Ophth. Drops:* 1–2 gtts Q4h	Monitor levels (peak and trough). Monitor renal status; may cause proximal tubule dysfunction. Watch for ototoxicity. Intrathecal or intraventricular administration is adjunctive to parenteral administration. Arachnoiditis and phlebitis are uncommon. **Therapeutic levels: 6–10 mg/L (peak); <2 mg/L (trough).** Eliminated more quickly in patients with cystic fibrosis, multiple sclerosis, or neutropenia. **Neonatal doses are the same for gentamicin and tobramycin. Amikacin dose is 3 times higher.**
Ibuprofen (Motrin, Medipren, Pediaprofen)	Suspension: 100 mg/5 ml Tabs: 200, 300, 400, 600, 800 mg	*Children:* Antipyretic: 20 mg/kg/d admin. Q8h PO JRA: 30–70 mg/kg/d admin. 6h–8h PO *Adults:* 400 mg/dose Q4–6h PO **Max. adult dose:** 2.4 gm/d	Side effects include GI distress (lessened with milk), rashes, ocular problems. Inhibits platelet aggregation. Use **caution** with aspirin hypersensitivity, or hepatic or renal insufficiency.
Iron Preparations	*Ferrous Sulfate (20% Elemental Fe):* Drops (Fer-In-sol): 75 mg (15 mg Fe)/0.6 ml (50 ml) Syrup (Fer-In-sol): 90 mg (18 mg/Fe)/5 ml Elixir (Feosol): 220 mg (44 mg Fe)/5 ml (355 ml) Caps and Tabs: 195 mg (39 mg Fe) 300 mg (60 mg Fe) 325 mg (65 mg Fe) *Ferrous Gluconate (12% Elemental Fe):* Elixir: 300 mg (35 mg Fe)/5 ml Tabs: 320 mg (37 mg Fe), 325 mg (38 mg Fe) Sustained-release Caps: 435 mg (50 mg Fe) Caps: 325 mg (38 mg Fe)	*Iron Deficiency Anemia:* 3–6 mg elemental Fe/kg/d admin. TID PO *Prophylaxis:* Children: PO/QD–TID Premature: 2 mg elemental Fe/kg/d Full-term: 1–2 mg elemental Fe/kg/d **Max. dose:** 15 mg/d elemental Fe Adults: 60–100 mg elemental Fe/d PO/QD–BID	Iron preparations are variably absorbed. **Do not** use in hemolytic disorders. Less GI irritation when given with or after meals. Vitamin C 200 mg per 30 mg iron may enhance absorption. Liquid iron preparations may stain teeth. Administer with dropper or straw. May produce constipation, dark stools, nausea, and epigastric pain. Iron and tetracycline inhibit each others' absorption. Antacids may decrease iron absorption.
Magnesium Citrate	Solution: (300 mg) 5 ml = 4–4.7 mEq/mg	*Children:* 4 ml/kg/dose PO repeat Q4–6h until liquid stool results **Max. dose:** 200 ml *Adults:* 240 ml OD PO PRN	Use with caution in renal insufficiency. May cause hypermagnesemia, hypotension, respiratory depression; up to about 20% of dose is absorbed.
Meperidine HCl (Demerol)	Tabs: 50, 100 mg Elixir: 50 mg/5 ml Inj: 25, 50, 75, 100 mg/ml	*PO, IM, IV, and SC* Children: 1–1.5 mg/kg/dose Q3–4h PRN. **Max. dose:** 100 mg Adults: 50–150 mg/dose Q3–4h PRN	**Contraindicated** in cardiac arrhythmias, asthma, increased intracranial pressure. Potentiated by MAO inhibitors, phenothiazines, other CNS-acting agents, and isoniazid. Lower dose if IV. May cause nausea, vomiting, respiratory depression, smooth muscle spasm, constipation, and lethargy. **Caution** in renal failure; accumulated metabolite has CNS effects. **75 mg IV meperidine = 10 mg IV morphine.** *Table continued on following page*

Drug	How Supplied	Dose and Route	Remarks
Metronidazole (Flagyl)	Tabs: 250, 500 mg Suspension†: 100 mg/5 ml, or 50 mg/ml Injection: 500 mg or 50 mg/ml ready to use	*Amebiasis:* Children: 35–50 mg/kg/d PO admin. TID × 10 days Adults: 750 mg/dose PO TID × 5–10 days *Anaerobic Infection:* Neonates: Loading dose: 15 mg/kg IV Maintenance: Pre-term: 7.5 mg/kg/dose IV Q12h beginning 48h after loading dose Term: 7.5 mg/kg/dose IV Q12h beginning 24h after initial dose Infants, Children, and Adults: Loading dose: 15 mg/kg IV Maintenance: 7.5 mg/kg/dose Q6h IV or PO. **Max. dose:** 4 gm/d *Gardnerella vaginalis Vaginitis:* 500 mg PO BID × 7 d *Giardiasis:* Children: 15 mg/kg/d PO admin. TID × 10 d *Pelvic Inflammatory Disease:* 1 gm BID PO or IV *Trichomonas* or *Vaginitis:* Children: 15 mg/kg/d PO admin. TID × 7 d Adults: 250 mg/dose PO TID × 7 d or 2 gm PO × 1 *Clostridium difficile:* (Adult) 0.75–2 gm/d PO admin. TID–QID × 7–14 d	Side effects include nausea, diarrhea, urticaria, dry mouth, leukopenia, vertigo. Candidiasis may worsen. Pts should not ingest alcohol for 24 h after dose (disulfuram-type reaction). Potentiates anticoagulants. IV infusion must be given slowly over 1 h. Except for amebiasis, safe use of metronidazole in children <12 yr has not been established.
Morphine Sulfate	Oral Sol'n: 2, 4, 20 mg/ml (30, 120 ml) Tabs: 10, 15, 30 mg Sustained-Release Tabs: 30 mg Inj: †1, 2, 4, 5, 8, 10, 15 mg/ml	*Analgesia/Tetralogy (Cyanotic) Spells:* *Child:* 0.1–0.2 mg/kg/dose SC, IV or IM Q2–4h PRN. **Max. dose:** 15 mg/dose Adults: PO: 10–30 mg Q4h PRN IV: 2–15 mg dose Q2–6h PRN *Continuous IV:* 0.025–2 mg/kg/hr begin with lower dose and titrate to effect	Causes dependence. CNS and respiratory depression, nausea, vomiting, constipation, hypotension, bradycardia, increased intracranial pressure, biliary or urinary tract spasm, allergy may occur. IM/IV dose equal to 6 × PO dose. Naloxone may be used to reverse effects, especially respiratory depression.
Naloxone (Narcan)	Inj: 0.4, 1 mg/ml Neonatal Inj: 0.02 mg/ml	*Children:* 5–10 mcg/kg/dose IM or IV Repeat as necessary Q3–5 min *Adults:* 0.4–2.0 mg/dose Q2–3 min × 1–3. May give 10-fold higher dose if needed for diagnosis or therapy *Continuous Infusion:* After titrating initial dose to effectiveness, add 75–100% of last effective dose to 1h of maintenance IV fluid to run over 1h. May wean in 50% increments over next 6–12h. (May need to wean over as long as 48h for methadone.) If symptoms recur, rebolus at 100% of dose **Max. dose:** 2 mg	Does not cause respiratory depression. Short duration of action may necessitate multiple doses. For very large ingestions, 100–200 mcg/kg have been necessary. Will produce narcotic withdrawal syndrome in patients with chronic dependence. Use with **caution** in patients with chronic cardiac disease.

Drug	How Supplied	Dose and Route	Remarks
Penicillin G Preparations: Potassium and Sodium	Potassium Tabs: 250,000, 400,000, 500,000, 800,000 Units Solution: 200,000, 400,000 Units/5 ml (100, 200 ml) Injection: 0.2, 0.5, 1, 5, 10, 20 million Units Sodium Injection: 5 million U	*Newborn:* (IV or IM) ≤7 days: <2 kg: 50,000–100,000 U/ kg/d admin. Q12h >2 kg: 50,000–150,000 U/ kg d admin. Q8h >7 days: <2 gm 75,000–150,000 U/ kg/d admin. Q8h >2 kg: 100,000–200,000 U/kg/d admin. Q6h *Children:* IV or IM: 100,000–300,000 U/kg/d admin. Q4–6h PO: 40,000–80,000 U/kg/d admin. 6h *Adults:* IV or IM: 100,000–250,000 U/kg/d admin. Q4–6h PO: 300,000–1.2 mil U/d admin. Q6h	1 mg = approx 1600 units. Contains 1.7 mEq of Na or K per 1 million units. Penicillin G must be taken 1–2h before or 2h after meals. Side effects: anaphylaxis, hemolyic anemia, interstitial nephritis. T½ = 30 min, may be prolonged by concurrent use of probenecid. For meningitis use at shorter dosing intervals.
Benzathine (Permapen, Bicillin L-A)	Inj: 300,000, 600,000 U/ml	*Newborns:* 50,000 U/kg ×1 IM *Infants/Children:* 50,000 U/kg × 1 IM. **Max. dose:** 2.4 ml U *Adults:* 1.2 ml U × 1 IM *Rheumatic Fever Prophylaxis:* 600,000 U Q2 wks or 1.2 million U Q month IM	Provides sustained levels for 2–4 wks. Do **not** administer IV.
Procaine (Duracillin, Wycillin)	Inj: 300,000, 500,000, 600,000 U/ml	*Infants and Children:* 25,000–50,000 U/kg/d admin. Q12–24h IM **Max. dose:** 4.8 million U/d *Adults:* 600,000–1 mil U/d admin. Q12–24h IM	Provides sustained levels for 2–4 days. May cause sterile abscess at injection site. Contains 120 mg procaine/300,000 Units—this may cause allergic reactions, CNS stimulation, seizures. Use with **caution** in neonates. Do **not** use IV.
Bicillin C-R	Tubex: 300,000 U Pen G Procaine + 300,000 U Pen G Benzathine/ml, or 150,000 U Pen G Procaine + 450,000 U Pen G Benzathine/ml	*Acute Streptococcal Infections* <14 kg: 600,000 U × 1 IM 14–27 kg: 900,000–1.2 mil U × 1 IM >27 kg: 2.4 million U × 1 IM	Provides early peak levels in addition to prolonged levels of penicillin in the blood.
Penicillin V Potassium (Pen-Vee K, V-Cillin-K)	Tabs: 125 mg (200,000 U) 250 mg (400,000 U) 500 mg (800,000 U) Oral Sol'n: 125, 250 mg/5 mg (100, 200 ml)	*Children:* 25–30 mg/kg/d admin. Q6h **Max. dose:** 3 gm/d *Adults:* 250–500 mg/dose PO Q6h *Rheumatic Fever/ Pneumococcal Prophylaxis:* <5 yr: 125 mg PO BID >5 yr: 250 mg PO BID	GI absorption is better than penicillin G. **Note:** Must be taken 1 h before or 2 h after meals.

Table continued on following page

Drug	How Supplied	Dose and Route	Remarks
Tetracycline HCl (Many brand names: Achromycin, Aureomycin, Panmycin, Sumycin, Terramycin)	Tabs: 250, 500 mg Caps: 100, 250, 500 mg Suspension: 125 mg/5 ml (473 ml) Ophth. Oint: 0.5%, 1% (3.5 gm) Ophth. Susp: 1% (4 ml) Cream: 1% Oint: 3% (15, 30 gm) Inj: (IV) 250, 500 mg; (IM) 100, 250 mg with 40 mg procaine/vial	**Do not use in children <8 yrs.** *Older Children* (**Max. dose:** 2 gm/d) PO: 25–50 mg/kg/d admin. Q6h IM: 15–25 mg/kg/d admin. Q8–12h **Max. dose:** 250 mg/d IV: 20–30 mg/kg/d admin. Q8–12h *Adults:* (**Max. dose:** 2 gm/d) PO: 1–2 gm/d admin. Q6h IM: 250–300 mg/d admin. Q8–12h IV: 250–500 mg/dose Q6–12h *Chlamydia Genital Infections:* 500 mg Q6h PO (see Chapter 15, p 249*) *Ophth:* 2 drops into affected eye BID-QID	**Not** recommended in patients <8 yr due to tooth staining and decreasing bone growth. Also **not** recommended for use in pregnancy because these side effects may occur in the fetus. May cause nausea and GI upset, hepatoxicity, stomatitis, rash, photosensitivity, fever. **Do not give** with dairy products or with any divalent cations (i.e., Fe + +, Ca + +, Mg + +). Give 1 h before or 2 h after meals.
Vancomycin (Vancocin)	Inj: 500, 1000 mg Caps: 125, 250 mg Solution: 1, 10 gm (reconstitute to 500 mg/6 ml)	*Neonates:* <7 days: <1 kg: 10 mg/kg Q24h IV 1–2 kg: 10 mg/kg Q18h IV >2 kg: 10 mg/kg Q12h IV >7 days: <1 kg: 10 mg/kg Q18h IV 1–2 kg: 10 mg/kg Q12h IV >2 kg: 10 mg/kg Q8h IV Give 15 mg/kg/dose if CNS involved. *Infants and Children:* CNS: 15 mg/kg/dose Q8h IV Other: 10 mg/kg/dose Q8h IV *Adults:* 2 gm/d admin. Q6–12h IV Colitis: *Children:* 40–50 mg/kg/d admin. Q6h PO **Max. dose:** 2 gm/d Adults: 0.5–2 gm/d admin. Q6h PO	Ototoxicity, nephrotoxicity, allergy may occur. "Red man syndrome" associated with rapid IV infusion. Infuse over 60 minutes. **Note:** diphenhydramine is used to treat "red man syndrome". Therapeutic Levels: Peak 25–40 mcg/ml Trough <10 mcg/ml

Oral Contraceptives: Combination, Sequential, and Microdose Progestins

From Hatcher RA. Contraceptive Technology 1990–1992. 15th revised ed. New York: Irvington Publishers, 1990, pp 262–263.

Year Introduced	Product	Manufacturer	Type	Progestin	Estrogen	Color(s)**
1960	Enovid 10	Searle	Comb.	10 mg norethynodrel	150 mcg mestranol	Pink
1962	Enovid 5	Searle	Comb.	5 mg norethynodrel	75 mcg mestranol	Pink
1963	Ortho-Novum 10	Ortho	Comb.	10 mg norethindrone	60 mcg mestranol	Purple
	Ortho-Novum 2	Ortho	Comb.	2 mg norethindrone	100 mcg mestranol	White
1964	Enovid-E	Searle	Comb.	2.5 mg norethindrone	100 mcg mestranol	Pink
	Norlestrin*	Parke-Davis	Comb.	2.5 mg norethindrone acetate	50 mcg ethinyl estradiol	Pink
	Norinyl 2	Syntex	Comb.	2 mg norethindrone	100 mcg mestranol	White
1965	Provest (discontinued 1970)	Upjohn	Comb.	10 mg medroxyprogesterone	50 mcg ethinyl estradiol	
	C-Quens (discontinued 1970)	Lilly	Seq.	2 mg chlormadinone	80 mcg mestranol	
	Oracon (discontinued 1970)	Mead Johnson	Seq.	25 mg dimethisterone	100 mcg ethinyl estradiol	
1966	Ovulen	Searle	Comb.	1 mg ethynodiol diacetate	100 mcg mestranol	White, Pink
	Ortho-Novum SQ (discontinued 1970)	Ortho	Seq.	2 mg norethindrone	80 mcg mestranol	
1967	Norinyl 1 + 50	Syntex	Comb.	1 mg norethindrone	50 mcg mestranol	White, Orange
	Ortho-Novum 1/50	Ortho	Comb.	1 mg norethindrone	50 mcg mestranol	Yellow, Green
	Norlestrin*	Parke-Davis	Comb.	1 mg norethindrone acetate	50 mcg ethinyl estradiol	Yellow, White
	Norquens (discontinued 1970)	Syntex	Seq.	1 mg norethindrone	80 mcg mestranol	
1968	Ovral	Wyeth	Comb.	0.5 mg dl-norgestrel	50 mcg ethinyl estradiol	White, Pink
	Ortho-Novum 1/80	Ortho	Comb.	1 mg norethindrone	80 mcg mestranol	White, Green
	Norinyl 1 + 80	Syntex	Comb.	1 mg norethindrone	80 mcg mestranol	Yellow, Orange
1970	Demulen	Searle	Comb.	1 mg ethynodiol diacetate	50 mcg ethinyl estradiol	White, Pink
1973	Micronor	Ortho	Prog.	0.35 mg norethindrone		Green
	Nor-Q.D.	Syntex	Prog.	0.35 mg norethindrone		Yellow
	Ovrette	Wyeth	Prog.	0.075 mg dl-norgestrel		Yellow
	Loestrin 1.5/30*	Parke-Davis	Comb.	1.5 mg norethindrone acetate	30 mcg ethinyl estradiol	Green*
	Loestrin 1/20*	Parke-Davis	Comb.	1 mg norethindrone acetate	20 mcg ethinyl estradiol	White*
1974	Zorane 1 + 20 (discontinued 1979)	Lederle	Comb.	1 mg norethindrone	20 mcg ethinyl estradiol	
	Zorane 1 + 50 (discontinued 1979)	Lederle	Comb.	1 mg norethindrone	50 mcg ethinyl estradiol	
	Zorane 1.5 + 30 (discontinued 1979)	Lederle	Comb.	1.5 mg norethindrone	30 mcg ethinyl estradiol	
1975	Lo/Ovral	Wyeth	Comb.	0.3 mg dl-norgestrel	30 mcg ethinyl estradiol	White, Pink
	Brevicon	Syntex	Comb.	0.5 mg norethindrone	35 mcg ethinyl estradiol	Blue, Orange
	Modicon	Ortho	Comb.	0.5 mg norethindrone	35 mcg ethinyl estradiol	White, Green
1976	Ovcon-35	Mead Johnson	Comb.	0.4 mg norethindrone	35 mcg ethinyl estradiol	Peach, Green
	Ovcon-50	Mead Johnson	Comb.	1 mg norethindrone	50 mcg ethinyl estradiol	Yellow, Green
1977	Loestrin Fe 1/20	Parke-Davis	Comb.	1 mg norethindrone acetate	20 mcg ethinyl estradiol	White, Brown*
	Loestrin Fe 1.5/30	Parke-Davis	Comb.	1.5 mg norethindrone acetate	35 mcg ethinyl estradiol	Green, Brown*
1980	Norinyl 1 + 35	Syntex	Comb.	1 mg norethindrone	35 mcg ethinyl estradiol	Green, Orange
	Ortho-Novum 1/35	Ortho	Comb.	1 mg norethindrone	35 mcg ethinyl estradiol	Orange, Green
1981	Demulen 35	Searle	Comb.	1 mg ethynodiol diacetate	35 mcg ethinyl estradiol	White, Blue
1982	Ortho-Novum 10/11	Ortho	Comb.	.5 mg norethindrone (days 1–10)	35 mcg ethinyl estradiol	White, Peach, Green
			Biphasic	1 mg norethindrone (days 11–21)	(all 21 days)	
	Nordette (Levlen - 1987)	Wyeth (Berlex)	Comb.	.15 mg levo-norgestrel	30 mcg ethinyl estradiol	Peach, Pink
1984	Ortho-Novum 7-7-7	Ortho	Comb.	.5 mg norethindrone (days 1–7)	35 mcg ethinyl estradiol	White
				.75 mg norethindrone (days 8–14)	(all 21 days)	Light Peach
				1.0 mg norethindrone (days 15–21)		Peach, Green
	Tri-Norinyl	Syntex	Comb.	0.5 mg norethindrone (days 1–7)	35 mcg ethinyl estradiol	Blue
				1.0 mg norethindrone (days 8–16)	(all days)	Green
				0.5 mg norethindrone (days 17–21)		Blue, Orange
	Triphasil (Tri-Levlen - 1986)	Wyeth (Berlex)	Comb.	0.05 mg levo-norgestrel (days 1–6)	30 mcg ethinyl estradiol	Brown
				0.075 mg levo-norgestrel (days 7–11)	40 mcg ethinyl estradiol	White
				0.125 mg levo-norgestrel (days 12–21)	30 mcg ethinyl estradiol	Yellow, Green

*Also available with 75 mg ferrous fumarate; pills are brown when they contain iron.
**Colors are presented for currently available OCs.

Index

Note: Numbers with an *i* indicate illustrations; those with a *t* indicate tables.

Abbe, Robert, 543
Abdominal pain. *See also* Pelvic pain.
  acute, 636–637
  endoscopy for, 244–245
  from psychogenic disorders, 246
  history for, 246–247
  recurrent, 234, 235t
  treatment of, 247–248
  trigger points for, 246
Abdominal wall, defects of, 617–619, 618i–620i
Abortion(s), consent to, 505–506
  legal aspects of, 501–503
  number of, 300t
Abscess, brain, 55t
  breast, 590–591
  tubo-ovarian, 462–463, 463i, 518
Absorptiometry, 131
Abuse. *See specific type, e.g.,* Child abuse; Sexual abuse.
Acanthosis nigricans, 212
Accidents. *See* Injury(ies).
Acetaminophen, 682t
Acetic acid, 239t
Achondroplasia, 25
Achromycin, 687t
Acne vulgaris, 70, 258, 258t, 270
  treatment for, 273
ACOG (American College of Obstetricians and
    Gynecologists), 3
Acquired immunodeficiency syndrome (AIDS), 356–359. *See
    also* Human immunodeficiency virus (HIV) *and* Sexually
    transmitted diseases (STDs).
  condoms and, 294–295
  cultural factors in, 280
  demographics of, 357t
  education about, 286–287, 358
  incidence of, 357t
  infants with, 358
  sexual abuse and, 329t, 329–330, 330t
  symptoms of, 358i, 358–359, 359i
  transmission of, 329–330
Acrodermatitis enteropathica, 209–210, 210i
Acromegaly, 57, 142t
ACTH. *See* Adrenocorticotropic hormone (ACTH).

Acupuncture, 239
Acyclovir, 327, 349, 682t
Adenitis, 233t
Adenocarcinoma, cervical, 603–604, 605i
  clear-cell, 227, 463–464, 464i
  diethylstilbestrol and, 601, 603
  renal cell, 578
Adenomyosis, 238t
Adjustment disorder, 418–420. *See also* Personality disorders
    and Depression.
Adnexal neoplasms, 220
Adnexal torsion, 461i, 649–650
Adrenal glands, hyperandrogenism and, 70, 263–264
  steroid biosynthesis and, 252i–254i, 252–254
  tumors of, 263–264
Adrenal hormones, 37–38, 40, 42
Adrenal hyperplasia, congenital. *See* Congenital adrenal
    hyperplasia (CAH).
Adrenal tumor, 60
Adrenarche, exaggerated, 260–261
  premature, 61t, 259–260, 260t
Adrenocorticotropic hormone (ACTH), 86–88
  eating disorders and, 403–404
  21-hydroxylase deficiency and, 262–263, 263i
  steroidogenic response to, 253i
Affective disorders. *See* Depression.
Agonadia, 95
AIDS. *See* Acquired immunodeficiency syndrome (AIDS).
AIDS-related complex (ARC), 356, 358. *See also* Human
    immunodeficiency virus (HIV).
Alcoholics Anonymous, 434, 438–440
  Twelve Steps of, 438t
Alcoholism. *See also* Substance abuse.
  depression and, 420, 422, 425
  suicide and, 434–435
  treatment of, 438t, 438–440
Alopecia, from hyperandrogenism, 258
  of pubic hair, 210, 212
Altchek, Albert, 2
Amastia, 585i. *See also* Breast(s).
Amcil, 682t
Amenorrhea. *See also* Dysmenorrhea *and* Menstruation.
  after irradiation, 472–475

Amenorrhea *(Continued)*
  causes of, 69–70
  contraception and, 487–488
  diet and, 482, 485i, 486i
  eating disorders and, 400
  exercise-induced, 480i, 480–481, 481i, 485i
  from estrogen therapy, 121
  hypothalamic, 68, 486i
  primary, 515i
  secondary, 228t, 487–488, 517i, 517–518, 518i, 539
American College of Obstetricians and Gynecologists
  (ACOG), 3
AMH (antimüllerian hormone), 78, 92
Amnion vaginoplasty, 549–550
Amoxicillin, 682t
Amphetamines, 435–436. *See also* Substance abuse.
Ampicillin, 683t
Androgen(s), 250–274
  action of, 256–258, 257i
  assays for, 659–660
  biosynthesis of, 250–252, 251i, 252i
  blood levels of, 256, 257t
  endogenous production of, 562
  excess of. *See* Hyperandrogenism.
  exogenous production of, 562
  growth control and, 37
  puberty and, 31t, 69
  regulation of, 252–256, 253i–255i
  short stature and, 40
  transport of, 256
Androgen insensitivity syndrome, 115–117, 116i, 561–564,
  564t
  delayed puberty and, 65t
  management of, 118i, 118–119
Androgen-binding gene, 93i
Androgen-binding receptor, 117i
Androstenedione, 677t
Anemia, 513, 514i
Anorexia nervosa, 397–399. *See also* Eating disorders.
  delayed puberty and, 65t, 67
  exercise and, 400, 486i, 487
  hypothalamic-pituitary-adrenal axis in, 403–404
  hypothalamic-pituitary-gonadal axis in, 400–401
  osteoporosis and, 408–409
  pregnancy and, 408
  treatment for, 410, 412–413
Anovulation, breast cancer and, 592
  dysfunctional uterine bleeding and, 227, 496
Anthropometry, 132
Antidepressants, 422, 438
  for eating disorders, 412
  for enuresis, 577
Antimüllerian hormone (AMH), 78, 92
Antisocial personality disorder, 424. *See also* Personality
  disorders.
Anus, fissures of, 374i
  injuries to, 530i, 530–531
    sexual abuse and, 372–374, 373t, 374t
    surgery for, 377
  perineal, 630–632, 631i, 632i
Aphthous ulcers, 213–214, 213t, 214i
Appendices vesiculosae, 9t, 10, 11i, 12i
Appendicitis, 233t
Arachidonic acid, 237i, 238i
Arrhenoblastoma, 518, 519i
Art therapy. *See* Expressive therapy.
Arthritis, 291t
Asherman's syndrome, 517

L-Asparaginase, 142t
Aspirator, vaginal, 183–184, 184i
Aspirin, 683t
Augmentin, 682t
Aureomycin, 687t
Avicenna, 543

Bacteriophages, 151–152
Bacteriuria, 567–568
Bactrim, 684t
Balbiani's vitelline body, 7, 8i
Bartholinitis, 338i
Bartholin's gland, 219, 220
Basal metabolic rate, 137
Battery, sexual, 381
Behçet's syndrome, 213, 213t
Bellotti v. Baird, 505
Bicillin, 687t
Binge eating, 403. *See also* Bulimia nervosa.
Biology, molecular, 151–161
Biosynthetic pathways, 86i
Blackouts, 433
Bladder. *See also* Urinary *entries.*
  embryology of, 12i
  homologies of, 9t
  "lazy," 578
  neurogenic dysfunction of, 574–575
BMI. *See* Body mass index (BMI).
Body composition. *See also* Lean body mass (LBM) *and*
  Weight.
  estimating of, 131–133, 134i, 134t
  exercise and, 481i, 482i
Body mass index (BMI), 129, 130i, 133, 134i, 134t
Bone, age of, 26–27
  assessment of, 410
  development of, 468–472, 469i
  physiology of, 409
Borderline personality disorder, 424, 426–427
Bowel, abnormalities of, 630–632, 631i, 632i
  inflammatory disease of, 65t, 67, 107, 244. *See also*
    Crohn's disease.
  obstruction of, 622–623
Bowlby, John, 417
Brachio-skeletal-genital syndrome, 90
Breast(s), 589i, 589–591, 590i. *See also* Nipple(s) *and*
  Thelarche.
  anomalies of, 584–585, 585i
  atrophy of, 590
  cyst of, 585, 591
  development of, 28i, 29i, 29t, 585–588, 586i, 586t, 587t,
    589i
  diseases of, 583–599, 591t
  during puberty, 588–589
  examination of, 583–584
  fibrocystic disease of, 591t, 592, 592i
  galactorrhea in, 591, 594
  hemangioma of, 585
  hypertrophy of, 590i
  infection of, 585
  malignancies in, 592–593, 593i
  mass in, 591–595
    evaluation of, 593–595, 594t
    imaging of, 595–598, 596i–599i
    unilateral, 585–586, 586i, 586t
  pain in, 590
  self-examination of, 584, 598–599

Breast(s) *(Continued)*
tuberous, 589i, 589–590
Bryans, Fred, 2
Bubo, from lymphogranuloma, 342i
Bulbourethral glands, 9t
Bulimia nervosa, 398–399. *See also* Eating Disorders.
exercise and, 486i, 487
hypothalamic-pituitary-adrenal axis in, 403–404
hypothalamic-pituitary-gonadal axis in, 401–403, 402i
premenstrual exacerbation of, 403
treatment for, 412–413
Bullous diseases, 214–220
chronic, 215–216, 216i
genital, 533t
vulvar, 214–220, 215i–216i, 215t, 217t, 218i–219i
Bullous pemphigoid, vulvar, 215t, 216

CAH. *See* Congenital adrenal hyperplasia (CAH).
Calcium channel blockers, 240
California laws, on medical consent, 503–504
Cancer therapy, delayed effects of, 467–476, 468t, 469i–476i
fertility after, 475
for dysgerminoma, 606–607, 607t
for rhabdomyosarcoma, 601–603, 602i, 603t, 605t
gonadal function after, 472–475, 473i
pregnancy after, 475
psychosocial factors of, 476
survival rates of, 468i, 468t, 470i
Candidiasis, diaper rash from, 208
oral, 358i
vulvovaginal, adolescents with, 198–200, 199i
children with, 193i, 193–194
symptoms of, 189t, 191
Capraro, Vincent, 2
Carboxylic acid, 239t
Carcinoma. *See also* Neoplasm(s).
breast, 592–593, 593i. *See also* Breast(s), mass in.
embryonal, 609i
endodermal, 226
mesonephric, 226–227
squamous cell, 220
vaginal, 225–227, 226i
Carey v. Population Services, 505
Carrington, Elsie, 1
Caruncles, urethral, 533t
Castration, 520, 522i
CBDC (chronic bullous disease of childhood), 215–216, 215t, 216i. *See also* Bullous diseases.
CCP (childhood cicatricial pemphigoid), 214t, 215–216
CDH (congenital diaphragmatic hernia), 619–621, 620i
Ceclor, 683t
Cefaclor, 683t
Celsus, Aulus Cornelius, 543
Centrioles, germ cell, 6, 7i
Cervical cap, 295
Cervicitis, mucopurulent, 341i
uterine bleeding and, 229t
Cervix, adenocarcinoma of, 603–604, 605i
agenesis of, 446, 448i, 639i
atresia of, 541–542
cancer of, 187, 194
chancre in, 345i
imaging of, 444–445
polyp in, 229t
rhabdomyosarcoma of, 604i
stenosis of, 238t, 639i

Cervix *(Continued)*
teratoma of, 623
tuberculosis of, 515
Chancre, 345i
Chemotherapy. *See* Cancer therapy.
Child abuse. *See also* Sexual abuse.
among teen parents, 300
forensics of, 657t
legal aspects of, 508, 510
prevention of, 657
Child protection laws, 365
Childhood cicatricial pemphigoid (CCP), 215t, 216
Chlamydial infection. *See also* Sexually transmitted diseases (STDs).
adolescent, 340–342, 341i, 342i
diagnosis of, 341
incidence of, 337, 340
symptoms of, 340
treatment for, 341–342
prepubertal, 316–320
demographics of, 316–317
diagnosis of, 319
presentation of, 317–318
transmission of, 318–319, 330
treatment for, 319–320
Chloride deficiency, 128
Cholesterol, steroid biosynthesis and, 251i, 252i
Cholesterol desmolase, 112t–113t, 114
Choriocarcinoma, 611i
Chorionic villus sampling, 557
Chronic bullous disease of childhood (CBDC), 215–216, 215t, 216i. *See also* Bullous diseases.
Ciprofloxacin, 683t
Circumcision, female, 518–520, 520i, 525
Cirrhosis, 229t
Cleocin, 683t
Clindamycin, 683t
Cliteromegaly, 70
Clitoris, 9t
Clitoroplasty, 559, 560i
Cloacal abnormalities, 633i, 633–634, 634i
Clofibrate, 142t
Clotrimazole, 683t
Coagulopathy, 229t
Cocaine, 435–436
Codeine, 683t
Colitis, ulcerative, 107, 233t, 244
Colorado laws, on child abuse, 508
on medical consent, 504
Columbo, Matteo Realdo, 543
Computed tomography (CT), 442. *See also* Diagnostic imaging.
for breast mass, 597–598, 599i
future trends in, 661t
Condoms, female, 296, 662
male, 294–295, 295t
periodic use of, 360
Conduct disorder, 425–426
Condyloma acuminatum, 321–326, 330t
demographics of, 321
diagnosis of, 323–324
presentation of, 321–322
transmission of, 322–323, 330t
treatment of, 324–326
vulvar, 209i, 220
Condyloma latum, 346i
Confidentiality, 501, 506–510. *See also* Legal issues.

Congenital adrenal hyperplasia (CAH), 59–60, 86–89, 91, 111–115, 557–562
  delayed puberty and, 65t
  diagnosis of, 557–559
  fertility and, 559–562
  precocious puberty and, 55t
  surgery for, 559–562, 560i–562i
  treatment for, 272
  virilizing, 261–263, 263i
Congenital anomalies. *See also specific organs, e.g., Vagina, agenesis of.*
  surgery for, 616–626
  teen pregnancies and, 304–305
Congenital diaphragmatic hernia (CDH), 619–621, 620i
Conjunctivitis, gonococcal, 315
Consent. *See also* Legal issues.
  parental, 500
  patient, 500–501
  to abortion, 505–506
  to contraception, 505
  to medical care, 500–501, 503–506
Constipation, 243, 574
Contamin, Robert, 2
Contraception, 289–298, 337i, 662
  art therapy and, 392
  athletes and, 487–488
  choice of, 290t
  condoms for, 294–295, 295t
  consent to, 505
  counseling for, 290–291
  for developmentally disabled, 496–497, 497t
  psychological factors of, 438
Contraceptives, oral, 690t
  contraindications to, 291t
  delayed puberty and, 71–73
  diabetes mellitus and, 291
  drug interactions with, 294t
  dysmenorrhea and, 239
  for developmentally disabled, 496, 497
  for uterine bleeding, 272–273
  genital tract infections and, 351
  health benefits of, 291t
  migraines and, 291
  osteoporosis and, 73
  side effects of, 293t, 293–294
  smoking and, 291
  thyroxine-binding globulin and, 142t
Corpora lutea, 458i
Corpus cavernosum clitoridis, 9t
Corpus cavernosum penis, 9t
Cortisol biosynthesis, disorders of, 111i, 111–115, 112t–113t
  treatment for, 114–115
  exercise and, 484i
Co-trimoxazole, 684t
Cowell, Carol, 2
Crack cocaine, 337, 361, 435–436. *See also* Substance abuse.
Craniopharyngioma, 55t, 65t
Creatinine clearance, 677t
Cretinism, 146–147
Crohn's disease. *See also* Inflammatory bowel disease.
  pelvic pain from, 244
  perianal abnormalities in, 374
  Turner syndrome and, 107
  vulvar disorders from, 210, 211i
CT. *See* Computed tomography (CT).
Cushing's disease, 40, 65t
Cushing's syndrome, 57, 65t
Cyst(s), arachnoid, 55t

Cyst(s) *(Continued)*
  breast, 585, 591
  follicular, 456–458, 457i–459i
  Gartner's duct, 455i
  hymenal, 455
  lutein, 456–458, 457i–459i
  mesosalpingeal, 458i
  ovarian, 455, 473i, 623–624. *See also* Polycystic ovary (PCO) syndrome.
    dysmenorrhea from, 238t
    fetal, 651i, 651–652
    oral contraceptives and, 291t
    pelvic pain from, 233t, 242
    precocious puberty and, 55t, 57
    prenatal diagnosis of, 623–624
  periurethral, 179i
  prenatal diagnosis of, 623
  suprasellar, 55t
  ultrasonography for, 596–598, 597i, 598i
  vaginal, 455i
  vulvar, 219
Cystadenoma, 465i. *See also* Neoplasm(s).
Cystic fibrosis, 65t, 67
Cystic hydroma, 623
Cystic teratoma, 455–456, 456i, 457i
Cystitis, 568
  pelvic pain from, 233t
  symptoms of, 568t
Cystosarcoma phylloides, 592
Cystourethrogram, 569
Cytomegalovirus, 21, 348
Cytotoxic drugs, hair loss with, 212

Darier's disease, 210, 215
Davydov's operation, 550, 551i, 552i
DDC (dideoxcytidine), 359
DDI (dideoxyinosine), 359
Dehydroepiandrosterone sulfate (DHEA), 88
  during puberty, 30t, 31t, 254i
  laboratory values for, 677t
  precocious puberty and, 60
Dehydroepiandrosterone sulfate (DHEAS), 677t
3β-ol-Dehydrogenase deficiency, 88, 91
Dementia, AIDS-related, 358
Demerol, 685t
Deoxyribonucleic acid (DNA), duplexes of, 154
  extraction of, 159
  "fingerprinting" with, 155–156, 156i, 157i, 159
  probes for, 152–153
  recombinant, 151–154, 159
  satellite, 155–156, 156i
  sequencing of, 155i
  storage of, 159t, 159–160
Depo-medroxyprogesterone acetate (DMPA), 496–497, 497t
Depression. *See also* Antidepressants, Dysthymia, *and* Suicide.
  abdominal pain from, 247
  adolescent, 422–427
    etiology of, 424
    indicators of, 422–423
    treatment for, 423–424, 427
  among developmentally disabled, 498
  anaclitic, 417, 419
  borderline personality with, 426–427
  childhood, 417–422
    etiology of, 420–421

Depression *(Continued)*
    indicators of, 417–419, 418t
    treatment for, 421–422
    types of, 418t, 418–419
  eating disorders and, 412
  from sexual abuse, 378
  substance abuse and, 420, 422, 425
  vaginal atresia and, 544
Dermatitis, 533t
  diaper, 205i
  perianal, 240
  seborrheic, 205i, 216
Dermatitis herpetiformis, 214t, 215, 215i
Dermatoses, vulvar, 217t
DES. *See* Diethylstilbestrol (DES).
17,20-Desmolase deficiency, 91–92
Developmentally disabled, contraception for, 496–497, 497t
  gynecologic examination for, 493t, 493–494
  health needs of, 492t, 492–498, 493t, 497t
  menstruation and, 494–496
  nutrition and, 492
  prevalence of, 490t, 491t
  seizures among, 492
  sexual abuse of, 497–498
  sexuality of, 494t, 495i
  sterilization of, 297–298, 494, 496t, 497, 509
  urologic problems in, 581
Dewhurst, John, 2
DGI (disseminated gonococcal infection), 338–339, 339i. *See also* Gonorrhea.
DHEA. *See* Dehydroepiandrosterone (DHEA).
Diabetes insipidus, 66–67
Diabetes mellitus, delayed puberty and, 65t, 67
  fetal growth and, 20
  oral contraceptives and, 291
Diagnostic imaging, 441–465. *See also specific types, e.g.,* Ultrasonography (USG).
  for urinary tract infections, 569
  future trends in, 660–661, 661t
  of benign disease, 455i–463i, 455–463
  of breast mass, 595–598, 596i–599i
  of cervix, 444–446, 448i
  of congenital abnormalities, 445–455, 446i–454i
  of endometrium, 444i, 445i
  of hydrocolpos, 445–446, 446i
  of hymen, 446, 447i
  of malignancies, 463–465, 464i, 465i
  of myometrium, 443–444
  of ovary, 445i
  of pelvis, 441–445, 443i–445i
  of pubertal disorders, 460–462, 462i
  of uterine agenesis, 446–449, 448i–450i
  of uterus, 443i–445i
  of vagina, 445
  of vaginal agenesis, 446–449, 448i–450i
  of vaginal septum, 446, 447i
Diagnostic tests, 659–660, 677t–680t
Diaper rash, 205i, 205–206, 206i
  from candidiasis, 208
  sexual abuse vs., 369i
  treatment for, 206i, 206–208, 207i
Diaphragm, contraceptive, 295t
Dideoxcytidine (DDC), 359
Dideoxyinosine (DDI), 359
Diet. *See also* Nutrition.
  exercise and, 482, 485i, 486i, 487
  fad, 138
Diethylstilbestrol (DES), 539, 601, 603

Dihydrotestosterone, 677t
Dimercaptosuccinic acid, 569
Disseminated gonococcal infection (DGI), 338–339, 339i. *See also* Gonorrhea.
DMPA (depo-medroxyprogesterone acetate), 496–497, 497t
DNA. *See* Deoxyribonucleic acid (DNA).
Döderlein's bacillus, 16–17
Dot blots, 154, 160
Down syndrome, growth chart for, 25
  hypothyroidism and, 25
  short stature and, 40
Doxycycline, 684t
Drash's syndrome, 90
Drugs, 682t–688t. *See also specific types, e.g.,* Amphetamines.
  abuse of, 432–440. *See also* Substance abuse.
  cancer. *See* Cancer therapy.
  cytotoxic, hair loss with, 212
  designer, 435–436
  future trends in use of, 661–662
  screening tests for, 437–438
DUB. *See* Dysfunctional uterine bleeding (DUB).
Ductus deferens, 9t
Duodenitis, 244–245
Dupuytren, Guillaume, 543
Duracillin, 687t
Dwarfism. *See also* Stature, short.
  camptomelic, 86
  pituitary, 97–98
Dysfunctional uterine bleeding (DUB), 227–231
  diagnosis of, 228–229, 229t
  evaluation of, 229t, 229–230
  treatment for, 230t, 230–231
Dysgerminoma, 464i. *See also* Neoplasm(s).
  ovarian, 605–607, 606i, 607t
  precocious puberty and, 55t
Dysmenorrhea, 235–241, 473–475. *See also* Amenorrhea *and* Menstruation.
  causes of, 235t, 238t
  diagnosis of, 237–238
  from uterine horn, 539, 540i
  history of, 236–237
  incidence of, 235–236, 236t
  oral contraceptives and, 291t
  pathogenesis of, 236–237
  prostaglandins and, 236–237, 237i, 238i
  severity of, 235–236, 236t
  treatment of, 238–241, 239t, 240t
  uterine anomalies and, 539
Dyspareunia, 285, 285t
Dysthymia. *See also* Depression.
  adolescent, 422, 423
  childhood, 418t
  conduct disorder with, 425–426
Dysuria, 580–581

Eating disorders, 397–413. *See also specific types, e.g.,* Anorexia nervosa.
  amenorrhea in, 400
  body composition and, 404–407, 405t, 406t
  hypothalamic-pituitary-adrenal axis in, 403–404
  hypothalamic-pituitary-thyroid axis in, 403
  infertility and, 407–408
  menstruation and, 400–403, 402i
  osteoporosis and, 408–411
  ovarian changes in, 407
  overexercise and, 400

Eating disorders *(Continued)*
  pregnancy and, 408
  purging and, 400
  sexual abuse and, 411–412
  treatment for, 410, 412–413
  uterine changes in, 407
Ectodermal anomalies, 86
Eczema, vulvar, 216–217
Ejaculation, premature, 284
Emans, S. Jean, 2
Embryology, 6–16, 7i–15i, 9t, 14t, 163–164
E-Mycin, 684t
Encephalitis, 55t
Endodermal sinus tumor, 607i, 607–609, 608t
Endometrial cancer, 291t
Endometrial shedding, 227t
Endometrioma, 459i
Endometriosis, 458–459, 459i, 637–644, 639i–642i, 641t, 643t
  development of, 637–638
  diagnosis of, 638–644, 641i, 642i
  dysmenorrhea from, 238, 238t
  pelvic pain from, 241–242
  symptoms of, 638, 641t
  uterine bleeding and, 229t
Endometrium, hyperplasia of, 463i
  imaging of, 444i, 445i
Endoscopy, 644i–651i, 644–652. *See also* Diagnostic imaging.
  for adnexal torsion, 649–650
  for ectopic pregnancy, 645–647
  for intraabdominal testes, 651i
  for ovarian cysts, 651–652
  for ovarian surgery, 647–649, 649i
  for pelvic inflammatory disease, 649
  for vaginal agenesis, 650–651
  new applications for, 661
Enolic acid, 239t
Enteritis, regional, 233t
Enterobius pruritus, 208
Enuresis. *See also* Incontinence.
  nocturnal, 575t, 575–577
    etiology of, 576
    evaluation of, 576
    treatment for, 576–577
Enzymes, restriction, 151–152
Ependymoma, 55t
Epidermolysis bullosa, 214i, 214t
Epididymis, 9t
Epilepsy, 245–246
Epithelium, coelomic, 6, 7i, 8
  tumors of, 220
Epoöphorantic duct, 9t
Epoöphoron, 9t, 11i, 12i
Epstein-Barr virus, 348
Erythromycin, 684t
Esophageal-facial-genital syndrome, 90
Esophagus, abnormalities of, 622i
  atresia of, 621i, 621–622, 622i
  inflammation of, 244–245
Estradiol, 119–120, 120t
  during puberty, 30i, 30t
  eating disorders and, 399
  laboratory values for, 678t
Estriol, 678t
Estrogen status, 177
Estrogen therapy, 71, 119–121, 120t
Estrogens, 292t
  during puberty, 30i, 30–31
  growth control and, 37

Estrogens *(Continued)*
  laboratory values for, 678t
  thyroxine-binding globulin and, 142t
Estropipate, 120t
''Euthyroid sick syndrome,'' 399, 403
Ewing's sarcoma, survival rate with, 469i
Exercise, body composition and, 481i, 482i
  bone density and, 409
  diet and, 482, 485i, 486i, 487
  hormonal changes with, 484i
  nutrition and, 658–659
  osteoporosis and, 485–486
  reproductive problems from, 478–488, 479i–486i
  stress of, 482–484, 483i, 485i, 486i
  weight loss from, 137
Expressive therapy, 383–394, 385i–395i
  applications of, 391–392
  contraception and, 392
  depression and, 421–422
  graphic development in, 389–391
  history of, 374
  human figure drawing in, 384–389, 385i–388i
  kinetic family drawing in, 389, 389i–391i

Fallopian tubes, 19t
  blocked, 518i
  tuberculous, 516
Fanconi's anemia, 229
Fédération Internationale de Gynécologie Infantile et Juvénile (FIGIJ), 2
Feminization, testicular, 92i, 92–94, 93i, 94i
Fenamic acid, 239t
Fertility. *See also* In vitro fertilization.
  after cancer therapy, 475
  congenital adrenal hyperplasia and, 559–562
  eating disorders and, 407–408
  hypogonadism and, 121–122
  müllerian anomalies and, 643t
  tuberculosis and, 515
  vaginal atresia and, 544
Fetal surgery, 625–626
Fibroadenoma, breast, 591t, 591–592
  ultrasonogram of, 598i
  unilateral, 585–586, 586i, 586t
Fibrocystic disease, 591t, 592, 592i
FIGIJ (Fédération Internationale de Gynécologie Infantile et Juvénile), 2
Fine needle aspiration, 592, 595
Fissure, perianal, 374i
Fistula, rectovaginal, 630–633, 631i, 632i
Fitz-Hugh-Curtis syndrome, 343
Flagyl, 686t
Florida laws, on medical consent, 504
Fludrocortisone (Florinef), 114, 684t
Fludrocortisone acetate, 684t
9α-Fluorohydrocortisone, 684t
5-Fluorouracil, 142t
Fluoxetine, 412
Follicle-stimulating hormone (FSH), androgens and, 254–256, 255i
  circadian variation in, 48–49, 49i
  deficiency of, 97
  during puberty, 29–30, 30i, 30t, 31
  eating disorders and, 399
  laboratory values for, 678t
  levels of, age and, 46i, 47i

Follicle-stimulating hormone (FSH) *(Continued)*
  midcycle surge of, 51
  precocious puberty and, 54i
Folliculitis, of pubic hair, 210
Forensics, DNA technology and, 159t, 159–161
  sexual abuse and, 657t
Fourchette, trauma to, 370i, 530i
Frank's procedure, 545i, 545–545, 546i
Fraser's syndrome, 99, 166
Freud, Sigmund, 384
Frye test, 161
FSH. *See* Follicle-stimulating hormone (FSH).

Galactorrhea, 591, 594
Galactosemia, 65t
Gamete intrafallopian transfer (GIFT), 80
Ganglioneuroma, 55t
Garamycin, 684t–685t
Gardnerella vaginalis, 189t, 197i
Gardner-Silengo-Wachtel syndrome, 86, 90
Gartner's duct, cyst of, 455i
  formation of, 10, 11i, 12i
  homologies of, 9t
Gastritis, 244–245
Gastroschisis, 617–619, 619i, 620i
Gene therapy, 662t
Genetics, sexual differentiation and, 163–167, 165i, 166i, 536
Genital ambiguity, 520–521, 523i, 524i, 557, 660
  management of, 117–119, 118i
Genital anomalies, endometriosis and, 638
Genital differentiation. *See* Sexual differentiation.
Genital ducts, disorders of, 98–99
Genital mutilation, 518–520, 520i, 521i, 525
Genital tract, anatomy of, 176i, 176–177
  anomalies of, 630–632, 631i, 632i
  embryology of, 535–536
  female, adnexa of, 10–13
    examination of. *See* Gynecologic examination.
    external, embryology of, 13i–15i, 13–15, 14t
    genetics and, 163–167, 165i, 166i
    homologies of, 9t
    internal, 19t
      embryology of, 7–13, 9t, 10i–14i, 80i
      malformations of, 10–13, 164–167, 165i, 166i
  histology of, 310–311, 311i
  infections of, 229t, 351
  lower, anomalies of, 542–564
  male, embryology of, 79i
    homologies of, 9t
  malformation patterns of, 90–91
  neoplasms of, 225–227, 226i, 226t, 229t
  of child, 16–19, 17t, 18i, 19t, 310–311
  of newborn, 16–19, 19t
  trauma to, 225, 225i, 528–534, 529i–534i, 533t
    evaluation of, 528t
    incidence of, 528
    treatment for, 528t, 529
  tuberculosis of, 513–518, 514i–518i, 514t
    types of, 514t
  upper, anomalies of, 536–542, 537i–541i
    chlamydial infection of, 340–341
Genital tubercle, 13i
Genital ulcer disease, 351
Genital warts, 219, 350i. *See also* Human papillomavirus (HPV).
Genitopalatocardiac syndrome, 86, 90

Gentamicin, 684t
Germ cell tumors, 605t, 605–611, 606i–611i, 607t–610t
Germ cells, 6–7, 7i, 77, 86
GH. *See* Growth hormone (GH).
Giardiasis, 243
Gidwani, Gita, 2
GIFT (gamete intrafallopian transfer), 80
Gigantism, 41t, 42
Gilbert-Dreyfus syndrome, 116
GISP (Gonococcal Isolate Surveillance Project), 339
Glanzmann's disease, 229
Glioma, 55t. *See also* Neoplasm(s).
Glucocorticoids, 114–115, 142t, 272, 409–410
GnRH. *See* Gonadotropin-releasing hormone (GnRH).
Goiter, endemic, 143t, 146–147
Goldfarb, Alvin, 3
Goldstein, Donald, 2
Gonadotropin, circadian variation in, 48–49, 49i
  deficiency of, 97
  developmental changes and, 48
  measurement of, 62
  midcycle surge of, 51
  pituitary, 48–50
  precocious puberty and, 54i
  regulation of, 45–48, 46i, 47i
  thyroid and, 141
Gonadotropin-releasing hormone (GnRH), modulators of, 48
  opiates and, 51
  polycystic ovary syndrome and, 267i
  precocious puberty and, 54i, 54–56, 55t, 56i
  puberty and, 44–47, 46i, 47i
Gonads. *See also specific types, e.g.,* Ovary(ies).
  dysgenesis of, 79, 85–86, 109–111, 110i
    asymmetric, 90
  fetal, 77–79, 78i, 79i
  function of, cancer therapy and, 472–475, 473i
  regulation of, 51
  steroid biosynthesis and, 252i
  streak, 79–80, 80i, 81i, 109, 110i, 462i
Gonococcal Isolate Surveillance Project (GISP), 339
Gonorrhea. *See also* Neisseria gonorrhoeae *and* Sexually transmitted diseases (STDs).
  adolescent, 337–340, 338i, 339i
    treatment for, 339
  chromosome-mediated–resistant, 339
  disseminated, 338–339, 339i
  prepubertal, 313i, 313–316
    biology of, 313
    demographics of, 313–314
    diagnosis of, 315–316
    presentation of, 314
    transmission of, 314–315, 330t
    treatment for, 316
  prevention of, 340
  tetracycline-resistant, 339
Gordon, Ronald, 2
Granuloma, 55t, 206i
Granulosa cell tumors, 464–465. *See also* Neoplasm(s).
  juvenile, 611–612, 612i, 612t
Graves' disease. *See* Hyperthyroidism, autoimmune.
Griswold v. Connecticut, 501
Growth, 20–27
  abnormal, 34–42, 149
  assessment of, 25–26, 131–136, 132i–135i, 134t, 136t
  childhood, 21–23, 22i, 23i
  control of, 34–38, 35i, 36t
  fetal, 20–21, 21i
  infant, 21, 23i

Growth *(Continued)*
  measurement of, 24–25, 25i
  pubertal, 23i, 23–24
    endocrinology of, 26–27
  rate of, vitamin A and, 128, 129i
Growth chart(s), fetal, 221i
  for boys, 667i, 669i, 671i, 672i, 675i
  for girls, 22i, 23i, 668i, 670i, 673i–675i
Growth hormone (GH), 35i
  deficiency of, 39, 65t
    cancer survivors and, 470–472, 472i
    treatment for, 108i, 119
    Turner syndrome and, 107
  during puberty, 26, 31–32
  insulin-like growth factor and, 32, 34–37, 35i, 36t
  laboratory values for, 379t
  tall stature and, 41
Gubernaculum, embryology of, 8, 10, 12i
Gynecologic examination, 170–186
  compliance with, 171–174, 172t
  consent to, 503–505, 510
  diagnostic, 171
  documentation of, 174–175, 175i
  educational, 170–171
  for developmentally disabled, 493t, 493–494
  positioning for, 172–173, 173i, 174i
  questionnaire for, 172
  special aspects of, 185i, 185–186, 186i
Gynecology, pediatric, history of, 1–3

Hailey-Hailey disease, 214t, 215
Hair, disorders of, 210, 212
Hallucinogens, 432t. *See also* Substance abuse.
Halofenate, thyroxine-binding globulin and, 142t
Hamartoma, 55t. *See also* Neoplasm(s).
Hashimoto's thyroiditis, 143t, 146–148, 148i
Head, trauma to, 55t
Health care, access to, 654–655
Health screening, 655–657, 656t
Helicobacter pylori, 244–245
Heller, R. H., 2
Helminths, 513, 514i
Hemangioma, breast, 585
  vulvar, 219, 219i, 225, 226i
Hematocolpos, 164, 178i, 242i, 554–557
  endometriosis and, 637
Hematoma, retroperitoneal, 530
  vulvar, 225i, 377i, 529i
Hematometra, 637
Hematometrocolpos, 447i
Hematuria, 578t, 578–579
Hepatitis, 142t
Hepatoblastoma, 623
Hermaphroditism, 95–97, 111, 660. *See also* Genital
  ambiguity *and* Pseudohermaphroditism.
Hernia, diaphragmatic, 619–621, 620i
Heroin, 142t. *See also* Substance abuse.
Herpes. *See also* Sexually transmitted diseases (STDs).
  genital, adolescents with, 347–349, 348i
    diagnosis of, 348
    first episode of, 348i
    HIV infection and, 348, 351
    prepubertal, 326–327, 330t
    treatment of, 327, 348–349
Herpes simplex virus (HSV), fetal growth and, 21
  incidence of, 337

Herpes simplex virus (HSV) *(Continued)*
  Stevens-Johnson syndrome and, 215
  vulvar disorders from, 208–209
Herpes zoster, 358i
Hidradenitis, 212–213
Hirschsprung's disease, 374
Hirsutism, from hyperandrogenism, 70, 258, 258t
  grading of, 259i
  treatment for, 273
Histiocytosis X, 210, 212i
Hodgkin's disease, 469i, 474
Hodgson v. Minnesota, 506–507
Homocystinuria, 41t, 42
Homosexuality, 285–286, 338
  HIV infection and, 358
  runaways and, 361
Hormone therapy, 119–121, 120t, 662
Hormones. *See specific types, e.g.,* Estrogens.
HPV. *See* Human papillomavirus (HPV).
HSV. *See* Herpes simplex virus (HSV).
Huffman, John, 2
Human immunodeficiency virus (HIV). *See also* Acquired
  immunodeficiency syndrome (AIDS) *and* Sexually
  transmitted diseases (STDs).
  adolescents with, 356–362
    incidence of, 359, 360i
    risk factors of, 360–361, 361i
  anogenital neoplasia and, 352
  children with, 329t, 329–330, 330t
  diagnosis of, 359
  herpes and, 348
  symptoms of, 358–359
  syphilis and, 345
  testing for, 121
  treatment for, 359
Human papillomavirus (HPV), 209, 660. *See also* Genital
  warts *and* Sexually transmitted diseases (STDs).
  adolescents with, 349–350
  condyloma acuminatum from, 321–326, 330t
  diagnosis of, 349–350, 350i
  incidence of, 337
  lesions of, 321t
  neoplasia from, 219, 351–352
  sexual abuse and, 373
  symptoms of, 349
  treatment for, 350t
  types of, 321t
  vulvovaginitis and, 187, 194
Hydatids of Morgagni, 10, 11i, 12i
Hydrocephalus, 55t
Hydrocolpos, 164, 445–446, 446i
Hydrocortisone, 114
Hydroma, cystic, 623
Hydronephrosis, 624
Hydrosalpinx, 462–463, 516i
3β-Hydroxydehydrogenase, 112t–113t, 113–114
11β-Hydroxylase, 112t–113t, 113
11β-Hydroxylase deficiency, 87–88
17α-Hydroxylase deficiency, 88, 91
17α-Hydroxylase/17,20 lyase, 112t–113t, 114
21-Hydroxylase, 111i, 111–113, 112t–113t
21-Hydroxylase deficiency, 87, 261–263, 263i
17-Hydroxyprogesterone (17-OHP), 379t
Hymen, configurations of, 178–183, 179i–183i
  cysts of, 455
  diameter of, 372t
  embryology of, 15–16, 16i, 17t
  homologies of, 9t

Hymen *(Continued)*
  imperforate, 164, 177i, 178i, 554–555, 639i
    amenorrhea from, 70
    delayed puberty and, 65t
    endometriosis and, 637
    imaging of, 446, 447i
  polyps on, 182i, 204i
  redundant, 180i, 182i
  septated, 178i
  trauma to, 530
    sexual abuse and, 371–372, 372t
  types of, 17t
  variations in, 177i–183i, 177–183
Hyperandrogenism, 70, 259–269, 557–564. *See also*
    Androgen(s).
  causes of, 259t
  diagnosis of, 269–271, 271i
  prognosis for, 273–274
  symptoms of, 258, 258t, 259i
  treatment for, 271–273
Hypercortisolism, 107
Hyperparathyroidism, 57
Hyperpigmentation, 212
Hyperplastic dystrophy (squamous cell hyperplasia), 217, 217t
Hyperprolactinemia, delayed puberty and, 65t, 66–67
  thyroid hormones and, 149
  uterine bleeding and, 229t
Hypertension, fetal growth and, 20
Hyperthyroidism, autoimmune, 144–146
  juvenile, 143t
  precocious puberty and, 57
  tall stature and, 41–42
  uterine bleeding and, 229t
Hypertrophy, virginal (juvenile), 590
Hypogonadism, fertility and, 121–122
  hormone replacement for, 119–121, 120t
  hypergonadotropic, 64–65, 65t
  hypogonadotropic, 40, 66–68, 67i, 97–98
  puberty and, 26
Hypogonadotropism, 65t
Hypomenorrhea, 228t
Hypopigmentation, 212, 212i–213i
Hypopituitarism, 65t
Hypospadias, 69, 95
Hypothalamic-pituitary-adrenal axis, 44–45, 45i, 139, 484
  abnormalities of, eating disorders and, 403–404
  in anorexia nervosa, 400–401
  in bulimia nervosa, 401–403, 402i
Hypothalamic-pituitary-gonadal axis, 484. *See also* Thyroid.
  delayed puberty and, 64
  oral contraceptives and, 293
  precocious puberty and, 54
  premature thelarche and, 58
  thyroid hormone and, 139–142, 140i, 142t
Hypothalamus, dysfunction of, 484–485, 485i, 486i
  hamartoma of, 55t
  hormones of, 44, 45i
  tumors of, 65t
Hypothyroidism, 146–148, 147t
  delayed puberty and, 65t, 68
  Down syndrome and, 25
  from irradiation, 471–472
  precocious puberty and, 55t
  puberty and, 149
  screening for, 656
  short stature and, 39i, 39–40
  thyroxine-binding globulin and, 142t
  Turner syndrome and, 107
  uterine bleeding and, 229t

Hysterosalpingography, 451–452, 452i
Hysteroscopy, 539, 541

Ibuprofen, 685t
Idiopathic thrombocytopenic purpura, 228–229, 229t
IGF. *See* Insulin-like growth factor (IGF).
Imaging. *See* Diagnostic imaging.
Impetigo, 204–205, 215t
Impotence, 284
In vitro fertilization. *See also* Fertility.
  for hypogonadism, 121–122
  monosomy X and, 80
  Turner syndrome and, 109
Incest. *See also* Sexual abuse.
  definition of, 365–366
  patterns of, 374
Incontinence, 573–575, 574i. *See also* Urologic problems.
  stress, 577
  treatment for, 575
Infantometer, 24
Infertile male syndrome, 563t
Infertility. *See* Fertility.
Inflammatory bowel disease, 65t, 67, 107, 244. *See also*
    Crohn's disease.
Inhalants, 432t, 436–437. *See also* Substance abuse.
Inhibin, 31
Injury(ies), anorectal, 530i, 530–531
  genital, 528t, 528–534, 529i–534i, 533t
    incidence of, 528
    lesions vs., 533i, 533t, 533–534, 534i
  perineal, 530i, 530–531
  sex-related, 531–533, 532i
  straddle, 528–530, 529i, 530i, 579
    treatment for, 528t
  urinary tract, 579
  vaginal, 530
Insulin-like growth factor (IGF), 20, 21
  androgen production and, 255i, 256
  during puberty, 26
  growth hormone and, 32, 34–37, 35i
  thyroid-stimulating hormone and, types of, 36t
Interferon, for condyloma acuminatum, 325
Intertrigo, 204
Intraepithelial neoplasia, vulva, 220
Intrauterine device (IUD), 296–297, 496, 497t, 662
  consent for, 505
  pelvic inflammatory disease and, 343
Intravenous pyelogram, 569
Iodine deficiency, 143t, 146–147
Iowa laws, on sexually transmitted diseases, 509
Iron, deficiency of, 128, 138, 291t
  preparations of, 685t
Irradiation. *See* Cancer therapy.
Irritable bowel syndrome, 244
Israels, Leon, 1
IUD. *See* Intrauterine device (IUD).

Jarisch-Herxheimer reaction, 347
Jones, Howard, 2
Jones' metroplasty, 539, 540i
Jung, Carl, 384
Juvenile dermatitis herpetiformis, 215–216, 215t
Juvenile hypertrophy, 590
Juvenile mole, 220

Kallmann's syndrome, 97
 delayed puberty and, 65t
 hypogonadism and, 66
 short stature and, 40
 tall stature and, 42
Kaplan-Meier estimates, 468t
Kaposi's sarcoma, 358, 359i. *See also* Acquired
 immunodeficiency syndrome (AIDS).
Kasabach-Merritt syndrome, 219
Kaufman-McKusick syndrome, 98
Keloids, Turner syndrome and, 107
Kentucky laws, on medical consent, 504
Kidney, agenesis of, 579–580
 anomalies of, 580
 embryology of, 6
Kinsey, Alfred C., 285
Klinefelter's syndrome, 42
Klippel-Feil syndrome, 543
Kramer, Edith, 384
Kwashiorkor, 130. *See also* Malnutrition.

Labia majora, homologies of, 9t
Labia minora, agglutination of, 370i
 fusion of, 164
 homologies of, 9t
Labial adhesions, treatment of, 206–208, 207i
Laboratory assays, 659–660, 677t–680t
Lactobacillus acidophilus, 16–17
Lactose malabsorption, 243
LAMB syndrome, 220
Lang, Warren, 1
Langerhans' cell histiocytosis, 210, 212i
Laparoscopy, 644i–647i, 644–645. *See also* Diagnostic
 imaging *and* Endoscopy.
Laurence-Moon-Biedl syndrome, 40, 65t, 68
Lauritzen, Christian, 2
Lean body mass (LBM). *See also* Body composition.
 body fat and, 133–137, 136t
 estimating of, 131
 exercise and, 137
 Prader-Willi syndrome and, 137
Legal issues. *See also* State laws.
 abortion and, 501–503
 child abuse and, 508
 confidentiality and, 501, 506–509
 medical billing and, 509
 minors and, treatment of, 499–510
 parental consent and, 500
 privacy and, 501–503
LeGuin, Ursula, 278
Leiomyoma, 229t
Lentigo, vulvar, 220
Lesbianism, 285–286. *See also* Homosexuality.
Leukemia. *See also* Neoplasm(s).
 breast, 593
 lymphoblastic, 469i
 non-lymphoblastic, 469i
 survival rate with, 486t
Levonorgestrel implants (Norplant), 297, 662
 contraindications to, 297t
Leydig cells, 77–78, 95
LGV (lymphogranuloma venereum), 342, 342i. *See also*
 Sexually transmitted diseases (STDs).
LH. *See* Luteinizing hormone (LH).
Lichen sclerosus, 217t, 217–219, 218i, 224i, 224–225, 533t
Lichen simplex, 217
Lichenification, 217

Lipoma, vulvar, 220
Lithium, 143t
Lotrimin, 683t
Low-birth-weight infants, 301–303. *See also* Pregnancy.
 nutrition and, 304
 race and, 301, 302t
Lubs' syndrome, 94, 116
Luteal phase defects, 479–480
Luteinizing hormone (LH), androgens and, 254–256, 255i
 circadian variation in, 48–49, 49i
 deficiency of, 97
 during puberty, 29–30, 30i, 30t
 eating disorders and, 399–403, 402i
 exercise and, 479–480, 484i
 laboratory values for, 379t
 levels of, age and, 46i, 47i
 midcycle surge of, 51
 precocious puberty and, 54i
 serum concentrations of, 402i
Lymphadenopathy, 358. *See also* Acquired immunodeficiency
 syndrome (AIDS).
Lymphangioma, vulvar, 219
Lymphogranuloma venereum (LGV), 342, 342i. *See also*
 Sexually transmitted diseases (STDs).
Lymphoma. *See also* Neoplasm(s).
 breast, 593
 HIV-associated, 358
 Hodgkin's, 469i, 474
 non-Hodgkin's, 469i, 486t

Magnesium citrate, 685t
Magnetic resonance imaging (MRI). *See also* Diagnostic
 imaging.
 for breast mass, 596–598, 597i, 598i
 for pelvis, 442–445, 445i, 650–651
 future trends in, 661t
Malignant melanoma, 220
Malnutrition, 64, 130, 513. *See also* Nutrition.
Mammography, 595–596, 596i
Marfan's syndrome, 41t, 42
Marijuana, 432t, 434. *See also* Substance abuse.
Masculinization, 111i. *See also* Virilization.
Mastitis, 590–591. *See also* Breast(s).
Masturbation, 498
Mayer-Rokitansky-Küster-Hauser (MRKH) syndrome, 98,
 446–449, 448i–450i
 delayed puberty and, 65t, 70, 71
 vaginal atresia in, 542–543, 545
McCune-Albright syndrome, 55t, 57i, 60, 143t
McDonough, Paul, 3
McIndoe vaginoplasty, 545–549, 547i–549i
McKusick-Kaufman syndrome, 98
Meckel-Gruber syndrome, 90
Meckel's diverticulitis, 233t, 245
Meckel's syndrome, 99, 536
Medipren, 685t
Medroxyprogesterone, 120, 121, 297
Melanocytic lesions, vulvar, 220
Melanoma, malignant, 220
Menarche. *See also* Menstruation *and* Puberty.
 age at, 27i, 27–28, 29i, 479i
 delayed, 69–70
  anorexia and, 398
  exercise and, 478–479, 479i
  fat content and, 404–407, 405t, 406t
  hyperthyroidism and, 143

Menarche *(Continued)*
  obesity and, 27
  pregnancy and, 32
  premature, 53, 60–61
Meningitis, 55t
Menometrorrhagia, 228t
Menorrhagia, 228t
Menstruation. *See also* Amenorrhea, Dysmenorrhea, *and*
  Menarche.
  developmentally disabled and, 494–496
  disorders of, 222, 227–231, 228t–230t
  endocrine factors in, 400–403, 402i
  fat content and, 404–407, 405t, 406t
  obstetric history and, 482
  tuberculosis and, 516–517
Mental retardation. *See* Developmentally disabled.
Meperidine, 685t
Mercuroacetylglycylglycylglycylglycine, 569
Mesovarium, homologies of, 9t
Messenger ribonucleic acid (mRNA), 152
Methadone, 142t
Methimazole, 144
Metronidazole, 686t
Metroplasty, 539–541, 540i, 541i
Metrorrhagia, 228t
Midgut malrotation, 245
Migraines, oral contraceptives and, 291
Mineralocorticoid deficiency, 114–115
''Minipill,'' 294. *See also* Contraceptives, oral.
Minors, treatment of, 499–510. *See also* Legal issues.
Mitotane, 142t
Mittelschmerz, 241, 637
Mole, juvenile, 220
Molecular biology, 151–161
Molluscum contagiosum, 209
Monosomy X, 79–81, 80i–82i, 82t
  pregnancy and, 80
  psychosocial aspects of, 81
  treatment for, 81
Mons pubis, development of, 13
  homologies of, 9t
''Morning-after'' pill, 294. *See also* Contraceptives, oral.
Morphine, 686t
Mosaicism, 45,X/46,XX, 81–83, 89–90, 110, 115, 521, 524i
  45,X/47,XXX, 81–83
MRI. *See* Magnetic resonance imaging (MRI).
MRKH syndrome. *See* Mayer-Rokitansky-Küster-Hauser
  (MRKH) syndrome.
mRNA (messenger ribonucleic acid), 152
Müllerian agenesis, 448i
Müllerian anomalies, 99, 165–166, 166i, 536, 537i
  classification of, 640i
  dysmenorrhea from, 238t
  endometriosis and, 637–638, 639i, 640i
  in males, 98–99, 166–167
  obstructive, 233t, 242, 242i
  pregnancy and, 643t
Müllerian aplasia, 98, 165i
Müllerian duct syndrome, 117
Muram, David, 3
Mycelex, 683t
Myomas, uterine, 238t
Myometrium, imaging of, 443–444

Naloxone, 686t
Narcan, 686t

Narcolepsy, 435
Narcotics Anonymous, 434, 438–440. *See also* Substance
  abuse.
National Center on Child Abuse and Neglect, 365, 366
Naumburg, Margaret, 384
Neisseria gonorrhoeae. See also Gonorrhea.
  pelvic inflammatory disease from, 341, 343
  penicillinase-producing, 339
  resistant, 339
Neoplasm(s). *See also specific types, e.g.,* Teratoma.
  adnexal, 220
  anogenital, 352
  breast, 591–595, 592i, 593i, 594t
    unilateral, 585–586, 586i, 586t
  delayed consequences of, 467–476, 468t, 469i–476i
  genital, 351–352
  germ cell, ovarian, 605t, 605–611, 606i–611i, 607t–610t
  human papillomavirus and, 351–352
  imaging of, 463–465, 464i, 465i. *See also* Diagnostic
    imaging.
  in offspring of survivors, 475–476
  malignant, treatment for. *See* Cancer therapy.
  nonepithelial, 218–219
  of urinary tract, 278–279
  ovarian, 464i, 464–465, 465i
    adnexal torsion and, 650
    children with, 226t
    oral contraceptives and, 291t
    precocious puberty and, 55t, 57, 60
    prognosis for, 274
    virilizing, 269
  prenatal diagnosis of, 623
  psychosocial adjustment to, 476
  renal, 579
  Sertoli-Leydig cell, 464i
  survival rates with, 468i, 468t, 470i
  thecal cell, 464–465
  uterine, 455i
  vaginal, 463–464, 464i
  vulvar, 219–220, 225–227, 226i, 226t
Nephrotic syndrome, 142t
Neuroblastoma. *See also* Neoplasm(s).
  breast, 593
  prenatal diagnosis of, 623
  survival rate with, 468t, 469i
Neuroendocrinology, pubertal, 44–51
Neurofibromatosis, precocious puberty and, 55t
  vulvar, 219
Nevus, 220
Nipple(s). *See also* Breast(s) *and* Thelarche.
  discharge from, 591
  during puberty, 29t
  inverted, 590
Nonepithelial neoplasms, 219
Non-neoplastic epithelial disorders, classification of, 217t
Nonoxynol-9, 296
Nonsteroidal anti-inflammatory drugs (NSAIDs), for
  dysmenorrhea, 239, 240t
  for pelvic pain, 641
  side effects of, 240t
Noonan's syndrome, 107
Norplant, 297, 662
Northern blotting, 153–154
NSAIDs. *See* Nonsteroidal anti-inflammatory drugs (NSAIDs).
Nutrition, 128–131. *See also* Diet *and* Malnutrition.
  amenorrhea and, 485i, 486i
  body mass index and, 129, 130i
  delayed puberty and, 130

Nutrition *(Continued)*
  developmentally disabled and, 492
  exercise and. *See* Exercise.
  growth rate and, 128
  pregnancy and, 304
  programs for, 659t
  sexual maturation and, 129–130
  somatomedin and, 130
  thyroid hormones and, 141

Obesity, 27, 136–137. *See also* Eating disorders.
Octoxynol–9, 296
Ohio v. Center for Reproductive Health, 506–507
Oligomenorrhea. *See* Amenorrhea, secondary.
Omphalocele, 617–619, 618i
Oocyte, donor. *See* In vitro fertilization.
  homologies of, 9t
  ultrastructure of, 7, 8i
Oophoritis, 65t
Oophoropexy, 472
Opiates, 51
Oral contraceptives. *See* Contraceptives, oral.
Orgasm, disorders of, 284–285, 285t
Osteopenia, amenorrhea and, 487
  eating disorders and, 408–411
Osteoporosis, after cancer therapy, 473
  eating disorders and, 408–411
  exercise and, 485–486
Osteosarcoma, 468t. *See also* Neoplasm(s).
Ovary(ies), 19t. *See also* Gonads.
  androgens and, 254–256, 255i
  cysts of. *See* Cyst(s), ovarian.
  differentiation of, 163
  disorders of, hyperandrogenism and, 264
  dysgenesis of, 79–86, 80i–86i
  embryology of, 8, 9t, 11i–14i
  function of, 255i, 543
    eating disorders and, 407
  hyperandrogenism and, 70
  imaging of, 445i
  neoplasms of. *See* Neoplasm(s), ovarian.
  polycystic. *See* Polycystic ovary (PCO) syndrome.
  streak, 79–80, 80i, 81i, 109, 110i, 462i
  supernumerary, 10
  surgery on, 647–649, 649i
  torsion of, 459–460, 461i
  tuberculosis of, 515
Ovotestis, 96i, 111, 521, 524i
Oxandrolone, 108
Oxicams, 239t

Panadol, 682t
Pancreatitis, 233t
Panmycin, 687t
Papanicolaou smears, 352
Papillomatosis, 593
Papillomavirus. *See* Human papillomavirus (HPV).
Paradidymis, homologies of, 9t
Parental consent, 500. *See also* Legal issues.
Paraöphoron, embryology of, 11i, 12i
  homologies of, 9t
Parry's disease. *See* Hyperthyroidism, autoimmune.
PCO. *See* Polycystic ovary (PCO) syndrome.
Pediamycin, 684t

Pediaprofen, 685t
Pediazole, 684t
Pelvic adhesions, 238t
Pelvic inflammatory disease (PID), 342–344, 637
  chlamydial infection and, 340–341, 343
  diagnosis of, 343–344, 344t
  dysmenorrhea from, 238t
  endoscopy for, 649
  hospitalization for, 344t
  intrauterine devices and, 343
  medical implications of, 351–352
  oral contraceptives and, 291t
  prevention of, 344
  risk factors for, 343t
  symptoms of, 343
  treatment for, 344t
Pelvic pain. *See also* Abdominal pain.
  acute, 233t, 233–234
  causes of, 241–246, 636t
  chronic, 234–235, 635–651, 636t, 639i–651i, 641t, 643t
  from constipation, 243
  from Crohn's disease, 244
  from giardiasis, 243
  from irritable bowel syndrome, 244
  from lactose malabsorption, 243
  history for, 246–247
  psychological aspects of, 636
  treatment for, 247–248
Pelvis, imaging of, 441–445, 443i–445i. *See also* Diagnostic imaging.
Pemphigoid, bullous, 215t, 216
  cicatricial, 215t, 216
Pemphigus vulgaris, 215, 215t
Penicillin, 687t
Perianal dermatitis, 204
Perianal fissures, 374i
Perineum, injuries to, 530i, 530–531
  of newborn, 15i
  of 10-year-old, 16i
Periurethral bands, 533, 534i
Permapen, 687t
Perphenazine, 142t
Personality disorders, 424–427
  sexual abuse and, 411
Peutz-Jeghers syndrome, 57
Phallus, cloaca with, 634i
  embryology of, 13–15
  homologies of, 9t
  trauma to, 521, 524i
Phenylbutazone, 142t
Phenylpropanolamine, 435
Phobia, of physician, 383
Phylloides tumor, 592, 593
Piaget, Jean, 391
PID. *See* Pelvic inflammatory disease (PID).
Pigmentation, disorders of, 212, 212i, 213i
Pill, contraceptive. *See* Contraceptives, oral.
Pilosebaceous units, 258
Pinworms, 190i
Pituitary, 48–50, 65t
Pityriasis versicolor, 208
Placenta, adequacy of, 20–21
Planned Parenthood Association of Kansas City v. Ashcroft, 505
Planned Parenthood v. Danforth, 505
Platelet-activating factor receptor, 154
Pneumocystis carinii, 358, 359. *See also* Acquired immunodeficiency syndrome (AIDS).

Polycillin, 683t
Polycystic ovary (PCO) syndrome, 70, 250, 459, 460i, 461i
  hyperandrogenism and, 264–269, 265i–267i
  pathophysiology of, 265i, 266i
  prognosis for, 274
  treatment for, 272–273
  uterine bleeding and, 229t
Polyhydramnios, 623
Polymastia, 585. *See also* Breast(s), anomalies of.
Polymenorrhea, 228t
Polymerase chain reaction, 156–159, 158i, 654, 655–656
Polyp, cervical, 229t
  hymenal, 182i, 204i
  uterine, dysmenorrhea from, 238t
Polythelia, 584i, 584–585
Porphyria, 142t, 245
Potter's syndrome, 579–580
Prader-Willi syndrome, delayed puberty and, 65t, 68
  lean body mass in, 137
  precocious puberty and, 55t
  short stature and, 40
Pregnancy, 299–307
  after chemotherapy, 475
  clinics for, 305–309
  cocaine and, 436
  complications of, 229t, 233t, 305
  congenital malformations and, 304–305, 643t
  eating disorders and, 408
  economics of, 306–307
  ectopic, 291t, 645–647, 647i, 648i
  education about, 657–658, 658t
  menarche and, 32
  nonmedical consequences of, 305
  nutrition and, 137–138, 304
  parity effects on, 303–304
  race and, 302t
  rates of, 289, 290i, 300t, 300–301
  risks of, 301–303
  sexually transmitted diseases and, 305
  smoking and, 305
  socioeconomic factors and, 301–303, 305
  substance abuse and, 305
  syphilis and, 347
  thyroxine-binding globulin and, 142t
Prenatal care, 305–306
Principen, 683t
Privacy, 501–503, 510. *See also* Legal issues.
Progesterone, 120, 379t
Progestin, 119, 120–121
  androgenic, 293t
  for contraceptives, 291t
Progestin-only ''minipill,'' 294
Prolactin, 31, 380t
Propionic acid, 239t
Propylthiouracil, 144
Prostaglandin synthetase inhibitors, 239t
Prostaglandins, 231, 236–237, 237i, 238i
Prostate, homologies of, 9t
Prostitution, 279, 361
Pruritus, 208
Pseudohermaphroditism. *See also* Genital ambiguity *and* Hermaphroditism.
  delayed puberty and, 69
  female, 86–89
  male, 89–95
Pseudohypoparathyroidism, 40
Pseudopuberty, 56–57
Psoriasis, diaper, 205–206, 206i

Psoriasis *(Continued)*
  vulvar, 216, 216i
Pubarche, 55t, 58–59, 259–260. *See also* Pubic hair.
Puberty, 23i, 23–24, 27–32. *See also* Menarche *and* Thelarche.
  androgens and, 31t
  body composition and, 27
  constitutional delay in, 32
  dehydroepiandrosterone and, 254i
  delayed, 64–73, 486–487
    causes of, 65t
    evaluation of, 71, 72t, 73i
    findings in, 72t
    nutrition and, 130
    psychosocial aspects of, 73, 109
    thyroid hormones and, 149
  disorders of, 460–462, 462i
  endocrinology of, 23i, 23–24
  estrogens and, 30–31
  gonadotropin and, 29–30, 30i, 30t, 45–50, 46i, 47i
  growth hormone and, 26, 31–32
  hormonal quiescence before, 49–50
  hypogonadism and, 26
  hypothyroidism and, 149
  in Third World, 513–525, 514i–524i
  inhibin and, 31
  neuroendocrinology of, 44–51
  onset of, 50–51
  physical changes in, 28–29, 29i, 29t
  precocious, 53–64
    causes of, 55t
    endometrial shedding and, 227
    evaluation of, 61t, 61–62
    findings in, 61t
    growth curve for, 63i
    incomplete, 57–61, 58i
    psychosocial aspects of, 63–64
    tall stature and, 42
    thelarche and, 586t, 586–588, 587t
    thyroid hormones and, 149
    treatment for, 62–63, 63i
  prolactin and, 31
  sex hormone–binding globulin and. *See* Sex hormone–binding globulin (SHBG).
  sexuality and, 282–283, 283t
  testosterone and, 30
  timing of, 27i, 27–28
Pubic hair, 28i, 29i, 58–59, 210, 212
Public health, future trends in, 654–659, 656t–659t
Purpura, 228–229, 229t, 245
Pyelonephritis, 233t, 568–570
  symptoms of, 568t
Pyococcal infection, 208
Pyosalpinx, tuberculous, 516
Pyrazolones, 239t

Rape, 159t, 159–161. *See also* Sexual abuse.
  definition of, 366, 381
  genital injuries from, 531–533, 532i
  substance abuse and, 433
Rectal inertia, syndrome of, 631
Rectum. *See also* Anus.
  homologies of, 9t
5α-Reductase deficiency, 95, 564
  clinical features of, 563t
  delayed puberty and, 65t

5α-Reductase deficiency *(Continued)*
  genital development and, 115
Reifenstein's syndrome, 93–94, 94i, 116, 563t
Renal agenesis, 579–580
Renal anomalies, 580
''Resistant ovaries'' syndrome, 65t
Retinoblastoma, 469i
Rey-Stocker, Irmi, 2
Rhabdomyosarcoma, 601–603, 602i–605i, 603t. *See also*
    Neoplasm(s).
  breast, 593
  pelvic, 464i
  survival rate with, 469i, 603t
  vaginal, 225–226, 226i
Rheumatoid arthritis, 65t
Ribonucleic acid, 152
Roe v. Wade, 501, 502, 505–506
Rubella, 21
Rudiger's syndrome, 99, 536

Salicylate, 142t
Salicylic acid, 239t
Salpingitis, tubercular, 515, 516
Salpingo-oophoritis, 229t
Sarcoma botryoides, 225–226, 226i, 602i. *See also*
    Rhabdomyosarcoma.
Schiller, Friedrich, 42
Schönlein-Henoch purpura, 245
Sclerosis, tuberous, 55t
Screening, health, 655–657, 656t
Scrotum, homologies of, 9t
Seborrheic dermatitis, 205i, 216
Septo-optic dysplasia, 55t
Septra, 684t
Sertoli cells, 77–78
Sex hormone–binding globulin (SHBG), 31, 256
Sex hormones, 261
Sex of rearing, determination for, 117–119, 118i
Sexual abuse, 365–382, 370i, 371i, 372t–375t, 374i. *See also*
    Child abuse.
  AIDS from, 329t, 329–330, 330t
  art therapy for, 392
  classification of, 369t
  colposcopy for, 368i, 368–369
  condyloma acuminatum from, 322
  confidentiality and, 366–367
  definitions of, 365–366, 381
  diaper rash vs., 369i
  eating disorders and, 411–412
  evidence collection in, 375i, 375–376, 376t
  family dynamics of, 279
  forensics of, 657t
  history for, 367t, 382
  human papillomavirus and, 373
  of developmentally disabled, 497–498
  physical examination for, 367–376
  precocious puberty and, 55t, 60
  prevention of, 657
  procedures for, 330t
  psychological support for, 377–378
  runaways and, 361
  sexually transmitted diseases and, 311–313, 377
  siblings and, 374–375, 375t
  symptoms of, nonspecific, 368t
  trauma from, 531–533, 532i
  treatment for, 376–378

Sexual abuse *(Continued)*
  vaginal trauma with, 367, 368i
  voiding and, 574
Sexual assault. *See* Rape.
Sexual differentiation, 13i, 13–15, 535–536, 660
  abnormal, 77–79, 79i, 557
    management of, 104–122, 118i
  genetics and, 163–167, 165i, 166i, 536
  molecular techniques for, 161–163
Sexual dysfunction, 284–285, 285t
Sexual maturation, 129–130
Sexuality, adolescent, 278–298
    development of, 280–281
    factors in, 278, 278t
  biology and, 279
  culture and, 279–280
  development of, family and, 279, 283–284
    intimacy and, 281
    peer influences on, 284
    personality and, 283
    poverty and, 283
    risk factors in, 282–284, 283t
  education about, 286–287
  media influence on, 284, 286
  of developmentally disabled, 494t, 495i
  race and, 282
  substance abuse and, 283
Sexually transmitted diseases (STDs). *See also specific types,*
    e.g., Gonorrhea.
  adolescent, 336–352
    epidemiology of, 336–337, 337i
    medical implications of, 350–352
  condoms and, 294
  education about, 286–287, 657–658, 658t
  in children, 193
  legal aspects of, 508–509
  minors and, 505, 510
  pregnancy and, 305
  prepubertal, 310–331
    causes of, 311–313
    testing for, 311
  sexual abuse and, 311–313, 377
  substance abuse and, 336
  urinary tract infection from, 580–581
Shauffler, Goodrich, 1
SHBG (sex hormone–binding globulin), 31, 256
Shigella vulvovaginitis, 192–193
Sickle cell disease, 65t
Skin graft, 545, 547i, 550
Skinfold thickness, measurement of, 132–133, 135i, 406t
Slot blots, 154
Smith-Lemli-Opitz type I syndrome, 90
Smoking, 432
  fetal growth and, 20
  genital neoplasia and, 351–352
  oral contraceptives and, 291
  pregnancy and, 305
Sodomy, definition of, 381
Somatomedin, 130
Somatotropin. *See* Growth hormone (GH).
Soranus of Ephesus, 543
Sotos's syndrome, 41t, 42
Southern blotting, 153, 154i, 156, 160
Spence, Jay, 2
Spermatozoa, homologies of, 9t
Spermicides, 296, 296t. *See also* Contraception.
Spitz nevus, 220
Sponge, 295–296. *See also* Contraception.

Sports, 478–488, 479i–486i. *See also* Exercise.
Squamous cell carcinoma, 220
Squamous cell hyperplasia, 217t
SSSS (staphylococcal scalded skin syndrome), 215, 215t
Stadiometer, 24–25, 25i
Staphylococcal infection, 208
Staphylococcal scalded skin syndrome (SSSS), 215, 215t
Starvation. *See* Eating disorders *and* Malnutrition.
State laws. *See also* Legal issues.
   minors and, treatment of, 499–500, 510
   on child abuse, 508
   on confidentiality, 506–509
   on medical consent, 503–506
   private institutions and, 502
Stature, assessment of, 131, 132i
   measurement of, 24–25, 25i
   short, 38–40. *See also* Dwarfism.
     causes of, 38t, 39–40, 81
   tall, 40–42
     causes of, 41t, 41–42
STDs. *See* Sexually transmitted diseases (STDs).
Sterilization, legal aspects of, 509
   of developmentally disabled, 297–298, 494, 496t, 497
Steroid-producing tumors, 60
Steroids, 142t, 251i, 252i
Stevens-Johnson syndrome, 214, 215t
Stimulants, 432t, 435–436, 438. *See also* Substance abuse.
Strassman's operation, 539, 540i
Stress, exercise-induced, 482–484, 483i, 485i, 486i
Stress incontinence, 577
Stringency, DNA duplexes and, 154
Substance abuse, adolescent, 352i, 432–440
   depression and, 420, 422
   fetal growth and, 20
   pregnancy and, 305, 436
   sexuality and, 283
   sexually transmitted diseases and, 336
   symptoms of, 432t, 432–433
   suicide and, 434–435
   treatment of, 438–440
Suicide, 422, 427–430. *See also* Depression.
   indicators of, 428–429
   prevention of, 429–430
   substance abuse and, 434–435
   vignette on, 428–429
Sumycin, 687t
Sweat glands, disorders of, 212–213
Swyer's syndrome, 110
Sympodia, 10
Synechiae, uterine, 517i
Syphilis, 345i, 345–347, 346i. *See also* Sexually transmitted
   diseases (STDs).
   diagnosis of, 347
   fetal growth and, 21
   latent, 346
   pregnancy and, 347
   prepubertal, 328–329, 330t
   primary, 345i
   secondary, 328, 345–346, 346i
   symptoms of, 345
   tertiary, 346–347
   treatment for, 347
Systemic disease, 209–210, 210i–212i

T_3. *See* Triiodothyronine (T_3).
T_4. *See* Thyroxine (T_4).

Tanner staging, 676i
Taylor, Stewart, 1
TBG (thyroxine-binding globulin), 142t
TDF (testis-determining factor), 77–78, 78i
Temperature conversion, 681t
Tempra, 682t
TEN (toxic epidermal necrolysis), 214, 215t
Teratoma. *See also* Neoplasm(s).
   cervical, 623
   cystic, benign, 455–456, 456i, 457i
   immature, 609–610, 610i, 610t
   malignant, 464
   prenatal diagnosis of, 623
   sacrococcygeal, 623i
Terramycin, 687t
Testicular feminization, 92i, 92–94, 93i, 94i, 563t
Testicular regression syndrome, 95
Testis, differentiation of, 163
   homologies of, 9t
   intraabdominal, 651i
Testis-determining factor (TDF), 77–78, 78i
Testosterone, action of, 256–258, 257i
   assay for, 660
   biosynthesis of, 91–92, 116i
   during puberty, 30
   fetal production of, 78
Tetracycline, 687t
Texas laws, on medical consent, 504–505
Thalassemia, 229
Thecal cell tumors, 464–465. *See also* Neoplasm(s).
Thelarche. *See also* Breast(s).
   delayed, 588–589
   premature, 55t, 58i, 61t, 586t, 586–588, 587t
Thyroid, 139–149. *See also* Hypothalamic-pituitary-gonadal
   axis.
Thyroid hormones, 37. *See also specific types, e.g.,* Thyroxine
   (T_4).
   and nutrition, 141
   deficiency of. *See* Hypothyroidism.
   excess of. *See* Hyperthyroidism.
   hypothalamic-pituitary-gonadal axis and, 139–142, 140i,
     142t
   illnesses affecting, 142t
   medications affecting, 142t
   synthesis of, 140i
Thyroiditis, 143t, 146–148, 148i
   symptoms of, 147t
Thyroid-stimulating hormone (TSH), 139–141, 140i, 230
   assay for, 659
Thyromegaly, 144, 145i
Thyrotoxicosis, 142–146, 144t
   autoimmune, 143t
   thyroxine-binding globulin and, 142t
Thyroxine (T_4), 139–142, 140i, 230
Thyroxine-binding globulin (TBG), 142t
Tissue expansion techniques, 554
Tissue growth factors, 38t
Tompkins' metroplasty, 539–541, 541i
Toxemia, 20
Toxic epidermal necrolysis (TEN), 214, 215t
Toxoplasmosis, 21
Trachea, abnormalities of, 622i
Transcutaneous electrical nerve stimulation (TENS), 239
Trauma. *See* Injury(ies).
Treponema pallidum, 328, 330t, 345
Triceps skinfold thickness, measurement of, 132–133, 135i
Trichomoniasis, 320–321, 330t
   symptoms of, 189t

Trichomoniasis *(Continued)*
vulvovaginitis and, 197t, 197–198, 198i
Triiodothyronine (T₃), 139–142, 140i
Trimethoprim-sulfamethoxazole, 684t
Trimox, 682t
Tuberculosis, genital, 513–518, 514i–518i, 514t
lesion sites of, 515–516
types of, 514t
menstrual disorders from, 516–517
Turner syndrome, 462i. *See also* Gonads, dysgenesis of.
delayed puberty and, 64, 66i, 589
differential diagnosis of, 107
features of, 106t
heart problems with, 107
keloids and, 107
management of, 105i, 105–109, 106t, 108i
psychosocial aspects of, 109
renal anomalies with, 107, 580
short stature and, 40, 41i, 81
treatment for, 106t, 107–108, 108i
Turner's stigmata, 79, 81
Tylenol, 682t

Ulcers, aphthous, 213–214, 213t, 214i
Ultrasonography (USG). *See also* Diagnostic imaging.
for breast mass, 591, 596–598, 597i, 598i
for uterine anomalies, 539
future trends in, 660–661, 661t
pelvic, 441–445, 443i–445i, 588
prenatal, 616–617, 617t
Undervirilized male syndrome, 563t
Urachus, homologies of, 9t
Ureter, calculus in, 233t
reimplantation of, 573
Ureteropelvic junction, obstructed, 246
Urethra, caruncles of, 533t, 534
homologies of, 9t
prolapse of, 55t, 223–224, 224i, 533t, 534, 580i
Urethral glands, homologies of, 9t
Urethritis, 314, 318, 580
Urinary tract, anomalies of, 543, 579–580, 624–625, 637
calculi in, 578
malignancies of, 578–579
Urinary tract infection (UTI), 567–570
bacteriology of, 569
diagnosis of, 569
evaluation of, 569
from sexually transmitted diseases, 580–581
prophylaxis for, 570
radiologic studies of, 569
symptoms of, 568t
treatment for, 570
Urologic problems, 567–581
USG. *See* Ultrasonography (USG).
Uterine horn, rudimentary, 539, 540i, 639i
Uterus, 19t
agenesis of, 446–449, 448i–450i
anomalous, classification of, 536, 537i, 538i
diagnosis of, 539
endometriosis and, 637
incidence of, 536
presentation of, 536–539
surgery for, 539–541, 540i, 541i
bicornuate, 448i, 453i, 454i
bleeding from. *See* Dysfunctional uterine bleeding (DUB).
changes in, eating disorders and, 407

Uterus *(Continued)*
communicating, 538i
didelphic, 242i, 448i, 453i
double, 448i, 450–455, 452i–454i, 518i
embryology of, 11i
homologies of, 9t
imaging of, 443i–445i
müllerian fusion of, 165–166, 166i
myoma in, 238t
neoplasms of, 455i
polyps in, 238t
prepubertal, 312i
septate, 448i
subseptate, 454i
synechiae of, 517i
tuberculosis of, 515
unicornuate, 448i, 449–450, 450i, 451i
UTI. *See* Urinary tract infection (UTI).
Utimox, 682t

Vagina, 19t, 192
adenocarcinoma of, 603–604, 605i
agenesis of, 446–449, 448i–450i, 639i
endoscopy for, 650–651
aspirator for, 183–184, 184i
atresia of. *See* Vaginal atresia.
bleeding from, 55t, 222–227, 223t
carcinoma of, 225–227, 226i
cysts of, 455i
discharge from, 190–191, 195
embryology of, 15–16, 16i
Enterobius infection of, 208
foreign bodies in, 223, 223i, 224i
histology of, 310–311, 311i
history for, 311, 312i
homologies of, 9t
imaging of, 445. *See also* Diagnostic imaging.
injuries to, 367, 368i, 530
instrumentation of, 183–185, 184i, 186i
laceration of, 371–372, 372t, 377
neoplasms of, 463–464, 464i
obstruction of, 554–557, 555i, 556i, 639i
rhabdomyosarcoma of, 604i
septum of. *See* Vaginal septum.
transverse fusion of, 554
trauma to, 367, 368i, 530
tuberculosis of, 515
unilateral, imperforate, 554
visualization of, 175i, 175–176
Vaginal atresia, 165i, 542–554, 545i–554i
diagnosis of, 543
etiology of, 542–543
incidence of, 542
ovarian function with, 543
psychological aspects of, 544
surgery for, 543–554, 545i–554i
Vaginal septum, endometriosis and, 637
longitudinal, 164–165
transverse, 98, 164, 446, 447i, 555i, 555–557, 556i, 639i
Vaginal smear, 189t
Vaginitis, 191–192, 568. *See also* Vulvovaginitis.
uterine bleeding and, 229t
Vaginoplasty, amnion, 549–550
flap, 550, 554i, 559, 562i
McIndoe, 545–549, 547i–549i

Vaginosis, 196–197, 197t. *See also* Sexually transmitted diseases (STDs).
  prepubertal, 327–328, 330t
Vancomycin, 688t
"Vanishing testes" syndrome, 116–117
Variable numbers of tandem repeats (VNTRs), 156, 160
Varicella zoster, 208, 348
Vecchetti technique, 554
Vesicoureteral reflux (VUR), 568, 570–573, 571i, 572i, 573t
  classification of, 571, 572i, 573t
  diagnosis of, 571
  etiology of, 571
  evaluation of, 571, 571i, 572i
  surgery for, 572–573, 573t
  symptoms of, 571–572
  treatment for, 572–573, 573t
Vestibular glands, homologies of, 9t
Vibramycin, 684t
Vincent's curtsey, 574i
Virginal hypertrophy, 590
Virilization. *See also* Masculinization.
  delayed puberty with, 65t
  from adrenal hyperplasia, 87, 261–263, 263i, 562
  from ovarian tumors, 269
Vitamin A, 128i–129i
Vitiligo, 212, 213i
VNTRs (variable numbers of tandem repeats), 156, 160
Voiding. *See also* Urologic problems.
  control of, 573
  dysfunction of, non-neurogenic, 573–574, 574i
    sexual abuse and, 574
    "suspected," 577–578
    treatment for, 575
Volvulus, 233t
Von Willebrand's disease, 228–229, 229t
Vulva, 192
  androgenization of, 557–564
  bleeding from, 223–224, 224i
  bullous pemphigoid of, 215t, 216
  cysts of, 219
  dermatoses of, 217t
  disorders of. *See* Vulvar disorders.
  eczema of, 216–217
  Enterobius infection of, 208
  genetic disorders of, 210
  hemangioma of, 219, 219i
  hematoma of, 225i, 377i, 529
  inflammation of, 182i. *See also* Vulvovaginitis.
  lacerations to, 529–530, 530i
  lichen sclerosus of, 217t, 217–219, 218i, 224i, 224–225
  lichen simplex of, 217
  lipoma of, 220
  lymphangioma of, 219
  neoplasms of, 219–220, 225–227, 226i, 226t
  neurofibromatosis of, 219
  psoriasis of, 216, 216i
  seborrheic dermatitis of, 216
  squamous cell carcinoma of, 220
  squamous cell hyperplasia of, 217t
  tuberculosis of, 515
  wart on, 209i, 220. *See also* Condyloma acuminatum.
Vulvar disorders, 203–220
  biopsy for, 203–204
  bullous diseases and, 214i–218i, 214t, 214–218, 217t
  evaluation of, 203
  infant with, 204i–207i, 204–208

Vulvoplasty, cut-back, 559, 561i
Vulvovaginitis, acute, 223i
  candidal, 198–200, 199i
    children with, 193i, 193–194
    recurrent, 199–200
    treatment for, 199
  examination for, 188–190, 189i, 189t, 196
  history for, 188, 195–196
  hormonal changes and, 190–191, 194–195
  in adolescents, 194–200
  in children, 187–194, 222–223, 223t
  management of, 191–194, 196–200, 197i–199t, 197t
  nonspecific, 370i
  papillomavirus and, 187, 194
  precocious puberty and, 55t, 60
  rarer causes of, 200
  risk factors for, 187, 188t, 195
  shigella, 192–193
  symptoms of, 187–188, 189t, 195
  treatment for, 189t
Vulvovaginoplasty, Williams', 550, 553i
VUR. *See* Vesicoureteral reflux (VUR).

Wart(s), genital. *See* Condyloma *entiries*.
Weaver's syndrome, 40
Weight. *See also* Body composition *and* Obesity.
  assessment of, 131, 132i
  gain of, 136–137
    growth chart for, 671i
    menarche and, 404–407, 405t, 406t
    pregnancy and, 304
  loss of, 136–137
    amenorrhea from, 485i, 486i
    exercise and, 137, 481i, 482i
Williams' vulvovaginoplasty, 550, 553i
Wilms' tumor, 90, 578. *See also* Neoplasm(s).
  prenatal diagnosis of, 623
  survival rate with, 469i
Wilson's disease, 67
Witch's milk, 584
Wolffian ducts, 6, 9t, 9–10, 10i–12i, 163
Wycillin, 687t
Wymox, 682t

X chromosome, abnormalities of, 83i, 83–84, 84i
  pseudoautosomal region of, 105i

Y chromosome, abnormalities of, 77, 78i, 84–85
  pseudoautosomal region of, 105i

Zachary, Robert, 2
ZFY (zinc finger Y), 77
Zidovudine, 359
ZIFT (zygote intrafallopian tube transfer), 54
Zinc deficiency, 210i
Zinc finger Y (ZFY), 77
Zovirax, 327, 349, 682t
Zygote intrafallopian tube transfer (ZIFT), 54